HANDBOOK OF PAIN ASSESSMENT

HANDBOOK OF PAIN ASSESSMENT

Second Edition

DENNIS C. TURK
RONALD MELZACK

Editors

THE GUILFORD PRESS

New York   London

© 2001 The Guilford Press
A Division of Guilford Publications, Inc.
72 Spring Street, New York, NY 10012
www.guilford.com

Printed in the United States of America

This book is printed on acid-free paper.

Last digit is print number: 9 8 7 6 5 4 3 2 1

Library of Congress Cataloging-in-Publication Data

Handbook of pain assessment / edited by Dennis C. Turk,
   Ronald Melzack.—2nd ed.
      p. ; cm.
   Includes bibliographical references and index.
   ISBN 1-57230-488-X
   1. Pain—Measurement—Handbooks, manuals, etc.   I. Turk, Dennis C.
II. Melzack, Ronald.
   [DNLM: 1. Pain—diagnosis. 2. Pain—psychology. 3. Pain Measurement.
WL 704 H243 2001]
RB127 .H355 2001
616′.0472—dc21   2001023116

To our wives, Lorraine Turk and Lucy Melzack,
who have inspired us throughout our careers.
We are grateful for their unconditional support,
understanding, and love.

About the Editors

Dennis C. Turk, PhD, is the John and Emma Bonica Professor of Anesthesiology and Pain Research at the University of Washington. He was the recipient of the American Psychological Association, Division of Health Psychology, Outstanding Scientific Contribution Award and the American Association of Pain Management's Janet Travell Award. An international survey published in 2000 identified Drs. Turk and Melzack as two of the "top 10 leaders in pain research and treatment development." He has over 300 publications and has written and edited 13 volumes. Dr. Turk is currently editor-in-chief of *The Clinical Journal of Pain*.

Ronald Melzack, PhD, studied psychology at McGill University. After he received his PhD in 1954, he spent 5 years carrying out physiological research at the University of Oregon Medical School; University College London, England; and the University of Pisa, Italy. Currently he is back at McGill University as a Professor in the Department of Psychology. Dr. Melzack developed the McGill Pain Questionnaire, which is now the most widely used measuring tool for research on pain in human subjects. In addition to more than 200 papers on research and theory, he has written and edited five books.

Contributors

Karen O. Anderson, PhD, Pain Research Group, Division of Anesthesiology and Critical Care, University of Texas M. D. Anderson Cancer Center, Houston, Texas

Frank Andrasik, PhD, Institute for Human and Machine Cognition, University of West Florida, Pensacola, Florida

Michele Crites Battié, PhD, Department of Physical Therapy, University of Alberta, Edmonton, Alberta, Canada

Laurence A. Bradley, PhD, Division of Clinical Immunology and Rheumatology, University of Alabama School of Medicine, University of Alabama at Birmingham, Birmingham, Alabama

Stephen Bruehl, PhD, Department of Anesthesiology, Vanderbilt University School of Medicine, Nashville, Tennessee

Charles S. Cleeland, PhD, Pain Research Group, Division of Anesthesiology and Critical Care, University of Texas M. D. Anderson Cancer Center, Houston, Texas

Kenneth D. Craig, PhD, Department of Psychology, University of British Columbia, Vancouver, British Columbia, Canada

Douglas E. DeGood, PhD, University of Virginia Health System Behavioral Medicine Center, University of Virginia School of Medicine, Charlottesville, Virginia; Augusta Pain Management Center, Fishersville, Virginia

Robert H. Dworkin, PhD, Department of Anesthesiology, University of Rochester School of Medicine and Dentistry, Rochester, New York

Samuel F. Dworkin, DDS, PhD, Departments of Oral Medicine and Psychiatry and Behavioral Sciences, University of Washington, Seattle, Washington

John T. Farrar, MD, Center for Clinical Epidemiology and Biostatistics and Department of Neurology, University of Pennsylvania Medical Center, Philadelphia, Pennsylvania

James A. Fauerbach, PhD, Department of Psychiatry and Behavioral Sciences, Johns Hopkins University School of Medicine, Baltimore, Maryland

Herta Flor, PhD, Neuropsychology and Clinical Psychology Unit, Central Unit of Mental Health, Mannheim, Germany

Lucia Gagliese, PhD, Department of Anesthesia, Toronto General Hospital and Mount Sinai Hospital, Toronto, Ontario, Canada

Bradley S. Galer, MD, Endo Pharmaceuticals, Inc., Chadds Ford, Pennsylvania

Robert D. Gerwin, MD, Department of Neurology, Johns Hopkins University School of Medicine, Baltimore, Maryland; Pain and Rehabilitation Medicine, Ltd., Bethesda, Maryland

Joanne Gillespie, MA, Department of Psychology, University of Western Ontario, London, Ontario, Canada

Ruth Eckstein Grunau, PhD, Department of Psychology, The British Columbia Children's Hospital, Vancouver, British Columbia, Canada

Thomas Hadjistavropoulos, PhD, Department of Psychology, University of Regina, Regina, Saskatchewan, Canada

R. Norman Harden, MD, Department of Physical Medicine and Rehabilitation, Rehabilitation Institute of Chicago and Northwestern University Medical School, Chicago, Illinois

Jennifer A. Haythornthwaite, PhD, Department of Psychiatry and Behavioral Sciences, Johns Hopkins University School of Medicine, Baltimore, Maryland

Roderick D. Hetzel, PhD, Department of Anesthesiology, University of Rochester School of Medicine and Dentistry, Rochester, New York

Quinn Hogan, MD, Department of Anesthesiology, Medical College of Wisconsin, Milwaukee, Wisconsin

Mary Casey Jacob, PhD, Departments of Psychiatry and Obstetrics and Gynecology, University of Connecticut Health Center, Farmington, Connecticut

Mark P. Jensen, PhD, Department of Rehabilitation Medicine, University of Washington, Seattle, Washington

Anthony Jones, MD, Pain Research Laboratory, Manchester University Rheumatic Diseases Centre, Salford, England

Paul Karoly, PhD, Department of Psychology, Arizona State University, Tempe, Arizona

Joel Katz, PhD, Acute Pain Research Unit, Department of Anesthesia, Toronto General Hospital, Toronto, Ontario, Canada; Departments of Public Health Sciences and of Anesthesia, University of Toronto, Toronto, Ontario, Canada

Francis J. Keefe, PhD, Department of Psychiatry and Behavioral Services, Duke University Medical School, Durham, North Carolina

Robert D. Kerns, PhD, Departments of Psychiatry, Neurology, and Psychology, Yale University, New Haven, Connecticut; Psychology Service, Department of Veterans Affairs Medical Center, West Haven, Connecticut

Laura May, PhD, PT, Department of Physical Therapy, University of Alberta, Edmonton, Alberta, Canada

Tom G. Mayer, MD, Department of Orthopedic Surgery, University of Texas Southwestern Medical Center, Dallas, Texas

Patricia A. McGrath, PhD, Pain Innovations, Inc., London, Ontario, Canada; Department of Pediatrics, University of Western Ontario, London, Ontario, Canada

Nancy L. McKendree-Smith, PhD, Division of Clinical Immunology and Rheumatology, University of Alabama School of Medicine, University of Alabama at Birmingham, Birmingham, Alabama

Ronald Melzack, PhD, Department of Psychology, McGill University, Montreal, Quebec, Canada

Elna M. Nagasako, BA, Department of Anesthesiology, University of Rochester School of Medicine and Dentistry, Rochester, New York

Richard Ohrbach, DDS, PhD, Department of Oral Diagnostic Sciences, State University of New York at Buffalo, Buffalo, New York

Akiko Okifuji, PhD, Department of Anesthesiology, University of Utah, Salt Lake City, Utah

Peter B. Polatin, MD, Department of Psychiatry, University of Texas Southwestern Medical Center, Dallas, Texas

Donald D. Price, PhD, Departments of Oral and Maxillofacial Surgery and of Neuroscience, University of Florida, Gainesville, Florida

Kenneth M. Prkachin, PhD, Department of Psychology, University of Northern British Columbia, Prince George, British Columbia, Canada

Joseph L. Riley III, PhD, Division of Public Health Service and Research, College of Dentistry, University of Florida, Gainesville, Florida

James P. Robinson, MD, PhD, Department of Rehabilitation Medicine, University of Washington, Seattle, Washington

Michael E. Robinson, PhD, Department of Clinical and Health Psychology, College of Health Professions, University of Florida, Gainesville, Florida

Joan M. Romano, PhD, Department of Psychiatry and Behavioral Sciences, University of Washington, Seattle, Washington

Karen B. Schmaling, PhD, Department of Psychiatry and Behavioral Sciences, University of Washington, Seattle, Washington

Jeffrey J. Sherman, PhD, Departments of Oral Medicine and of Anesthesiology, University of Washington, Seattle, Washington

Suzanne J. Smith, BA, Department of Psychology, Ohio University, Athens, Ohio

Herbert G. Steger, PhD, Department of Anesthesiology, University of Kentucky College of Medicine, Lexington, Kentucky

Mark D. Sullivan, MD, PhD, Department of Psychiatry and Behavioral Sciences, University of Washington, Seattle, Washington

Karen L. Syrjala, PhD, Fred Hutchinson Cancer Research Center and Department of Psychiatry and Behavioral Sciences, University of Washington School of Medicine, Seattle, Washington

Raymond C. Tait, PhD, Department of Psychiatry, St. Louis University School of Medicine, St. Louis, Missouri

Dennis C. Turk, PhD, Department of Anesthesiology, University of Washington, Seattle, Washington

Carl von Baeyer, PhD, Department of Psychology, University of Saskatchewan, Saskatoon, Saskatchewan, Canada

Michael Von Korff, ScD, Center for Health Studies, Group Health Cooperative of Puget Sound, Seattle, Washington

Gordon Waddell, DSc, MD, FRCS, Orthopaedic Department, The Glasgow Nuffield Hospital, Glasgow, Scotland, United Kingdom

James B. Wade, PhD, Department of Psychiatry, Medical College of Virginia, Virginia Commonwealth University, Richmond, Virginia

Ursula Wesselmann, MD, Departments of Neurology, Neurological Surgery, and Biomedical Engineering, Johns Hopkins University School of Medicine, Baltimore, Maryland

David A. Williams, PhD, Department of Psychiatry, Georgetown University Medical Center, Washington, DC

Preface

Pain is an integral part of life and plays an important protective function. It is also the primary symptom that prompts people to seek medical attention. We now know that uncontrolled and prolonged pain can alter both the peripheral and central nervous systems through processes of neural plasticity and central sensitization and thus become a disease itself. The person's mood (fear, depression, anger) can amplify or diminish the experience substantially. Pain is also influenced by one's social environment. How people and systems, including health care professionals and the compensation system, respond to patients' reports has been shown to have a profound influence on perceived pain intensity, response to treatments, and disability.

There is no question that the presence of pain greatly compromises the quality of life. Recognition of the significance of pain has become a growing feature of health care. There has been a movement in the United States to consider pain as the "fifth vital sign" (along with blood pressure, temperature, heart rate, and respiration) that warrants assessment and which patients have a "right" to have adequately controlled. In January 2001, U.S. President Bill Clinton signed into law a bill declaring the decade 2001–2010 as the Decade of Pain Control and Research.

Despite the prevalence of pain, there remains much that we do not understand about it. Everyone knows what pain is, but no one can truly know another's experience of pain. Pain has many perplexing characteristics. Why do two people with ostensibly the same degree of physical pathology sometimes report such different intensities of pain? Why do patients treated by the same methods to control pain show different results? What causes pain in the absence of peripheral tissue damage, as in the case of spinal cord injuries or strokes? Why are so many chronic pain syndromes more prevalent in women?

Pain is a perception that is experienced by a conscious person, whereas nociception is neural transmission resulting from sensory transduction of mechanical, thermal, or clinical energy impinging on specialized nerve endings. The nerves involved convey information about tissue damage to the central nervous system. The association between nociception and pain is far from perfect. According to the International Association for the Study of Pain (IASP) (1986), "Pain is an unpleasant sensory and emotional experience associated with actual or potential tissue damage or described in terms of such damage" (p. 217). This definition underscores the inherent subjectivity of pain. The definition acknowledges the importance of emotional as well as sensory factors.

To understand and adequately treat pain, we need to be able to measure it. This seems at first to be quite a simple task. All that is required is that the individual responds to the question, "How much does it hurt?" Unfortunately, as is illustrated throughout this volume, the problem is not as simple as this question might suggest. Many factors contribute to the individual's response. This is the primary rationale for this volume. There does not appear to be a simple isomorphic relationship between the amount of pain and the extent of tissue damage. As noted in the previously cited definition, psychological factors are involved in the pain experience. A number of cultural, economic, social, demographic, and environmental factors, along with the person's unique history, situational factors, interpretation of the symptoms and resources, current psychological state, as well as physical pathology, all contribute to the response to the question, "How much does it hurt?"

The complexity of pain has been revealed in recent decades. Investigators and clinicians have learned that a diverse range of factors need to be examined in the hope of understanding the response to the simple question of how much it hurts. In the first edition of this volume, published almost a decade ago, we asked a group of internationally acknowledged experts to provide a description of the available instruments and procedures for assessing people's pain. In addition, we asked contributors to evaluate existing methods and to provide practical information about their merits, thereby assisting clinical investigators or health care providers to make informed decisions regarding the most appropriate methods to assess the person who is experiencing pain. We also included contributions that provided more general discussion of the issues that need to be considered in selection from the array of instruments and procedures that are available. From the time the first edition was published, our knowledge of pain has increased exponentially. Many of the advances have been directly related to improved methods of assessment. This second edition is greatly expanded and it is more than one third larger to accommodate recent knowledge and developments.

This handbook is divided into six parts, with an introduction and a closing chapter by the editors (Dennis C. Turk and Ronald Melzack). The first part, *Measurement of Pain*, includes chapters that address the assessment of pain per se. This part includes chapters on self-report scales used with adults (Mark P. Jensen and Paul Karoly; Ronald Melzack and Joel Katz), children and adolescents (Patricia A. McGrath and Joanne Gillespie), and the elderly (Lucia Gagliese). The chapter prepared by Donald D. Price, Joseph L. Riley III, and James B. Wade covers a range of methodological issues regarding self-reports that transcend the population being targeted.

Psychophysiological methods have greatly advanced since the first edition of this volume. Herta Flor provides practical information about both traditional and innovative methods for using physiological data to assess people with persistent pain. There is an important, new chapter in this part on assessing pain in persons with limited ability to communicate (Thomas Hadjistavropoulos, Carl von Baeyer, and Kenneth D. Craig), groups that, unfortunately, are often neglected. The chapters by Flor and Hadjistavropoulos and colleagues bridge the second part of this volume: behaviors connoting pain.

The second part focuses specifically on behavioral expressions of pain. In addition to self-report, other important modes of communicating are characterized by facial expressions, nonverbal sounds (e.g., sighs, moans), and characteristic movements, postures, and soothing efforts (e.g., rubbing a painful body part)—all observable behaviors. Kenneth D. Craig, Kenneth M. Prkachin, and Ruth Eckstein Grunau provide an elegant discussion of the potential to make use of facial expression to make inferences about pain. Facial expressions (action patterns) are universal in humans (and other primates) and specific patterns appear to be unique to the experience of pain. Thus, they provide a more objective measure of pain than in self-report measures, which are open to distortion by a range of biases and can be consciously manipulated. The chapter by Francis J. Keefe, David A. Williams, and Suzanne J. Smith describes methods to observe, record, and quantify a range of movements in addition to facial expression and nonverbal sounds: pain behaviors.

What is of central importance here is not only that these behaviors can be carefully monitored and assessed by health care providers; they are also observable by patients' significant others. These behaviors, then, not only communicate about the subjective experience of pain, they are capable of eliciting responses. Thus, in contrast to the facial action patterns of pain that appear to be relatively hard-wired, pain behaviors are subject to the changing influences of environmental contingencies.

The third part, *Medical and Physical Evaluation of Patients with Pain*, includes chapters that focus on diagnostic methods for assessing people with pain. Peter B. Polatin and Tom G. Mayer describe the use of a detailed protocol to quantify function as well as making use of electronic recording devices. In a new chapter in this edition, Michele Crites Battié and Laura May describe the range of physical and occupational therapy methods incorporating both physical and self-report measures of functioning, including activities of daily living. Both general and disorder-specific methods are described.

In another new chapter in Part III, Quinn Hogan critiques the potential use of diagnostic injections. He discusses both the uses and abuses of these methods and describes the inferences that are appropriate from these diagnostic procedures. The final chapter in this part deals with the important but very difficult and controversial topic of disability evaluation. James P. Robinson describes the intricacies of different compensation systems and provides useful suggestions regarding how an evaluator can conduct impairment and disability evaluations that address the ambiguities while meeting the demands inherent in these imperfect compensation systems.

In Part IV, *Psychological Evaluation of Patients with Pain*, chapters address psychiatric disorders that are prevalent in people with chronic pain patients (Mark D. Sullivan), assessment methods to evaluate emotional distress (Laurence A. Bradley and Nancy L. McKendree-Smith), and assessment of patients' beliefs and coping strategies (Douglas E. DeGood and Raymond C. Tait).

People with persistent pain do not live in isolation. Thus there has been an increasing recognition that the unit of assessment is not only the identified patient but his or her social context. One important contextual factor is the family environment. In a new chapter in Part IV, Joan M. Romano and Karen B. Schmaling describe methods for assessing couples and families. Mary Casey Jacob and Robert D. Kerns expand the discussion beyond couples and family to consider methods of assessing the patient within his or her environment more broadly.

A number of advanced surgical and neuroaugmentation procedures have been developed since the publication of the first edition of this volume. Despite technical advances, there is growing evidence that psychosocial factors have an important role to play in treatment response. Detailed assessment methods have been developed to screen patients prior to receiving these treatments. In another new chapter in Part IV, Michael E. Robinson and Joseph L. Riley III describe the components of presurgical psychological screening. In the final chapter in this part, Dennis C. Turk and Akiko Okifuji demonstrate that there are subgroups of chronic pain patients based on psychosocial and behavioral characteristics that appear to be independent of physical pathology or medical diagnosis. They make a cogent argument for the potential of improving outcomes by tailoring treatments to match the patient subgroup characteristics.

Part V, *Specific Pain States and Syndromes*, includes a set of chapters that describe unique features of diagnosing and assessing patients with acute pain (Jennifer A. Haythornthwaite and James A. Fauerbach) and the most prevalent chronic pain syndromes: back pain (Gordon Waddell and Dennis C. Turk), headache (Frank Andrasik), facial pain (Samuel F. Dworkin and Richard Ohrbach), myofascial pain syndromes (Robert D. Gerwin), and pain associated with cancer (Karen O. Anderson, Karen L.

Syrjala, and Charles S. Cleeland). In addition to the updates of these chapters that appeared in the first edition, diagnosis and assessment of several other common pain syndromes are included in this edition, namely, neuropathic pain (Robert H. Dworkin, Elna M. Nagasako, and Bradley S. Galer), complex regional pain syndrome (formerly reflex sympathetic dystrophy, or RSD) (Stephen Bruehl, Herbert G. Steger, and R. Norman Harden), and chronic pelvic pain (Ursula Wesselmann).

Assessment is performed for one or more purposes: to establish incidence, prevalence, and trends; to arrive at a diagnosis; for decision making; to communicate; to perform outcome assessment; and to conduct program evaluation. In order to accomplish each of these purposes in a satisfactory fashion, careful attention must be given to research design. The final part of this volume, *Methodological Issues*, includes a set of chapters discussing important methodological topics that transcend the topic of assessment.

The chapters making up Part VI include updated and expanded discussions of epidemiological and survey methods (Michael Von Korff) and psychometrics (Samuel F. Dworkin and Jeffrey J. Sherman) that were covered in the first edition. Three new chapters have been added to this part. There have been increasing demands for outcomes to substantiate treatment claims. Practitioners' time for such efforts is limited, but program evaluation is essential. Akiko Okifuji and Dennis C. Turk provide suggestions (a survival guide) for outcome evaluation that can be performed efficiently in busy clinical practices. Robert H. Dworkin, Elna M. Nagasako, Roderick D. Hetzel, and John T. Farrar discuss important issues in the conduct of formal clinical trials that will permit valid conclusions regarding the effectiveness of any treatment. There has been an explosion of interest in the use of sophisticated imaging technologies. In another new chapter, Anthony Jones provides a primer on state-of-the-art imaging methods and offers some suggestions for the future of these technologies.

In our introductory and summary chapters, we provide an overview of concepts of pain assessment and attempt to identify current trends as well as future directions. We hope that this volume reflects the advances in assessment methods that have contributed so much to the increased understanding of pain, the person with pain, and the evaluation of new treatments. Furthermore, our intent for this edition, as in the previous one, is that it will (1) provide a practical guide to currently available instruments and procedures, (2) suggest areas in which currently available procedures are inadequate, and (3) serve as an impetus for research to improve upon existing instruments and procedures. The achievement of these goals should further enhance our understanding of pain and lead to more successful treatment. Our ultimate aim in this volume is to contribute to decreased suffering and improvement in the quality of life of those who experience pain.

DENNIS C. TURK
RONALD MELZACK

REFERENCE

International Association for the Study of Pain (IASP) Subcommittee on Taxonomy & Merskey, H. (Eds.). (1986). Classification of chronic pain syndromes and definitions of pain terms. *Pain* (Suppl. 3), S1–S226.

Contents

HANDBOOK OF PAIN ASSESSMENT

INTRODUCTION

Chapter 1

The Measurement of Pain and the Assessment of People Experiencing Pain

DENNIS C. TURK
RONALD MELZACK

> Just as "my pain" belongs in a unique way only to me, so I am utterly alone with it. I cannot share it. I have no doubt about the reality of the pain experience, but I cannot tell anybody what I experience. I surmise that others have "their" pain, even though I cannot perceive what they mean when they tell me about them. I am certain about the existence of their pain only in the sense that I am certain of my compassion for them. And yet, the deeper my compassion, the deeper is my certitude about the other person's utter loneliness in relation to his experience.
> —ILLICH (1976, pp. 147-148)

> . . . the investigator who would study pain is at the mercy of the patient, upon whose ability and willingness to communicate he is dependent.
> —LASAGNA (1960, p. 28)

Pain is the primary symptom that motivates people to seek medical treatment, accounting for over 35 million new office visits to physicians (Knapp & Koch, 1984) and over 70 million (80%) of all office visits to physicians each year in the United States (Koch, 1986). Pain medications are the second most frequently prescribed medications (after cardiac–renal drugs) during visits to physicians' offices and emergency rooms (Schappert, 1998). Almost one in five adult Americans (a total of 50 million) experiences chronic pain (Joranson & Lietman, 1994); 17% of patients in the United States seen by primary care physicians suffer from persistent pain (Gureje, 1998);

and 4.9 million people seek treatment for chronic pain each year (Marketdata Enterprises, 1999). More than 23 million surgical procedures are performed each year in the United States, with significant pain accompanying the majority of these procedures (Peebles & Schneidman, 1991). Annually, in the United States there are over 50 million trauma injuries, many associated with high levels of pain (Chapman & Turner, 1986). Furthermore, approximately 3.5 million people in the United States have cancer, with moderate to severe pain reported by 35%–45% at the intermediate state of the disease and 60%–85% in advanced stages (Raj, 1990).

The statistics cited above are derived from physician and hospital records, but they probably reflect only the tip of the iceberg when it comes to the prevalence of pain. Many people who experience pain self-manage their pain without seeking medical attention. Von Korff, Dworkin, LeResche, and Kruger (1988) conducted an epidemiological study of common pain conditions among adults enrolled in a health maintenance organization in Seattle, Washington (see also Von Korff, Chapter 31, this volume). They reported that the prevalence of recurrent episodes of pain was 37%, with 8% reporting severe, persistent pain. They also reported that 2.7% of the sample indicated that they experienced 7 or more days of pain during which they were unable to carry out their usual activities in the 6 months preceding the survey.

The direct costs for the treatment of pain and indirect costs related to indemnity costs, retraining, and lost tax revenues are astronomical. For example, over 250,000 lumbar surgeries are performed each year, the majority to ameliorate back pain, at a cost of $25,000 (J. D. Loeser, personal communication, February 7, 2000) for each surgery totaling $8.75 billion annually. In 1995, over 176,000 patients with chronic pain were treated in pain treatment centers at an average cost of $8,100 (Marketdata Enterprises, 1995) totaling over $1.4 billion. Turk, Okifuji, and Kaluaokalani (1999) have estimated that the combined direct and indirect costs may exceed $125 billion per year.

Given the statistics cited above, it might be expected that pain would be well understood. Unfortunately, this is not the case. Most forms of chronic pain are poorly understood, and even when they are understood, the severity may not be adequately managed.

A central impediment to increased understanding and appropriate treatment of pain is the result of the inherent subjectivity of pain. It is difficult to describe pain, and there may be little commonality in the language used by two people attempting to describe what might objectively be viewed as the same phenomenon. Similarly, the language used by a patient to describe his or her subjective experience to a health care provider may be difficult to communicate because the patient and health care provider have different languages, different experiences, and different frames of reference. The problem is even more acute for infants (see McGrath & Gillespie, Chapter 6) and for others with limited abilities to communicate (e.g., patients who have suffered a stroke or are mentally impaired; see Hadjistavropoulos, von Baeyer, & Craig, Chapter 8, and Craig, Prkachin, & Grunau, Chapter 9). The person is the

"experiencer," whereas the physician or investigator can only be an observer (note the quote by Illich with which we introduce this chapter). In short, pain is a subjective experience, a complex perceptual phenomenon. Thus, by its very nature, pain can only be assessed indirectly. However, in order to communicate there needs to be a common language, whether verbal or nonverbal (see Craig et al., Chapter 9, and Keefe, Williams, & Smith, Chapter 10), and a classification system that can be used in a meaningful and consistent fashion.

CLASSIFYING PAIN

One common way to classify pain is to consider it along a continuum of duration. Thus, pain associated with tissue damage, inflammation, or a disease process that is of relatively brief duration (i.e., hours, days, or even weeks), regardless of its intensity, is frequently referred to as *acute pain* (e.g., postsurgical pain—see Haythornthwaite & Fauerbach, Chapter 22). Pain that persists for extended periods of time (i.e., months or years), that accompanies a disease process (e.g., rheumatoid arthritis), or that is associated with an injury that has not resolved within an expected period of time (e.g., myofascial pain syndromes—see Gerwin, Chapter 26; complex regional pain syndrome—see Bruehl, Steger, & Harden, Chapter 28; and chronic pelvic pain—see Wesselmann, Chapter 29) is referred to as *chronic pain*. This duration continuum is inadequate, as it does not include acute recurrent pain (e.g., migraine headaches, sickle cell anemia); it tends to ignore pain associated with progressive diseases, such as chronic obstructive pulmonary disease and metastatic cancer; and it does not cover pain induced in a laboratory context. In the case of acute recurrent pain, people may suffer from episodes of acute pain interspersed with periods of being totally pain-free. In the case of pain associated with progressive diseases, certain unique features of the pain are influenced by the nature of the disease and need to be considered. Finally, in the laboratory a number of contextual factors need to be considered before extrapolations can be made to the clinical context. Using these five discrete classifications of pain (i.e., acute, acute recurrent, chronic, chronic progressive, and laboratory-induced) comprises a categorical approach to classification rather than a simple continuum based on duration.

Another way to classify pain is based on diagnosis. For example, pain associated with headaches (see Andrasik, Chapter 24), orofacial pain (see Dworkin & Ohrbach, Chapter 25), and low back pain (see Polatin & Mayer, Chapter 11) has been contrasted with pain associated with neuropathic pain (see Dworkin, Nagasako, & Galer, Chapter 27) and pain associated with cancer (see Anderson, Syrjala, & Cleeland, Chapter 30). Related to diagnosis, but more specific, are recent calls for classification based on underlying mechanisms (see, e.g., Woolf et al., 1998).

Yet another continuum used to discuss pain is one based on the ages of the sufferers. For example, there has been much debate whether children experience pain in the same way as adults do (see Chapter 6). At the other end of the life span, there has been considerable discussion regarding alterations in sensory sensitivity of people in the later stages of life, and the impact of age-related physical changes on pain perception (see Gagliese, Chapter 7).

The classifications described above are only a few examples and are definitely not exhaustive (Turk & Okifuji, 2001). There is, however, no one system for classifying pain patients that has been universally accepted by clinicians or researchers.

Regardless of the way one classifies pain and people with pain, there appears to be a number of commonalities that transcend the age of the sufferer, the duration of pain, or the diagnosis. However, before we can hope to understand pain, we need to consider how to measure this elusive phenomenon (Turk, 1989).

MEASUREMENT OF PAIN

The measurement of pain is essential for the study of pain mechanisms and for the evaluation of methods to control pain. There is no simple thermometer that can objectively record how much pain an individual experiences. As we have noted, all that can be determined about the intensity of a person's pain is based on what the patient verbally or nonverbally communicates about his or her subjective experience. Often patients are asked to quantify their pain by providing a single general rating of pain: "Rate your *usual* level of pain on a scale from 0 to 10, where 0 equals no pain and 10 is the worst pain you can imagine." Here a patient is being asked to quantitate and average his or her experience of pain over time and situations. These ratings are retrospective, and a number of studies have reported that patients significantly overestimate their pain when asked to recall previous levels of pain (e.g., Linton & Gotestam, 1983). Moreover, pain intensity is likely to vary over time and depends upon what the patient is doing. It has also been demonstrated that

present levels of pain tend to influence memory; consequently, present pain levels may serve as anchors that influence the averaging of pain (Eich, Reeves, Jaeger, & Graff-Radford, 1984; see Haythornthwaite & Fauerbach, Chapter 22). Furthermore, it is possible that patients may be unable to discriminate reliably between the points on a scale, and for some the points may not even be on the same dimensions. The anchor words of the scale may also influence the distribution of responses. Many of these points are discussed by Jensen and Karoly in Chapter 2 of this volume.

Despite the concerns noted, intensity of pain is without a doubt the most salient dimension of pain, and a variety of procedures have been developed to measure it. There have been tremendous interest in developing, and efforts to develop, reliable and valid measures for quantifying pain intensity (see Jensen & Karoly, Chapter 2, and Price, Riley, & Wade, Chapter 4) and for objectively identifying the causes of pain (see Battié & May, Chapter 12; Hogan, Chapter 13; and Dworkin & Sherman, Chapter 32). However, pain is a complex, multidimensional, subjective experience. The report of pain is related to numerous variables, such as cultural background, past experience, the meaning of the situation, personality variables, attention, arousal level, emotions, and reinforcement contingencies (Melzack & Wall, 1983; Turk, Meichenbaum, & Genest, 1983; see Sullivan, Chapter 15; Bradley & McKendree-Smith, Chapter 16; DeGood & Tait, Chapter 17; Romano & Schmaling, Chapter 18; and Jacob & Kerns, Chapter 19). Using a single dimension, such as intensity, will inevitably fail to capture the many qualities of pain (Melzack, 1975; Melzack & Katz, Chapter 3, this volume). In short, pain intensity, although frequently used in clinical practice to quantify the disorder, is inadequate. Moreover, pain intensity itself does not provide a good reflection of either psychological or physical disruption caused by specific disorder (Naliboff, Cohen, Swanson, Bonebakker, & McArthur, 1985; and as noted in many chapters in this volume).

Considerable attention has been devoted to developing measures of physical functioning. A number of attempts have relied on people's self-reports of their abilities to engage in a range of functional activities (e.g., Bergner, Bobbitt, Carter, & Gilson, 1981; Millard, 1989) and the pain experienced upon performance of those activities (e.g., Jette, 1987). Although many investigators are skeptical of the validity of self-report measures and prefer more objective measures, studies have revealed a high level of concordance among self-report and disease characteristics, physicians' or physical therapists' ratings of functional abilities, and objective functional performance (e.g., Deyo & Diehl, 1983; Jette, 1987). Despite obvious limitations of bias, self-report instruments have several advantages. They are economical; enable the assessment of a wide range of behaviors that are relevant to the patient; and permit emotional, social, and mental functioning to be assessed. Investigators have also developed systematic procedures for physical examination and evaluation of functional capacity that directly assess the individual's physical limitations and capabilities (see Polatin & Mayer, Chapter 11, and Battié & May, Chapter 12).

In an effort to avoid the many problems inherent in self-reports of pain severity, some investigators and many clinicians suggest that the report of pain should be ignored, since it is a symptom rather than an "objective" sign (which is believed to be more reliable and valid). For example, the Social Security Administration in the United States bases disability determination solely on physical examination and on imaging and laboratory diagnostic tests. It is only when these objective findings are identified that subjective report of pain is considered (see Robinson, Chapter 14).

Physicians are often wary of patients' self-reports and may prefer more "objective" measures. Moreover, some physicians are skeptical about the validity of questionnaire techniques in general. Biomedical research and advanced technology have been used in an attempt to identify the physical basis of the report of pain. The implicit assumption of this research seems to be that there is an isomorphic relationship between the report of pain and tissue pathology. Thus, once the extent of tissue pathology is identified, the intensity of pain can be known. Using objective physical assessment, diagnostic nerve blocks and sophisticated imaging, and laboratory diagnostic procedures to identify the nature and extent of pathology is assumed to provide direct knowledge of the subjective state (see Polatin & Mayer, Chapter 11, and Hogan, Chapter 13). To date, this research has been disappointing (see Polatin & Mayer, Chapter 11). Little information is available on how to integrate effectively and appropriately the information derived from multiple physical examinations, diagnostic imaging, and laboratory tests. Moreover, the relationships among pathology, physical measurements of muscle strength and range of motion, behavior, and reports of pain have not been firmly established, and these factors appear to be only weakly correlated (Deyo, 1986; Nachemson, 1976). A number of studies demonstrate significant pathology in

subjects who have little or no pain (e.g., Boden, Davis, Dina, Patronas, & Wiesel, 1990; Hitselberger & Witten, 1968; Jensen, Brant-Zawadski, Obuchowski, Modic, & Malkasian Ross, 1994; Wiesel, Tsourmas, & Feffer, 1984), but, conversely, little identifiable pathology in patients who report severe pain (e.g., White & Gordon, 1982).

In short, the association between physical abnormalities and patients' reports of pain is often ambiguous or weak. In addition, physical pathology has been reported not to be predictive of disability (Cats-Baril & Frymoyer, 1991; Hagglund, Haley, Reveille, & Alarcon, 1989; Waddell, 1987; see Robinson, Chapter 14), of return to work after an injury (Bigos et al., 1991), or of treatment outcome (see, e.g., Cairns, Mooney, & Crane, 1983). One possible factor contributing to the apparent lack of correlation between pathology, symptoms, and outcome is the observation that the reliability of many physical examination procedures is questionable (see, e.g., Matyas & Bach, 1985; Waddell et al., 1982; see also Waddell & Turk, Chapter 23, and Dworkin & Sherman, Chapter 32). In addition, although physical examination measurements such as flexibility and strength may be objective, they are influenced in many cases by patients' motivation, effort, and psychological state.

In many patients, objective physical findings to support their complaints of pain are absent. Thus reliable and valid measures of pain and function must be developed. A number of studies have demonstrated that self-report questionnaires can be highly valid measures of functional status (see, e.g., Deyo & Diehl, 1983). Physical and laboratory measures are useful primarily to the degree that they correlate with symptoms and functional ability (see Flor, Chapter 5). However, self-report functional status instruments seek to quantify symptoms, function, and behavior directly, rather than inferring them (Deyo, 1988).

A number of physicians have tried to develop systematic approaches to physical assessment, and have suggested that sophisticated laboratory and imaging techniques should form the basis of pain assessment (see Battié & May, Chapter 12; Hogan, Chapter 13; Waddell & Turk, Chapter 23; Andrasik, Chapter 24; Dworkin & Ohrbach, Chapter 25; Gerwin, Chapter 26; Dworkin et al., Chapter 27; Bruehl et al., Chapter 28; Wesselmann, Chapter 29). However, a preponderance of research has demonstrated that there is no isomorphic association between physical pathology and pain. Many factors seem to mediate this association in both acute pain (Bonica, 1990) and chronic pain (Waddell,

Bircher, Finlayson, & Main, 1984), as well as pain associated with terminal illnesses (Turk & Fernandez, 1990).

Identification of pain-specific physiological response has also met with mixed success (cf. Sternbach, 1968; Turk, 1989). The reliability of many psychophysiological parameters has been questioned (see, e.g., Arena, Blanchard, Andrasik, Cotch, & Myers, 1983, see Price et al., Chapter 4, and Flor, Chapter 5). As Sternbach (1968) noted, "Because of the variability of response elicited by different pain stimuli, and because of the additional variance contributed by individual differences in response-stereotype, it is difficult to specify a pattern of physiological responses characteristic of pain" (p. 259).

Psychologists have also been concerned with the development of assessment procedures that do not rely on self-reports to evaluate patients with pain. Fordyce (1976) provided an important contribution by emphasizing the important role of environmental contingencies on the communication of pain, distress, and suffering. Patients experiencing pain display a broad range of observable manifestations that communicate to others the fact that they are feeling pain—that they are distressed and suffering. These behaviors, termed *pain behaviors*, include verbal report, paralinguistic vocalizations, motor activity, facial expressions, gesticulations, and postural adjustments (Fordyce, 1976). Because pain behaviors, unlike pain per se, are observable, they are susceptible to conditioning and learning influences. Patients have many opportunities to learn that the display of pain behaviors may lead to reinforcing consequences, such as attention, and the opportunity to avoid unwanted responsibilities. In some cases, these pain behaviors may be maintained by their reinforcing consequences long after the normal healing time for injury.

According to operant theory, behavior is controlled to a great extent by its consequences. With an initial injury or pathological state, these behaviors may be reflexive responses (in the language of behavioral theory, *respondents*); however, over time these initially reflexive responses may be maintained by reinforcement contingencies. That is, attention or financial gain may be positively reinforcing and thereby contribute to the maintenance of the behaviors long after the initial cause of pain has been resolved. These insights have led to an emphasis on the assessment of these pain behaviors (see Keefe et al., Chapter 10), as well as treatments designed to extinguish maladaptive pain behaviors and to increase activity (i.e., adaptive or well behaviors).

Typically, methods used to assess pain behaviors have relied on patients' self-reports of their ac-

tivities. For example, patients have been asked to indicate in general how much time they spend engaging in specific activities such as sitting, standing, and walking (*uptime*), or to complete daily monitoring forms that record the frequency of such activities. Some studies, however, have reported that patients are not accurate in their self-reports of activities, and thus challenge the validity of them (e.g., Kremer, Block, & Gaylor, 1981). Keefe and his colleagues (for a review, see Keefe et al., Chapter 10) have developed specific behavioral observation methods to assess pain behaviors that are not dependent on patients' self-reports.

Unfortunately, none of the pain behaviors appear to be uniquely or invariably associated with the experience of pain. Craig and his colleagues (see Craig et al., Chapter 9) have made a strong case for the priority of nonverbal facial expression of pain for making judgments about the pain experienced by others. These investigators have conducted fine-grained observations of the facial musculature that is associated with pain. As noted previously, assessment of pain based on nonverbal communication may be particularly important for those who have restrictions in their ability to communicate.

Interestingly, Flor and Turk (1988), among others (e.g., Waddell, 1987), have found that although physical impairment is related to disability, it bears a much smaller association with self-reported pain. Council, Ahern, Follick, and Kline (1988) found that the actual physical performance of patients with back pain was best predicted by their *beliefs of their capabilities* and not by pain per se. Turk and colleagues (Flor & Turk, 1988; Turk, Okifuji, Sinclair, & Starz, 1996) examined the relationship among general and specific pain-related thoughts, convictions of personal control, pain severity, and disability levels in patients with chronic back pain, rheumatoid arthritis, and fibromyalgia. The general and situation-specific convictions of uncontrollability and helplessness were more highly related to pain and disability than disease status for the patients with back pain and rheumatoid arthritis. For the patients with fibromyalgia, there was only a low correlation between what they *said* they were able to do and their actual activities. These data suggest that it is important not only to assess how much patients report they hurt and what they say they are able to do, but also how much they actually do.

The failure to find a relationship between reported pain and pathology has resulted in the suggestion that personality factors may be the cause of pain or may influence reports of pain that are disproportionate to the identified pathology. The search for a "pain-prone personality" (see, e.g., Blumer & Heilbronn, 1982) and for "psychogenic pain" has proven to be futile (see Sullivan, Chapter 15). The many variables that have been perceived to be part of a personality constellation related to psychogenic pain may actually be reactions to illness independent of psychiatric diagnosis. A number of investigators have begun to examine the predictive power of individual-difference measures to predict response to diverse treatments for pain. Many third-party payers are beginning to require presurgical screening prior to surgery or use of implantable devices (i.e., spinal cord stimulators, pumps; see Robinson & Riley, Chapter 20). However, many of the commonly used psychological instruments have not demonstrated clear utility in either diagnostic or treatment outcome predictions (Turk, 1989). This is an area that holds promise for improving outcomes but calls for additional research to confirm the predictive validity of the assessment protocols.

A BROADER PERSPECTIVE ON THE PAIN SUFFERER

Over the past 35 years, major research advances have greatly increased knowledge of the anatomy and physiology of nociception. The landmark papers by Melzack and his colleagues (Melzack & Casey, 1968; Melzack & Wall, 1965) formulating the *gate control* theory of pain expanded the conceptualization of pain from a purely sensory phenomenon to a multidimensional model that integrates motivational-affective and cognitive-evaluative components with sensory-physiological ones. The gate control model served as an important impetus to physiological research and research on identifying and demonstrating the modulation of pain perception by psychological variables. The gate control model emphasizes that pain is not exclusively sensory and that simple measures of pain intensity are inadequate to understand it. In the 1970s, Melzack and colleagues (Melzack, 1975; Melzack & Torgerson, 1971) developed the first assessment instrument, the McGill Pain Questionnaire, designed to measure the three components of pain postulated by the gate control theory (see Melzack & Katz, Chapter 3).

Since Melzack and his colleagues' pioneering work on pain assessment, a number of investigators have emphasized that pain that extends over time (i.e., chronic pain, acute recurrent pain, pain associated with progressive diseases) has an important impact on all domains of the sufferer's life. Persistent pain is so prepotent that psychological factors may come

to play an even greater role influencing the subjective experience, report, and responses. Physicians have long recognized that disease categories provide minimal information about the impact of illness upon patients' experiences. A diagnosis is important because it may identify a cause of symptoms and suggest a course of treatment. Yet within each specific diagnosis, patients differ considerably in how they are affected (see, e.g., Turk & Rudy, 1990) and how they respond to treatment (see Turk & Okifuji, Chapter 21). Consequently, appropriate assessment of these patients requires assessment of much more than just the direct components of pain; it also calls for assessment of mood, attitudes, beliefs, coping efforts, resources, and the impact of pain on patients' lives (see Bradley & McKendree-Smith, Chapter 16, and DeGood & Tait, Chapter 17). Moreover, because people do not live in isolation, chronic pain influences interpersonal relationships and is influenced by them. Thus it is important to consider contextual as well as individual patient characteristics (Jacob & Kerns, Chapter 19).

In conclusion, health care providers have long considered pain as being synonymous with nociceptive stimulation and pathology. It is important, however, to make a distinction among *nociception*, *pain*, *pain behavior*, and *suffering*. Nociception is the processing of stimuli that are defined as related to the stimulation of nociceptors and capable of being experienced as pain. Pain, because it involves conscious awareness, selective abstraction, appraisal, ascribing meaning, and learning, is best viewed as a perceptual process comprised of the integration and modulation of a number of afferent and efferent processes (Melzack & Casey, 1968). Thus the experience of pain should not be equated with peripheral stimulation. Suffering, which includes interpersonal disruption, economic distress, occupational problems, and a myriad of other factors associated with pain's impact on life functioning, is largely associated with the interpretive processes and subsequent response to the perception of pain. Reesor and Craig (1988) demonstrated that cognitive processes appear to amplify or distort patients' experience of pain and suffering. In sharp contrast to the nociceptive model, operant pain behaviors can occur in the absence of and thus may be independent of nociception.

Although biomedical factors appear to instigate the initial report of pain in the majority of cases, psychosocial and behavioral factors may serve over time to exacerbate and maintain levels of pain and subsequent disability. It is important to acknowledge that disability is not solely a function of the extent of physical pathology or reported pain severity (see, e.g.,

70

Fordyce et al., 1984; Naliboff et al., 1985; Waddell et al., 1984). Disability is a complex phenomenon that incorporates the tissue pathology, the total individual's response to that physical insult, and environmental factors that can serve to maintain the disability and associated pain even after the initial physical cause has resolved. Pain that persists over time should be viewed not as the result of either solely physical or solely psychological causes, but rather as a set of biomedical, psychosocial, and behavioral factors contributing to the total experience of pain.

CHANGES IN HEALTH CARE

Over the past few years, there has been a marked change in health care. Much greater attention is being given to evidence for not only the clinical effectiveness but the cost-effectiveness of treatments. Health care providers are being asked—actually, challenged—to provide evidence of the effectiveness of the treatment they propose to perform. Many decisions regarding reimbursement are based on the availability of convincing data that the treatment results in positive outcomes—ones that are important to third-party payers (i.e., reduction in health care consumption, reduction in indemnity payments, return to gainful employment) and are less costly than alternatives. To be responsive to these demands, it has become incumbent on health care providers to make available information supporting the effectiveness of their treatments and demonstrating that they achieve positive outcomes in their practices. Effective dissemination of evidence of treatment outcomes is also becoming crucial. Thus health care providers will need to give greater attention to the performance of clinical trials, to program evaluation, and to effective communication of their own and others' published results of relevant outcome studies and epidemiological research (see Von Korff, Chapter 31; Okifuji & Turk, Chapter 33; and Dworkin, Nagasako, Hetzel, & Farrar, Chapter 34). In selecting measures to use for communication, for treatment decision making, for the interpretation of published results, and for the evaluation of their own practices, they need to be aware of the basic requirements of psychometrics (see Dworkin & Sherman, Chapter 32).

SOME PROSPECTIVE CAVEATS

In this volume, detailed discussions are presented and descriptions are provided of a broad range of assessment techniques, methods, and measures. At this point, it seems appropriate to provide some cautions that may serve to inoculate the reader. One of us (DCT) is reminded of the examination question that he gave to graduate students in the course on tests and measurements that he taught: "Imagine that you read a journal article describing a new assessment battery, and you believe it is the answer to your prayers for the research study that you are proposing in a grant application. Describe how you would go about convincing your collaborators and the grant reviewers that this battery is appropriate and should be used."

We must balance the tendency to focus on variables for which there are existing reliable and valid measures against the need to examine what is truly important. Clinicians and researchers should also guard against picking instruments blindly "off the shelf" simply because they are well known, are popular, or have received extensive validation. It is essential that the instrument or procedure under consideration has been standardized on the population of interest. We should not assume that because an instrument or procedure has been demonstrated to have good psychometric properties in one population, it can be applied to another population without a demonstration of the instrument's psychometric properties in the new population.

Currently there is no single agreed-upon method for evaluating patients with pain. Many competing instruments, procedures, and methods are available. Each investigator or clinician develops his or her own set by selecting from the many available techniques or developing personalized assessment instruments—often without giving sufficient attention to the psychometric properties of the instruments used. This practice makes it difficult to compare results across studies. There needs to be some agreement with regard to what set of instruments and procedures will be used as the standards for each relevant domain of assessment. This is something of a double-edged sword, and we must be careful not to preclude using some new measures that may provide important new information.

Developing assessment instruments and procedures that have appropriate psychometric properties is necessary, but not sufficient. Given the complexities inherent in the construct of subjective pain, there is a need to obtain a diversity of assessment information that must then be integrated to understand the patient's pain and to contribute to treatment decision making.

Most of what is known about patients with chronic pain has been learned from studying patients referred to specialized pain clinics. These patients represent a very small percentage of patients who experience chronic pain—those who have gone through a selective filtering process (Turk & Rudy, 1990). The degree to which this segment of patients is representative of the larger population of people with chronic pain is highly questionable. As epidemiological surveys seem to suggest, the pain clinic samples may differ in many ways from community samples. For example, the association between psychological findings and pain frequently noted in pain clinics is less frequently observed in epidemiological studies (Crook, Weir, & Tunks, 1989).

The primary purpose of this volume is to provide a comprehensive and practical review of the advances in the measurement of pain and the assessment of patients with pain, and to recommend the most appropriate tests and procedures, given the current state of knowledge. Our hope is that the reader will, upon examination of each of the contributions, be in a better situation to provide psychometrically acceptable and sufficiently comprehensive approaches to the problem to be investigated.

ACKNOWLEDGMENTS

Preparation of this chapter was supported in part by grants from the National Institute of Arthritis and Musculoskeletal and Skin Diseases (No. AR/AI44724) and the National Institute of Child Health and Human Development (No. HD33989) awarded to Dennis C. Turk.

REFERENCES

Arena, J. G., Blanchard, E. B., Andrasik, F., Cotch, P. A., & Meyers, P. E. (1983). Reliability of psychophysiological assessment. *Behaviour Research and Therapy, 21*, 447–460.

Bergner, M., Bobbitt, R. A., Carter, W. B., & Gilson, B. S. (1981). The Sickness Impact Profile: Development and final revision of a health status measure. *Medical Care, 19*, 787–805.

Bigos, S. J., Battié, M. C., Spengler, D. M., Fisher, L. D., Fordyce, W. E., Hansson, T. H., Nachemson, A. C., & Wortley, M. D. (1991). A prospective study of work perceptions and psychosocial factors affecting the report of back injury. *Spine, 16*, 1–6.

Blumer, D., & Heilbronn, D. (1982). Chronic pain as a variant of depressive disease: The pain-prone disorder. *Journal of Nervous and Mental Disease, 170*, 381–406.

Boden, S. D., Davis, D. O., Dina, T. S., Patronas, N. J., & Wiesel, S. W. (1990). Abnormal magnetic-resonance scans of the lumbar spine in asymptomatic subjects. *Journal of Bone and Joint Surgery, 72A*, 403–408.

Bonica, J. J. (1990). Postoperative pain. In J. J. Bonica, J. D. Loeser, C. R. Chapman, & W. E. Fordyce (Eds.), *The management of pain* (Vol. 1, pp. 461–480). Philadelphia: Lea & Febiger.

Cairns, D., Mooney, V., & Crane, P. (1982). Spinal pain rehabilitation: Inpatient and outpatient treatment results and development of predictors for outcome. *Spine, 9*, 91–95.

Cats-Baril, W. L., & Frymoyer, J. W. (1991). Identifying patients at risk of becoming disabled because of low back pain: The Vermont Engineering Center Predictive Model. *Spine, 16*, 605–607.

Chapman, C. R., & Turner, J. A. (1986). Psychological control of acute pain in medical settings. *Journal of Pain and Symptom Management, 1*, 9–20.

Council, J. R., Ahern, D. K., Follick, M. J., & Kline, C. L. (1988). Expectancies and functional impairment in chronic low back pain. *Pain, 33*, 323–331.

Crook, J., Weir, R., & Tunks, E. (1989). An epidemiological follow-up survey of persistent pain sufferers in a group family practice and specialty pain clinic. *Pain, 36*, 49–61.

Deyo, R. A. (1986). The early diagnostic evaluation of patients with low back pain. *Journal of General Internal Medicine, 1*, 328–338.

Deyo, R. A. (1988). Measuring the functional status of patients with low back pain. *Archives of Physical Medicine and Rehabilitation, 69*, 1044–1053.

Deyo, R. A., & Diehl, A. K. (1983). Measuring physical and psychosocial function in patients with low-back pain. *Spine, 8*, 635–642.

Eich, E., Reeves, J., Jaeger, B., & Graff-Radford, S. B. (1985). Memory for pain: Relation between past and present pain intensity. *Pain, 23*, 375–379.

Flor, H., & Turk, D. C. (1988). Chronic back pain and rheumatoid arthritis: Predicting pain and disability from cognitive variables. *Journal of Behavioral Medicine, 11*, 251–265.

Fordyce, W. E. (1976). *Behavioral methods for chronic pain and illness.* St. Louis, MO: Mosby.

Fordyce, W. E., Lansky, D., Calsyn, D. A., Shelton, J. L., Stolov, W. C., & Rock, D. L. (1984). Pain measurement and pain behavior. *Pain, 18*, 53–69.

Gureje, O. (1998). Persistent pain and well-being: A World Health Organization study in primary care. *Journal of the American Medical Association, 280*, 147–151.

Hagglund, K. J., Haley, W. E., Reveille, J. D., & Alarcon, G. S. (1989). Predicting individual impairment among patients with rheumatoid arthritis. *Arthritis and Rheumatism, 32*, 851–858.

Hitselberger, W. E., & Witten, R. M. (1968). Abnormal myelograms in asymptomatic patients. *Journal of Neurosurgery, 28*, 204–206.

Illich, I. (1976). *Medical nemesis: The exploration of health.* Harmondsworth, England: Penguin Books.

Jensen, M. C., Brant-Zawadski, M. N., Obuchowski, N., Modic, M. T., & Malkasian Ross, J. S. (1994). Magnetic resonance imaging of the lumbar spine in people with back pain. *New England Journal of Medicine, 331*, 69–73.

Jette, A. M. (1987). The Functional Status Index: Reliability and validity of a self-report functional disability measure. *Journal of Rheumatology, 14*(Suppl. 14), 15–19.

Joranson, D. E., & Lietman, R. (1994). *The McNeil National Pain Study.* New York: Louis Harris & Associates.

Knapp, D. A., & Koch, H. (1984). *The management of new pain in office-based ambulatory care: National and Ambulatory Medical Care Survey, National Center for Health Statistics, 1980 and 1981* (Advance Data from Vital and Health Statistics, No. 97; DHHS Publication

No. PHS 84-1250). Hyattsville, MD: U.S. Public Health Service.

Koch, H. (1986). *The management of chronic pain in office-based ambulatory care: National Ambulatory Medical Care Survey* (Advance Data from Vital and Health Statistics, No. 123; DHHS Publication No. PHS 86-1250). Hyattsville, MD: U.S. Public Health Service.

Kremer, E. F., Block, A., & Gaylor, M. S. (1981). Behavioral approaches to treatment of chronic pain: The inaccuracy of patient self-report measures. *Archives of Physical Medicine and Rehabilitation, 62,* 188-191.

Lasagna, L. (1960). Clinical measurement of pain. *Annals of the New York Academy of Sciences, 86,* 28-37.

Linton, S. J., & Gotestam, K. G. (1983). A clinical comparison of two pain scales: Correlation, remembering chronic pain and a measure of compliance. *Pain, 17,* 57-66.

Marketdata Enterprises. (1995). *Chronic pain management programs: A market analysis.* Valley Stream, NY: Author.

Marketdata Enterprises. (1999). *Pain management programs: A market analysis.* Tampa, FL: Author.

Matyas, T. A., & Bach, T. M. (1985). The reliability of selected techniques in clinical arthrometrics. *Australian Journal of Physiotherapy, 31,* 173-197.

Melzack, R. (1975). The McGill Pain Questionnaire: Major properties and scoring methods. *Pain, 1,* 277-299.

Melzack, R., & Casey, K. L. (1968). Sensory, motivational, and central control determinants of pain: A new conceptual model. In D. Kenshalo (Ed.), *The skin senses* (pp. 423-443). Springfield, IL: Charles C. Thomas.

Melzack, R., & Torgerson, W. S. (1971). On the language of pain. *Anesthesiology, 34,* 50-59.

Melzack, R., & Wall, P. D. (1965). Pain mechanisms: A new theory. *Science, 150,* 971-979.

Melzack, R., & Wall, P. D. (1983). *The challenge of pain.* New York: Basic Books.

Millard, R. W. (1989). The Functional Assessment Screening Questionnaire: Application for evaluating pain-related disability. *Archives of Physical Medicine and Rehabilitation, 70,* 303-307.

Nachemson, A. L. (1976). The lumbar spine: An orthopedic challenge. *Spine, 1,* 59-71.

Naliboff, B. D., Cohen, M. J., Swanson, G. A., Bonebakker, A. D., & McArthur, D. L. (1985). Comprehensive assessment of chronic low back pain patients and controls: Physical abilities, level of activity, psychological adjustment and pain perception. *Pain, 23,* 121-134.

Peebles, R. J., & Schneiderman, D. S. (1991). *Socioeconomic fact book for surgery, 1991-1992.* Chicago: American College of Surgeons.

Raj, P. P. (1990). Pain relief: Fact or fancy? *Regional Anesthesia, 15,* 157-169.

Reesor, K. A., & Craig, K. D. (1988). Medically incongruent chronic back pain: Physical limitations, suffering, and ineffective coping. *Pain, 32,* 35-45.

Schappert, S. M. (1998, February). Ambulatory care visits to physicians offices, hospital outpatient departments,

and emergency departments: United States, 1996. *Vital and Health Statistics,* Series 13 (134), 1-80.

Sternbach, R. (1968). *Pain: A psychophysiological analysis.* New York: Academic Press.

Turk, D. C. (1989). Assessment of pain: The elusiveness of latent constructs. In C. R. Chapman & J. D. Loeser (Eds.), *Advances in pain research and therapy: Vol. 12. Issues in pain measurment* (pp. 267-279). New York: Raven Press.

Turk, D. C., & Fernandez, E. (1990). On the putative uniqueness of cancer pain: Do psychological principles apply? *Behaviour Research and Therapy, 28,* 1-13.

Turk, D. C., Meichenbaum, D., & Genest, M. (1983). *Pain and behavioral medicine: A cognitive-behavioral perspective.* New York: Guilford Press.

Turk, D. C., & Okifuji, A. (2001). Pain terms and taxonomies. In J. D. Loeser, C. R. Chapman, S. D. Butler, & D. C. Turk (Eds.), *Bonica's management of pain* (3rd ed., pp. 17-25). Philadelphia: Lippincott Williams & Wilkins.

Turk, D. C., Okifuji, A., & Kalauokalani, D. (1999). Clinical outcome and economic evaluation of multidisciplinary pain centers. In A. R. Block, E. F. Kremer, & E. Fernandez (Eds.), *Handbook of pain syndromes: Biopsycosocial perspectives* (pp. 77-98). Mahwah, NJ: Erlbaum.

Turk, D. C., Okifuji, A., Sinclair, J. D., & Starz, T. W. (1996). Pain, disability, and physical functioning in subgroups of fibromyalgia patients. *Journal of Rheumatology, 23,* 1255-1262.

Turk, D. C., & Rudy, T. E. (1990). Neglected factors in chronic pain treatment outcome studies: Referral patterns, failure to enter treatment, and attrition. *Pain, 43,* 7-26.

Von Korff, M., Dworkin, S. G., LeResche, L., & Kruger, A. (1988). An epidemiologic comparison of pain complaints. *Pain, 32,* 33-40.

Waddell, G. (1987). A new clinical method for the treatment of low back pain. *Spine, 12,* 632-644.

Waddell, G., Bircher, M., Finlayson, D., & Main, C. J. (1984). Symptoms and signs: Physical disease or illness behavior? *British Medical Journal, 289,* 739-741.

Waddell, G., Main, C. J., Morris, E. W., Venner, R. M., Rae, P. S., Sharmy, S. H., & Galloway, H. (1982). Normality and reliability in the clinical assessment of backache. *British Medical Journal, 284,* 1519-1523.

White, A. A., & Gordon, S. L. (1982). Synopsis: Workshop on idiopathic low-back pain. *Spine, 7,* 141-149.

Wiesel, S. W., Tsourmas, N., & Feffer, H. (1984). A study of computer-assisted tomography: 1. The incidence of positive CAT scans in an asymptomatic group of patients. *Spine, 9,* 549-551.

Woolf, C., Bennett, G. J., Doherty, M., Dubner, R., Kidd, B., Koltzenburg, M., Lipton, R., Loeser, J., Payne, R., & Torebjork, E. (1998). Towards a mechanism-based classification of pain. [Editorial] *Pain, 77,* 227-229.

Part I

MEASUREMENT
OF PAIN

Chapter 2

Self-Report Scales and Procedures for Assessing Pain in Adults

MARK P. JENSEN
PAUL KAROLY

Pain and suffering are private, internal events that cannot be directly observed by clinicians or assessed via bioassays. Assessment of the pain experience is therefore frequently built upon the use of patient self-reports. The purpose of this chapter is to critically evaluate the available self-report measures of pain. Our hope is that the chapter will assist clinicians and researchers to select the procedures that best serve their purposes. We begin with a brief discussion of issues relevant to the use of self-report pain scales. We then describe and critique the methods currently available for assessing four aspects of the pain experience: pain intensity, pain affect, pain quality, and pain location.

THEORETICAL AND ASSESSMENT MODEL

Because decisions about the choice of pain assessment procedures are usually based on one's model or conceptualization of pain, it is important to make explicit the model or concept that we use to guide our understanding of pain. We label our assumptive framework the *pain context model* (Karoly, 1985, 1991; Karoly & Jensen, 1987). Like those of others (see Flor, Birbaumer, & Turk, 1990; Keefe & France, 1999), our model is based on the assumption that the pain experience can be examined at several levels, and that the data obtained can be

influenced by numerous psychological, medical, and social factors.

In the pain context model, pain is considered to be a construct (see Cleeland, 1986, 1989; Rudy, 1989; Turk, 1989). A *construct* is a label for categorizing a related group of observations. Pain is similar to other psychological constructs, such as depression, anxiety, and intelligence, in that it is not directly observable, but rather is inferred from varied observations.

Even the best measures or indicants of a construct are not always closely related to one another (Cleeland, 1986). This is because the different observations or components that make up a construct do not always co-occur in time or in the same configuration in all people. For example, even though pain may be assessed via behavioral observation or self-report, one person may display nonverbal pain behaviors without complaining of pain; another may complain bitterly of pain and yet display no nonverbal pain activities; and a third person may display pain behaviors and report intense pain and suffering (see also Craig, Prkachin, & Grunau, Chapter 9, and Keefe, Williams, & Smith, Chapter 10, this volume). Because of the multidimensionality of pain, no single measure can adequately assess the totality of the pain construct. An important preliminary task in pain assessment is therefore to define the dimensions of pain relevant to one's evaluation purposes, and to demonstrate that the selected dimensions are related to adjustment and well-being.

A considerable amount of work has already gone into defining the dimensions of subjective pain. Although there is more work to be done, at this point at least four dimensions or categories of the pain experience can be assessed in nearly all pain patient populations: *pain intensity*, *pain affect*, *pain quality*, and *pain location*.

Pain intensity may be defined as *how much* a person hurts. Patients are usually able to provide quantitative pain intensity estimates relatively quickly, and most measures of pain intensity tend to be closely related to one another statistically (Jensen, Karoly, & Braver, 1986; Jensen, Karoly, O'Riordan, Bland, & Burns, 1989). These findings suggest that pain intensity is a fairly homogeneous dimension, and one that is relatively easy for adults to identify and gauge.

Pain affect, on the other hand, appears to be more complex than pain intensity. We define pain affect as the degree of emotional arousal or changes in action readiness caused by the sensory experience of pain. This arousal is often felt as distressing or frightening, and can lead to interference in daily activities and habitual modes of response. Pain affect is thus a mental state triggered by an implicit or explicit appraisal of threat. In chronic pain, the emotional aspects (or fear appraisals) can come to dominate the clinical picture.

Measures of pain affect have been shown to be statistically distinct from measures of pain intensity, but pain affect and pain intensity are rarely if ever independent (Fernandez & Turk, 1992; Gracely, 1992). Furthermore, measures of pain affect do not appear to be as homogeneous as measures of pain intensity; they are less likely than measures of pain intensity to be strongly related to one another. This finding indicates that the affective component of pain consists of a variety of emotional reactions (Morley, 1989; Morley & Pallin, 1995). Thus pain experience is probably similar to other sensory/perceptual experiences, such as those involved in the perception of light or sound. The color intensity or brightness reflecting off a painting may be relatively easy to rate, whereas judgments regarding how that color makes one feel may require considerably more reflection. Affective responses probably also require more than a single word or number to describe adequately. We believe that pain affect operates in a fashion similar to color or sound affect.

Pain quality refers to the specific physical sensations associated with pain. Because pain can be felt (and described) in so many ways, this category of pain contains a variety of constructs, such as perceived temperature (e.g., "cold" vs. "hot") and sharpness (e.g., "dull" vs. "sharp"), among many others (see Melzack & Katz, Chapter 3).

Pain location can be defined as the perceived location(s) of pain sensation that patients experience on or in their bodies. Clinicians have learned to pay attention to several aspects of patient descriptions of pain location. Where patients describe pain, the number of locations indicated, and the way in which patients describe the location(s) of their pain all appear to be related to physical and psychosocial functioning.

ON THE MULTIPLE CONTEXTS OF PAIN MEASUREMENT

The pain context model directs one's attention to the degree to which the pain experience is embedded in its surroundings. Pain is a dynamic, developmental process, not a single event or simple quantifiable product (see also Chapman, Nakamura, & Flores, 1999). Thus, when we and others talk of "objective" measures or "quantifiable" indices, the reader should understand that we do not intend to depict pain as a static, all-or-none, unidimensional, body-centered occurrence that exists somehow independently of time, place, the patient's states of consciousness, or the observer's presuppositions. We have elsewhere noted: "As pain assessors, we are coparticipants, not merely observers and, therefore, although there is no single best way to interpret pain, we can probably serve our patients better if we acknowledge that we are jointly engaged in creating the pain dimensions we seek to measure" (Karoly & Jensen, 1987, p. 7).

Language habits and cultural conventions sometimes force us to further decontextualize the pain experience by addressing separately an individual's awareness of pain (e.g., "My arm hurts"), emotional reactivity (e.g., "The pain in my arm is killing me"), and behavioral (motor) responses (e.g., the tendency to use the other arm or to keep the arm in a sling). However, it is critical to remember that thought, action, and emotion are inextricably bound together in the sentient organism—and that they are separable only for the sake of convenience. Moreover, pain experience *emerges* from the dynamic interplay of thought, action, and emotion in context.

Research from a number of sources and with different populations provides strong evidence that many factors influence communication about pain. A brief review of this research will help to illustrate this important pain.

Levine and De Simone (1991) assigned college students to be in the presence of an attractive male or female while holding their hand in ice water and rating pain. Based on gender role expectations, Levine and De Simone predicted that males would report less pain in the presence of the female as opposed to the male experimenter. This was exactly what they found. Female students, on the other hand, were not significantly influenced by the gender of the experimenter. In another study, Craig and Weiss (1971) found that modeling of pain tolerance influences the report of pain. Subjects who observed people modeling high pain tolerance reported higher pain tolerance (in response to electric shock) than subjects who observed people modeling low pain tolerance. Dworkin and Chen (1982) showed that changing the environment influenced pain report. Their subjects reported that tooth pulp stimulation hurt more when it was administered in a dental clinic than when it was administered in a research laboratory setting. Even a person's history of injury can alter how that person responds to painful stimuli. Dar, Ariely, and Frank (1995) found that veterans who had been severely injured reported a higher pain threshold (more stimulation was necessary before they interpreted the stimuli as painful) and higher pain tolerance than veterans who had not been severely injured. Finally, research indicates that relatively subtle changes, such as altering the orientation of a scale (presenting the same scale either horizontally or vertically) or making slight changes in the descriptive endpoints of scales, can alter the responses to those measures (Ogon, Krismer, Söllner, Kanter-Rumplmair, & Lampe, 1996; Seymour, Simpson, Charlton, & Phillips, 1985; Sriwatanakul et al., 1983).

Research also indicates that the time of day is related to pain intensity ratings. Folkard, Glynn, and Lloyd (1976) asked patients with chronic pain to rate their pain intensity every 2 hours from 8:00 A.M. to 10:00 P.M. On average, reported pain demonstrated an increase over the course of a day, with "peaks" occurring at noon and 6:00 P.M. However, there was much variation between patients regarding their diurnal variation in pain report. Similarly, Jamison and Brown (1991) found that pain intensity reports changed in a predictable pattern throughout the course of a day for the majority of patients with chronic pain, although the specific temporal pattern varied from individual to individual.

There are two implications of the above-cited findings for assessing and interpreting self-report pain data. First, the findings illustrate that self-reports of pain do not stand in a one-to-one relationship to nociception. (*Nociception* is the activation of sensory transduction in receptors or nerves that convey information about tissue damage.) In addition, although it is likely that people attempt to report their subjective pain experience honestly in most situations, there are no guarantees that what people say about their pain accurately reflects their current or past pain experience. These considerations have caused some clinicians and investigators to advocate the elimination of self-report data. Although we do not agree with such an extreme position, we strongly advise clinicians and researchers to be wary of relying solely on decontextualized subjective pain reports when attempting to understand an individual's pain problem (see also Craig et al., Chapter 9).

A second implication of this body of research is that clinicians and researchers should take into account the factors known to influence self-report of pain. The conditions under which self-reports of pain are made should be as similar as possible between comparison groups or between assessment periods. Attempts should be made, for example, to have patients rate their pain at the same time of day, in the same place, and in the presence of the same people at each assessment period. It is also necessary to use the same measures, with the same endpoint descriptors, across time. A decision to aggregate multiple measures across time and/or across measures (e.g., taking the average of several pain measures) will help to minimize the influence of extraneous or irrelevant contextual factors, and may have a greater impact in increasing the reliability and validity of pain assessment than any other decision that a clinician or researcher makes, including decisions about specific pain measures. In support of this practice, aggregated pain measures have been shown to be more reliable (Andrasik & Holroyd, 1980; Jensen & McFarland, 1993; Jensen, Turner, Romano, & Fisher, 1999) and more sensitive to treatment effects (Max, 1991) than single items. It is also possible to allow the respondent him- or herself to aggregate pain experience by providing a rating of "average" pain over the course of a specific time period (say, during the past week). Although such estimates are adequately valid in many situations (Jensen et al., 1996; Salovey,

Smith, Turk, Jobe, & Willis, 1993), memory of previous pain is biased (to some degree) by current pain experience—that is, people tend to rate their previous pain as worse if they are experiencing more pain at the time they are asked to recall previous pain than if they are experiencing less pain when rating previous pain (Jensen et al., 1996; Salovey et al., 1993). Therefore, more accurate estimates of actual average pain can be obtained by averaging multiple measures (of current pain) over time than by asking patients to recall and rate their average pain (Jensen et al., 1996).

We have briefly discussed some theoretical and practical issues related to the assessment of the subjective experience of pain in order to provide the reader with a context within which to use and understand self-report data. Given this background, we are now ready to describe and critique the available self-report measures of the pain experience. The next four sections discuss the procedures that may be used to assess the dimensions of the pain experience introduced above: pain intensity, pain affect, pain quality, and pain location.

ASSESSING PAIN INTENSITY

Pain intensity is a quantitative estimate of the severity or magnitude of perceived pain. The three most commonly used methods to assess pain intensity are Verbal Rating Scales (VRSs), Visual Analogue Scales (VASs), and Numerical Rating Scales (NRSs). Less common measures include various versions of a picture (or face) scale, and the Descriptor Differential Scale of Pain Intensity (DDS-I).

Verbal Rating Scales

A VRS consists of a list of adjectives describing different levels of pain intensity. An adequate VRS of pain intensity should include adjectives that reflect the extremes of this dimension (e.g., from "no pain" to "extremely intense pain"), and sufficient additional adjectives to capture the gradations of pain intensity that may be experienced. Patients are asked to read over the list of adjectives and select the word or phrase that best describes their level of pain on the scale. Many different VRS lists have been created, and some of the most common are presented in Table 2.1.

VRSs are usually scored by listing the adjectives in order of pain severity, and assigning each one a score as a function of its rank. In the 4-point

TABLE 2.1. Verbal Rating Scales (VRSs) of Pain Intensity

4-point scale[a]	4-point scale[c]
No pain	No pain at all
Mild	Some pain
Moderate	Considerable pain
Severe	Pain that could not be more severe

5-point scale[b]	15-point scale[d]
None	Extremely weak
Mild	Very weak
Moderate	Weak
Severe	Very mild
Very severe	Mild
	Very moderate
	Slightly moderate
	Moderate
	Barely strong
	Slightly intense
	Strong
	Intense
	Very strong
	Very intense
	Extremely intense

[a]From Seymour, R. A. (1982). The use of pain scales in assessing the efficacy of analgesics in post-operative dental pain. *European Journal of Clinical Pharmacology*, 23, 441–444. Copyright 1982 by the *European Journal of Clinical Pharmacology*. Reprinted by permission.

[b]From Frank, A. J. M., Moll, J. M. H., and Hort, J. F. (1982). A comparison of three ways of measuring pain. *Rheumatology and Rehabilitation*, 21, 211–217. Copyright 1982 by the British Association of Rheumatology and Rehabilitation. Reprinted by permission.

[c]From Joyce, C. R. B., Zutshi, D. W., Hrubes, V., and Mason, R. M. (1975). Comparison of fixed interval and visual analogue scales for rating chronic pain. *European Journal of Clinical Pharmacology*, 8, 415–420. Copyright 1975 by the *European Journal of Clinical Pharmacology*. Reprinted by permission.

[d]Reprinted from *Pain, 5*, R. H. Gracely, P. McGrath, and R. Dubner, Ratio scales of sensory and affective verbal pain descriptors, 5–18. Copyright 1978, with permission from Elsevier Science.

VRS used by Seymour (1982), for example, no pain would be given a score of 0, mild pain a score of 1, moderate pain a score of 2, and severe pain a score of 3. The number associated with the adjective chosen by the patient would constitute his or her pain intensity score.

A criticism frequently raised with respect to the rank-scoring method is that it assumes equal intervals between the adjectives, even though it is extremely unlikely that equal perceptual intervals exist. That is, the interval between no pain and mild pain may be much smaller than that between moderate pain and severe pain, yet each interval is scored as if the difference were equivalent. This characteristic of rank-scoring procedures can pose several problems when one is interpreting VRS data. For example, rank scores do not allow for adequate interpretations of the magnitude of any differences found. A change from 3 to 2 (on a 4-point scale) might represent a 10% change in perceived pain or a 50% change, depending on the perceived interval represented by the words on the list. In addition, some investigators have raised the objection that ranked data should not be analyzed with the more common (and usually more powerful) parametric statistics. However, it has become increasingly recognized that most parametric techniques (such as analysis of variance and the *t*-test) are still valid when used with data that do not represent equal-interval values, especially if the number of categories on the scale is five or more (Cicchetti, Showalter, & Tyrer, 1985; Philip, 1990; Rasmussen, 1989; see also Baker, Hardyck, & Petrinovich, 1966).

Cross-modality matching procedures have been used as a means of transforming VRS ratings to scale scores that are more likely to have ratio properties—that is, to scores with equivalent intervals (Gracely, McGrath, & Dubner, 1978a, 1978b; see also Price, Riley, & Wade, Chapter 4). The matching procedure involves asking each patient to indicate the severity that each word represents in reference to one or more other modalities (such as the loudness of a tone, the length of a line, or handgrip force). The rating that the patient gives to a particular word (or the average of several, if the patient rates each word more than once) is then used as the score for that word. Because the modalities used by patients to match pain descriptors to can themselves be indexed via ratio scales, the numbers or scores derived from such a procedure are believed likely to have ratio properties and to reflect actual perceived differences in magnitudes.

There are two major limitations of cross-modality matching procedures. First, such procedures are time-consuming and can be tedious, both of which can adversely affect patient compliance (Ahles, Ruckdeschel, & Blanchard, 1984). One way around this problem is to assign standardized scores for each word based on data from groups of previously tested individuals (see Gracely et al., 1978a; Tursky, Jamner, & Friedman, 1982; and Urban, Keefe, & France, 1984, for standardized scores for specific words). Second, most of the standardized scores have been developed using nonpatients in response to experimental pain. There

is evidence that patients with chronic pain may rate the intensity of pain words differently than do patients with acute (i.e., postoperative) pain (Wallenstein, Heidrich, Kaiko, & Houde, 1980). Even within diagnostic subgroups, the score given to a word by one patient has been shown to vary from that given by other patients, indicating that standardized scores for VRS adjectives may be less reliable than originally hoped (Urban et al., 1984).

Moreover, VRS scores obtained through cross-modality procedures may correlate so highly with those obtained by using the ranking method that they contain essentially the same degree of useful information (Hall, 1981; Levine & De Simone, 1991). Similarly, VRS scores created by either of the two methods show the same patterns of associations to other pain measures, again suggesting that the information contained in the scores derived from the two methods is comparable (Jensen et al., 1989). Therefore, we recommend that the simpler ranking method be used when relationships between pain intensity and other factors are examined. The more sophisticated cross-modality matching procedures should be used only when ratio-like scaling is needed (i.e., when one needs to know the specific magnitude of differences in pain ratings across time or between groups).

The strengths of VRSs include the ease with which they can be administered and scored, provided that scores are calculated using the ranking method or from data developed from previous cross-modality matching experiments. Because they are generally easy to comprehend, compliance rates for VRSs are as good and often better than those for other measures of pain intensity (Jensen et al., 1986, 1989). Also, VRSs have consistently demonstrated their validity as indicants of pain intensity. They are related positively and significantly to other measures of pain intensity (see, e.g., Jensen et al., 1986; Kremer, Atkinson, & Ignelzi, 1981; Ohnhaus & Adler, 1975; Paice & Cohen, 1997). VRSs also consistently demonstrate sensitivity to treatments that are known to have an impact on pain intensity (Fox & Melzack, 1976; Ohnhaus & Adler, 1975; Rybstein-Blinchik, 1979).

Despite these strengths, we hesitate to recommend VRSs as the method of choice if only one index is employed. One weakness of VRSs is that patients need to read over, or be familiar with, the entire list of pain adjectives before they can select the one that most closely describes their pain. For a longer list (e.g., 15 or more items), this requirement can make the task time-consuming, and the clinician or researcher cannot be assured that the patient or subject has adequately reviewed the entire list of adjectives. Also, because VRSs require patients to select from a finite number of descriptors, patients may be unable to find one that accurately describes their perceived pain intensity (Joyce, Zutshi, Hrubes, & Mason, 1975). Among illiterate patients, VRSs are less reliable than other pain intensity measures (Ferraz et al., 1990). Finally, a clinician or researcher using a VRS must select a scoring procedure; and, as already discussed, each scoring method has its drawbacks. Possibly because of the relative weaknesses of VRSs, and the availability of other measures of pain intensity, VRSs are being used less often than they have previously been in pain treatment outcome research.

Visual Analogue Scales and Graphic Rating Scales

A VAS consists of a line, usually 10 cm long, whose ends are labeled as the extremes of pain (e.g., "no pain" to "pain as bad as it could be"). A VAS may have specific points along the line that are labeled with intensity-denoting adjectives or numbers. Such a scale is called a graphic rating scale (GRS). Patients are asked to indicate which point along the line best represents their pain intensity. The distance from the no pain end to the mark made by the patient is that patients' pain intensity score. Figure 2.1 illustrates a VAS and two GRSs.

As for VRSs, there is much evidence supporting the validity of VASs for pain intensity. Such scales demonstrate positive relations to other self-

report measures of pain intensity (Jensen et al., 1986; Kremer et al., 1981; Paice & Cohen, 1997; Seymour, 1982) as well as to observed pain behavior (Gramling & Elliot, 1992; Teske, Daut, & Cleeland, 1983). They are sensitive to treatment effects (Joyce et al., 1975; Seymour, 1982; Turner, 1982), and are distinct from measures of other subjective components of pain (Ahles et al., 1984). The scores from VASs appear to have the qualities of ratio data for groups of people (Price & Harkins, 1987; Price, McGrath, Rafii, & Buckingham, 1983). This means that differences in pain intensity (for groups, not necessarily for individuals) as measured by VASs represent actual differences in magnitude. For example, a significant change in average pain intensity from 60 to 30 in a group of individuals who received a treatment not only would reflect a decrease in pain intensity, but would specifically indicate that perceived pain intensity was halved. Another advantage of VASs over some other pain intensity scales is the high number of response categories of VASs. Since they are usually measured in millimeters, a 10-cm VAS can be considered as having 101 response levels. This high number of response categories makes the VAS potentially more sensitive to changes in pain intensity than measures with limited numbers of response categories.[1] Although research that compares the VAS to other measures indicates minimal differences in sensitivity to change most of the time, when differences are found, the VAS is usually more sensitive than other measures, especially those with a limited number of response categories (i.e., seven or fewer; Bolton & Wilkinson, 1998; Joyce et al., 1975; Max, Schafer, Culnane, Dubner, & Gracely, 1987; Sriwatanakul et al., 1983).

One of the problems with VASs is that scoring is more time-consuming and involves more steps (and therefore more opportunity for error) than scoring for the other measures of pain intensity. To address this problem, several investigators have created mechanical VASs (see, e.g., Choinière & Amsel, 1996; Gaston-Johansson, 1996; Grossi et al., 1983; Grossman et al., 1992; Price, Bush, Long, & Harkins, 1994; Thomas & Griffiths, 1982). A mechanical VAS is usually a laminated paper or plastic VAS with a sliding marker that patients use to rate their pain intensity. Commonly, one side of the scale, which a patient sees, just lists the pain endpoints (e.g., "no pain" to "unbearable pain"). For some mechanical VASs, an additional cue—such as gradations of color from a pale pink (on the "no pain" side) to a dark red (on the "un-

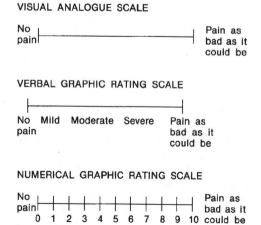

FIGURE 2.1. A Visual Analogue Scale (VAS) and two graphic rating scales (GRSs) of pain intensity.

bearable pain" side; Grossi et al., 1983)—is provided. The other side of the mechanical VAS usually indicates (numerically), usually in millimeters, how far the patient has slid the marker from the "no pain" end toward the extreme pain end. After the patient rates his or her pain, all the researcher or clinician need do is examine the other side of the scale to obtain the intensity score. Mechanical VASs have been shown to be strongly associated with classic paper-and-pencil VASs (Choinière & Amsel, 1996; Grossi et al., 1983; Grossman et al., 1992; Thomas & Griffiths, 1982) and have been shown to have good test–retest reliability over a 2-hour period (Gaston-Johansson, 1996). In addition, like paper-and-pencil VASs, mechanical VASs appear to have ratio qualities (Price et al., 1994).

One drawback to both the paper-and-pencil and mechanical VASs is that they require the respondent to have a minimum level of motor abilities to use the scale. Any study that uses these measures must therefore exclude persons with significant motor disabilities (see Hadjistavropoulos, von Baeyer, & Craig, Chapter 8). Also (and perhaps of greater concern), research consistently shows that VASs are more difficult to understand than other measures of pain intensity—especially among persons at risk for cognitive difficulties, such as some elderly individuals or persons on high doses of opioid analgesics (Jensen et al., 1986; Kremer et al., 1981; Paice & Cohen, 1997; Walsh, 1984). This may explain the preference that patients tend to have for the more straightforward NRSs or VRSs (Choinière & Amsel, 1996). Comprehension difficulties place further limits on the populations for whom a VAS can be considered valid and reliable. Therefore, unless a particular clinician or researcher has a strong rationale for using a VAS (e.g., he or she may require a scale more likely to have ratio qualities), and providing that the population being studied is limited to persons who are at low risk for cognitive difficulties, we recommend against using the VAS as a primary (or sole) measure of pain intensity. If an investigator plans to use a VAS, careful explanation and patient practice with the scale may decrease the failure rate (Scott & Huskisson, 1976), although high failure rates can still occur despite careful explanations (Walsh, 1984).

Numerical Rating Scales

A NRS involves asking patients to rate their pain from 0 to 10 (11-point scale), from 0 to 20 (21-point scale), or from 0 to 100 (101-point scale), with the understanding that the 0 represents one end of the pain intensity continuum (i.e., no pain) while the 10, 20, or 100 represents the other extreme of pain intensity (i.e., pain as bad as it could be). Verbal NRSs do not require paper and pencil. The patient is simply asked to verbally state his or her pain intensity on a 0–10 (or 0–20, or 0–100) scale. Nonetheless, a number of paper-and-pencil NRSs exist. One simply asks patients to record the number that best represents their pain intensity (see, e.g., Jensen et al., 1986, 1989). Another presents the numbers in ascending order with the endpoint descriptors near the 0 and the highest number of the scale, and asks patients to circle the number that best represents their pain intensity (e.g., the pain intensity scales of the Brief Pain Inventory; Cleeland & Ryan, 1994). Yet another version of the NRS is a box scale, which consists of 11 numbers (0 through 10) presented in ascending order and surrounded by boxes (Downie et al., 1978). For the box scale, patients are asked to place an "X" through the number that represents their pain. For all of these scales, the patient's pain intensity score is simply the number the patient has indicated.

The validity of NRSs has been well documented. They demonstrate positive and significant correlations with other measures of pain intensity (Jensen et al., 1986, 1989; Kremer et al., 1981; Seymour, 1982; Wilkie, Lovejoy, Dodd, & Tesler, 1990). They have also demonstrated sensitivity to treatments that are expected to have an impact on pain intensity (Chesney & Shelton, 1976; Keefe, Schapira, Williams, Brown, & Surwit, 1981; Paice & Cohen, 1997; Stenn, Mothersill, & Brooke, 1979). NRSs are likewise extremely easy to administer and score, so they can be used with a greater variety of patients (e.g., geriatric patients, patients with marked motor difficulties) than is possible with a VAS. Because a verbal NRS does not require special materials (e.g., pencil and printed cards or paper), it can be administered over the phone. The simplicity of the measure may be one of the reasons for the high rate of comparative compliance with the measurement task. Moreover, older people do not appear to have as much difficulty with NRSs as they do with the traditional VAS (Jensen et al., 1986; Paice & Cohen, 1997). Also, if an investigator wishes to maximize the number of response categories, he or she may use a 101-point NRS.

The primary weakness of NRSs is that they may not have ratio qualities (Price et al., 1994), especially when compared to VASs, which do appear to have ratio qualities. Although this may not affect the reliability, validity, or sensitivity of NRSs to treatment outcome, an evaluator cannot necessarily conclude that a change in perceived pain from 9.0 to 6.0 as measured by a NRS represents a 33% decrease in perceived pain. On the other hand, the only type of scale that has been shown to have ratio qualities (the VAS) has other weaknesses not shared by NRSs. Taking all these issues into consideration, we choose 0–10 NRSs over other measures because we work with a great diversity of patients.

Other Intensity Measures

Picture or Face Scales

Picture or face scales employ photographs or line drawings that illustrate facial expressions of persons experiencing different levels of pain severity (e.g., Beyer & Knott, 1998; Frank, Moll, & Hort, 1982; Keck, Gerkensmeyer, Joyce, & Schade, 1996; Wong & Baker, 1988). Patients are asked to indicate which one of the illustrations best represents their pain experience. Each face has a number representing the rank order of pain illustrated, and the number associated with the picture chosen by the patient represents that individual's pain inten-

sity score. Figure 2.2 illustrates the facial expressions used in one of the picture scales (Frank et al., 1982).

Because picture and face scales do not require patients to be literate, they provide an option for individuals who have difficulty with written language. This makes such scales particularly useful in pediatric populations, for whom the scales have demonstrated validity through their association with other measures of pain intensity (Beyer & Knott, 1998; Bieri, Reeve, Champion, Addicoat, & Ziegler, 1990; West et al., 1994; see also McGrath & Gillespie, Chapter 6), and through their ability to detect the effects of analgesia (Beyer & Knott, 1998). Picture and face scales also appear to be preferred by children over other intensity measures (West et al., 1994; Wong & Baker, 1988). There is also evidence that picture and face scales are valid for use with adults, as demonstrated by their association with other measures of pain intensity (see Frank et al., 1982; Stuppy, 1998). Picture and face scales seem an ideal option for those situations where the clinician or researcher has a question about the literacy of the patient/ subject population he or she is working with. Nonetheless, Picture or face scales need to be *explained* to patients, implying a degree of comprehension

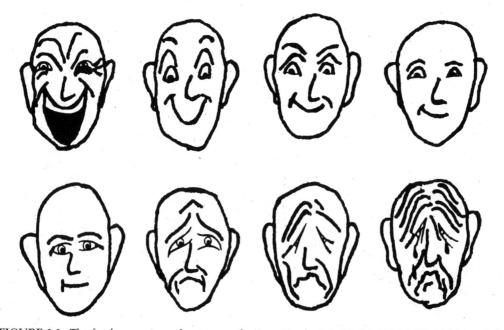

FIGURE 2.2. The facial expressions of a picture scale. From Frank, A. J. M., Moll, J. M. H., and Hurt, J. F. A. (1982). A comparison of three ways of measuring pain. *Rheumatology and Rehabilitation, 21,* 211–217. Copyright 1982 by the British Association of Rheumatology and Rehabilitation. Illustrations by J. M. H. Moll. Reprinted by permission.

that may be lacking in very young children or in the cognitively impaired (see McGrath & Gillespie, Chapter 6, and Hadjistavropoulos et al., Chapter 8).

Descriptor Differential Scale of Pain Intensity

The DDS-I consists of a list of adjectives describing different levels of pain intensity (Gracely & Kwilosz, 1988). Patients are asked to rate the intensity of their pain as being more or less than each word on the list (see Table 2.2). If their experienced pain is greater than that described by the word, they place a check mark to the right of the word in proportion to how much greater their pain is. If their pain is less than that described by the word, they place a check mark to the left of the word. If the word exactly describes their pain level, they place a check mark directly below the descriptor. There are 10 points along which patients can rate their pain intensity to the right and left of each word, so pain is rated along a 21-point scale for each word. Pain intensity is defined as the mean of the ratings, and therefore can range from 0 to 20.

The DDS-I has many strengths. Because it is a multiple-item measure, it is possible to assess the internal consistency of the scale, and this consistency appears to be very high (Gracely & Kwilosz, 1988). Test–retest stability has also been shown to be very high (Gracely & Kwilosz, 1988). The scale is strongly associated with other measures of pain intensity (Williams et al., 1998) and is sensitive to treatment effects (Atkinson et al., 1998). Another advantage of the scale is that the consistency with which people use it (compared to themselves on different occasions or compared to other individuals) can be assessed. Patients who are using the measure in an inconsistent fashion can be eliminated from study trials, therefore increasing the potential power of controlled treatment outcome studies. The DDS-I has been shown to be sensitive to very small changes in painful (electrical) stimulation and more sensitive than a VAS (Doctor, Slater, & Atkinson, 1995). It has also been shown to have ratio scale qualities (Doctor et al., 1995).

The major weakness of the scale is its complexity, especially relative to other existing measures of pain intensity. It is possible, even likely, that the same patients who might have difficulty understanding and using a VAS might have trouble with the DDS-I. The utility of the measure with patient populations at risk for cognitive difficulties (e.g., older patients) is not known.[2] Finally, the scale

TABLE 2.2. Descriptor Differential Scale of Pain Intensity (DDS-I)

Instructions: Each word represents an amount of sensation. Rate your sensation in relation to each word with a check mark.

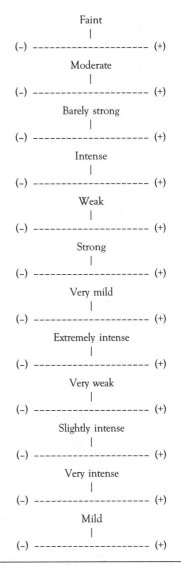

Note. Reprinted from *Pain, 35,* R. H. Gracely and D. M. Kwilosz, The Descriptor Differential Scale: Applying psychophysical principles to clinical pain assessment, 279–288. Copyright 1988, with permission from Elsevier Science.

may require more time to complete than other pain intensity measures. Overall, we view the DDS-I as being less useful than other pain intensity measures in most situations. However, there are clearly situations when the DDS-I would be the measure of choice. It would be particularly useful in clinical trials where maximum sensitivity and ability to detect inconsistent responders is desired, assuming that the subject population understands the measure and that there is time to instruct the patients in the use of the scale. The DDS-I would also be useful if a clinician seeks to track pain intensity in an individual patient over time, since the multiple-item nature of the scale increases its reliability.

Summary and Recommendations Regarding Pain Intensity Measures

A summary of the strengths and weaknesses of the five types of pain intensity measures described above is presented in Table 2.3. Because pain intensity is a relatively easy dimension of pain experience for patients to report, most self-report measures of pain intensity are strongly related to one another, and so most of these measures can be used in most situations. However, each procedure has its particular strengths and weaknesses, and these should be considered when one is choosing among measures.

ASSESSING PAIN AFFECT

There is evidence for an affective component of pain that is conceptually and empirically distinct from pain intensity (Gracely et al., 1978a, 1978b; Jensen et al., 1989; Jensen, Karoly, & Harris, 1991; Melzack & Wall, 1983; Tursky, 1976), although it is important to remember that pain affect is not completely independent of pain intensity (Fernandez & Turk, 1992; Gracely, 1992). Whereas pain intensity may be defined as how much a person hurts, pain affect may be defined as the emotional arousal and disruption engendered by the pain experience. Because people's feelings about events can be mixed, it is likely that the domain of pain affect consists of multiple, coactivated dimensions, which may be closely related to one another (Morley, 1989; Morley & Pallin, 1995). However, it is still unclear whether pain affect is most usefully and reliably assessed as a single global response to sensory arousal, as multiple responses, or as both a global construct and a set of related affect dimensions (cf. Cacioppo & Berntson, 1999).

By far the most widely used measure of pain affect is the Affective subscale of the McGill Pain Questionnaire (MPQ; Melzack, 1975a, 1975b).

This subscale (along with the other subscales of the MPQ) is described in detail by Melzack and Katz in Chapter 3 of this volume, and so is not discussed in detail here. Four additional methods of assessing pain affect are VRSs, VASs, the Descriptor Differential Scale of Pain Affect (DDS-A), and the Affective subscale of the Pain-O-Meter (POM). Each of these assesses pain affect as a single global dimension. To date, no multiple-dimension measure of pain affect has been developed.

Verbal Rating Scales

VRSs have been developed to assess the suffering component of pain; one of these is illustrated in Table 2.4 on page 26. Similar to VRSs for pain intensity, VRSs for pain affect consist of adjectives describing increasing amounts of discomfort and suffering. Respondents select a single word from the list that best describes the degree of unpleasantness of their pain. Like VRS intensity measures, VRS affect measures may be scored in three ways: (1) the ranking method, (2) the cross-modality matching method, or (3) the standardized score method (using scores developed from cross-modality matching procedures with a standardization group). The advantages and disadvantages of these methods have already been discussed with respect to VRSs of pain intensity, and therefore we offer the same cautions here. That is, we recommend the simpler ranking method if the investigator wishes to examine the relation between pain intensity and other constructs, and the use of standardized scores developed from cross-modality matching procedures if the investigator requires a measure more likely to have ratio properties.

Evidence for the validity of VRSs of pain affect is mixed. On the positive side, VRSs of pain affect appear to be more sensitive than measures of pain intensity to treatments designed to impact the emotional component of pain (Fernandez & Turk, 1994; Gracely, Dubner, & McGrath, 1979; Gracely et al., 1978a, 1978b; Heft, Gracely, & Dubner, 1984). On the other hand, factor-analytic and correlational investigations among patients with chronic pain, patients with postoperative pain, and laboratory volunteers indicate that VRSs designed to measure pain affect are not always distinct from measures of pain intensity (Jensen et al., 1989; Jensen & Karoly, 1987; Levine & De Simone, 1991). This pattern of overlap may have something to do with the relatively low level of reliability of

TABLE 2.3. The Strengths and Weaknesses of Five Types of Pain Intensity Measures

Scale	Strengths	Weaknesses
VRS	• Easy to administer. • Easy to score. • Good evidence for construct validity. • Compliance with measurement task is high. • May approximate ratio scaling if cross-modality matching methods (or scores developed from such methods) are used.	• Can be difficult for persons with limited vocabulary. • Relatively few response categories compared to the VAS or 101-point NRS.[a] • If scored via the ranking method, the scores do not necessarily have ratio qualities. • People are forced to choose one word, even if no word on the scale adequately describes their pain intensity.
VAS	• Easy to administer. • Many ("infinite") response categories. • Scores can be treated as ratio data. • Good evidence for construct validity.	• Extra step in scoring the paper-and-pencil version can take more time and adds an additional source of error.
NRS	• Easy to administer. • Many response categories if 101-point NRS is chosen. • Easy to score. • Good evidence for construct validity.	• Limited number of response categories if 11-point NRS is used. • Compliance with measurement task is high. • Scores cannot necessarily be treated as ratio data.
Picture or face scale	• Easy to administer. • Easy to score.	• No evidence regarding relative compliance rates. • Limited number of response categories. • Scores cannot necessarily be treated as ratio data.
DDS-I	• Because the scale has several items, it may be more reliable than single-item rating scales. • Allows for estimates of the consistency with which people complete the measure.	• Some patients may have difficulty comprehending the measure. • Limited research on the validity and sensitivity of the measure. • Completion of the scale takes more time than other measures.

[a]There is no evidence to suggest that VRSs with 15 or more items are less sensitive to treatment effects than VASs or NRSs, but evidence does suggest that VRSs with 5 or fewer categories may be less sensitive in some situations.

single-item measures. Alternatively, a lack of independence between measures of pain intensity and those of pain affect may reflect the simple fact that these two dimensions are not completely independent; some degree of pain intensity is necessary for there to be pain affect, and presumably pain affect should increase as pain intensity increases. Pain intensity and pain affect may be conceptually distinct, but often closely related to one another in the same way that height and weight are distinct but closely associated with each other (Gracely, 1992). Another drawback to VRSs for pain affect is that they force respondents to choose only one descriptor, even when none of the available descrip-

tors (or more than one of the available descriptors) captures their affective response to pain.

Visual Analogue Scales

VASs for pain affect are very similar to VASs for pain intensity; only the endpoint descriptors are different. Examples of the extremes used in VAS affect measures are "not bad at all" and "the most unpleasant feeling possible for me" (Price, Harkins, & Baker, 1987). A great deal of evidence supports the validity of VAS affect measures. They are more sensitive than VAS intensity measures to treatments

TABLE 2.4. A 15-Point VRS of Pain Affect

Bearable	Frightful
Distracting	Dreadful
Unpleasant	Horrible
Uncomfortable	Agonizing
Distressing	Unbearable
Oppressive	Intolerable
Miserable	Excruciating
Awful	

Note. Reprinted from *Pain, 5,* R. H. Gracely, P. McGrath, and R. Dubner, Ratio scales of sensory and affective verbal pain descriptors, 5–18. Copyright 1978, with permission from Elsevier Science.

that should influence pain affect more than pain intensity (Price, Barrell, & Gracely, 1980; Price et al., 1987). They appear to have the qualities of ratio scales (Price & Harkins, 1987; Price et al., 1983). Also, they are sensitive to treatment effects (Price & Barber, 1987; Price, Harkins, Rafii, & Price, 1986; Price, Von der Gruen, Miller, Rafii, & Price, 1985).

The weaknesses of VAS affect measures are likely to be similar to those of VAS intensity measures. Most of the research using these measures has been conducted with young or middle-aged subjects. The utility of such measures in geriatric populations has not yet been examined; it may be that older people have difficulty with VAS affect measures, as they do with VAS intensity measures. Because VAS affect measures are single-item scales, they may be less reliable and less valid for examining the full spectrum of affective responses relative to multiple-item measures, such as the Affective subscales of the MPQ or the POM, described below. Also, there is limited research comparing VAS affect measures to other measures of pain affect. A single experiment suggests that VAS affect measures may be less able then VRS affect measures to discriminate between pain intensity and pain affect (Duncan, Bushnell, & Lavigne, 1989), perhaps because words are so often used to describe emotional reaction, whereas VASs (and NRSs, for that matter) may pull for more of the intensity (magnitude) component of the pain experience.

Descriptor Differential Scale of Pain Affect

The DDS-A is similar to the DDS-I, but uses different descriptors (see Table 2.5). Although the scale has not yet undergone thorough evaluations

TABLE 2.5. Descriptor Differential Scale of Pain Affect (DDS-A)

Instructions: Each word represents an amount of sensation. Rate your sensation in relation to each word with a check mark.

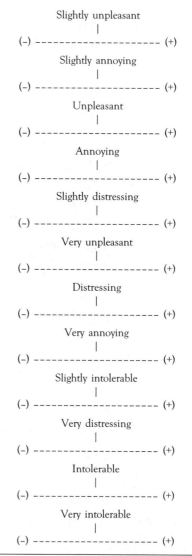

Note. Reprinted from *Pain, 35,* R. H. Gracely and D. M. Kwilosz, The Descriptor Differential Scale: Applying psychophysical principles to clinical pain assessment, 279–288. Copyright 1988, with permission from Elsevier Science.

of its psychometric properties, it shares the advantages of the DDS-I. It is a multiple-item measure, and so may provide more reliable and valid assessments of pain affect than single-item scales. It demonstrates excellent test–retest stability and internal consistency (Gracely & Kwilosz, 1988). Also, investigators may compare an individual's response at one time to his or her response at another time (or to group responses), in order to assess how consistently a particular person is performing on the assessment task.

Another potential advantage of the DDS-A relates to the ability of respondents to rank their pain affect as either being greater than or less than the target word. No other measure of pain affect allows for this level of specificity. For example, a person with a pain that is more than what he or she would have considered "exhausting," "terrifying," or "unbearable" would be unable to communicate this on the MPQ (where these words represent the highest levels of specific affective lists). The DDS-A permits respondents not only to indicate whether their affective response to pain is more than the specific descriptors, but to indicate how much more (or less). Despite the potential drawbacks to using the DDS-A, we strongly encourage additional research with this measure, as we feel it has excellent potential for assessing pain affect.

Affective Scale of the Pain-O-Meter

The POM includes a mechanical VAS and two lists of pain descriptors, which are subsets of words selected from the MPQ (Gaston-Johansson, 1996). Eight of the 11 words on the Affective subscale of the POM (POM Affective) were selected from the MPQ Affective subscale, and the other 3 words were taken from the MPQ Miscellaneous subscale ("nagging," "agonizing," "torturing"), although these latter words clearly have affective valance. Patients indicate which of the 11 words may be used to describe their pain. Each word has an intensity value associated with it (range = 1–5), and these values are summed to give the total POM Affective score. For the most part, the POM Affective scale may be considered a brief version of the MPQ Affective scale (but not as brief as the short form of the MPQ; see Melzack & Katz, Chapter 3). Thus it probably shares many of the strengths and weakness of the MPQ Affective scale.

On the positive side, the POM Affective scale has been shown to be adequately reliable, and sensitive to analgesic treatment (Gaston-Johansson, 1996). It has also been shown to discriminate patients with acute myocardial infarction from patients with chest pain but no diagnosis of a myocardial infarction. Patients diagnosed with a myocardial infarction reported a much higher affective component to their pain than patients who did not receive such a diagnosis (Gaston-Johansson, Hofgren, Watson, & Herlitz, 1991).

On the down side, research suggests that the POM Affective scale may be less strongly related to other measures of affective disturbance (e.g., measures of anxiety and depression) than the POM Sensory scale or the VAS measure of pain intensity on the POM (Gaston-Johansson, Franco, & Zimmerman, 1992). Also, to date, no research has directly compared the POM Affective scale with the MPQ Affective scale. Given the proven validity of the MPQ Affective scale (see Melzack & Katz, Chapter 3), such research is needed in order to demonstrate that the use of fewer items from the MPQ Affective scale in the POM Affective scale does not also involve a loss of validity or reliability. At this point, we conclude that the POM Affective scale shows promise as a measure of the affective component of pain, but until research shows that it is at least as valid and reliable as the MPQ Affective scale, the MPQ Affective scale should probably be selected over the POM Affective scale.

Summary and Recommendations for Assessing Pain Affect

Pain affect is more complex than pain intensity, and there are fewer measures available to assess this construct. In addition, there are several unresolved questions regarding the construct of pain affect. In view of the multidimensional nature of pain affect, is it reasonable to use a global measure of the distress associated with pain, or is there a need for separate indices that tap distinct affective dimensions of pain? Are single-item measures of pain affect less reliable than multiple-item measures, as would be suggested by the complexity of pain affect? These and other basic questions will need to be addressed in future research.

In the meantime, investigators have several options for the assessment of pain affect. Among the single-item measures are VRSs and VASs for affect. Both of these types of procedures have demonstrated discriminant validity (from pain intensity) in some treatment outcome studies. However, both also appear closely related to single-item measures of pain intensity in other situations. A multiple-item scale, the DDS-A, shows great promise. Unfortunately, more research is needed to clarify the strengths and weaknesses of this scale. Additional research is also needed to clarify the specific dimensions of pain affect (Morley & Pallin,

1995, have gotten a good start in this effort), in order then to develop pain affect measures that best capture these dimensions. Until additional research is performed, clinicians and researchers may wish to use both single-item and multiple-item measures and perform psychometric analyses to determine which measure(s) are most useful in their particular situation.

ASSESSING PAIN QUALITY

Pain has many sensory qualities, in addition to its intensity and affective components (Melzack & Casey, 1968). For many years, there was only one primary measure of this component of pain—the Sensory scale from the MPQ. However, Melzack (1987) then published a description of a brief version of the MPQ that also included a Sensory subscale. Because both of these scales are described in detail elsewhere (see Melzack & Katz, Chapter 3), they are not described here, except as compared to a new measure of pain quality, the Neuropathic Pain Scale (NPS; Galer & Jensen, 1997; see also Dworkin, Nagasako, & Galer, Chapter 27).

The NPS begins with instructions that cue patients to note that pain can have many different qualities, and then asks the respondents to rate their pain along 10 of these. Two of the descriptors are global ratings of pain intensity and unpleasantness. The remaining eight descriptors were selected based on their high rate of use among persons with neuropathic pain conditions: "sharp," "hot," "dull," "cold," "sensitive," "itchy," "deep," and "surface." Patients are asked to rate the severity of each of these pain qualities on 0-10 NRSs, with 0 = "no pain" (or "not sharp," "not dull," etc.) and 10 = "the most intense (sharp, dull, etc.) pain sensation imaginable." The NPS also includes items allowing patients to indicate the extent to which their pain fluctuates over time.

A primary difference between the NPS and the MPQ or MPQ short form is that the items of the NPS are scored individually. That is, the 10 NPS items result in 10 pain scores. The MPQ and short-form MPQ Sensory scales, on the other hand, are scored to create global estimates of sensory pain (although it should be noted that either of these scales could be scored to create individual pain descriptor scores). Support for not combining the NPS items into a single composite measure of sensory pain came from correlation analyses revealing that many of the associations between the NPS items were weak (18, or 40%, of the correlation

coefficients were less than .20; 39, or 87%, of the coefficients were less than .50; Galer & Jensen, 1997). Combining item ratings in such a situation would lead to a composite score that would have limited meaning. For example, such a composite score would contain information about both the number and magnitude of different pain sensations that the patient was experiencing, but would be unable to capture the relative contribution of each of these components to the total score. A person could obtain a moderately high score for reporting a relatively few sensations at a very large magnitude, or for reporting a large variety of sensations at moderate magnitudes. Thus Galer and Jensen (1997) recommend against combining the NPS items, and argue for examining the profile of sensations described by each patient.

Support for this profile approach was found in the ability of the NPS items to discriminate between groups of persons with different neuropathic pain diagnoses. For example, persons with postherpetic neuralgia pain describe their pain as more "sharp" than do persons with complex regional pain syndrome, type 1 (also known as reflex sympathetic dystrophy), diabetic neuropathy, peripheral nerve injury, or Charcot-Marie-Tooth disease, whereas persons with Charcot-Marie-Tooth disease describe their pain as less "sensitive" than persons with the other disorders (Carter et al., 1998; Galer & Jensen, 1997). (See also Dworkin et al., Chapter 27, and Bruehl, Steger, & Harden, Chapter 28.)

One of the strengths of the NPS is its brevity. It is able to capture the most common pain qualities of neuropathic pain using just 10 descriptors (as opposed to the 78 descriptors of the MPQ). Although the short-form MPQ also has relatively few descriptors (15), some of the pain qualities common in persons with neuropathic pain conditions (such as "dull," "cold," "sensitive," "itchy," "deep," and "surface") are not listed on the short-form MPQ. In addition, the NPS allows the patient to rate each descriptor along a 0-10 scale—using more levels for each individual descriptor than either the MPQ or short-form MPQ. This option may provide greater sensitivity to treatment effects and greater accuracy in each patient's ratings.

The primary weakness of the NPS is that is was developed for use with persons with neuropathic pain conditions. This makes the scale less useful for other pain conditions. However, the basic approach underlying the scale could certainly be extended to other conditions. All that would be required would be to identify the most common pain qualities associated with the specific pain condition or pain population, and create a series of 0–10 rating scales for each of these pain qualities. In this way, a series of pain quality scales (e.g., a Low Back Pain Scale, a Headache Scale) could be fashioned. Of course, each of these would be specialized for use with certain populations of persons with pain, rendering comparisons across pain conditions very difficult. For such comparisons, a more global measure of pain sensations, such as the MPQ, is necessary.

Summary and Recommendations for Assessing Pain Quality

At this point, there are relatively few measures of pain quality: the MPQ, the short form MPQ, and the NPS. We see the MPQ or short-form MPQ as being more appropriate than the NPS for assessing pain quality in persons who do not have neuropathic pain, or in heterogeneous samples of persons with pain. Both the MPQ and short-form MPQ have support for their reliability and validity, and assess many, if not most, of the possible qualities of pain. For neuropathic pain conditions, the NPS should be strongly considered. It assesses those qualities of pain most likely to be reported by persons with neuropathic pain, and therefore may provide a more efficient assessment of pain quality in this population.

ASSESSING PAIN LOCATION

A fourth dimension of subjective experience is the location of pain. The instrument most commonly used to assess pain location is the pain drawing. This procedure usually involves a line drawing of the front and back of the human body. Sometimes line drawings of the face, head, and neck are also presented for patients experiencing localized pain. Patients are asked to indicate the location of their pain on the surface of the drawings. It is possible to vary the instructions regarding how patients are to indicate their pain to suit the purposes of the investigator. Patients may be asked to distinguish between various sensations of their pain experience, and to indicate the location of these sensations by means of different symbols. For example, the letters "E" and "I" have been used for external (surface) and internal (deep somatic) pain, respectively (Melzack, 1975b). Similarly, "–" has been used for numbness, "oo" for pins and needles, "xx" for

burning pain, and "//" for stabbing pain (Ransford, Cairns, & Mooney, 1976). The most common procedure is to ask a patient simply to shade in the areas of his or her body that are "in pain."

Toomey, Gover, and Jones (1983) divided line drawings of the human body into 32 regions, and gave their patients a score equal to the number of regions that were shaded (see Figure 2.3 for an example of a pain drawing scoring template). This score was found to be related to many important pain-related constructs, such as dimensions of the MPQ (number of words chosen, MPQ Sensory, and MPQ Total scores); self-report of time spent reclining; interference of pain with basic activities such as walking, working, socializing, and recreation; number of health care professionals consulted; and medication use. Interestingly, the number of pain sites shaded was unrelated to pain intensity, duration of the pain problem, and pain affect. Other investigators have similarly found pain extent (or the percentage of body surface in pain) to show moderate associations with disability, pain severity, and tendency to focus on and report physical symptoms (Öhlund, Eek, Palmblad, Areskoug, & Nachemson, 1996; Tait, Chibnall, & Margolis, 1990; Toomey, Mann, Abashian, & Thompson-Pope, 1991). Pain extent scores derived from pain drawings among patients with recent-onset low back pain have also predicted return to work (Öhland et al., 1996). Evidence for the pre-

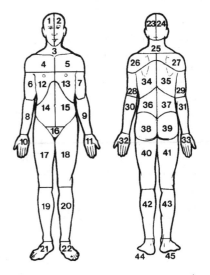

FIGURE 2.3. Scoring template for a pain drawing. From *Pain, 24*, R. B. Margolis, R. C. Tait, and S. J. Krause, A rating system for use with patient pain drawings, 57–65. Copyright 1986, with permission from Elsevier Science.

dictive validity of specific pain site was found by Toomey, Gover, and Jones (1984), who demonstrated that patients with low back pain (or low back pain plus head and neck pain) were more likely than other patients to report interference of pain with life's activities. The reliability of data from pain drawings has also been established. Test–retest stability is high and does not appear to decrease even after 3 months (Margolis, Chibnall, & Tait, 1988). Scoring for "inappropriate" drawings (see below), as well as for total body area in pain, appears to be extremely reliable from person to person (Chan, Goldman, Ilstrup, Kunselman, & O'Neill, 1993; Margolis, Tait, & Krause, 1986; Parker, Wood, & Main, 1995; Udén, Åström, & Bergenudd, 1988).

Some clinicians have suggested that information regarding psychopathology may be contained in the manner by which patients complete pain drawings. To examine this hypothesis, Ransford and colleagues (1976) developed a system for rating the normality versus abnormality of pain drawings. These investigators found patients with abnormal drawings to have higher Hysteria and Hypochondriasis scale scores on the Minnesota Multiphasic Personality Inventory, suggesting that exaggerated pain drawing may reflect a tendency toward somatic preoccupation. Similarly, Gil, Phillips, Abrams, and Williams (1990) found that pain drawing responses of persons with sickle cell disease that were rated as "inconsistent" with sickle cell disease had significantly higher Somatization subscale scores on the Symptom Checklist 90–R (Derogatis, 1983). High scores on this subscale reflect a tendency to be focused on somatic symptoms. Although the relationship between abnormal pain drawings and various measures of psychopathology has continued to be positive in subsequent research, the magnitude of the relationship has generally been shown to be weak (Ginzburg, Merskey, & Lau, 1988; Hildebrandt, Franz, Choroba-Mehnen, & Temme, 1988; Parker et al., 1995; Schwartz & DeGood, 1984; von Baeyer, Bergstrom, Brodwin, & Brodwin, 1983).

Summary and Recommendations for Assessing Pain Location

The assessment of pain location is a necessary part of any thorough pain evaluation. Although research suggests that in some patients, scores derived from pain drawings predict disability, pain interference, medication use, return to work, and psychological functioning, this same body of research indicates that these associations are not consistent and are rarely strong. Therefore, we do not recommend that pain drawings be relied upon as proxy measures of psychopathology or disability (see Sullivan, Chapter 15, and Bradley & McKendree-Smith, Chapter 16). Although drawings that appear overly detailed or exaggerated may raise questions about possible hypochondriacal tendencies or greater disability, it is possible that a detailed drawing may reflect a person's wish to be extremely thorough in providing data. Caution should be extended in any attempt to overinterpret data from pain drawings. In short, pain drawings should primarily be used to assess what they measure well—patients' reports of the sensory distribution of pain.

GENERAL SUMMARY AND CONCLUSION

The assessment of pain intensity, pain affect, pain quality, and pain location continues to be important to clinicians and researchers alike. Self-report is the most direct way to access these pain dimensions. Although additional research is needed to answer important questions regarding the nature and dimensionality of pain experience, most of the measures that are now available have demonstrated adequate to excellent reliability and validity. Clinicians and researchers should select measures with full knowledge of their psychometric strengths and weaknesses, as well as in keeping with their explicit conceptual model(s) of pain. In this chapter, we have attempted to provide investigators with some of the information necessary to make informed decisions regarding the use of self-report measures of pain in adults.

NOTES

1. There is probably an upper limit to the number of response categories necessary to fully characterize different levels of perceived pain intensity. For example, 1,000,001 response categories (i.e., "choose a number between 0 and 1,000,000 that best represents your pain intensity") are unlikely to be more sensitive than 101 response categories. Laboratory research indicates that people are unable to identify more than 21 noticeable differences between weak and intolerable experimental pain (Hardy, Wolff, & Goodell, 1952). Based on these findings, scale sensitivity is likely to be maximal if a measure has at least 22 levels.

2. Preliminary research suggests that the DDS-I may be difficult for naive chronic pain patients to complete, but that patients can learn to use the measure with minimal training (Good, Slater, & Doctor, 1991).

REFERENCES

Ahles, T. A., Ruckdeschel, J. C., & Blanchard, E. B. (1984). Cancer-related pain: II. Assessment with visual analogue scales. *Journal of Psychosomatic Research, 28,* 121-124.

Andrasik, F., & Holroyd, K. A. (1980). Reliability and concurrent validity of headache questionnaire data. *Headache, 20,* 44-46.

Atkinson, J. H., Slater, M. A., Williams, R. A., Zisook, S., Patterson, T. L., Grant, I., Wahlgren, D. R., Abranson, I., & Garfin, S. R. (1998). A placebo-controlled randomized clinical trial of nortriptyline for chronic low back pain. *Pain, 76,* 287-296.

Baker, B. O., Hardyck, C. D., & Petrinovich, L. F. (1966). Weak measurement vs. strong statistics: An empirical critique of S. S. Stevens' prescriptions on statistics. *Educational and Psychological Measurement, 26,* 291-309.

Beyer, J. E., & Knott, C. B. (1998). Construct validity estimation for the African-American and Hispanic versions of the Oucher Scale. *Journal of Pediatric Nursing, 13,* 20-31.

Bieri, D., Reeve, R. A., Champion, G. D., Addicoat, L., & Ziegler, J. B. (1990). The Faces Pain Scale for the self-assessment of the severity of pain experienced by children: Development, initial validation, and preliminary investigation for ratio scale properties. *Pain, 41,* 139-150.

Bolton, J. E., & Wilkinson, R. C. (1998). Responsiveness of pain scales: A comparison of three pain intensity measures in chiropractic patients. *Journal of Manipulative and Physiological Therapeutics, 21,* 1-7.

Cacioppo, J. T., & Berntson, G. G. (1999). The affect system: Architecture and operating characteristics. *Current Directions in Psychological Science, 8,* 133-137.

Carter, G. T., Jensen, M. P., Galer, B. S., Kraft, G. H., Crabtree, L. D., Beardsley, R. M., Abresch, R. T., & Bird, T. D. (1998). Neuropathic pain in Charcot-Marie-Tooth disease. *Archives of Physical Medicine and Rehabilitation, 79,* 1560-1564.

Chan, C. W., Goldman, S., Ilstrup, D. M., Kunselman, A. R., & O'Neill, P. I. (1993). The pain drawing and Waddell's nonorganic physical signs in chronic low-back pain. *Spine, 18,* 1717-1722.

Chapman, C. R., Nakamura, Y., & Flores, L. Y. (1999). Chronic pain and consciousness: A constructivist perspective. In R. J. Gatchel & D. C. Turk (Eds.), *Psychosocial factors in pain* (pp. 35-55). New York: Guilford Press.

Chesney, M. A., & Shelton, J. L. (1976). A comparison of muscle relaxation and electromyogram biofeedback treatments for muscle contraction headache. *Journal of Behavior Therapy and Experimental Psychiatry, 7,* 221-225.

Choinière, M., & Amsel, R. (1996). A visual analogue thermometer for measuring pain intensity. *Journal of Pain and Symptom Management, 11,* 299-311.

Cicchetti, D. V., Showalter, D., & Tyrer, P. J. (1985). The effect of number of rating scale categories on levels of interrater reliability: A Monte Carlo investigation. *Applied Psychological Measurement, 9,* 31-36.

Cleeland, C. S. (1986). How to treat a "construct." *Journal of Pain and Symptom Management, 1,* 161-162.

Cleeland, C. S. (1989). Measurement of pain by subjective report. In C. R. Chapman & J. D. Loeser (Eds.), *Advances in pain research and therapy* (Vol. 12, pp. 391-403). New York: Raven Press.

Cleeland, C. S., & Ryan, K. M. (1994). Pain assessment: Global use of the Brief Pain Inventory. *Annals of the Academy of Medicine, 23,* 129-138.

Collins, F. L., & Thompson, J. K. (1979). Reliability and standardization in the assessment of self-reported headache pain. *Journal of Behavioral Assessment, 1,* 73-86.

Craig, K. D., & Weiss, S. M. (1971). Vicarious influences on pain-threshold determinations. *Journal of Personality and Social Psychology, 19,* 53-59.

Dar, R., Ariely, D., & Frank, H. (1995). The effect of past injury on pain threshold and tolerance. *Pain, 60,* 189-193.

Derogatis, L. R. (1983). *SCL-90-R: Administration, scoring and procedures manual II.* Towson, MD: Clinical Psychometric Research.

Doctor, J. N., Slater, M. A., & Atkinson, J. H. (1995). The Descriptor Differential Scale of Pain Intensity: An evaluation of item and scale properties. *Pain, 61,* 251-260.

Downie, W. W., Leatham, P. A., Rhind, V. M., Wright, V., Branco, J. A., & Anderson, J. A. (1978). Studies with pain rating scales. *Annals of the Rheumatic Diseases, 37,* 378-381.

Duncan, G. H., Bushnell, M. C., & Lavigne, G. J. (1989). Comparison of verbal and visual analogue scales for measuring the intensity and unpleasantness of experimental pain. *Pain, 37,* 295-303.

Dworkin, S. F., & Chen, A. C. N. (1982). Pain in clinical and laboratory contexts. *Journal of Dental Research, 6,* 772-774.

Fernandez, E., & Turk, D. C. (1992). Sensory and affective components of pain: Separation and synthesis. *Psychological Bulletin, 112,* 205-217.

Fernandez, E., & Turk, D. C. (1994). Demand characteristics underlying differential ratings of sensory versus affective components of pain. *Journal of Behavioral Medicine, 17,* 375-390.

Ferraz, M. B., Quaresma, M. R., Aquino, L. R. L., Atra, E., Tugwell, P., & Goldsmith, C. H. (1990). Reliability of pain scales in the assessment of literate and illiterate patients with rheumatoid arthritis. *Journal of Rheumatology, 17,* 1022-1024.

Flor, H., Birbaumer, N., & Turk, D. C. (1990). The psychobiology of chronic pain. *Advances in Behaviour Research and Therapy, 12,* 47-84.

Folkard, S., Glynn, C. J., & Lloyd, J. W. (1976). Diurnal variation and individual differences in the perception of intractable pain. *Journal of Psychosomatic Research, 20,* 289-301.

Fox, E. J., & Melzack, R. (1976). Transcutaneous electrical stimulation and acupuncture: Comparison of treatment for low-back pain, *Pain, 2,* 141-148.

Frank, A. J. M., Moll, J. M. H., & Hort, J. F. (1982). A comparison of three ways of measuring pain. *Rheumatology and Rehabilitation, 21*, 211–217.

Galer, B. S., & Jensen, M. P. (1997). Development and preliminary validation of a pain measure specific to neuropathic pain: The Neuropathic Pain Scale. *Neurology, 48*, 332–338.

Gaston-Johansson, F. (1996). Measurement of pain: The psychometric properties of the Pain-O-Meter, a simple, inexpensive pain assessment tool that could change health care practices. *Journal of Pain and Symptom Management, 12*, 172–181.

Gaston-Johansson, F., Franco, T., & Zimmerman, L. (1992). Pain and psychological distress in patients undergoing autologous bone marrow transplantation. *Oncology Nursing Forum, 19*, 41–48.

Gaston-Johansson, F., Hofgren, C., Watson, P., & Herlitz, J. (1991). Myocardial infarction pain: Systematic description and analysis. *Intensive Care Nursing, 7*, 3–10.

Gil, K. M., Phillips, G., Abrams, M. R., & Williams, D. A. (1990). Pain drawings and sickle cell disease pain. *Clinical Journal of Pain, 6*, 105–109.

Ginzburg, B. M., Merskey, H., & Lau, C. L. (1988). The relationship between pain drawings and the psychological state. *Pain, 35*, 141–146.

Good, A. B., Slater, M. A., & Doctor, J. (1991, November). *Validation of the Descriptor Differential Scale for pain measurement.* Poster presented at the 10th Annual Meeting of the American Pain Society, New Orleans, LA.

Gracely, R. H. (1992). Evaluation of multi-dimensional pain scales. *Pain, 48*, 297–300.

Gracely, R. H., Dubner, R., & McGrath, P. A. (1979). Narcotic analgesia: Fentanyl reduces the intensity but not the unpleasantness of painful tooth pulp sensations. *Science, 203*, 1261–1263.

Gracely, R. H., & Kwilosz, D. M. (1988). The Descriptor Differential Scale: Applying psychophysical principles to clinical pain assessment. *Pain, 35*, 279–288.

Gracely, R. H., McGrath, P., & Dubner, R. (1978a). Ratio scales of sensory and affective verbal pain descriptors. *Pain, 5*, 5–18.

Gracely, R. H., McGrath, P., & Dubner, R. (1978b). Validity and sensitivity of ratio scales of sensory and affective verbal pain descriptors: Manipulation of affect by diazepam. *Pain, 5*, 19–29.

Gramling, S. E., & Elliot, T. R. (1992). Efficient pain assessment in clinical settings. *Behaviour Research and Therapy, 30*, 71–73.

Grossi, E., Borghi, C., Cerchiari, E. L., Della Puppa, T., & Francucci, B. (1983). Analogue Chromatic Continuous Scale (ACCS): A new method for pain assessment. *Clinical and Experimental Rheumatology, 1*, 337–340.

Grossman, S. A., Sheidler, V. R., McGuire, D. B., Geer, C., Santor, D., & Piantadosi, S. (1992). A comparison of the Hopkins Pain Rating Instrument with standard visual analogue and verbal descriptor scales in patients with cancer pain. *Journal of Pain and Symptom Management, 7*, 196–203.

Hall, W. (1981). On "Ratio scales of sensory and affective verbal pain descriptors." *Pain, 4*, 101–107.

Hardy, J. D., Wolff, H. G., & Goodell, H. (1952). *Pain sensations and reactions.* Baltimore: Williams & Wilkins.

Heft, M. W., Gracely, R. H., & Dubner, R. (1984). Nitrous oxide analgesia: A psychophysical evaluation using verbal descriptor scaling. *Journal of Dental Research, 63*, 129–132.

Hildebrandt, J., Franz, C. E., Choroba-Mehnen, B., & Temme, M. (1988). The use of pain drawings in screening for psychological involvement in complaints of low-back pain. *Spine, 13*, 681–685.

Jamison, R. N., & Brown, G. K. (1991). Validation of hourly pain intensity profiles with chronic pain patients. *Pain, 45*, 123–128.

Jensen, M. P., & Karoly, P. (1987). *Assessing the subjective experience of pain: What do the scale scores of the McGill Pain Questionnaire measure?* Poster presented at the Eighth Annual Scientific Sessions of the Society of Behavioral Medicine, Washington, DC.

Jensen, M. P., Karoly, P., & Braver, S. (1986). The measurement of clinical pain intensity: A comparison of six methods. *Pain, 27*, 117–126.

Jensen, M. P., Karoly, P., & Harris, P. (1991). Assessing the affective component of chronic pain: Development of the Pain Discomfort Scale. *Journal of Psychosomatic Research, 35*, 149–154.

Jensen, M. P., Karoly, P., O'Riordan, E. F., Bland, F., Jr., & Burns, R. S. (1989). The subjective experience of acute pain: An assessment of the utility of 10 indices. *Clinical Journal of Pain, 5*, 153–159.

Jensen, M. P., & McFarland, C. A. (1993). Increasing the reliability and validity of pain intensity measurement in chronic pain patients. *Pain, 55*, 195–203.

Jensen, M. P., Turner, L. R., Turner, J. A., & Romano, J. M. (1996). The use of multiple item scales for pain intensity measurement in chronic pain patients. *Pain, 67*, 35–40.

Jensen, M. P., Turner, J. A., Romano, J. M., & Fisher, L. (1999). Comparative reliability and validity of chronic pain intensity measures. *Pain, 83*, 157–162.

Joyce, C. R. B., Zutshi, D. W., Hrubes, V., & Mason, R. M. (1975). Comparison of fixed interval and visual analogue scales for rating chronic pain. *European Journal of Clinical Pharmacology, 8*, 415–420.

Karoly, P. (1985). The assessment of pain: Concepts and issues. In P. Karoly (Ed.), *Measurement strategies in health psychology* (pp. 1–43). New York: Wiley.

Karoly, P. (1991). Assessment of pediatric pain. In J. P. Bush & S. W. Harkins (Eds.), *Children in pain: Clinical and research issues from a developmental perspective* (pp. 59–82). New York: Springer-Verlag.

Karoly, P., & Jensen M. P. (1987). *Multimethod assessment of chronic pain.* New York: Pergamon Press.

Keck, J. F., Gerkensmeyer, J. E., Joyce, B. A., & Schade, J. G. (1996). Reliability and validity of the faces and word descriptor scales to measure procedural pain. *Journal of Pediatric Nursing, 11*, 368–374.

Keefe, F. J., & France, C. R. (1999). Pain: Biopsychosocial mechanisms and management. *Current Directions in Psychological Science, 8*, 137–141.

Keefe, F. J., Schapira, B., Williams, R. B., Brown, C., & Surwit, R. S. (1981). EMG-assisted relaxation training in the management of chronic low back pain. *American Journal of Clinical Biofeedback, 4*, 93–103.

Kremer, E., Atkinson, J. H., & Ignelzi, R. J. (1981). Measurement of pain: Patient preference does not confound pain measurement. *Pain, 10*, 241–248.

Levine, F. M., & De Simone, L. L. (1991). The effects of experimenter gender on pain report in male and female subjects. *Pain, 44*, 69–72.

Margolis, R. B., Chibnall, J. T., & Tait, R. C. (1988). Test-retest reliability of the pain drawing instrument. *Pain, 33,* 49-51.

Margolis, R. B., Tait, R. C., & Krause, S. J. (1986). A rating system for use with patient pain drawings. *Pain, 24,* 57-65.

Max, M. B. (1991). Neuropathic pain syndromes. In M. Max, R. Portenoy, & E. Laska (Eds.), *Advances in pain research and therapy* (Vol. 18, pp. 193-219). New York: Springer.

Max, M. B., Schafer, S. C., Culnane, M., Dubner, R., & Gracely, R. H. (1987). Association of pain relief with drug side effects in postherpetic neuralgia: A single-dose study of clonidine, codeine, ibuprofen, and placebo. *Clinical Pharmacology and Therapeutics, 43,* 363-371.

Melzack, R. (1975a). The McGill Pain Questionnaire. In R. Melzack (Ed.), *Pain measurement and assessment* (pp. 41-47). New York: Raven Press.

Melzack, R. (1975b). The McGill Pain Questionnaire: Major properties and scoring methods. *Pain, 1,* 277-299.

Melzack, R. (1987). The short-form McGill Pain Questionnaire. *Pain, 30,* 191-197.

Melzack, R., & Casey, K. L. (1968). Sensory, motivational, and central control determinants of pain: A new conceptual model. In D. Kenshalo (Ed.), *The skin senses* (pp. 423-439). Springfield, IL: Charles C. Thomas.

Melzack, R., & Wall, P. D. (1983). *The challenge of pain.* New York: Basic Books.

Morley, S. (1989). The dimensionality of verbal descriptors in Tursky's pain perception profile. *Pain, 37,* 41-49.

Morley, S., & Pallin, V. (1995). Scaling the affective domain of pain: A study of the dimensionality of verbal descriptors. *Pain, 62,* 39-49.

Ogon, M., Krismer, M., Söllner, W., Kantner-Rumplmair, W., & Lampe, A. (1996). Chronic low back pain measurement with visual analogue scales in different settings. *Pain, 64,* 425-428.

Öhlund, C., Eek, C., Palmblad, S., Areskoug, B., & Nachemson, A. (1996). Quantified pain drawing in subacute low back pain. *Spine, 21,* 1021-1031.

Ohnhaus, E. E., & Adler, R. (1975). Methodological problems in the measurement of pain: A comparison between the verbal rating scale and the visual analogue scale. *Pain, 1,* 379-384.

Paice, J. A., & Cohen, F. L. (1997). Validity of a verbally administered numeric rating scale to measure cancer pain intensity. *Cancer Nursing, 20,* 88-93.

Parker, H., Wood, P. L. R., & Main, C. J. (1995). The use of the pain drawing as a screening measure to predict psychological distress in chronic low back pain. *Spine, 20,* 236-243.

Philip, B. K. (1990). Parametric statistics for evaluation of the visual analog scale. *Anesthesia and Analgesia, 71,* 710.

Price, D. D., & Barber, J. (1987). An analysis of factors that contribute to the efficacy of hypnotic analgesia. *Journal of Abnormal Psychology, 96,* 46-51.

Price, D. D., Barrell, J. J., & Gracely, R. H. (1980). A psychophysical analysis of experiential factors that selectively influence the affective dimension of pain. *Pain, 8,* 137-149.

Price, D. D., Bush, F. M., Long, S., & Harkins, S. W. (1994). A comparison of pain measurement charac-teristics of mechanical visual analogue and simple numerical rating scales. *Pain, 56,* 217-226.

Price, D. D., & Harkins, S. W. (1987). Combined use of experimental pain and visual analogue scales in providing standardized measurement of clinical pain. *Clinical Journal of Pain, 3,* 1-8.

Price, D. D., Harkins, S. W., & Baker, C. (1987). Sensory-affective relationships among different types of clinical and experimental pain. *Pain, 28,* 297-307.

Price, D. D., Harkins, S. W., Rafii, A., & Price, C. (1986). A simultaneous comparison of fentanyl's analgesic effects on experimental and clinical pain. *Pain, 24,* 197-203.

Price, D. D., McGrath, P. A., Rafii, A., & Buckingham, B. (1983). The validation of visual analogue scales as ratio scale measures for chronic and experimental pain. *Pain, 17,* 45-56.

Price, D. D., Von der Gruen, A., Miller, J., Rafii, A., & Price, C. (1985). A psychophysical analysis of morphine analgesia. *Pain, 22,* 261-269.

Ransford, A. O., Cairns, D., & Mooney, V. (1976). The pain drawing as an aid to the psychologic evaluation of patients with low-back pain. *Spine, 1,* 127-134.

Rasmussen, J. L. (1989). Analysis of Likert-scale data: A reinterpretation of Gregoire and Driver. *Psychological Bulletin, 105,* 167-170.

Rudy, T. E. (1989). Innovations in pain psychometrics. In C. R. Chapman & J. D. Loeser (Eds.), *Advances in pain research and therapy* (Vol. 12, pp. 51-61). New York: Raven Press.

Rybstein-Blinchik, E. (1979). Effects of different cognitive strategies on chronic pain experience. *Journal of Behavioral Medicine, 2,* 93-101.

Salovey, P., Smith, A. F., Turk, D.C., Jobe, J.B., & Willis, G. B. (1993). The accuracy of memory for pain: Not so bad most of the time. *American Pain Society Journal, 2,* 184-191.

Schwartz, D. P., & DeGood, D. E. (1984). Global appropriateness of pain drawings: Blind ratings predict patterns of psychological distress and litigation status. *Pain, 19,* 383-388.

Scott, J., & Huskisson, E. C. (1976). Graphic representation of pain. *Pain, 2,* 175-184.

Seymour, R. A. (1982). The use of pain scales in assessing the efficacy of analgesics in post-operative dental pain. *European Journal of Clinical Pharmacology, 23,* 441-444.

Seymour, R. A., Simpson, J. M., Charlton, J. E., & Phillips, M. E. (1985). An evaluation of length and end-phrase of visual analogue scales in dental pain, *Pain, 21,* 177-185.

Sriwatanakul, K., Kelvie, W., Lasagna, L., Calimlim, J. F., Weis, O. F., & Mehta, G. (1983). Studies with different types of visual analog scales for measurement of pain. *Clinical Pharmacology and Therapeutics, 34,* 235-239.

Stenn, P. G., Mothersill, K. J., & Brooke, R. I. (1979). Biofeedback and a cognitive behavioral approach to treatment of myofascial pain dysfunction syndrome. *Behavior Therapy, 10,* 29-36.

Stuppy, D. J. (1998). The Faces Pain Scale: Reliability and validity with mature adults. *Applied Nursing Research, 11,* 84-89.

Tait, R. C., Chibnall, J. T., & Margolis, R. B. (1990). Pain extent: Relations with psychological state, pain severity, pain history, and disability. *Pain, 41,* 295-301.

Teske, K., Daut, R. L., & Cleeland, C. S. (1983). Relationships between nurses' observations and patients' self-reports of pain. *Pain, 16*, 289-296.

Thomas, T. A., & Griffiths, M. J. (1982). A pain slide rule. *Anaesthesia, 37*, 960-961.

Toomey, T. C., Gover, V. F., & Jones, B. N. (1983). Spatial distribution of pain: A descriptive characteristic of chronic pain. *Pain, 17*, 289-300.

Toomey, T. C., Gover, V. F., & Jones, B. N. (1984). Site of pain: Relationship to measures of pain description, behavior and personality. *Pain, 19*, 389-397.

Toomey, T. C., Mann, J. D., Abashian, S., & Thompson-Pope, S. (1991). Relationship of pain drawing scores to ratings of pain description and function. *Clinical Journal of Pain, 7*, 269-274.

Turk, D. C. (1989). Assessment of pain: The elusiveness of latent constructs. In C. R. Chapman & J. D. Loeser (Eds.), *Advances in pain research and therapy* (Vol. 12, pp. 267-279). New York: Raven Press.

Turner, J. A. (1982). Comparison of group progressive-relaxation training and cognitive-behavioral group therapy for chronic low back pain. *Journal of Consulting and Clinical Psychology, 50*, 757-765.

Tursky, B. (1976). The development of a pain perception profile: A psychophysical approach. In M. Weisenberg & B. Tursky (Eds.), *Pain: New perspectives in therapy and research* (pp. 171-194). New York: Plenum Press.

Tursky, B., Jamner, L. D., & Friedman, R. (1982). The pain perception profile: A psychophysical approach to the assessment of pain report. *Behavior Therapy, 13*, 376-394.

Udén, A., Åström, M., & Bergenudd, H. (1988). Pain drawings in chronic back pain. *Spine, 13*, 389-392.

Urban, B. J., Keefe, F. J., & France, R. D. (1984). A study of psychophysical scaling in chronic pain patients. *Pain, 20*, 157-168.

von Baeyer, C. L., Bergstrom, K. J., Brodwin, M. G., & Brodwin, S. K. (1983). Invalid use of pain drawings in psychological screening of back pain patients. *Pain, 16*, 103-107.

Wallenstein, S. L., Heidrich, G., III, Kaiko, R., & Houde, R. W. (1980). Clinical evaluation of mild analgesics: The measurement of clinical pain. *British Journal of Clinical Pharmacology, 10*, 319S-327S.

Walsh, T. D. (1984). Practical problems in pain measurement. *Pain, 19*, 96-98.

West, N., Oakes, L, Hinds, P. S., Sanders, L, Holden, R., Williams, S., Fairclough, D., & Bozeman, P. (1994). Measuring pain in pediatric oncology ICU patients. *Journal of Pediatric Oncology Nursing, 11*, 64-68.

Wilkie, D., Lovejoy, N., Dodd, M., & Tesler, M. (1990). Cancer pain intensity measurement: Concurrent validity of three tools—finger dynamometer, pain intensity number scale, visual analogue scale. *Hospice Journal, 6*, 1-13.

Williams, R. A., Pruitt, S. D., Doctor, J. N., Epping-Jordan, J. E., Wahlgren, D. R., Grant, I., Patterson, T. L., Webster, J. S., Slater, M. A., & Atkinson, J. H. (1998). The contribution of job satisfaction to the transition from acute to chronic low back pain. *Archives of Physical Medicine and Rehabilitation, 79*, 366-374.

Wong, D. & Baker, C. (1988). Pain in children: Comparison of assessment scales. *Pediatric Nursing, 14*, 9-17.

Chapter 3

The McGill Pain Questionnaire: Appraisal and Current Status

RONALD MELZACK
JOEL KATZ

Pain is a personal, subjective experience influenced by cultural learning, the meaning of the situation, attention, and other psychological variables (Melzack & Wall, 1996). Pain processes do not begin with the stimulation of receptors. Rather, injury or disease produces neural signals, which enter an active nervous system that is the substrate of our past experience, culture, anxiety, and depression. These brain processes actively participate in the selection, abstraction, and synthesis of information from the total sensory input. Pain, then, is not simply the end product of a linear sensory transmission system; rather, it is a dynamic process that involves continuous interactions among complex ascending and descending systems.

DIMENSIONS OF PAIN EXPERIENCE

Since the beginning of the 20th century, research on pain has been dominated by the concept that pain is purely a sensory experience. Yet pain also has a distinctly unpleasant, affective quality. It becomes overwhelming, demands immediate attention, and disrupts ongoing behavior and thought. It motivates or drives the organism into activity aimed at stopping the pain as quickly as possible. To consider only the sensory features of pain and ignore its motivational-affective proper-

ties is to look at only part of the problem. Even the concept of pain as a perception, with full recognition of past experience, attention, and other cognitive influences, still neglects the crucial motivational dimension.

These considerations led Melzack and Casey (1968) to suggest that there are three major psychological dimensions of pain: sensory-discriminative, motivational-affective, and cognitive-evaluative. They proposed, moreover, that these dimensions of pain experience are subserved by physiologically specialized systems in the brain. The sensory-discriminative dimension of pain is influenced primarily by the rapidly conducting spinal systems; the powerful motivational drive and unpleasant affect characteristic of pain are subserved by activities in reticular and limbic structures that are influenced primarily by the slowly conducting spinal systems; neocortical or higher central nervous system processes, such as evaluation of the input in terms of past experience, exert control over activity in both the discriminative and motivational systems.

It is assumed that these three categories of activity interact with one another to provide *perceptual information* on the location, magnitude, and spatiotemporal properties of the noxious stimuli; *a motivational tendency* toward escape or attack; and *cognitive information* based on past experience and probability of outcome of different response strategies (Melzack & Casey, 1968). All three forms of activity can then influence motor mechanisms responsible for the complex pattern of overt responses that characterize pain.

THE LANGUAGE OF PAIN

Clinical investigators have long recognized the varieties of pain experience. Descriptions of the burning qualities of pain after peripheral nerve injury, or the stabbing, cramping qualities of visceral pains, frequently provide the key to diagnosis and may even suggest the course of therapy. Despite the frequency of such descriptions, and the seemingly high agreement that they are valid descriptive words, studies of their use and meaning are relatively recent.

Anyone who has suffered severe pain and tried to describe the experience to a friend or to the doctor often finds him- or herself at a loss for words. The reason for this difficulty in expressing pain experience, actually, is not because the words do not exist. As we shall soon see, there is an abundance of appropriate words. Rather, the main reason is that, fortunately, they are not words we have occasion to use often. Another reason is that the words may seem absurd. We may use descriptors such as "splitting," "shooting," "gnawing," "wrenching," or "stinging" as useful metaphors, but there are no external objective references for these words in relation to pain. If we talk about a blue pen or a yellow pencil, we can point to an object and say, "That is what I mean by yellow," or "This color of the pen is blue." But what can we point to to tell another person precisely what we mean by "smarting," "tingling," or "rasping"? A person who suffers terrible pain may say that the pain is "burning" and add, "It feels as if someone is shoving a red-hot poker through my toes and slowly twisting it around." These "as if" statements are often essential to convey the qualities of the experience.

If the study of pain in people is to have a scientific foundation, it is essential to measure it. If we want to know how effective a new drug is, we need numbers to say that the pain decreased by some amount. Yet, while overall intensity is important information, we also want to know whether the drug specifically decreased the burning quality of the pain, or whether the especially miserable, tight, cramping feeling is gone.

TRADITIONAL MEASURES OF PAIN INTENSITY

Until recently, the methods that were used for pain measurement treated pain as though it were a single unique quality that varies only in intensity (Beecher, 1959). These methods include Verbal Rating Scales (VRSs), Numerical Rating Scales (NRSs), and Visual Analogue Scales (VASs). These simple methods have all been used effectively in hospital clinics, and have provided valuable information about pain and analgesia. VRSs, NRSs, and VASs provide simple, efficient, and minimally intrusive measures of pain intensity which have been used widely in clinical and research settings where a quick index of pain intensity is required and to which a numerical value can be assigned. These scales, which are outlined below, are described in detail elsewhere in this volume (see Jensen & Karoly, Chapter 2, and Price, Riley, & Wade, Chapter 4).

Verbal and Numerical Rating Scales

VRSs typically consist of a series of verbal pain descriptors ordered from least to most intense (e.g., "no pain," "mild," "moderate," "severe") (see Jensen & Karoly, Chapter 2). The patient reads the list and chooses the one word that best describes the intensity of his or her pain at the moment. A score of 0 is assigned to the descriptor with the lowest rank; a score of 1 is assigned to the descriptor with the next lowest rank; and so on. NRSs typically consist of a series of numbers ranging from 0 to 10 or 0 to 100, with endpoints intended to represent the extremes of the possible pain experience and labeled "no pain" and "worst possible pain," respectively. The patient chooses the number that best corresponds to the intensity of his or her pain at the moment. Although VRSs and NRSs are simple to administer and have demonstrated reliability and validity, the advantages associated with VASs (see below) make VASs the measurement instrument of choice when a unidimensional measure of pain is required. However, this may not be true when assessing chronic pain in the elderly. At least one study indicates that elderly patients make fewer errors on a VRS than on a VAS (Gagliese & Melzack, 1997).

Visual Analogue Scales

The most common VAS consists of a 10-cm horizontal or vertical line with the two endpoints labeled "no pain" and "worst pain ever" (or similar verbal descriptors; see Jensen & Karoly, Chapter 2). The patient is required to place a mark on the 10-cm line at a point that corresponds to the level of pain intensity he or she presently feels. The distance in centimeters (or millimeters) from the low end of the VAS to the patient's mark is used as a numerical index of the severity of pain. VASs for pain affect have been developed in an effort to include domains of measurable pain experience other than the sensory intensity dimension. The patient is asked to rate the unpleasantness of the pain experience (i.e., how disturbing it is). End-points are labeled "not bad at all" and "the most unpleasant feeling imaginable."

The major disadvantage of VASs is the assumption that pain is a unidimensional experience that can be measured with a single-item scale (Melzack, 1975). Although intensity is without a doubt a salient dimension of pain, it is clear that the word "pain" refers to an endless variety of qualities that are categorized under a single linguistic label, not to a specific, single sensation that varies only in intensity or affect. The development of VASs to measure pain affect or unpleasantness has partially addressed the problem, but the same shortcoming applies within the affective domain. Each pain has unique qualities. Unpleasantness is only one such quality. The pain of a toothache is obviously different from that of a pinprick, just as the pain of a coronary occlusion is uniquely different from the pain of a broken leg. To describe pain solely in terms of intensity or affect is like specifying the visual world only in terms of

light flux, without regard to pattern, color, texture, and the many other dimensions of visual experience.

THE McGILL PAIN QUESTIONNAIRE

Development and Description

Melzack and Torgerson (1971) made a start toward specifying qualities of pain. In the first part of their study, physicians and other university graduates were asked to classify 102 words, obtained from the clinical literature, into small groups that describe distinctly different aspects of the experience of pain. On the basis of the data, the words were categorized into three major classes and 16 subclasses (Figure 3.1). The classes are (1) words that describe the sensory qualities of the experience in terms of temporal, spatial, pressure, thermal, and other properties; (2) words that describe affective qualities in terms of tension, fear, and autonomic properties that are part of the pain experience; and (3) evaluative words that describe the subjective overall intensity of the total pain experience. Each subclass, which was given a descriptive label, consists of a group of words that were considered by most subjects to be qualitatively similar. Some of these words are undoubtedly synonyms; others seem to be synonymous but vary in intensity; and many provide subtle differences or nuances (despite their similarities) that may be of importance to a patient who is trying desperately to communicate to a physician.

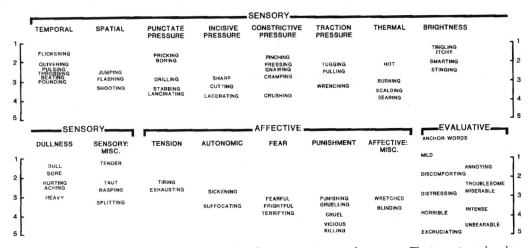

FIGURE 3.1. Spatial display of pain descriptors based on intensity ratings by patients. The intensity scale values range from 1 ("mild") to 5 ("excruciating"). Copyright 1971 Ronald Melzack and Warren S. Torgerson.

The second part of the Melzack and Torgerson (1971) study was an attempt to determine the pain intensities implied by the words within each subclass. Groups of physicians, patients, and students were asked to assign an intensity value to each word, using a numerical scale ranging from "least (or mild) pain" to "worst (or excruciating) pain." When this was done, it was apparent that several words within each subclass had the same relative intensity relationships in all three sets. For example, in the spatial subclass, "shooting" was found to represent more pain than "flashing," which in turn implied more pain than "jumping." Although the precise intensity scale values differed for the three groups, all three agreed on the positions of the words relative to each other. The scale values of the words for patients, based on the precise numerical values listed in Melzack and Torgerson, are shown in Figure 3.1.

Because of the high degree of agreement on the intensity relationships among pain descriptors by subjects from different cultural, socioeconomic, and educational backgrounds, a pain questionnaire (Figure 3.2) was developed as an experimental tool for studies of the effects of various methods of pain management. In addition to the list of pain descriptors, the questionnaire contains line drawings of the body to show the spatial distribution of the pain, words that describe temporal properties of pain, and descriptors of the overall Present Pain Intensity (PPI). The PPI is recorded as a number from 1 to 5, in which each number is associated with the following words: 1, "mild"; 2, "discomforting"; 3, "distressing"; 4, "horrible"; 5, "excruciating." The mean scale values of these words, which were chosen from the evaluative category, are approximately equally far apart, so that they represent equal scale intervals and thereby provide "anchors" for the specification of the overall pain intensity (Melzack & Torgerson, 1971).

In a preliminary study, the pain questionnaire consisted of the 16 subclasses of descriptors shown in Figure 3.1, as well as the additional information deemed necessary for the evaluation of pain. It soon became clear, however, that many of the patients found certain key words to be absent. These words were then selected from the original word list used by Melzack and Torgerson (1971), were categorized appropriately, and ranked according to their mean scale values. A further set of words ("cool," "cold," "freezing") was used by patients on rare occasions, but was indicated to be essential for an adequate description of some types of pain. Thus four supplementary—or "miscella-neous"—subclasses were added to the word lists of the questionnaire (Figure 3.2). The final classification, then, appeared to represent the most parsimonious and meaningful set of subclasses without at the same time losing subclasses that represent important qualitative properties. The questionnaire, which is known as the McGill Pain Questionnaire (MPQ; Melzack, 1975), has become a widely used clinical and research tool (Melzack, 1983; Reading, 1989; Wilkie, Savedra, Holzemier, Tesler, & Paul, 1990).

Measures of Pain Experience

The descriptor lists of the MPQ are read to a patient with the explicit instruction that he or she choose only those words that describe his or her feelings and sensations at that moment. Three major indices are obtained:

1. The Pain Rating Index (PRI), based on the rank values of the words. In this scoring system, the word in each subclass implying the least pain is given a value of 1; the next word is given a value of 2; and so forth. The rank values of the words chosen by a patient are summed to obtain separate scores for the Sensory (subclasses 1–10), Affective (subclasses 11–15), Evaluative (subclass 16), and Miscellaneous (subclasses 17–20) subscales, in addition to providing a Total score (subclasses 1–20). Figure 3.3 on page 40 shows MPQ scores (Total scores from subclasses 1–20) obtained by patients with a variety of acute and chronic pains.

2. The Number of Words Chosen (NWC).

3. The PPI, which is the number–word combination chosen as the indicator of overall pain intensity at the time of administration of the questionnaire.

Alternate Procedures for Scoring

Several additional procedures for scoring the MPQ have been suggested (Charter & Nehemkis, 1983; Hartman & Ainsworth, 1980; Melzack, Katz, & Jeans, 1985). Hartman and Ainsworth (1980) have proposed transforming the MPQ data into a pain ratio or fraction: The "pain ratio was calculated for each session by dividing the post-session rating by the sum of the pre- and post-session ratings" (p. 40). Kremer, Atkinson, and Ignelzi (1982) suggested dividing the sum of the obtained ranks within each dimension by the total possible score

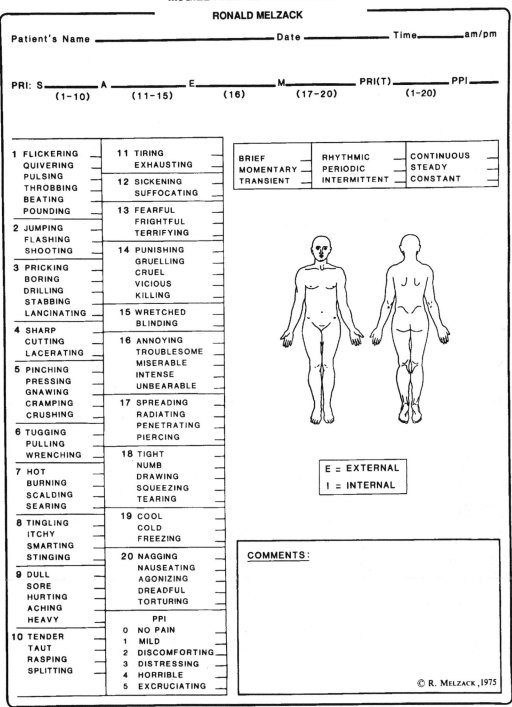

FIGURE 3.2. The McGill Pain Questionnaire (MPQ). The descriptors fall into four major groups: Sensory, 1 to 10; Affective, 11–15; Evaluative, 16; and Miscellaneous, 17–20. The rank value for each descriptor is based on its position in the word set. The sum of the rank values is the pain rating index (PRI). The present pain intensity (PPI) is based on a scale of 0 to 5. Copyright 1975 Ronald Melzack.

MEASUREMENT OF PAIN

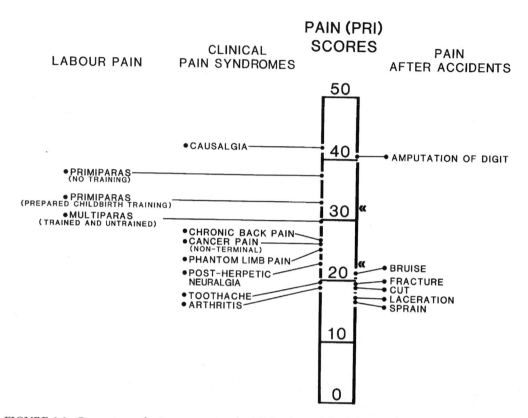

FIGURE 3.3. Comparison of pain scores using the MPQ, obtained from women during labor (Melzack et al., 1981) and from patients in a general hospital pain clinic (Melzack, 1975), and an emergency department (Melzack et al., 1982). The pain score for causalgic pain is reported by Tamoush (1981). Copyright 1975, 1981, 1982 Ronald Melzack.

for a particular dimension, thus making differences among the Sensory, Affective, Evaluative, and Miscellaneous dimensions more interpretable.

A final form of computation (Melzack et al., 1985) may be useful, since it has been argued (Charter & Nehemkis, 1983) that the MPQ fails to take into account the true relative intensity of verbal descriptors, because the rank-order scoring system loses the precise intensity of the scale values obtained by Melzack and Torgerson (1971). For example, Figure 3.1 shows that the affective descriptors generally have higher scale values than the sensory words. This is clear when we consider the fact that the words "throbbing" and "vicious" receive a rank value of 4, but have scale values of 2.68 and 4.26, respectively, indicating that the latter descriptor implies considerably more pain intensity than the former. A simple technique was developed (Melzack et al., 1985) to convert rank values to weighted rank values that more closely approximate the original scaled values obtained by Melzack and Torgerson. Use of this procedure may

provide enhanced sensitivity in some statistical analyses (Melzack et al., 1985). In general, the system of rank value scoring has been sufficiently sensitive to evaluate the effectiveness of a variety of pain-relieving procedures, as well as to discriminate among different pain syndromes. The correction by weighted ranks may not be necessary for most research studies, but can be valuable when results are statistically marginal by maximizing the sensitivity of the MPQ. The weights for each descriptor subclass are as follows: 1 (0.69), 2 (1.38), 3 (0.93), 4 (1.59), 5 (0.81), 6 (1.19), 7 (1.28), 8 (0.70), 9 (0.72), 10 (0.95), 11 (1.74), 12 (2.22), 13 (1.87), 14 (1.32), 15 (2.33), 16 (1.01), 17 (1.22), 18 (0.82), 19 (1.0), 20 (1.15).

Usefulness

The most important requirement of a measure is that it be valid, reliable, consistent, and—above all—useful. The MPQ appears to meet all of these requirements (Melzack, 1983; Reading, 1989; Wilkie et al., 1990) and provides a relatively rapid way of measuring subjective pain experience (Melzack, 1975). When it is administered to a patient by an evaluator reading each subclass, it can be completed in about 5 minutes. It can also be filled out by the patient in a more leisurely way as a paper-and-pencil test, though the scores are somewhat different (Klepac, Dowling, Rokke, Dodge, & Schafer, 1981).

Since its introduction in 1975, the MPQ has been used in over 350 studies of acute, chronic, and laboratory-produced pains. It has been translated into several languages and has also spawned the development of similar pain questionnaires in other languages (Table 3.1).

Because pain is a private, personal experience, it is impossible for us to know precisely what someone else's pain feels like. No man can possibly know what it is like to have menstrual cramps or labor pain. Nor can a psychologically healthy person know what a psychotic patient is feeling when the patient says he or she has excruciating pain (Veilleux & Melzack, 1976). But the MPQ provides us with an insight into the qualities that are experienced. Recent studies indicate that each kind of pain is characterized by a distinctive constellation of words. There is a remarkable consistency in the choice of words by patients suffering the same or similar pain syndromes (Graham, Bond, Gerkovitch, & Cook, 1980; Grushka & Sessle, 1984; Katz, 1992; Katz & Melzack, 1991; Melzack, Taenzer, Feldman, & Kinch, 1981; Van Buren & Kleinknecht, 1979). For example, in a study of amputees with phantom limb pain (group PLP) or nonpainful phantom limb sensations (group PLS), every MPQ descriptor chosen by 33% or more of subjects in group PLS was also chosen by 33% or more subjects in group PLP, although there were other descriptors the latter group endorsed with greater frequency (Katz & Melzack, 1991). These data indicated that the phantom limb experiences of the two groups have in common a paresthetic quality (e.g., "tingling," "numb"), although painful phantoms consist of more than this shared component.

Reliability and Validity

Reading, Everitt, and Sledmere (1982) investigated the reliability of the groupings of adjectives in the MPQ by using different methodological and statistical approaches. Subjects sorted each of the 78

TABLE 3.1. Pain Questionnaires in Different Languages Based on the MPQ

Language	Authors
Amharic (Ethiopia)	Hiwot et al. (in press)
Arabic	Harrison (1988)
Chinese	Hui & Chen (1989)
Czech (SF-MPQ)	Šolcová et al. (1990) Knotek et al. (2000)
Danish	Drewes et al. (1993)
Dutch (and Flemish)	Vanderiet et al. (1987) Verkes et al. (1989) van Lankveld et al. (1992) van der Kloot et al. (1995)
English	Melzack (1975, 1987)
Finnish	Ketovuori & Pöntinen (1981)
French	Boureau et al. (1984, 1992)
German	Kiss et al. (1987) Radvila et al. (1987) Stein & Mendl (1988)
Greek	Georgoudis et al. (in press)
Hungarian	Bende et al. (1993)
Italian	De Benedittis et al. (1988) Ferracuti et al. (1990) Maiani & Sanavio (1985)
Japanese	Satow et al. (1990) Hasegawa et al. (1996, in press)
Norwegian	Strand & Wisnes (1991) Kim et al. (1995)
Polish	Sedlak (1990)
Portuguese	Pimenta & Teixeiro (1996)
Slovak	Bartko et al. (1984)
Spanish	Laheurta et al. (1982) Bejarano et al. (1985) Lázaro et al. (1994) Escalante et al. (1996)
Swedish (SF-MPQ)	Burckhardt & Bjelle (1994)

words of the MPQ into groups that described similar pain qualities. The mean number of groups was 19 (with a range of 7 to 31), which is remarkably close to the MPQ's 20 groups. Moreover, there were distinct subgroups for sensory and affective-evaluative words. Since the cultural backgrounds of subjects in this study and in Melzack and Torgerson's (1971) were different, and the methodology and data analysis were dissimilar, the degree of correspondence is impressive. More recently, Gaston-Johansson, Albert, Fagan, and Zimmerman (1990) reported that subjects with diverse ethnic/cultural and educational backgrounds use similar MPQ adjectives to describe commonly used words such as "pain," "hurt," and "ache." Nevertheless, interesting differences between the studies were found, which suggest alternative approaches for future revisions of the MPQ.

Evidence for the stability of the MPQ was provided by Love, Leboeuf, and Crisp (1989), who administered the MPQ to patients with chronic low back pain on two occasions (separated by several days) prior to receiving treatment. Their results show very strong test–retest reliability coefficients for the MPQ PRIs, as well as for some of the 20 categories. The lower coefficients for the 20 categories may be explained by the suggestion that many clinical pains show fluctuations in quality over time, yet still represent the "same" pains to the persons who experience them.

Studies of the validity of the three-dimensional framework of the MPQ are numerous and have been reviewed by Reading (1989). Generally, the distinction between the Sensory and Affective dimensions has held up extremely well, but there is still considerable debate on the separation of the Affective and Evaluative dimensions. Nevertheless, several excellent studies (Holroyd et al., 1992; McCreary, Turner, & Dawson, 1981; Prieto et al., 1980; Reading, 1979) have reported a discrete Evaluative factor. The different factor-analytic procedures that were used undoubtedly account for the reports of four factors (Holroyd et al., 1992; Reading, 1979), five factors (Crockett, Prkachin, & Craig, 1977), six factors (Burckhardt, 1984), or seven factors (Leavitt, Garron, Whisler, & Sheinkop, 1978). The major source of disagreement, however, seems to be the different patient populations that are used to obtain data for factor analyses. The range includes patients with brief laboratory-induced pains, dysmenorrhea, back pain, and cancer pain. In some studies, relatively few words are chosen, while large numbers are selected in others. It is not surprising, then, that factor-analytic studies based on such diverse populations have confused rather than clarified some of the issues.

Turk, Rudy, and Salovey (1985) examined the internal structure of the MPQ by using techniques that avoided the problems of most earlier studies and confirmed the three (Sensory, Affective, and Evaluative) dimensions. In a later study, Lowe, Walker, and McCallum (1991) again confirmed the three-factor structure of the MPQ, using elegant statistical procedures and a large number of subjects. Finally, a paper by Chen, Dworkin, Haug, and Gerhig (1989) presents data on the remarkable consistency of the MPQ across five studies using the cold pressor task; and Pearce and Morley (1989) provided further confirmation of the construct validity of the MPQ, using the Stroop color-naming task with patients who had chronic pain.

Sensitivity

Various studies show that MPQ is sensitive to interventions designed to reduce pain (Briggs, 1996; Burchiel et al., 1996; Eija, Tasmuth, & Pertti, 1996; Nikolajsen et al., 1996; Pozehl, Barnason, Zimmerman, Nieveen, & Crutchfield, 1995; Tesfaye et al., 1996). The relative sensitivity of the MPQ to change in postoperative pain following administration of oral analgesics was evaluated by comparing it with VAS and VRS measures of pain intensity (Jenkinson et al., 1995). While all three measures of pain revealed the same pattern of change over time, effect sizes for the MPQ were consistently related to self-reported change in pain, directly assessed with a VRS. These findings probably underestimate the MPQ's sensitivity to change, since the benchmark for change was a VRS. In support of this, the MPQ appears to provide a more sensitive measure of mild postoperative pain than does a simple VAS that assesses pain intensity only, since patients can be more precise in describing their experience by selecting appropriate descriptors (Katz et al., 1994). This increased ability of the MPQ to detect differences in pain at the low end of the pain continuum is most likely a function of the multidimensional nature of the MPQ and the large number of descriptors from which to choose.

Discriminative Capacity

One of the most exciting features of the MPQ is its potential value as an aid in the differential diagnosis between various pain syndromes. The first study to demonstrate the discriminative capacity of the MPQ was carried out by Dubuisson and Melzack (1976), who administered the questionnaire to 95 patients suffering from one of eight known pain syndromes: postherpetic neuralgia, phantom limb pain, metastatic carcinoma, toothache, degenerative disc disease, rheumatoid arthritis or osteoarthritis, labor pain, and menstrual pain. A multiple-group discriminant analysis revealed that each type of pain is characterized by a distinctive constellation of verbal descriptors (Figure 3.4). Furthermore, when the descriptor set for each patient was classified into one of the eight diagnostic categories, a correct classification was made in 77% of cases. Table 3.2 shows the pain descriptors most characteristic of the eight clinical pain syndromes in the Dubuisson and Melzack (1976) study.

Descriptor patterns can also provide the basis for discriminating between two major types of low back pain. Some patients have clear physical causes for pain, such as degenerative disc disease, while others suffer from low back pain even though no physical causes can be found. Using a modified version of the MPQ, Leavitt and Garron (1980) found that patients whose pain had physical ("organic") causes used distinctly different patterns of words from patients whose pain

TABLE 3.2. Descriptions Characteristic of Clinical Pain Syndromes

Menstrual pain (n = 25)	Arthritic pain (n = 16)	Labor pain (n = 11)	Disc disease pain (n = 10)	Toothache (n = 10)	Cancer pain (n = 8)	Phantom limb pain (n = 8)	Postherpetic pain (n = 6)
Sensory							
Cramping (44%) Aching (44%)	Gnawing (38%) Aching (50%)	Pounding (37%) Shooting (46%) Stabbing (37%) Sharp (64%) Cramping (82%) Aching (46%)	Throbbing (40%) Shooting (50%) Stabbing (40%) Sharp (60%) Cramping (40%) Aching (40%) Heavy (40%) Tender (50%)	Throbbing (50%) Boring (40%) Sharp (50%)	Shooting (50%) Sharp (50%) Gnawing (50%) Burning (50%) Heavy (50%)	Throbbing (38%) Stabbing (50%) Sharp (38%) Cramping (50%) Burning (50%) Aching (38%)	Sharp (84%) Pulling (67%) Aching (50%) Tender (83%)
Affective							
Tiring (44%) Sickening (56%)	Exhausting (50%)	Tiring (37%) Exhausting (46%) Fearful (36%)	Tiring (46%) Exhausting (40%)	Sickening (40%)	Exhausting (50%)	Tiring (50%) Exhausting (38%) Cruel (38%)	Exhausting (50%)
Evaluative							
	Annoying (38%)	Intense (46%)	Unbearable (40%)	Annoying (50%)	Unbearable (50%)		
Temporal							
Constant (56%)	Constant (44%) Rhythmic (56%)	Rhythmic (91%)	Constant (80%) Rhythmic (70%)	Constant (60%) Rhythmic (40%)	Constant (100%) Rhythmic (88%)	Constant (88%) Rhythmic (63%)	Constant (50%) Rhythmic (50%)

Note. Only those words chosen by more than one-third of the patients are listed, and the percentages of patients who chose each word are shown below the word. From Dubuisson and Melzack (1976). Copyright 1976 Ronald Melzack.

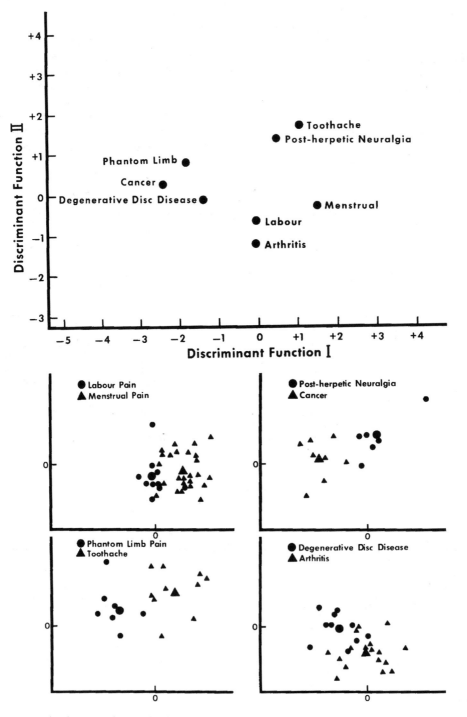

FIGURE 3.4. (*Top*) Centroids of eight diagnostic groups in the space of the first two discriminant functions, reported by Dubuisson and Melzack (1976). (*Bottom*) Individual patients' scores on the first two discriminant functions, for each diagnostic group. Large circle or triangle represents group centroid; small circles and triangles represent individual scores. Copyright 1976 Ronald Melzack.

had no detectable cause and was labeled as "functional." A concordance of 87% was found between established medical diagnosis and classification based upon the patients' choice of word patterns from the MPQ. Along similar lines, Perry, Heller, and Levine (1988, 1991) reported differences in the pattern of MPQ subscale correlations in patients with and without demonstrable organic pathology.

Further evidence of the discriminative capacity of the MPQ was furnished by Melzack, Terrence, Fromm, and Amsel (1986), who differentiated between the pain of trigeminal neuralgia and atypical facial pain. Fifty-three patients were given a thorough neurological examination that led to a diagnosis of either trigeminal neuralgia or atypical facial pain. Each patient rated his or her pain using the MPQ, and the scores were submitted to a discriminant analysis. Ninety-one percent of the patients were correctly classified with seven key descriptors. To determine how well the key descriptors were able to predict either diagnosis, the discriminant function derived from the 53 patients was applied to MPQ scores obtained from a second, independent validation sample of patients with trigeminal neuralgia or atypical facial pain. The results showed a correct prediction for 90% of the patients.

Specific verbal descriptors of the MPQ have also been shown to discriminate between reversible and irreversible damage of the nerve fibers in a tooth (Grushka & Sessle, 1984), and between leg pain caused by diabetic neuropathy and leg pain arising from other causes (Masson, Hunt, Gem, & Boulton, 1989). Jerome and colleagues (1988) further showed that the MPQ discriminates between cluster headache pain and other vascular (migraine and mixed) headache pain. Cluster headache is more intense and distressing than the others and is characterized by a distinct constellation of descriptors.

It is evident, however, that the discriminative capacity of the MPQ has limits. High levels of anxiety and other psychological disturbance, which may produce high Affective scores, may obscure the discriminative capacity (Kremer & Atkinson, 1983). Moreover, certain key words that discriminate among specific syndromes may be absent (Reading, 1982). Nevertheless, it is clear that there are appreciable and quantifiable differences in the way various types of pain are described, and that patients with the same disease or pain syndrome tend to use remarkably similar words to communicate what they feel.

Modifications

In general, modifications to the MPQ have involved the development of alternate scoring methods (as described above) and reclassification of the original pain descriptors (Clark, Fletcher, Janal, & Carroll, 1995; Fernandez & Towery, 1996; Towery & Fernandez, 1996). Efforts to modify the MPQ have led to a parsimonious subset of verbal descriptors from the sensory subcategories (Fernandez & Towery, 1996; Towery & Fernandez, 1996). In two separate studies, university students were asked to classify the MPQ descriptors and provide an estimate of the intensity of each descriptor, using a 0–10 rating scale. A three-step decision rule was applied to each descriptor to determine its inclusion or exclusion in the modified subset of words. Thirty-two out of the 84 descriptors (38%) met the criteria for inclusion. Interestingly, the intensity ratings of the modified descriptors correlated significantly ($r = .91$) with that of the original descriptors in the Melzack and Torgerson (1971) study attesting to the reliability of the MPQ. Although these efforts have yielded a more parsimonious subset of adjectives, the decision to limit the descriptors to the sensory subcategories means that the resulting scale is unidimensional; the Affective and Evaluative dimensions of pain have been omitted. The decision to exclude important descriptors that may have diagnostic utility (e.g., "numb," "tingling") because they were deemed ambiguous seems excessively strict. Comparisons with the MPQ in clinical and experimental settings will determine whether there is any incremental utility associated with the modified set of descriptors over the original MPQ.

THE SHORT-FORM MPQ

The short-form McGill Pain Questionnaire (SF-MPQ; Melzack, 1987; see Figure 3.5) was developed for use in specific research settings when the time to obtain information from patients is limited and when more information is desired than that provided by intensity measures such as the VAS or PPI. The SF-MPQ consists of 15 representative words from the Sensory ($n = 11$) and Affective ($n = 4$) categories of the standard MPQ. The PPI and a visual analogue scale are included to provide indices of overall pain intensity. The 15 descriptors making up the SF-MPQ were selected on the basis of their frequency of endorsement by patients with a variety of acute, intermittent, and

SHORT-FORM McGILL PAIN QUESTIONNAIRE
RONALD MELZACK

PATIENT'S NAME: _____   DATE: _____

	NONE	MILD	MODERATE	SEVERE
THROBBING	0) ____	1) ____	2) ____	3) ____
SHOOTING	0) ____	1) ____	2) ____	3) ____
STABBING	0) ____	1) ____	2) ____	3) ____
SHARP	0) ____	1) ____	2) ____	3) ____
CRAMPING	0) ____	1) ____	2) ____	3) ____
GNAWING	0) ____	1) ____	2) ____	3) ____
HOT-BURNING	0) ____	1) ____	2) ____	3) ____
ACHING	0) ____	1) ____	2) ____	3) ____
HEAVY	0) ____	1) ____	2) ____	3) ____
TENDER	0) ____	1) ____	2) ____	3) ____
SPLITTING	0) ____	1) ____	2) ____	3) ____
TIRING-EXHAUSTING	0) ____	1) ____	2) ____	3) ____
SICKENING	0) ____	1) ____	2) ____	3) ____
FEARFUL	0) ____	1) ____	2) ____	3) ____
PUNISHING-CRUEL	0) ____	1) ____	2) ____	3) ____

NO PAIN ├──────────────────────────────────────┤ WORST POSSIBLE PAIN

PPI

0	NO PAIN	____
1	MILD	____
2	DISCOMFORTING	____
3	DISTRESSING	____
4	HORRIBLE	____
5	EXCRUCIATING	____

© R. Melzack, 1984

FIGURE 3.5. The short-form McGill Pain Questionnaire (SF-MPQ). Descriptors 1–11 represent the Sensory dimension of pain experience, and 12–15 represent the Affective dimension. Each descriptor is ranked on an intensity scale of 0 = "none," 1 = "mild," 2 = "moderate," 3 = "severe." The PPI of the standard MPQ and the VAS are also included to provide overall pain intensity scores. Copyright 1984 Ronald Melzack.

chronic pains. An additional word—"splitting"—was added because it was reported to be a key discriminative word for dental pain (Grushka & Sessle, 1984). Each descriptor is ranked by the patient on an intensity scale of 0 = "none," 1 = "mild," 2 = "moderate," 3 = "severe."

The SF-MPQ correlates very highly with the major PRIs (Sensory, Affective, and Total) of the MPQ (Dudgeon, Ranbertas, & Rosenthal, 1993; Melzack, 1987), and is sensitive to clinical change brought about by various therapies—analgesic drugs (Harden, Carter, Gilman, Gross, & Peters, 1991;

Melzack, 1987), epidurally or spinally administered agents (Harden et al., 1991; Melzack, 1987;
Serrao, Marks, Morley, & Goodchild, 1992), transcutaneous electrical nerve stimulation (Melzack,
1987), and low-power light therapy (Stelian et al.,
1992). In addition, concurrent validity of the
SF-MPQ was reported in a study of patients with
chronic pain due to cancer (Dudgeon et al., 1993).
On each of three occasions separated by at least a
3-week period, the major PRI scores correlated
highly with scores on the MPQ.

Figure 3.6 shows SF-MPQ scores obtained
by patients with a variety of acute and chronic
pains. As can be seen, the SF-MPQ has been used
in studies of chronic pain (al Balawi, Tariq, &
Feinmann, 1996; Burckhardt, Clark, & Bennett,
1992; Dudgeon et al., 1993; Gagliese & Melzack,
1997; Grönblad, Lukinmaa, & Konttinen, 1990;
Stelian et al., 1992) and acute pain (Harden et al.,
1991; King, 1993; McGuire et al., 1993; Melzack,

1987; Thomas, Heath, Rose, & Flory, 1995) of
diverse etiology, and has been used to evaluate pain
and discomfort in response to medical interventions (Backonja et al., 1998; Fowlow, Price, &
Fung, 1995; Miller & Knox, 1992; Rowbotham,
Harden, Stacey, Bernstein, & Magnus-Miller, 1998).
Furthermore, initial data (Melzack, 1987) suggest
that the SF-MPQ may be capable of discriminating
among different pain syndromes, which is an important property of the standard MPQ. A Czech
version (Šolcová, Jacoubek, Sýkora, & Hník, 1990)
and a Swedish version (Burckhardt & Bjelle, 1994)
of the SF-MPQ have been developed.

A recent study of patients with chronic arthritis suggests that the SF-MPQ may be appropriate
for use with geriatric patients who experience pain
(Gagliese & Melzack, 1997). In this study, the frequency of failing to complete the SF-MPQ appropriately did not differ among young, middle-aged,
and elderly patients. In addition, the subscales
showed high intercorrelations and consistency.
Although elderly patients endorsed fewer adjectives
than their younger counterparts, there was a consistency among the three age groups in the most
frequently chosen pain descriptors. These results
suggest that pain patients across the life span approach the SF-MPQ in a similar manner. Future
studies are required to demonstrate the reliability
and validity of the SF-MPQ when used with elderly patients.

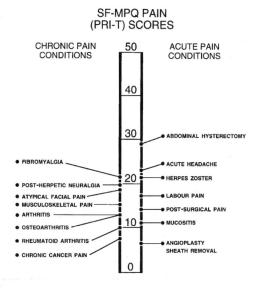

FIGURE 3.6. Comparison of Total PRI (PRI-T) scores
using the SF-MPQ for acute and chronic pain conditions. References for the various pain conditions are as
follows: labor pain, musculoskeletal pain, and postsurgical pain (Melzack, 1987), abdominal hysterectomy
(Thomas et al., 1995), acute headache (Harden et al.,
1991), herpes zoster and postherpetic neuralgia (King,
1993), mucositis (McGuire et al., 1993), angioplasty
sheath removal (Fowlow et al., 1995), fibromyalgia and
rheumatoid arthritis (Burckhardt & Bjelle, 1994), atypical facial pain (al Balawi et al., 1996), arthritis (Gagliese
& Melzack, 1997), osteoarthritis (Stelian et al., 1992),
and chronic cancer pain (Dudgeon et al., 1993). Copyright 1999 Joel Katz and Ronald Melzack.

MULTIDIMENSIONAL PAIN EXPERIENCE

Turk and colleagues (1985) and Holroyd and colleagues (1992) have evaluated the theoretical structure of the MPQ, using factor-analytic methods to
analyze their data. Turk and colleagues concluded
that the three-factor structure of the MPQ—Sensory,
Affective, and Evaluative—is strongly supported by
the analyses; Holroyd and colleagues' "most clearly
interpretable structure" was provided by a four-factor solution obtained by oblique rotation in which
two Sensory factors were identified in addition to
an Affective and an Evaluative factor.

Like most others who have used the MPQ,
Turk and colleagues (1985) and Holroyd and colleagues (1992) found high intercorrelations among
the factors. However, these authors have then argued that because the factors measured by the MPQ
are highly intercorrelated, they are therefore not
distinct. They conclude that the MPQ does not
discriminate among the factors, and, according to

Turk and colleagues (1985), only the Total PRI should be used. It is fallacious and potentially misleading to argue that the MPQ lacks discriminative capacity and clinical utility because factor-analytic studies reveal significant intercorrelations among the identified factors (Gracely, 1992). There is, in fact, considerable evidence that the MPQ is effective in discriminating among the three factors, despite the high intercorrelations.

First, Gracely (1992) has convincingly argued that factor-analytic methods may be inappropriate for assessing the factor structure of the MPQ, although they provide useful information about patient characteristics. Torgerson (1988) distinguished between *semantic meaning* (how the MPQ descriptors are arranged) and *associate meaning* (how patients arrange the MPQ descriptors) to emphasize that factor analysis provides a context-dependent structure of the latter; that is, the outcome depends on how specific patient samples make use of the MPQ descriptors. Gracely (1992) elaborated further on the difference between semantic and associative meaning and concluded that factor-analytic techniques do not directly evaluate the semantic structure of the questionnaire.

Second, a high correlation among variables does not necessarily imply a lack of discriminant capacity. Traditional psychophysics has shown repeatedly that in the case of vision, increasing the intensity of light produces increased capacity to discriminate color, contours, texture, and distance (Kling & Riggs, 1971). Similarly, in the case of hearing, increases in volume lead to increased discrimination of timbre, pitch, and spatial location (Kling & Riggs, 1971). In these cases, there are clearly very high intercorrelations among the variables in each modality. But this does not mean that we should forget about the differences between color and texture, or between timbre and pitch, just because they intercorrelate highly. This approach would lead to the loss of valuable, meaningful data (Gracely, 1992).

Third, many papers have demonstrated the discriminant validity of the MPQ. Reading and Newton (1977) showed, in a comparison of primary dysmenorrhea and intrauterine device (IUD)-related pain, that the "pain intensity scores were reflected in a larger sensory component with IUD users, whereas with dysmenorrhea the affective component predominated" (p. 265). In a later study, Reading (1982) compared MPQ profiles of women experiencing chronic pelvic pain and postepisiotomy pain, and showed that "acute-pain patients displayed greater use of sensory word

groups, testifying to the pronounced sensory input from the damaged perineum. Chronic pain patients used affective and reaction subgroups with greater frequency" (p. 185).

In a study of hypnosis and biofeedback, Melzack and Perry (1975) found that there were significant decreases in both the sensory and affective dimensions, as well as the overall PRI, but that the affective dimension shows the largest decrease. In studies on labor pain, Melzack and his colleagues (Melzack, Kinch, Dobkin, Lebrun, & Taenzer, 1984; Melzack et al., 1981) found that distinctly different variables correlate with the Sensory, Affective, and Evaluative dimensions. Prepared childbirth training, for example, correlates significantly with the Sensory and Affective dimensions but not the Evaluative one. Menstrual difficulties correlate with the Affective but not with the Sensory or Evaluative dimension. Physical factors, such as mother's and infant's weight, also correlate selectively with one or another dimension.

Similarly, a study of acute pain in emergency ward patients (Melzack, Wall, & Ty, 1982) has revealed a normal distribution of sensory scores but very low affective scores compared to patients with chronic pain. Finally, Chen and colleagues (1989) have consistently identified a group of pain-sensitive and pain-tolerant subjects in five laboratory studies of tonic (prolonged) pain. Compared with pain-tolerant subjects, pain-sensitive subjects show significantly higher scores on all PRIs except the Sensory dimension. Atkinson, Kremer, and Ignelzi (1982) are undoubtedly right that high Affective scores tend to diminish the discriminant capacity of the MPQ, so that at high levels of anxiety and depression, some discriminant capacity is lost. However, the MPQ still retains good discriminant function even at high levels of anxiety.

One study is of particular interest because it examined laboratory models of phasic (brief) and tonic (prolonged) pain, and compared them by using the MPQ. Chen and Treede (1985) found a very high Sensory loading for phasic pain and relatively few choices of Affective and Evaluative words. In contrast, tonic pain was characterized by much higher scores in the Affective and Evaluative dimensions. Furthermore, they found that when tonic pain is used to inhibit the phasic pain, "the sensory component is reduced by 32%, whereas the affective component vanishes almost completely" (p. 72).

In brief, therefore, high intercorrelations among psychological variables do not mean that they are all alike and can therefore be lumped into a single variable such as intensity; rather, certain biological and psychological variables can covary to a high degree yet represent distinct, discriminable entities. Moreover, the MPQ has been shown in many studies to be capable of discriminating among the three component factors.

SUMMARY

Pain is a personal, subjective experience influenced by cultural learning, the meaning of the situation, attention, and other psychological variables. Approaches to the measurement of pain include VRSs, NRSs, behavioral observation scales, and physiological responses. The complex nature of the experience of pain suggests that measurements from these domains may not always show high concordance. But because pain is subjective, the patient's self-report provides the most valid measure of the experience. The VAS and the MPQ are probably the most frequently used self-rating instruments for the measurement of pain in clinical and research settings. The MPQ is designed to assess the multidimensional nature of pain experience and has been demonstrated to be a reliable, valid, and consistent measurement tool. The SF-MPQ is available for use in specific research settings when the time to obtain information from patients is limited and when more information than simply the intensity of pain is desired. Further development and refinement of pain measurement techniques will lead to increasingly accurate tools with greater predictive powers.

ACKNOWLEDGMENTS

The writing of this chapter was supported by Grant No. A7891 from the Natural Sciences and Engineering Research Council of Canada to Ronald Melzack; by a Scientist Award from the Medical Research Council of Canada (MRC) to Joel Katz; by MRC Grant No. MT-12052 to Joel Katz; and by National Institute of Neurological Disorders and Stroke Grant No. NS35480 to Joel Katz.

REFERENCES

al Balawi, S., Tariq, M., & Feinmann, C. (1996). A double-blind, placebo-controlled, crossover study to evaluate the efficacy of subcutaneous sumatriptan in the treat-ment of atypical facial pain. *International Journal of Neuroscience, 86*(3–4), 301–309.

Atkinson, J. H., Kremer, E. F., & Ignelzi, R. J. (1982). Diffusion of pain language with affective disturbance confounds differential diagnosis. *Pain, 12,* 375–384.

Backonja, M., Beydoun, A., Edwards, K. R., Schwartz, S. L., Fonseca, V., Hes, M., LaMoreaux, L., & Garofalo, E. (1998). Gabapentin for the symptomatic treatment of painful neuropathy in patients with diabetes mellitus: A randomized controlled trial. *Journal of the American Medical Association, 280,* 1831–1836.

Bartko, D., Kondos, M., & Jansco, S. (1984). Slovak version of the McGill–Melzack's Questionnaire on pain. *Ceskoslovenska Neurologie a Neurochirurgie, 47,* 113–121.

Beecher, H. K. (1959). *Measurement of subjective responses.* New York: Oxford University Press.

Bejarano, P. F., Noriego, R. D., Rodriguez, M. L., & Berrio, G. M. (1985). Evaluación del dolor: Adaptación del cuestionario de McGill [Evaluation of pain: Adaptation of the McGill Pain Questionnaire. *Revista Columbia Anestesia, 13,* 321–351.

Bende, J., Menesi, R., Beno, U., Baltas, B., Lencz, L., Szegesdi, I., & Troidl, H. (1993). Hungarian version of McGill Pain Questionnaire. *Aneszteziologia es Intenziv Terapia, 23,* 99–103.

Boureau, F., Luu, M., & Doubrère, J. F. (1992). Comparative study of the validity of four French McGill Pain Questionnaire (MPQ) versions. *Pain, 50,* 59–65.

Boureau, F., Luu, M., Doubrère, J. F., & Gay, C. (1984). Elaboration d'un questionnaire d'auto-évaluation de la douleur par liste de qualicatifs [Development of a self-evaluation questionnaire comprising pain descriptors.]. *Thérapie, 39,* 119–129.

Briggs, M. (1996). Surgical wound pain: A trial of two treatments. *Journal of Wound Care, 5*(10), 456–460.

Burchiel, K. J., Anderson, V. C., Brown, F. D., Fessler, R. G., Friedman, W. A., Pelofsky, S., Weiner, R. L., Oakley, J., & Shatin, D. (1996). Prospective, multicenter study of spinal cord stimulation for relief of chronic back and extremity pain. *Spine, 21*(23), 2786–2794.

Burckhardt, C. (1984). The use of the McGill Pain Questionnaire in assessing arthritis pain. *Pain, 19,* 305–314.

Burckhardt, C. S., & Bjelle, A. (1994). A Swedish version of the short-form McGill Pain Questionnaire. *Scandinavian Journal of Rheumatology, 23*(2), 77–81.

Burckhardt, C. S., Clark, S. R., & Bennett, R. M. (1992). A comparison of pain perceptions in women with fibromyalgia and rheumatoid arthritis: Relationship to depression and pain extent. *Arthritis Care and Research, 5*(4), 216–222.

Charter, R. A., & Nehemkis, A. M. (1983). The language of pain intensity and complexity: New methods of scoring the McGill Pain Questionnaire. *Perceptual and Motor Skills, 56,* 519–537.

Chen, A. C. N., Dworkin, S. F., Haug, J., & Gerhig, J. (1989). Human pain responsivity in a tonic pain model: Psychological determinants. *Pain, 37,* 143–160.

Chen, A. C. N., & Treede, R. D. (1985). McGill Pain Questionnaire in assessing the differentiation of phasic and tonic pain: Behavioral evaluation of the "pain inhibiting pain" effect. *Pain, 22,* 67–79.

Clark, W. C., Fletcher, J. D., Janal, M. N., & Carroll, J. D. (1995). Hierarchical clustering of pain and emotion descriptors: Toward a revision of the McGill Pain Questionnaire. In B. Bromm & J. E. Desmedt (Eds.), Advances in pain research and therapy (Vol. 22, pp. 319-330). New York: Raven Press.

Crockett, D. J., Prkachin, K. M., & Craig, K. D. (1977). Factors of the language of pain in patients and normal volunteer groups. Pain, 4, 175-182.

De Benedittis, G., Massei, R., Nobili, R., & Pieri, A. (1988). The Italian Pain Questionnaire. Pain, 33, 53-62.

Drewes, A. M., Helweg-Larsen, S., Petersen, P., Brennum, J., Andreasen, A., Poulsen, L. H., & Jensen, T. S. (1993). McGill Pain Questionnaire translated into Danish: Experimental and clinical findings. Clinical Journal of Pain, 9(2), 80-87.

Dubuisson, D., & Melzack, R. (1976). Classification of clinical pain descriptors by multiple group discriminant analysis. Experimental Neurology, 51, 480-487.

Dudgeon, D., Ranbertas, R. F., & Rosenthal, S. (1993). The short-form McGill Pain Questionnaire in chronic cancer pain. Journal of Pain and Symptom Management, 8, 191-195.

Eija, K., Tasmuth, T., & Pertti, N. J. (1996). Amitriptyline effectively relieves neuropathic pain following treatment of breast cancer. Pain, 64(2), 293-302.

Escalante, A., Lichtenstein, M. J., Rios, N., & Hazuda, H. P. (1996). Measuring chronic rheumatic pain in Mexican Americans: Cross-cultural adaptation of the McGill Pain Questionnaire. Journal of Clinical Epidemiology, 49(12), 1389-1399.

Fernandez, E., & Towery, S. (1996). A parsimonious set of verbal descriptors of pain sensation derived from the McGill Pain Questionnaire. Pain, 66(1), 31-37. (Published erratum appears in Pain, 1996, 68(2-3), 437.)

Ferracuti, S., Romeo, G., Leardi, M. G., Cruccu, G., & Lazzari, R. (1990). New Italian adaptation and standardization of the McGill Pain Questionnaire. Pain (Suppl. 5), S300.

Fowlow, B., Price, P., & Fung, T. (1995). Ambulation after sheath removal: A comparison of 6 and 8 hours of bedrest after sheath removal in patients following a PTCA procedure. Heart and Lung, 24(1), 28-37.

Gagliese, L., & Melzack, R. (1997). Age differences in the quality of chronic pain: A preliminary study. Pain Research and Management, 2, 157-162.

Gaston-Johansson, F., Albert, M., Fagan, E., & Zimmerman, L. (1990). Similarities in pain descriptors of four different ethnic-culture groups. Journal of Pain and Symptom Management, 5, 94-100.

Georgoudis, G., Oldham, J. A., & Watson, P. J. (in press). Reliability and sensitivity measures of Greek version of the short-form McGill Pain Questionnaire. European Journal of Pain.

Gracely, R. H. (1992). Evaluation of multi-dimensional pain scales. Pain, 48, 297-300.

Graham, C., Bond, S. S., Gerkovitch, M. M., & Cook, M. R. (1980). Use of the McGill Pain Questionnaire in the assessment of cancer pain: Replicability and consistency. Pain, 8, 377-387.

Grönblad, M., Lukinmaa, A., & Konttinen, Y. T. (1990). Chronic low-back pain: Intercorrelation of repeated measures for pain and disability. Scandinavian Journal of Rehabilitation Medicine, 22, 73-77.

Grushka, M., & Sessle, B. J. (1984). Applicability of the McGill Pain Questionnaire to the differentiation of "toothache" pain. Pain, 19, 49-57.

Harden, R. N., Carter, T. D., Gilman, C. S., Gross, A. J., & Peters, J. R. (1991). Ketorolac in acute headache management. Headache, 31, 463-464.

Harrison, A. (1988). Arabic pain words. Pain, 32, 239-250.

Hartman, L. M., & Ainsworth, K. D. (1980). Self-regulation of chronic pain. Canadian Journal of Psychiatry, 25, 38-43.

Hasegawa, M., Hattori, S., Ishizaki, K., Suzuki, S., & Goto, F. (1996). The McGill Pain Questionnaire, Japanese version, reconsidered: Confirming the reliability and validity. Pain Research and Management, 1, 233-237.

Hasegawa, M., Mishima, M., Matsumoto, I., Sasaki, T., Kimura, T., Baba, Y., Senami, K., Kanemura, K., Takano, O., & Shibata, T. (in press). McGill Pain Questionnaire, Japanese version reconsidered: Confirming the theoretical structure of the Japanese version of the McGill Pain Questionnaire in chronic pain. Pain Research and Management, 6.

Hiwot, M. G., Arega, A., Molla, M., Samson, S., Seyoum, N., Ressom, S., Worku, S., Mulatu, M., Egale, T., & Aboud, F. E. (in press). The McGill Pain Questionnaire in Amharic: Some data on the experience of pain. Ethiopian Medical Journal.

Holroyd, K. A., Holm, J. E., Keefe, F. J., Turner, J. A., Bradley, L. A., Murphy, W. D., Johnson, P., Anderson, K., Hinkle, A. L., & O'Malley, W. B. (1992). A multi-center evaluation of the McGill Pain Questionnaire: Results from more than 1700 chronic pain patients. Pain, 48, 301-311.

Hui, Y. L., & Chen, A. C. (1989). Analysis of headache in a Chinese patient population. Ma Tsui Hsueh Tsa Chi, 27, 13-18.

Jenkinson, C., Carroll, D., Egerton, M., Frankland, T., McQuay, H., & Nagle, C. (1995). Comparison of the sensitivity to change of long and short form pain measures. Quality of Life Research, 4(4), 353-357.

Jerome, A., Holroyd, K. A., Theofanous, A. G., Pingel, J. D., Lake, A. E., & Saper, J. R. (1988). Cluster headache pain vs. other vascular headache pain: Differences revealed with two approaches to the McGill Pain Questionnaire. Pain, 34, 35-42.

Katz, J. (1992). Psychophysical correlates of phantom limb experience. Journal of Neurology, Neurosurgery and Psychiatry, 55, 811-821.

Katz, J., Clairoux, M., Kavanagh, B. P., Roger, S., Nierenberg, H., Redahan, C., & Sandler, A. N. (1994). Preemptive lumbar epidural anaesthesia reduces postoperative pain and patient-controlled morphine consumption after lower abdominal surgery. Pain, 59, 395-403.

Katz, J., & Melzack, R. (1991). Auricular TENS reduces phantom limb pain. Journal of Pain and Symptom Management, 6, 73-83.

Katz, J., & Melzack, R. (1999, April). Measurement of pain. In A. N. Sandler (Ed.), The Surgical Clinics of North America [Special issue]. Pain Control in the Perioperative Period, 79(2), 231-252.

Ketovuori, H., & Pöntinen, P. J. (1981). A pain vocabulary in Finnish: The Finnish Pain Questionnaire. Pain, 11, 247-253.

Kim, H. S., Schwartz-Barcott, D., Holter, I. M., & Lorensen, M. (1995). Developing a translation of the

McGill Pain Questionnaire for cross-cultural comparison: An example from Norway. *Journal of Advanced Nursing, 21*(3), 421–426.

King, R. B. (1993). Topical aspirin in chloroform and the relief of pain due to herpes zoster and postherpetic neuralgia. *Archives of Neurology, 50*(10), 1046–1053.

Kiss, I., Müller, H., & Abel, M. (1987). The McGill Pain Questionnaire—German version: A study on cancer pain. *Pain, 29*, 195–207.

Klepac, R. K., Dowling, J., Rokke, P., Dodge, L., & Schafer, L. (1981). Interview vs. paper-and-pencil administration of the McGill Pain Questionnaire. *Pain, 11*, 241–246.

Kling, J. W., & Riggs, L. A. (1971). *Experimental psychology.* New York: Holt, Rinehart & Winston.

Knotek, P., Blahuš, P., Šolcová, I., & Žalskey, M. (2000). Standard Czech version of the Short Form McGill Pain Questionnaire. *Bolest, 5*, 113–117.

Kremer, E., & Atkinson, J. H. (1983). Pain language as a measure of affect in chronic pain patients. In R. Melzack (Ed.), *Pain measurement and assessment* (pp. 119–127). New York: Raven Press.

Kremer, E., Atkinson, J. H., & Ignelzi, R. J. (1982). Pain measurement: The affective dimensional measure of the McGill Pain Questionnaire with a cancer pain population. *Pain, 12*, 153–163.

Lahuerta, J., Smith, B. A., & Martinez-Lage, J. L. (1982). An adaptation of the McGill Pain Questionnaire to the Spanish language. *Schmerz, 3*, 132–134.

Lázaro, C., Bosch, F., Torrubia, R., & Baños, J. E. (1994). The development of a Spanish questionnaire for assessing pain: Preliminary data concerning reliability and validity. *European Journal of Psychological Assessment, 10*, 145–151.

Leavitt, F., & Garron, D. C. (1980). Validity of a back pain classification scale for detecting psychological disturbance as measured by the MMPI. *Journal of Clinical Psychology, 36*, 186–189.

Leavitt, F., Garron, D. C., Whisler, W. W., & Sheinkop, M. B. (1978). Affective and sensory dimensions of pain. *Pain, 4*, 273–281.

Love, A., Leboeuf, D. C., & Crisp, T. C. (1989). Chiropractic chronic low back pain sufferers and self-report assessment methods: Part I. A reliability study of the visual analogue scale, the pain drawing and the McGill Pain Questionnaire. *Journal of Manipulative and Physiological Therapeutics, 12*, 21–25.

Lowe, N. K., Walker, S. N., & McCallum, R. C. (1991). Confirming the theoretical structure of the McGill Pain Questionnaire in acute clinical pain. *Pain, 46*, 53–60.

Maiani, G., & Sanavio, E. (1985). Semantics of pain in Italy: The Italian version of the McGill Pain Questionnaire. *Pain, 22*, 399–405.

Masson, E. A., Hunt, L., Gem, J. M., & Boulton, A. J. M. (1989). A novel approach to the diagnosis and assessment of symptomatic diabetic neuropathy. *Pain, 38*, 25–28.

McCreary, C., Turner, J., & Dawson, E. (1981). Principal dimensions of the pain experience and psychological disturbance in chronic low back pain patients. *Pain, 11*, 85–92.

McGuire, D. B., Altomonte, V., Peterson, D. E., Wingard, J. R., Jones, R. J., & Grochow, L. B. (1993). Patterns of mucositis and pain in patients receiving preparative chemotherapy and bone marrow transplantation. *Oncology Nursing Forum, 20*(10), 1493–1502.

Melzack, R. (1975). The McGill Pain Questionnaire: major properties and scoring methods. *Pain, 1*, 277–299.

Melzack, R. (Ed.). (1983). *Pain measurement and assessment.* New York: Raven Press.

Melzack, R. (1987). The short-form McGill Pain Questionnaire. *Pain, 30*, 191–197.

Melzack, R., & Casey, K. L. (1968). Sensory, motivational, and central control determinants of pain: A new conceptual model. In D. Kenshalo (Ed.), *The skin senses* (pp. 423–443). Springfield, IL: Charles C Thomas.

Melzack, R., Katz, J., & Jeans, M. E. (1985). The role of compensation in chronic pain: Analysis using a new method of scoring the McGill Pain Questionnaire. *Pain, 23*, 101–112.

Melzack, R., Kinch, R., Dobkin, P., Lebrun, M., & Taenzer, P. (1984). Severity of labour pain: Influence of physical as well as psychologic variables. *Canadian Medical Association Journal, 130*, 579–584.

Melzack, R., & Perry, C. (1975). Self-regulation of pain: The use of alpha-feedback and hypnotic training for the control of chronic pain. *Experimental Neurology, 46*, 452–469.

Melzack, R., Taenzer, P., Feldman, P., & Kinch, R. A. (1981). Labour is still painful after prepared childbirth training. *Canadian Medical Association Journal, 125*, 357–363.

Melzack, R., Terrence, C., Fromm, G., & Amsel, R. (1986). Trigeminal neuralgia and atypical facial pain: Use of the McGill Pain Questionnaire for discrimination and diagnosis. *Pain, 27*, 297–302.

Melzack, R., & Torgerson, W. S. (1971). On the language of pain. *Anesthesiology, 34*, 50–59.

Melzack, R., & Wall, P. D. (1996). *The challenge of pain* (2nd ed.). London: Penguin Books.

Melzack, R., Wall, P. D., & Ty, T. C. (1982). Acute pain in an emergency clinic: Latency of onset and description patterns related to different injuries. *Pain, 14*, 33–43.

Miller, R. M., & Knox, M. (1992). Patient tolerance of ioxaglate and iopamidol in internal mammary artery arteriography. *Catheterization and Cardiovascular Diagnosis, 25*, 31–34.

Nikolajsen, L., Hansen, C. L., Nielsen, J., Keller, J., Arendt-Nielsen, L., & Jensen, T. S. (1996). The effect of ketamine on phantom pain: A central neuropathic disorder maintained by peripheral input. *Pain, 67*(1), 69–77.

Pearce, J., & Morley, S. (1989). An experimental investigation of the construct validity of the McGill Pain Questionnaire. *Pain, 39*, 115–121.

Perry, F., Heller, P. H., & Levine, J. D. (1988). Differing correlations between pain measures in syndromes with or without explicable organic pathology. *Pain, 34*, 185–189.

Perry, F., Heller, P. H., & Levine, J. D. (1991). A possible indicator of functional pain: Poor pain scale correlation. *Pain, 46*, 191–193.

Pimenta, C. A., & Teixeiro, M. J. (1996). [Proposal to adapt the McGill Pain Questionnaire into Portuguese]. *Revista da Escola de Enfermagem Da USP, 30*(3), 473–483.

Pozehl, B., Barnason, S., Zimmerman, L., Nieveen, J., & Crutchfield, J. (1995). Pain in the postoperative coronary artery bypass graft patient. *Clinical Nursing Research, 4*(2), 208–222.

Prieto, E. J., Hopson, L, Bradley, L. A., Byrne, M., Geisinger, K. F., Midax, D., & Marchisello, P. J. (1980). The language of low back pain: Factor structure of the McGill Pain Questionnaire. *Pain, 8,* 11–19.

Radvila, A., Adler, R. H., Galeazzi, R. L., & Vorkauf, H. (1987). The development of a German language (Berne) pain questionnaire and its application in a situation causing acute pain. *Pain, 28,* 185–195.

Reading, A. E. (1979). The internal structure of the McGill Pain Questionnaire in dysmenorrhea patients. *Pain, 7,* 353–358.

Reading, A. E. (1982). An analysis of the language of pain in chronic and acute patient groups. *Pain, 13,* 185–192.

Reading, A. E. (1989). Testing pain mechanisms in persons in pain. In P. D. Wall & R. Melzack (Eds.), *Textbook of pain* (2nd ed., pp. 269–283). Edinburgh: Churchill Livingstone.

Reading, A. E., Everitt, B. S., & Sledmere, C. M. (1982). The McGill Pain Questionnaire: A replication of its construction. *British Journal of Clinical Psychology, 21,* 339–349.

Reading, A. E., & Newton, J. R. (1977). On a comparison of dysmenorrhea and intrauterine device related pain. *Pain, 3,* 265–276.

Rowbotham, M., Harden, N., Stacey, B., Bernstein, P., & Magnus-Miller, L. (1998). Gabapentin for the treatment of postherpetic neuralgia: A randomized controlled trial. *Journal of the American Medical Association, 280,* 1837–1842.

Satow, A., Nakatani, K., Taniguchi, S., & Higashiyama, A. (1990). Perceptual characteristics of electrocutaneous pain estimated by the 30-word list and visual analog scale. *Japanese Psychological Review, 32,* 155–164.

Sedlak, K. (1990). A Polish version of the McGill Pain Questionnaire. *Pain* (Suppl. 5), S308.

Serrao, J. M., Marks, R. L., Morley, S. J., & Goodchild, C. S. (1992). Intrathecal midazolam for the treatment of chronic mechanical low back pain: A controlled comparison with epidural steroid in a pilot study. *Pain, 48,* 5–12.

Šolcová, I., Jacoubek, B., Sýkora, J., & Hník, P. (1990). Characterization of vertebrogenic pain using the short form of the McGill Pain Questionnaire. *Casopis Lekaru Ceskych, 129,* 1611–1614.

Stein, C., & Mendl, G. (1988). The German counterpart to McGill Pain Questionnaire. *Pain, 32,* 251–255.

Stelian, J., Gil, I., Habot, B., Rosenthal, M., Abramovici, I., Kutok, N., & Kahil, A. (1992). Improvement of pain and disability in elderly patients with degenerative osteoarthritis of the knee treated with narrowband light therapy. *Journal of the American Geriatrics Society, 40,* 23–26.

Strand, L. I., & Wisnes, A. R. (1991). The development of a Norwegian pain questionnaire. *Pain, 46,* 61–66.

Tahmoush, A. J. (1981). Causalgia: Redefinition as a clinical pain syndrome. *Pain, 10,* 187–197.

Tesfaye, S., Watt, J., Benbow, S. J., Pang, K. A., Miles, J., & MacFarlane, I. A. (1996). Electrical spinal-cord stimulation for painful diabetic peripheral neuropathy. *Lancet, 348,* 1698–1701.

Thomas, V., Heath, M., Rose, D., & Flory, P. (1995). Psychological characteristics and the effectiveness of patient-controlled analgesia. *British Journal of Anaesthesia, 74*(3), 271–276.

Torgerson, W. S. (1988). Critical issues in verbal pain assessment: Multidimensional and multivariate issues. *American Pain Society Abstracts.*

Towery, S., & Fernandez, E. (1996). Reclassification and rescaling of McGill Pain Questionnaire verbal descriptors of pain sensation: A replication. *Clinical Journal of Pain, 12*(4), 270–276.

Turk, D. C., Rudy, T. E., & Salovey, P. (1985). The McGill Pain Questionnaire reconsidered: Confirming the factor structures and examining appropriate uses. *Pain, 21,* 385–397.

Van Buren, J., & Kleinknecht, R. (1979). An evaluation of the McGill Pain Questionnaire for use in dental pain assessment. *Pain, 6,* 23–33.

van der Kloot, W. A., Oostendorp, R. A., van der Meij, J., & van den Heuvel, J. (1995). [The Dutch version of the McGill Pain Questionnaire: A reliable pain questionnaire]. *Nederlands Tijdschrift voor Geneeskunde, 139*(13), 669–673.

van Lankveld, W., van 't Pad Bosch, P., van de Putte, L., van der Staak, C., & Naring, G. (1992). [Pain in rheumatoid arthritis measured with the visual analogue scale and the Dutch version of the McGill Pain Questionnaire]. *Nederlands Tijdschrift voor Geneeskunde, 136*(24), 1166–1170.

Vanderiet, K., Adriaensen, H., Carton, H., & Vertommen, H. (1987). The McGill Pain Questionnaire constructed for the Dutch language (MPQ-DV): Preliminary data concerning reliability and validity. *Pain, 30,* 395–408.

Veilleux, S., & Melzack, R. (1976). Pain in psychotic patients. *Experimental Neurology, 52,* 535–563.

Verkes, R. J., Van der Kloot, W. A., & Van der Meij, J. (1989). The perceived structure of 176 pain descriptive words. *Pain, 38,* 219–229.

Wilkie, D. J., Savedra, M. C., Holzemier, W. L., Tesler, M. D., & Paul, S. M. (1990). Use of the McGill Pain Questionnaire to measure pain: A meta-analysis. *Nursing Research, 39,* 36–41.

Chapter 4

Psychophysical Approaches to Measurement of the Dimensions and Stages of Pain

DONALD D. PRICE
JOSEPH L. RILEY III
JAMES B. WADE

Current methods for measurement and assessment of pain have historical roots in *psychophysics*, the branch of psychology concerned with the relationships of physical stimulus properties to behavioral responses and sensory perceptions. The psychophysics of pain has been critical for improvements in pain measurement, particularly for providing methods for differential measurement of the different psychological dimensions of pain experience. Both of these applications of psychophysics have important relevance for the treatment and management of acute and chronic pain. The psychophysics of pain has a pivotal role in clarifying the mechanisms of pain and in providing a scientific basis for modern methods of pain measurement and assessment. With this psychophysical perspective in mind, we pursue two interrelated objectives in this chapter. The first is to briefly review modern approaches for the measurement of pain and to explain how psychophysical methods can be applied to measurement and assessment of both clinical and laboratory pain. The second objective is to review an approach for assessment and measurement of the different dimensions and stages of pain processing.

APPLICATION OF PSYCHOPHYSICAL METHODS TO THE MEASUREMENT OF PAIN

Measurement of pain, similar to optometrists' measurements of visual acuity, is directly dependent on the person who experiences the pain. Someone who is having pain is asked to match the perceived intensity of that pain to a scale. This can be done in a variety of ways. For example, one can match words or numbers to pain intensity, or match an intensity of experimental pain to that of clinical pain, or use more than one of these procedures. In all such methods, the critical observer is someone experiencing pain. The clinician or investigator also has a crucial role in pain measurement. This person provides the scaling procedures, records the reported values, and uses a measurement method that has been shown to be reliable and valid.

People who are experiencing pain can be asked to scale different dimensions of their experience. Thus they can judge the relative intensity of the painful sensation, the degree of its immediate unpleasantness, spatial distribution, and qualities.

These separate judgments are by no means exclusive to pain and have a long history in the psychophysics of smell, taste, audition, vision, and somatosensory modalities. For example, with some instruction and training, it is possible to make separate and highly reliable judgments of intensity, pitch, timbre, volume, and density of the same sound stimuli, as well as of their pleasantness or unpleasantness.

Criteria for Pain Measurement

Assessments of human pain have evolved from extensive reliance on threshold and tolerance measures to the use of a wide variety of psychological and physiological methods that explicitly recognize that pain experience and pain behavior have multiple dimensions. Despite this diversity of approaches, all methods share a common goal of accurately representing the human pain experience. Although these approaches have different emphases, there is general agreement as to the principal criteria for an ideal pain measurement procedure. The following criteria include those originally suggested by Gracely and Dubner (1981), and two others (1 and 9) that we have added. An ideal method would:

1. Have ratio scale properties.
2. Be relatively free of biases inherent in different psychophysical methods.
3. Provide immediate information about the accuracy and reliability of the subjects' performance of the scaling responses.
4. Be useful for both experimental and clinical pain and allow for reliable comparison between both types of pain.
5. Be reliable and generalizable.
6. Be sensitive to changes in pain intensity.
7. Be simple to use for patients/subjects with and without pain in both clinical and research settings.
8. Separately assess the sensory intensive and affective dimensions of pain.
9. Separately assess the multiple stages of pain-related affect and the meanings that support them.

The goal of current methods of human pain measurement is to fulfill all or most of these criteria. Several general approaches to pain measurement are briefly described in terms of their historical role in pain measurement and the capacity for each method to fulfill the criteria above. Emphasis is placed on direct scaling methods, because they are likely to have the most direct and practical value in research and clinical pain assessment.

Three basic and commonly used approaches to quantifying pain are discussed next. These include (1) methods that define a threshold for pain and measure changes in pain threshold; (2) ordinal rating scale methods, in which people rate pain intensity on scales with clearly defined numerical limits and intervals on verbal rating scales whose words indicate a rank order; and (3) visual analogue scale (VAS) procedures, in which direct judgments of sensation intensity or unpleasantness are made by representing perceived magnitude by length along continuous scales. Considerable emphasis is given to the latter two methods, because they have become extensively used in both experimental and clinical pain studies.

Alternative Methods of Pain Measurement

Pain Threshold Measurements

There are two general procedures for obtaining pain threshold—the method of limits and the method of constant stimuli (Guilford, 1954). In the former, stimulus intensity is gradually increased to a point where the person being tested perceives the stimulus as painful and then gradually decreased to a point where it is no longer painful. The stimulus intensity midway between these two limits is considered threshold. Multiple trials of this procedure can be carried out to improve accuracy. In the method of constant stimuli, stimulus intensity is increased in steps to a level at which the person being tested perceives one-half the stimuli as painful (Guilford, 1954). Regardless of which procedure is employed, people are required to identify the point on the stimulus continuum that distinguishes painful from nonpainful experience.

Pain threshold measures are commonly used to infer someone's sensitivity to pain and changes in pain sensitivity. In combination with other measures of pain, they can be useful measurements. However, pain threshold measures cannot directly provide information about pain intensity or ratios of pain intensity (criterion 1). Pain threshold can be strongly influenced by attentional, motivational, emotional, and sensory factors unrelated to pain (e.g., touch), as well as by whether the threshold is defined in sensory or affective terms (related to criterion 2). Pain threshold measurements require a stimulus continuum that is controllable by the tester, and therefore they are more applicable to experimental pain than to clinical pain measurements. Nevertheless, clinical pain thresholds can sometimes be very important, as in the assessment of tender muscle points. Given adequate instructions, pain thresholds can be reliable, generalizable across groups of people (criterion 5), and simple to obtain (criterion 7). However, under some experimental conditions, they have been shown to be relatively insensitive to effects of clinically proven drugs (criterion 6), for reasons related to physiological mechanisms (Hardy, Wolff, & Goodell, 1940, 1952; Price, 1988; Price, von der Gruen, Miller, Rafii, & Price, 1985). Stimuli used to test pain thresholds in humans and other animals are typically brief and have a rapid rise time. Rapid, brief nociceptive stimuli produce neural responses mediated by peripheral $A\delta$ nociceptive afferents. These responses are less sensitive to opioid analgesics than are slowly rising and/or sustained nociceptive stimuli that evoke tonic impulse discharge in C nociceptive afferents. Clearly, the latter are more likely to be relevant to most forms of persistent clinical pain states. Finally, depending on instructions that define the perceptual endpoint, pain thresholds can be obtained separately for sensory (e.g., pricking pain threshold) or affective (e.g., unpleasantness) dimensions of pain (criterion 8) (Blitz & Dinnerstein, 1968; Price, 1999).

Ordinal Rating Scale Methods

Ordinal rating scales are relatively simple and consequently are often used in clinical studies of pain and even in many experimental pain studies. Numbers on ordinal scales refer only to rank ordering and cannot be used to reflect ratios of magnitude (criterion 1). For example, if someone rates his or her pain as an 8 and then later rates it as a 2, one can conclude that the pain has reduced in intensity, but not that it has reduced by 75%. One type of ordinal rating scale is a category scale whose categories clearly denote rank ordering. An example is a scale designed by Melzack and Torgerson (1971) which has five categories: "mild," "discomforting," "distressing," "horrible," and "excruciating." Other ordinal scales are simple numerical scales (e.g., 1–5 or 1–10) that are anchored by descriptors indicative of extremes such as no pain and severe pain. One major advantage of ordinal rating scales is that they can be used to determine quickly whether pain intensity has changed (crite-

rion 6), and so they have relative simplicity (criterion 7). Health care professionals commonly use ordinal scales to assess pain and effects of pain treatments. Both health care professionals and patients easily understand and can respond to a 1–5 pain scale where 5 denotes severe pain. Ordinal scales can be used to quickly assess both experimental and clinical pain (criterion 4), and they are reliable and generalizable (criterion 5). Similar to VASs, they can be adapted to assess both sensory-intensive and affective dimensions of pain (criterion 8) (Price & Harkins, 1987; Price, Harkins, & Baker, 1987; Price, Long, & Harkins 1994).

Unfortunately, ordinal scales have methodological problems, and they are widely misused and misinterpreted by both health care professionals and researchers. One problem is that when pain intensity is classified into categories of scales, the category boundaries are not known, and the assignment of equal numerical intervals between the categories is often assumed without supportive evidence. For example, assigning numbers 1–5 to the categories of the scale devised by Melzack and Torgerson (1971) (described above) would not necessarily provide information about ratios or proportions of pain intensity. The numbers would only provide information about rank order, and any data collected through the use of such scales should be analyzed with nonparametric statistics. This requirement is especially essential in view of Heft and Parker's (1984) demonstration that category boundaries of pain category scales are not equally spaced.

Direct Magnitude Scaling Methods

Direct magnitude scaling techniques rely on the capacity of human observers to represent the perceived intensity of one type of sensation by making responses on another physical continuum. For example, patients can adjust a sound intensity to represent perceived intensity of a pain sensation. An unlimited number of sound intensities can be used to represent pain intensity. Similarly, patients can use a relatively unlimited number of line lengths or distances along a VAS to quickly represent their pain intensity.

With the development of psychophysical techniques of cross-modality matching and other direct scaling procedures, it has become apparent that one given kind of sensory continuum can be matched to another sensory continuum and to numbers. For example, perceived length is a precisely linear function of actual length and numerical ratings of length are also precisely linear. Power function exponents for both perceived length and perceived numerical extent are 1.0. This means very simply, for example, that people numerical rate 6 feet and 3 feet in such a manner that the ratings have a ratio of 2:1, regardless of whether a given individual uses a 0–10 scale or a 0–100 scale. This potential for matching perceived numerical extent to perceived length and vice versa is critical for both validating the power functions that relate perceived magnitudes to stimulus intensity (Marks, 1974; Stevens, 1975) and to the development of ratio scales. Ratio scales have true zero points, and magnitudes along ratio scales reflect true proportions or ratios. A ratio scale is a type of scale most useful to science. Since measurement on a ratio scale is the first criterion for ideal pain measurement on the list given above, and since direct scaling techniques have the potential for producing ratio scales, methods for direct scaling of pain require careful consideration.

An example of a pain scale that at least approximates a ratio scale level of measurement is the VAS. VASs have become extremely popular in pain research and in clinical pain assessment, partly as a result of this property and the fact that they are relatively simple to use (criterion 7). A critical test of whether a VAS has ratio scale properties is to have subjects rate different intensities of painful stimuli and then have them adjust different stimulus intensities to reflect ratios of intensity (Price, McGrath, Rafii, & Buckingham, 1983; Price et al., 1994). The ratings of painful stimuli and the independent judgments of ratios should be in quantitative agreement if the rating method represents a ratio scale. In one study, subject ratings of 5-second nociceptive temperature stimuli provided a stimulus–response curve, as shown in Figure 4.1 (top). After this stimulus–response curve was obtained, the same individuals were given a standard test stimulus (i.e., 47°C) after which they chose a stimulus intensity that was perceived as *twice as intense* as this standard. According to the stimulus–response regression curve, one would predict that they would choose 49.8°C as the stimulus perceived as twice as intense as 47°C. The mean temperature chosen as twice as intense as the 47°C standard was 49.6°C—a value in nearly precise agreement with that predicted from VAS ratings of a broad range of stimulus temperatures (Figure 4.1, top). This same test was replicated using other standard temperatures within the nociceptive range. Of further importance was the

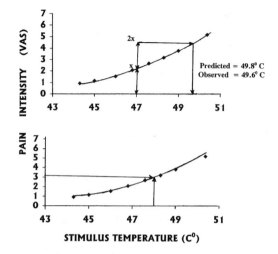

FIGURE 4.1. *Top*: Temperature stimulus–VAS rating function predicts separate judgments of ratios of stimulus intensity. The regression line was derived in double logarithmic coordinates and is displayed here in linear coordinates. The vertical arrows intersecting the functions represent the standard temperature (47°C), and the temperature predicted from the function as twice as intense as the standard. The predicted temperature is 49.8°C, and the average temperature actually chosen by subjects was 49.6°C. It closely corresponds to the VAS rating function. The data are from Price et al. (1994).

Bottom: The triangulation procedure carried out for 10 patients with chronic pain. The intersection (i.e., the "match point") of the mean temperature match (vertical arrow) and mean VAS rating of clinical pain (horizontal arrow) occurs on the temperature stimulus–pain VAS rating curve. The consistency of these three responses demonstrates that the VAS is an internally consistent measure of clinical and experimental pain.

simultaneous demonstration that a 0–10 numerical rating scale, a common type of scale used by health care professionals, did *not* have ratio scale properties.

As mentioned above, numerical scales and some verbal descriptor scales can only measure the rank order of different pain intensities. However, the verbal descriptor scale developed by Gracely, McGrath, and Dubner (1978) may have ratio scale characteristics, because virtually identical nociceptive stimulus–response functions have been shown for both VAS and verbal descriptor scales when used by the same subjects (Duncan, Bushnell, & Levigne, 1989). That people are able to rate pain in a manner that reflects their separate judgments of ratios of perceived intensities indirectly supports the likelihood of a true zero point for the scale. It is also not too much of a stretch of the imagination to think that a pain scale anchored at the low end as "no pain" or "no pain sensation intensity" has a true zero point. If someone were to ask you to rate the pain on your forehead right at this moment, it is very likely that you would mark the left verbal anchor of the VAS, the zero point of the scale. The consistent power functions obtained with VAS scaling of nociceptive stimuli, combined with their capacity to predict ratios of pain intensity simultaneously, demonstrate that the scaling method is relatively bias-free (criterion 2) and at least closely approximates a ratio scale level of measurement (criterion 1).

However, it is important to point out that not all pain VASs are likely to be bias-free or to be ratio scales. Studies that have compared different types of VASs have shown that the sensitivity and reliability of these scales are influenced by the words used to anchor the endpoints, the length of the VASs, and other factors (Seymour, Simpson, Charlton, & Phillips, 1985). Those VASs that most clearly delineate extremes (e.g., "the worst pain," "the most intense pain sensation imaginable") and have sufficient length (≥10 cm) have been shown to have the greatest sensitivity and are the least vulnerable to distortions. In contrast, a VAS anchored on the right with a weak superlative such as "intense pain" or even "maximum pain" is likely to generate pain ratings that are more concentrated toward the right end of the scale rather than being distributed throughout the scale, as in a normal distribution.

When painful contact heat stimuli of varying intensity are randomly applied to the forearm, the stimulus–response functions obtained from VAS ratings and verbal descriptor scaling are found to be power functions with exponents greater than 2.0, as shown in Figure 4.1. These functions have been found to be very similar across diverse groups, despite the fact that the different groups consisted of pain-free participants, patients with low back pain, and patients with myofascial pain dysfunction patients (Price et al., 1983; Price & Harkins, 1987; Price et al., 1994). The same stimulus–response curve was generated within each of these three groups across different times and studies, thereby demonstrating the reliability of the rating method for groups of participants. The reliability and repeatability of individual subjects' VAS ratings are also high. Kiernan, Dane, Phillips, and Price (1995) demonstrated a test–retest reliability of $r = .90$ for participant VAS ratings within an experimental session wherein mean group ratings did

not change across stimulus trials. In that study, pain was evoked by electric shock—a form of stimulation that is optimal for testing the test–retest reliability of a pain scale, because it produces a highly reliable stimulus. Such a highly reliable stimulus does not confound the test of reliability of the pain scale itself. However, even for heat-induced pain tested at weekly intervals, VAS ratings of the same painful skin temperature stimuli (45°, 46°, 47°, 48°, and 49°C) differed by an average of 0.7 to 1.2 VAS units on a 10-unit scale (Rosier, Iadarola, & Coghill, 1999). This level of repeatability is acceptable, considering that sources of variability are likely to include slight variations in stimulus intensity (related to different sites on the forearm) and physiological and/or psychological reasons for actual changes in pain intensity. In support of this interpretation, when the same participants used a VAS to rate grey stimuli (for which stimulus intensity was constant across sessions), an even smaller average difference of about 0.6 VAS unit was obtained. Finally, verbal descriptor scale ratings were found to have statistically larger mean differences across weekly experimental sessions, ranging 1.3 to 1.6 units on a 10-unit scale.

The test–retest reliabilities of VASs used to assess pain-related emotional feelings, also have been shown to be high, with r values ranging from .70 to .90 (Wade, Price, Hamer, Schwartz, & Hart, 1990). These ratings were obtained from patients with clinical pain who were tested over weeks without an intervening treatment. Taken together, these similar stimulus–response functions across groups of patients with pain and pain-free subjects, combined with high reliability and repeatability of individual subjects' ratings, demonstrate the fulfillment of generalizability and reliability of VASs (criterion 5).

It has been shown that patients use verbal descriptor scales (Heft, Gracely, Dubner, & McGrath, 1980) and VASs in a very consistent manner to rate quite different types of pain, including low back myofascial pain, jaw muscle pain, and even experimental pain (Price & Harkins, 1987; Price et al., 1983, 1994). A specific psychophysical procedure has been developed to determine whether patients use verbal descriptor scales or VASs as common psychological scales to rate clinical and experimental pain (Gracely & Dubner, 1981; Heft et al., 1980; Price et al., 1983, 1994), termed the *triangulation procedure*. The procedure tests the internal consistency of three response tasks, as shown in Figure 4.1 (bottom). First, patients make verbal descriptor or VAS ratings of various intensities of painful experimental stimuli, for which a regression line is plotted. Second, they directly match the stimulus intensity of the experimental pain to that of their clinical pain. Third and finally, they make direct verbal descriptor or VAS ratings of their clinical pain. If these three tasks are performed in an internally consistent manner, then the direct stimulus match to clinical pain on the X axis and the direct rating of clinical pain on the Y axis should intersect very close to the regression line of the stimulus intensity–rating scale response function. That such internal consistency has in fact been demonstrated indicates that the specific type of scale in question (e.g., VAS) represents a common psychological scale by which to compare intensities of very different types of pain, including experimental pain.

If different types of patients with pain use a particular rating scale in an internally consistent manner to rate clinical and experimental pain, and if different types of patients and pain-free subjects have the same nociceptive stimulus–pain intensity curve, then this curve can serve as a reference standard. Pain intensities of very different types of clinical and experimental pain can then be compared on a common scale—one that has been demonstrated to approach a ratio scale level of measurement. The significance of a common scale and standard of pain intensity is that it could provide a basis for quantitative comparison of different types of pain and different types of pain-reducing treatments. These comparisons could occur both within and across different studies. Comparisons of magnitudes of pain reduction from different studies are often difficult to make, because different investigators use radically different and usually quite simplistic pain measurement methods such as category scales or other simple ordinal scales.

The direct rating of pain can be a sensitive way of measuring the relative efficacies of different pain treatments if the rating method provides for a broad range of possible pain intensities and if the rating scale is not too constrained by a small number of possible responses. Some verbal descriptor scales and a continuous scale such as a VAS fulfill this criterion because of the large number of possible responses along the scales. However, the empirical demonstration of the sensitivity of a VAS to pain-reducing treatments comes from studies that tested low to moderate doses of opioid analgesics. In one study, low (0.06 mg/kg–0.08 mg/kg) doses

of intravenous morphine produced statistically reliable reductions in VAS ratings of 45°–51°C temperature stimuli (Price, von der Gruen, et al., 1985). In a second similarly designed study in patients with chronic low back pain, low (0.8 mg/kg) to moderate (1.1 mg/kg) doses of fentanyl produced significant reductions in both experimental and clinical pain (Price, Harkins, Rafii, & Price, 1986). The sensory intensities of clinical pain and experimental pain were reduced by an internally consistent amount. Presently, experimental demonstrations of opioid analgesia have moved well beyond the mere establishment of analgesic effects. Demonstrations have been made of dose–response relationships, effects of infusion rates, effects of real or simulated potentiation, influence of central summation mechanisms, and the relationship between subjective report and neurophysiological indices (see Gracely, 1994, for an excellent review). Experimental models of pain-reducing treatments offer considerable promise for testing and screening new analgesic drugs and procedures.

Pain scales can be adapted to measure pain sensation intensity and pain unpleasantness separately (Gracely, 1994; Price, 1999). When subjects are properly instructed and when the two scales have verbal descriptors or verbal anchors that clearly distinguish these pain dimensions, reliably different ratings of nociceptive stimulus temperatures are obtained for pain sensation intensity and pain unpleasantness, as is illustrated in Figure 4.2 (top) on page 60. Mean VAS unpleasantness ratings were found to be significantly lower than mean VAS sensory ratings for each of the five temperatures between 43° and 51°C. In this experiment, the two types of VASs had the same length and differed only in the use of verbal anchor points— for example, "the most intense pain sensation imaginable" and "the most unpleasant imaginable" in the case of the sensory and affective dimensions, respectively. That systematically different mean intensities of pain unpleasantness than of pain sensation intensity occur for the same type of pain provides evidence for the existence of two measurably separate dimensions of pain. The dimensions are separate despite the facts that *both* pain unpleasantness and pain sensation dimensions have precise psychophysical relationships to stimulus intensity, and that both relationships are highly sensitive to small changes in stimulus intensity.

Nevertheless, pain-related sensation and pain-related unpleasantness demonstrate reliably different relationships to nociceptive stimulus intensity. Moerover, pain unpleasantness can be separately influenced by various psychological factors (Gracely, 1979, 1994; Gracely & Dubner, 1981; Gracely et al., 1978; Price, 1999; Price and Harkins, 1987; Price, McHaffie, & Stein, 1992; Price et al., 1983, 1987; Rainville, Carrier, Hofbauer, Bushnell, & Duncan, 1999; Rainville, Duncan, Price, Carrier, & Bushnell, 1997; Rainville, Feine, Bushnell, & Duncan, 1992). Thus the ratios of pain intensity to pain unpleasantness differ systematically for different types of experimental pain (Rainville et al., 1992) and for different types of clinical pain (Price et al., 1987), as shown in Figure 4.2 (top). These systematic differences are not a consequence of instructions, because exactly the same instructions for rating these dimensions are given to all participants within each study. Lower ratings for very brief pain are likely the results of assurances made to participants that the stimuli are to be brief, not damaging to tissue, and within tolerable limits. Very different ratings would probably have been made if these assurances had not been given or if the stimuli had not been so brief. In support of this latter possibility, Rainville et al. (1992) showed that ratios of affective to sensory ratings of brief experimental pain stimuli (electric shock, 5-second heat pulses) were systematically less than 1.0, whereas those of long duration pain stimuli (ischemia, cold pressor) were 1.0 or greater. Thus systematic differences in ratios of affective to sensory ratings of nociceptive stimulus intensity occur as a predicted consequence of simple factors, such as stimulus duration and presence or absence of assurances. These differences constitute one line of evidence for measurably separate dimensions of pain sensation and pain affect.

STAGES OF PAIN-RELATED AFFECT AND THEIR MEASUREMENT

The division of pain into sensory and affective dimensions, though critically important in many experimental and clinical contexts, is somewhat overly simplistic because the affective dimension of pain consists of multiple stages or levels of processing. We suggest that successful measurement of these stages is a final criterion (9) for ideal pain measurement. The rationale for its inclusion requires considerable explanation, which is presented in this section. First of all, the affective dimension of pain is the end product of multiple contributing processes, including the pain sensation itself, arousal, autonomic and somatomotor activation, and (finally and most critically) cognitive appraisals or meanings. It is

readily apparent from reflection about the experience of pain itself that there are two quite different stages of the affective dimension of pain (Figure 4.3 on page 62). The first stage is related to immediate first-order appraisals associated with the sensory features of the pain, with autonomic and somatomotor activation, and with perception of the immediate context in which pain is present. The second stage is fueled by the first stage and yet is additionally related to reflection about the *longer-term implications* of having a persistent pain condition. Support for the multistage model of pain processing shown in Figure 4.3 is provided by considering the psychological nature of pain affect and by reviewing psychological studies of experimental and clinical pain. Finally, the implications of this view for clinical pain assessment are discussed.

The Psychological Nature of Affect

Prior to discussing the stages of the affective dimension of pain, we must briefly consider the psychological nature of emotions in order to understand how pain-related affect fits into the larger schema of pain experience. As Buytendyck (1961) has pointed out, an adequate theory of pain requires an adequate theory of emotions in general. Therefore, we first consider current theories of emotions and the roles of arousal, bodily responses, and cognitive evaluation in human emotions. Our subsequent discussion focuses on how pain-related emotional feelings can be explained in terms of what is known about general mechanisms of emotions.

Modern Views of Emotion Mechanisms

Damasio (1994) provides a modern view of emotional feelings that takes into account classical theories of emotions but extends them by more precise explanation of the interrelationships between cognition and profiles of psychophysiological responses. According to his view, an emotional feeling requires that neural signals from viscera, muscles, joints, and neurotransmitter nuclei, all of which are activated during the process of an emotion, reach certain subcortical nuclei and the cerebral cortex. Endocrine and other chemical signals are said to be additional inputs to the central nervous system via the bloodstream and other routes. Thus the felt changes in the body produced by these means accompany specific thoughts or meanings.

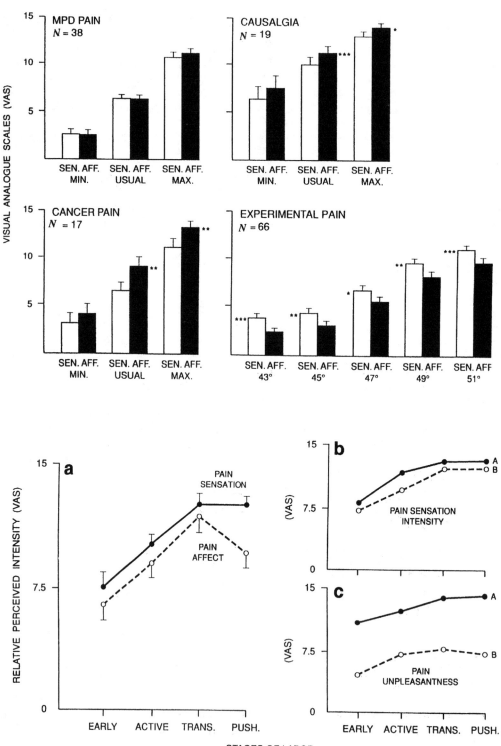

For Damasio, "the essence of feeling an emotion is the experience of such changes in juxtaposition to the mental images that initiated the cycle" (p. 145). In his view, emotional feelings derive from somatic representations of the self and the body. In subsequent work, Damasio (1999) relates body representations to emotions and to two kinds of consciousness. The first kind of consciousness is termed *core consciousness*. It can be conceptualized as the moment by moment awareness of the state of the body and self and the perceptual aspects of what it taking place in the present. The other kind of consciousness is *extended consciousness*, and it is largely autobiographical. It is based on extended awareness of the past and the future, and it links present perceptions to memories and reflections. It is sustained by core consciousness. Different emotional feeling states reflect these two kinds of consciousness to some extent, and they provide the felt sense of meanings, particularly as they relate to what is desired and expected by the organism.

A Concept and Definition of Emotions

Emotions require both cognitive appraisals and physiological activation in an interdependent manner. Cognitive appraisals, in turn, are often comprised of two general dimensions—significance or desire, and expectation or level of perceived fulfillment. As Arnold (1970) has pointed out, emotionally related significance or desire is often in relationship to something "good for me" or "bad for me"—that is, as something to be approached or avoided. Profiles of bodily states during emotions reflect these factors. For example, the feeling of unlikely fulfillment of a desire may be accompanied by felt body tension if one focuses on the intention to remove the obstacle to fulfillment. Similarly, feelings of weakness or heaviness accompany the meaning of hopelessness of acting on one's desires during episodes of depression. The *extent* of physiological arousal will generally increase with significance or desire. The *pattern* of physiological response is codetermined by the nature of one's intentions, attitudes, and expectations of fulfillment. For example, an intense emotional feeling of frustration may arise when a patient with chronic pain experiences a low expectation of being able to carry out an important physical task. The felt sense of this frustration is one of bodily tension accompanied by an urge to remove the source of the interruption. The patterns of physiological arousal, including both autonomic and somatomotor activation, help to provide the felt sense of the emotion (Damasio, 1994; Price, 1999; Price, Barrell, & Barrell, 1985). The felt sense of an emotional feeling comes from the body. Thus an emotional feeling is the felt sense of a cognitive appraisal that occurs in relation to something of personal significance, often in relation to desire and expectation. Similar to some classical theories of emotion, modern explanations of emotion mechanisms recognize the interaction between meanings and physiological activation patterns, yet provide a more precise explanation of their interactions.

The Immediate Affective Dimension of Pain

Emotional feelings are integral components of pain experience for two major reasons. The first is related to the fact that qualities of painful sensations are distinctive in that they dispose us to perceive

---

FIGURE 4.2. *Top:* VAS sensory (white bars) and VAS affective (black bars) ratings (and 1 *SEM*) for three types of clinical and one type of experimental pain. VAS ratings of patients with chronic pain were obtained at minimum (MIN.), usual (USUAL), and maximum (MAX.) levels experienced during the week prior to their clinical visit. VAS affective and VAS sensory ratings were compared using paired *t*-tests (*$p < .05$, **$p < .02$, ***$p < .001$). Asterisks to the right of the black bars indicate higher affective ratings, and asterisks to the left of the white bars indicate higher sensory ratings. MPD, myofascial pain dysfunction. Adapted from *Pain, 28,* D. D. Price, S. W. Harkins, and C. Baker, Sensory–affective relationships among different types of clinical and experimental pain, 297–307. Copyright 1987, with permission from Elsevier Science.
Bottom: (a) Mean VAS sensory and VAS affective ratings of pain of 23 patients in labor at various phases of labor (vertical lines are standard errors). (b) VAS sensory ratings of women who focused mainly on pain or avoiding pain (group A) compared to women who focused mainly on the impending birth (group B). Note that both groups gave very similar VAS sensory ratings. (c) VAS affective ratings of groups A and B. Note that VAS affective ratings of group B are approximately one-half those of group A. Adapted from *Pain, 28,* D. D. Price, S. W. Harkins, and C. Baker, Sensory–affective relationships among different types of clinical and experimental pain, 297–307. Copyright 1987, with permission from Elsevier Science.

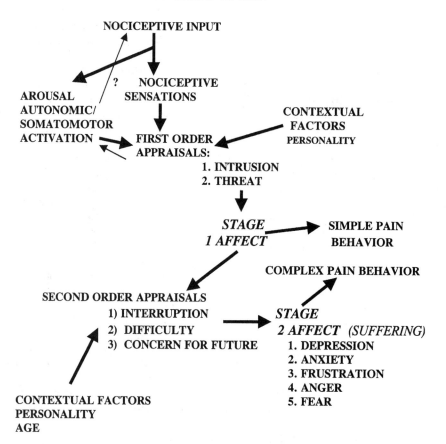

FIGURE 4.3. A schematic used to illustrate interactions between different dimensions and stages of pain.

them as unpleasant. Thus, similar to states of nausea and dizziness, the sensory features of pain dispose us to experience them as unpleasant. Experiencing them as unpleasant, in turn, disposes us to engage in behaviors that seek to avoid or escape the pain-evoking stimulus or conditions. One component of immediate pain affect is the unpleasantness associated with somatosensory components of pain. A second reason why pain is unpleasant is that it is often threatening for reasons other than the pain sensation itself. For example, pain may be part of an integrated perception, as in the case of acute trauma wherein the person perceives the cause or the potential cause of tissue injury. Pain is immediately unpleasant partly as a consequence of the sensory qualities of pain, and partly because the overall integrated perception of pain involves the sense of harm or threat. Both of these components of pain unpleasantness are often accompanied by *desires* to terminate, reduce, or escape pain, as well as *expectations* as to what behaviors are

necessary to do so. For these reasons, pain experiences can contain a large variety of unpleasant emotional feelings about what is going on in the present. These feelings are about the pain sensations and the contexts in which they occur. The *immediate* affective dimension of pain is a stage consisting of the moment-by-moment unpleasantness of pain, as well as other emotional feelings that pertain to the present or short-term future, such as distress, annoyance, or fear. The immediate affective stage of pain is often closely linked with the intensity of the painful sensation and its accompanying arousal. The causal interactions between pain sensation and pain unpleasantness can be both immediate and cumulative over time. Thus, enduring a pain for a few moments may be unpleasant because of the qualities of the sensation and the experienced arousal, somatomotor (e.g., startle, withdrawal), and autonomic responses associated with an acute pain. However, the pain may be even more unpleasant if one has to endure it for several hours, despite the fact that arousal, autonomic, and somato-motor responses have subsided to some extent.

Aside from the qualities of painful sensation, other psychological and physiological components may contribute to pain unpleasantness. These include components associated with coping with or attempting to reduce, escape, or deny the pain. Several additional psychophysiological components can be a part of immediate pain affect. These include arousal, an immediate shift of attention to the bodily area of concern, motoric orientation to this area, and autonomic responses. It is important to point out that to the extent one experiences one's own arousal, changes in attention, autonomic reactions, and motoric orientation in response to a nociceptive stimulus, these processes may be integral to one's affective reactions during pain. Indeed, just as multiple exteroceptive stimuli (sight, sound) can be integrated into the overall perception of bodily threat, interoceptive inputs related to autonomic and somatomotor responses can also influence this perception. For example, Barrell and Price (1975) found that the unpleasantness of painful electrical shock depended not only on the intensity of the evoked sensation, but also on the unpleasantness of experiencing ones own startle response. The magnitude of both startle and unpleasantness were, in turn, largely determined by the psychological set at the time of stimulus presentation. The point here is that even the *immediate* affective dimension of pain may be synthesized from nociceptive and other exteroceptive (e.g., sight, sound) and interoceptive (e.g., startle, increased autonomic nervous system evoked activity) sensory processes. Pain sensation may be a salient but not sole determinant of the affective state during pain. Thus, consistent with modern views of mechanisms of emotional feelings formulated by Damasio (1994, 1999), Arnold (1970), and Price, Barrell, and Barrell (1985), the emotional state that accompanies the immediate unpleasantness of pain represents a synthesis from several psychophysiological sources. These include pain sensation, arousal, autonomic, neuroendocrine, and somatomotor responses, all in relationship to meanings of the pain and to the context in which pain presents itself.

The first stage of pain affect, immediate pain unpleasantness, is about what is going on in the present and is sustained by Damasio's *core consciousness* as described above. Evidence is now presented for the separate contributions of nociceptive sensations and cognitive processes to immediate pain unpleasantness.

The Contribution of Nociceptive Sensations to Pain Unpleasantness

Pain-related sensations may not only be intense and persisting, but can be perceived as spreading, penetrating, and sometimes summating. They are experienced as an invasion of both the body and consciousness because their intensity and qualities are perceived as intense and/or penetrating (Bakan, 1968; Buytendyck, 1961). Therefore, a frequent meaning given to painful sensations is that of *intrusion*, a meaning that requires little reflection and occurs somewhat though not entirely automatically. It is the meaning conveyed by someone who says, "It bothers me because it hurts!" Similar to states of nausea, dizziness, intense thirst, and intense hunger, part of the affective dimension of pain is closely linked to the nature of the sensations themselves. This being the case, both neural and psychological processes related to pain-related sensation can be conceived as important causal links in the production of pain-related emotional disturbance. The qualities and intensities of pain sensations themselves dispose us to perceive them as immediately unpleasant under most conditions. The painful sensation of a bee sting, for example, is unpleasant partly because it is experienced as an intense, sharply penetrating, and spatially spreading sensation. Its persistence over time results in increased unpleasantness. Thus sensations evoked by nociceptive stimuli are among the immediate causes of pain-related emotional feelings, in the same way that sensations of dizziness or nausea are direct causes of unpleasant affective states.

A study by Rainville and colleagues (1999) helps to further establish the direction of causation between pain sensation intensity and immediate pain unpleasantness. The study was a hypnotic analgesia experiment in which pain was induced in subjects by immersing their left hands in a moderately painful water bath heated to 47°C. Two types of experiments were compared. In the first, hypnotic suggestions were targeted specifically toward enhancing or decreasing pain unpleasantness. In the second, the hypnotic suggestions were targeted specifically toward enhancing or decreasing pain sensation intensity. Pain unpleasantness ratings, but not pain sensation intensity ratings, were changed in the directions suggested in the first experiment—an effect consistent with the view that pain affect is the result rather than the cause of pain sensation. However, both pain sensation intensity and pain unpleasantness ratings changed in parallel in the second experiment, despite the fact that the suggestions *did not mention pain unpleasantness*. The combination of these results helps to establish the direction of causation: Pain sensation is one of the immediate causes of pain unpleasantness, and not vice versa.

The Contribution of Cognitive Evaluation to Immediate Pain Unpleasantness

Part of the confusion about pain as having two separate dimensions, sensory and affective, may stem from the fact that pain-related sensation intensity and pain unpleasantness are often closely linked under controlled laboratory conditions. In fact, both dimensions bear strong psychophysical relationships to nociceptive stimulus intensity. Both dimensions are very sensitive to small stimulus intensity differences, and both show power function relationships. However, pain unpleasantness can be powerfully and selectively modulated by psychological manipulations (such as hypnotic suggestions) or by contextual factors (such as the degree of threat that is present within the experimental setting). Common to all instances of pain-related affect is the perception of threat, either to one's body or to one's consciousness or both. As pointed out above, the immediate emotional disturbance associated with an acute pain episode is often part of a more integrated perception of threat, which is accompanied by a desire to eliminate the source of pain and expectations as to how this can be done. As such, one would expect that the intensity of immediate pain unpleasantness could be modulated by cognitive factors, such as expectations.

In addition to the component of pain unpleasantness that is closely linked to sensations of pain, another component of pain unpleasantness relates to one's immediate desire to terminate the pain, as well as expectations about what actions to take to do so. This requires cognitive appraisals of the meanings of the pain in relation to one's overall context. It can include resistance to the pain itself and efforts to cope with, deny, or avoid the pain-evoking situation. As Levine (1979) has pointed out, much of what we consider pain is our resistance to this phenomenon. And often the resistance is more unpleasant than that of the original sensation. In the same way, when we experience tiredness, boredom, or fear, part of what we experience is our resistance to these states. Thus a second component of immediate pain unpleasantness is related to evaluation of its immediate impact on our body and state of mind.

The Influence of Expectancy on the Affective Dimension of Experimental Pain

Evidence that desires and expectations are integral components of pain experience comes from studies of experimental pain wherein manipulations are explicitly directed toward changing expectation. In one such study, a psychophysical analysis was made of experiential factors that influence the affective but not sensory-discriminative dimension of heat-induced pain (Price, Barrell, & Gracely, 1980). Trained participants made cross-modality matching judgments of both pain sensation intensity and unpleasantness. Non-noxious (35°–42°C) and noxious (45°–51°C) skin temperature stimuli (5-second duration) were randomly interspersed during each experimental session. Changes in expectation of receiving painful stimulation were induced by preceding one-half of all the noxious stimuli by a warning signal. The mean responses of these participants clearly indicated that noxious temperatures were experienced as less unpleasant when preceded by a warning signal. In contrast, pain sensation magnitudes, evoked by the same stimulus temperatures, were completely unaffected by the warning signal. Moreover, the selective lowering of pain unpleasantness by the warning signal was greatest toward the lowest end of the noxious temperature range (i.e., 45°C) and was minimal or ineffective at the highest end of the stimulus range (i.e., 51°C). Apparently, subjects prefer knowing that the next stimulus will be painful, as compared to being taken by surprise. The uncertainty of knowing whether the next stimulus will be painful, is likely to produce anxiety. However, if the intensity of stimulation is high (i.e., 51°C), then it makes little difference whether or not someone is warned.

This interpretation of the antianxiety effects of a warning signal is supported by other experiments that reduce anxiety associated with experimental pain, either via an antianxiety drug or via placebo saline. Gracely and colleagues (1978) demonstrated that 5 mg of intravenous diazepam, a common tranquilizer, significantly reduced affective descriptor responses to painful electrocutaneous shock without altering sensory descriptor responses. Similar to the expectancy manipulation of providing a warning signal, the reductions were greatest for low-intensity noxious stimuli. In another study by Gracely (1979), a very similar pattern was found for intravenous saline placebo injection. The results of all of these studies can be parsimoniously explained as a selective lowering of pain unpleasantness by reduction in anxiety. Part of pain unpleasantness is the anxiety associated with anticipating and receiving a noxious stimulus. Anxiety represents a state of wanting to avoid negative consequences combined with an experienced uncertainty of avoiding them (Price, Barrell, & Barrell, 1985). Regardless of whether anxiety is reduced by a drug or by a cognitive manipulation that modifies expectation, the result is that of selectively reducing pain unpleasantness, with the largest effects occurring for mildly painful intensities.

Expectations about the qualitative nature of pain sensations also have been shown to selectively influence pain affect. Johnson (1973) found that subjects who received a description of the painful sensations produced by ischemia of the forearm had lowered levels of distress compared to subjects who only received a description of the procedure. As in the Price and colleagues (1980) study, pain sensation intensities were unaffected by this difference in description. Thus it is apparent that different kinds of expectations—either about the time of occurrence of pain or about the types of sensations that will occur—can alter experienced unpleasantness without changing the intensity of experimentally induced painful sensation.

It is also important to recognize that expectancy can modulate pain sensation intensity and unpleasantness under some circumstances. Recent studies have unequivocally demonstrated that nonverbal manipulations of expectancy, such as repeated exposure to a pain-reducing agent, have stronger effects than verbal manipulations of expectancy (Amanzio & Benedetti, 1999; Benedetti, Arduino, & Amanzio, 1999; Montgomery & Kirsch, 1996; Price et al., 1999; Voudouris, Peck, & Coleman, 1990). All of these studies used conditioning trials in which a cream applied to the skin under the guise of a local analgesic was combined with surreptitious lowering of intensity of painful stimulation. Although all of these studies demonstrated placebo analgesic effects after the stimulus intensity was restored to the original baseline value. These placebo analgesic effects were shown in different ways to be mediated by expectancy (Amanzio and Benedetti, 1999; Benedetti et al., 1999; Montgomery & Kirsch, 1996; Price et al., 1999).

In summary, based on consideration of studies of experimental pain, it is apparent that expectations about different aspects of pain and about the contextual conditions in which pain is present influence pain differently. Expectations about when the pain will occur and what it means once it does occur may have relatively selective effects on the immediate unpleasantness of pain. However, strong manipulations designed to modulate expectations about pain sensation intensity can have at least a modest influence on perceived pain intensity. Thus, among the numerous cognitive factors that can modulate pain unpleasantness, different types of expectation appear to have reliable and systematic influences.

The Influence of Cognitive Factors on the Immediate Unpleasantness of Clinical Pain

In general, the factors of desire for relief and expectation would appear to have a greater influence on pain-related affect in the case of clinical pain, because the implications of having clinical pain in general are likely to be perceived as more openended and threatening than those of experimental pain. Unfortunately, there have been few explicit attempts to directly assess the role of expectancy in clinical pain. Nevertheless, such a role is strongly supported by at least indirect evidence largely consistent with the idea that a significant component of clinical pain affect is that of anxiety. Thus one study hypothesized that affective ratings of clinical pain would be higher in patients whose pain was likely to be associated with a serious threat to health or life, in comparison to patients whose pain was likely to be less threatening (Price et al., 1987). Patients with cancer pain and patients with labor pain were chosen as representative of the former and latter, respectively. As a corollary to this hypothesis, it was proposed that women in labor who focused mainly on the birth of their children would have lower ratings of pain unpleasantness than women who focused mainly on pain or on avoiding pain. Sensory and unpleasantness ratings of experimental pain were also compared to those of various types of clinical pain.

Patients with labor pain and those with cancer pain used separate VASs to rate their levels of pain sensation intensity and degree of unpleasantness that occurred at different times during their clinical condition. Patients with cancer pain were distinguished by the fact that their VAS unpleasantness ratings were higher than their VAS sensory ratings, whereas the reverse was true for patients with labor pain, as shown in Figure 4.2. Furthermore, significant differences in pain VAS affect ratings were observed among patients with labor pain as a function of whether the patients focused primarily on pain or avoiding pain, as compared to focusing on having their babies. Patients who focused primarily on having their babies rated their experienced magnitude of pain unpleasantness as approximately one-half that of patients who focused primarily on pain or avoiding pain (Figure 4.2, bottom, c). This difference occurred for each stage of labor. In contrast, no significant differences in mean VAS pain sensory ratings occurred between these two groups of patients at any stage of labor (Figure 4.2, bottom upper right, b).

The combination of all these results indirectly indicates that a person's goals, desires, and expectations about outcomes strongly influence emotional feelings associated with different clinical pain conditions. The influence of these factors is most apparent when divergent psychological orientations exist within a clinical pain condition. Thus the unpleasantness brought about by the immediate implications of cancer pain, including the reminder that pain sensation is a signal for the presence of a progressive disease, appears to add to that which is directly related to the pain sensations. One of the implications of having labor pain, on other hand, is that birth of a baby is imminent. The positive emotional consequence of this implication appears to offset to some degree the unpleasantness of labor pain. This interpretation is further supported by the much greater degree of labor pain unpleasantness among women who focus on avoiding pain as compared to those who focus on the birth of their babies. Part of what constitutes pain unpleasantness is the *immediate* implication of the pain condition. The implication, in turn, is related to a goal, a desire, and an expectation associated with that goal.

Results obtained in studies of experimental and clinical pain demonstrate that cognitive evaluations can selectively and sometimes powerfully modulate the immediate unpleasantness of pain. Some of these manipulations can be quite simple, such as stimulus duration or the presence or absence of a warning signal. Others may be much more complex and relate to the context and meanings associated with pain, such as experiencing pain as meaning that childbirth is imminent or that tissue damage has occurred.

The Secondary Stage of Pain Affect

Like many types of biological threat, pain sometimes contains both immediate and long-term implications. Cognitive appraisals of these implications constitute the link between the sensory features of pain and emotional feelings and their expressions. Cognitive appraisals, in turn, are often

associated with specific and complex desires and expectations, and therefore with complex emotional feelings. An understanding of these feelings must take into account the meanings that are common to the experience of pain and pain-related suffering.

Both empirical studies of experiential factors of pain and consideration of the experience of pain itself indicate that there are two stages of pain-related emotional feeling (Price, 1999; Wade, Dougherty, Archer, & Price, 1996). A sequential processing model of pain proposes two stages of pain-related affect that are distinguished by the time frame over which cognitive appraisals are directed. These stages and their interrelationships with nociception, arousal, and cognitive appraisals are illustrated schematically in Figure 4.3. The first, discussed already, is the *immediate* affective stage, consisting of the moment-by-moment unpleasantness, distress, and possible annoyance that is often closely linked with the intensity of the painful sensation and its accompanying arousal. The *secondary* stage of pain-related affect is based on more elaborate reflection and is related to that which one remembers or imagines. These involve meanings directed toward the long-term implications of having pain. These meanings are related to perceptions of how pain has interfered or will interfere with different aspects of one's life, reflections on how difficult it is or has been to endure the pain over time, and concern for the long-term future consequences of having pain. Persistent pain can be experienced as a serious threat to one's freedom, to the significance of one's life, and ultimately to one's self-esteem (Bakan, 1968; Buytendyck, 1961). Whereas the immediate affective stage is based on the present and short-term future, the secondary stage is based on the past and long-term future. Thus one may be fearful, anxious, or annoyed about the short-term implications of having pain, or chronically anxious or depressed about the long-term implications. Pain is often experienced not only as an immediate threat to one's body, comfort, or activity, but also to one's well-being and life in general. Therefore, the cognitions and accompanying negative emotions related to the meanings of how pain influences one's life activities and future are what constitute much of the second stage of pain-related affect—a stage that may be thought of as *suffering*. The secondary stage of pain affect is related to Damasio's concept of *extended consciousness*, as described above. It is largely autobiographical and is concerned with memories and reflections that sustain the identity of the individual—one that includes a sense of one's history and self. As the term implies, extended consciousness is directed toward the long-term past and long-term future.

A psychological distinction that helps further clarify the two stages of pain affect is that of *state* and *trait* manifestations of emotions—anxiety, for example. Whereas state anxiety is the anxiety someone is feeling in the moment, trait anxiety refers to a person's general disposition to feel anxious or to have anxious feelings about one's life in general. Similarly, whereas immediate pain unpleasantness contains those negative affective feelings associated with pain in the present or immediate future, secondary pain-related affect contains those feelings about pain as they relate to the long-term future or to one's life in general.

The sequential processing model of pain indicates that immediate pain unpleasantness is the proximate cause of the secondary stage of pain affect (see Figure 4.3). To use spatial metaphors of "vertical" and "horizontal" causation, pain unpleasantness causes secondary pain affect in two ways. It causes secondary pain affect because over an extended period of time (days, weeks, or months), pain unpleasantness provokes reflection and meanings related to suffering; that is, the causal interaction is horizontal. Most brief acute pains and almost all experimentally evoked pains contain only the sensory discriminative and the immediate unpleasantness stages of pain, because time is required for the development of more complex meanings and future implications. However, pain unpleasantness can also serve as an immediate cue for the meanings related to the secondary stage of pain affect once these meanings have been established over time. That is, it can act "vertically" as well. The sudden exacerbation of pain intensity in a patient with low back pain can serve as an instant reminder of how long he or she has had to endure the interruption of normal life activities and the unlikely prospects of relief in the future. The secondary stage of pain affect is often a component of pain experience itself. Thus, for our patient with low back pain, the experience of the pain sensations, immediate unpleasantness, and meanings and emotions of suffering can exist simultaneously as a coherent integrated structure.

The second stage of pain-related affect is based on three potential meanings (Buytendyck, 1962; Price, 1999). The first is that the painful condition has and will continue to interrupt ones ability to live, such as ones ability to function or to live a meaningful life. The second is that the painful condition and its accompanying domination of consciousness constitute a burden that one

has endured over a long time. Finally, the condition of persistent pain may mean that something permanently harmful might happen or has happened.

The meaning of intrusion during immediate pain unpleasantness and the meanings of life interruption, enduring anxiety, and concern for the future in the second stage of pain affect are directed toward the painful sensations, the context in which they occur, and the implications of avoiding harm. Each of these meanings, in turn, is easily related to a desire to avoid or remove the interruption, burden, or negative future consequences. Numerous contextual factors that relate to information about the nature of the painful condition and about potential means of avoiding or reducing the pain and its associated negative consequences converge to determine one's level of expectation that pain and its associated negative consequences will or can be reduced. As such, emotional feelings associated with the first and second stages of pain-related affect may be determined to an extent by desires and expectations, in the same way that many common human emotions are determined by these two factors (Price, Barrell, & Barrell, 1985). The following discussion provides empirical support for the construct of the secondary stage of pain affect and for the types of negative emotional feelings that constitute this stage of pain processing.

Measurement of the Second Stage of Pain Affect

Since the number and types of cognitive appraisals during pain are a function of both the intensity of the painful sensation and several psychological contextual factors, it is not surprising that the number and types of negative emotional feelings experienced during pain are also diverse. Thus patients in pain may feel anxiety, frustration, depression, anger, despair, or fear to different degrees, depending on the nature of the appraisals and the time frame toward which they are directed. The prevalence and relative magnitudes of these emotional feelings are illustrated for patients with different types of pain in Figure 4.4 (Price, 1988). Patients were instructed to rate these feelings as they specifically pertained to their chronic pain and not to problems unrelated to their pain. Moreover, except for patients with labor pain, they were asked to rate how strong these feelings had been over the previous week, approximately analogous to a "trait"

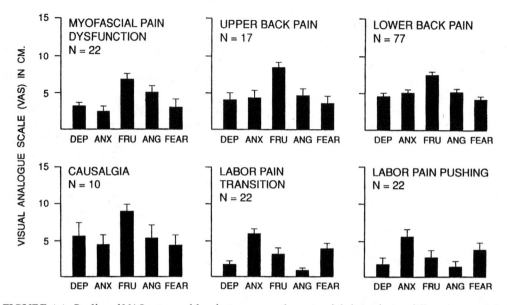

FIGURE 4.4. Profiles of VAS ratings of five distinct types of emotional feelings during different types of clinical pain. Adapted from Price, D. D. (1988). *Psychological and neural mechanisms of pain.* New York: Raven Press. Copyright 1988 by Raven Press, Ltd. Reprinted by permission of Lippincott Williams & Wilkins.

assessment of these emotional feelings. Whereas chronic frustration was the predominant emotional feeling of patients with musculoskeletal types of pain, *both* depression and frustration were predominant feelings of patients with complex regional pain syndrome. Anxiety and fear were found to be the most common negative feelings of patients with labor pain. In addition, these emotions in patients with labor pain were more reflective of immediate pain affect because they pertained to how they were feeling at the time (i.e. a "state" assessment). Importantly, all five emotional feelings were present in patients with different types of pain, to varying degrees.

The secondary stage of pain processing has been assessed by administering a VAS for each of the five pain-related negative emotions (see Figure 4.4) and for cognitive factors that are likely to mediate these emotions (Bush, Harkins, Harrington, & Price, 1993; Harkins, Price, & Braith, 1989; Wade et al., 1990, 1992, 1996). The combined ratings of these five emotions and ratings of interruption, difficulty of enduring the pain, and concern for future consequences have been shown to represent a psychological stage that is unique and separate from that of immediate pain unpleasantness (Harkins et al., 1989; Wade et al., 1990, 1996; Wade, Dougherty, Hart, & Price, 1992). The evidence for this separately measurable stage con-

sists of three types of studies. The first showed associations between these VAS measures and other indices of emotional disturbance, such as the Beck Depression Inventory (Wade et al., 1990). The second directly tested the sequential model shown below in Figures 4.5–4.7, using the method of linear structural equation modeling (LISREL) (Wade et al., 1996). The third showed selective effects of personality traits or demographic factors on VAS measures of secondary pain affect (Harkins et al., 1989; Wade et al., 1992).

Testing the Sequential Model with LISREL

One kind of evidence for this sequential model of pain processing comes from multivariate (LISREL) analysis (Wade et al., 1996). Path analysis with patients who had chronic pain demonstrated that VAS could be used to assess pain sensation intensity, pain-related unpleasantness, and pain-related suffering (secondary affect), and that a structured interview could assess pain-related behavior. Pain-related behavior was conceptualized as a final stage of pain processing. This stage reflects the activities of daily living that are influenced by pain (e.g., number of hours spent in bed during the day due to pain). This stage can be evaluated by self-report inventories and by structured observation methods. Both exploratory analysis of data from 506 patients

MODEL 1: $\chi^2(61) = 223.4$; $\chi^2/df = 3.7$

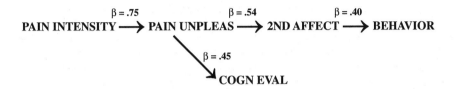

MODEL 2: $\chi^2(61) = 211.7$; $\chi^2/df = 3.5$

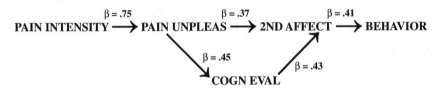

MODEL 3: $\chi^2(60) = 169.3$; $\chi^2/df = 2.8$

FIGURE 4.5. Three alternative LISREL models of pain processing.

and confirmatory analysis of data from a second sample of 502 patients confirmed a high goodness of fit for sequential model 1 in Figure 4.5 (Wade et al., 1996). However, Figure 4.5 is based on the original 1,008 patients originally studied by Wade and colleagues (1996) plus an additional 639 patients. The demographics of these 1,647 patients were very similar to that of the original study. This more recent analysis used the LISREL-8 statistical program (Joreskog & Sorbom, 1993). Both the previous study by Wade and colleagues and this recent analysis support the sequential model originally proposed on the basis of other types of data (Harkins et al., 1989; Price, 1988; Wade et al., 1992). However, Wade and colleagues found that the model's goodness of fit slightly improved when cognitive evaluation was removed from the sequence.

However, there are strong theoretical reasons for including cognitive evaluation as a mediating factor in producing pain-related emotions. Cognitive evaluation as a dimension of pain (e.g., perception of impact of pain on lifestyle) represents a secondary appraisal that could mediate the relationship between pain unpleasantness and secondary pain affect. Such a conceptualization is consistent with cognitive-behavioral models of pain and depression, which suggest that pain unpleasantness should have a significant indirect effect on secondary pain affect through an individual's perception of the impact of pain on his or her lifestyle (Rudy, Kerns, & Turk, 1988).

Thus we compared three alternative models to further clarify the possible mediating role of cognitive evaluation (Figure 4.5). The strongest test of a model is not just that the data support it, but that it fits better than a competing model. A covariance matrix was generated and used to test the path models, and pain duration was used as a control variable. The first two (models 1 and 2) are similar to those compared by Wade and colleagues (1996). As the latter study originally demonstrated, removing cognitive evaluation from the linear sequence (as represented by model 2) increased the goodness of fit beyond that provided by model 1. For this second model, we accepted the assumption that an individual's cognitive evaluation of his or her pain follows from pain unpleasantness and retained this path in the model. However, we did not make the assumption at this point that cognitive evaluation was a mediator. Consequently, we deleted the path from cognitive evaluation to secondary pain affect (Figure 4.5). Leaving cognitive evaluation in the model allowed us to test directly for statistical improvements in model fit. In this way, any change in the chi-square statistic would be a function of changes in the model's paths, not in changes attributable to elimination of measurement error from our measurement of cognitive evaluation. Thus model 2 represents Wade and colleagues' final four-stage model, with cognitive evaluation *not* in the linear sequence, but as a parallel consequence of pain unpleasantness. The goodness of fit improved still further when cognitive evaluation was then specified as a mediator of secondary pain affect and when a parallel alternative path between pain unpleasantness and secondary pain affect was retained, as shown for model 3 (Figure 4.5). The difference in chi-square between models 1 and 3, $\Delta\chi^2$ (1) = 54.12, $p < .05$ and between models 2 and 3, $\Delta\chi^2$ (1) = 42.40, $p < .05$, indicates that model 3 is statistically better than either models 1 or 2.

The differences in chi-square among models 1, 2, and 3 represent statistical tests indicating improvement of fit (Figure 4.5). Importantly, the beta value between cognitive evaluation and secondary pain affect remained significant in the face of adding the direct path between pain unpleasantness and secondary pain affect. Comparison of model 3 to models 1 and 2 shows that the measures of cognitive evaluation used are likely to at least partly mediate the relationship between pain unpleasantness and secondary pain affect. However, this comparison also indirectly suggests that there may exist other mediating cognitive factors that we have not measured, and/or that there are direct influences between pain unpleasantness and secondary pain affect. These possibilities are evident in two ways. First, there is a small reduction in the path coefficient between cognitive evaluation and secondary pain affect, from $\beta = .52$ (model 1) to $\beta = .43$ (model 3), when the direct path between pain unpleasantness and secondary pain affect is included in the model. Second, the direct path from pain unpleasantness to secondary pain affect is also significant ($\beta = .37$). This path could include other contextual factors (e.g., beliefs about the nature of the pain), as well as types of pain coping (e.g., use of social support).

Effects of Extraversion and Neuroticism

A second and more powerful line of evidence supporting this multistage model is the demonstration of *selective* effects of demographic variables (such as age) and personality factors (such as neuroticism) on later stages of pain processing. This type of demonstration is similar in principle to the study by Rainville and colleagues (1999), which found that pain unpleasantness was selectively modulated in one experimental context and passively modulated in parallel with pain intensity in another. Two separate studies have shown that personality traits exert their largest effects on the secondary stage of pain affect. The differential influence of two personality traits, neuroticism and extraversion, on pain sensation intensity (the immediate unpleasantness stage) and the secondary stage of pain-related affect were assessed in a group of patients with myofascial pain dysfunction (Harkins et al., 1989). Eysenck and Eysenck's (1975) personality inventory was used to measure neuroticism and extraversion, and VASs were used to measure the various dimensions and stages of pain. The five pain-related emotion VASs were used as an overall measure of the secondary stage of pain affect. Canonical correlation and multiple-regression methods had previously demonstrated significant associations between the composite of these five VASs and other indices of depression (i.e., Beck Depression Inventory, Minnesota Multiphasic Personality Inventory depression scales). At the same time, this analysis demonstrated that each emotion VAS assessed a unique and separate emotional feeling (Wade et al., 1990). Importantly, it was determined that the emotion VASs were not simply redundant measures of the *immediate* unpleasantness of pain as assessed by the unpleasantness VASs.

Neuroticism is a personality trait characterized by Eysenk (1967) as high emotionality and arousability, as well as a predisposition to engage in maladaptive behaviors and negative emotions. First, neither the personality traits of extraversion nor those of neuroticism had any influence on VAS sensory ratings of experimental heat pain in these patients. Patients with high and low scores on these two personality dimensions had nearly identical nociceptive temperature–VAS sensory rating curves. Second, these high- and low-scoring groups of patients did not significantly differ with respect to their VAS sensory ratings of their clinical pain (Figure 4.6). Therefore, these two personality traits do not appear to influence the first stage of pain,

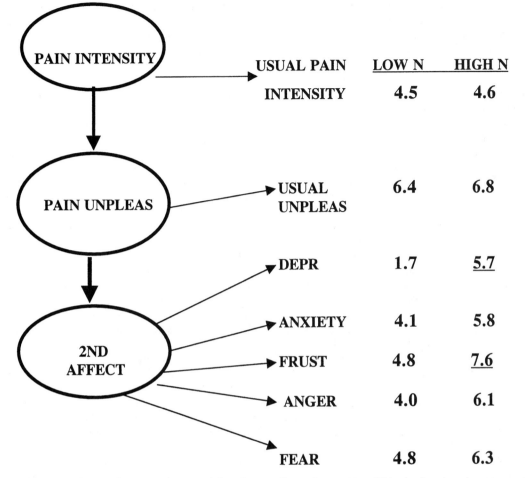

FIGURE 4.6. Stages of pain processing and the selective effects of neuroticism (N in the figure) on later stages of pain. Mean VAS ratings of patients with myofascial pain dysfunction who scored high and low on neuroticism; the ratings were made in response to judgments of magnitudes of pain sensation intensity, pain unpleasantness, depression (Depr), anxiety (Anx), frustration (Frust), anger, and fear. Patients with high neuroticism scores rated depression and frustration higher than did patients with low neuroticism scores. Underlined numbers are significantly different at $p < .05$. The data are from Harkins, Price, and Braith (1989).

sensory discrimination. Third, neuroticism but not extraversion was associated with a modest but statistically significant enhancement of VAS unpleasantness ratings of experimental heat pain as well as their clinical pain (Figure 4.6). Thus neuroticism appears to exert a small but reliable effect on the immediate stage of pain-related affect—an effect that was consistent for *both* experimental and clinical pain.

Finally, it was at the secondary stage of pain-related affect that the personality trait of neuroticism but not extraversion appeared to exert its

largest influences (Figure 4.6). As hypothesized, patients with high neuroticism scores evidenced more intense emotions related to suffering (i.e., depression, frustration, anxiety, etc.) as compared to patients with low neuroticism scores. Extraverts and introverts did not differ in their ratings of these emotions. Precisely the same overall pattern of results was replicated in a study by Wade and colleagues (1992) in which canonical correlation analysis was used to assess the influence of neuroticism and extraversion on these stages of pain in 205 patients with chronic pain. This study differed from that of Harkins and colleagues (1989) in that the NEO Personality Inventory (Costa & McCrae, 1985) was used to assess neuroticism and extraversion, and that the patients had a variety of types of chronic pain. These included low back pain, reflex sympathetic dystrophy, and other types. Despite these differences, the results again clearly demonstrated that neuroticism (and not extraversion) exerted its largest influences not on early stages of pain sensory processing and immediate unpleasantness, but on the secondary stage related to higher order cognitive processes and suffering.

Although several studies (BenDebba, Torgerson, & Long, 1997; Harkins et. al., 1989; Wade et al., 1992) suggest that extraversion is also related to suffering, its relationship is weaker than that of neuroticism. In the Wade and colleagues (1992) study, assertiveness, a facet score of extraversion, was the most important predictor of pain suffering. Both assertiveness and activity level were the only facet scores associated with illness behavior. The relationship between extraversion and behavior is a complicated one. It appears that highly assertive subjects manifested more pain behavior at home and during clinical interviews when they were unobtrusively observed. In contrast, they also reported less lifestyle disruption (i.e., sickness impact) and fewer incidents of solicitous behavior (e.g., receiving less secondary gain from family members). Several reports (Eysenck, 1967; Gordon & Hitchcock, 1983; Harkins et al., 1989) provide support for the finding that extraverts express their suffering more frequently than introverts.

Effects of Age

Studies examining the relationship between age and pain have focused primarily on the first stage of pain processing, pain sensation intensity (see Harkins & Price, 1992, for a review). Although studies using simplistic measures of pain threshold and/or tolerance have yielded somewhat contradictory results, other studies (Harkins, Price, & Martelli, 1986; Harkins, Davis, Bush, & Kasberger, 1996) using direct scaling techniques to evaluate threshold and suprathreshold levels of experimental pain sensitivity demonstrate much stronger similarities than differences in pain sensitivity across the life span. A minor exception is the demonstration of selective reduction of heat-induced "first pain" in the elderly (Harkins et al., 1996).

With the limitations of most previous demographic studies of pain in mind, the extent to which age influenced the magnitude of the various stages of pain processing was examined in 1,712 patients with chronic pain (Riley, Wade, Robinson, & Price, 2000). As shown in Figure 4.7, no effects of age were evident for pain sensation ratings or immediate unpleasantness ratings, consistent with previous results obtained for experimental pain (Harkins et al., 1986). Thus no age effects were observed in the first two stages of pain processing. However, age had large (>1.5 VAS unit) and selective effects on the secondary stage of pain affect and illness behavior, with older patients (>65 years of age) manifesting lower mean ratings of negative emotional feelings as compared to younger patients. Older patients had considerably lower ratings of anxiety, frustration, anger, and fear (Figure 4.7) and significantly lower composite ratings of the five pain-related emotional feelings. Harkins and Price (1992) also observed a large and selective effect of age on the secondary stage of pain affect. The highly selective and relatively potent effect of age on the secondary stage of pain affect may be related to lower lifestyle disruption and less concern for future consequences in the elderly. For example, older patients with pain are less likely to be dealing with concerns such as the interaction of pain with their employment, their children's college tuition, or other midlife issues. Older adults may view pain as having less of a long-term threat, resulting in less suffering. Similar to the studies of personality factors on the stages of pain processing, the selective impact of age on secondary pain affect further validates the sequential model of pain processing by showing a selective impact of a factor on the secondary stage of pain affect.

Personality factors and age have their greatest influence on later stages (suffering and illness behavior) of pain processing. This reinforces the uniqueness of these later-stage pain components and highlights the separateness of these pain dimensions. Although this literature demonstrates an association between measures of normal personality (mainly neuroticism and extraversion) and pain-related suffering, it does not clearly assign a causal relationship between these variables. One possibility is that lifelong depression and enduring anxiety contribute to a pattern of catastrophizing that serves to exacerbate emotional disturbance in patients with chronic pain. An alternate explanation is that increasing lifestyle disruption resulting from pain leads to an intensification of suffering. The latter hypothesis is particularly plausible as an explanation for age effects on secondary pain affect. Thus, although pain sensation and immediate pain unpleasantness may be similar across age

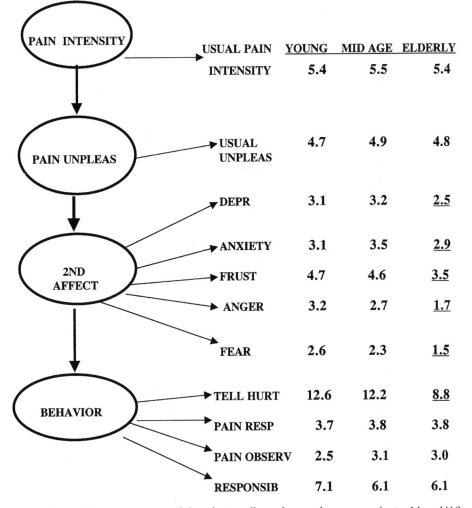

		YOUNG	MID AGE	ELDERLY
PAIN INTENSITY	USUAL PAIN INTENSITY	5.4	5.5	5.4
PAIN UNPLEAS	USUAL UNPLEAS	4.7	4.9	4.8
2ND AFFECT	DEPR	3.1	3.2	<u>2.5</u>
	ANXIETY	3.1	3.5	<u>2.9</u>
	FRUST	4.7	4.6	<u>3.5</u>
	ANGER	3.2	2.7	<u>1.7</u>
	FEAR	2.6	2.3	<u>1.5</u>
BEHAVIOR	TELL HURT	12.6	12.2	<u>8.8</u>
	PAIN RESP	3.7	3.8	3.8
	PAIN OBSERV	2.5	3.1	3.0
	RESPONSIB	7.1	6.1	6.1

FIGURE 4.7. Stages of pain processing and the selective effects of age on later stages of pain. Mean VAS ratings of young (<45 years of age), middle-aged (45–64 years of age), and elderly (65 years and older) patients with pain; the ratings were made in response to judgments of magnitudes of pain sensation intensity, pain unpleasantness, depression (Depr), anxiety (Anx), frustration (Frust), anger, and fear. Elderly patients rated depression, anxiety, and frustration lower than did young or middle-aged patients. Underlined numbers are significantly different at $p < .01$. From Riley et al. (2000). "Tell Hurt" refers to answers to a questionnaire that assesses how others are able to determine whether the patient is in pain (Wade et al., 1996).

groups, less lifestyle disruption and consequently less suffering may occur in the elderly.

Implications of the Sequential Processing Model for Pain Measurement and Assessment

If pain consists of different dimensions and stages of processing, and if there are psychological, pharmacological, and physiological factors that can se-lectively influence a given stage of processing or dimension, then measurement and assessment of pain should ideally address each of these dimensions and stages. For example, just as some personality traits and age strongly and selectively influence the secondary stage of pain affect, so might some psychological therapeutic interventions exert their greatest influence at this level. Multidimensional measurement and assessment are most critical for chronic pain management. If chronic pain is multidimensional and multiple treatments are used in its management, then its assessment likewise needs separate measures of nociception, immediate pain unpleasantness or affective disturbance, emotional feelings reflective of pain-related suffering, and overt pain behavior.

As discussed earlier, patients with cancer pain have been shown to give significantly higher VAS affect ratings of their pain than VAS sensory ratings, whereas the reverse is true for women in labor. Thus simple antinociceptive treatments that are directed mechanistically toward reducing the sensation of pain may not be adequate pain control for some patients with cancer, because any amount of pain may carry a strongly negative implication. Therefore, psychological therapies may be especially important in pain management in such patients. Similarly, personality traits such as neuroticism may operate to enhance the overall sense of hopelessness and anxiety associated with living with chronic pain. In such cases, group therapies and support groups may enable patients to examine and become aware of the processes by which different individuals develop meanings associated with the secondary stage of pain affect. However, even when a strictly antinociceptive treatment is given to a patient with chronic pain, its impact on the several stages of pain processing may vary as a function of several possible intervening psychological factors. Consequently, the assessment of various stages of pain is of paramount importance in patients with chronic pain, even when the treatments given for such pain are directed only toward reducing nociceptive processing. Studies of the secondary stage of pain-related affect can only be carried out in patients with pain, since this stage involves more reflective cognitive processes that occur during suffering. The secondary stage of pain-related affect, which is based on cognitive processes directed toward long-term implications and more elaborate meanings, is of considerable importance for patients with cancer pain and for patients with severe, debilitating chronic pain. Just as there are pharmacological and psychological factors that can reduce pain sensation intensity and immediate pain unpleasantness, so there may be factors that selectively reduce the secondary stage of pain-related affect.

REFERENCES

Amanzio, M., & Benedetti, F. (1999). Neuropharmacological dissection of placebo analgesia: Expectation-activated opioid systems versus conditioning-activated specific subsystems. *Journal of Neuroscience, 19*, 484–494.

Arnold, M. B. (1970). *Feelings and emotions.* New York: Academic Press.

Bakan, D. (1968). *Disease, pain, and sacrifice.* Chicago: University of Chicago Press.

Barrell, J. J., & Price, D. D. (1975). The perception of first and second pain as a function of psychological set. *Perception and Psychophysics, 17*, 163–166.

BenDebba, M., Torgerson, W. S., & Long, D. M. (1997). Personality traits, pain duration and severity, functional impairment, and psychological distress in patients with persistent low back pain. *Pain, 72*, 115–125.

Benedetti, F., Arduino, C., & Amanzio, M. (1999). Somatotopic activation of opioid systems by target-directed expectations of analgesia. *Journal of Neuroscience, 19*(9), 3639–3648.

Bush, F. M., Harkins, S. W., Harrington, W. G., & Price, D. D. (1993). Analysis of gender effects on pain perception and symptom presentation in temporomandibular pain. *Pain, 53*, 73–80.

Buytendyck, F. J. J. (1961). *Pain.* London: Hutchinson.

Blitz, B. & Dinnerstein, A. J. (1968). Effects of different types of instructions on pain parameters. *Journal of Abnormal Psychology, 73*, 276–280.

Costa, P. T., & McCrae, R. R. (1985). *The NEO Personality Inventory Manual.* Odessa, FL: Psychological Assessment Resources.

Damasio, A. (1994). *Descartes' error.* New York: Avon Books.

Damasio, A. (1999). *The feeling of what happens.* New York: Avon Books.

Duncan, G., Bushnell, M. C., & Levigne, G. (1989). Comparison of verbal and visual analogue scales for measuring the intensity and unpleasantness of experimental pain. *Pain, 38*, 295–303.

Eysenck, H. J. (1967). *The biological basis of personality.* Springfield, IL: Charles C Thomas.

Eysenck, H. J., & Eysenck, S. B. G. (1975). *The manual of the Eysenck Personality Questionnaire.* London: Hodder & Stoughton.

Gordon, A., & Hitchcock, E.R. (1983). Illness behaviour and personality in intractable facial pain syndromes. *Pain, 17*(3), 267–276.

Gracely, R. H. (1979). Psychophysical assessment of human pain. In J. J. Bonica, J. C. Liebeskind, & D. G. Albe-Fessard (Eds.), *Advances in pain research and therapy* (Vol. 3, pp. 211–229). New York: Raven Press.

Gracely, R. H. (1994). Studies of pain in normal man. In P. D. Wall & R. Melzack (Eds.), *Textbook of pain* (3rd ed., pp. 315–336). Edinburgh: Churchill-Livingstone.

Gracely, R. H., & Dubner, R. (1981). Pain assessment in humans: A reply to Hall. *Pain, 11*, 109–120.

Gracely, R. H., McGrath, P. A., & Dubner, R. (1978). Validity and sensitivity of ratio scales of sensory and affective verbal pain descriptors: Manipulation of affect by diazepam. *Pain, 5*, 19–29.

Guilford, J. P. (1954). *Psychometric methods,* New York: McGraw-Hill.

Hardy, J. D., Wolff, H. G., & Goodell, H. (1940). Studies on pain. A new method for measuring pain threshold: Observations on spatial summation of pain. *Journal of Clinical Investigations, 19*, 649–657.

Hardy, J. D., Wolff, H. G., & Goodell, H. (1952). *Pain sensations and reactions.* Baltimore: Williams & Wilkins.

Harkins, S. W., Davis, M. D., Bush, F. M., & Kasberger, J. (1996). Suppression of first pain and slow temporal summation of second pain in relation to age. *Journals of Gerontology: Series A. Biological Sciences and Medical Sciences, 51,* 260-265.

Harkins, S. W., & Price, D. D. (1992). Assessment of pain in the elderly. In D. Turk & R. Melzack (Eds.), *Handbook of pain assessment* (pp. 315-331). New York: Guilford Press.

Harkins, S. W., Price, D. D., & Braith, J. (1989). Effects of extraversion and neuroticism on experimental pain, clinical pain, and illness behavior. *Pain, 36,* 209-318.

Harkins, S. W., Price, D. D., & Martelli, M. (1986). Effects of age on pain perception: Thermonociception. *Journal of Gerontology, 41,* 58-63.

Heft, M. W., Gracely, R. H., Dubner, R., & McGrath, P. A. (1980). A validation model for verbal descriptor scaling of human clinical pain. *Pain, 9,* 363-373.

Heft, M. W., & Parker, S. R. (1984). An experimental basis for revising the graphic rating scale for pain. *Pain, 19,* 153-161.

Kiernan, B. D., Dane, J. R., Phillips, L., & Price, D. D. (1995). Hypnotic analgesia reduces R-III nociceptive reflex: Further evidence concerning the multifactorial nature of hypnotic analgesia. *Pain, 60,* 39-47.

Johnson, J. E. (1973). Effects of accurate expectations about sensations on the sensory and distress components of pain. *Journal of Personality and Social Psychology, 27,* 261-275.

Joreskog, K. G., & Sorbom, D. (1993). *LISREL 8: A guide to the program and applications,* Chicago: SPSS.

Levine, S. (1979). *A gradual awakening.* New York: Anchor Press.

Marks, L. W. (1974). *Sensory processes: The new psychophysics.* New York: Academic Press.

Melzack, R., & Torgerson, W. S. (1971). On the language of pain. *Anesthesiology, 34,* 50-59.

Montgomery, G. H., & Kirsch, I. (1996). Classical conditioning and the placebo effect. *Pain, 72,* 103-113.

Price, D. D. (1988). *Psychological and neural mechanisms of pain.* New York: Raven Press.

Price, D. D. (1999). *Psychological mechanisms of pain and analgesia.* Seattle, WA: International Association for the Study of Pain Press.

Price, D. D., Barrell, J. E., & Barrell, J. J. (1985). A quantitative–experiential analysis of human emotions. *Motivation and Emotions, 9,* 19-38.

Price, D. D., Barrell, J. J., & Gracely, R. H. (1980). A psychophysical analysis of experiential factors that selectively influence the affective dimension of pain. *Pain, 8,* 137-179.

Price, D. D., & Harkins, S. W. (1987). The combined use of visual analogue scales and experimental pain in providing standardized assessment of clinical pain. *Clinical Journal of Pain, 3,* 3-11.

Price, D. D., Harkins, S. W., & Baker, C. (1987). Sensory-affective relationships among different types of clinical and experimental pain. *Pain, 28,* 297-307.

Price, D. D., Harkins, S. W., Rafii, A., & Price, C. (1986). A simultaneous comparison of fentanyl's analgesic effects on experimental and clinical pain. *Pain, 24,* 197-203.

Price, D. D., Long, S., & Harkins, S. W. (1994). A comparison of pain measurement characteristics of mechanical visual analogue and simple numerical rating scales of pain. *Pain, 56,* 217-226.

Price, D. D., McGrath, P. A., Rafii, A., & Buckingham, B. (1983). The validation of visual analogue scales as ratio scale measures for chronic and experimental pain. *Pain, 17,* 45-56.

Price, D. D., McHaffie, J. G., & Stein, B. E. (1992). The psychophysical attributes of heat-induced pain and their relationships to neural mechanisms. *Journal of Cognitive Neuroscience, 4,* 1-14.

Price, D. D., Milling, L. S., Kirsch, I., Duff, A., Montgomery, G., & Nicholls, S. S. (1999). An analysis of factors that contribute to the magnitude of placebo analgesia in an experimental paradigm. *Pain, 83,* 147-156.

Price, D. D., von der Gruen, A., Miller, J., Rafii, A., & Price, C. (1985). A psychophysical analysis of morphine analgesia. *Pain, 22,* 320-330.

Rainville, P., Carrier, B., Hofbauer, R. K., Bushnell, M. C., & Duncan, G. H. (1999). Dissociation of sensory and affective dimensions of pain using hypnotic modulation. *Pain, 82,* 159-171.

Rainville, P., Duncan, G. H., Price, D. D., Carrier, B., & Bushnell, M. C. (1997). Pain affect encoded in human anterior cingulate but not somatosensory cortex. *Science, 277,* 968-971.

Rainville, P., Feine, J. S., Bushnell, M. C., & Duncan, G. H. (1992). A psychophysical comparison of sensory and affective responses to four modalities of experimental pain. *Somatosensory and Motor Research, 9,* 265-277.

Riley, J. R. III, Wade, J. B., Robinson, M. E., & Price, D. D. (2000). The stages of pain processing across the adult lifespan. *Journal of Pain, 1(2),* 162-170.

Rosier, E., Iadarola, M., & Coghill, R. C. (1999). Reproducibility of pain measurement and perception. *Abstracts of 18th Annual Meeting of the American Pain Society,* 140.

Rudy, T. E., Kerns, R. D., & Turk, D. C. (1988). Chronic pain and depression: Toward a cognitive-behavioral mediation model. *Pain, 35,* 129-140.

Seymour, R. A., Simpson, J. M., Charlton, J. E., & Phillips, M. E. (1985). An evaluation of length and end-phrase of visual analogue scales in dental pain. *Pain, 21,* 177-186.

Stevens, S. S. (1975). *Psychophysics. Introduction to its perceptual, neural, and social prospects.* New York: Wiley.

Voudouris, N. J., Peck, C. L., & Coleman, G. (1990). The role of conditioning and expectancy in the placebo response. *Pain, 43,* 121-128.

Wade, J. B., Dougherty, L. M., Archer, C. R., & Price, D. D. (1996). Assessing the stages of pain processing: A multivariate analytical approach. *Pain, 68,* 157-167.

Wade, J. B., Dougherty, L. M., Hart, R. P., & Price, D. D. (1992). A canonical correlation analysis of the influence of neuroticism and extroversion on chronic pain, suffering, and pain behavior. *Pain, 51,* 67-74.

Wade, J. B., Price, D. D., Hamer, R. M., Schwartz, S. M., & Hart, R. P. (1990). An emotional component analysis of chronic pain. *Pain, 40,* 303-310.

Chapter 5

Psychophysiological Assessment of the Patient with Chronic Pain

HERTA FLOR

In recent decades, psychophysiological assessment methods have gained importance for both somatic and psychological disorders (Cacioppo, Tassinary, & Berntson, 2000; Turpin, 1989). They are used primarily as tools for determining the influence of psychological factors on bodily functioning, and specifically for assessing their contribution to the initiation and maintenance of symptoms. In many chronic pain syndromes, psychophysiological factors play a major role in the development and/or maintenance of the problems (see, e.g., Flor & Birbaumer, 1991; Flor & Turk, in press; Turk & Flor, 1999). The purpose of this chapter is to provide an overview of the role of psychophysiological assessments in clinical pain syndromes, and to suggest a framework for the integration of psychophysiological assessment data within the comprehensive interdisciplinary assessment and treatment of pain. An overview of the use of psychophysiological measures in laboratory pain assessments is provided by Handwerker and Kobal (1993). This chapter is divided into two major sections; the first section discusses peripheral psychophysiological measures that are of primary importance in the assessment of chronic pain syndromes, whereas the second focuses on central psychophysiological measures that have so far only found limited applications to chronic pain. I discuss them here because they have been found to be of increasing importance in the understanding of the causes of chronic pain syndromes and for treatment planning.

Early attempts to assess psychophysiological concomitants of pain were undertaken in the 1950s (e.g., Malmo, Shagass, & Davis, 1950), but such efforts became more accepted in the 1960s when biofeedback methods came into wider use. Over the past 30 years, a great deal of evidence for the interaction of psychological and physiological variables in pain has been obtained (Wall & Melzack, 2000), and thus psychophysiological concepts of pain have gained increased importance (Flor & Birbaumer, 1994; Keefe & Gil, 1986). Furthermore, the quality of the measurements has been enhanced, due to significant progress made in electronics and computer technology. Despite these advances, much of the research related to the psychophysiology of pain still lacks adequate theoretical foundation and methodological rigor (Flor & Turk, 1989). Thus only few conclusive results have been obtained with respect to the psychophysiology of pain.

Psychophysiological data serve a number of useful functions in the assessment of chronic and acute pain states. They provide evidence of the role of psychological factors in maladaptive physiological functioning in specific patients. Moreover, results of psychophysiological recordings may be used for the differential indication of intervention methods. For example, we (Flor & Birbaumer, 1991) have employed psychophysiological responses to personal and general stress in order to classify patients as biofeedback responders versus responders to operant or cognitive-behavioral therapy (see also Flor & Turk, in press). Psychophysiological assessments are, moreover, a necessary prerequisite for the use of biofeedback treatment. Psychophysiological measurements during treatment and following treatment help to document the efficacy of the intervention, as well as generalization and transfer. They may also serve as predictors of treatment outcome (Blanchard et al., 1983; Flor & Birbaumer, 1993). Another important aspect of psychophysiological measurements is their motivational character. Patients may learn from the results of the assessment that they are able to influence bodily processes by their own thoughts, emotions, and actions. Thus feelings of helplessness may be reduced and the acceptance of psychological interventions may be increased, not only in the patients but also in referring physicians, to whom psychophysiological assessment data should be made available. In experimental pain research, psychophysiological data have been used to examine physiological concomitants of anxiety and general arousal associated with pain, and they have served as measures of central processes related to the pain experience (see the section on central measures).

PERIPHERAL MEASURES IN THE ASSESSMENT OF PAIN

Electromyographic Recordings

Basic Issues

Elevated levels of muscle tension have been discussed as an etiological factor in a number of chronic pain syndromes (e.g., tension headache, temporomandibular pain and dysfunction [TMPD], low back pain). Furthermore, it has been assumed that in any type of pain syndrome, reflex muscle spasm may develop that further increases pain (Zimmermann, 1993). Thus the surface electromyogram (EMG) is a frequently used psychophysiological parameter with patients who have chronic pain. In order to obtain EMG measures, muscle action potentials summed over a large area of the muscle are recorded as a voltage difference between adjacent sites. In contrast to a neurological EMG (using needle vs. surface electrodes), which mainly serves the purpose of testing the function of motor neurons, psychophysiological EMG assessments are designed to record muscle tension related to psychological factors that may contribute to the pain experience. EMG evaluations are especially indicated for musculoskeletal pain syndromes such as

chronic back pain, headache, or pain in the jaw and neck region.

Several aspects of muscular function may be measured in psychophysiological assessment: elevated baseline levels, asymmetry of bilateral muscle tension, hyperreactivity to physical or psychological stress, time to return to baseline after stress, irregularities during movement, or aberrant frequency spectra (Flor & Turk, 1989; Schwartz & Associates, 1995). These characteristics may be assessed by themselves, or they may appear in combination. It must be noted that a causal role of muscular dysfunctions has so far not been demonstrated for pain disorders. There is, however, conclusive evidence that pain may be maintained or exacerbated by increases in muscle tension (e.g., Jensen, 1999; Larsson, Oberg, & Larsson, 1999).

Whereas previously the frontalis muscle has most often been the target of measurements—based on the assumption that generalized hyperarousal is present in patients with chronic pain—today more emphasis is placed on localized increases in muscle tension levels. Therefore, measurements tend to be site-specific. For example, the masseter and temporalis muscles are used with patients who suffer from chronic TMPD; the erector spinae muscles are used in patients with lower back pain; the trapezius muscle is used in patients with upper back pain; and the splenius capitis, occipitalis, trapezius, and/or frontalis muscles are used for patients with muscle tension headache. There has also been a trend to assess several muscle groups simultaneously, because this procedure yields information on the prime location of increased tension and permits an assessment of the generality or specificity of the response.

Methodological Considerations

Most physiological signals are quite weak and thus need sufficient amplification. The amplification factor of the EMG is usually around 100. An amplification that is too low can lead to misinterpretations of the signal, because relevant EMG changes may not be detected (Cobb, deVries, Urban, Leukens, & Bagg, 1975). Because of the high "noise" level present in unshielded clinical settings (where most assessments are made), differential amplifiers with a high common mode rejection (80–100 dB) are required. Thus signals are suppressed that act symmetrically on the electrodes, which would lead to artifacts. It is necessary for the impedance between the surface of the skin and the electrode not to exceed 10 kΩ. The use of nonpolarizing Ag-AgCl electrodes is recommended. Amplifiers with very high input impedance allow for less strict skin preparation and permit the use of lower-quality electrodes (see the section on muscle scanning, below). The amplifiers also need to have an adequate filtering range. Many biofeedback machines have a range of 100–200 Hz only, which is not sufficient for EMG dysfunction assessment. As was shown by Cram and Garber (1986), such a limited signal range leads to an underestimation of true activity in the muscles tested, and thus to incorrect treatment decisions.

The raw EMG signal must be processed in order to receive adequate information about the state of muscle tension. Usually a root mean square integrated EMG is calculated from the raw data. It is important not to use integration intervals that are too long, because these will then disguise artifacts related to movements or other intrusions in the recording process. The raw EMG should always be displayed in order to detect artifacts. Another important aspect is the sampling rate of the signal. It must be at least two times higher than the highest frequency of the signal. If this requirement is not met, the signal will be distorted ("aliasing"). Cheaper biofeedback equipment usually does not have this high-speed sampling capability. Further details on recording sites, skin preparation, and other technical considerations may be found in Basmajian (1986), Coles, Gratton, Kramer, and Miller (1986), Fridlund and Cacioppo (1986), and Schwartz and Associates (1995).

Resting Baseline Levels

In our critical review of 60 psychophysiological studies on chronic headache, back pain, and TMPD, we (Flor & Turk, 1989) noted that elevated resting baseline levels have sometimes been found, but they are not a prime characteristic of patients with chronic pain. Overall, the evidence for permanently elevated baseline levels in patients suffering from chronic musculoskeletal pain problems has been scarce. Although normative data for the EMG levels of various muscle groups have been established (see, e.g., Cram, 1988, 1990; Flor & Turk, in press), resting baseline levels must be interpreted with caution. Elevated levels may not always be considered as abnormal, nor may low values be interpreted as normal. Even though low baseline levels may be present, abnormal responses may be detected during movement or during psychological or physical stress. On the other hand, Wolf, Wolf, and Segal (1989) have shown that resting values

may be inflated by slight changes in posture that are difficult to control. Tests that used the induction of acute pain and measured EMG resting levels found no significant relationship between increases in pain and resting muscle tension (see, e.g., Svensson, Graven-Nielsen, Matre, & Arendt-Nielsen, 1998). There are also doubts about the reliability of measurement in certain muscle groups (see, e.g., Arena, Blanchard, Andrasik, Cotch, & Myers, 1983), although the assessment of low back muscle tension in different postures has been demonstrated as reliable (Arena, Sherman, Bruno, & Young, 1990; Cram, Lloyd, & Cahn, 1994).

Stress Reactivity

A possibly more important physiological parameter than the baseline value is the reactivity of the muscle during physical or psychological stress. The EMG is assessed while the person is exposed to a somatic stressor (e.g., a certain body position, writing on a computer keyboard) or a psychological stressor (e.g., stressful imagery, discussion of an emotionally involving event). The stressor should have personal relevance for the individual. The superiority of personally relevant stressors has been demonstrated in various experiments (e.g., Arntz, Merckelbach, Peters, & Schmidt, 1991; Ohrbach, Blascovich, Gale, McCall, & Dworkin, 1998). Studies that used general stressors or only healthy controls often failed to find the proposed pain–tension relationship (see, e.g., Bansevicius, Westgaard, & Jensen, 1997). However, it is quite possible that a certain vulnerability, as predicted by the diathesis–stress model of chronic pain (Flor, Birbaumer, & Turk, 1990), is a prerequisite for tension and pain levels to rise.

Several studies have shown that the EMG stress response is symptom-specific. In patients with chronic back pain, the erector spinae muscles are most responsive to stress; in patients with TMPD, the masseter muscle is most reactive (see, e.g., Flor, Birbaumer, Schugens, & Lutzenberger, 1992). In stress reactivity assessments, the question of norms and criteria for a stress response is still open. The best procedure is to employ both neutral and general as well as stressful stimuli, and to assess person-specific differences in the response to all three types of stimuli. Stress reactivity seems to be especially high in patients with high levels of fear of movement or reinjury (cf. Vlaeyen et al., 1999), as predicted by the diathesis–stress model of chronic pain (see, e.g., Flor et al., 1990; Turk & Flor, 1999).

Overall, a number of empirical studies have demonstrated symptom-specific EMG hyperreactivity in chronic back pain (Arntz et al., 1991; Burns, 1997; Flor, Birbaumer, et al., 1992; DeGood, Stewart, Adams, & Dale, 1994). Similar results have been obtained for TMPD (Flor, Birbaumer, Schulte, & Roos, 1991; Gramling, Grayson, Sullivan, & Schwartz, 1997). There is also convincing evidence that symptom-specific responses are present in patients with chronic headache. In 29 of 37 studies that we reviewed (Flor & Turk, 1989), at least one significant difference was found with respect to the muscular reactivity of patients with chronic headache as compared to healthy controls. Significant differences are especially present if the EMG is recorded from several muscles and personal relevant (e.g., socially involving situations) or physical stressors are used (see, e.g., Clark et al., 1997; Jensen, 1999). It must be noted that the reactivity is symptom-specific and not general, as has been shown by the assessment of additional physiological parameters, such as heart rate, blood pressure, and skin conductance.

Return to Baseline

An additional parameter, the time to return to baseline after the induction and termination of a stressor, has so far not been sufficiently assessed. Traue, Bischof, and Zenz (1985), as well as Pritchard and Wood (1984), reported a slower return to baseline of the trapezius and frontalis EMG in patients with chronic tension headache, but these results could not be replicated in other studies (Feuerstein, Bush, & Corbisiero, 1982; Kröner, 1984). We (Flor & Turk, 1989) presented a detailed analysis of the methodological problems, as well as suggestions for improved recording methods. Subsequent, better-controlled studies frequently observed extended returns to baseline (e.g., Flor, Birbaumer, et al., 1992; Moulton & Spence, 1992).

Posture and Dynamic Movement

Wolf and Basmajian (1978) first reported that patients with chronic back pain often show abnormal static posture. Similar results have been noted by Magnusson and colleagues (1996) and Cassisi, Robinson, O'Conner, and MacMillan (1999), but there have also been negative results (e.g., Miller, 1995). So far, it is not known whether the changes in posture maintain pain problems, elicit them, or are merely consequences of or adaptations to the

pain. It is also unclear whether too high or too low EMG levels during certain postures are the main problem. This is aggravated by the fact that normative data on static postures in healthy controls are sparse (cf. Roy et al., 1997). In addition, evidence from experimental studies as well as ambulatory monitoring suggests that EMG alterations related to postural abnormalities may be consequences rather than antecedents of the experience of pain (e.g., Arendt-Nielsen, Graven-Nielsen, Svarrer, & Svensson, 1996; Jalovaara, Niinimaki, & Vanharanta, 1995). Differences in posture-related EMG also seem to be based on diagnostic subgroups. Arena, Sherman, Bruno, and Young (1989, 1991) showed that although patients with low back pain in general display higher EMG levels in a standing position, patients with intervertebral disk disorder are significantly different from other patients with back pain and from healthy controls, in that they exhibit higher EMG levels during supported sitting. This points to the necessity of a differential diagnostic assessment in these patients, and supports the assumption that these postural EMG abnormalities may be of a reactive nature.

Wolf, Nacht, and Kelly (1982), as well as Wolf and colleagues (1989), have reported the presence of abnormal patterns of movement in patients with chronic back pain. Follow-up studies confirmed that abnormal body motion patterns are present in patients with chronic pain (e.g., Cassisi et al., 1999), with most studies reporting deficient tension levels during movement. Based on these results, the authors suggested the use of biofeedback training to correct these posture and movement abnormalities (Jones & Wolf, 1980; Wolf et al., 1982). It is, however, not clear to what extent abnormal movement patterns are etiological factors or just consequences of suffering from a chronic pain problem.

Muscle Scanning

EMG scanning is a quick and easy method to detect abnormal levels of muscle activity in patients with chronic pain (Cram & Engstrom, 1988; Cram & Steger, 1983). An evaluator using hand-held electrodes can scan 22 muscle sites in about 15 minutes. Bilateral recordings in a sitting and standing posture with scan times of at least 2 seconds are suggested. The values obtained are then compared to normative integrated EMG values from healthy controls. Due to the use of high-quality differential amplifiers, the necessity of extensive skin abrasion is reduced. Test–retest reliability (Cram et al., 1994; Thompson, Erickson, Madson, & Offord, 1989) and validity (Thompson, Madson, & Erickson, 1991; Traue, Kessler, & Cram, 1992) of the measurements have been demonstrated. As noted above, the relationship of these elevated EMG levels to pain and psychological antecedents of pain has not been clarified, and thus the value of EMG scanning for the selection of psychological intervention methods still needs to be established.

Analysis of EMG Frequency Patterns

Several authors have suggested that changes in the predominant EMG frequency may be more important for the development of back pain and other musculoskeletal disorders than alterations in integrated EMG levels (Lundblad, Elert, & Gerdle, 1998; Mannion, Connolly, Wood, & Dolan, 1997; Oddson et al., 1997). Using this spectral analysis of EMG patterns, Lundblad and colleagues (1998) showed that shifts in EMG frequency during certain movement tasks were correlated with pain complaints and that higher shifts were associated with fewer complaints.

Discrimination of Muscle Tension

Several authors have emphasized that the inadequate perception of bodily states, specifically muscle tension levels, may contribute to the maintenance of chronic pain problems (e.g., Appelbaum, Blanchard, & Andrasik, 1984; Flor et al., 1990). We have examined the perception of physical symptoms and of muscle tension in patients with chronic back pain, TMPD, and tension headache (Flor, Fürst, & Birbaumer, 1999; Flor, Schugens, & Birbaumer, 1992). Patients with chronic pain were shown to be notoriously unable to perceive muscle tension levels correctly at the affected muscle, but also at a muscle unrelated to the pain problem. On the other hand, they greatly overestimated physical symptoms related to the tension production tasks, rated the tasks as more aversive, and experienced more pain upon tensing their muscles. This inability to estimate current muscle tension levels correctly may contribute to the continued maintenance of high muscle tension levels after stressors have subsided. The intense focus on bodily symptoms and their overestimation may contribute to the perception of pain even at low levels of stimulation.

In psychophysiological assessments, a simple method can be used to estimate tension perception ability. Patients are presented with a bar of varying height on a video monitor and are asked to tense a muscle in accordance with the height of the bar—in other words, to produce low tension with a low bar and high tension when the bar is high. Subsequently, the integrated EMG activity during the tension production procedure can be correlated with the height of the bar. Good tension discrimination yields a correlation over .80; bad tension discrimination ranges around .50 or lower.

Relationship of EMG and Pain Levels

It is important to note that pain intensity and EMG levels are usually not systematically correlated at any given point in time (Arena et al., 1991; Mense & Hoheisel, 1999). It has, however, been shown that an elevation of muscle tension over an extended period of time leads to pain induction or an enhancement of already existing pain in the facial, back, or head muscles (e.g., Borgeat, Hade, Elie, & Larouche, 1984; Christensen, 1986a, 1986b). In order to understand the relationship of pain and EMG levels better, extended EMG assessments with concurrent assessment of pain levels are necessary, preferably through the use of ambulatory monitoring devices. Several attempts in this direction have been reported (see Arena et al., 1994; Geisser, Robinson, & Richardson, 1995; Sherman, Arena, Searle, & Ginther, 1991). A naturalistic examination of supermarket cashiers with frequent pain problems revealed significantly elevated stress values at work, accompanied by elevated EMG levels, in those with more musculoskeletal pain (Lundberg et al., 1999). In general, muscular work patterns seem to be predictive of future pain problems (see, e.g., Veiersted, Westgaard, & Andersen, 1993). Several studies have also provided evidence that pain may be induced by experimentally produced increases of muscle tension (e.g., Bakke, Tfelt-Hansen, Olson, & Moller, 1982; Borgeat et al., 1984), and that there may be lag times of several days between the increase of muscle tension and the induction of pain (e.g., Feuerstein, Bartolussi, Houle, & Labbé, 1983), thus precluding high pain–tension correlation at the same point in time.

Autonomic Measures

Autonomic measures seem to be of little relevance in pain syndromes of a musculoskeletal nature. They may, however, play a major role in vascular pain problems (such as migraine headache or Raynaud's disease), as well as in pain syndromes related to sympathetic dysfunction (such as complex regional pain syndromes). They have also been used in laboratory investigations with acute pain stimuli. Several methods are available to assess cardiovascular parameters: namely, the electrocardiogram (ECG) to measure heart rate; photoplethysmography, laser Doppler flowmetry, or sonographic Doppler flowmetry to assess changes in blood flow; thermistor recordings or thermography to measure changes in skin temperature; and blood pressure recordings.

Measures of Blood Flow

Photoplethysmography involves the measurement of the volume of blood vessels, using a light source directed at the vessel and a photosensitive plate that records the reflected light. When blood flow increases, the saturation with red blood cells increases, and less light is reflected. Tonic measurements involve the changes in blood flow over time (blood volume recordings); phasic measurements are related to beat-to-beat variations in the force of flow (pulse volume recordings). Both, blood and pulse volume are reduced with certain emotional responses (see, e.g., Coles, Donchin, & Porges, 1986). Photoplethysmographic measures, however, have the disadvantage that they can only display relative changes in volume, not absolute values.

Changes in blood volume are of special interest in migraine headaches because of etiological theories that assume an important role of vasomotor processes in the development of pain. Comparable to the results of EMG recordings in patients with tension headache, most controlled studies have not found baseline differences in vascular parameters in patients with migraine as compared to healthy controls (for a summary, see Flor & Turk, 1989). It was interesting to note that few specific differences with respect to EMG baseline values and vascular parameters have been reported for the different types of headaches (see, e.g., Arena, Blanchard, Andrasik, Appelbaum, & Myers, 1985). In migraine patients, migraine attacks could even be elicited by inducing spasms in the head muscles (Bakke et al., 1982). The authors reported a high correlation between the onset of pain and peaks in EMG readings. This finding suggests that in migraine pain, a muscular component may be relevant as well.

Studies on stress reactivity in patients with migraine point toward a functional abnormality of the major head arteries, particularly the temporal artery, especially if personally relevant stressors were used (e.g., Arena et al., 1985; Rojahn & Gerhards, 1986). The empirical results with respect to a slower return to baseline after stressors are controversial (see Flor & Turk, 1989, for a summary). Photoplethysmography of the temporal artery in patients with migraine was used in several studies as a biofeedback and assessment method. Patients were trained to reduce vascular contraction in order to block excessive dilation shortly before and during attacks. In a study of children with migraine headache, Hermann and Blanchard (1998) found no significant differences between patients and healthy controls with respect to several measures of autonomic reactivity; they have suggested that assessments in children may provide a clearer picture of the psychophysiology of migraine headache because many chronicity-related factors are not yet present.

Peripheral sympathetic reflexes related to noxious stimulation as measured by photoplethysmography may be valid indicators of painful experiences. Significant abnormalities were observed in patients with complex regional pain syndrome (Birklein, Riedel, Neundörfer, & Handwerker, 1998). Measurement of blood flow velocity with ultrasound Doppler sonography in migraine reveals abnormally increased flow velocity after presentation of stressful stimuli in patients with migraine, but not in controls (Rieke et al., 1993). Doppler sonography uses high-frequency sound waves (above 20 kHz; for large vessels, 4–5 MHz) directed toward the vessels. The frequency of the reflection of the two slightly distant sound sources is proportional to the blood flow velocity (Anliker, Casty, Friedl, Kubli, & Keller, 1977). Laser Doppler flowmetry has been introduced as an alternative method (see, e.g., Magerl, Szolcsanyi, Westerman, & Handwerker, 1987). The interpretation of vascular parameters in clinical practice may be problematic, because the signals are very much prone to artifact. Body temperature, the temperature of the environment, or the position of the body may all influence the recordings. Additional data on cerebral blood flow and pain are reported in the section on neuroimaging below.

Skin Temperature

Skin temperature is largely dependent on peripheral circulation. Vasoconstriction is associated with lower, and vasodilation with higher, skin temperature. Usually temperature-sensitive thermistors are used that measure temperature changes and convert them to changes in electrical resistance. However, recordings with thermistors are highly prone to artifact, especially because they are easily disturbed by slight changes in temperature or air circulation in a room. Skin temperature does respond to stress. This is of special relevance in Raynaud's disease, which has been found to be associated with pain related to cold extremities. In a series of studies, Freedman and his coworkers (e.g., Freedman, Ianni, & Wenig, 1983; Jennings et al., 1999) have shown that emotional as well as physical stressors lead to more local vasoconstriction in patients who suffer from Raynaud's disease than in healthy controls. Consequently, temperature biofeedback has proven to be a very efficient treatment method for these patients (Freedman, 1991).

In studies of patients with phantom limb pain, Sherman and his colleagues identified subgroups of patients based on their psychophysiological responses (Sherman & Bruno, 1987; Sherman, Griffin, Evans, & Grana, 1992). Whereas burning, throbbing, and tingling phantom limb pain seemed to covary with reduced temperature in the stump, cramping phantom limb pain was found to be related to and often preceded by decreases in muscle tension in the residual limb. These findings suggest differential treatments for these two subgroups of patients.

Although temperature biofeedback has often been used for patients with migraine, the usefulness of temperature recordings has not yet been demonstrated for migraine headaches. The procedure is based on the observation that migraine attacks may improve with hand-warming biofeedback in attack-free periods. The studies assessing the role of temperature and temperature reactivity in migraine headaches have not provided empirical evidence for a specific role in the therapeutic effect (for a summary, see Flor & Turk, 1989; for a more recent report, see Blanchard et al., 1997).

In thermography, infrared photography of the body surface is used to measure vascular abnormalities related to pain. Abnormally high as well as low temperatures may be associated with pain. Thermography has been widely used as an assessment instrument, as well as in the documentation of treatment-related changes (see, e.g., Fergason, 1964; Uematsu, Hendeler, & Hungerford, 1981). Thermography is especially used in the asssessment of pain caused by inflammatory processes such as rheumatoid arthritis (MacDonald, Land, & Sturrock, 1994). Its usefulness as a psychophysiological research method has not yet been adequately as-

sessed. Thermographic recordings have tended to suffer from inadequate analyses and may have little specificity (Leclaire, Esdaile, Hanley, Rossignol, & Bourdouxhe, 1996; Mills, Davies, Getty, & Conay, 1986), although computerized thermographic recordings have yielded more reliable results (Bruehl, Lubenow, Nath, & Ivankovich, 1996; Sherman, Woerman, & Karstetter, 1996).

Thermographic recordings have also been used in the analysis of facial temperature in migraine patients as well as patients with facial pain. In patients with TMPD, high thermal asymmetry of the temporomandibular joint region was found as compared to healthy controls (see, e.g., Graff-Radford, Ketelaer, Gratt, & Solberg, 1995). Drummond and Lance (1984) did not report resting baseline differences in facial temperature between patients with migraine and healthy controls, but they found lower temperature in the patients following pressure on the temporal artery. Thus reactivity measures may be a better indicator of dysfunction than resting levels and should be studied more carefully.

Heart Rate and Blood Pressure

The recording of heart rate is often used in psychophysiology, because heart rate is very easy to measure. Usually the number of R-waves of the ECG is converted into beats per minute. Although the ECG is frequently used in acute laboratory pain assessments, there is little research on the relationship of heart rate and chronic pain, and even less research on the relationship of blood pressure and chronic pain. Most of the research available is inconclusive. For example, two studies (Collins, Cohen, Naliboff, & Schandler, 1982; Flor, Turk, & Birbaumer, 1985) reported no differences in heart rate during resting baseline or during various stressors (brief cold pressor, mental math, discussion of personally relevant stress and pain episodes) between patients with chronic back pain and healthy controls. On the other hand, Arntz and colleagues (1991) found lower heart rate reactivity to an extended cold pressor test; we (Flor, Birbaumer, et al., 1992) noted lower heart rate reactivity to personally relevant stress images in patients with chronic back pain compared to healthy controls; and Kappel, Glaros, and McGlynn (1989) also reported less reactivity in patients with TMPD than in healthy controls. Both Arntz and colleagues (1991) and we (Flor, Birbaumer, et al., 1992) interpreted these findings as indicative of a lack of active coping in the patients as compared to the controls. This hypothesis is based on Obrist's (1976) findings of a coupling of somatic and cardiovascular responses during active coping and a decoupling during passive coping. This assumption is corroborated by the high negative correlation between heart rate reactivity and passive coping (catastrophizing) we reported (Flor, Birbaumer, et al., 1992).

Heart rate has also frequently been used as a physiological correlate of acute pain intensity (Sternbach, 1968). However, increases in tonic heart rate have been more closely related to subjective pain ratings than to objective characteristics of the nociceptive stimulus (cf. Hampf, 1990; Möltner, Hölzl, & Strian, 1990). In studies of postoperative pain, cardiovascular measures have been used to document the effects of postoperative pain as well as the favorable effects of psychological interventions. Both, blood pressure and heart rate reductions have been reported in patients who underwent psychological coping training as compared to patients not involved in these procedures (see, e.g., Wallace, 1984).

In experimental pain studies, a negative correlation of blood pressure and pain experience has been established for subjects with elevated tonic blood pressure, whereas this correlation is positive for normotensives (Larbig, Elbert, Rockstroh, Lutzenberger, & Birbaumer, 1985). The induction of elevated blood pressure levels by the use of baroreceptor stimulation leads to a reduction in pain sensitivity in patients with borderline hypertension and to an increase of pain sensitivity in normotensive individuals (Dworkin et al., 1994). Similar blood-pressure-related changes in pain sensitivity have also been reported for patients with chronic pain, but their practical relevance has not yet been established (cf. Bruehl, McCubbin, & Harden, 1999).

Skin Conductance Measures

Skin conductance may be viewed as a measure of general arousal. It changes with the activation of the sweat glands that are responsive to psychological stimuli (Fowles, 1986). Sweat gland activity is mediated by the sympathetic nervous system. Parameters of the sympathetic activity of the skin include the tonic skin conductance level and the phasic skin conductance response. Acute pain is associated with both increased heart rate and skin conductance levels (Dowling, 1983; Sternbach, 1968). In certain pain syndromes, autonomic dysfunction seems to be of some importance (e.g., in

complex regional pain syndromes or phantom limb pain). Here, measures of the activity of the sympathetic system such as skin conductance level seem indicated (Cronin & Kirshner, 1982; Howe, 1983). However, results on the significance of skin conductance measures for chronic pain have been controversial. Collins and colleagues (1982) and Peters and Schmidt (1991) reported increased skin conductance levels in response to stress in patients with low back pain, but these results were not confirmed (Flor et al., 1985; Flor, Birbaumer, et al., 1992). Jamner and Tursky (1987) as well as Salamy, Wolk, and Shucard (1983) reported that patients with pain show increased electrodermal activity in response to words that are relevant to their pain syndrome. The authors' suggestion to use this measure in the detection of deception in medicolegal cases is questionable and has not been followed up.

Overall, responses to painful stimuli seem to be associated with characteristic peripheral physiological responses in the muscular and vascular systems, as well as the eccrine system (e.g., Myrtek & Spital, 1986). Further research is needed to determine the role of peripheral psychophysiological variables in chronic pain.

Recommendations

Based on the methodological suggestions we have made (Flor & Turk, 1989), several guidelines for the assessment of psychophysiological variables in chronic pain syndromes may be established (see Table 5.1 on the next page). First, the type of pain problem should be clearly described, and a differential diagnosis should be made. Only in conjunction with a multiaxial evaluation of the patient with chronic pain (cf. Turk & Rudy, 1987) can psychophysiological assessment data be interpreted in a valid manner. Moreover, the multiaxial assessment is necessary to identify the physical or psychosocial stressors that are relevant for a given patient and can subsequently be used to test psychophysiological reactivity.

Psychophysiological measurements should be tailored to the assumed etiology of the pain problem. Thus EMG recordings seem to be of primary importance in chronic musculoskeletal pain problems, vascular and muscular measures in migraine headaches and Raynaud's disease, and vascular combined with skin conductance measures in neuropathic pain syndromes. As we do not yet know enough about the role of symptom-specific

TABLE 5.1. Recommendations for Psychophysiological Assessment

- Use multiaxial classification of patients, to identify specific somatic and psychosocial characteristics of the patients.
- If possible, use normative data from controls.
- Control for pain status (i.e., test in a pain-free and a painful state, if possible).
- Control for medication (i.e., make sure patient has not taken analgesic or psychotropic medication for several days, if possible).
- Use sites both proximal and distal to the painful site.
- Make sure that the measures selected are relevant for the specific type of pain being studied (e.g., temperature recordings for Raynaud's syndrome, rather than EMG levels).
- Use ecologically valid methods of stress induction (i.e., use self-selected stressors; test stressfulness by assessing subjective stress rating, heart rate, or skin conductance levels).
- Use sufficiently long adaptation phases and baselines.
- Use a syndrome-specific and a general autonomic measure.

and general arousal in patients with chronic pain, at least one specific and one general activation measure (skin conductance, heart rate) should be used. Following Dolce and Raczynski (1985), I recommend that EMG assessments should be accompanied by the recording of autonomic responses, in order to identify patients who are generally overaroused and could profit from nonspecific stress management and relaxation. In patients with specific local dysfunctions, such as heightened stress reactivity of the back muscles or heightened vascular reactivity of the extremities, specific biofeedback is indicated (see, e.g., Flor & Birbaumer, 1991; Freedman, 1991). It has been shown that feedback that includes stress exposure has a more favorable outcome than feedback that is only aimed at resting levels (see, e.g., Freedman et al., 1983). Laboratory measures should be supplemented by field recordings in the natural environment with portable equipment.

One of the major problems in psychophysiological pain assessments is the frequent use of test stimuli that may not be relevant for the patient that is being tested. Whereas mental arithmetic may be a personally relevant stressor for a student, this type of stressor is most likely of no significance to a homemaker or a blue-collar worker. I have found it most useful to identify physical and psychological stressors from the pain assessment interview and then have the patient produce or report them dur-

ing the assessment. It is also important to determine whether the stress induction was successful. This can be achieved by using subjective ratings of the stressfulness and the personal relevance of the stressor. The validity of these ratings may be verified by the additional use of measures that represent autonomic activation, such as heart rate or skin conductance levels.

Recordings from several muscles seem to be especially important, because several muscles may be involved in the disorder. In addition, recordings from a distal site should be made, because this allows conclusions about the site specificity of the dysfunction and again has treatment implications. When one is choosing muscles to record from, it is important to use a muscle site close to the site of pain, as well as a more distant muscle in order to obtain comparison values about the generality or specificity of the response. Although EMG may often be the measure of choice in chronic pain syndromes, sometimes other variables may be more relevant for a specific pain syndrome. For example, in Raynaud's disease, peripheral temperature is a much more relevant variable to indicate deficient peripheral circulation. In patients with phantom limb pain, Sherman (1997) has reported that changes in temperature of the stump may be related to throbbing, burning phantom limb pain, whereas increases in muscle tension may precede cramping, aching types of phantoms as discussed above.

Sufficient adaptation to the laboratory situation (about 15 minutes) and sufficiently long intertrial intervals (5–10 minutes) are required to allow for measures to return to baseline. Pretrial baselines should be recorded in order to take into account resting baseline changes due to different postures or lack of return to baseline on previous trials. Patients should refrain from taking analgesic and muscle-relaxing medication at least on the day of the assessment.

If possible, normative data from controls should be used to determine to what extent a given level of psychophysiological reactivity is actually deviant. Published norms are available for a large number of patient samples and situations (cf. Flor & Turk, in press; Schwartz & Associates, 1995). A comparison of several tasks within a patient may also be useful. It is also important to control for pain status. Ideally, patients with intermittent pain should be assessed in a pain-free and a painful state. This allows for the determination of the effect of pain on muscle tension levels and the significance of tonically elevated tension levels or heightened reactivity in pain-free states. Level of medication also needs to be controlled; as noted, both analgesic and psychotropic medication can influence muscle tension levels and lead to distorted recordings. Table 5.1 summarizes these assessment guidelines.

Case Study

The following case is presented in order to demonstrate the integration of verbal/subjective, somatic/motor, and physiological/organic data into a comprehensive assessment profile that allows for specific treatment prescriptions.

Mr. F, a 55-year-old married blue-collar worker with a high school diploma, attended the outpatient pain clinic with a complaint of facial pain. The pain had begun 5 years ago when he was involved in an accident at his work site. Since then, his ability to work was greatly reduced (he missed many days at work) and he was informed that he might lose his job even though he was quite willing to work. After a comprehensive pain interview, the following assessment instruments were used: the West Haven–Yale Multidimensional Pain Inventory (WHYMPI; Kerns, Turk, & Rudy, 1985), the Pain-Related Self-Statements and Pain-Related Convictions of Control Scales (Flor & Turk, 1988), the Brief Stress Questionnaire (Flor, 1991), and the Tübingen Pain Behavior Check List (Flor & Turk, in press).

The analysis of the questionnaires and the interview data indicated that the patient's pain and interference levels were very high, compared to those of other patients in the pain clinic. Both affective distress and depression scores were low. Life control a well as active coping with the pain were low; tendencies to catastrophize and to assume a helpless attitude toward the pain were high. Mr. F's spouse was supportive but showed little tendency to reinforce pain behaviors that were overall unremarkable. The patient experienced a high level of stress in his everyday life. He also noticed that anger or stress—especially at the work site—increased his pain. Additional factors that influenced the pain were heat and cold, changes in light, changes in mood, and high levels of concentration on a task. Overall, the patient attempted to ignore the pain or control it by rest and medication (narcotics and antidepressants). He reported sleep disturbances he attributed to the pain. However, the patient seemed to be eager to work, despite his incapacitating pain problem.

The psychophysiological assessment consisted of bilateral EMG measurements at the masseter, frontalis, and trapezius muscles, as well as the recording of heart rate and skin conductance level. Following a 10-minute adaptation and a 2-minute baseline, the patient imagined personally relevant pain and stress situations and a neutral situation, participated in extended (10-minute) mental arithmetic, and completed a 10-minute movement task. Each phase had 1-minute pre- and postbaseline recordings.

The resting values of the masseter, trapezius, and frontalis were significantly elevated (EMG values > 15 μV), with a marked asymmetry, especially at the frontalis muscle (related to damage during the accident). EMG levels at other sites, as well as heart rate and skin conductance levels, were not remarkable.

During stress testing, a marked response to the stressors was noted, with a very high reactivity for the pain episode. Overall, the assessment revealed that the patient showed elevated facial muscle tension levels both in the resting state and during exposure to relevant stressors as compared to healthy controls (see Figure 5.1 on the next page). These increases in muscle tension are most likely a reaction to the pain problem, which was additionally exacerbated and maintained by them. This elevated tension also extended to the upper back, but not to the erector spinae muscles.

Based on these findings, the primary goal of the treatment was viewed as the reduction of tension in the relevant muscles and the alteration of the patient's response to aversive stimulation. The patient received EMG biofeedback training that focused on alternative ways of dealing with stressful situations. The patient imagined the aversive situations and simultaneously observed his EMG response in the masseter muscle and a "control" muscle of the lower back. Real-life exposure, such as aggressive verbalization from the therapist, was also combined with the task of bringing the EMG response of the masseter back to the normal level of the "control" muscle as quickly as possible. Homework included the recording of stress episodes, the patient's response to them, and the generation of alternative responses.

CENTRAL MEASURES OF THE PAIN EXPERIENCE

Neuroimaging and Neurophysiological Methods

Several blood-flow-based neuroimaging methods have been used in identifying the neuroanatomical correlates of pain. These measures include positron

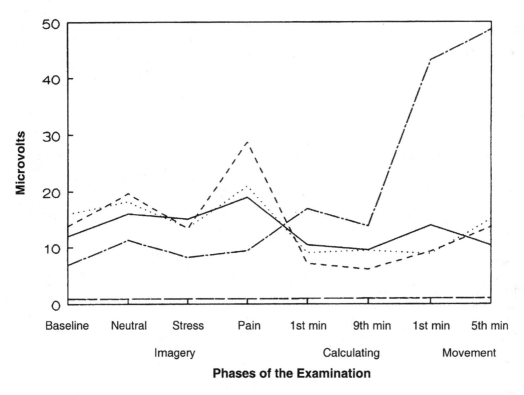

FIGURE 5.1. EMG profile of Mr. F.

emission tomography (PET), single-photon emission computerized tomography (SPECT), and functional magnetic resonance imaging (fMRI). PET is based on the use of radio tracers such as $H_2[^{15}O]$ or [O]-butanol, which are usually introduced into the bloodstream and whose concentration is subsequently measured by a scanner that detects positrons emitted by the radioactive molecules. This permits the determination of which brain regions have taken up a radioactive substance and are thus active during a certain type of stimulation. A drawback of the PET technique is, however, is its relatively low temporal resolution, which is related to the fact that changes in metabolic activity occur only very slowly (in the range of seconds) and that fairly long interstimulus intervals are needed to allow for return to baseline (several minutes). Moreover, the use of radioactive markers generally precludes repeat measurements in the same patient. PET is usually based on the analysis of group data. The relationship of blood flow changes and neuronal signals—which are the actual targets of the measurement—has not yet been sufficiently clarified.

SPECT is similar to PET in that it also uses radio tracers such as $[^{123}]$iodoamphetamin, which emit signals that can be measured by photosensitive equipment. It has lower resolution and longer acquisition times than PET, but has the advantage that no cyclotrone is needed to produce the radioisotopes.

fMRI is a relatively new method that is rapidly gaining acceptance (see Belliveau et al., 1991). fMRI is based on the application of a strong magnetic field through a person's head; this leads to a spin of nuclei in hydrogen molecules with a particular orientation. Through application of high-frequency impulses, the relaxation times of the hydrogen protons can subsequently be measured. The relaxation times are dependent on the molecule density of the tissue. The most commonly used fMRI technique is based on the blood-oxygenation-level-dependent contrast, where a stimulus-associated reduction in the local concentration of deoxyhemoglobin is used as the measure of brain activation. The temporal resolution of fMRI is much better than that of PET, ranging around 2 seconds; the spatial resolution is in the range of several millimeters (Villringer, 1997).

Neuroelectric and neuromagnetic methods (i.e., electroencephalographic [EEG] and magnetoencephalographic [MEG] recordings) have the advantage of assessing neuronal activity rather than reflections of neuronal activity in metabolic changes. They do have very high temporal resolution. Thus they are uniquely suited to measure quickly changing brain processes, but have the disadvantage of a lower spatial resolution. The combination of multichannel EEG and MEG measurements with magnetic resonance imaging (MRI) has led to the development of neuroelectric and neuromagnetic source imaging methods with a resolution of a few millimeters (2–5 mm, depending on the activity and measure used; cf. Hari & Forss, 1999; Kristeva-Feige et al., 1997).

The EEG reflects fluctuations of voltages caused by changes of the summed ionic currents of the many billions of pyramidal cells of the cerebral cortex. Their dendrites in the apical layers (layers I and II) of the cerebral cortex and their soma in the deeper brain structures (i.e., layers III to V) generate an electrical dipole when there is input from thalamic or other brain structures. Thousands of pyramidal cells are simultaneously activated and create the potential changes on the cortical surface. The amplitude of the EEG is attenuated by the skull and the scalp, so that the normal EEG activity recorded from external electrodes ranges somewhere between 1 μV and several hundred microvolts. The EEG assesses changes in the electric potential of the cerebral cortex, which may be related to subcortical activations whose activity is conducted as field potentials. The basis of neuroelectric source imaging of pain is the measurement of pain-related electric potentials. These values must be extracted from the spontaneous EEG by averaging, and therefore require multiple stimulus presentations. After the EEG is averaged to a stimulus, a complex sequence of waves results that represents various physiological and psychophysiological events (Niedermeyer & Lopez da Silva, 1998).

Three types of evoked potentials have been identified as correlates of pain perception (they cannot be called measures of pain, because they are influenced by a number of factors such as attention and general activation): brainstem potentials (10 to 15 milliseconds [msec] after the application of the stimulus); potentials of short latency (15 to 20 msec after the application of the stimulus) that are probably based on thalamo-cortical sources; and long-latency potentials (50 to 200 msec after the stimulus), that have a cortical basis (Chapman & Jacobson, 1984). Subjective pain perception correlates with the amplitude of the evoked potential in the 150- to 260-msec range that may

provide information in addition to the subjective pain rating (Chapman et al., 1985). Dowman (1996) computed a difference potential between the evoked response at pain threshold and that at noxious levels in the time range 75–240 msec after the stimulus (sural nerve evoked potentials) and found evidence that these potentials reflects exclusively Aδ fiber activity.

The EEG power spectrum provides a measure of the relative "power" of the EEG waves within a certain frequency band. Usually four bands are discriminated: delta (0.5 to 3.5 Hz—profound sleep and pathology); theta (3.5 to 7.5 Hz—deep sleep, but also focused attention if localized in the frontal area); alpha (8 to 12 Hz—relaxed wakefulness with eyes closed); and beta (13 to 30 hz—eyes open, attentiveness).

New methods of EEG analysis, such as nonlinear dimensional analysis (Elbert et al., 1994), are other possible applications of central nervous system recordings in the quantification of pain processing in the human brain. The use of nonlinear ("chaos") deterministic models allows for the dimensional reduction of the EEG trace into a few basic factors (fractal dimensions) that determine the actual time series.

MEG assesses magnetic fields in the brain that are based on electric potentials. Highly sensitive detectors—so-called "SQUIDS" (superconducting quantum interference devices), which are positioned about 10–15 mm from the skull—are able to detect the weak magnetic fields generated by electric dipoles of the brain. Like in EEG measurements, activity peaks are usually determined by averaging over many stimulations. Since MEGs can be recorded without electrodes and are not distorted by skull and fluids, this procedure is more accurate and convenient for patient studies. However, it has the disadvantage that only tangential components of the signal (i.e., those that are perpendicular to the surface of the cortex) can be detected have been measured. EEG and MEG have excellent time resolution, but also quite good spatial resolution (1–4 mm for early components); however, the location of the signal sources has to be reconstructed via mathematical models.

Neuronal Changes Related to Chronic Pain Syndromes

A number of studies suggest that patients with chronic pain show more pronounced cerebral responses to painful stimulation or pain-related stimuli than healthy controls do. Lower heat thresholds at the hand, as well as lower mechanical thresholds at the tender points and control sites, were associated with higher peak-to-peak amplitudes of the CO_2 laser-evoked cortical responses at pain threshold as well as at 1.5 times pain threshold intensity in patients with fibromyalgia (Gibson, Littlejohn, Gorman, Helme, & Granges, 1994). In addition, these patients displayed larger mechanically induced neurogenic flare responses. Similarly, Lorenz (1998) and Lorenz, Grasedyck, and Bromm (1996) reported increased N170 and P390 components of the evoked potential related to painful laser stimulation. In addition, a lower laser intensity was needed to reach pain threshold in patients with fibromyalgia syndrome. By contrast, auditory evoked potentials were unaltered suggesting that it is nociceptive not aversive processing in general that is enhanced in patients with chronic fibromyalgia.

My colleagues and I studied patients with chronic back pain (Flor, Knost, & Birbaumer, 1997) and patients with subchronic back pain (Knost, Flor, Braun, and Birbaumer, 1997) for their cortical responses to pain-related as compared to neutral and body-related words. We assumed that pain-related words should have acquired the status of cues for pain through classical conditioning and should elicit pain-related peripheral and central responses. As predicted, the patients with chronic pain responded with increased muscle tension as well as increased early components (N150) of the evoked potential to the pain-relevant words. This enhanced brain response was also observed in the patients with subacute pain, but not in the healthy controls; nor was it found in response to the body-related words (thus there was no generalization) or the neutral words. Later components of the evoked response (e.g., the P300 or late positive complex) were found to be generally enhanced in patients with chronic pain (see, e.g., Flor, Knost, & Birbaumer, 1997; Knost et al., 1997; Larbig et al., 1996) suggesting that the experience of chronic pain might chronically disregulate inhibitory brain mechanisms. In a related study, we (Montoya, Larbig, Pulvermüller, Flor, & Birbaumer, 1996) used a classical conditioning paradigm in healthy subjects to test the hypothesis that neutral words (the conditioned stimuli) could acquire characteristics of the pain stimulus (the unconditioned stimulus) with which they were paired. They observed an enhanced N150 response to the word stimuli that had previously been paired with painful electric shock, thus confirming the assumption (Flor, Knost, & Birbaumer, 1997) that the observed evoked response to pain-

related words might have been the consequence of prior respondent conditioning.

The effects of operant conditioning on pain-related cortical responses have also been studied. Miltner, Larbig, and Braun (1988) showed that the pain-related brain potential can be modified by operant conditioning, and that the increased or decreased amplitude of the N150/P260 is also reflected in increased or decreased pain ratings. Dowman (1996), however, could not replicate these earlier reports that the operantly conditioned P200 component of the somatosensory evoked potential is correlated with altered pain ratings and altered nociceptive reflexes. We (Knost, Flor, & Birbaumer, in press) used operant conditioning of verbal pain reports to study effects of this procedure on the processing of pain-related responses in the brain. Both patients with chronic pain and healthy controls showed good up-conditioning (increased pain) and down-conditioning (decreased pain) of verbal pain reports when they were selectively reinforced. The patients with chronic pain, however, maintained elevated N150 components of the evoked potential during the extinction session, whereas the healthy controls quickly changed their brain potentials back to baseline when pain increases were no longer reinforced. These data suggest that patients with chronic pain may be more prone to lasting effects of operant conditioning of pain behaviors, and may thus be more inclined to maintain learned pain responses.

In a recent study, we (Flor, Lutzenberger, Knost, & Birbaumer, 2000) tested the extent to which spouses' responses to pain influence patients' brain responses. Chronic pain patients participated in a laboratory pain assessment while their spouses were either present or absent. The spouses were classified into a group of "solicitous" spouses (who routinely reinforced the pain behaviors of the patients) and "nonsolicitous" spouses (who never reinforced the patients' pain behaviors), based on the WHYMPI (Kerns et al., 1985). During the assessment, the patients received painful electric stimuli to the back (pain-relevant site) or the finger (pain-irrelevant site) while the evoked cortical responses to these stimuli were recorded. The global field power, which reflects the summed activity over all electrodes, was approximately three times higher when the spouses were present as compared to the spouse-absent condition in the patients with solicitous spouses. This increased brain response to painful stimulation was specific for the site of pain; it did not occur when the finger was stimulated. These data suggest that psychosocial processes may have a direct influence on the brain response to pain and can thus directly modify physiology.

Analysis of the dimensional complexity of the spontaneous EEG trace in humans during the actual experience of and memory for a pain episode showed that patients with chronic pain, compared to healthy controls, process memories of painful events with a much greater complexity; this suggests that more pain-related networks are activated when pain-related stimuli are presented (Lutzenberger, Flor, & Birbaumer, 1997).

MEG and EEG measures have also been used to study characteristics of patients with headache, especially persons who suffer from migraine headaches. In general, studies were conducted during the prodromal phase, during the migraine attack, after an attack, or in the interictal phase. Most studies did not find abnormalities in evoked potentials or fields. For example, Rieke and colleagues (1993) found no abnormalities in somtosensory evoked magnetic fields in patients with migraine as compared to healthy controls when they were tested in a headache-free phase. Using a P300 and contingent negative variation (CNV) paradigm, Evers, Bauer, Grotemeyer, Kurlemann, and Husstedt (1998) studied children and adolescents who suffered from migraine and found no differences except for a slower habituation of the P300 component. Similar reports on delayed habituation have also been reported by Gerber and his colleagues (e.g., Siniatchkin, Gerber, Kropp, & Vein, 1998), who assume that heightened CNV amplitudes are predictive of the onset of a migraine attack (Kropp & Gerber, 1998). By contrast, Oelkers and colleagues (1999) found no evidence for delayed habituation using a visual evoked potential paradigm, but observed prolonged N200 latency when very small checkerboards were presented. They suggested that precortical visual processing might be affected in patients with migraine. A transcranial magnatic stimulation study found enhanced excitability of occipital cortex neurons in patients with migraine who experienced an aura, suggesting that this hyperexcitability might predispose those patients to spreading depression (Aurora, Ahmad, Welch, Bhardhwaj, & Ramadan, 1998).

Metabolic Changes Related to Chronic Pain

Whereas neurophysiological measures have yielded highly variable results, blood-flow-based imaging studies have revealed fairly consistent changes of cerebral blood flow in patients with migraine; these changes are indicative of hypoperfusion in the phase before an attack and the interictal phase, and suggest hyperperfusion during the attack. The data are also consistent with the idea of spreading depression as a cause of migraine headaches. Several studies (e.g., Cutrer et al., 1998; LaSpina, Vignati, & Porazzi, 1997; Sanchez del Rio et al., 1999) found significantly reduced blood flow (mostly in the occipital region) during the aura phase, and Mirza and colleagues (1998) observed impaired vascular autoregulation also in the headache-free phase. Cao, Welch, Aurora, and Vikinstad (1999) showed that the onset of a migraine attack was accompanied by neuronal suppression, which was associated with a pronounced increase in vasodilatation and hyperoxygenation that might activate the migraine attack. They observed this pattern in occipital cortex after visual stimulation, using fMRI. Increases of activity in the brainstem have been observed during migraine headache (Diener, 1997), and increased activation of the hypothalamus was found during cluster headache (May, Bahra, Büchel, Frackowiak, & Goadsby, 1998), suggesting that there may be subcortical headache generators (Diener & May, 1996).

Overall, these studies suggest a vascular mechanism underlying migraine headache. Unfortunately, none of the studies examined the effect of psychological variables on these blood flow changes either preceding or during a headache episode. Studies on metabolic changes in other pain syndromes are fairly scarce and not consistent. Metabolic changes related to acute and tonic painful stimulation in healthy humans have been extensively studied and are reviewed in Gracely (1999).

Cortical Reorganization and Chronic Pain

The phenomenon of *cortical reorganization* refers to changes in the functional and structural architecture of the primary sensory and motor areas of the cortex as a consequence of the loss or increase of peripheral input (Kaas & Florence, 1997). Such changes were previously thought to be possible only in early stages of development. Neuroscientific research has shown that such changes also occur in the adult brain. The structure that is of special importance for chronic pain is the primary somatosensory (SI) cortex, with its point-to-point representation of the surface of the body in specific anatomical locations, referred to as *somatosensory homunculus*. We have observed an expansion of the representation of the lower back in SI cortex in patients with long-standing chronic back pain (Flor, Braun, Elbert, & Birbaumer, 1997). The longer the pain duration, the more of this type of reorganizational change was detected using magnetic source imaging (see Figure 5.2). The representation of the unaffected digits remained unchanged. Since the size of the cortical representation and sensory acuity are very highly correlated, it is possible that these cortical changes underlie the heightened pain sensitivity often reported by patients with chronic pain. Spinal and thalamic changes may, of course, also contribute to this phenomenon.

Similar changes have been observed in patients with phantom limb pain. We (e.g., Flor et al., 1995, 1998; Lotze et al., 1999) found that phantom limb pain is highly significantly related to an altered somatosensory and motor cortical representation of the mouth and hand zone in patients with upper-extremity amputations. In patients with phantom limb pain, the cortical representation of the deafferented hand or arm was found to be invaded by the adjacent representation of the mouth. The larger the cortical shift, the more

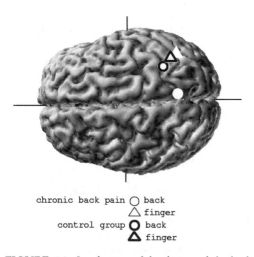

chronic back pain   ○ back
                     △ finger
control group   ● back
                ▲ finger

FIGURE 5.2. Localization of the digits and the back in patients with back pain and healthy controls in primary somatosensory cortex. Stimulation was on the left side of the body; the representations are on the hemisphere contralateral to the stimulation side. Please note the shift of the back representation of the patients with back pain into a more medial position (i.e., toward the leg representation). The shift amounted to about 2–3 cm. Data from Flor, Braun, Elbert, and Birbaumer (1997).

severe the phantom limb pain. These cortical changes seem to be maintained by peripheral factors in some, but not all, patients with phantom limb pain. Brachial plexus anesthesic blockers abolished phantom limb pain and cortical reorganization in 50% of the patients with upper-extremity amputations who were studied, while in 50% neither cortical reorganization nor phantom limb pain was affected (Birbaumer et al., 1997). An analysis of cortical reorganizational changes, along with an analysis of peripheral psychophysiological changes, can help to determine whether more centrally acting or more peripheral treatments for phantom limb pain should be used.

Case Study

Mrs. M was a 55-year-old female who sustained an arm amputation due to a car accident 14 years prior to the psychophysiological assessment. She suffered from intense phantom limb pain, which she described as constant, with intermittent attacks of burning and tingling pain, and of a mean intensity of 48 on a visual analogue scale ranging from 0 to 100 (her mean WHYMPI pain score was 3.4). Occasionally, a peak pain intensity of 100 was reached. She did not have stump pain or unpleasant stump or phantom sensations. The remaining WHYMPI scale scores were unremarkable and much below comparable scores in patients with chronic back pain. The psychophysiological assessment of the stump included the application of capsaicin to test C-fiber activity and its relationship to phantom limb pain, temperature, and EMG recordings. The application of capsaicin did not lead to an increase in phantom limb pain activity. In addition, muscle tension was unremarkable in the stump as compared to the contralateral arm, both in the resting state and during imagery of pain-provoking stimuli (e.g., the imagery of movement). Temperature recordings did not show a significant change in blood flow in the stump in general, but revealed patches of reduced activity.

Cortical reorganization was assessed by neuroelectric source imaging that used somatosensory potentials from 61 electrodes combined with structural MRI. The first and fifth digit and the mouth on the intact side, and the mouth on the amputation side, were stimulated. The analysis of the sources of the evoked electric activity on the patient's MRI (see Figure 5.3) revealed substantial reorganization of SI cortex. Based on the fairly unremarkable peripheral findings, a tactile discrimi-

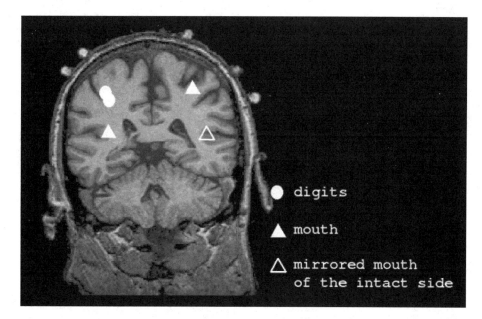

FIGURE 5.3. Representation of the mouth on the intact side, the digits of the intact hand, and the mouth on the amputation side in Mrs. M. Note the shift of the mouth region into the hand region. "Mirrored mouth" denotes the position where the mouth should be located, based on the representation of the intact side (assuming symmetrical locations on the hemispheres).

nation training was prescribed; this was to consist of the application of various high-intensity but nonpainful stimuli to the patient's residual limb, with the instruction to locate the location, the intensity, or the frequency of the stimulation. The purpose of the training was to supply the de-afferented cortical area with behaviorally relevant input and to restore its original function. It was assumed that this procedure would reduce both cortical reorganization and phantom limb pain. The treatment is still ongoing.

SUMMARY

The purpose of this chapter has been to demonstrate the usefulness of psychophysiological recording methods in the assessment of clinical pain syndromes. Whereas peripheral measures—especially the EMG and vascular parameters—have been widely used in the assessment of chronic pain, the use of central measures such as the spontaneous EEG, event-related potentials, PET, and fMRI has so far mainly been limited to laboratory pain assessments. An integration of peripheral and central measures in clinical applications would be desirable. Furthermore, the relationship of physio-

logical measures and psychological processes should be further investigated. Many clinicians and researchers limit their endeavors to the assessment of abnormalities in physiological functioning of pain patients without relating them to psychological processes. A truly multidimensional assessment of pain must assess both physiological and psychological parameters of the pain experience, and—most importantly—must elucidate their mutual interrelationship.

ACKNOWLEDGMENT

The completion of this chapter was facilitated by a grant from the Deutsche Forschungsgemeinschaft (No. Fl 156/16).

REFERENCES

Anliker, M., Casry, N., Friedl, P., Kubli, R., & Keller, H. (1977). Noninvasive measurement in blood flow. In N. H. Hwang & N. A. Norman (Eds.), *Cardiovascular flow dynamics and measurement* (pp. 177–198). Baltimore: University Park Press.

Appelbaum, K. A., Blanchard, E. B., & Andrasik, F. (1984). Muscle discrimination ability at three muscle sites in three headache groups. *Biofeedback and Self-Regulation, 9,* 421–430.

Arena, J. G., Blanchard, E. B., Andrasik, F., Appelbaum, K., & Myers, P. E. (1985). Psychophysiological comparisons of three kinds of headache subjects during and between headache states: Analysis of poststress adaptation periods. *Journal of Psychosomatic Research, 29,* 427–441.

Arena, J. G., Blanchard, E. B., Andrasik, F., Cotch, P. A., & Myers, P. E. (1983). Reliability of psychophysiological assessment. *Behaviour Research and Therapy, 21,* 447–460.

Arena, J. G., Bruno, G. M., Brucks, A. G., Searle, J. R., Sherman, R. A., & Meador, K. J. (1994). Reliability of an ambulatory electromyographic activity device for musculoskeletal pain disorders. *International Journal of Psychophysiology, 17,* 153–157.

Arena, J. G., Sherman, R. A., Bruno, G. M., & Young, T. R. (1989). Electromyographic recordings of five types of low back pain subjects and non-pain controls in different positions. *Pain, 37,* 57–65.

Arena, J. G., Sherman, R. A., Bruno, M., & Young, T. R. (1990). Temporal stability of paraspinal electromyographic recordings in low back pain. *International Journal of Psychophysiology, 9,* 31–37.

Arena, J. G., Sherman, R. A., Bruno, M., & Young, T. R. (1991). Electromyographic recording of low back pain subjects and non-pain controls in six different position: Effect of pain levels. *Pain, 45,* 23–28.

Arendt-Nielsen, L., Graven-Nielsen, T., Svarrer, H., & Svensson, P. (1996). The influence of low back pain on muscle activity and coordination during gait: A clinical and experimental study. *Pain, 64,* 231–240.

Arntz, A., Merckelbach, H., Peters, M. C., & Schmidt, A. J. M. (1991). Chronic low back pain, response specifity and habituation to painful stimuli. *Journal of Psychophysiology, 5,* 177–188.

Aurora, S. K., Ahmad, B. K., Welch, K. M., Bhardhwaj, P., & Ramadan, N. M. (1998). Transcranial magnatic stimulation confirms hyperexcitability of occipital cortex in migraine. *Neurology, 50,* 1111–1114.

Bakke, M., Tfelt-Hansen, P., Olsen, J., & Moller, E. (1982). Action of some pericranial muscles during provoked attacks of common migraine. *Pain, 14,* 121–135.

Bansevicius, D., Westgaard, R. H., & Jensen, C. (1997). Mental stress of long duration: EMG activity, perceived tension, fatigue, and pain development in pain-free subjects. *Headache, 37,* 499–510.

Basmajian, J. V. (1986). The musculature. In M. G. H. Coles, E. Donchin, & S. W. Porges (Eds.), *Psychophysiology: Systems, processes, and applications* (pp. 97–106). New York: Guilford Press.

Belliveau, J. W., Kennedy, D. N., Jr., McKinstry, R. C., Buchbinder, B. R., Weisskoff, R. M., Cohen, M. S., Vevea, J. M., Brady, T. J., & Rosen, B. R. (1991). Functional mapping of the human visual cortex by magnetic resonance imaging. *Science, 254,* 716–719.

Birbaumer, N., Lutzenberger, W., Montoya, P., Larbig, W., Unertl, K., Töpfner, S., Grodd, W., Taub, E., & Flor, H. (1997). Effects of regional anesthesia on phantom limb pain are mirrored in changes in cortical reorganization. *Journal of Neuroscience, 17,* 5503–5508.

Birklein, F., Riedl, B., Neundörfer, B., & Handwerker, H. O. (1998). Sympathetic vasoconstrictor reflex patterns in patients with complex regional pain syndrome. *Pain, 75,* 93–100.

Blanchard, E. B., Andrasik, F., Arena, J. G., Neff, D. F., Saunders, N. L., Jurish, S. E., Teders, S. J., & Rodichok, L. D. (1983). Psychophysiological responses and predictors of response to behavioral treatment of chronic headache. *Behavior Therapy, 14,* 357–374.

Blanchard, E. B., Peters, M. L., Hermann, C., Turner, S. M., Buckley, T. C., Barton, K., & Dentinger, M. P. (1997). Direction of temperature control in the thermal biofeedback treatment of vascular headache. *Applied Psychophysiology and Biofeedback, 22,* 227–245.

Borgeat, F., Hade, B., Elie, R., & Larouche, L. M. (1984). Effects of voluntary muscle tension increases in tension headache. *Headache, 24,* 199–202.

Bruehl, S., Lubenow, T. R., Nath, H., & Ivankovich, O. (1996). Validation of thermography in the diagnosis of reflex sympathetic dystrophy. *Clinical Journal of Pain, 12,* 316–325.

Bruehl, S., McCubbin, J. A., & Harden, R. N. (1999). Theoretical review: Altered pain regulatory systems in chronic pain. *Neuroscience and Biobehavioral Reviews, 23,* 877–890.

Burns, J. (1997). Anger management style and hostility: Predicting symptom-specific physiological reactivity among chronic low back pain patients. *Journal of Behavioral Medicine, 20,* 505–522.

Cacioppo, J. T., Tassinary, L. G., & Berntson, G. G. (Eds.). (2000). *Handbook of psychophysiology* (2nd ed.). Cambridge, England: Cambridge University Press.

Cao, Y., Welch, K. M., Aurora, S., & Vikinstad, E. M. (1999). Functional MRI-BOLD of visually triggered headache in patients with migraine. *Archives of Neurology, 56,* 548–554.

Cassisi, J. E., Robinson, M. E., O'Conner, P., & MacMillan, M. (1999). Trunk strength and lumbar paraspinal muscle activity during isometric exercise in chronic low back pain patients and controls. *Spine, 18,* 245–251.

Chapman, C. R., Casey, K. L., Dubner, R., Foley, K. M., Gracely, R. H., & Reading, A. E. (1985). Pain measurement: An overview. *Pain, 22,* 1–31.

Chapman, C. R., & Jacobson, R. C. (1984). Assessment of analgesic states: Can evoked potentials play a role? In B. Bromm (Ed.), *Pain measurement in man: Neurophysiological correlates of pain* (pp. 233–255). Amsterdam: Elsevier.

Christensen, L. V. (1986a). Physiology and pathophysiology of skeletal muscle contraction: Part 1. Dynamic activity. *Journal of Oral Rehabilitation, 13,* 451–461.

Christensen, L. V. (1986b). Physiology and pathophysiology of skeletal muscle contraction: Part 2. Static activity. *Journal of Oral Rehabilitation, 13,* 463–477.

Clark, G. T., Sakai, S., Merrill, R., Flack, V. F., McArthur, D., & McCreary, C. (1997). Waking and sleeping temporalis EMG levels in tension-type headache patients. *Journal of Orofacial Pain, 11,* 298–306.

Cobb, C. R., deVries, H. A., Urban, R. T., Leukens, C. A., & Bagg, R. J. (1975). Electrical activity in muscle pain. *American Journal of Physical Medicine, 54,* 80–87.

Coles, M. G. H., Donchin, E., & Porges, S. W. (Eds.). (1986). *Psychophysiology: Systems, processes, and applications.* New York: Guilford Press.

Coles, M., G. H., Gratton, G., Kramer, A. I., & Miller, G. A. (1986). Principles of signal acquisition and analysis. In M. G. H. Coles, E. Donchin, & S. W. Porges (Eds.), *Psychophysiology: Systems, processes, and applications* (pp. 183–226). New York: Guilford Press.

Collins, G. A., Cohen, M. J., Naliboff, B. D., & Schandler, S. L. (1982). Comparative analysis of paraspinal and frontalis EMG, heart rate and skin conductance in chronic low back pain patients and normals to various postures and stress. *Scandinavian Journal of Rehabilitation Medicine, 14*, 39–46.

Cram, J. R. (1988). Surface EMG recordings and pain-related disorders: A diagnostic framework. *Biofeedback and Self-Regulation, 13*, 123–138.

Cram, J. R. (Ed.). (1990). *Clinical EMG surface recordings* (Vol. 2). Bothell, WA: Clinical Resources.

Cram, J. R., & Engstrom, D. (1986). Patterns of neuromuscular activity in pain and non pain patients. *Clinical Biofeedback and Health, 9*, 106–116.

Cram, J. R., & Garber, A. (1986). The relationship between narrow and wide bandwidth filter settings during an EMG-scanning procedure. *Biofeedback and Self-Regulation, 11*, 105–114.

Cram, J. R., Lloyd, J., & Cahn, T. S. (1994). The reliability of EMG muscle scanning. *International Journal of Psychosomatics, 41*, 41–45.

Cram, J. R., & Steger, J. S. (1983). EMG scanning and the diagnosis of chronic pain. *Biofeedback and Self-Regulation, 8*, 229–242.

Cronin, K. D., & Kirshner, R. L. F. (1982). Diagnosis of reflex sympathetic dysfunction: Use of the skin potential response. *Anaesthesia, 37*, 848–852.

Cutrer, F. M., Sorensen, A. G., Weisskoff, R. M., Ostergaard, L., Sanchez del Rio, M., Lee, E. J., Rosen, B. R., & Moskowitz, M. A. (1998). Perfusion-weighted imaging defects during spontaneous migrainous aura. *Annals of Neurology, 43*, 25–31.

DeGood, D. E., Stewart, W. R., Adams, L. E., & Dale, J. A. (1994). Paraspinal EMG and autonomic reactivity of patients with back pain and controls to personally relevant stress. *Perceptual and Motor Skills, 79*, 1399–1409.

Diener, H. C. (1997). Positron emission tomography studies in headache. *Headache, 37*, 622–625.

Diener, H. C., & May, A. (1996). New aspects of migraine pathophysiology: Lessons learned from positron emission tomography. *Current Opinion in Neurology, 9*, 199–201.

Dolce, J. J., & Raczynski, J. M. (1985). Neuromuscular activity and electromyography in painful backs: Psychological and biomechanical models in assessment and treatment. *Psychological Bulletin, 97*, 502–520.

Dowling, J. (1983). Autonomic measures and behavioral indices of pain sensitivity. *Pain, 16*, 193–200.

Dowman, R. (1996). Effects of operantly conditioning the amplitude of the P200 peak of the SEP on pain sensitivity and the spinal nociceptive withdrawal reflex in humans. *Psychophysiology, 33*, 252–261.

Drummond, P. D., & Lance, J. W. (1984). Facial temperature in migraine, tension–vascular and tension headache. *Cephalalgia, 4*, 149–158.

Dworkin, B. R., Elbert, T., Rau, H., Birbaumer, N., Pauli, P., Droste, C., & Brunia, C. H. (1994). Central effects of baroreceptor activation in humans: Attenuation of skeletal reflexes and pain perception. *Proceedings of the National Academy of Sciences USA, 91*, 6329–6333.

Elbert, T., Ray, W. J., Kowalik, Z. J., Skinner, J. E., Graf, K. E., & Birbaumer, N. (1994). Chaos and physiology: Deterministic chaos in excitable cell assemblies. *Physiological Reviews, 74*, 1–47.

Evers, S., Bauer, B., Grotemeyer, K. H., Kurlemann, G., & Husstedt, I. W. (1998). Event-related potentials (P300) in primary headache in childhood and adolescence. *Journal of Child Neurology, 13*, 322–326.

Fergason, J. L. (1964). Liquid crystals. *Scientific American, 211*, 76–82.

Feuerstein, M., Bortolussi, L., Houle, M. & Labbé, E. (1983). Stress, temporal artery activity, and pain in migraine headache: A prospective analysis. *Headache, 23*, 296–304.

Feuerstein, M., Bush, C., & Corbisiero, R. (1982). Stress and chronic headache: A psychophysiological analysis of mechanisms. *Journal of Psychosomatic Research, 26*, 167–182.

Flor, H. (1991). *Psychobiologie des Schmerzes [Psychobiology of pain]*. Bern: Huber.

Flor, H., & Birbaumer, N. (1991). Comprehensive assessment and treatment of chronic back pain patients without physical disabilities. In M. Bond (Ed.), *Proceedings of the VIth World Congress on Pain* (pp. 229–234). Amsterdam: Elsevier.

Flor, H., & Birbaumer, N. (1993). Comparison of the efficacy of electromyographic biofeedback, cognitive-behavioral therapy, and conservative medical interventions in the treatment of chronic musculoskeletal pain. *Journal of Consulting and Clinical Psychology, 61*, 653–658.

Flor, H., & Birbaumer, N. (1994). Psychophysiological methods in the assessment and treatment of chronic musculoskeletal pain. In J. G. Carlson, A. S. Seifert, & N. Birbaumer (Eds.), *Clinical applied psychophysiology* (pp. 171–184). New York: Plenum Press.

Flor, H., Birbaumer, N., Schugens, M. M., & Lutzenberger, W. (1992). Symptom-specific psychophysiological responses in chronic pain patients. *Psychophysiology, 29*, 452–460.

Flor, H., Birbaumer, N., Schulte, W., & Roos, R. (1991). Stress-related EMG responses in chronic temporomandibular pain patients. *Pain, 46*, 125–142.

Flor, H., Birbaumer, N., & Turk, D. C. (1990). The psychobiology of chronic pain. *Advances in Behaviour Research and Therapy, 12*, 47–87.

Flor, H., Braun, C., Elbert, T., & Birbaumer, N. (1997). Extensive reorganization of primary somatosensory cortex in chronic back pain patients. *Neuroscience Letters, 224*, 5–8.

Flor, H., Elbert, T., Knecht, S., Wienbruch, C., Pantev, C., Birbaumer, N., Larbig, W., & Taub, E. (1995). Phantom limb pain as a perceptual correlate of cortical reorganization. *Nature, 357*, 482–484.

Flor, H., Elbert, T., Mühlnickel, W., Pantev, C., Wienbruch, C., & Taub, E. (1998). Cortical reorganization and phantom phenomena in congenital and traumatic upper extremity amputees. *Experimental Brain Research, 119*, 205–212.

Flor, H., Fürst, M., & Birbaumer, N. (1999). Deficient discrimination of EMG levels and overestimation of perceived tension in chronic pain patients. *Applied Psychophysiology and Biofeedback, 24*, 55–66.

Flor, H., Knost, B., & Birbaumer, N. (1997). Processing of pain-related information in chronic pain patients: Electrocortical and peripheral correlates. *Pain, 73,* 413-421.

Flor, H., Lutzenberger, W., Knost, B., & Birbaumer, N. (2000). *Spouse presence alters brain processing of painful stimuli in chronic pain patients.* Manuscript submitted for publication.

Flor, H., Schugens, M. M., & Birbaumer, N. (1992). Discrimination of muscle tension in chronic pain patients and healthy controls. *Biofeedback and Self-Regulation, 17,* 165-177.

Flor, H., & Turk, D.C. (1988). Chronic back pain and rheumatoid arthritis: Relationship of pain-related cognitions, pain severity, and pain behaviors. *Journal of Behavioral Medicine, 11,* 251-265.

Flor, H., & Turk, D. C. (1989). Psychophysiology of chronic pain: Do chronic pain patients exhibit symptom-specific psychophysiological responses? *Psychological Bulletin, 105,* 215-259.

Flor, H., & Turk, D. C. (in press). *A biobehavioral perspective of chronic pain and its management.* Washington, DC: American Psychological Association Press.

Flor, H., Turk, D. C., & Birbaumer, N. (1985). Assessment of stress-related psychophysiological reactions in chronic back pain patients. *Journal of Consulting and Clinical Psychology, 53,* 354-364.

Fowles, D. (1986). The eccrine system and electrodermal activity. In M. G. H. Coles, E. Donchin, & S. W. Porges (Eds.), *Psychophysiology: Systems, processes, and applications* (pp. 51-96). New York: Guilford Press.

Freedman, R. R. (1991). Physiological mechanisms of temperature biofeedback. *Biofeedback and Self-Regulation, 16,* 95-115.

Freedman, R. R., Ianni, P., & Wenig, P. (1983). Behavioral treatment of Raynaud's disease. *Journal of Consulting and Clinical Psychology, 51,* 539-549.

Fridlund, A. J., & Cacioppo, J. T. (1986). Guidelines for human electromyographic research. *Psychophysiology, 23,* 567-589.

Geisser, M. E., Robinson, M. E., & Richardson, C. (1995). A time series analysis of the relationship between ambulatory EMG, pain, and stress in chronic low back pain. *Biofeedback and Self-Regulation, 20,* 339-355.

Gibson, S. J., Littlejohn, G. O., Gorman, M. M., Helme, R. D., & Granges, G. (1994). Altered heat pain thresholds and cerebral event-related potentials following painful CO2 laser stimulation in subjects with fibromyalgia syndrome. *Pain, 58,* 185-193.

Gracely, R. H. (1999). Pain measurement. *Acta Anaesthesiologica Scandinavica, 43,* 897-908.

Graff-Radford, S. B., Ketelaer, M. C., Gratt, B. M., & Solberg, W. K. (1995). Thermographic assessment of neuropathic facial pain. *Journal of Orofacial Pain, 9,* 138-146.

Gramling, S. E., Grayson, R. L., Sullivan, T. N., & Schwartz, S. (1997). Schedule-induced masseter EMG in facial pain subjects versus no-pain controls. *Physiology and Behavior, 61,* 301-309.

Hampf, G. (1990). Influence of cold pain in the hand on skin impedance, heart rate, and skin temperature. *Physiology and Behavior, 47,* 217-218.

Handwerker, H. O., & Kobal, G. (1993). Psychophysiology of experimentally induced pain. *Physiological Reviews, 73,* 639-671.

Hari, R., & Forss, N. (1999). Magnetoencephalography in the study of human somatosensory cortical processing. *Philosophical Transactions of the Royal Society of London: Series B. Biological Sciences, 354,* 1145-1154.

Hermann, C., & Blanchard, E. B. (1998). Psychophysiological reactivity in pediatric migraine patients and healthy controls. *Journal of Psychosomatic Research, 44,* 229-240.

Howe, F. (1983). Phantom limb pain: A reafferentiation syndrome. *Pain, 15,* 101-107.

Jalovaara, P., Niinimaki, T., & Vanharanta, H. (1995). Pocket-size, portable EMG device in the differentiation of low back pain patients. *European Spine Journal, 4,* 210-212.

Jamner, L. D., & Tursky, B. (1987). Discrimination between intensity and affective pain descriptors: A psychophysiological evaluation. *Pain, 30,* 271-283.

Jennings, J. R., Maricq, H. R., Canner, J., Thompson, B., Freedman, R. R., Wise, R., & Kaufmann, P. G. (1999). A thermal vascular test for distinguishing between patients with Raynaud's phenomenon and healthy controls: Raynaud's Treatment Study investigators. *Health Psychology, 18,* 421-426.

Jensen, R. (1999). Pathophysiological mechanisms of tension type headache: A review of epidemiological and experimental studies. *Cephalalgia, 19,* 602-621.

Jones, A., & Wolf, S. (1980). Treating chronic low back pain: EMG biofeedback-training during movement. *Physical Therapy, 60,* 58-63.

Kaas, J. H., & Florence, S. L. (1997). Mechanisms of reorganization in sensory systems of primates after peripheral nerve injury. *Advances in Neurology, 73,* 47-58.

Kapel, L, Glaros, A. G., & McGlynn, F. D. (1989). Psychophysiological dysfunction syndrome. *Journal of Behavioral Medicine, 12,* 397-406.

Keefe, F. J., & Gil, K. M. (1986). Behavioral concepts in the analysis of chronic pain syndromes. *Journal of Consulting and Clinical Psychology, 54,* 776-783.

Kerns, R. D., Turk, D. C., & Rudy, T. E. (1985). The West Haven-Yale Multidimensional Pain Inventory (WHYMPI). *Pain, 23,* 345-356.

Knost, B., Flor, H., & Birbaumer, N. (in press). The role of operant conditioning in chronic pain: An experimental investigation. *Pain.*

Knost, B., Flor, H., Braun, C., & Birbaumer, N. (1997). Cerebral processing of words and the development of chronic pain. *Psychophysiology, 34,* 474-481.

Kristeva-Feige, R., Grimm, C., Huppertz, H. J., Otte, M., Schreiber, A., Jager, D., Feige, B., Buchert, M., Hennig, J., Mergner, T., & Lücking, C. H. (1997). Reproducibility and validity of electric source localisation with high-resolution electroencephalography. *Electroencephalography and Clinical Neurophysiology, 103,* 652-660.

Kröner, B. (1984). Psychophysiologische Korrelate chronischer Kopfschmerzen [Psychophysiological correlates of chronic headache]. *Zeitschrift für Experimentelle und Angewandte Psychologie, 31,* 610-639.

Kropp, P., & Gerber, W. (1998). Prediction of migraine attacks using a slow cortical potential, the contingent negative variation. *Neuroscience Letters, 27,* 73-76.

Larbig, W., Elbert, T., Rockstroh, B., Lutzenberger, W., & Birbaumer, N. (1985). Elevated blood pressure and reduction of pain sensitivity. In J. F. Orlebeke, G. Mulder, & L. J. P. van Doornen (Eds.), *Psycho-*

physiology of cardiovascular control (pp. 350–365). New York: Plenum Press.

Larbig, W., Montoya, P., Flor, H., Bilow, H., Weller, S., & Birbaumer, N. (1996). Evidence for a change in neural processing in phantom limb pain patients. *Pain, 67,* 275–283.

Larsson, R., Oberg, P. A., & Larsson, S. E. (1999). Changes of trapezius muscle blood flow and electromyography in chronic neck pain due to trapezius myalgia. *Pain, 79,* 45–50.

LaSpina, I., Vignati, A., & Porazzi, D. (1997). Basilar artery migraine: Transcranial Doppler, EEG and SPECT from the aura phase to the end. *Headache, 37,* 43–47.

Leclaire, R., Esdaile, J. M., Hanley, J. A., Rossignol, M., & Bourdouxhe, M. (1996). Diagnostic accuracy of technologies used in low back pain assessment: Thermography, triaxial dynamometry, spinoscopy, and clinical examination. *Spine, 21,* 1325–1330.

Lorenz, J. (1998). Hyperalgesia or hypervigilance?: An evoked potential approach to the study of fibromyalgia syndrome. *Zeitschrift für Rheumatologie, 57*(Suppl. 2), 19–22.

Lorenz, J., Grasedyck, K., & Bromm, B. (1996). Middle and long latency somatosensory evoked potentials after painful laser stimulation in patients with fibromyalgia syndrome. *Electroencephalography and Clinical Neurophysiology, 100,* 165–168.

Lotze, M., Grodd, W., Birbaumer, N., Erb, M., Huse, E., & Flor, H. (1999). Does use of a myoelectric prosthesis reduce cortical reorganization and phantom limb pain? *Nature Neuroscience, 2,* 501–502.

Lundberg, U., Dohns, I. E., Melin, B., Sandsjo, L., Palmerud, G., Kadefors, R., Ekstrom, M., & Parr, D. (1999). Psychophysiological stress responses, muscle tension, and neck and shoulder pain among supermarket cashiers. *Journal of Occupational Health Psychology, 4,* 245–255.

Lundblad, I., Elert, J., & Gerdle, B. (1998). Worsening of neck and shoulder complaints in humans are correlated with frequency parameters of electromyogram recorded 1-year earlier. *European Journal of Applied Physiology, 79,* 7–16.

Lutzenberger, W., Flor, H., & Birbaumer, N. (1997). Enhanced dimensional complexity of the EEG during memory for personal pain in chronic pain patients. *Neuroscience Letters, 266,* 167–170.

MacDonald, A. G., Land, D. V., & Sturrock, R. D. (1994). Microwave thermography as a noninvasive assessment of disease activity in inflammatory arthritis. *Clinical Rheumatology, 13,* 589–592.

Magerl, W., Szolcsanyi, J., Westerman, R. A., & Handwerker, H. O. (1987). Laser Doppler flowmetry measurements of skin vasodilatation elicited by percutaneous electrical stimulation of nociception in humans. *Neuroscience Letters, 82,* 349–354.

Magnusson, M. L., Alkesiev, A., Wilder, D. G., Pope, M. H., Spratt, K., Lee, S. H., Goel, V. K., & Weinstein, J. N. (1996). Unexpected load and asymmetric posture as etiologic factors in low back pain. *European Spine Journal, 5,* 23–35.

Malmo, R. B., Shagass, C., & Davis, F. H. (1950). Symptom specificity and bodily reactions during psychiatric interview. *Psychosomatic Medicine, 12,* 362–372.

Mannion, A. F., Connolly, B., Wood, K., & Dolan, P. (1997). The use of surface EMG power spectral analysis in the evaluation of back muscle function. *Journal of Rehabilitation Research Development, 34,* 427–439.

May, A., Bahra, A., Büchel, C., Frackowiak, R. S., & Goadsby, P. J. (1998). Hypothalamic activation in cluster headache attacks. *Lancet, 325,* 275–278.

Mense, S., & Hoheisel, U. (1999). New developments in the understanding of the pathophysiology of muscle pain. *Journal of Musculoskeletal Pain, 7,* 13–24.

Miller, D. J. (1995). Comparison of electromyographic activity in the lumbar paraspinal muscles of subjects with and without chronic low back pain. *Physical Therapy, 65,* 1347–1354.

Mills, G. H., Davies, G. K., Getty, C. J., & Conay, J. (1986). The evaluation of liquid crystal thermography in the investigation of nerve root compression due to lumbosacral lateral spinal stenosis. *Spine, 11,* 420–432.

Miltner, W., Larbig, W., & Braun, C. (1988). Biofeedback of somatosensory event-related potentials: Can individual pain sensations be modified by biofeedback-induced self-control of event-related potentials? *Pain, 35,* 205–213.

Mirza, M., Tutus, A., Erdogan, F., Kula, M., Tomar, A., Silov, G., & Koseglu, E. (1998). Interictal SPECT with Tc-99m HMPAO studies in migraine patients. *Acta Neurologica Belgica, 98,* 190–194.

Möltner, A., Hölzl, R., & Strian, F. (1990). Heart rate changes as an autonomic change measure of the pain response. *Pain, 43,* 81–89.

Montoya, P., Larbig, W., Pulvermüller, F., Flor, H., & Birbaumer, N. (1996). Cortical correlates of classical semantic conditioning of pain. *Psychophysiology, 33,* 644–649.

Moulton, B., & Spence, S. H. (1992). Site-specific muscle hyper-reactivity in musicians with occupational upper limb pain. *Behaviour Research and Therapy, 30,* 375–386.

Myrtek, M., & Spital, S. (1986). Psychophysiological response patterns to single, double, and triple stressors. *Psychophysiology, 23,* 663–671.

Niedermeyer, E., & Lopez da Silva, F. (1998). *Electroencephalography: Basic principles, clinical applications, and related fields* (4th ed.). Philadelphia: Lippincott Williams & Wilkins.

Obrist, P. A. (1976). The cardiovascular–behavioral interaction—as it appears today. *Psychophysiology, 13,* 95–107.

Oddson, L. I., Giphart, J. E., Buijs, R. J., Roy, S. H., Taylor, H. P., & De Luca, C. J. (1997). Development of new protocols and analysis procedures for the assessment of LBP by surface EMG techniques. *Journal of Rehabilitation Research and Development, 43,* 415–426.

Oelkers, R., Grosser, K., Lang, E., Geisslinger, G., Kobal, G., Brune, K., & Lotsch, J. (1999). Visual evoked potentials in migraine patients: Alterations depend on pattern spatial frequency. *Brain, 122,* 1147–1155.

Ohrbach, R., Blascovich, J., Gale, E. N., McCall, W. D., Jr., & Dworkin, S. F. (1998). Psychophysiological assessments of stress in chronic pain: Comparison of stressful stimuli and of response systems. *Journal of Dental Research, 77,* 1840–1850.

Peters, M., & Schmidt, A. J. (1991). Psychophysiological responses to repeated acute pain stimulation in chronic low back pain patients. *Journal of Psychosomatic Research, 35,* 59–74.

Pritchard, D. W., & Wood, M. M. (1984). EMG levels
in the occipito-frontalis muscles under an experimental
stress condition. *Biofeedback and Self-Regulation, 8,*
165-175.

Rieke, K., Gallen, C. C., Baker, L., Dalessio, D. J.,
Schwartz, B. J., Torruella, A. K., & Otis, S. M. (1993).
Transcranial Doppler ultrasound and magnetoencephalography in migraine. *Journal of Neuroimaging,
3,* 109-114.

Rojahn, J., & Gerhards, F. (1986). Subjective stress sensitivity and physiological responses to an aversive auditory stimulus in migraine and control subjects. *Journal of Behavioral Medicine, 9,* 203-212.

Roy, S. H., De Luca, C. J., Emley, M., Oddson, L. I., Buijs,
R. J., Levins, J. A., Newcombe, D. S., & Jabre, J. F.
(1997). Classification of back muscle impairment
based on the surface electromyographic signal. *Journal of Rehabilitation Research and Development, 34,*
405-414.

Salamy, J. G., Wolk, D. J., & Shucard, D. W. (1983).
Psychophysiological assessment of statements about
pain. *Psychophysiology, 20,* 579-584.

Sanchez del Rio, M., Bakker, D., Wu, O., Agosti, R.,
Mitsikostas, D. D., Ostergaard, L., Wells, W. A.,
Rosen, B. R., Sorensen, G., Moskowitz, M. A., &
Cutrer, F. M. (1999). Perfusion weighted imaging
during migraine: Spontaneous visual aura and head-
ache. *Cephalalgia, 19,* 701-707.

Schwartz, M., & Associates. (1995). *Biofeedback: A practitioner's guide* (2nd ed.). New York: Guilford Press.

Sherman, R. A. (1997). *Phantom limb pain.* New York:
Plenum Press.

Sherman, R. A., Arena, J. G., Searle, J. R., & Ginther,
J. R. (1991). Development of an ambulatory recorder
for evaluation of muscle tension related low back pain
and fatigue in soldiers normal environment. *Military
Medicine, 156,* 245-248.

Sherman, R. A., & Bruno, G. M. (1987). Concurrent
variation of burning phantom limb and stump pain
with near surface blood flow in the stump. *Orthopedics, 10,* 1395-1402.

Sherman, R. A., Griffin, V. D., Evans, C. B., & Grana,
A. S. (1992). Temporal relationships between changes
in phantom limb pain intensity and changes in surface electromyogram of the residual limb. *International
Journal of Psychophysiology, 13,* 71-77.

Sherman, R. A., Woerman, A., & Karstetter, K. W. (1996).
Comparative effectiveness of videothermography, contact thermography, and infrared beam thermography
for scanning relative skin temperature. *Journal of Rehabilitation Research and Development, 33,* 377-386.

Siniatchkin, M., Gerber, W. D., Kropp, P., & Vein, A.
(1998). Contingent negative variation in patients with
chronic daily headache. *Cephalalgia, 18,* 565-569.

Sternbach, R. A. (1968). *Pain: A psychophysiological analysis.* New York: Academic Press.

Svensson, P., Graven-Nielsen, T., Matre, D., & Arendt-
Nielsen, L. (1998). Experimental muscle pain does not
cause long-lasting increases in resting electromyographic activity. *Muscle and Nerve, 21,* 1382-1389.

Thompson, J. M., Erickson, R. P., Madson, T. J., &
Offord, K. P. (1989). Stability of hand-held surface
electrodes. *Biofeedback and Self-Regulation, 14,* 55-62.

Thompson, J. M., Madson, T. J., & Erickson, R. P. (1991).
EMG muscle scanning: Comparison to attached surface electrodes. *Biofeedback and Self-Regulation, 16,*
167-179.

Traue, H. C., Bischoff, C., & Zenz, H. (1985). Sozialer
Streß, Muskelspannung und Spannungskopfschmerz
[Social stress, muscle tension, and tension headache].
Zeitschrift für Klinische Psychologie, 15, 57-70.

Traue, H. C., Kessler, M., & Cram, J. R. (1992). Surface
EMG topography and pain distribution in pre-chronic
back pain patients. *International Journal of Psychosomatics, 39,* 18-27.

Turk, D. C., & Flor, H. (1999) Chronic pain: A bio-
behavioral perspective. In R. J. Gatchel & D. C. Turk
(Eds.), *Psychosocial factors in pain* (pp. 18-34). New
York: Guilford Press.

Turk, D. C., & Rudy, T. E. (1987). Toward a comprehensive assessment of chronic pain patients. *Behaviour
Research and Therapy, 25,* 237-249.

Turpin, G. (Ed.). (1989). *Handbook of clinical psychophysiology.* Chichester, England: Wiley.

Uematsu, S., Hendeler, N., & Hungerford, D. (1981).
Thermography and electromyography in the differential diagnosis of chronic pain syndrome and reflex
sympathetic dystrophy. *Electromyography and Clinical
Neurophysiology, 21,* 165-182.

Veiersted, K. B., Westgaard, R. H., & Andersen, P. (1993).
Electromyographic evaluation of muscular work pattern as a predictor of trapezius myalgia. *Scandinavian
Journal of Work and Environmental Health, 19,* 284-
290.

Villringer, A. (1997). Understanding functional neuroimaging methods based on neurovascular coupling.
Advances in Experimental Medicine and Biology, 413,
177-193.

Vlaeyen, J. W., Seelen, H. A., Peters, M., de Jong, P.,
Arntz, E., Beisiegel, E., & Weber, W. E. (1999). Fear
of movement/(re)injury and muscular reactivity in
chronic low back pain patients: An experimental investigation. *Pain, 82,* 297-304.

Wall, P. D., & Melzack, R. (Eds.). (2000). *Textbook of pain*
(4th ed.). Edinburgh: Churchill Livingstone.

Wallace, L. M. (1984). Psychological preparation as a
method of reducing the stress of surgery. *Journal of
Human Stress, 10,* 62-77.

Wolf, S. L., & Basmajian, J. V. (1978). Assessment of
paraspinal electromyographic activity in normal subjects and in chronic back pain patients using a muscle
biofeedback device. In E. Asmussen & K. Jorgenson
(Eds.), *Biomechanics: VI. Proceedings of the Sixth International Congress of Biomechanics* (pp. 319-324).
Baltimore: University Park Press.

Wolf, S. L., Nacht, M., & Kelly, J. L. (1982). EMG feedback training during dynamic movement for low back
pain patients. *Behavior Therapy, 13,* 395-496.

Wolf, S. L., Wolf, L. B., & Segal, R. L. (1989). The relationship of extraneous movements to lumbar paraspinal muscle activity: Implications for EMG biofeedback training applications to low back pain patients.
Biofeedback and Self-Regulation, 14, 63-73.

Zimmermann, M. (1993). Pathophysiological mechanisms
of fibromyalgia. *Clinical Journal of Pain, 7*(Suppl 1),
S8-S15.

Chapter 6

Pain Assessment in Children and Adolescents

PATRICIA A. McGRATH
JOANNE GILLESPIE

Although pain assessment is an intrinsic component of pain management, few health care providers routinely use objective methods to evaluate children's pain. Anecdotal information suggests several reasons for the disparity between acknowledging the importance of regular pain assessment in theory and failing to assess pain in clinical practice. First, pain is a subjective experience, and some health care providers still assume that children cannot reliably provide meaningful information about their pain. Other providers perceive pain scales as a cumbersome addition to already overwhelming responsibilities. Still other providers are unsure which of the myriad pain measures are best to use. Different measures may be used in different units throughout a hospital, so that there is no common language for interpreting the resulting pain scores and communicating meaningful information about children's pain or pain relief. Even when a child's pain score is charted, staff members often disregard the pain score when making decisions about pain management.

Pain assessment is further compromised at some centers by a lack of commitment at the executive board and administrative levels. Although dedicated to comprehensive (and often family-centered) child care and responsive to quality assurance guidelines, the delivery of effective and continuous pain control may not be a major priority of the hospital. Instead, this responsibility is diffused to

different groups with no clear accountability for identifying gaps in care and ensuring that the most efficient therapies are used. Administration may also not provide support for required education on how to select the most appropriate pain scales, or how to administer pain measures consistently so that the resulting pain scores are valid. Thus the health care environment does not support the interest and efforts of individual staff members to incorporate pain measurement into clinical practice.

Despite the attitudinal, logistic, and administrative reasons for why pain assessment in children has been better supported in theory than in practice, many health care providers are now attempting to change practice. They are interested in using "state-of-the-art" pain scales for monitoring children, interpreting pain scores to guide therapeutic decisions, and documenting treatment effectiveness. Yet accurate pain assessment requires careful consideration of the nature of a child's pain perception, as well as knowledge of the available pain scales and their appropriateness for different types of pain and ages of children.

THE NATURE OF A CHILD'S PAIN

A child's pain system was once believed to be a relatively rigid and straightforward nervous system, in that any tissue damage initiated a sequence of neural events, which inevitably produced pain. Moreover, the strength of the subsequent pain was believed to be predetermined by the intensity of the tissue damage. However, this belief has been refuted during the past two decades by an impressive array of anatomical, physiological, neurochemical, medical, and psychological research (for reviews, see Bush & Harkins, 1991; McGrath, 1990; Ross & Ross, 1988; Schechter, Berde, & Yaster, 1993). We now know that the nociceptive system functions as an active and complex integrative mechanism, not as a fixed and rigid system that passively relays information.

The nociceptive system is plastic because it has the capacity to respond differently to the same amount of tissue damage. The neural activity initiated by tissue damage can be modified by a diverse array of physical and psychological factors, so that a child's pain cannot be predicted solely by the nature of his or her damage. Even routine muscular injections do not necessarily cause the same pain for all children. Instead, a child's age, sex, developmental level, prior pain experience, and relevant contextual and psychological factors will affect how his or her nociceptive system responds to tissue damage. Children can experience different pains, depending on the context in which they receive the injections. When children use a simple coping strategy or are actively involved in preparing an injection site (e.g., choosing the arm, cleaning site with an alcohol swab), they will generally experience less pain.

A model depicting the factors that affect a child's pain perception is shown in Figure 6.1. Some factors are relatively stable for a child, such as sex, age, cognitive level, and family background (shown in the closed box). These child characteristics shape how children generally interpret and experience the various sensations evoked by tissue damage. In contrast, the cognitive, behavioral, and emotional factors (shown in the shaded boxes) are not stable. They represent a unique interaction between the child experiencing pain and the context in which the pain is experienced (McGrath, 1990; Ross & Ross, 1988). These situational factors can vary dynamically, depending on the specific circumstances in which children experience pain. Even though the pain source may remain constant, the particular set of situational factors is unique for each occurrence of pain. Moreover, unlike the stable child characteristics, health care providers can change these factors and lessen children's pain dramatically.

What children understand, what they do, and how they feel have a profound impact on their pain experience. Differences in situational factors may account for why the same tissue damage can evoke

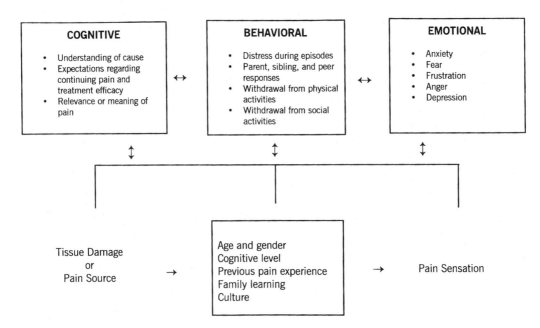

FIGURE 6.1. A model of the cognitive, behavioral, and emotional factors that affect a child's pain.

pains that vary in intensity, and may partially explain why proven analgesics can vary in effectiveness for different children and for the same child at different times. In addition, some situational factors are the primary causes of certain recurrent and persistent pains in otherwise pain-free and healthy children (McGrath & Hillier, 2001).

The gradual recognition that a child's pain is not simply and directly related to the nature and extent of tissue damage has profound implications for the assessment and management of children's pain. Clinical emphasis shifts from an exclusive focus on the source of tissue damage to a more comprehensive focus, not only on the source of tissue damage, but also on the relevant situational factors that modify nociceptive processing. Pain assessment is inextricably linked to pain management. Unless we assess the factors that modify a child's pain, our attempts to control it will necessarily be inadequate. Because the same noxious stimulus, whether invasive procedure, disease, or trauma, does not produce equivalent pain in all children, we cannot control pain by gearing our interventions solely to the type of tissue damage.

DEVELOPMENTAL CONSIDERATIONS

From birth, infants exhibit an array of distress behaviors and physiological changes in response to tissue damage. Some of these overt distress responses seem to be general for all pain situations, while other responses may be more specifically related to the particular type of tissue damage (Craig & Grunau, 1993). The magnitude and nature of distress responses change as infants mature, so that there are developmental differences in behavioral responses and pain expression for neonates, infants, toddlers, children, and adolescents. Although it is possible to assess distress and pain from infancy throughout adolescence, developmental differences influence our selection of pain measures.

At a very early age, children recognize that pain is an unpleasant sensory and emotional experience. Their understanding and descriptions of pain naturally depend on their age, cognitive level, and previous pain experience. They learn to judge the strength and unpleasantness of pain in comparison to sensations that they have already experienced. As is the case for adults, the nature and diversity of children's pain experience form their frame of reference for perceiving all new pain. Yet, whereas adults generally have a wide frame of reference of pain experience, children's frames of reference are constantly changing as they mature and sustain more diverse types of tissue damage. Table 6.1 lists samples of the minimum and maximum pains that children report. As shown, young children usually report childhood injuries for their "least" and "most" pains that generally do not differ very much in the severity of tissue damage. As children mature and experience more pains, they report injuries that do differ greatly. We must remember that they use a pain scale based on their experience. When young children use the upper end of a scale to rate their pain, they are indicating its strength to them. Older children and adults may rate the same injury or procedure as less painful because they have experienced a wider variety of pains. For young children, a particular injury or procedure may cause their strongest pain to date.

Children learn to describe the various aspects of their pain sensations (temporal, quality, spatial, and intensity) in the same manner that they learn specific words to describe the different sounds,

TABLE 6.1. Children's Minimum and Maximum Pain Experiences

Sex	Age	Minimum	Maximum
Female	6	"Fell down running."	"Fell off bike . . . had great big scab on knee . . . bled a lot and hurt."
Male	10	"I stubbed my toe."	"I got hit by a hardball by a fast pitch on the thigh."
Female	14	"Got bitten by an ant."	"Got glass pieces in my foot and had 10 stitches (age 4)."
Male	17	"Paper cut."	"Being beaten up."
Female	17	"Scratch from my kitten, not deep."	"Breaking my elbow really badly, I had an operation on it."

Note. Data from McGrath (1990).

tastes, smells, and colors they experience. Most children can communicate meaningful information about their pain. But their ability to describe specific pain features—the quality (aching, burning, pounding, sharp), intensity (mild to severe), duration and frequency (a few seconds to years), location (diffuse location on surface of the skin to more precise localization internally), and unpleasantness (mild annoyance to an intolerable discomfort)—develops as they mature. Their understanding of pain and the pain language that they learn develop through their exposure to the words and expressions used by their families and peers, as well as to characters depicted in books, videos, and movies.

Children naturally differ in the words they use to describe their pains because of differences in their backgrounds, previous pain experiences, and learning. Yet, although the sophistication and ingenuity of their pain descriptions (like the quality and diversity of their pain experiences) vary idiosyncratically, all children seem to understand both the intrinsic physical and emotional aspects of hurting. Table 6.2 lists the definitions of pain for the same five children whose responses to "What is the least and most pain you have experienced?" are shown in Table 6.1. The sophistication of their definitions parallels their chronological age.

TABLE 6.2. Children's Definitions of Pain

Sex	Age	Definition
Female	6	"When you fell, did you have a big scab or a little scab?"
Male	10	"An uncomfortable feeling when something is injured."
Female	14	"A feeling of hurt physically or mentally by something."
Male	17	"Either physical or emotional. The physical is self-explanatory and is healed naturally, while the emotional is attained by life circumstances which sadden, anger, and disturb. It is not healed naturally, but must be healed with an effort or fade with time."
Female	17	"The sensation completely opposite to comfort. It can be physical or emotional. When my father died, I felt deep emotional pain that was stronger than any physical discomfort I had ever experienced."

Note. Data from McGrath (1990).

Younger children use concrete examples in response to "What is pain?" As children mature, their definitions change from a primarily physical understanding to a more abstract understanding, composed of both physical and psychological components (Gaffney, 1988; Gaffney & Dunne, 1986, 1987; Harbeck & Peterson, 1992).

Children's level of cognitive development determines how they are able to understand pain. The recognition that children's concepts of pain follow a consistent developmental pattern provides a framework not only for evaluating their understanding of pain, but also for selecting pain measures that are age-appropriate. It is essential to use children's own terminology in communicating with children about pain. Most toddlers (approximately 2 years of age) can communicate the presence of pain, using words learned from their parents to describe the sensations they feel when they hurt themselves. They use concrete analogies to describe their perceptions. Gradually children learn to differentiate and describe three levels of pain intensity—basically "a little," "some" or "medium," and "a lot." By the age of 5, most children can differentiate a wider range of pain intensities and they can use simple quantitative scales to rate their pain intensity.

Thus administration of a pain measure for children requires a basic appreciation of children's different developmental stages and their cognitive levels. Basic interviewing skills are required to ensure that children are comfortable and truly understand the questions. Questions should be spaced so that difficult and emotionally arousing items are interspersed with easier items. When children are asked to rate a specific dimension of pain (e.g., its intensity), they should first complete a brief calibration task to ensure that they understand the particular concept (e.g., rating its magnitude). A brief calibration task enables the clinician to assess whether a child can use the scale and make meaningful judgments about his or her perceptions. Table 6.3 shows a calibration task that we use in our clinical practice and research program.

We explain the pain measure in simple words. In Table 6.3, the intensity measure is the Coloured Analogue Scale (CAS), introduced with the following instructions:

"This scale is like a ruler. The bottom, where it is small and there is hardly any color at all, means no pain at all. The top, where it is large, very red and a long way from the bottom means the most pain. I want you to slide the marker up the scale to show me how much your pain hurts."

TABLE 6.3. Calibration Instructions to Evaluate Whether Children Can Use a Pain Intensity Scale

Informal method

To obtain a child's pain rating, introduce scale with simple instructions.

For the CAS, start with the marker at 0. Say: "This scale is like a ruler. The bottom, where it is small and there is hardly any color at all, means no pain at all. The top, where it is large, very red, and a long way from the bottom, means the most pain. I want you to slide the marker up the scale to show me how much your pain hurts."

To ensure that children know how to use the scale, ask children to use it to rate the pain caused by a few common injuries (which should cause pains of different strengths). When children have moved the marker to indicate their pain level, turn the scale over and record the number. When children say that they have no pain, still have them use the scale ("Show me where that is").

Formal method

Ask children: "Have you . . .	If yes, how much did it hurt?
1. ". . . fallen off your bike and banged your leg?"	—
2. ". . . had a bee sting?"	—
3. ". . . had a headache?"	—
4. ". . . had a little bruise?"	—
5. "By the way, what was the strongest pain you ever had?"	
6. "How much did it hurt?"	—

When administering the pain scale

Introduce it in a consistent manner. For the CAS, present the scale with the marker set at the bottom of the scale. Never influence children's responses. Document a child's pain score on his or her chart.

As shown in Table 6.3, the calibration task begins with practice questions about events that most children have experienced. For these and all questions, children indicate whether they have experienced the event. If so, they are asked whether it hurt, and if so, how strong the pain felt. Children use the CAS to rate the pain strength and the Facial Affective Scale to rate the unpleasant quality. The events listed represent common childhood pain experiences; children's pain ratings should show that they can discriminate among items by different pain scores. Visual inspection of the scatter of their ratings, with higher ratings for items that usually cause stronger tissue damage, demonstrates that children can use the measure. For a more rigorous evaluation of children's calibration responses, a child's pain ratings may be compared to age- and gender-normative responses. (Note: These normative data will be supplied upon request.)

PAIN MEASURES FOR CHILDREN

Many different types of pain measures have been developed and validated for use with infants, children, and adolescents. (For reviews, see Beyer & Wells, 1989; Champion, Goodenough, von Baeyer, & Thomas, 1998; McGrath, 1990; McGrath, 1998; Royal College of Nursing Institute, 1999; Ross & Ross, 1988; Sweet & McGrath, 1998.) Because space limitations preclude a comprehensive description of each measure, our focus is on the measures available for clinical use. Particular emphasis is placed on those measures that are appropriate for assessing pain intensity and versatile for use in different hospital units. (For reviews of the analysis of cry and facial expressions as pain measures, please see Craig & Grunau, 1993; Fuller, Conner, & Horii, 1990; Grunau & Craig, 1990; Johnston & O'Shaughnessy, 1988; see also Craig, Prkachin, & Grunau, Chapter 9, this volume.)

The criteria for an accurate pain measure for children are similar to those required for any measuring instrument. A pain measure must be valid, in that it unequivocally measures a specific dimension of a child's pain, so that changes in a child's pain ratings reflect meaningful differences in a child's pain experience. The measure must be reliable, in that it provides consistent and trustworthy pain ratings regardless of the time of testing, the clinical setting, or who is administering the measure. The measure must be relatively free from bias, in that children use it similarly regardless of differences in how they may wish to please adults. The pain measure should be practical and versatile for assessing different types of pain and for use in diverse clinical settings.

Children's pain measures are classified as physiological, behavioral, and psychological, depending on what is monitored—physical parameters, such as heart or respiration rate; distress behaviors, such as crying or facial expression; or children's own descriptions of what they are experiencing. Both physiological and behavioral measures provide indirect estimates of pain, because the presence or strength of pain is inferred solely from the type and magnitude of responses to a noxious stimulus. In contrast, psychological measures can provide direct estimates for many different dimensions of pain—intensity, quality, affect, duration, frequency—and provide valuable information on the impact of pain and suffering.

Behavioral Pain Measures

Most behavioral pain measures have been designed to obtain concise records of how children respond when they experience pain. Usually trained staff members observe children in some painful situation (e.g., during invasive medical procedures, after surgery, or throughout a designated time period for children with chronic pain) and document any behaviors that seem caused by the pain. The distress behaviors that are observed in many children are subsequently identified as pain behaviors. Itemized behavioral checklists/scales are then developed listing the behaviors specific for each type of pain. Clinicians complete such a checklist by noting which behaviors occur and by ranking their intensity on a 0–2 or 0–4 scale. The rationale is that an objective evaluation of children's pain behaviors should provide an accurate estimate of the strength of their pain experiences. The vast majority of behavioral scales were developed for acute procedural or postoperative pain in otherwise healthy children. More recently, behavioral scales are being developed in consultation with parents and caregivers for special populations, such as children who are cognitively or physically impaired (Hunt, Goldman, Mastroyannopoulou, & Seers, 1999).

The intensity scores for each of the behaviors are then added to produce a composite pain score for a child. In some scales, researchers have assigned specific weights to the various behaviors that reflect different pain strengths (e.g., crying at needle insertion may have a higher weight as a pain behavior than just grimacing). In these scales, the weighted scores for each observed behavior are summed to obtain a composite pain score.

The major behavioral measures available for infants and children are shown below in Tables 6.4 and 6.5, respectively. Each table lists the formal scale name, acronym, type of pain that was monitored in developing the scale, behaviors that are monitored, and type of pain score obtained. The amount of time required to monitor children's behavior, the different pains used to develop scales, the intensity ratings for each pain behavior, the range of possible pain scores, and the amount of training required for health care providers all vary greatly for the different scales. At present, no one scale is appropriate for all children and for all situations in which they experience pain. Instead, scales should be selected first on the basis of the type of pain (acute injury, acute procedural, acute postoperative, or persistent) that will be monitored. Then the specific clinical objectives will guide the choice among scales validated for that type of pain.

When multiple staff members intend to monitor children to evaluate their pain levels at regular intervals during their hospitalization, then they require a relatively simple and straightforward scale (a few distress behaviors to note, a brief time period for observation, and an easy calculation of a pain score). When staff members are investigating the effectiveness of varied pain control therapies, then they may require a more sophisticated scale with many subcategories of distress behaviors and physiological parameters, with clearly delineated descriptions of which changes in behavior match the different intensity ratings that can be applied, and a more complicated scoring system of both subcategories and a global pain score. Specially trained raters may be needed to monitor pain at frequent intervals to determine the temporal pattern of pain and pain relief. This methodology should be more sensitive to subtle changes in children's pain experience, which might go undetected with a scale that is adequate for routine clinical use.

Regardless of the specific pain scale used, it is also important to note the context in which infants are suffering. Their disease or health condition, concomitant drug therapy, and the other distress sources in the health care environment may limit their responsivity and affect the validity of the pain score as a meaningful index of their pain. It is essential that health care providers use their content expertise to carefully consider the type of distress behaviors in a selected pain scale, to ensure that these behaviors are likely to be unaffected by the context and thus sensitive primarily to changes in a child's pain experience.

Behavioral Pain Scales for Infants

Fourteen behavioral pain scales for infants are listed in Table 6.4. The validity, reliability, or both of each scale have been demonstrated in at least one study. Although most scales assess general vocalizations, expressive body movements, and facial expressions during a presumed period of pain (e.g., during an injection or postoperatively), some include an assessment of physiological parameters or the infant's consolability and interactions with caregivers.

Several methods have been used to demonstrate the validity and/or reliability of infant pain scales. Each of the studies listed in Table 6.4 includes some demonstration of these properties. The construct or content validity is often demonstrated initially by comparing pain scores before and after infants experience a painful stimulus (e.g., heel stick, surgery) or before and after they receive an analgesic. The concurrent validity is often demonstrated by comparing pain scores on the new scale with ratings on another established scale. The reliability of behavioral methods is usually determined by comparing the pain scores obtained by different raters for the same infant (interrater reliability) and by correlating the scores among the individual behavioral items (internal consistency).

For example, the validity of the Postoperative Pain Scale was demonstrated initially when infants' pain scores decreased after small doses of intraoperative opioids (Barrier, Attia, Mayer, Amiel-Tison, & Shnider, 1989). The COMFORT Scale was developed as a behavioral measure for those infants and children whose behaviors were restricted due to their medical care (Ambuel, Hamlett, Marx, & Blumer, 1992). The interrater reliability was high, and the concurrent validity (COMFORT pain scores in comparison to score on a global visual analogue scale) was high. The construct validity of the Premature Infant Pain Profile was demonstrated by comparing the pain scores for an invasive heel stick in comparison to those for a sham procedure, and its internal consistency was good (Stevens, Johnston, Petryshen, & Taddio, 1996). The validity of the Toddler–Preschooler Postoperative Pain Scale was demonstrated initially when children's pain scores decreased after administration of postoperative analgesics, and its interrater reliability was good (Tarbell, Cohen, & Marsh, 1992).

Behavioral Pain Scales for Children

Ten behavioral pain scales for children are listed in Table 6.5 on page 106. These scales have been developed to measure children's acute pain during invasive procedures, postoperative pain, disease-related cancer pain, and acute injury pain caused by normal childhood play activities. As shown in Table 6.5, some scales are very similar. Since our understanding of how children express pain (through their words and behaviors) is continually increasing, pain scales are often revised to reflect our increased knowledge, so that there may be revised versions developed by the same team of investigators or new scales that are essentially modified versions by different investigators. The number of revised scales may initially complicate the selection of a pain measure, particularly when different scales have similar or almost identical names. Thus, after a scale has been selected, it is important to check that the version is current and that it (not just the original) has been validated in at least one study.

As shown in the "Pain Behaviors" column in Table 6.5, some behaviors may also reflect children's fear, anxiety, and overall distress as well as their pain. In essence, these scales provide reliable, valid, and quantitative indices of children's overt distress. They enable health care providers to evaluate children's distress objectively, with minimal response bias. Some behavioral scales provide well-defined descriptions of different types of distress behavior as a foundation, so that health care providers can more easily use uniform criteria (rather than only their interpretation of the children's distress) when they observe children and rate their pain.

Similar to infant pain scales, several methods have been used to demonstrate the validity and/ or reliability of behavioral pain scales in children. For example, the concurrent validity of the Observational Scale of Behavioral Distress was shown by correlating it with children's ratings on self-report pain scales and with changes in children's heart rate (Jay, Elliot, Woody, & Siegal, 1991). The construct validity of the FLACC was initially demonstrated by comparing pain scores before and after opioid administration (Merkel, Voepel-Lewis, Shayevitz, & Malviya, 1997). The preliminary validation of the Child Facial Coding System included a comparison of the facial action summary scores with an observer's visual analogue scale rating of the child's pain level (Gilbert et al., 1999).

Most behavioral scales are more appropriate for use with children aged 6 to 10 than with ado-

TABLE 6.4. Behavioral Pain Scales for Infants and Toddlers (Listed in Chronological Order)

Name	Pain type	Method/time	Pain behaviors	Pain score	Comments
Infant Pain Behavior Rating Scale (IPBRS; Craig et al., 1984)	Procedural (injection)	Phase sampling (three periods in procedure)	Four, with 13 subcategories (main–vocalizations, facial expressions, torso and limb)	Mean percentage of intervals during which pain behaviors are observed	Also records nurse and parent behaviors
Objective Pain Scale (OPS) or Pain Discomfort Scale (Broadman et al., 1988)	Postoperative	Time sampling (5-min intervals)	Five: cry, movement, agitation, posture, arterial blood pressure	Behaviors rated 0–2 in intensity; pain score calculated for each interval, max. 10	Also for children
Postoperative Pain Scale (POPS; Attia et al., 1987; Barrier et al., 1989)	Postoperative	Time sampling	Ten: sleep, facial expression, quality of cry, consolability, sociability, sucking, spontaneous excitability, spontaneous motor activity, flexion of fingers and toes, tone	Behaviors rated 0–2 in intensity, max. 20	Infants 1–7 mos
Nursing Assessment of Pain Intensity (NAPI; Joyce et al.; Stevens, 1990, 1994)	Postoperative	Time sampling	Four: verbal/vocal, body movement, facial expression, touching of surgical site	Behaviors rated 0–2 in intensity, max. 8	Adapted from CHEOPS (see Table 6.5)
Neonatal Infant Pain Scale (NIPS; Lawrence et al., 1991)	Procedural	Phase sampling (three 1-min periods in procedure)	Six: facial expression, cry, breathing, arm movement, leg movement, arousal state	Five behaviors rated 0–1 in intensity, cry rated 0–2, max. 7	For preterm and full-term neonates
Pain Rating Scale (PRS; Joyce et al., 1994; Rafferty & Moser, 1991)	Postoperative	Time sampling	Six constellations of behaviors stratified to reflect different levels of pain, based on infants' global behaviors and interactions with caregivers	Constellations rated 0–6 in intensity, max. 6	Developed for infants from 1 mo to 1 yr
COMFORT Scale (Ambuel et al., 1992)	Distress in pediatric ICU patients	Time sampling (2 min)	Eight: arterial blood pressure, heart rate, muscle tone, facial tension, alertness, calmness/agitation, respiratory behavior, physical movement	Behaviors rated 0–5 in intensity, max. 40	Infants to adolescents

Scale	Purpose	Method	Behaviors	Scoring	Population
CRIES (Krechel & Bildner, 1995)	Postoperative	Time sampling	Five: cry, oxygen saturation levels, heart rate, blood pressure, and sleeplessness	Behaviors rated 0–2 in intensity, max. 10	Neonates
Premature Infant Pain Profile (PIPP; Stevens et al., 1996)	Procedural and postoperative	Time sampling (15–30 sec)	Seven: gestational age, behavioral state, heart rate, O_2, brow bulge, eye squeeze, nasolabial furrow	Behaviors rated 0–4 in intensity	Premature infants
Modified Infant Pain Scale (MIPS; Buchholz et al., 1998)	Postoperative	Time sampling (5 min)	Thirteen: sleep, facial expression, quality of cry, spontaneous motor activity, excitability, flexion of fingers and toes, sucking, tone, consolability, sociability, physiological changes (heart rate, blood pressure, O_2)	Behaviors rated 0–2 in intensity, max. 26	Infants
Toddler-Preschooler Postoperative Pain Scale (TPPPS; Tarbell, Cohen, & Marsh, 1992)	Postoperative	Time sampling (5-min period)	Seven: verbal pain (cry, groan) facial expression (open mouth, squint, brow bulge) bodily expression (restless motor behavior, rub or touch painful area)	Each behavior scored as 0 (absent) or 1 (present), max. 7	Children 1–5 yrs
Scale for Use in Newborns (SUN; Blauer & Gerstmann, 1998)	Procedural	Time sampling (7 min)	Seven: central nervous system state, breathing, movement, tone, face, heart rate, and mean blood pressure changes	Behaviors rated 0–4 in intensity, max. 28	Neonates
Preverbal, Early Verbal Pediatric Pain Scale (PEPPS; Schultz et al., 1999)	Postoperative	Time sampling (2–3 min)	Seven: body posture, heart rate, facial, cry, consolability/state of restfulness, sociability, sucking/feeding	Six behaviors rated 0–4 in intensity, sucking rated 0–2, max. 26	Toddlers, 12–24 mos
Children's and Infants' Postoperative Pain Scale (CHIPPS; Büttner & Finke, 2000)	Postoperative (report of 7 studies)	Time sampling (5–10 min intervals for 1 hr)	Five: crying, facial expression, posture of the trunk, posture of the legs, motor restlessness	Five behaviors rated 0–2 in intensity, max. 10	Infants and children, 1–5 yrs

TABLE 6.5. Behavioral Pain Measures for Children

Name	Pain type	Method/time	Pain behaviors	Pain score	Comments
Procedural Behavioral Rating Scale–Revised (PBRS-R; Katz, Kellerman, & Siegel, 1980)	Procedural (LP and BMA)[a]	Phase sampling (three periods in procedure)	Thirteen: muscle tension, screaming, crying, restraint used, pain verbalized, anxiety verbalized, verbal stalling, physical resistance, trembling, groaning, wincing, flinching, nausea/vomit	Composite score based on number of observed behaviors, max. 13	Children 6–10 yrs
Observational Scale of Behavioral Distress (OSBD; Jay, Ozolins, Elliott, & Caldwell, 1983)	Procedural (BMA)	Continual observation	Eleven: cry (1.5), scream (4.0), physical restraint (4.0), verbal resistance (2.5), requests emotional support (2.0), muscular rigidity (2.5), verbal fear (2.5), verbal pain (2.5), flail (4.0), nervous behavior (1.0), information seeking (1.5)	Weighted scores for each behavior, 0–4	Children 6–10 yrs; revised version of PBSR-R
Procedure Behavior Checklist (PBCL; LeBaron & Zeltzer, 1984)	Procedural (LP and BMA)	Phase sampling (three periods in procedure)	Eight: muscle tension, screaming, crying, restraint used, pain verbalized, anxiety verbalized, verbal stalling, physical resistance	Behaviors rated 1–5 in intensity, subscores for each period, max. 40	Children and adolescents, 6–18 yrs
Children's Hospital of Eastern Ontario Pain Scale (CHEOPS; P. J. McGrath et al., 1985)	Postoperative	Time sampling (multiple 30-sec periods)	Six: cry, facial, verbal, torso, touch behavior, legs	Behaviors rated 0–2 or 0–3 in intensity	Toddlers and children 1–7 yrs
Douleur de l'Enfant Goustave–Roussy (DEGR; Gauvain-Piquard et al., 1987)	Cancer pain	Time sampling (4-hr period)	Seven: pain (e.g., somatic complaint) Six: depression (e.g., lack of expressiveness) Four: anxiety (e.g., moodiness)	Behaviors rated 0–4 in intensity	Children 2–6 yrs

Instrument	Setting	Sampling	Behaviors/items	Scoring	Age
Princess Margaret Hospital Pain Assessment Tool (PMH-PAT; Robertson, 1993)	Postoperative	Time sampling	Five: facial expression, nurse's assessment, position in bed, sounds, self-assessment	Behaviors rated 0–2 in intensity, max. 10	Children 7–14 yrs
Postoperative Pain Measure for Parents (Chambers et al., 1996)	Postoperative	Period sampling (morning, afternoon, evening)	A 29-item checklist, reduced to 15 based on correlations with child-rated pain	Behaviors scored when present, max. 15	Children 7–12 yrs
FLACC (Facial expression, Leg movement, Activity, Cry, Consolability; Merkel et al., 1997)	Postoperative	Time sampling (5 min)	Five, as listed in scale name	Behaviors rated 0–2 in intensity, max. 10	Children 2–7 yrs; also for infants
Child Facial Coding System (CFCS; Gilbert et al., 1999)	Postoperative and procedural	Time sampling (multiple 20-sec periods)	Thirteen: brow lower, eye squeeze, eye squint, blink, nasolabial furrow, nose wrinkler, flared nostril, cheek raiser, open lips, upper lip raiser, lip corner puller, horizontal mouth stretch, vertical mouth stretch	Ten behaviors rated 0–2 in intensity, max. 23	Toddlers and children 1–6 yrs
Pain Observation Scale for Young Children (POCIS; Bolen-van der Loo et al., 1999)[b]	Postoperative	Time sampling (2-min periods)	Nine: facial, cry, breath, movement of torso, movement of arms/fingers, movement of legs/toes, state of arousal, child's verbal response, touching the painful spot	Behaviors scored when present, max. 9	Children 1–4 yrs

[a]LP, lumbar puncture; BMA, bone marrow aspiration.

[b]Derived from CHEOPS and NIPS

lescents, because adolescents usually display different and often more subtle distress behaviors. Yet it is essential to recognize that all children do not consistently display the same type of distress behavior in direct proportion to the intensity of their pain experience. Behavioral pain scores do not always correlate with children's own pain ratings (Beyer, McGrath, & Berde, 1990; Glebe-Gage, McGrath, & Kissoon, 1991). Some children may behave stoically but still experience pain, whereas other children may exhibit many distress behaviors in clinics even before a scheduled painful treatment. The relationship between children's pain and their behaviors is influenced by the situational factors shown in Figure 6.1 on page 98. Thus it is important to interpret children's pain scores within the context in which they experience pain and within the limitations of the behaviors they can display. Only recently have investigators tackled the difficult problem of beginning to develop behavioral scales for children with physical impairments, who may respond very differently from otherwise healthy children when they experience pain.

Physiological Pain Measures

Many physiological parameters have been monitored in infants and children as potential pain measures; they include heart rate, respiration rate, blood pressure, palmar sweating, cortisol and cortisone levels, O_2 levels, vagal tone, and endorphin concentrations (Anders, Sachar, Kream, Roffwarg, & Hellman, 1971; Campos, 1991; Gunnar, Isensee, & Fust, 1987; Harpin & Rutter, 1982, 1983; Jay et al., 1983; Johnston & Strada, 1986; Katz et al., 1982; Owens &Todt, 1984; Porter & Porges, 1991; Szyfelbein, Osgood, Atchison, & Carr, 1987). Like behavioral pain measures, these physiological responses reflect a generalized and complex response to pain and to stress. They provide valuable information about children's distress states and are important, but more work is required to develop a sensitive system for interpreting how these parameters reflect the quality or intensity of children's pain experience. The unprecedented recent advances in brain imaging may lead to the development of instrumentation that can be used to monitor children's pain physiologically. At present, though, physiological parameters are not specific pain measures for children and are not yet available for clinical practice. Thus they are not reviewed individually in this chapter.

Psychological Pain Measures

Psychological pain measures include a broad spectrum of projective techniques, interviews, questionnaires, qualitative descriptive scales, and quantitative rating scales used to capture the subjective experience of pain. Thus these measures potentially provide the most comprehensive information about children's pain. Projective techniques allow children to express their feelings about pain through their drawings, choice of colors, and interpretation of pictures or cartoons. Although these methods are useful for young children or children who are unable to express their feelings verbally, standardized techniques with age-appropriate guidelines for interpreting children's responses are not yet available for clinical use.

In contrast, much psychometric and clinical research has focused on developing standardized self-report pain measures for children. A diverse array of self-report measures can provide valuable diagnostic information about the causes and contributing factors for children's pain. Quantitative rating scales provide health care providers with practical tools for regularly assessing pain intensity to ensure that children receive adequate pain control.

Self-Report Pain Measures–Interviews

Children's interviews are ideally suited to the assessment of children's understanding of their pain, as well as the factors that influence it. Health care providers should interview all children (when possible) to obtain information about the sensory dimensions of their pain (location, quality, intensity, duration or frequency) and the primary situational factors that modify it. As part of the usual clinical examination, a few basic questions can be asked in a consistent manner, with different follow-up questions depending on the child's information. This semistructured format enables health care providers to obtain the same information from children with consistency and yet flexibility, so that any individually relevant aspects of a pain problem may be discussed in depth with each child, but health care providers are still able to make meaningful comparisons among children. Several structured and semistructured interviews have been designed to assess children's knowledge about pain and to evaluate the language they use to describe pain (Abu-Saad, 1984a, 1984b; Abu-Saad, Kroonen, & Halfens, 1990; Gaffney, 1988; Harbeck & Peterson, 1992; Harrison, Badran, Ghalib, &

Rida, 1991; McGrath, 1990; McGrath, Speechley, Seifert, & Gorodzinsky, 1997; Ross & Ross, 1984b; 1988; Savedra, Gibbons, Tesler, Ward, & Wegner, 1982; Savedra, Tesler, Holzemer, Wilkie, & Ward, 1989; Savedra, Tesler, Ward, Wegner, & Gibbons, 1981; Schultz, 1971; Varni, Katz, & Dash, 1987; Wilkie et al., 1990).

As shown in Table 6.6 on the next page, five interview questionnaires are used in clinical practice to assess multiple dimensions of children's pain experience. In addition, Belter, McIntosh, Finch, and Saylor (1988), Gaffney and Dunne (1986, 1987), Lollar, Smits, and Patterson (1982), McGrath and colleagues (1997, 2001), Ross and Ross (1984b), and Savedra and colleagues (1982) have conducted excellent interviews on children's general pain experiences that provide valuable information about children's understanding. Two of these interviews are based on pictorial representations of situations depicting different types of pain (Belter et al., 1988; Lollar et al., 1982). Two interviews were designed as survey instruments for epidemiological studies on childhood pain: the Pain Knowledge Interview to capture information on how children acquired knowledge about the different sensory features of pain and the impact of pain (McGrath et al., 1997), and the Pain Experiences Interview to capture prevalence information about a child's acute, recurrent, and chronic pain experiences (McGrath et al., 2000).

The Varni–Thompson Pediatric Pain Questionnaire includes visual analogue scales, color-coded rating scales, and verbal descriptors to provide information about a child's pain history; socioenvironmental factors that may influence the pain; and the sensory, affective, and evaluative dimensions of a child's chronic pain (Varni, Thompson, & Hanson, 1987). The Adolescent Pediatric Pain Tool includes a body outline (children color it to denote the location of their pain), a combined analogue and Likert scale (children mark the line to denote pain intensity), and a verbal descriptor scale (children select among 56 words to choose those that best describe the qualitative, affective, evaluative, and duration qualities of their pain) (Savedra et al., 1993). The Children's Comprehensive Pain Questionnaire is a semistructured interview used for assessing children with recurrent or chronic pain (McGrath, 1990). After a decade of use in various research studies and in the pain clinic, the authors refined and revised the global interview to more efficiently capture information about pain characteristics and about the primary and secondary causes of different types of

recurrent and chronic pain in children and adolescents (McGrath & Hillier, 2001). The Children's Headache Interview is an assessment interview designed to obtain objective information about headache activity and about the cognitive, behavioral, and emotional factors that cause or exacerbate headaches (McGrath & Hillier, 2001; McGrath & Koster, 2001). This assessment interview provides the basic information required to develop a treatment plan for children—a plan that addresses not only the primary pain source, but also the secondary contributing factors (Hillier & McGrath, 2001).

Pain Intensity Rating Scales

Children can use many quantifiable scales to rate the strength of their pain experience. As shown in Tables 6.7 and 6.8, several analogue, facial, and verbal rating scales have been developed for toddlers, children, and adolescents. Children are asked to choose a level on such a scale that best matches the strength of their own pain (i.e., a level on a number or thermometer scale, a number of objects, a mark on a visual analogue scale, a face from a series of faces varying in emotional expression, a particular word from lists describing different intensities). These scales are easy to administer, requiring only a few minutes for children to rate their pain intensity.

However, the resulting pain scores from different intensity scales are not equivalent. In some scales, adult investigators selected the number scores associated with different pain intensity levels (e.g., no hurt equals 0, mild pain equals 1, moderate pain equals 2, strong pain equals 3). Yet a child's perceived change in pain from a score of 1 to 2 (mild to moderate) may not be the same as the change from 2 to 3 (moderate to strong). Similarly, when a child's pain is rated as 4, the level may not really be 4 times the strength of the pain he or she rates as a 1. Nevertheless, the numbers are often interpreted as if they represent absolute and accurate amounts of pain. Pain scores are usually treated as if they represent numbers on equal-interval or ratio scales.

The four types of measurement scales (nominal, such as the numbers designating players on a sports team; ordinal, such as the rank ordering of children according to height; interval, such as the Fahrenheit temperature scale; and ratio, such as a yardstick) refer to four different relationships between the properties of an event or perception (e.g., pain intensity score) and the number or metric

TABLE 6.6. Pain Questionnaires for Children

Name	Pain type	Method	Pain characteristic	Scale type/pain score	Comments
Varni–Thompson Pediatric Pain Questionnaire (PPQ; Varni et al., 1987)	Chronic pain (arthritis)	Questionnaire with visual analogue scale, color-coded rating scales, and word descriptors	Sensory, affective, and evaluative dimensions	Descriptive information on multiple aspects, with some pain features scored on interval and ratio scales	Children and adolescents ages 4–19 yrs
Adolescent Pediatric Pain Tool (APPT; Savedra et al., 1989; Tesler et al., 1991)	Postoperative	Questionnaire with body outline, analogue scale, and adjective pain descriptor scale	Pain location, intensity, and quality	Descriptive information on multiple aspects, with some pain features scored on interval and ratio scales	Children and adolescents ages 8–17 yrs
Children's Comprehensive Pain Questionnaire (CCPQ; McGrath, 1990)	Recurrent pain syndromes, chronic pain	Semistructured interview with visual analogue scale, rating scales, and word descriptors	Sensory, affective, and evaluative dimensions; situational factors that intensify pain	Descriptive information on multiple aspects, with some pain features scored on interval and ratio scales	Children and adolescents ages 5–19 yrs
Abu-Saad Paediatric Pain Assessment Tool (Abu-Saad et al., 1990, 1994)	Postoperative	Dutch questionnaire with analogue scale, words, and questions on impact of pain	Intensity, quality, and affect	Descriptive information, with some pain features scored on interval scales	Children and adolescents ages 5–15 yrs
Children's Headache Interview (McGrath & Hillier, 2001; McGrath & Koster, 2001)	Recurrent migraine and tension-type headache	Semistructured interview with quantitative and word descriptor scales, and questions on impact of pain and disability	Sensory and affective dimensions, location, intensity, duration, quality, frequency, and affect; pain-related disability	Descriptive information on cognitive, behavioral, and emotional factors that affect headache, pain features scored on interval and ratio scales	Children and adolescents ages 5–19 yrs

system. Ratio scales have all the properties of the three other scales: They represent a set position or order between numbers, the magnitude of the difference between numbers is the same, and the numbers reflect actual ratios of magnitude. Since each scale has a certain number of permissible mathematical calculations that are valid, it is important to know the specific scale type when measuring a child's pain or evaluating analgesic efficacy. Conclusions about how much more intense one type of pain is than another or how much pain is reduced are valid only when ratio scales are used (Price, 1999).

The most common methods for validating pain intensity scales are to compare pain scores on the proposed new measure with those on an accepted scale (concurrent validity) or to verify that pain scores on the proposed scale decrease after analgesic administration (construct validity). Some studies have compared several of the rating scales listed in Tables 6.7 and 6.8 to determine the correlations among different measures and to explore whether one measure may represent a more valid index of pain than another (Abu-Saad, Pool, & Tulkens, 1994; Beyer et al., 1990; Fogel-Keck, Gerkensmeyer, Joyce, & Schade, 1996; Fradet, McGrath, Kay, Adams, & Luke, 1990; Goodenough et al., 1997; Stein, 1995; Tesler et al., 1991; Tyler, Tu, Douthit, & Chapman, 1993; Van Cleve, Johnson, & Pothier, 1996; Vessey, Carlson, & McGill, 1994). The results of most studies show good correlations among tools, with no unequivocal demonstration of one particular scale's superiority. Thus the choice of scale can be based on the type of pain, age of child, and specific clinical or research objectives.

The major pain intensity scales developed for children and adolescents for clinical use are shown in Tables 6.7 and 6.8. Each table lists the formal scale name, type of pain used to develop the scale initially, scale methodology, pain characteristics measured, scale type, and type of pain score obtained. At present, no one scale is appropriate for all children and for all situations in which they experience pain. However, visual and colored analogue scales are ideal for most children above 5 years of age. In addition to excellent psychometric properties, these scales are versatile for use with acute, recurrent, and chronic pain, and provide convenient and flexible pain assessment tools for use in hospital and at home.

Many analogue scales are variants of the traditional visual analogue scale—a black 100-mm line with endpoints designated as "no pain" and "strongest pain imaginable." Children mark the line to show their pain level; the length of the line from the left endpoint to a child's mark represents the strength of his or her pain. These scales were developed for adults and children to enable us to understand how changes in perception (e.g., brightness, loudness, pain) corresponded with changes in physical stimuli (e.g., light intensity, sound level, noxious stimulation). Generally children over 5 years of age are able to use these scales in a valid and reliable manner to rate their pain intensity (Abu-Saad, 1984a; McGrath, 1990; Zeltzer, Anderson, & Schechter, 1990). The CAS, described earlier in this chapter, is the pain intensity scale that we generally use for children above 5 years of age. In addition to its psychometric properties (McGrath et al., 1996) and construct validity (McGrath et al., 1999), the scale is convenient to administer, easy for children to understand, versatile for many clinical settings, and beneficial for parents to monitor children's pain at home.

As shown in Table 6.7 on the next page, some object scales (involving the use of poker chips, red balls, or partially filled glasses) have been developed for use with young children (appropriate for older children) or for children who are visually impaired. The concrete physical features of the two poker chip scales and the limited range (four chips) should appeal to young children as clear indices of four different intensity levels (Hester, 1979; St. Laurent-Gagnon, Bernard-Bonnin, & Villeneuve, 1999). The Tactile Scale, with a larger range of nine balls, might be equally suited to young and older children (who would probably use the entire range of intensity levels).

As listed in Table 6.8 on page 113, five facial scales have been developed as measures of pain intensity, pain affect, or anxiety for children. Although similar in that they consist of six or seven faces varying in emotional expression, each of these scales has different properties and the resulting numbers are not equivalent. The Faces Pain Scale displays only the seven faces (Bieri, Reeve, Champion, Addicote, & Ziegler, 1990). The Faces Pain Rating Scale displays six faces, but the instructions to children link a specific face with a particular amount of hurt (Wong & Baker, 1988; Wong et al., 1999). In contrast, the Oucher Scale depicts six photographs of a child expressing increasing levels of distress; the photographs are positioned at equal intervals along a 0–100 numerical scale (Beyer, 1984). The author carefully stipulates that the number and facial scales are distinct, with the numbers representing an in-

TABLE 6.7. Analogue Pain Scales for Children

Name	Pain type	Method	Pain characteristic	Scale type/pain score	Comments
Eland Color Tool (Eland, 1974; Eland & Anderson, 1977)	Postoperative	Projective rating scale on body outline	Intensity, location	Quantitative (probably interval)	Children select colors to represent three levels of pain and shade body outline
Poker Chip Tool (Hester, 1979)	Acute pain (immunization)	Object scale consisting of four poker chips	Intensity	Quantitative, interval scale; pain scores 0–4	Children ages 4–7 yrs
Visual Analogue Scale (VAS; Abu-Saad, 1984a; McGrath, 1987; McGrath, deVeber, & Hearn, 1985)	Acute, recurrent, and chronic pain	Analogue scale, vertical with endpoints designated as "no pain" and "strongest pain" (100 and 150 cm)	Intensity, affect, and emotions caused by pain	Quantitative, ratio scale properties; pain scores 0–100	Children ages 5 and older
Pain Thermometer (Jay et al., 1983; Szyfelbein et al., 1985)	Treatment (Burn dressing change)	Analogue scale, shaped like thermometer	Intensity	Quantitative, may be interval or ratio scale; pain scores 0–10	Children and adolescents, ages 8–17
Glasses Rating Scale (Whaley & Wong, 1987)	Hypothetical pain situations	Object scale consisting of six glasses, filled to different levels	Intensity	Quantitative, may be ordinal or interval scale, pain scores 0–6	Children and adolescents, ages 3–18
Coloured Analogue Scale (CAS; McGrath et al., 1996, 2000; McGrath & Hillier, 2001)	Acute trauma, postoperative, recurrent, chronic pain	Analogue scale, varying in length, hue, and area	Intensity	Quantitative, ratio scale properties; pain scores 0–10	Psychometric properties demonstrated; children ages 5 yrs and older; versatility demonstrated for clinical and home use
Pain Ladder (Hester, Foster, & Kristensen, 1990)	Acute pain	Analogue scale, depicted as ladder	Intensity	Quantitative, may be ordinal or interval scale; pain scores 0–10	Children ages 5–13 yrs
Children's Global Rating Scale (CGRS; Carpenter, 1990)	Procedural (venipuncture)	Number and pictorial scale, with pain levels depicted by progressively wavy lines along the number scale	Intensity and fear	Quantitative, may be ordinal or interval scale; pain scores 0–4	Younger children select the wavy lines to match their pain, while older children use the numerical scale
Tactile Scale (TaS; Westerling, 1999)	Postoperative pain	Object scale consisting of nine red balls in graduated sizes	Intensity and nausea	Quantitative, may be ordinal or interval scale; pain scores 0–9	Children who are visually impaired
Multiple Size Poker Chip Tool (MSPCT; St. Laurent-Gagnon, Bernard-Bonnin, & Villeneuve, 1999)	Procedural (immunization)	Object scale consisting of four poker chips, varying in size (2–3.8 cm)	Intensity	Quantitative, interval scale; pain scores 0–4	Children ages 4–6 yrs

TABLE 6.8. Facial and Word Pain Scales for Children

Name	Pain type	Method	Pain feature	Scale type/pain score	Comments
The Oucher (Beyer, 1984; Beyer & Aradine, 1986; African American and Hispanic versions available (Beyer, Denyes, & Villarruel, 1992; Villarruel & Denyes, 1991)	Postoperative pain	Number and pictorial scales; children's pictures postioned at regular intervals along number scale	Intensity	Numbers: Interval scale; pain scores 0–100. Pictures: Ordinal or interval scale; pain scores 0–5	Two scales should not be combined; numbers are for older children, while pictures are for younger children
Facial Affective Scale (FAS; McGrath, 1990; McGrath et al., 2000; McGrath & Hillier, 2001; McGrath, deVeber, & Hearn, 1985)	Acute, recurrent, and chronic pain	Discrete pictorial scale, consisting of nine faces varying in emotional expression	Affect	Interval scale; pain scores 0–97	Intended to measure the affect associated with pain for children aged 5 yrs and older; affective values for faces were determined by children's own ratings, and not assigned by adults
Faces Pain Scale (Bieri et al., 1990; Goodenough et al., 1997)	Hypothetical levels, procedural	Discrete pictorial scale, consisting of seven adult faces varying in emotional expression	Intensity, affect	Interval scale, pain scores 0–7	Children and adolescents ages 3–15 yrs; initially developed to measure pain intensity, subsequently studied as measure of pain affect
Faces Pain Rating Scale (Wong & Baker, 1988; Wong et al., 1999)	Procedural	Discrete pictorial scale, consisting of six faces varying in emotional expression	Intensity	May be ordinal or interval scale; pain scores 0–6	Children and adolescents ages 3–18 yrs; instructions link each face to a different amount of hurt
Children's Anxiety and Pain Scale (CAPS; Kuttner & LePage, 1989)	Postoperative pain, acute injury	Two sets of five faces, depicting increasing levels of anxiety and pain	Anxiety, pain intensity	Interval scales; anxiety and pain scores 0–5	Children ages 4–10 yrs
Word-Descriptor Scale (Whaley & Wong, 1987); Simple Descriptor Scale (SDS; Wong & Baker, 1988)	Varied painful events for hospitalized children	Combined number, word, and analogue scale	Intensity	Interval scale; pain scores 0–5	Children and adolescents ages 3–18 yrs
Word–Graphic Rating Scale (WGRS), a component of the APPT (see Table 6.6) (Sinkin-Feldman, Tesler, & Savedra, 1997; Tesler et al., 1991)	Postoperative pain, pain in hospitalized children	Analogue and word scale	Intensity	Interval scale, may have ratio properties	Children and adolescents ages 8–18 yrs

113

terval scale and the faces representing only an ordinal scale. Subsequent versions of the scale have been developed for African American children (Beyer, Denyes, & Villarruel, 1992) and Hispanic children (Villarruel & Denyes, 1991).

The Facial Affective Scale was designed to capture the affective dimension of pain. Preliminary studies showed that children ages 5–8 had difficulty using the same analogue scale (e.g., a simple visual analogue scale with the endpoints changed to reflect pain intensity or pain affect) to measure different dimensions of pain. Thus an artist sketched nine faces representing different levels of distress and joy; children rated the unpleasantness depicted by each face to determine its number or affective value (McGrath, 1990; McGrath, deVeber, & Hearn, 1985). The Children's Anxiety and Pain Scale consists of two sets of five drawings of children's faces, each set displaying increasing levels of either anxiety or pain (Kuttner & LePage, 1989).

Although children provide essential information about their pain in their own words, verbal scales of pain intensity are not widely used. Only two formal scales are available, as listed in Table 6.8. We have used a five-level word scale in some of our studies, using adjectives that children have used in our clinical program to describe their pain. The scale includes "very little," "a little bit," "medium," "a lot," and "a real lot" for children less than 7 years of age and "slight," "mild," "moderate," "strong," and "intense" for children 7 and older. The scale has face validity; we are now obtaining children's numerical ratings for each of the levels. This scale is similar to the words listed in the revised Word–Graphic Rating Scale (WGRS; Tesler et al., 1991): "no pain," "little pain," "medium pain," "large pain," "worst possible pain." In the WGRS, the words are spaced at approximately equidistant intervals along a line from 0 to 100 mm. Although subsequent research has shown that children do not rate the words at equal intervals, their use of the scale to measure their pain should still be valid because they mark the line (similar to an analogue scale) rather than simply circling the words.

GUIDELINES FOR SELECTING A PAIN MEASURE

Although no one pain measure is equally appropriate for all children or for all types of pain, the 40+ measures listed in this chapter provide a versatile repertoire of clinical pain measures for almost any situation. The critical issue is how to select the most appropriate measure for the age and cognitive level of the child, and one that satisfies the evaluator's clinical objectives. Many simple, easy-to-use pain scales provide meaningful values that reflect a child's pain intensity and are ideal measures for evaluating treatment effectiveness throughout a child's treatment. But they are not adequate for teaching us about the nature of a child's pain or for identifying the primary and secondary situational factors that affect pain. In contrast, a more lengthy semistructured interview or questionnaire is an essential component of a thorough pain assessment for children with recurrent pain syndrome or a chronic pain condition, but is rarely required for children treated for acute pain problems in hospitals or outpatient clinics.

Thus health care providers who treat a wide range of children's pain problems need a flexible pain measurement inventory consisting of some simple pain intensity scales and a more comprehensive assessment instrument. Only previously validated instruments should be used in clinical practice, unless clinicians are willing to conduct the rigorous research necessary to prove that a measure is valid and reliable.

At present, we must rely on behavioral and physiological distress indices to infer the presence and severity of pain in infants. Although caution must always be used when interpreting children's pain solely from their scores on these scales, because children's behaviors are not simply passive reflections of their pain intensity, these indices are also valuable adjunct tools for toddlers, children, and adolescents. Because a child's pain behaviors naturally vary in relation to the type of pain experienced, different behavioral scales must be used for children with acute, recurrent, and chronic pain. Behavioral observation and monitoring provide a broader base of information about the factors that affect a child's pain—knowledge that is essential for optimal pain control. For example, the behavioral responses of parents and teachers to children with recurrent pains must be evaluated to design a treatment program where children are encouraged to use positive pain-reducing strategies and to minimize disability behaviors.

Self-report measures represent the "gold standard" in pediatric pain measurement, because they are the only direct source for obtaining information about a child's full pain experience. As described previously, many rating scales are available as valid and reliable measures of pain intensity.

Concrete physical scales, such as the poker chip scales, are ideally suited for children under 5 years of age. However, some of these children may also use a simple word rating scale, such as "not there," "a little," "medium," and "a lot." Children 5 years of age and older can use all of the analogue and facial scales shown in Tables 6.7 and 6.8. Most of these measures are convenient and practical methods for assessing pain intensity; children can easily complete the scales in the clinic and at home.

Both quantitative and qualitative assessment tools are needed for children with recurrent or chronic pain. Comprehensive pain assessments for these children begin with the recognition that the causative and contributing factors must be evaluated, in addition to pain intensity. A standardized assessment inventory should include a semi-structured interview to evaluate the factors shown in Figure 6.1, and then subsequent regular assessments of pain intensity or pain behaviors via brief quantitative scales. Although pain diaries and pain logs are not formally reviewed in this chapter, many scientists and health care providers use diaries and logs to monitor specific aspects of a child's pain during therapy (for a review, see McGrath, 1990). These can be flexible instruments to fit the needs of the specific therapy program. For example, health care providers may monitor school attendance, physical activity, peer activities, medication use, and use of nondrug strategies, using a simple observation form that they develop.

In summary, evaluating a child's pain requires an integrated approach. Health care providers should always ask a child directly about his or her pain experience, and should determine precisely the sensory characteristics to facilitate an accurate diagnosis. They should also assess relevant cognitive, behavioral, and emotional factors to determine their potential pain-exacerbating impact. And they should regularly measure a child's pain intensity to monitor the effectiveness of their therapy.

REFERENCES

Abu-Saad, H. H. (1984a). Assessing children's responses to pain. *Pain, 19,* 163–171.

Abu-Saad, H. H. (1984b). Cultural group indicators of pain in children. *American Journal of Maternal and Child Nursing, 13,* 187–196.

Abu-Saad, H. H., Kroonen, E., & Halfens, R. (1990). On the development of a multidimensional Dutch pain assessment tool for children. *Pain, 43,* 249–256.

Abu-Saad, H. H., Pool, H., & Tulkens, B. (1994). Further validity testing of the Abu-Saad Paediatric Pain Assessment Tool. *Journal of Advanced Nursing, 19,* 1063–1071.

Ambuel, B., Hamlett, K. W., Marx, C. M., & Blumer, J. L. (1992). Assessing distress in pediatric intensive care environments: The COMFORT scale. *Journal of Pediatric Psychology, 17,* 95–109.

Anders, T. F., Sachar, E. J., Kream, J., Roffwarg, H., & Hellman, L. (1971). Behavioral state and plasma cortisol response in the human newborn. *Pediatrics, 46,* 532–537.

Attia, J., Amiel-Tison, C., Mayer, M. N., Shnider, S. M., & Barrier, G. (1987). Measurement of postoperative pain and narcotic administration in infants using a new clinical scoring system. *Anesthesiology, 67,* A532.

Barrier, G., Attia, J., Mayer, M. N., Amiel-Tison, C. L., & Shnider, S. M. (1989). Measurement of postoperative pain and narcotic administration in infants using a new clinical scoring system. *Intensive Care Medicine, 15,* S37–S39.

Belter, R. W., McIntosh, J. A., Finch, A. J., Jr., & Saylor, C. F. (1988). Preschoolers' ability to differentiate levels of pain: Relative efficacy of three self-report measures. *Journal of Clinical Child Psychology, 17,* 329–335.

Beyer, J. E. (1984). *The Oucher: A user's manual and technical report.* Evanston, IL: Judson.

Beyer, J. E., & Aradine, C.R. (1986). Content validity of an instrument to measure young children's perceptions of the intensity of their pain. *Journal of Pediatric Nursing, 1,* 386–395.

Beyer, J. E., Denyes, M. J., & Villarruel, A. M. (1992). The creation, validation and continuing development of the Oucher: A measure of pain intensity in children. *Journal of Pediatric Nursing, 7,* 335–346.

Beyer, J. E., McGrath, P. J., & Berde, C. B. (1990). Discordance between self-report and behavioral pain measures in children aged 3–7 years after surgery. *Journal of Pain and Symptom Management, 5,* 350–356.

Beyer, J. E., & Wells, N. (1989). The assessment of pain in children. *Pediatric Clinics of North America, 36,* 837–854.

Bieri, D., Reeve, R. A., Champion, G. D., Addicoat, L., & Ziegler, J. B. (1990). The Faces Pain Scale for the self-assessment of the severity of pain experienced by children: Development, initial validation, and preliminary investigation for ratio scale properties. *Pain, 41,* 139–150.

Blauer, T., & Gerstmann, D. (1998). A simultaneous comparison of three neonatal pain scales during common NICU procedures. *Clinical Journal of Pain, 14,* 39–47.

Boelen-van der Loo, W. J. C., Scheffer, E., de Haan, R. J., & de Groot, C. J. (1999). Clinimetric evaluation of the pain observation scale for young children in children aged between 1 and 4 years after ear, nose, and throat surgery. *Developmental and Behavioral Pediatrics, 20,* 222–227.

Broadman, L. M., Rice, L. J., & Hannallah, R. S. (1988). Testing the validity of an objective pain scale for infants and children. *Anesthesiology, 69,* A770.

Buchholz, M., Karl, H. W., Pomietto, M., & Lynn, A. (1998). Pain scores in infants: A Modified Infant Pain Scale versus visual analogue. *Journal of Pain and Symptom Management, 15,* 117–124.

Bush, J. P., & Harkins, S. W. (Eds.). (1991). *Children in pain: Clinical and research issues from a developmental perspective*. New York: Springer-Verlag.

Büttner, W., & Finke, W. (2000). Analysis of behavioural and physiological parameters for the assessment of postoperative analgesic demand in newborns, infants and young children: A comprehensive report on seven consecutive studies. *Pediatric Anesthesiology, 10*, 303–318.

Campos, R. G. (1991). Temperament and soothing responses to pain-induced distress. *Journal of Pain and Symptom Management, 6*, 195.

Carpenter, P. J. (1990). New method for measuring young children's self-report of fear and pain. *Journal of Pain and Symptom Management, 5*, 233–240.

Chambers, C. T., Reid, G. J., McGrath P. J., & Finley, G. A. (1996). Development and preliminary validation of a Postoperative Pain Measure for Parents. *Pain, 68*, 307–313.

Champion, G. D., Goodenough, B., von Baeyer, C. L., & Thomas, W. (1998). Measurement of pain by self-report. In G. A. Finley & P. J. McGrath (Eds.), *Measurement of pain in infants and children* (pp. 123–160). Seattle, WA: IASP Press.

Craig, K. D., & Grunau, R. V. E. (1993). Neonatal pain perception and behavioral measurement. In K. J. S. Anand & P. J. McGrath (Eds.), *Pain in neonates* (pp. 67–105). Amsterdam: Elsevier.

Craig, K. D., McMahon, R. J., Morison, J. D., & Zaskow, C. (1984). Developmental changes in infant pain expression during immunization injections. *Social Science and Medicine, 19*, 1331–1337.

Eland, J. M. (1974). *Children's communication of pain*. Unpublished master's thesis, University of Iowa.

Eland, J. M., & Anderson, J. E. (1977). The experience of pain in children. In A. K. Jacox (Ed.), *Pain: A source book for nurses and other health professionals* (pp. 453–471). Boston: Little, Brown.

Fogel-Keck, J., Gerkensmeyer, J. E., Joyce, B. A., & Schade, J. G. (1996). Reliability and validity of the Faces and Word Descriptor Scales to measure procedural pain. *Journal of Pediatric Nursing, 11*, 368–374.

Fradet, C., McGrath, P. J., Kay, J., Adams, S., & Luke, B. (1990). A prospective survey of reactions to blood tests by children and adolescents. *Pain, 40*, 53–60.

Fuller, B. F., Conner, D., & Horii, Y. (1990). Potential acoustic measures of infant pain and arousal. In D. C. Tyler & E. J. Krane (Eds.), *Advances in pain research and therapy* (Vol. 15, pp. 137–145). New York: Raven Press.

Gaffney, A. (1988). How children describe pain: A study of words and analogies used by 5–14 year-olds. In R. Dubner, G. F. Gebhart, & M. R. Bond (Eds.), *Pain research and clinical management* (Vol. 3, pp. 341–347). Amsterdam: Elsevier.

Gaffney, A., & Dunne, E. A. (1986). Developmental aspects of children's definitions of pain. *Pain, 26*, 105–117.

Gaffney, A., & Dunne, E. A. (1987). Children's understanding of the causality of pain. *Pain, 29*, 91–104.

Gauvain-Piquard, A., Rodary, C., Rezvani, A., & Lemerle, J. (1987). Pain in children aged 2–6 years: A new observational rating scale elaborated in a pediatric oncology unit—preliminary report. *Pain, 31*, 177–188.

Gilbert, C. A., Lilley, C. M., Craig, K. D., McGrath, P. J., Court, C. A., Bennett, S. M., & Montgomery, C. J.

(1999). Postoperative pain expression in preschool children: Validation of the Child Facial Coding System. *Clinical Journal of Pain, 15*, 192–200.

Glebe-Gage, D., McGrath, P. A., & Kissoon, N. (1991). Children's responses to painful procedures in the emergency department. In M. R. Bond, J. E. Charlton, & C. J. Woolf (Eds.), *Proceedings of the VIth World Congress on Pain* (pp. 437–442). Amsterdam: Elsevier.

Goodenough, B., Addicoat, L., Champion, G. D., McInerney, M., Young, B., Juniper, K., & Ziegler, J. B. (1997). Pain in 4- to 6-year-old children receiving intramuscular injections: A comparison of the Faces Pain Scale with other self-report and behavioral measures. *Clinical Journal of Pain, 13*, 60–73.

Grunau, R. V. E., & Craig, K. D. (1990). Facial activity as a measure of neonatal pain expression. In D. C. Tyler & E. J. Krane (Eds.), *Advances in pain research and therapy* (Vol. 15, pp. 147–155). New York: Raven Press.

Gunnar, M. R., Isensee, J., & Fust, L. S. (1987). Adrenocortical activity and the Brazelton Neonatal Assessment Scale: Moderating effects of the newborn's biobehavioral status. *Child Development, 58*, 1448–1458.

Harbeck, C., & Peterson, L. (1992). Elephants dancing in my head: A developmental approach to children's concepts of specific pains. *Child Development, 63*, 138–149.

Harpin, V. A., & Rutter, N. (1982). Development of emotional sweating in the newborn infant. *Archives of Disease in Childhood, 57*, 691–695.

Harpin, V. A., & Rutter, N. (1983). Making heel pricks less painful. *Archives of Disease in Childhood, 58*, 226–228.

Harrison, A., Badran, S., Ghalib, R., & Rida, S. (1991). Arabic children's pain descriptions. *Pediatric Emergency Care, 7*, 199–203.

Hester, N. K. (1979). The preoperational child's reaction to immunization. *Nursing Research, 28*, 250–255.

Hester, N. K., Foster, R., & Kristensen, K. (1990). Measurement of pain in children: Generalizability and validity of the Pain Ladder and the Poker Chip Tool. In D. C. Tyler & E. J. Krane (Eds.). *Pediatric pain. Advances in pain research and therapy* (Vol. 15, pp. 79–84). New York: Raven Press.

Hillier L. M., & McGrath, P. A. (2001). A cognitive-behavioral program for treating recurrent headache. In P. A. McGrath & L. M. Hillier (Eds.), *The child with headache: Diagnosis and treatment* (pp. 183–220). Seattle, WA: IASP Press.

Hunt, A. M., Goldman, A., Mastroyannopoulou, K., & Seers, K. (1999). Identification of pain cues of children with severe neurological impairment [Abstract]. *Proceedings of the 9th World Congress on Pain* (pp. 84–85). Seattle, WA: IASP Press.

Jay, S. M., Elliot, C. H., Woody, P. D., & Siegel, S. (1991). An investigation of cognitive-behavior therapy combined with oral valium for children undergoing painful medical procedures. *Health Psychology, 10*, 317–322.

Jay, S. M., Ozolins, M., Elliott, C. H., & Caldwell, S. (1983). Assessment of children's distress during painful medical procedures. *Health Psychology, 2*, 133–147.

Johnston, C. C., & O'Shaughnessy, D. (1988). Acoustical attributes of infants pain cries: Discriminating features. In R. Dubner, G. F. Gebhart, & M. R. Bond

(Eds.), *Pain research and clinical management* (Vol. 3, pp. 336–340). Amsterdam: Elsevier.

Johnston, C. C., & Strada, M. E. (1986). Acute pain response in infants: A multidimensional description. *Pain, 24,* 373–382.

Joyce, B. A., Schade, J. G., Keck, J. F., Gerkensmeyer, J., Raftery, T., Moser, S., & Huster, G. (1994). Reliability and validity of preverbal pain assessment tools. *Issues in Comprehensive Pediatric Nursing, 17,* 121–135.

Katz, E. R., Kellerman, J., & Siegel, S. E. (1980). Behavioral distress in children with cancer undergoing medical procedures: Developmental considerations. *Journal of Consulting and Clinical Psychology, 48,* 356–365.

Katz, E. R., Sharp, B., Kellerman, J., Marston, A. R., Hershman, J. M., & Siegel, S. E. (1982). Beta-endorphin immunoreactivity and acute behavioral distress in children with leukemia. *Journal of Nervous and Mental Disease, 170,* 72–77.

Krechel, S. W., & Bildner, J. (1995). CRIES: A new neonatal postoperative pain measurement score. Initial testing of validity and reliability. *Paediatric Anaesthesia, 5,* 53–61.

Kuttner, L., & LePage, T. (1989). Face scales for the assessment of paediatric pain: A critical review. *Canadian Journal of Behavioural Sciences, 21,* 198–209.

Lawrence, J., Alcock, D., Kay, J., & McGrath, P. J. (1991). The development of a tool to assess neonatal pain. *Journal of Pain and Symptom Management, 6,* 194.

LeBaron, S., & Zeltzer, L. (1984). Assessment of acute pain and anxiety in children and adolescents by self-reports, observer reports, and a behavior checklist. *Journal of Consulting and Clinical Psychology, 52,* 729–738.

Lollar, D. J., Smits, S. J., & Patterson, D. L. (1982). Assessment of pediatric pain: An empirical perspective. *Journal of Pediatric Psychology, 7,* 267–277.

McGrath, P. A. (1987). The multidimensional assessment and management of recurrent pain syndromes in children and adolescents. *Behaviour Research and Therapy, 25,* 251–262.

McGrath, P. A. (1990). *Pain in children: Nature, assessment, and treatment.* New York: Guilford Press.

McGrath, P. A., deVeber, L. L., & Hearn, M. T. (1985). Multidimensional pain assessment in children. In H. L. Fields, R. Dubner, & F. Cervero (Eds.), *Advances in pain research and therapy* (Vol. 9, pp. 387–393). New York: Raven Press.

McGrath, P. A., Girvan, D. P., Hillier, L. M., & Seifert, C. E. (1999). Post-operative pain in children: Can parents integrate assessment and management? [Abstract]. In *Proceedings of the 9th World Congress on Pain* (p. 201). Seattle, WA: IASP Press.

McGrath, P. A., & Hillier, L. M. (1996). Controlling children's pain. In R. J. Gatchel & D. C. Turk (Eds.), *Psychological approaches to pain management: A practitioner's handbook* (pp. 331–370). New York: Guilford Press.

McGrath, P. A., & Hillier, L. M. (Eds.). (2001). *The child with headache: Diagnosis and treatment.* Seattle, WA: IASP Press.

McGrath, P. A., & Koster, A. L. (2001). Headache measures for children: A practical approach. In P. A. McGrath & L. M. Hillier (Eds.), *The child with headache: Diagnosis and treatment* (pp. 29–56). Seattle, WA: IASP Press.

McGrath, P. A., Seifert, C. E., Speechley, K. N., Booth, J. C., Stitt, L., & Gibson, M. C. (1996). A new analogue scale for assessing children's pain: An initial validation study. *Pain, 64,* 435–443.

McGrath, P. A., Speechley, K. N., Seifert, C. E., Biehn, J. T., Cairney, A. E. L., Gorodzinsky, F. P., Dickie, G. L., McCusker, P. J., & Morrisy, J. R. (2000). A survey of children's acute, recurrent, and chronic pain: Validation of the Pain Experience Interview. *Pain, 87,* 59–73.

McGrath, P. A., Speechley, K. N., Seifert, C. E., & Gorodzinsky, F. P. (1997). A survey of children's pain experience and knowledge: Phase 1. In T. S. Jensen, J. A. Turner, & Z. Wiesenfeld-Hallin (Eds.), *Proceedings of the 8th World Congress on Pain: Progress in pain research and management* (pp. 903–916). Seattle, IASP Press.

McGrath, P. J. (1998). Behavioral measures of pain. In G. A. Finley & P. J. McGrath (Eds.), *Measurement of pain in infants and children* (pp. 83–102). Seattle, WA: IASP Press.

McGrath, P. J., Johnson, G., Goodman, J. T., Schillinger, J., Dunn, J., & Chapman, J. (1985). CHEOPS: A behavioral scale for rating postoperative pain in children. In H. L. Fields, R. Dubner, & F. Cervero (Eds.), *Advances in pain research and therapy* (Vol. 9, pp. 395–402). New York: Raven Press.

Merkel, S. I., Voepel-Lewis, T., Shayevitz, J. R., & Malviya, S. (1997). The FLACC: A behavioral scale for scoring postoperative pain in young children. *Pediatric Nursing, 23,* 293–297.

Owens, M. E., & Todt, E. H. (1984). Pain in infancy: Neonatal reaction to a heel lance. *Pain, 20,* 77–86.

Porter, F. L., Porges, S. W., & Marshall, R. E. (1988). Newborn cries and vagal tone: Parallel changes in response to circumcision. *Child Development, 59,* 495–505.

Price, D. D. (1999). *Psychological mechanisms of pain and analgesia.* Seattle, WA: IASP Press.

Rafferty, T., & Moser, S. (1991). [Pilot study of Short Stay Unit Pain Rating Scale]. Unpublished raw data.

Royal College of Nursing Institute. (1999). *Clinical guideline for the recognition and assessment of acute pain in children: Recommendations.* London: Author.

Robertson, J. (1993). Pediatric pain assessment: Validation of a multidimensional tool. *Pediatric Nursing, 19,* 209–213.

Ross, D. M., & Ross, S. A. (1984a). Childhood pain: The school-aged child's viewpoint. *Pain, 20,* 179–191.

Ross, D. M., & Ross, S. A. (1984b). The importance of type of question, psychological climate and subject set in interviewing children about pain. *Pain, 19,* 71–79.

Ross, D. M., & Ross, S. A. (1988). *Childhood pain: Current issues, research, and management.* Baltimore: Urban & Schwarzenberg.

Savedra, M. C., Gibbons, P. T., Tesler, M. D., Ward, J. A., & Wegner, C. (1982). How do children describe pain?: A tentative assessment. *Pain, 14,* 95–104.

Savedra, M. C., Holzemer, W. L., Tesler, M. D., & Wilkie, D. J. (1993). Assessment of postoperation pain in children and adolescents using the Adolescent Pediatric Pain Tool. *Nursing Research, 42,* 5–9.

Savedra, M. C., Tesler, M. D., Holzemer, W. L., Wilkie, D. J., & Ward, J. A. (1989). Pain location: Validity and reliability of body outline markings by hospitalized children and adolescents. *Research in Nursing and Health, 12,* 307–314.

Savedra, M., Tesler, M., Ward, J., Wegner, C., & Gibbons, P. (1981). Description of the pain experience:

A study of school-age children. *Issues in Comprehensive Pediatric Nursing, 5,* 373–380.

Schechter, N. L., Berde, C. B., & Yaster, M. (Eds.). (1993). *Pain in infants, children and adolescents.* Baltimore: Williams & Wilkins.

Schultz, A. A., Murphy, E., Morton, J., Stempel, A., Messenger-Rioux, C., & Bennett, K. (1999). Preverbal, Early Verbal Pediatric Pain Scale (PEPPS): Development and early psychometric testing. *Journal of Pediatric Nursing, 14,* 19–27.

Schultz, N. V. (1971). How children perceive pain. *Nursing Outlook, 19,* 670–673.

Sinkin-Feldman, L., Tesler, M., & Savedra, M. (1997). Word placement on the Word-Graphic Rating Scale by pediatric patients. *Pediatric Nursing, 23,* 31–34.

St. Laurent-Gagnon, T., Bernard-Bonnin, A. C., & Villeneuve, E. (1999). Pain evaluation in preschool children and by their parents. *Acta Paediatrics, 88,* 422–427.

Stein, P. (1995). Indices of pain intensity: Construct validity among preschoolers. *Pediatric Nursing, 21,* 119–123.

Stevens, B. (1990). Development and testing of a pediatric pain management sheet. *Pediatric Nursing, 16,* 543–548.

Stevens, B., Johnston, C., Petryshen, P., & Taddio, A. (1996). Premature Infant Pain Profile: Development and initial validation. *Clinical Journal of Pain, 12,* 13–22.

Sweet, S. D., & McGrath, P. J. (1998). Physiological measures of pain. In G. A. Finley & P. J. McGrath (Eds.), *Measurement of pain in infants and children* (pp. 59–81). Seattle, WA: IASP Press.

Szyfelbein S. K., Osgood, P. F., Atchison, N. E., & Carr, D. B. (1987). Variations in plasma beta-endorphin and cortisol levels in acutely burned children. *Pain* (Suppl. 4), S234.

Szyfelbein, S. K., Osgood, P. F., & Carr, D. B. (1985). The assessment of pain and plasma beta-endorphin immunoactivity in burned children. *Pain, 22,* 173–182.

Tarbell, S. E., Cohen, I. T., & Marsh, J. L. (1992). The Toddler–Preschooler Postoperative Pain Scale: An observational scale for measuring postoperative pain in children aged 1–5. Preliminary report. *Pain, 50,* 273–280.

Tesler, M. D., Savedra, M. C., Holzemer, W. L., Wilkie, D. J., Ward, J. A., & Paul, S. M. (1991). The Word-Graphic Rating Scale as a measure of children's and adolescents' pain intensity. *Research in Nursing and Health, 14,* 361–371.

Tyler, D. C., Tu, A., Douthit, J., & Chapman, C. R. (1993). Toward validation of pain measurement tools for children: A pilot study. *Pain, 52,* 301–309.

Van Cleve, L., Johnson, L., & Pothier, P. (1996). Pain responses of hospitalized infants and children to venipuncture and intravenous cannulation. *Journal of Pediatric Nursing, 11,* 161–168.

Varni, J. W., Katz, E. R., & Dash, J. (1982). Behavioral and neurochemical aspects of pediatric pain. In D. C. Russo & J. W. Varni (Eds.), *Behavioral pediatrics: Research and practice* (pp. 177–224). New York: Plenum Press.

Varni, J. W., Thompson, K. L., & Hanson, V. (1987). The Varni-Thompson Pediatric Pain Questionnaire: I. Chronic musculoskeletal pain in juvenile rheumatoid arthritis. *Pain, 28,* 27–38.

Vessey, J. A., Carlson, K. L., & McGill, J. (1994). Use of distraction with children during an acute pain experience. *Nursing Research, 43,* 369–372.

Villarruel, A. M., & Denyes, M. J. (1991). Pain assessment in children: Theoretical and empirical validity. *Advances in Nursing Science, 14,* 32–41.

Westerling, D. (1999). Postoperative recovery evaluated with a new, tactile scale (TaS) in children undergoing ophthalmic surgery. *Pain, 83,* 297–301.

Whaley, L., & Wong, D. L. (1987). *Nursing care of infants and children.* St. Louis: Mosby.

Wilkie, D. J., Holzemer, W. L., Tesler, M. D., Ward, J. A., Paul, S. M., & Savedra, M. C. (1990). Measuring pain quality: Validity and reliability of children's and adolescents' pain language. *Pain, 41,* 151–159.

Wong, D. L, & Baker, C. M. (1988). Pain in children: Comparison of assessment scales. *Pediatric Nursing, 14,* 9–17.

Wong, D. L., & Whaley, L. F. (1999). *Whaley and Wong's nursing care of infants and children* (6th ed.). St. Louis, MO: Mosby/Year Book.

Zeltzer, L., Anderson, C. M., & Schechter, N. L. (1990). Pediatric pain: Current status and future directions. *Current Issues in Pediatrics, 20,* 415–486.

Chapter 7

Assessment of Pain in Elderly People

LUCIA GAGLIESE

There has been a steady increase of research into pain in elderly persons over the past decade. This is in part a reaction to the growing numbers of elderly individuals in society and the demand this group will create for effective pain management (Ferrell, 1996). Although information regarding age-related patterns of pain, disability, and psychological distress is now more readily available, many gaps in our knowledge remain, and the need for further research is clear. For instance, the fundamental issue of how best to measure the relevant variables (or constructs) in samples of elderly people and across age groups has yet to be resolved. Despite this, studies have employed measures that were developed for younger adults or for healthy, community-dwelling elderly individuals. The appropriateness of these scales for elderly people with pain has not always been demonstrated. Consequently, the interpretation of the rapidly accumulating data is limited until we know whether these data are in fact valid. Fortunately, some preliminary evidence is available.

In this chapter, I review the evidence regarding the reliability and validity of several of the measures of pain, functional impairment, and emotional distress most commonly employed with elderly individuals. Where possible, I make recommendations regarding those tools most appropriate for use with elderly patients and in research designed to measure age differences. I also review data regarding pain measurement in a highly selected sample of elderly people—those with cognitive impairment. Throughout the text, I highlight those issues that remain to

be resolved or have yet to be addressed, in an effort to stimulate further research.

MEASUREMENT OF PAIN IN THE GENERAL ELDERLY POPULATION

Self-Report Measures

Measures of Pain Intensity

The most frequently assessed component of pain is intensity—how much it hurts (see Jensen & Karoly, Chapter 2, this volume). Commonly used measures of pain intensity include Visual Analogue Scales (VASs), Verbal Rating Scales (VRSs), and Numerical Rating Scales (NRSs) (see Jensen & Karoly, Chapter 2, for reviews). Preliminary data regarding the psychometric properties of these types of instruments in samples of the elderly have become available only recently. These studies have assessed elderly persons' ability to complete the scales, their preferences among them, and the consistency of intensity estimates obtained from different measures.

Significant attention has been paid to age differences in the ability to complete various pain tools. Failure has been defined as providing responses that cannot be scored (e.g., leaving a question blank, choosing more than one option on a VRS or NRS, or circling the anchors or line on a VAS). Interestingly, increasing age has been associated with a higher frequency of incomplete or unscorable responses on a VAS (Gagliese & Melzack, 1997; Jensen, Karoly, & Braver, 1986; Kremer, Atkinson, & Ignelzi, 1981), but not on a VRS (Gagliese & Melzack, 1997; Jensen et al., 1986), a behavioral rating scale (BRS) (Gagliese & Melzack, 1997; Jensen et al., 1986), or an NRS (Jensen et al., 1986). These studies have reported failure rates on a VAS of between 7% and 30% of elderly subjects (Gagliese & Melzack, 1997; Herr & Mobily, 1993). Kremer and colleagues (1981) suggested that elderly people may have deficits in abstract reasoning that make use of a VAS difficult, but the nature of these difficulties has not been elucidated.

Preferences among various types of pain intensity scales have also been measured. This represents an aspect of face validity, as subjects are asked which type of scale they prefer, which is the easiest to complete, and which is the best representation of their pain. Consistent with data regarding scale failure, the elderly report that VASs are more difficult to complete and are poorer descriptions of pain than VRSs (Benesh, Szigeti, Ferraro, & Gullicks, 1997; Herr & Mobily, 1993). These data suggest that even among those who are able to complete a VAS, this type of scale is difficult and of questionable face validity. This raises concerns regarding subject compliance, especially for studies requiring repeated or independent completion of the VAS.

Generally, studies of elderly subjects' preferences have found that a VRS (Herr & Mobily, 1993; Kremer et al., 1981) and a pain thermometer, in which gradations are marked with verbal descriptors (Benesh et al., 1997), are rated as the easiest measures to complete, the best or most accurate measures of pain, and the most preferred for future use. Despite one failed replication (Benesh et al., 1997), a VAS is generally the least preferred type of measure among elderly samples (Herr & Mobily, 1993; Kremer et al., 1981). The conclusions that can be drawn from these data are limited, because the samples were small and age differences in scale preferences and face validity have not been assessed.

One indication of a measure's concurrent validity is the extent to which it correlates positively with other measures of the same construct (Anastasi, 1988). As such, one would expect that various measures of pain intensity would at least be moderately correlated with each other. Several studies have assessed the intercorrelation of various pain intensity tools in elderly samples. Generally, these studies involve completing the tools in immediate succession with appropriate controls for the effects of subject fatigue, scale order, or practice (Benesh et al., 1997; Herr & Mobily, 1993). Although there have been reports suggesting only modest correlation between the VAS and the VRS ($r = .40-.58$) (Helme, Katz, Gibson, & Corran, 1989; Herr & Mobily, 1993), other studies have found a high level of correlation between these scales ($r = .88-.90$) (Benesh et al., 1997; Herr & Mobily, 1993). High levels of correlation ($r = .84-.98$) have been reported between other types of pain scales, including VASs, pain thermometers with verbal descriptors, NRSs, electronic NRS ratings, and VRSs (Benesh et al., 1997; Herr & Mobily, 1993; Lewis, Lewis, & Cumming, 1995). Although these results are encouraging, only limited conclusions may be drawn. The samples in these studies were small. Detailed description of the protocol for test administration was not provided, and age differences have not been assessed. A highly sophisticated, but post hoc, statistical analysis by Svensson (1998) suggested that a VAS is not appropriate for the evaluation of changes in pain intensity in elderly samples. Despite the clear need for further work on this question, the preliminary data available support the use of pain intensity measures in elderly samples, although the reliability and validity of VASs remain to be clearly established.

Another approach to the assessment of concurrent validity of different pain intensity tools has been to convert scores to percentages and then compare across scales. This methodology has identified another potential difficulty with a VAS—namely, lack of agreement with other measures in estimates of pain intensity levels. Specifically, within the same group of elderly individuals, VAS scores may be significantly different from scores on other intensity measures, including a VRS and BRS, which do not differ from each other (Gagliese & Melzack, 1997; Herr & Mobily, 1993). This pattern is not found in young and middle-aged patients with chronic pain (Gagliese & Melzack, 1997). However, VAS ratings may not differ from electronic NRS ratings of pain intensity made by elderly patients with chronic pain (Lewis et al., 1995). Methodological differences between these studies limit comparison.

Because of the special challenges present in the assessment of pain in elderly individuals, especially the possibility of impaired verbal expression and abstract reasoning, Harkins and Price (1992) suggested, in the first edition of this volume, that scales originally designed for use with children may be appropriate for this population. Facial scales, which use a series of facial expressions to depict varying levels of pain intensity, have been advocated as appropriate for use with elderly samples. Herr, Mobily, Kohout, and Wagenaar (1998) showed that the Faces Pain Scale (Bieri, Reeve, Champion, Addicoat, & Ziegler, 1990) has strong ordinal properties and test–retest reliability in a sample of healthy, community-dwelling elderly persons. Nonetheless, approximately 12% of this sample of cognitively intact elderly people were unable to use this scale to quantify the intensity of their pain. Using a different facial scale, Fernandez-Galinski, Rue, Moral, Castells, and Puig (1996) found only a moderate correlation between the Faces Scale and VAS ratings of postoperative pain intensity, with scores on the Faces Scale indicating more intense pain than VAS scores did. The greatest limitation to the use of this type of scale among the elderly is the questionable level of construct validity. Specifically, the faces used in these scales are often interpreted as expressing negative emotions, such as sadness, in addition to pain. Therefore, ratings may reflect both pain intensity and emotional distress (Herr et al., 1998). Nonetheless, when these limitations are kept in mind, these studies provide interesting data regarding the psychometric properties of this type of scale. It is easy to imagine that such a scale may be especially useful among the elderly with language impairments. However, data are needed to support the use of such scales among this subpopulation of elderly people.

Taken together, these data provide important preliminary evidence regarding the use of pain intensity measures in elderly samples. For the most part, the data are encouraging. It appears that intensity measures, especially those made up of verbal descriptors, may be appropriate for use with the elderly. On the other hand, these preliminary data also raise important problems for the use of VASs with the elderly. As many as 30% of cognitively intact elderly may be unable to complete this type of scale (Gagliese & Melzack, 1997). Furthermore, among those who can complete VASs, intensity estimates may be significantly different from those obtained using VRSs, NRSs, or facial expression scales. Reasons for this, and strategies to improve the validity and reliability of VASs in the elderly, require further study.

Interestingly, elderly people also experience difficulties in using a VAS to measure constructs other than pain (Tiplady, Jackson, Maskrey, & Swift, 1998). The source of these difficulties remains elusive, although Tiplady and colleagues (1998) suggested that the difficulties may be specific to ratings of subjective attributes or internal states, but not to ratings of the attributes of external, concrete objects (e.g., size of animals). Clearly, a systematic research program is needed to examine (both within elderly samples and across age groups) the full range of psychometric properties of the various pain tools available, in order to develop a valid and reliable pain intensity assessment protocol for clinical and research use.

The McGill Pain Questionnaire

Unidimensional single-item scales such as those described above give an indication of only one element of the pain experience/intensity. Multidimensional measures, on the other hand, provide a more comprehensive picture of an individual's pain. The McGill Pain Questionnaire (MPQ; Melzack, 1975) is the most widely used multidimensional pain inventory (Wilke, Savedra, Holzemer, Tesler, & Paul, 1990; see Melzack & Katz, Chapter 3, this volume). It consists of 20 sets of adjectives that are divided into four subscales for the Sensory, Affective, Evaluative, and Miscellaneous components of pain. Subjects endorse those words that describe their feelings and sensations at that moment. There is much evidence for the validity, reliability, and discriminative abilities of the MPQ when used with younger adults (Katz & Melzack, 1999).

Herr and Mobily (1991) have suggested that the MPQ may be too complex and time-consuming for elderly persons. They argue that this group may have difficulty understanding some of the pain descriptors and may be overwhelmed by the large number of choices. These authors do not present data to support this claim, however. Although reliable use of the MPQ does require basic reading and comprehension abilities, these demands are similar across age groups. The concerns of Herr and Mobily may pertain more directly to issues of educational level, reading level, or cognitive impairment than to age. Furthermore, recent evidence regarding the use of the MPQ in elderly samples suggests that their concerns may not be well founded.

Although the evidence is preliminary, it appears that the psychometric properties of the MPQ may not be age-related. Specifically, we (Gagliese, Stratford, Hickey, Gamsa, & Melzack, 1998) have found that the latent structure, internal consistency, and pattern of subscale correlations of the MPQ are very similar in young and elderly patients with chronic pain who have been matched for pain diagnosis, location, and duration, and gender. Similar results have also been found in middle-aged and older men when the MPQ was used to assess post-operative pain following radical prostatectomy (Gagliese, Wowk, Sandler, & Katz, 1999). In both studies, elderly patients endorsed fewer adjectives than younger patients did, although the same adjectives were chosen the most frequently regardless of age. This raises the important, but not tested possibility, that the discriminative abilities of the MPQ are also not age-related. Although further studies are needed, these results suggest that the MPQ is indeed appropriate for use with older patients with both chronic and acute pain. It appears to measure the same constructs in the same way across the adult life span.

The short form of the MPQ (SF-MPQ; Melzack, 1987; see Melzack & Katz, Chapter 3), which measures Sensory and Affective dimensions of pain, may also be appropriate for use with elderly individuals. Error rates on this scale do not differ between age groups (Gagliese & Melzack, 1997). Internal consistency, a measure of reliability, is high ($\alpha = .90$) (LeFort, Murray, & Ribeiro, 1996), and the subscales provide comparable estimates of pain levels within elderly samples (Gagliese & Melzack, 1997). As on the full-scale MPQ, elderly people endorse fewer words overall than younger people, but regardless of age, the same adjectives are chosen most frequently to describe the same type of pain (e.g., arthritis pain) (Gagliese & Melzack, 1997). These findings must be replicated in larger samples with more detailed psychometric analyses before conclusions can be drawn.

Pain Scale Sensitivity

In order to be valid, scores on a pain scale must change in predicted ways (Jensen, 1997). For instance, scores on valid pain scales should decrease over time following surgery. There is preliminary evidence to suggest that this is indeed the case in elderly patients when pain is measured with the MPQ, VRSs, and VASs (Gagliese, Jackson, Ritvo, Wowk, & Katz, 2000; Gagliese, Wowk, et al., 1999; Oberle, Paul, Wry, & Grace, 1990). However, similarity in the magnitude of the decrease over the first 3 postoperative days across pain scales and age groups has not been consistently reported (Gagliese et al., 2000; Gagliese, Wowk, et al., 1999; Oberle et al., 1990). This may reflect age differences in the properties of the scales, but also in the pattern of healing and recovery following surgery. This issue urgently requires more systematic study.

Pain scale sensitivity is also demonstrated through changes in pain levels following manipulations known to reduce pain such as the administration of analgesics (Jensen, 1997). This issue has not been adequately assessed. One study suggests that the sensitivity of VRSs is superior to that of VASs (Frank, Moll, & Hort, 1982). Grant, Bishop-Miller, Winchester, Anderson, and Faulkner (1999) reported that the magnitude of change found following physical therapies was the same, whether it was measured with a VAS or the Nottingham Health Profile. Similarly, Lewis and colleagues (1995) found moderate correlations between VAS and MPQ scores, and between these scales and a clinical assessment of function following various pain management conditions. Studies designed to systematically address the issue of the sensitivity of various scales for elderly samples and age differences in scale sensitivity are lacking.

Pain Location and Distribution

In addition to descriptors of pain qualities, the MPQ includes line drawings of the body (a pain map) on which to indicate the spatial distribution of pain (Melzack, 1975). Although the interpretation of pain maps remains unclear (see Jensen & Karoly, Chapter 2), a valid and reliable scoring method has been developed for younger adults (Margolis, Tait, & Krause, 1986), but the validity of this method for elderly samples has not been demonstrated. Escalante, Lichtenstein, White, Rios, and Hazuda (1995) have developed a scoring system specifically for assessing arthritis pain in the elderly. The preliminary psychometric data are promising. This scoring system is associated with a high level of interrater and intrarater reliability (Escalante et al., 1995). Test–retest reliability is also good, and acceptable levels of internal consistency have been reported (Lichtenstein, Dhanda, Cornell, Escalante, & Hazuda, 1998). Interestingly, in this administration method, elderly subjects point to the painful area on the drawing, and the interviewers make the markings on it (Escalante et al., 1995)—a scoring method originally developed for use with children (Savedra, Tesler, Holzemer, Wilkie, & Ward, 1989). It is not clear whether similar results would be obtained if elderly subjects were to complete the pain maps independently.

The relationship of this measure to MPQ and VRS scores has been inconsistent, with reports of weak (Lichtenstein et al., 1998) and strong (Escalante et al., 1995) correlations. This inconsistency should not be taken as a challenge to the usefulness of a pain map. There is no obvious a priori reason to expect a strong relationship between pain location and intensity or qualities. It is easy to imagine that one could experience highly localized severe pain, highly localized mild pain, diffuse severe pain, and diffuse mild pain. Each of these situations would lead to a different correlation between pain location and intensity. Although preliminary, these data suggest that the elderly are able to use a pain map to indicate the location of their pain. This method of scoring the pain map has not been tested in younger adults.

Summary

As this review has made clear, much more work is needed in order to establish the appropriateness of various self-report measures of pain for use with elderly people. The preliminary data available support the following tentative conclusions. The assessment of pain in cognitively intact, elderly people should include a VRS measure of pain intensity and either the MPQ or SF-MPQ. This combination of scales also would be the most appropriate for the assessment of age differences in pain. Pain maps appear to provide useful data regarding the location and spatial distribution of pain, although none of the available scoring methods has been tested across age groups. There appear to be several potential problems with the use of a VAS by elderly people. These include high failure rates, low face validity, and as yet unclear levels of reliability and sensitivity. Future work should examine the factors that hinder appropriate use of a VAS by elderly persons, as well as the age-related sensitivity of each of these scales to experimental or therapeutic manipulations. Larger studies are needed to assess more adequately the psychometric properties of the scales discussed above across the adult life span. These scales have been used extensively, although data on their psychometric properties in elderly samples are limited. As a result, the validity of this research remains unclear until it is shown that these tools are appropriate for use with elderly individuals.

Observational/Nonverbal Methods

Pain Behaviors

Considerable attention has been devoted to the development of valid and reliable protocols for the assessment of pain behaviors. *Pain behaviors* are actions, both verbal and nonverbal, that communicate pain to others (see Keefe, Williams, & Smith, Chapter 10). They include, but are not limited to, grimacing, rubbing the painful area, limping, and groaning (Keefe et al., 1987). As with the self-report measures reviewed above, these standardized protocols were developed for use with younger people, and their appropriateness for elderly samples remains to be established.

Keefe and colleagues (Keefe, 1982; Keefe et al., 1987) have provided extensive evidence for the reliability and validity of a standardized protocol for the assessment of pain due to arthritis. This protocol requires that individuals perform, in random order, activities such as sitting, standing, and walking. The occurrence and frequency of pain behaviors during the activities are used to determine a total pain behavior score. The speed of movements is also scored. Using this protocol, Keefe et al. (1987) found that increasing age was associated with slower movements and increased pain behaviors. The authors point out that it is impossible to determine whether the increased pain behavior score is related to pain or aging (Keefe et al., 1987). This represents a serious difficulty for the use of this protocol in the assessment of pain behaviors in elderly individuals, and especially for the assessment of age differences in pain behaviors. It would be interesting to compare behaviors during this protocol in elderly individuals with and without chronic pain.

Pain behaviors observed during the protocol developed by Keefe and colleagues (1987) (traditional) were compared to those displayed following a more rigorous protocol made up of movements that simulate activities of daily living (ADLs) in a sample of elderly people with low back pain (Weiner, Peiper, McConnell, Martinez, & Keefe, 1996). Interrater reliability was acceptable in both conditions. However, the ADLs protocol was more strongly correlated with self-report measures of pain and disability than the traditional protocol. Despite these promising preliminary results, several limitations must be considered. The ADLs protocol was much more rigorous than the traditional protocol, and although the sample in this study was made up of independent adults, approximately 8% were unable to complete the ADLs protocol because it triggered severe pain (Weiner et al., 1996). It is reasonable to expect that this proportion would be higher among a sample of frail elderly patients with chronic pain.

Evidence regarding the use of standardized behavioral protocols for the assessment of pain behaviors in elderly people remains scant. Systematic studies with larger, more representative samples are needed. In addition, the manner in which pain behaviors may change with age needs to be examined independently of pain intensity. Age differences in the reliability and validity of the pain behavior protocols have not been assessed. A further limitation, not specific to the elderly, concerns the clinical utility of these protocols. Their use requires videotaping and careful scoring by well-trained observers. This may not always be feasible in the clinical setting.

Facial Expression of Pain

Facial expressions have been shown to be reliable nonverbal indicators of painful states (see Craig, Prkachin, & Grunau, Chapter 9). However, their role in the assessment of pain in elderly people is less clear. There may be age-related changes in facial structure and expression that make it more difficult to interpret the facial expressions of elderly people than of younger people (Malatesta, Fiore, & Messina, 1987; Malatesta, Izard, Culver, & Nicolich, 1987). The validity and reliability of facial expressions of pain in elderly individuals has received very little attention. There are no reports of the appropriateness of the Facial Action Coding System, a standardized, objective assessment of the facial expression of pain (Ekman & Friesen, 1978), in cognitively intact elderly persons with pain; nor have age differences using this scoring system been studied.

Another strategy has been to have judges rate perceived pain of subjects videotaped during painful experiences. A study using this methodology found that elderly individuals were judged to be experiencing more intense pain than younger individuals, despite comparable self-report ratings of pain intensity. This was true when both young and older judges rated pain intensity. It is not clear whether the higher pain ratings ascribed to older faces were due to objective changes in facial expression, to biases held by the judges that elderly people experience more pain, or to an interaction of both (Matheson, 1997). Certainly, this study requires replication before the results can be accepted. Nonetheless, it raises an important issue regarding the validity of observer ratings of nonverbal expressions of pain in elderly people, and it highlights the need for more research into this question.

Self-Report versus Observational and Nonverbal Measures

The advantages and disadvantages of self-report and observational and nonverbal measures of pain have been debated in the literature (Jensen, 1997) and are not reviewed here except to point out that there may be problems with both types of assessment in elderly patients. Further insight into this issue may be obtained from studies that directly compare self-reports with health care workers' and significant others' judgments of pain. Because of the inherently subjective nature of pain, it is extremely difficult for an observer to accurately rate the pain being experienced by someone else. This may limit the utility of nonverbal pain measures. In the clinical setting, nevertheless, others' subjective judgments are the norm, and the majority of this work suggests that health care workers (usually nurses) underestimate the prevalence and intensity of pain experienced by younger patients (see, e.g., Allcock, 1996). This can have serious implications, because the administration of pain treatment often relies largely on health care workers' judgments of patients' pain.

Observer ratings of pain among cognitively intact elderly patients have recently begun to receive empirical attention. Weiner, Peterson, Ladd, McConnell, and Keefe (1999) studied pain ratings made by patients, staff members, and family members of elderly adults attending an adult day care center. Patients completed VRS ratings of present pain and least and most pain in the preceding 2 weeks. The composite pain intensity measure derived from these ratings had a high level of internal consistency ($\alpha = .90$). Unfortunately, proxy ratings were made only for severity of pain over the past 2 weeks; a more serious problem was that the ratings by the various informants were made up to one month apart. Despite these limitations, a moderate level ($\kappa = .38-.44$) of concordance between raters was found, with a tendency for family members to overestimate pain intensity. Interestingly, regression analysis suggested that ratings provided by both the patients and informants could by predicted by the presence of musculoskeletal disease and number of medications. In addition, patients' self-reports were associated with levels of depressive symptomatology. This suggests that observers make use of more objective attributes to judge someone else's pain, whereas self-report of pain is influenced by both objective attributes and subjective states that are not readily apparent to an observer. Age differences in levels of concordance have not been documented.

Hall-Lord, Larsson, and Steen (1998) compared the intensity of pain reported in an intensive care setting by elderly patients and their nurses, using a five-item Likert scale. They found that patients and nurses reported comparable levels of pain. However, interventions designed to relieve pain were judged less effective by patients than by nurses. Taken together, these studies suggest that in both acute and chronic care settings, informants and elderly patients provide comparable reports of pain with at least a moderate level of concordance. Generally, nurses tend to underestimate pain experienced by younger patients (see, e.g., Allcock, 1996). It may be that the bias to attribute more pain to elderly individuals reported by Matheson (1997) may actually result in greater concordance between different raters of pain in elderly persons. This issue, as well as age differences in these factors, requires greater study.

Assessment of Pain-Related Disability and Functional Limitations

Both chronic pain (Brattberg, Thorslund, & Wikman, 1989) and increasing age (Forbes, Hatward, & Agwani, 1991) have been associated with impairment in functional abilities and the performance of ADLs. In fact, it has been proposed that high rates of comorbidity, deconditioning, polypharmacy, and social isolation may make elderly patients more susceptible than younger patients to impairments associated with pain (Kwentus, Harkins, Lignon, & Silverman, 1985). Therefore, a comprehensive pain assessment must incorporate measures of the impact and associated features of pain. This can include, but is certainly not limited to, the assessment of physical disability, interference of pain in the performance of daily and desired activities, and psychological distress. Self-report and objective measures of many of these constructs have been developed and are in frequent use in both the research and clinical setting. However, comparable to the measurement of pain, few of these measures have been validated for samples of elderly individuals with pain.

Several measures have been developed for the assessment of pain-specific disability or interference in the performance of activities. Among the most frequently used of these tools is the Pain Disability Index (PDI), a self-report measure of the extent to which the performance of daily activities is limited by pain (Pollard, 1984). The PDI has demonstrated good psychometric properties in younger individuals (Tait, Chibnall, & Krause, 1990). There is limited evidence regarding the psychometric properties of this scale for elderly individuals. Ross and Crook (1998) found adequate levels of internal consistency ($\alpha = .79$) and moderate but significant correlations with scores on the SF-MPQ within a sample of frail community-dwelling senior citizens. Interestingly, neither the PDI nor a generic measure of disability differentiated subjects with chronic pain from those without pain, suggesting that impairment measured by these scales was not specific to pain (Ross & Crook, 1998). The psychometric properties of other pain-specific measures of interference and disability (e.g., the West Haven–Yale Multidimensional Pain Inventory [WHYMPI]; Kerns, Turk, & Rudy, 1985) when used with elderly samples have not been reported.

Several generic measures of impairment due to chronic illness, not specific to pain, have demonstrated good psychometric properties in patients with chronic pain. In addition, some preliminary work has focused on the application of these scales to elderly persons. For the purposes of the present chapter, I discuss only those measures that have been studied in samples of elderly patients with chronic pain. Unfortunately, studies that directly compare these scales across age groups could not be located. The most extensively studied scales are the Sickness Impact Profile (SIP; Bergner, Bobbitt, Kressel, et al., 1976; Bergner, Bobbitt, Pollard, Martin, & Gilson, 1976), the Human Activity Profile (HAP; Fix & Daughton, 1988), and the Physical Activity Scale for the Elderly (PASE; Washburn, Smith, Jette, & Janney, 1993). Generally, these scales have been found to have good levels of internal consistency, as well as moderate correlations with measures of pain. The SIP is a 136-item inventory of the extent to which health problems interfere with physical and psychosocial functioning (Bergner, Bobbitt, Kressel, et al., 1976; Bergner, Bobbitt, Pollard, et al., 1976). It has been shown to have good psychometric properties across various samples, including younger adults with chronic pain, and older people with a variety of health problems in community, acute, and institutional settings (Morishita et al., 1995). Item-scaling analysis has shown that younger and older people do not differ significantly in the perception of the severity of dysfunction assessed by each item (Marchionni et al., 1997). The SIP has been shown to have comparable properties within elderly samples, whether administered as part of an in-person or a telephone interview (Morishita et al., 1995), although comparability with independent completion has not been assessed. Among elderly people with chronic hip and knee pain, the Physical and Psychosocial subscales have been found to be moderately correlated (Hopman-Rock, Odding, Hofman, Kraaimaat, & Bijlsma, 1996).

A second measure that has been validated for use with elderly patients who have chronic pain is the HAP (Fix & Daughton, 1988). This questionnaire assesses the overall, current, and past performance of 94 activities. A subscale factor structure has been identified based on a sample of elderly patients seen at a pain clinic (Farrell, Gibson, & Helme, 1996). In addition, this scale has shown good levels of internal consistency, high test–retest reliability over a 2-week interval, significant correlation with the Physical subscale of the SIP, and sensitivity to treatment effects in this sample (Farrell, Gibson, & Helme, 1996). Total HAP scores are weakly but significantly correlated with the Affective but not the Sensory subscale of the SF-MPQ, suggesting only a weak relationship between measures of pain and activity in elderly patients (Farrell, Gibson, & Helme, 1995). Although the total scores of the HAP have been validated for younger patients with chronic pain, the subscales identified by Farrell, Gibson, and Helme (1996) have yet to be replicated and contrasted across age groups.

The PASE has shown promising psychometric properties for elderly patients with chronic pain (Washburn et al., 1993). This self-report or interview-based measure was developed specifically for elderly individuals. It is made up of 12 items that assess frequency, duration, and intensity of participation in leisure, household, and occupational physical activities over the previous week. A weighted scoring system that reflects the amount of energy required to perform each activity is available. Among healthy elderly persons, this scale has been shown to correlate with the SIP and self-assessed health status and to have moderate to good levels of test–retest reliability in intervals ranging from 3 to 7 weeks. Among elderly persons with daily knee pain secondary to osteoarthritis, PASE scores are significantly correlated with performance on a walking test and measures of knee strength, but not with measures of pain intensity or frequency (Martin et al., 1999). The PASE has not been validated for younger individuals.

Clearly, far more work is needed to determine which measure of activity level or disability due to pain is the most appropriate for elderly samples and for the assessment of age differences. Each of the scales described above measures a slightly different aspect of functioning, and the lack of data comparing them in a systematic way makes it difficult to recommend one over the others. The SIP has the most empirical evidence favoring its use; however, it is a very long questionnaire and may represent considerable burden to patients, especially if repeated administration is necessary. The HAP and PASE are shorter and less burdensome, and have demonstrated limited but favorable psychometric properties. However, their comparability and their relationship to pain-specific measures of disability have not been assessed. There is an urgent need for research into these questions.

Measures of Health-Related Quality of Life

Increasingly, it has been recognized that functional limitations constitute only one aspect of perceived overall health, well-being, and quality of life. Several measures have been developed to assess quality of life, although there is still considerable debate regarding which of these is most appropriate for elderly samples (Bowling, 1998). The most widely used is undoubtedly the Medical Outcome Study 36-Item Short-Form Health Survey (SF-36), a generic, multidimensional measure of functioning and well-being (McHorney, Ware, & Raczek, 1993). The subscales include Physical Functioning; Role Limitations due to Physical Problems; Social Functioning; Bodily Pain; General Mental Health; Role Limitations due to Emotional Problems; Vitality; and General Health Perceptions (McHorney et al., 1993). Concerns have been raised regarding the relevance of some of the items in this scale to the lives of the elderly, and several authors have noted a high level of item nonresponse on this scale (e.g., Bowling, 1998).

The SF-36 has been shown to have acceptable psychometric properties for community-dwelling elderly people (Sherman & Reuben, 1998). Its subscales have demonstrated acceptable levels of internal consistency (Carver, Chapman, Thomas, Stadnyk, & Rockwood, 1999; Sherman & Reuben, 1998) and good test–retest reliability with a 3-week intertest interval (Carver et al., 1999). In addition, responses on the Physical Functioning subscale, but not the Emotional Problems and General Mental Health subscales, are moderately correlated with performance-based and self-report measures of physical functioning, suggesting convergent and divergent validity (Sherman & Reuben, 1998). Scores on the SF-36 are also moderately correlated with scores on the SIP (Weinberger et al., 1991). However, several of the subscales have demonstrated floor and ceiling effects, possibly limiting sensitivity to treatment effects. In addition, principal-components analysis has been unable to replicate the proposed factor structure (Carver et al., 1999).

The difficulties noted above become even more pronounced among frail elderly respondents. In this group, approximately one-third of patients are unable to answer all the items of the SF-36, whereas 25% provide inconsistent responses. There are also substantial floor and ceiling effects (Andresen, Gravitt, Aydelotte, & Podgorski, 1999; Stadnyk, Calder, & Rockwood, 1998). Nonetheless, the internal consistency of the subscales is moderate to high, with acceptable test–retest reliability (Andresen et al., 1999; Stadnyk et al., 1998). In addition, researchers using a multitrait–multimethod correlation matrix have found evidence for acceptable levels of convergent and divergent validity (Andresen et al., 1999; Stadnyk et al., 1998).

Despite its widespread, if somewhat controversial, use among elderly samples, only two studies that have assessed the psychometric properties of the SF-36 in the elderly with pain are available at this writing. In one, moderate to high levels of internal consistency and a gradient of scores reflecting increasingly poor health were found among elderly individuals with chronic pain in community and institutional settings (Murray, LeFort, & Ribeiro, 1998). Nonetheless, the face validity of the SF-36 was questionable, and the authors recommend caution in the interpretation of responses (Murray et al., 1998). Mangione and colleagues (1993) compared the SF-36 in middle-aged and elderly patients undergoing elective surgery. They found similar levels of subscale internal consistency across age groups, but significant age differences in the magnitude of subscale correlations. Most importantly, the correlation of overall health perception and pain was almost twice as high in the middle-aged as in the elderly patients. These authors suggest that the determinants of health-related quality of life may differ by age, and that the SF-36 may not assess those that are most important to elderly individuals (Mangione et al., 1993). Taken together, data regarding the use of the SF-36 in elderly persons with pain or across age groups are not very encouraging. However, much more work is needed before firm conclusions can be drawn or recommendations for or against use of this scale can be made.

Assessment of the Affective Dimension of Chronic Pain

The affective dimension of chronic pain is most often conceptualized in terms of depression and/or anxiety. Despite evidence of significant anxiety among geriatric patients with chronic pain (Casten, Parmelee, Kleban, Lawton, & Katz, 1995), very little attention has been paid to its assessment. Fortunately, more attention has been paid to the assessment of depression in the elderly.

As in younger individuals, there is significant comorbidity of pain and depression in the elderly. In fact, there is convincing evidence that the prevalence and intensity of depression among patients with chronic pain is similar across age groups (Gagliese, Katz, & Melzack, 1999). Clinical differentiation of these states among the elderly may be difficult (Herr & Mobily, 1991), especially since many of the most common symptoms of depression, such as sleep and appetite disturbance, may be part of normal aging (Parmelee, 1997). In addition, elderly patients are more likely to have atypical presentation of both pain (Gagliese et al., 1999) and depression (Gallo & Rabins, 1999).

There are several well-validated instruments for the assessment of depression in the elderly (Brink et al., 1982). In addition, several scales originally developed for use with younger samples have been studied with elderly respondents. In order to be useful, these scales must be able to identify clinically significant levels of depressive symptomatology with acceptable sensitivity and specificity (Papassotiropoulos & Heun, 1999). In other words, these scales must accurately identify cases of depression while not misidentifying individuals (i.e., false positives and false negatives). Not surprisingly, high levels of comorbidity and atypical presentation of depression among elderly individuals present significant problems for these measures. Generally, the use of cutoff scores developed with younger samples is associated with a high rate of false positives, or overestimation of depression, leading several authors to suggest raising the cutoff for definition of "caseness" among elderly individuals. There also may be problems with using these scales to estimate absolute levels of symptomatology across age groups. Many of the items assess the vegetative or somatic symptoms of depression, which may also be associated with age-related increases in comorbidity that are independent of depression. This would inflate the scores obtained on these scales by elderly persons (Bourque, Blanchard, & Saulnier, 1992; Irwin, Artin, & Oxman, 1999; Papassotiropoulos & Heun, 1999).

Unfortunately, studies that specifically assess the psychometric properties of these scales in samples made up of individuals with chronic pain of various ages are not available. This is extremely important because chronic pain, regardless of age, may necessitate a change in the application of these scales for many of the same reasons described above (Turk & Okifuji, 1994). Therefore, the extent to which these scales can be used in the case of elderly patients with chronic pain remains questionable. Nonetheless, these scales have been used in this population. Although their psychometric properties have not been documented, it has been suggested that scores on the Center for Epidemiologic Studies–Depression (CES-D) scale (Radloff, 1977), the Beck Depression Inventory (BDI; Beck, 1978), and the Geriatric Depression Scale (GDS; Yesavage, 1988) differentiate between elderly respondents with and without chronic pain. The interpretation of these findings is limited, however. For instance, Parmelee, Katz, and Lawton (1991) reported that among institutionalized elderly patients, GDS scores indicative of minor or no depression were correlated with a measure of pain intensity, but that GDS scores indicative of major depression were not. This is a very intriguing pattern of results, but interpretation is limited, because the psychometric properties of the GDS for institutionalized elderly patients with chronic pain have not been reported.

Another very provocative finding was reported by Turk, Okifuji, and Scharff (1995). They found that the patterns of association between levels of depressive symptomatology measured on the CES-D and the impact of pain measured on the WHYMPI (Kerns et al., 1985) were different in younger and older patients. The meaning of these differences is difficult to ascertain, because neither of these measures has been well validated for use among elderly patients with chronic pain. The interpretation of studies designed to identify profiles or clusters of elderly patients with chronic pain based on responses to various self-report measures (Corran, Farrell, Helme, & Gibson, 1997) is similarly limited. Clearly, these data are needed so that both our theoretical and clinical understanding of the relationship between depression, pain, and impairment in patients of various ages with chronic pain can advance.

ASSESSMENT OF PAIN IN COGNITIVELY IMPAIRED ELDERLY PEOPLE

The assessment of pain in the cognitively impaired elderly population has recently begun to receive empirical attention. This population presents many additional challenges to those outlined above, and a reliable and valid assessment protocol for this population remains to be developed (see Hadjistavropoulos, von Baeyer, & Craig, Chapter 8). This work is hindered by many inherent challenges. Among cognitively impaired elderly patients who are capable of verbal report, memory and language impairments may confound reports of pain, especially if such patients are asked, for instance, to recall pain in the previous 2 weeks (Farrell, Katz, & Helme, 1996). Furthermore, studies based on self-report do not provide evidence that the cognitively impaired subjects understood the demands of the task. Specifically, it is not clear that the protocols assessed each subject's understanding of the concept of pain or of the method used to quantify intensity. Studies rarely include modified pain assessment tools that accommodate for the cognitive limitations of the respondents. For instance, scales designed for children may be more appropriate for this population (Harkins & Price, 1992), but these scales have not been tested in a systematic fashion.

The effect of mild to moderate cognitive impairment on the completion of pain scales has been studied. Not surprisingly, high failure rates have been reported. For instance, in a sample of cognitively impaired patients who were able to report pain verbally, only 32% could complete all five of the pain scales employed, while 17% were unable to complete any one of them (Ferrell, Ferrell, & Rivera, 1995). Failure rates were lowest for Present Pain Intensity (a VRS) from the MPQ (35%) and the highest for a horizontal VAS (56%) (Ferrell et al., 1995). Among those who were able to complete more than one scale, moderate to strong interclass correlations were found among the ratings on the various tools (Ferrell et al., 1995). Unfortunately, the relationship between degree of cognitive impairment and the ability to complete the scales was not explored (Ferrell et al., 1995). Feldt, Ryden, and Miles (1998) reported that test–retest reliability with almost immediate readministration of a VRS rating of postoperative pain was excellent ($r = .94$) among intact elderly individuals, but only fair among cognitively impaired individuals ($r = .31$). In addition, while all of the intact elderly persons were able to complete this scale, over 20% of the cognitively impaired persons could not.

Within a sample of acutely confused elderly individuals, Miller and colleagues (1996) found a failure rate of 73% on a vertical VAS even with repeated cueing. A colored VAS that has a triangular shape corresponding to increased pain intensity may be easier to conceptualize and use than a standard VAS, but is still associated with a 54% failure rate among cognitively impaired elderly subjects (Hadjistavropoulos, Craig, Martin, Hadjistavropoulos, & McMurtry, 1997). Weiner and colleagues (1999) found a 20% to 42% failure rate on an NRS, but a moderate to good level of test–retest reliability with a 1-month intertest interval. Promising data were reported regarding the use of pain maps in this group (Weiner, Peterson, & Keefe, 1998). When administration procedures tested in cognitively intact elderly individuals (Escalante et al., 1995) were used, there were no failures and good to excellent levels of test–retest reliability over a 1-hour interval (Weiner et al., 1998). Interestingly, scores on the pain map were correlated with pain thermometer scores but not with NRSs of intensity in this sample (Weiner et al., 1998). Reasons for this dissociation are not clear. Taken together, these data highlight the difficulties of using self-report scales in this population. The challenge of developing a reliable, quantitative pain assessment instrument for use with this population remains.

An alternative to self-report may be to rely on the observation of pain behaviors or facial expressions. This may be especially important as dementia progresses and patient self-report becomes impossible. At this point, valuable information may be obtained from significant others (Werner, Cohen-Mansfield, Watson, & Pasis, 1998) or through direct observation of behavior, especially abrupt changes in behavior or disruption in usual functioning (Marzinski, 1991). Hurley, Volicer, Hanrahan, Houde, and Volicer (1992) have developed a scale to measure behavioral indicators of discomfort in noncommunicative patients with advanced Alzheimer's disease. The properties of this scale have been tested in verbal but acutely confused elderly patients with acute pain (Miller et al., 1996). In this sample, high levels of internal consistency and good interrater reliability were found, although observers reported that items pertaining to facial expression (i.e., "sad," "frowning") were very difficult to judge. These items achieved only fair levels of interrater reliability

and were omitted from a revised version of the scale. Others have reported that moderate correlations are found between VRS ratings and pain behavior checklists, with the magnitude of correlation quite similar in cognitively intact and impaired groups (Feldt et al., 1998). Interestingly, the cognitively impaired patients displayed more frequent pain behaviors than the cognitively intact ones (Feldt et al., 1998).

The level of agreement between caretakers' (usually nurses') and cognitively impaired patients' identification and rating of pain intensity has only been fair to moderate (Feldt et al., 1998; Weiner et al., 1998, 1999). However, detailed analysis of the pattern of discrepancy leads to some surprising conclusions. Generally, errors in both directions are made (i.e., nurses both over- and underestimate the intensity of pain as compared to patients' ratings) but when an error does occur, a nurse is more likely to overestimate than to underestimate the intensity of a patient's pain (Weiner et al., 1999). As yet, it is not clear which pain behaviors are most important for these people; nor has work addressed how pain behaviors change with the progression of dementia. Although a promising start has been made, clearly more work is required.

Facial expressions may be reliable indicators of painful states among nonverbal populations (see Craig et al., Chapter 9). However, there is little information regarding the facial expression of pain among demented elderly individuals. In three small studies, an increase in the number of facial movements during exposure to noxious stimuli was found, but the responses were highly variable (Asplund, Norberg, Adolfsson, & Waxman, 1991; Hadjistavropoulos et al., 1997; Porter et al., 1996). Specific facial movements associated with pain could not be identified, and complex facial expressions, which are indicators of emotion (Collier, 1985), were not seen (Asplund et al., 1991; Hadjistavropoulos et al., 1997; Porter et al., 1996).

Hadjistavropoulos and colleagues (1997) reported that observer ratings of facial expression of pain, but not VAS ratings made by a cognitively impaired elderly sample, were significantly correlated with objective measures of facial activity in response to venipuncture. The meaning of this dissociation is not clear. Interestingly, in response to venipuncture, cognitively impaired elderly people demonstrated blunted physiological responses (heart rate) but increased facial expressiveness during the actual needle puncture compared to cognitively intact elderly people (Porter et al., 1996). The authors speculate that this may have been related to the impaired elderly subjects' inability to prepare for the aversive event, leading to greater "surprise" (and expression of this reaction) during the event than was experienced by the cognitively intact elderly subjects. On the other hand, the apparent dissociation between physiological and facial responses may be related to generalized emotional disinhibition rather than pain perception per se among cognitively impaired elderly individuals (Porter et al., 1996). Much more work is needed in order to develop systematic guidelines for the assessment of pain in nonverbal demented elderly patients.

CONCLUSIONS

The proportion of elderly people in our society is rapidly increasing. These people will require effective assessment and management of both acute and chronic pain. This will be necessary across various settings, including inpatient, community, and long-term institutional care, and among people with highly variable levels of disability and cognitive functioning. Each of these sources of variability adds a layer of complexity to the task of pain assessment, and it has become increasingly clear that it is not always possible to generalize findings across these disparate groups of elderly people. There is an urgent need for systematic research designed to identify the most valid methods of pain assessment for the elderly. As we have seen, this work is still at a very early stage. There are large gaps in our knowledge, and many inconsistencies remain to be resolved. This is a serious hindrance to the progress of the field of pain and aging. It is impossible to interpret studies regarding the mechanisms of age-related changes in pain, the effectiveness of pain management strategies, and the interaction of pain with other highly prevalent disorders of aging until these data are available. Put simply, how can we know whether data regarding pain in the elderly are valid if we do not yet know how to measure pain in this group?

It has been my goal throughout this chapter to present the preliminary evidence that is available and to highlight the gaps in our knowledge while proposing directions for future work. In addition, a critical stance has been adopted in the hope of stimulating further research, so that we will be able to meet the challenge presented by the increasing numbers of elderly patients who will require effective pain control.

ACKNOWLEDGMENTS

This work was supported by a Medical Research Council of Canada Postdoctoral Fellowship. Special thanks to Drs. Joel Katz and Ronald Melzack for helpful discussion of the material.

REFERENCES

Allcock, N. (1996). Factors affecting the assessment of postoperative pain: A literature review. *Journal of Advanced Nursing, 24*, 1144–1151.

Anastasi, A. (1988). *Psychological testing* (6th ed.). New York: Macmillan.

Andresen, E. M., Gravitt, G. W., Aydelotte, M. E., & Podgorski, C. A. (1999). Limitations of the SF-36 in a sample of nursing home residents. *Age and Ageing, 28*, 562–566.

Asplund, K., Norberg, A., Adolfsson, R., & Waxman, H. M. (1991). Facial expressions in severely demented patients: A stimulus–response study of four patients with dementia of the Alzheimer type. *International Journal of Geriatric Psychiatry, 6*, 599–606.

Beck, A. T. (1978). *Beck Depression Inventory.* Philadelphia: Center for Cognitive Therapy.

Benesh, L. R., Szigeti, E., Ferraro, F. R., & Gullicks, J. N. (1997). Tools for assessing chronic pain in rural elderly women. *Home Healthcare Nurse, 15*, 207–211.

Bergner, M., Bobbitt, R. A., Kressel, S., Pollard, W. E., Gilson, B. S., & Morris, J. R. (1976). The Sickness Impact Profile: Conceptual formulation and methodology for the development of a health status measure. *International Journal of Health Services, 6*, 393–415.

Bergner, M., Bobbitt, R. A., Pollard, W. E., Martin, D. P., & Gilson, B. S. (1976). The Sickness Impact Profile: Validation of a health status measure. *Medical Care, 14*, 57–67.

Bieri, D., Reeve, R. A., Champion, G. D., Addicoat, L., & Ziegler, J. B. (1990). The Faces Pain Scale for the self-assessment of the severity of pain experienced by children: Development, initial validation, and preliminary investigation for ratio scale properties. *Pain, 41*, 139–150.

Bourque, P., Blanchard, L., & Saulnier, J. (1992). L'impact des symptômes somatiques dans l'evaluation de la dépression chez une population gériatrique. *Revue Canadienne des Sciences du Comportement, 24*, 118–128.

Bowling, A. (1998). Measuring health related quality of life among older people. *Aging and Mental Health, 2*, 5–6.

Brattberg, G., Thorslund, M., & Wikman, A. (1989). The prevalence of pain in a general population: The results of a postal survey in a county of Sweden. *Pain, 37*, 215–222.

Brink, T. L., Yesavage, J. A., Lum, O., Heersema, P. H., Adey, M., & Rose, T. L. (1982). Screening tests for geriatric depression. *Clinical Gerontologist, 1*, 37–43.

Carver, D. J., Chapman, C. A., Thomas, V. S., Stadnyk, K. J., & Rockwood, K. (1999). Validity and reliability of the Medical Outcomes Study Short Form—20 questionnaire as a measure of quality of life in elderly people living at home. *Age and Ageing, 28,* 169-174.

Casten, R. J., Parmelee, P. A., Kleban, M. H., Lawton, M. P., & Katz, I. R. (1995). The relationships among anxiety, depression, and pain in a geriatric institutionalized sample. *Pain, 61,* 271-276.

Collier, G. (1985). *Emotional expression.* Hillsdale, NJ: Erlbaum.

Corran, T. M., Farrell, M. J., Helme, R. D., & Gibson, S. J. (1997). The classification of patients with chronic pain: Age as a contributing factor. *Clinical Journal of Pain, 13,* 207-214.

Ekman, P., & Friesen, W. (1978). *Investigator's guide to the Facial Action Coding System.* Palo Alto, CA: Consulting Psychologists Press.

Escalante, A., Lichtenstein, M. J., White, K., Rios, N., & Hazuda, H. P. (1995). A method for scoring the pain map of the McGill Pain Questionnaire for use in epidemiologic studies. *Aging (Milano), 7,* 358-366.

Farrell, M. J., Gibson, S. J., & Helme, R. D. (1995). The effect of medical status on the activity level of older pain clinic patients. *Journal of the American Geriatrics Society, 43,* 102-107.

Farrell, M. J., Gibson, S. J., & Helme, R. D. (1996). Measuring the activity of older people with chronic pain. *Clinical Journal of Pain, 12,* 6-12.

Farrell, M. J., Katz, B., & Helme, R. D. (1996). The impact of dementia on the pain experience. *Pain, 67,* 7-15.

Feldt, K. S., Ryden, M. B., & Miles, S. (1998). Treatment of pain in cognitively impaired compared with cognitively intact older patients with hip-fracture. *Journal of the American Geriatrics Society, 46,* 1079-1085.

Fernandez-Galinski, D., Rue, M., Moral, V., Castells, C., & Puig, M. M. (1996). Spinal anesthesia with bupivacaine and fentanyl in geriatric patients. *Anesthesia and Analgesia, 83,* 537-541.

Ferrell, B. A. (1996). Overview of aging and pain. In B. R. Ferrell & B. A. Ferrell (Eds.), *Pain in the elderly* (pp. 1-10). Seattle, WA: International Association for the Study of Pain Press.

Ferrell, B. A., Ferrell, B. R., & Rivera, L. (1995). Pain in cognitively impaired nursing home residents. *Journal of Pain and Symptom Management, 10,* 591-598.

Fix, A. J., & Daughton, D. M. (1988). *Human Activity Profile: Professional manual.* Odessa, FL: Psychological Assessment Resources.

Forbes, W. F., Hatward, L. M., & Agwani, N. (1991). Factors associated with the prevalence of various self-reported impairments among older people residing in the community. *Canadian Journal of Public Health, 82,* 240-244.

Frank, A. J., Moll, J. M., & Hort, J. F. (1982). A comparison of three ways of measuring pain. *Rheumatology and Rehabilitation, 21,* 211-217.

Gagliese, L., Jackson, M., Ritvo, P., Wowk, A., & Katz, J (2000). Age is not an impediment to effective use of patient-controlled analgesia by surgical patients. *Anesthesiology, 93,* 601-610.

Gagliese, L., Katz, J., & Melzack, R. (1999). Pain in the elderly. In P. D. Wall & R. Melzack (Eds.), *Textbook of pain* (4th ed., pp. 991-1006) . Edinburgh: Churchill Livingstone.

Gagliese, L., & Melzack, R. (1997). Age differences in the quality of chronic pain: A preliminary study. *Pain Research and Management, 2,* 157-162.

Gagliese, L., Stratford, J. G., Hickey, D., Gamsa, A., & Melzack, R. (1998). The psychometric properties of the McGill Pain Questionnaire in young and elderly chronic pain patients. *Pain Research and Management, 3,* 58.

Gagliese, L., Wowk, A., Sandler, A. N., & Katz, J. (1999). Pain and opioid self-administration following prostatectomy in middle-aged and elderly men. *Abstracts of the 9th World Congress of Pain,* 77.

Gallo, J. J., & Rabins, P. V. (1999). Depression without sadness: Alternative presentations of depression in late life. *American Family Physician, 60,* 820-826.

Grant, D. J., Bishop-Miller, J., Winchester, D. M., Anderson, M., & Faulkner, S. (1999). A randomized comparative trial of acupuncture versus transcutaneous electrical nerve stimulation for chronic back pain in the elderly. *Pain, 82,* 9-13.

Hadjistavropoulos, T., Craig, K. D., Martin, N., Hadjistavropoulos, H., & McMurtry, B. (1997). Toward a research outcome measure of pain in frail elderly in chronic care. *The Pain Clinic, 10,* 71-79.

Hall-Lord, M. L., Larsson, G., & Steen, B. (1998). Pain and distress among elderly intensive care unit patients: Comparison of patients' experiences and nurses' assessments. *Heart and Lung, 27,* 123-132.

Harkins, S. W., & Price, D. D. (1992). Assessment of pain in the elderly. In D.C. Turk & R. Melzack (Eds.), *Handbook of pain assessment* (pp. 315-331). New York: Guilford Press.

Helme, R. D., Katz, B., Gibson, S., & Corran, T. (1989). Can psychometric tools be used to analyse pain in a geriatric population? *Clinical and Experimental Neurology, 26,* 113-117.

Herr, K. A., & Mobily, P. R. (1991). Complexities of pain assessment in the elderly: Clinical considerations. *Journal of Gerontological Nursing, 17,* 12-19.

Herr, K. A., & Mobily, P. (1993). Comparison of selected pain assessment tools for use with the elderly. *Applied Nursing Research, 6,* 39-46.

Herr, K. A., Mobily, P. R., Kohout, F. J., & Wagenaar, D. (1998). Evaluation of the Faces Pain Scale for use with the elderly. *Clinical Journal of Pain, 14,* 29-38.

Hopman-Rock, M., Odding, E., Hofman, A., Kraaimaat, F. W., & Bijlsma, J. W. (1996). Physical and psychosocial disability in elderly subjects in relation to pain in the hip and/or knee. *Journal of Rheumatology, 23,* 1037-1044.

Hurley, A. C., Volicer, B. J., Hanrahan, P. A., Houde, S., & Volicer, L. (1992). Assessment of discomfort in advanced Alzheimer patients. *Research in Nursing and Health, 15,* 369-377.

Irwin, M., Artin, K. H., & Oxman, M. N. (1999). Screening for depression in the older adult: Criterion validity of the 10-item Center for Epidemiological Studies Depression Scale (CES-D). *Archives of Internal Medicine, 159,* 1701-1704.

Jensen, M. P. (1997). Validity of self-report and observation measures. In T. S. Jensen, J. A. Turner, & Z. Wiesenfeld-Hallin (Eds.), *Proceedings of the 8th World Congress on Pain* (pp. 637-662). Seattle, WA: International Association for the Study of Pain Press.

Jensen, M. P., Karoly, P., & Braver, S. (1986). The measurement of clinical pain intensity: A comparison of six methods. *Pain, 27,* 117-126.

Katz, J., & Melzack, R. (1999). Measurement of pain. *Surgical Clinics of North America, 79,* 231-252.

Keefe, F. J. (1982). Behavioral assessment and treatment of chronic pain: Current status and future directions. *Journal of Consulting and Clinical Psychology, 50*, 896–911.

Keefe, F. J., Caldwell, D. S., Queen, K., Gil, K. M., Martinez, S., Crisson, J. E., Ogden, W., & Nunley, J. (1987). Osteoarthritic knee pain: A behavioral analysis. *Pain, 28*, 309–321.

Kerns, R. D., Turk, D. C., & Rudy, T. E. (1985). The West Haven–Yale Multidimensional Pain Inventory (WHYMPI). *Pain, 23*, 345–356.

Kremer, E., Atkinson, J. H., & Ignelzi, R. J. (1981). Measurement of pain: Patient preference does not confound pain measurement. *Pain, 10*, 241–249.

Kwentus, J. A., Harkins, S. W., Lignon, N., & Silverman, J. J. (1985). Current concepts in geriatric pain and its treatment. *Geriatrics, 40*, 48–57.

LeFort, S., Murray, M., & Ribeiro, V. (1996, November). *Chronic pain in the elderly: Experiences and coping. A preliminary report of pain assessment instruments.* Paper presented at Research into Healthy Aging: Challenges in Changing Times, Dartmouth, Nova Scotia, Canada.

Lewis, B., Lewis, D., & Cumming, G. (1995). Frequent measurement of chronic pain: An electronic diary and empirical findings. *Pain, 60*, 341–347.

Lichtenstein, M. J., Dhanda, R., Cornell, J. E., Escalante, A., & Hazuda, H. P. (1998). Disaggregating pain and its effect on physical functional limitations. *Journals of Gerontology: Series A. Biological Sciences and Medical Sciences, 53*, M361–M371.

Malatesta, C. Z., Fiore, M. J., & Messina, J. J. (1987). Affect, personality, and facial expressive characteristics of older people. *Psychology and Aging, 2*, 64–9.

Malatesta, C. Z., Izard, C. E., Culver, C., & Nicolich, M. (1987). Emotion communication skills in young, middle-aged, and older women. *Psychology and Aging, 2*, 193–203.

Mangione, C. M., Marcantonio, E. R., Goldman, L, Cook, E. F., Donaldson, M. C., Sugarbaker, D. J., Poss, R., & Lee, T. H. (1993). Influence of age on measurement of health status in patients undergoing elective surgery. *Journal of the American Geriatrics Society, 41*, 377–383.

Marchionni, N., Ferrucci, L., Baldasseroni, S., Fumagalli, S., Guralnik, J. M., Bonazinga, M., Cecchi, F., & Masotti, G. (1997). Item re-scaling of an Italian version of the Sickness Impact Profile: Effect of age and profession of the observers. *Journal of Clinical Epidemiology, 50*, 195–201.

Margolis, R. B., Tait, R. C., & Krause, S. J. (1986). A rating system for use with patient pain drawings. *Pain, 24*, 57–65.

Martin, K. A., Rejeski, W. J., Miller, M. E., James, M. K., Ettinger, W. H., Jr., & Messier, S. P. (1999). Validation of the PASE in older adults with knee pain and physical disability. *Medicine and Science in Sports and Exercise, 31*, 627–633.

Marzinski, L. R. (1991). The tragedy of dementia: Clinically assessing pain in the confused, nonverbal elderly. *Journal of Gerontological Nursing, 17*, 25–28.

Matheson, D. H. (1997). The painful truth: Interpretation of facial expressions of pain in older adults. *Journal of Nonverbal Behavior, 21*, 223–238.

McHorney, C. A., Ware, J. E., Jr., & Raczek, A. E. (1993). The MOS 36-Item Short-Form Health Survey (SF-36): II. Psychometric and clinical tests of validity in measuring physical and mental health constructs. *Medical Care, 31*, 247–263.

Melzack, R. (1975). The McGill Pain Questionnaire: Major properties and scoring methods. *Pain, 1*, 277–299.

Melzack, R. (1987). The short-form McGill Pain Questionnaire. *Pain, 30*, 191–197.

Miller, J., Neelon, V., Dalton, J., Ng'andu, N., Bailey, D., Jr., Layman, E., & Hosfeld, A. (1996). The assessment of discomfort in elderly confused patients: A preliminary study. *Journal of Neuroscience Nursing, 28*, 175–182.

Morishita, L., Boult, C., Ebbitt, B., Rambel, M., Fallstrom, K., & Gooden, T. (1995). Concurrent validity of administering the Geriatric Depression Scale and the Physical Functioning dimension of the SIP by telephone. *Journal of the American Geriatrics Society, 43*, 680–683.

Murray, M., LeFort, S., & Ribeiro, V. (1998). The SF-36: Reliable and valid for the institutionalized elderly? *Aging and Mental Health, 2*, 24–27.

Oberle, K., Paul, P., Wry, J., & Grace, M. (1990). Pain, anxiety and analgesics: A comparative study of elderly and younger surgical patients. *Canadian Journal of Aging, 9*, 13–22.

Papassotiropoulos, A., & Heun, R. (1999). Screening for depression in the elderly: A study on misclassification by screening instruments and improvement of scale performance. *Progress in Neuro-Psychopharmacology and Biological Psychiatry, 23*, 431–446.

Parmelee, P. A. (1997). Pain and psychological function in late life. In J. Lomranz & D. I. Mostofsky (Eds.), *Handbook of pain and aging* (pp. 207–226). New York: Plenum Press.

Parmelee, P. A., Katz, I. R., & Lawton, M. P. (1991). The relation of pain to depression among institutionalized aged. *Journal of Gerontology: Psychological Science, 46*, P15–P21.

Pollard, C. A. (1984). Preliminary validity study of the Pain Disability Index. *Perceptual and Motor Skills, 59*, 974.

Porter, F. L., Malhorta, K. M., Wolf, C. M., Morris, J. C., Miller, J. P., & Smith, M. C. (1996). Dementia and the response to pain in the elderly. *Pain, 68*, 413–421.

Radloff, L. S. (1977). The CES-D scale: A self-report depression scale for research in the general population. *Applied Psychological Measurement, 1*, 385–401.

Ross, M. M., & Crook, J. (1998). Elderly recipients of home nursing services: Pain, disability and functional competence. *Journal of Advanced Nursing, 27*, 1117–1126.

Savedra, M. C., Tesler, M. D., Holzemer, W. L., Wilkie, D. J., & Ward, J. A. (1989). Pain location: Validity and reliability of body outline markings by hospitalized children and adolescents. *Research in Nursing and Health, 12*, 307–314.

Sherman, S. E., & Reuben, D. (1998). Measures of functional status in community-dwelling elders. *Journal of General Internal Medicine, 13*, 817–823.

Stadnyk, K., Calder, J., & Rockwood, K. (1998). Testing the measurement properties of the Short Form-36 Health Survey in a frail elderly population. *Journal of Clinical Epidemiology, 51*, 827–835.

Svensson, E. (1998). Ordinal invariant measures for individual and group changes in ordered categorical data. *Statistics in Medicine, 17*, 2923–2936.

Tait, R. C., Chibnall, J. T., & Krause, S. (1990). The Pain Disability Index: Psychometric properties. *Pain, 40,* 171–182.

Tiplady, B., Jackson, S. H., Maskrey, V. M., & Swift, C. G. (1998). Validity and sensitivity of visual analogue scales in young and older healthy subjects. *Age and Ageing, 27,* 63–66.

Turk, D. C., & Okifuji, A. (1994). Detecting depression in chronic pain patients: Adequacy of self-reports. *Behaviour Research and Therapy, 32,* 9–16.

Turk, D. C., Okifuji, A., & Scharff, L. (1995). Chronic pain and depression: Role of perceived impact and perceived control in different age cohorts. *Pain, 61,* 93–101.

Washburn, R. A., Smith, K. W., Jette, A. M., & Janney, C. A. (1993). The Physical Activity Scale for the Elderly (PASE): Development and evaluation. *Journal of Clinical Epidemiology, 46,* 153–162.

Weinberger, M., Samsa, G. P., Hanlon, J. T., Schmader, K., Doyle, M. E., Cowper, P. A., Uttech, K. M., Cohen, H. J., & Feussner, J. R. (1991). An evaluation of a brief health status measure in elderly veterans. *Journal of the American Geriatrics Society, 39,* 691–694.

Weiner, D., Peiper, C., McConnell, E., Martinez, S., & Keefe, F. J. (1996). Pain measurement in elders with chronic low back pain: Traditional and alternative approaches. *Pain, 67,* 461–467.

Weiner, D., Peterson, B., & Keefe, F. J. (1998). Evaluating persistent pain in long term care residents: What role for pain maps? *Pain, 76,* 249–257.

Weiner, D., Peterson, B., Ladd, K., McConnell, E., & Keefe, F. J. (1999). Pain in nursing home residents: An exploration of prevalence, staff perspectives, and practical aspects of measurement. *Clinical Journal of Pain, 15,* 92–101.

Werner, P., Cohen-Mansfield, J., Watson, V., & Pasis, S. (1998). Pain in participants of adult day care centers: Assessment by different raters. *Journal of Pain and Symptom Management, 15,* 8–17.

Wilke, D. J., Savedra, M. C., Holzemer, W. L., Tesler, M. D., & Paul, S. M. (1990). Use of the McGill Pain Questionnaire to measure pain: A meta-analysis. *Nursing Research, 39,* 36–41.

Yesavage, J. A. (1988). Geriatric Depression Scale. *Psychopharmacology Bulletin, 24,* 709–711.

Chapter 8

Pain Assessment in Persons with Limited Ability to Communicate

THOMAS HADJISTAVROPOULOS
CARL VON BAEYER
KENNETH D. CRAIG

People who accept responsibility for the care of persons with a limited ability to communicate subjective states of pain confront a considerable predicament: The communication challenge does not spare such persons from the sources of pain that could afflict anyone. If the person is to be spared pain and suffering, pain assessment is necessary.

A tragic illustration of an assessment challenge received considerable attention in the late 1990s in the Canadian media (McGrath, 1998). The focus of the case was Tracy Latimer, a 12-year-old girl with severe cerebral palsy who had very limited ability to communicate as a result of cognitive and motor impairment. Although there is little doubt that she had pain caused by the neuromuscular pathologies of cerebral palsy and by surgery to release contractures, systematic assessment posed a real challenge and apparently was not undertaken. Tracy's father decided to end her life because of what he described as her unremitting pain and suffering. The basis for his assessment of Tracy's pain and pain-related suffering is unclear, but it was probably his observation of her behavior, conjecture, and inference. He was subsequently convicted of murder. A main component of his legal defense was that he chose to kill Tracy in order to alleviate her continuous suffering. Mr. Latimer said he had been told that nothing could be done to relieve her pain.

The Supreme Court of Canada heard the case and ruled that Mr. Latimer must spend at least 10 years in jail for killing his severely disabled daughter. Mr. Latimer has received support from persons arguing that unremitting, unendurable pain justifies active euthanasia. But opponents have presented the case for the availability of systematic pain control, even in severe cases such as Tracy's. They have also raised objections to euthanasia, and expressed concern for vulnerable children and adults who cannot effectively express themselves. Regardless of the viewpoint taken, valid methods of pain assessment are needed to contest either position. McGrath (1998) has observed that the media attention focused on the right to live or die, whereas the most important issue behind the case was missed—namely, the right of people with severe communication difficulties to have adequate pain management and health care. Inadequate methods of assessing pain in those with communication difficulties will impede the ability to exercise these rights.

MAGNITUDE OF THE PROBLEM

The problem of pain assessment and management for those with communication difficulties is substantial, because a remarkably extensive set of categories of individuals is represented within the general rubric of communication impairment. Table 8.1 provides a classification of human conditions often associated with communication difficulties. This chapter focuses primarily on pain in persons with cognitive impairments, including children with cerebral palsy, adults with severe intellectual disabilities, and elderly persons with dementia. These populations can serve as illustrations of the problems that can be generalized to others with communication difficulties. The extent of the problem can be understood by examining these conditions as examples of the others delineated in Table 8.1.

Tracy Latimer's suffering was not unusual. Cerebral palsy, a disorder of motor function related to perinatal trauma that commonly involves neuro-

TABLE 8.1. Categories of Persons and Conditions That May Be Associated with a Limited or Reduced Capacity to Communicate about Pain

1. Central nervous system (CNS) immaturity
   a. Infants, toddlers, and preschool children
2. CNS abnormalities and/or damage—persistent
   a. Developmental/intellectual disabilities and disorders (e.g., Down's syndrome)
   b. Acquired brain damage (pervasive and specific)
   c. Brain diseases (e.g., Alzheimer's or multi-infarct dementia)
   d. Specific speech or language impairment
   e. Neuromuscular disorders (e.g., cerebral palsy, multiple sclerosis)
3. CNS impairment—temporary
   a. General anesthesia
   b. Toxic conditions producing delirium
   c. Muscle-paralyzing agents
   d. Use of CNS depressants (e.g., barbiturates, sedatives)
   e. Abuse of "recreational" drugs (e.g., alcohol, opiates)
4. Psychosocial conditions
   a. Inability to speak the language
   b. Speech disorders
   c. Voluntary mutism
   d. Voluntary exaggeration or suppression of reports
   e. Behavior disorders (anxiety, depression, psychotic conditions)
   f. Motivational deficits

Note. The categories are not mutually exclusive. For example, cerebral palsy can be associated with brain damage, reducing cognitive functioning as well as neuromuscular control. Some of the conditions are transitory (e.g., being an infant or young child), and others are reversible (e.g., toxic conditions, or deficits due to brain damage following healing and/or rehabilitation programs).

cognitive impairment, often leads to painful spasticity that can progress over the life span. Treatments of cerebral palsy symptoms are often invasive and painful (see, e.g., McGrath, 1998). Surgery such as selective posterior rhizotomy involves the severing of dorsal nerve rootlets (Abbott, Forem, & Johan, 1989), is designed to reduce spasticity, and is followed by painful physical rehabilitation (Miller, Johann-Murphy, & Cate, 1997). Moreover, cerebral palsy can lead to hip dislocations, scoliosis, contractures, painful spasms, ulcers, and skin breakdown (Dormans & Pellegrino, 1988; Gooch & Sandell, 1996; Miller et al., 1997).

These and other children with neurological disorders represent a commonplace and complex problem (Oberlander, O'Donnell, & Montgomery, 1999). Estimates of the incidence of births involving cerebral palsy range from 2 per 1,000 (MacKenzie & Lignor, 1994) to 6 per 1,000 (Kolb & Whishaw, 1985). This translates to hundreds of thousands of affected persons in the Western world alone and tens of millions worldwide. Cognitive deficits are common in this general population. Numerous other congenital conditions (e.g., Down's syndrome) also produce intellectual disability. The overall percentage of persons with mental retardation in the population is 2.5%, and approximately 5%–6% of such individuals can be classified as having severe and profound mental retardation (American Psychiatric Association, 1994).

Elderly people are at risk not only for accidents due to falls (Ferrell, 1991); as the body ages, the incidence of a number of painful illnesses increases (see, e.g., Helme & Gibson, 1999; Melding, 1991). Hence, the likelihood of an elderly person's suffering from a painful condition is substantial, whether or not he or she has communication impairments (see Gagliese, Chapter 7, this volume). More specifically, a recent epidemiological study found that about 80% of persons over 65 years of age reported a pain problem in the year preceding the survey. Many reported multiple pain complaints. The most common type of pain was joint pain (Mobily, Herr, Clark, & Wallace, 1994).

It is noteworthy that although many types of chronic pain are experienced more frequently by older persons, the increased likelihood does not continue after the seventh decade unless institutionalization has occurred (Helme, 1996). Roy and Thomas (1986) found that 83% of elderly persons in nursing homes and day hospitals reported having pain problems, mostly due to connective tissue diseases. Nonetheless, pain patterns across age levels vary for different types of pain. Headaches, for example, tend to be less prevalent among elderly people, whereas the experience of facial pain and pain associated with connective tissue is more frequent (Cook & Thomas, 1994). A substantial proportion of those suffering painful conditions associated with aging will also have an impaired capacity to communicate their pain.

It is estimated that 8% of persons aged over 65 meet the criteria for dementia, including Alzheimer's disease and vascular dementia (Canadian Study on Health and Aging Working Group, 1994), with the incidence increasing in older populations. Because pain is frequent among elderly individuals, it must be common among the millions of these individuals who have dementia around the world. Senile dementia often co-occurs with those painful conditions and accidents that are more common in late life (e.g., arthritis, hip fractures). The existing evidence suggests that pain identification among those with dementia is difficult. Parmelee, Smith, and Katz (1993) found a significant negative association between levels of cognitive impairment and self-reported pain, even after the number of health problems was controlled for. Sengstaken and King (1993) found that the pain problems of elderly patients with neurological disorders were often missed by physicians. Thus it is not surprising that a considerable proportion of nursing home residents who report pain receive no treatment for their pain (Roy & Thomas, 1986).

Accounts of common conditions associated with impaired ability to communicate should include not only children, adults with intellectual disability, and elderly persons with dementia, but also the considerable number of younger adults who sustain head injuries. In fact, cerebral trauma is the commonest form of brain damage in people younger than 40 years (Kolb & Whishaw, 1985). Many of these injuries are severe and cause substantial impairments in ability to communicate. In the United States alone, the reported incidence of head injuries ranges from 500,000 to 1.9 million per year (Berrol, 1989; Frankowski, Annegers, & Whitman, 1985; Gennarelli, 1983). Cognitive deficits are very common among people who sustain head injuries, and about 10% of victims sustain severe injuries (Lezak, 1995). A large majority of these severely traumatized victims are unable to return to fully independent living. The incidence of injuries to other parts of the body among those who sustain head trauma is very high, given that approximately half of these patients are injured in motor vehicle accidents (Spivack & Balicki, 1990). Consequently, adequate pain assessment and management is critical for these populations, and particularly challenging for those who are cognitively impaired.

It is believed that the lack of adequate pain assessment in populations with cognitive impairments has led to medical catastrophes (Biersdorff, 1991). Death due to intestinal obstruction, for example, is approximately 34 times more common among persons with intellectual disabilities (Roy & Simon, 1987), and this may be the result of failure of early detection. There is also evidence that persons with cognitive impairments receive fewer medications than those who are cognitively intact (see, e.g., Kaasalainen et al., 1998).

A CONCEPTUAL BASIS FOR PAIN ASSESSMENT IN COMMUNICATION-RESTRICTED POPULATIONS

An appreciation of the assessment challenges requires an understanding of the processes whereby one person's pain becomes known to others. From a communication's perspective (Craig, Lilley, & Gilbert, 1996; Prkachin & Craig, 1995), the sensory, affective, and evaluative components of the experience of pain remain private unless they are encoded in activity that can be decoded by observers as expressive of the subjective state. In the non-limited person, the inference can be based upon a specifiable domain of information sources: (1) language; (2) paralinguistic qualities of speech, including speech timbre, dynamics, and temporal features; (3) nonverbal vocalizations such as crying and moaning; (4) nonvocal behavior, including facial expression and bodily activities; and (5) physiological activity, ranging from that which is visible (e.g., breathing, pallor, flushing, sweating, or muscle tension) to other indices requiring psychophysiological transduction instrumentation (e.g., autonomic measures, brain imaging, endocrine measures).

Information sources can be categorized by the extent to which they represent a biological adaptation that was successful in the communication of important information. Some have evolved because they convey useful personal information to others, who may intervene on the individual's behalf or act in their own interests. Mr. Latimer claimed, for instance, that he had knowledge of his daughter's pain and that he acted in her best interest. Language is certainly important in the communication of distress. Facial expression also has a primary and powerful role in interpersonal communication (see Craig, Prkachin, & Grunau, Chapter 9, this volume). But facial activity also has nonsocial functions (e.g., narrowing the eyes to protect them) or represents vestigial remnants of earlier behavior that had adaptive functions (e.g., baring the teeth to make them available for attack would also signal a capacity for retaliation to predators, or brow lowering would reflect use of the same muscles as were required to orient the ears forward for better hearing) (Fridlund, 1991). The communicative value of other actions appears to be quite secondary to other functions.

Bodily activity, other than facial expression, most often serves the purpose of permitting escape or avoidance from pain and physical harm. Others can cue in on these actions, and it is possible to dissimulate them to deceive others, but these uses appear to be secondary to the instrumental value of the behaviors in controlling sources of pain. Physiological activity appears either to serve homeostatic functions or to facilitate escape or avoidance of physically dangerous or harmful environments. Its communicative role is minimal, although astute observers may interpret autonomic or musculoskeletal activity as indicative of pain. No specific physiological measure of pain has emerged in humans, in part because most of the measures that have been evaluated reflect stress reactions more broadly. All pain is stressful, but not all stress is painful. Thus physiological measures have proven sensitive but not specific to pain.

The most common form of communication deficit in the categories provided above is loss of the facility to use language. Although the capacity to communicate pain via language evolved as a uniquely human attribute, there is no reason to believe that persons who do not have this capacity should be impaired in either the capacity to experience pain or in the use of other communication modalities to convey their pain to others. Although other sources of information may remain intact, the loss of language represents a particular challenge, given the emphasis among practitioners, investigators, and others on the use of self-report in pain assessment. It is often assumed that because the experience of pain is a subjective state, the only means whereby it can be tapped is through the suffering person's verbalizations. It is not unusual to read or hear assertions that the only way to assess another person's pain is through self-report (McCaffery & Beebe, 1989). The current

definition of pain (Merskey & Bogduk, 1994), which emphasizes the use of self-description, can be taken to imply that states of pain and suffering cannot be understood in nonverbal persons (Anand & Craig, 1996). This position limits attention to the availability and usefulness of nonverbal expression (Anand, 1997; Craig, 1992).

HOW IS PAIN EXPERIENCED BY PERSONS WITH COMMUNICATION DISABILITIES?

The diverse neurocognitive impairments capable of influencing the experience and expression of pain differ considerably in their nature and extent. Damage to the central nervous system may have an impact on the perception of pain, the elaborated experience of pain, and the manner in which pain is expressed in manifest behavior. Focusing upon afferent systems responsible for the sensory/discriminative qualities of pain, pain insensitivity could result from abnormal or deficient sensory neurons, as well as from disruptions in sensory pathways (Biersdorff, 1994). It is generally acknowledged that a reasonably good understanding has emerged of sensory afferent systems providing input to the brain (Rosenzweig, Leiman, & Breedlove, 1999). However, the neurophysiological systems involved in the affective and cognitive modulation of pain are less well understood (Pinel, 1997). It is generally appreciated that afferent input undergoes substantial processing in higher cortical systems to yield the manifestation of the complex experience of pain (Melzack & Wall, 1965). Damage to the somatosensory cortex and its connections apparently have a demonstrable impact on the response to noxious stimuli (Bassetti, Bogousslavsky, & Regali, 1993; Berthier, Starkstein, & Leiguarda, 1988; Farrell, Katz, & Helme, 1996), but brain systems involved in advanced processing of nociceptive input are far more complex (Casey & Minoshima, 1997).

The impact of diseases and damage to the brain would be expected to depend upon their location, extent, and nature. It is conceivable that certain conditions may produce pain insensitivity (diminished sensation), whereas others may produce pain indifference (no variation in the perception of sensory/discriminative qualities, but diminished affective distress and escape motivation). For example, Farrell and colleagues (1996) have pointed out that Alzheimer's disease is a disorder of the neocortex that leaves the somatosensory cortex relatively unaffected. Thus we might expect that the sensory/discriminative aspect of pain may be preserved in patients with Alzheimer's disease, although distortions in perception (related to parietal lobe dysfunction) may occur. Farrell and colleagues also observed that emotional components of pain may be affected in Alzheimer's disease, due to neuronal loss in the prefrontal cortex and limbic system. Similarly, in frontal lobe dementia and in other damage to the frontal lobe, disinhibited pain reactions may be observed.

Gibson, Voukelatos, Bradbeer, and Helme (1996) have shown that elderly patients suffering from Alzheimer's disease do not differ in pain thresholds but are less reliable in reporting them. Nonetheless, Benedetti and colleagues (1999) showed that pain tolerance in patients with Alzheimer's disease increases, whereas stimulus detection and pain thresholds are unchanged. The alterations in pain tolerance are consistent with the proposition that Alzheimer's disease has effects on motivational and affective processes.

Based largely on case study evidence (Comings & Amromin, 1974; Winkelmann, Lambert, & Hayles, 1962), it has been argued that the incidence of pain insensitivity and indifference in younger persons with intellectual disabilities is high. Recent work with such persons indicates that this general proposition does not hold for the group as a whole, despite evidence of occasional insensitivity or indifference. Facial reactions to acute phasic pain do not correlate with intelligence quotients and do not vary as a function of cognitive status (see, e.g., Hadjistavropoulos et al., 1998; LaChapelle, Hadjistavropoulos, & Craig, 1999; see also Craig et al., Chapter 9), suggesting no alteration in the subjective experience for these persons using this nonverbal measure. It is conceivable that there is as broad a range of individual differences in pain experience and behavior in this population as there is in the population at large, and that it would be wrong to develop general stereotypes based upon case studies that represent individual anomalies. Thus, although a blunting of pain reactions may occur among certain individuals with significant neurological impairments, as reported by Oberlander, Gilbert, Chambers, O'Donnell, and Craig (1999), this cannot be assumed for large numbers of persons with limited ability to communicate.

When one is considering the nature of pain experience in people with cognitive impairments, it would be parsimonious to assume that only brain systems for cognitive functioning are impaired.

Such an individual may have greater difficulty cognizing the meaning of events, remembering related experiences, anticipating what is likely to happen, or engaging in cognitive and behavioral problem solving and coping. The corollary assumption would be that the capacity to experience the affective/motivational components of the pain experience remains intact. Because capacities for planning, coping, perceiving opportunities for establishing control, and establishing a sense of self-efficacy are fundamental to maintaining control over pain, cognitive impairment may leave greater confusion, frustration, and distress than is the case in nonimpaired persons.

ASSESSMENT METHODS

All available avenues of communication should be considered when assessment of pain in persons with communication impairments is being planned. Methods may include self-report (when possible), observational methods, proxy reports, and physiological reactions.

Self-Report

Self-report measures require a substantial capacity for abstract thinking and have met with only partial success in populations with communication difficulties. Although adaptations of commonly used self-report procedures show promise for use among those with mild to moderate cognitive impairment (e.g., Hadjistavropoulos et al., 1998), there are documented problems with their use among persons with profound to severe communication problems. Investigators have established, for instance, that many adults with severe, lifelong intellectual disabilities are unable to respond to a simple question concerning the self-report of pain. LaChapelle and colleagues (1999) found that 35% of such persons were not able to respond (i.e., they could not understand the question). Their findings also suggested that many of those who responded to the simple self-report question did not provide reliable pain ratings. Similar findings were obtained in elderly patients with severe dementia (Hadjistavropoulos, Craig, Martin, Hadjistavropoulos, & McMurtry, 1997). Nonetheless, when the cognitive impairment is milder, self-report procedures such as the Coloured Analogue Scale (CAS; McGrath et al., 1996) appear to have some validity (Hadjistavropoulos et al., 1998; see also

McGrath & Gillespie, Chapter 6). This scale was developed to provide a practical clinical measure for young children with marginal self-report skills and was found to be easier to administer than a standard visual analogue scale (VAS) (McGrath et al., 1996). In our experience, self-report assessment of pain should be attempted, even when difficulties are anticipated, and rejected only after it has been demonstrated that the individual cannot use the measure reliably.

The standard VAS has been used extensively with seniors (Harkins & Price, 1992; see also Gagliese, Chapter 7), but modifications may facilitate use by persons who have cognitive deficits. Pain is rated on the CAS by moving a plastic glide along a 14.5-cm-long grid, varying in width and color from 1 cm wide and a light pink color at the bottom, to 3 cm wide and a deep red color at the top. The ends of the scale are anchored with the words "no pain" (bottom) and "most pain" (top). Patients are thus presented with visible cues for scaling pain severity: length of the scale and anchoring words, along with variations in width and changes in hue from pink to red. The CAS has been found to be reliable and to satisfy validity criteria (Hadjistavropoulos et al., 1998; McGrath et al., 1996). It is notable that elderly persons are more likely to have difficulty using unidimensional self-report instruments (e.g., a VAS) correctly than are younger adults (Gagliese & Melzack, 1997).

Attempts to use self-report procedures in children with cerebral palsy and cognitive impairment have met with little success. Miller and colleagues (1997), for example, attempted to use a modified version of the Faces Scale (LeBaron & Zeltzer, 1984; see also McGrath & Gillespie, Chapter 6) in a sample of children with cerebral palsy who varied in age and level of cognitive functioning. The children were asked to choose from among five line drawings of facial displays depicting increasing severities of distress. Fully 60% of the sample failed a validity test designed to assess their understanding of the procedure. Developing technologies in the use of facial rating scales might warrant further exploration of their usefulness (Chambers, Giesbrecht, Craig, Bennett, & Huntsman, 1999). Similarly, a broader range of self-report scales deserves careful evaluation. It would be of interest to know which components of cognitive functioning contribute to the ability to use self-report scales reliably. Given the limitations of self-report, various observational procedures have been studied.

Observational Procedures

Nonverbal manifestations of pain can be a rich source of information in pain assessment (see also Craig et al., Chapter 9). Observational procedures can be categorized as global (namely, ratings made using general integrative judgments of observers—e.g., pain vs. no pain), behaviorally focused (e.g., ratings of intensity of crying, frequency of facial grimaces, etc.), and fine-grained (i.e., systems that identify series of behaviorally defined pain behaviors—e.g., specific facial actions). (See Craig et al., Chapter 9, and Keefe, Williams, & Smith, Chapter 10.) Undoubtedly, global judgments are relied upon most frequently in clinical and family settings, with behaviorally focused or fine-grained measures favored in research studies.

The behaviorally focused Dalhousie Everyday Pain Scale (DEPS; Fearon, McGrath, & Achat, 1996) has been used with success to examine differences in the pain behavior of children with and without developmental delays (Gilbert-MacLeod, Craig, Rocha, & Mathias, 2000). The DEPS (see Appendix 8.A) is a brief observational instrument that includes subscales designed to assess the intensity and duration of distress, the intensity and duration of anger, the nature and the duration of protective behaviors (e.g., holding or favoring the injured part), and the nature of the child's social reaction (e.g., whether the child approached or withdrew from others). Children with developmental delays displayed less intense distress relative to nondelayed children, and a smaller proportion of the former engaged in help-seeking behaviors following the painful event. These observations are notable, because differences in the style of responding to painful events are likely to exist with at least some people who have developmental and communication problems.

Observational procedures have been used with children diagnosed with cerebral palsy. Koh and Fanurik (1997), for instance, used the behaviorally focused Children's Hospital of Eastern Ontario Pain Scale (CHEOPS; McGrath et al., 1985) with a sample of children who had borderline to profound cognitive impairment and who had undergone surgery. The CHEOPS involves assignment of weighted values on a scale of increasing pain to crying, facial grimace, verbal complaint, torso position, touch behavior, and leg position (see Appendix 8.B). Koh and Fanurik found no differences in CHEOPS scores assigned to children with and without cognitive impairment. The magnitude of the correlations of CHEOPS scores acquired through parental observation, nurses' observation, and the children's self-reported numerical ratings (where available) were comparable for the two groups of children. Although the CHEOPS appeared promising in this population, the authors acknowledged that idiosyncratic behaviors of cognitively impaired children could have interfered with adequate measurement.

Schade, Joyce, Gerkensmeyer, and Keck (1996) utilized the Nursing Assessment of Pain Intensity (Stevens, 1990), a shortened version of the CHEOPS, with a group of children (of varying ages) diagnosed with cerebral palsy. These researchers also administered the Postoperative Pain Scale (POPS; Barrier, Attia, Mayer, Amiel-Tison, & Shnider, 1989) and the Riley Infant Pain Scale (RIPS; Rafferty & Moser, 1991). In using the RIPS, nurses rate pain behaviors along 3-point scales. The seven behavior categories rated are facial, body movement, sleep, verbal or vocal, consolability, and response to movement and touch. Using the POPS, the observer scores the following 10 behavioral responses conceptually associated with pain: sleep, facial expression, quality of cry, consolability, sociability, sucking, spontaneous excitability, spontaneous motor activity, constant and excessive tension of fingers and toes, and a global evaluation of muscle tone. Schade and colleagues reported difficulties with reliability in their sample with cerebral palsy. As the sample was relatively small (n = 20) and heterogeneous in age, more research on the utility of these instruments in assessing pain among those with communication difficulties would be useful.

Miller and colleagues (1997) used a slightly modified version of the Observation Scale of Behavioral Distress (OSBD; Elliott, Jay, & Woody, 1987) with children with cerebral palsy who varied in age and level of cognitive functioning. The scale provides a list of 15 operationally defined behaviors designed to measure anxiety and pain (e.g., cry, scream), but does not differentiate between these states. Interrater reliability was satisfactory. Consistent with the researchers' hypothesis, scores decreased as rehabilitation progressed. This provided support for the validity of the scale as an index of distress, but not necessarily of pain. However, scores on the scale were significantly correlated with global ratings of pain completed by a physiotherapist and a psychologist. Although this also supports the use of global ratings, it must be noted that a substantial portion of the Miller and colleagues sample consisted of cognitively intact children. Their inclusion could have increased the

overall reliability and validity of the measurements. It would be of interest to determine whether interrater reliability and validity of the measures used by Miller and colleagues would have been affected if the sample had consisted exclusively of children with severe cognitive deficits and communication impairments.

Giusiano, Jimeno, Collignon, and Chau (1995) studied an observational procedure developed specifically for children with profound mental retardation (Collignon et al., 1993). The procedure is based on 22 items originally proposed by physicians as likely to reflect pain in children with cerebral palsy (e.g., groans or silent tears, abrupt or spontaneous crying). The researchers concluded that there was variability in the manner in which children express pain. This would support the development of individualized approaches to pain assessment for children with cognitive impairments and physical handicaps. The utility and reliability of the tool studied by Giusiano and colleagues merits additional study.

At present, it may be premature to recommend the routine clinical use of any one of the aforementioned observational scales with children who have serious neurological impairments, because their utility with such populations has not been studied adequately. Work is underway at the time of writing at several centers in Europe and North America on development, validation, and field testing of instruments designed for this purpose. It is hoped that one or a few such instruments will emerge by 2002 with solid validation and demonstrated utility. Until such time, we would encourage the use of the aforementioned scales for research purposes.

Observational assessment tools have also been used for the measurement of discomfort in seniors with dementia. Hurley, Volicer, Hanrahan, Houde, and Volicer (1992) developed a discomfort scale for use with elderly patients who have communication difficulties. Nurses rate patients' discomfort by assigning VAS ratings to nine behavioral indicators (e.g., frown, noisy breathing). The scale, which was also used by Miller, Moore, Schofield, Ng'andu, and Sedlak (1996), while useful, is not pain-specific. That is, it includes items such as "sad facial expressions" and was validated during episodes of intercurrent illness, typically involving fever. Simons and Malabar (1995) attempted to validate a more pain-specific observational approach. Nurses provided the frequencies with which certain behaviors occurred (e.g., "crying," "looks unresponsive," "relaxed," and "awake") before and after "pain intervention" and concluded that the frequencies changed in the predicted direction. A limitation of this study was that statistical analyses were not reported. Moreover, the nurses, who completed the ratings, may not have been unaware of whether or not the "pain intervention" had taken place.

Fine-grained measures of pain involving facial displays have been discussed widely in the pain literature (e.g., Craig, 1992; Hale & Hadjistavropoulos, 1997; Prkachin, 1992; see Craig et al., Chapter 9) and have received particular attention in the study of pain in infants and young children (Craig, 1998; Craig & Grunau, 1993; see McGrath & Gillespie, Chapter 6). As a result of their visibility and rapid transmission time, nonverbal pain expressions are especially important when self-report is lacking.

Several studies have demonstrated the utility of examining facial reactions in the assessment of seniors with dementia (Hadjistavropoulos et al., 1997, 1998; Hadjistavropoulos, LaChapelle, MacLeod, Snider, & Craig, 2000; Porter et al., 1996), younger adults with severe intellectual disabilities (LaChapelle et al., 1999), and adolescents with significant neurological impairment (Oberlander et al., 1999). These studies have examined facial reactions to routine invasive procedures causing acute, phasic pain (e.g., venipuncture and injection).

The Facial Action Coding System (FACS; Ekman & Friesen, 1978; see Craig et al., Chapter 9) has been the prime research instrument used to study facial reactions of pain, because it is objective, comprehensive, anatomically based, and reliable. With the aid of slow-motion video, qualified coders systematically identify each possible facial action using rigorous, explicit criteria. Generally, the findings show that the facial reactions of both cognitively intact and cognitively impaired elderly persons intensify (compared to a brief baseline period) even in response to very minor pain (Hadjistavropoulos et al., 1997, 1998). The intensity of facial actions, rather than their frequency, has been particularly responsive to invasive events. The findings indicate that pain is not diminished by dementia in elderly populations. Indeed, there is some evidence to suggest even more vigorous pain reactions in elderly persons with cognitive impairment when pain is exacerbated (Hadjistavropoulos, LaChapelle, MacLeod, et al., 2000). However, particularly severe brain damage has been associated with virtually no response to invasive procedures (Oberlander, O'Donnell, & Montgomery, 1999), indicating that variation in

the impact of neurocognitive impairment is to be expected and requires further investigations.

The advantage of the FACS approach has been that it minimizes subjective judgment, whereas its main disadvantage for use in clinical settings is the time-consuming nature of both the training and application of the system. The FACS also requires slow-action video and does not allow for real-time coding. Nonetheless, measures based on the FACS seem to be well suited for use in clinical trials that investigate the effectiveness of pain management interventions.

Studies of global judgments of pain, relative to the FACS measure of pain, suggest the global judgments have criterion validity. Hadjistavropoulos and colleagues (1997, 1998) studied elderly patients with dementia who were undergoing injections and venipuncture. The results indicated that global judgments provided by untrained university students and nurses (obtained using a VAS and based on the observation of facial reactions) were highly correlated with indices of pain based upon the FACS measure. This suggests that simple facial-reaction-based ratings can be useful in clinical settings, and that health professionals can be instructed to attend to the face as a rich source of information about pain experienced. Interestingly, Hadjistavropoulos and colleagues (1998) found that the nurses provided significantly lower pain ratings than did the students, possibly because repeated exposure to situations involving patient discomfort could have desensitized them. This is consistent with earlier literature showing that nurses' perception of the intensity of patients' pain declines with experience (Davitz & Davitz, 1981). It is worth noting, however, that the nurses' ratings had a higher correspondence to patient scores than the students' ratings, and may thus carry more validity. This possibility is open for further study.

A disadvantage of such global measures is that they can potentially be affected by factors such as stereotypes based on patients' age (Hadjistavropoulos, LaChapelle, Hale, & MacLeod, 2000), sex, and physical appearance (Hadjistavropoulos, McMurtry, & Craig, 1996). Nonetheless, although such stereotypes have been found to affect ratings of pain in cognitively intact individuals, LaChapelle and colleagues (1999) showed that global ratings of the pain reactions of young persons with intellectual disabilities were unaffected by the degree to which a patient's appearance and mannerisms were indicative of intellectual disabilities.

Other nonverbal behaviors have been studied. Hadjistavropoulos, LaChapelle, MacLeod, and colleagues (2000) investigated a fine-grained observational procedure (Pain Behavior Measurement), developed and validated by Keefe and Block (1982; see Keefe et al., Chapter 10) in elderly patients undergoing physical rehabilitation. Some of the patients who were studied had significant (mild to moderate) cognitive impairments, and some did not. Trained coders observed the frequency of occurrence of clearly defined pain-related behaviors (e.g., guarding, bracing, and grimacing) while the individuals were undergoing structured activities, including walking, standing, sitting, reclining and transferring from one activity to another. It was found that pain-related behaviors occurred more frequently during more physically demanding activities than during more passive ones. Patient cognitive status did not affect the occurrence of these behaviors, suggesting that these activities could be used for pain assessment in persons with cognitive impairment. Of particular usefulness appeared to be guarding that was defined as "abnormally stiff, interrupted or rigid movement while moving from one position to another" (Keefe & Block, 1982, p. 366). Guarding appeared to provide the most sensitive Pain Behavior Measurement index of pain for seniors, although it might better be interpreted as reflecting fear of pain (Asmundson, Norton, & Norton, 1999).

Overall, the results from observational studies suggest that global observational procedures can be satisfactory indices of pain and tend to be correlated with behaviorally focused and fine-grained ratings. Nonetheless, global observational procedures can be affected by individual factors such as observers' background (e.g., nurses vs. students) or prior experience with pain. As well, significant correlations do not provide information on under- or overestimation of pain, and additional investigation of measures of agreement is needed (cf. Chambers, Reid, Craig, McGrath, & Finley, 1998). Behaviorally focused and fine-grained approaches vary in the degree to which they are useful and often need to be tailored to the specific population studied. Some of these procedures are resource-intensive (e.g., the FACS), despite their substantial information yield. Although their use in clinical settings can be difficult because of such practical considerations, they are particularly suited to research (e.g., clinical trials).

Proxy Measures

In contrast to observational procedures that require trained coders or health care professionals, proxy

approaches to measurement involve caregivers who are familiar with a person's day-to-day behavior and can report on this (e.g., increases and decreases in sleeping). The approach has yielded information concerning how children with cognitive impairments experience and cope with pain. McGrath, Rosmus, Camfield, Campbell, and Hennigar (1998) asked caregivers of 20 children with intellectual disabilities to recall two incidents of short, sharp pain and two instances of longer-lasting pain for each child, and then to describe the child's behavior. Thirty-one behaviors were extracted from these reports. Although the specific behaviors varied from child to child, the categories of behavior (vocal, eating or sleeping, facial expression, social and personality, physiological, body, and limps) were common to all children. Breau, McGrath, Camfield, Rosmus, and Finley (1998) provided some validity evidence for the checklist (see Appendix 8.C) and expanded its use to children with autism and other pervasive developmental disorders. Caregivers of children with such conditions completed the checklist in a retrospective fashion, and were also asked to report for each child on two pain incidents, one incident of frustration, and one incident during which the child was calm. The scale showed satisfactory internal consistency and could differentiate the pain incidents from the frustration and calm incidents through the endorsement of more items for the pain incidents. The approach appears promising, and further investigation of its clinical utility is warranted.

Physiological Measures

Porter, Porges, and Marshall (1988) found that infant heart rate increases and that respiratory sinus arrhythmia (i.e., an oscillation in the cardiac cycle length mediated by the vagus nerve) decreases with increased stimulus invasiveness. These findings led Porter and colleagues (1996) to attempt to measure pain in elderly persons with and without dementia using these physiological measures. Findings indicated that mean heart rate increased during venipuncture (as compared to the preparatory phase), although respiratory sinus arrhythmia did not differentiate venipuncture from the preparatory phase. Nonetheless, the investigators concluded that dementia is associated with a blunting of the physiological response. A limitation of this procedure is that the autonomic response to pain is difficult to discriminate physiologically from other states of arousal or distress. More research is needed to determine the utility of this approach in the assessment of chronic or recurrent pain.

It is noteworthy that considerable progress has been made in imaging the neurophysiological representation of pain. Casey and Minoshima (1997) reviewed the pertinent literature and concluded that 50% or more of the relevant studies of normal participants revealed pain-related activations of the ventral posterior thalamus, the medial dorsal midbrain, and the cerebellum, as well as contralateral insular and anterior cingulate cortex (see also Flor, Chapter 5). The heterogeneity that did exist in the various studies (see Casey & Minoshima, 1997, for a review) was attributed to variability in pain induction methods, data acquisition procedures, and analysis techniques. Although the study of pain imaging is just beginning, its certainly very promising and worth investigating in the assessment of special populations.

Individualized Procedures

Given the wide range of effects that central nervous system damage can have on pain reactivity, individualized and multidimensional approaches to pain assessment must be considered when the well-being of an individual is at stake. McGrath and colleagues (1998) observed that there were individual differences in the apparent manifestations of pain among children with intellectual disabilities. Similarly, physical and cognitive impairments unique to the person (e.g., paralysis, contractures, impaired memory, etc.) may need to be considered. When Miller and colleagues (1997) tailored the OSBD (Elliott et al., 1987) for children with cerebral palsy who were undergoing physiotherapy, they added an extra behavior, "reaching for pain." Reaching for pain was defined as "any extension of the hand toward the area of the body which is being treated/manipulated" (p. 694). They characterized this behavior an important expression of these children's distress that was not captured by the original instrument. This specific behavior occurred in 39% of their sample. This supports the value of tailoring existing instruments to suit the needs of the individuals under study.

Two approaches are suggested: individually tailored behavior checklists, and individually anchored global rating scales. In the first approach, lists of pain-relevant behaviors that are specific to each individual patient are devised. Knowledge of individuals with similar problems (either through clinical experience or the preexisting literature) would be helpful in developing each individualized approach. Pain-relevant behaviors could be obtained from caregivers familiar with the patients (see Romano & Schmaling, Chapter 18), as well as from the observation of patients during discomforting (but necessary) medical procedures. They could also be obtained through observation of the patients during periods of suffering from known medical conditions. The approach effectively avoids the possibility that idiosyncratic behaviors such as exaggerated vocalizations (e.g., screaming or moaning) or facial grimaces or peculiarities would lead to exaggeration in pain ratings by those unfamiliar with a person's typical behavior (Fanurik, Koh, Schmitz, Harrison, & Conrad, 1999). In the second approach (Philpott, 1997), a global rating scale (e.g., a 0–5 scale) would be further defined by parents' adding individualized behavioral descriptors for their child for each pain level.

Although such individualized approaches have obvious advantages, their reliability and validity remain to be demonstrated. Although we consider these approaches useful, we would recommend that they should not be the only method of pain assessment.

FUTURE DIRECTIONS

Preparation of this chapter rapidly led us to conclude that the development of assessment instruments that will contribute to a better understanding of pain in the populations of interest is in its infancy. The observation applies both to clinical management and to scientific investigation. Assessment is rarely systematic, as there are few well-designed research or clinical instruments for these specific populations. Moreover, unsubstantiated beliefs concerning the nature of pain in particular populations, rather than evidence-based knowledge, often dictate care; as a result, care is frequently inadequate. As the foregoing should indicate, there are some initial self-report, observational, proxy, and physiological measures that show promise. A database is needed on the psychometric properties of these measures. In the interest of avoiding proliferation of casually designed and unvalidated measures, proposals for new measures should demonstrate that they represent improvements on existing ones. Similarly, practitioners working with any of the populations of interest should be trained in the best instruments available, and their application should be routine in any facility for persons with limited ability to communicate. This would also encourage systematic evaluation of the efficacy of pain control interventions in these populations.

ACKNOWLEDGMENTS

The preparation of this chapter was supported in part by a Health Services Utilization and Research Commission grant to Thomas Hadjistavropoulos, and by a grant from the Social Sciences and Humanities Research Council of Canada to Kenneth D. Craig.

REFERENCES

Abbott, R., Forem, S. L., & Johann, M. (1989). Selective posterior rhizotomy for the treatment of spasticity: A review. *Child's Nervous System, 5*, 337–346.

American Psychiatric Association (1994). *Diagnostic and statistical manual of mental disorders* (4th ed.). Washington, DC: Author.

Anand, K. J. (1997). Long term effects of pain in neonates and infants. In T. S. Jensen, J. A. Turner, & Z. Wiesenfeld-Hallins (Eds.), *Proceedings of the 8th World Congress on Pain* (pp. 881–892). Seattle, WA: International Association for the Study of Pain Press.

Anand, K. J., & Craig, K. D. (1996). New perspectives on the definition of pain [Editorial]. *Pain, 67,* 3–6.

Asmundson, G. J. G., Norton, P. J., & Norton, G. R. (1999). Beyond pain: The role of fear and avoidance in chronicity. *Clinical Psychology Review, 19,* 97–119.

Barrier, P. J., Attia, J., Mayer, M. N., Amiel-Tison, C., & Shnider, S. M. (1989). Measurement of post-operative pain and narcotic administration in infant using a new clinical scoring system. *Intensive Care Medicine, 15,* S37–S39.

Bassetti, C., Bogousslavsky, J., & Regali, F. (1993). Sensory syndromes in parietal stroke. *Neurology, 43,* 1942–1949.

Benedetti, F., Vighetti, S., Ricco, C., Lagna, E., Bergamasco, B., Pinessi, L., & Rainero, I. (1999). Pain threshold and tolerance in Alzheimer's disease. *Pain, 80,* 377–382.

Berrol, S. (1989). Moderate head injury. In P. Bach y Rita (Ed.), *Traumatic brain injury* (pp. 31–40). New York: Demos.

Berthier, M., Starkstein, S., & Leiguarda, R. (1988). Asymbolia for pain: A sensory limbic disconnection syndrome, *Annals of Neurology, 24,* 41–49.

Biersdorff, K. K. (1991). Pain insensitivity and indifference: Alternative explanations for some medical catastrophes. *Mental Retardation, 29,* 259–262.

Biersdorff, K. K. (1994). Incidence of significantly altered pain experience among individuals with developmental disabilities. *American Journal of Mental Retardation, 98,* 619–631.

Breau, L., McGrath, P., Camfield, C., Rosmus, C., & Finley, G. A. (1998). Preliminary validation of the Non-Communicating Children's Pain Checklist. *Pain Research and Management, 3,* 40.

Canadian Study on Health and Aging Working Group. (1994). Canadian Study on Health and Aging: Study methods and prevalence of dementia. *Canadian Medical Association Journal, 150,* 899–913.

Casey, K. L., & Minoshima, S. (1997). Can pain be imaged? In T. S. Jensen, J. A. Turner & Z. Wiesenfelde-Halin (Eds.), *Proceedings of the 8th World Congress on Pain* (pp. 855–866). Seattle, WA: International Association for the Study of Pain Press.

Chambers, C. T., Giesbrecht, K., Craig, K. D., Bennett, S. M., & Huntsman, E. (1999). A comparison of faces scales for the measurement of pediatric pain: Children's and parent's ratings. *Pain, 83,* 25–35.

Chambers, C. T., Reid, G. J., Craig, K. D., McGrath, P. J., & Finley, G. A. (1998). Agreement between child and parent reports of pain. *Clinical Journal of Pain, 14,* 336–342.

Cook, A., & Thomas, M. (1994). Pain and the use of health services among the elderly. *Journal of Aging and Health, 6,* 155–172.

Comings, D. E., & Amromin, G. D. (1974). Autosomal dominant insensitivity to pain with hyperplastic myelinopathy and autosomal dominant indifference. *Neurology, 24,* 838–848.

Collignon, P., Giusiano, B., Jimeno, M. T., Combe, J. C., Thirion, X., & Porsmoguer, E. (1993). Une echelle d' heteroevaluation de la douleur chez l'enfant polyhandicape. In A. Gauvin-Piquard, I. Murat, & G. Pons (Eds.), *La douleur chez l'enfant: Echelles de evaluation. Traitments medicamenteux* (pp. 11–20). Paris: Springer-Verlag.

Craig, K. D. (1992). The facial expression of pain: Better than a thousand words. *American Pain Society Journal, 1,* 153–162.

Craig, K. D., & Grunau, R. V. E. (1993). Neonatal pain perception and behavioral measurement. In K. J. S. Arnand & P. J. McGrath (Eds.) *Neonatal pain and distress. Pain research and clinical management* (Vol 4., pp. 67–105). Amsterdam: Elsevier Science.

Craig, K. D., Lilley, C., & Gilbert, C. A. (1996). Social barriers to optimal pain management in children. *Clinical Journal of Pain, 17,* 147–259.

Davitz, J. R., & Davitz, L. L. (1981). *Inferences of patients' pain and psychological distress.* New York: Springer.

Dormans, J. P., & Pellegrino, L. (1988). *Caring for children with cerebral palsy.* Baltimore: Paul H. Brookes.

Ekman, P., & Friesen, W. (1978). *Investigator's guide to the Facial Action Coding System.* Palo Alto, CA: Consulting Psychologists Press.

Elliott, C. H., Jay, S. M., & Woody, P. (1987). An observation scale for measuring children's distress during medical procedures. *Journal of Pediatric Psychology, 12,* 543–551.

Fanurik, K., Koh, J. L., Schmitz, M. L., Harrison, R. D., & Conrad, T. M. (1999). Children with cognitive impairment: Parent report of pain and coping. *Journal of Developmental and Behavioral Pediatrics, 20,* 228–234.

Farrell, M. J., Katz, B., & Helme, R. D. (1996). The impact of dementia on the pain experience. *Pain, 67,* 7–15.

Ferrell, B. A. (1991). Pain management in elderly people. *Journal of the American Geriatrics Society, 39,* 1897–1903.

Fearon, I., McGrath, P. J., & Achat, H. (1996). "Booboos": The study of everyday pain among young children. *Pain*, 68, 55–62.

Frankowski, R. F., Annegers, J. F., & Whitman, S. (1985). The descriptive epidemiology of head trauma in the United States. In D. P. Becker & J. T. Povlishock (Eds.), *Central nervous system trauma: Status report, 1985* (pp. 33–43). Bethesda, MD: National Institutes of Health.

Fridlund, A. J. (1991). Evolution and facial action in reflex, social motive and paralanguage. *Biological Psychology*, 32, 3–100.

Gagliese, L., & Melzack, R. (1997). Age differences in the quality of chronic pain: A preliminary study. *Pain Research and Management*, 2, 157–162.

Gennarelli, T. A. (1983). Head injury in man and experimental animals: Clinical aspects. *Acta Neurochirugica*, Suppl. 32, 1–13.

Gibson, S. J., Voukelatos, X., Bradbeer, M., & Helme, R. D. (1996). Pain perception in the cognitively impaired elderly. *Abstracts of the 8th World Congress on Pain*, 281.

Gilbert-MacLeod, C. A., Craig, K. D., Rocha, E. M., & Mathias, M. D. (2000). Everyday pain in children with developmental delays. *Pediatric Psychology*, 25, 301–308.

Giusiano, B., Jimeno, M. T., Collignon, P., & Chau, Y. (1995). Utilization of a neural network in the elaboration of an evaluation scale for pain in cerebral palsy. *Methods of Information in Medicine*, 34, 498–502.

Gooch, J. L., & Sandell, T. V. (1996). Botulism toxin for spasticity and athetosis in children with cerebral palsy. *Archives of Physical Medicine and Rehabilitation*, 77, 508–511.

Hadjistavropoulos, T., Craig, K. D., Martin, N., Hadjistavropoulos, H. D., & McMurtry, B. (1997). Toward a research outcome measure of pain in frail elderly in chronic care. *The Pain Clinic*, 10, 71–79.

Hadjistavropoulos, T., LaChapelle, D., Hale, C., & MacLeod, F. (2000). Age- and appearance-based stereotyping about patients undergoing a painful medical procedure. *The Pain Clinic*, 12, 25–33.

Hadjistavropoulos, T., LaChapelle, D., MacLeod, F., Hale, C., O'Rourke, N., & Craig, K. D. (1998). Cognitive functioning and pain reactions in hospitalized elders. *Pain Research and Management*, 3, 145–151.

Hadjistavropoulos, T., LaChapelle, D., MacLeod, F., Snider, B., & Craig, K. D. (2000). Measuring movement exacerbated pain in cognitively impaired frail elders. *Clinical Journal of Pain*, 16, 54–63.

Hadjistavropoulos, T., McMurtry, B., & Craig, K. D. (1996). Beautiful faces in pain: Biases and accuracy in the perception of pain. *Psychology and Health*, 64, 435–443.

Hale, C., & Hadjistavropoulos, T. (1997). Emotional components of pain. *Pain Research and Management*, 2, 217–225.

Harkins, S. W., & Price, D. D. (1992). Assessment of pain in the elderly. In D. C. Turk & R. Melzack (Eds.), *Handbook of pain assessment* (pp. 315–331). New York: Guilford Press.

Helme, R. D. (1996). Pain in the elderly. *Abstracts of the 8th World Congress on Pain* (p. 434). Seattle, WA: International Association for the Study of Pain Press.

Helme, R. D., & Gibson, S. J. (1999). Pain in older people. In I. K. Crombie, P. R. Croft, S. J. Linton, L. LeResche, & M. Von Korff (Eds.), *Epidemiology of pain*

(pp. 103–112). Seattle, WA: International Association for the Study of Pain Press.

Hurley, A. C., Volicer, B. J., Hanrahan, P. A., Houde, S., & Volicer, L. (1992). Assessment of discomfort in Alzheimer patients. *Research in Nursing and Health*, 15, 369–377.

Kaasalainen, S., Middleton, J., Knezacek, S., Hartley, T., Stewart, N., Ife, C., & Robinson, L. (1998). Pain and cognitive status in institutionalized elderly: Perceptions and interventions. *Journal of Gerontological Nursing*, 24, 24–31.

Keefe, F. J., & Block, A. R. (1982). Development of an observation method for assessing pain behavior in chronic low back pain patients. *Behavior Therapy*, 13, 363–375.

Koh, J. L., & Fanurik, D. (1997). *Post-operative pain assessment in children with cognitive impairment*. Poster presented at the convention of the American Pain Society, New Orleans, LA.

Kolb, B., & Whishaw, I. Q. (1985). *Fundamentals of human neuropsychology* (2nd ed.). New York: Freeman.

LaChapelle, D., Hadjistavropoulos, T., & Craig, K. D. (1999). Pain measurement in persons with intellectual disabilities. *Clinical Journal of Pain*, 15, 13–23.

LeBaron, S., & Zeltzer, L. (1984). Assessment of acute pain and anxiety in children and adolescents by self-report, observer reports, and a behavior checklist. *Journal of Consulting and Clinical Psychology*, 48, 356–365.

Lezak, M. D. (1995). *Neuropsychological assessment* (3rd ed.). New York: Oxford University Press.

MacKenzie, L., & Lignor, A. (Eds.). (1994). *The complete directory for people with chronic illness*. Lakeville, CT: Grey House.

McCaffery, M., & Beebe, A. (1989). Pain in the elderly. In M. McCaffery & A. Beebe (Eds.), *Pain: Clinical manual for nursing* (pp. 308–323). St. Louis, MO: Mosby.

McGrath, P. A., Seifert, S. E, Speechley, K. N., Booth, J. C., Stitt, L., & Gibson, M. C. (1996). A new analogue scale for assessing children's pain. *Pain*, 64, 435–443.

McGrath, P. J. (1998). We all failed the Latimers. *Journal of Paediatrics and Child Health*, 3, 153–154.

McGrath, P. J., Johnson, G., Goodman, J. T., Schillinger, J., Dunn, J., & Chapman, J. A. (1985). CHEOPS: A behavioral scale for rating post-operative pain in children. In H. L. Fields, R. Dubner, & F. Cervero (Eds.), *Advances in pain research and therapy* (Vol. 9, pp. 395–402). New York: Raven Press.

McGrath, P. J.. Rosmus, C., Camfield, C., Campbell, M. A., & Hennigar, A. (1998). Behaviors caregivers use to determine pain in non-verbal, cognitively impaired children. *Developmental Medicine and Child Neurology*, 40, 340–343.

Melding, P. (1991). Is there such a thing as geriatric pain? *Pain*, 46, 119–121.

Merskey, H., & Bogduk, N. (1994). *Classification of chronic pain: Descriptions of chronic pain syndromes and definitions of pain terms*. Seattle, WA: International Association for the Study of Pain Press.

Melzack, R., & Wall, P. D. (1965). Pain mechanisms: A new theory. *Science*, 150, 971–979.

Miller, A. C., Johann-Murphy, M., & Cate, I. M. (1997). Pain, anxiety, and cooperativeness in children with rhizotomy: Changes throughout rehabilitation. *Journal of Pediatric Psychology*, 22, 689–705.

Miller, J., Moore, K., Schofield, A., Ng'andu, N., & Sedlak, C. (1996). A study of discomfort and confusion among elderly surgical patients. *Orthopaedic Nursing, 15,* 27–34.

Mobily, P., Herr, K., Clark, K., & Wallace, R. (1994). An epidemiological analysis of pain in the elderly. *Journal of Aging and Health, 6,* 139–154.

Oberlander, T. F., Gilbert, C. A., Chambers, C. T., O'Donnell, M. E., & Craig, K. D. (1999). Biobehavioral responses to acute pain in adolescents with significant neurological impairment. *Clinical Journal of Pain, 15,* 201–209.

Oberlander, T. F., O'Donnell, M. E., & Montgomery, C. J. (1999). Pain in children with significant neurological impairment. *Journal of Developmental and Behavioral Pediatrics, 20,* 235–243.

Parmelee, P. A., Smith, B., & Katz, I. R. (1993). Pain complaints and cognitive status among elderly institution residents. *Journal of the American Geriatrics Society, 41,* 517–522.

Philpott, B. (1997). *A pain assessment for children with special needs.* Paper presented at the Fourth International Symposium on Pediatric Pain, Helsinki, Finland.

Pinel, J. P. J. (1997). *Biopsychology* (4th ed.). Boston: Allyn & Bacon.

Porter, F. L., Malhotra, K. M., Wolf, C. M., Morris, J. C., Miller, J. P., & Smith, M. (1996). Dementia and response to pain in the elderly. *Pain, 68,* 413–421.

Porter, F. L., Porges, S. W., & Marshall, R. E. (1988). Newborn pain cries and vagal tone: Parallel changes in response to circumcision. *Child Development, 59,* 495–505.

Prkachin, K., & Craig, K. D. (1995). Expressing pain: The communication and interpretation of facial pain signals. *Journal of Nonverbal Behavior, 19,* 191–205.

Rafferty, T., & Moser, S. (1991). [Pilot study of Short Stay Unit Pain Rating Scale]. Unpublished raw data.

Rosenzweig, M. R., Leiman, A. L., & Breedlove, S. M. (1999). *Biological psychology* (2nd ed.). Sunderland, MA: Sinauer Associates.

Roy, A., & Simon, G. B. (1987). Intestinal obstruction as a cause of death in the mentally handicapped. *Journal of Mental Deficiency Research, 31,* 193–197.

Roy, R., & Thomas, M. A. (1986). A survey of chronic pain in elderly populations. *Canadian Family Physician, 32,* 513–516.

Schade, J. G., Joyce, B. A., Gerkensmeyer, J., & Keck, J. (1996). Comparison of three preverbal scales for postoperative pain assessment in a diverse pediatric sample. *Journal of Pain and Symptom Management, 12,* 348–359.

Sengstaken, E. A., & King, S. A. (1993). The problems of pain and its detection among geriatric nursing home residents. *Journal of the American Geriatrics Society, 41,* 541–544.

Simons, W., & Malabar, R. (1995). Assessing pain in elderly patients who cannot respond verbally. *Journal of Advanced Nursing, 22,* 663–669.

Spivack, M., & Balicki, M. (1990). Scope of the problem. In D. Corthell (Ed.), *Traumatic brain injury and vocational rehabilitation* (pp. 1–20). Menomonie: Research and Training Center, University of Wisconsin-Stout.

Stevens, B. (1990). Development and testing of a pediatric pain measurement scale. *Pediatric Nursing, 16,* 543–548.

Winkelmann, R. K., Lambert, E. H., & Hayles, A. B. (1962). Congenital absence of pain. *Archives of Dermatology, 85,* 325–339.

APPENDIX 8.A. DALHOUSIE EVERYDAY PAIN SCALE (DEPS)

Date: _____   Observer: _____
Time: _____   Subject's Name: _____
Class: _____   Age: _____ (mos)
                                                              ID#: _____

Location   Code: _____

Outside: playground / park / other
Inside: library / block area / art area / housekeeping / kitchen / gym / other

Behavioral context

Activity level   1---------2---------3---------4---------5
                                  low   medium   high

Tone   1---------2---------3---------4---------5
                                  calm   agitated

Number of participants   1   2   3–5   6 or more

Level of personal control   1---------2---------3---------4---------5
                                  high   low

Description of incident

Body location (a code number could be used) _____

Hurt caused by: self   other   child   adult   object

Perceived severity of hurt   0---------1---------2---------3---------4
                                  no hurt   severe hurt

Subject's response

Intensity of distress   0---------1---------2---------3---------4---------5
                            none   facial   verbal   sobbing   crying   screaming
                                    expression comment

    Duration of distress _ (sec)

Intensity of anger   1---------2---------3---------4---------5
                                  none   facial   angry   verbal   physical
                                          expression behavior aggression aggression

    Aggression directed toward: object   hurter   helper   other person

Protective behaviors   none   holding   favoring   reduction of activity

    Duration of protective behaviors _ (sec)

Social response   withdrawal   neutral   help seeking

Adult response   none   distraction   verbal   physical   first aid
                                                          comfort   comfort

Comments

Note. The DEPS allows for the systematic recording of information pertaining to pain incidents. From Fearon, I., McGrath, P. J., and Achat, H. (1996). "Booboos": The study of everyday pain among young children. *Pain, 68,* 55–62. Copyright 1996 by the International Association for the Study of Pain. Reprinted by permission.

APPENDIX 8.B. BEHAVIORAL DEFINITIONS AND SCORING OF THE CHILDREN'S HOSPITAL OF EASTERN ONTARIO PAIN SCALE (CHEOPS)

Item	Behavior	Score	Definition
Cry	No cry	1	Child is not crying.
	Moaning	2	Child is moaning or quietly vocalizing, silent cry.
	Crying	2	Child is crying, but the cry is gentle or whimpering.
	Scream	3	Child is full-lunged cry, sobbing; may be scored with complaint or without complaint.
Facial	Composed	1	Neutral facial expression.
	Grimace	2	Score only if definite negative facial expression.
	Smiling	0	Score only if definite positive facial expression.
Child verbal	None	1	Child is not talking.
	Other complaints	1	Child complains, but not about pain, e.g., "I want to see mommy," or "I am thirsty."
	Pain complaints	2	Child complains about pain.
	Both complaints	2	Child complains about pain and about other things, e.g., "It hurts; I want mommy."
	Positive	0	Child makes any positive statement or talks about other things without complaint.
Torso	Neutral	1	Body (not limbs) is at rest; torso is inactive.
	Shifting	2	Body is in motion in a shifting or serpentine fashion.
	Tense	2	Body is arched or rigid.
	Shivering	2	Body is shuddering or shaking involuntarily.
	Upright	2	Child is in a vertical or upright position.
	Restrained	2	Body is restrained.
Touch	Not touching	1	Child is not touching or grabbing at wound.
	Reach	2	Child is reaching for but not touching wound.
	Touch	2	Child is gently touching wound or wound area.
	Grab	2	Child is grabbing vigorously at wound.
	Restrained	2	Child's arms are restrained.
Legs	Neutral	1	Legs may be in any position but are relaxed; includes gentle swimming or serpentine-like movements.
	Squirming/kicking	2	Definitive uneasy or restless movements in the legs and/or sinking out with foot or feet.
	Drawn up/tensed	2	Legs tensed and/or pulled up tightly to body and kept there.
	Standing	2	Standing, crouching, or kneeling.
	Restrained	2	Child's legs are being held down.

Note. The range of total scores is 4 to 13 for each time period sampled. Higher scores are indicative of increased pain. From McGrath, P. J., Johnson, G., Goodman, J. T., Schillinger, J., Dunn, J., & Chapman, J. A. (1985). CHEOPS: A behavioral scale for rating postoperative pain in children. In H. L. Fields, R. Dubner, & F. Cervero (Eds.), *Advances in pain research and therapy* (Vol. 9, pp. 395–402). New York: Raven Press. Copyright 1985 by Raven Press, Ltd. Reprinted by permission of Lippincott Williams & Wilkins.

APPENDIX 8.C. THE NON-COMMUNICATING CHILDREN'S CHECKLIST

Name of child: _____   Completed by: _____

How often has this child shown these behaviours in the last 10 minutes? Please circle a number for each behaviour.

	Not at all	Just a little	Fairly often	Very often
Moaning, whining, whimpering (fairly soft)	1	2	3	4
Crying (moderately loud)	1	2	3	4
Screaming/yelling (very loud)	1	2	3	4
A specific sound or word for pain (for example: a word, cry, or type of laugh)[a]	1	2	3	4
Eating less, not interested in food	1	2	3	4
Increase in sleep	1	2	3	4
Decrease in sleep	1	2	3	4
Not co-operating, cranky, irritable, unhappy	1	2	3	4
Less interaction with others, withdrawn	1	2	3	4
Seeking comfort or physical closeness	1	2	3	4
Being difficult to distract, not able to satisfy or pacify	1	2	3	4
A furrowed brow	1	2	3	4
A change in eyes, including: squinching of eyes, eyes opened wide; eyes frowning	1	2	3	4
Turning down of mouth, not smiling	1	2	3	4
Lips puckering up, tight, pouting or quivering	1	2	3	4
Clenching or grinding teeth, chewing or thrusting tongue out	1	2	3	4
Not moving, less active, quiet	1	2	3	4
Jumping around, agitated, fidgety	1	2	3	4
Floppy	1	2	3	4
Stiff, spastic, tense, rigid	1	2	3	4
Gesturing to or touching part of the body that hurt	1	2	3	4
Protecting, favouring or guarding part of the body that hurts	1	2	3	4
Flinching or moving the body part away, being sensitive to touch	1	2	3	4
Moving the body in specific way to show pain (e.g. head back, arms down, curls up, etc.)[a]	1	2	3	4
Shivering[a]	1	2	3	4
Change in colour, pallor	1	2	3	4
Sweating, perspiring	1	2	3	4
Tears	1	2	3	4
Sharp intake of breath, gasping	1	2	3	4
Breath holding[a]	1	2	3	4

Note. Ongoing work is aimed at evaluating the utility of the scale using these instructions (i.e., "How often has this child shown these behaviors in the last 10 minutes?") (Lynn Breau, personal communication, November 26, 1999). The Non-Communicating Children's Checklist was developed by McGrath, P. J., Rosmus, C., Camfield, C., Campbell, M. A., and Hennigar, A. (1998). Behaviours caregivers use to determine pain in non-verbal, cognitively impaired children. *Developmental Medicine and Child Neurology, 40,* 340-343. The items could also be classified into categories (e.g., vocal, physical signs). The McGrath and colleagues (1998) article does not include a copy of the scale, but its items appear as part of their Table 3. The version of the scale above does not include one of the original items ("cringe or grimace") because it was considered to be subjective (Breau et al., 1998). The information in this appendix is reprinted with the kind permission of the developers of the scale as well as of MacKeith Press. Permission for future reproductions of the scale should be obtained from the original copyright holders.

[a]There is some evidence that the omission of these items could improve the internal consistency of the scale (Breau et al., 1998).

Part II

ASSESSMENT OF THE BEHAVIORAL EXPRESSION OF PAIN

Chapter 9

The Facial Expression of Pain

KENNETH D. CRAIG
KENNETH M. PRKACHIN
RUTH ECKSTEIN GRUNAU

Pain is a private experience with complex qualities that must be measured if people in distress are to be helped. Sensations, feelings, and thoughts may be salient for the sufferer, but they are incomprehensible to others without observable manifestations. Fortunately, behavioral information, both verbal and nonverbal, often permits valid inferences about a person's pain. This chapter examines how a primary and powerful form of nonverbal communication—facial expression—allows clinicians, investigators, and others to formulate judgments about another person's pain, whether or not the person can use words to communicate.

NONVERBAL DETERMINANTS OF JUDGMENTS OF ANOTHER'S PAIN

People in pain are capable of communicating their experience through a remarkable variety of actions, ranging from the use of language to diverse nonverbal actions. The latter include (1) paralinguistic vocalizations, such as crying or moaning; (2) other nonverbal qualities of speech, such as volume, hesitancies, or timbre; (3) visible physiological activity, such as pallor, flushing, sweating, or muscle tension; (4) bodily activity, including involuntary reflexes and purposeful action; and (5) facial expressions.

The communicative value of these behaviors may be secondary to other functions. For example,

limb and bodily activities primarily serve to avoid and terminate injury or to prevent abrupt escalation in pain, although they often provide convincing evidence of distress or invalid status. In contrast, speech and facial expression can control pain only indirectly. They function, above all, as social communications that convey distress and may recruit the help of others.

The observer confronts a challenge in attempting to extract from this potential flood of information a synthesis of the cues that will establish the presence of pain, its severity, and its qualitative features. Judgments will also be affected by the observer's understanding of physical trauma and disease, additional biomedical information, input from others, and other contextual information. The information that may be specific to pain also needs to be sorted from information signaling other life activities. The problem of separating signal from noise can be considerable. Despite these complexities, the behavioral parameters are what provide the key to understanding another's subjective experience, with the others serving as important context for evaluating the information.

Nonverbal expression has uniquely important properties that may be unavailable in other cues concerning pain. It often remains accessible when the capacity for speech is not available (see Hadjistavropoulos, von Baeyer, & Craig, Chapter 8, this volume). For some patients and in certain situations, nonverbal indices of pain may be the only information available. This is the case with infants and very young children, who do not have a capacity for verbal report, although their capacity for communicating subjective states through vocalizations and nonverbal behavior is considerable. People with intellectual disabilities, language disorders, acquired brain damage, or dementia also have varying capacities for communicating pain through speech, and caregivers may have to rely exclusively upon nonverbal communication. Patients who are recovering from anesthetics, impaired by toxic substances, or refusing to report pain illustrate a situationally determined need to rely on nonverbal expressions of pain.

But nonverbal expression is also a valuable source of information from people who can use language, and the likelihood that observers will use it is very strong. Observers tend to rely upon a mix of nonredundant sources of information. Appraisals of others' distress are often more heavily weighted by nonverbal activity than by self-report (Craig, 1992; Poole & Craig, 1992). The importance of nonverbal information is well established in clinical practice, as the successful physical examination and ongoing care often depend upon sensitivity to nonverbal response on the part of the examiner. Jacox (1980) reported that nurses found nonverbal behaviors and physiological signs to be more salient and easier to use in pain assessment than patient verbalizations about their pain. There also are times when a clinician does not want to ask to avoid alarming the patient or when one is otherwise occupied.

Observers often favor nonverbal expression, relative to self-report, in their judgments of others, because of its apparent greater credibility (Craig, Hill, & McMurtry, 1999). People do not monitor nonverbal actions as attentively as they do their speech (Craig & Prkachin, 1980); hence nonverbal expressions are less subject to purposeful distortion than verbalizations. In a review of research, von Baeyer, Johnson, and McMillan (1984) noted that "nonverbal behaviors may be a more accurate source of information than verbal reports because they are less subject to 'motivated dissimulation'" (p. 1319). The tendency to trust nonverbal information more than self-report is widespread. People judging the emotional significance of another's actions appear to assume that nonverbal behavior is less amenable to dissimulation than self-report is (Ekman & Friesen, 1969), and consider it more important when self-report and nonverbal behavior are discordant (De Paulo, Rosenthal, Eisenstat, Rogers, & Findelstein, 1978). Kraut (1978) concluded that accuracy in the detection of others' attempts to deceive is enhanced when nonverbal behavior is available. Of course, people can purposefully misrepresent themselves as being in pain by conveying this verbally and nonverbally through an assumed role, as actors effectively demonstrate. Even untrained people are quite successful in convincing others that their pain is genuine (Poole & Craig, 1992). However, the likelihood remains greater that nonverbal expression will be more spontaneous and less subject to purposeful manipulation than self-report.

A PRIMARY ROLE FOR FACIAL ACTIVITY

The prominence of the face as a source of information among the various channels of nonverbal communication is well established (Collier, 1985; Ekman & Rosenberg, 1997; Russell & Fernandez-Dols, 1997). People's facial expressions tend to be readily accessible and highly plastic, as they can change very rapidly to display a remarkable variety of discriminable patterns (Ekman & Friesen, 1969). One can often appreciate features of another person's emotions, motives, thoughts, attention, and intentions by scanning his or her face. People who fail to monitor and correctly interpret the ongoing dynamic pattern of others' facial activity are vulnerable to social deficits (Custrini & Feldman, 1989). There tends to be added value even when others are communicating verbally, as the information disclosed by the facial display is unlikely to be entirely redundant with the content of speech.

The usefulness of attending to others' facial displays is intuitively appreciated, as there is a powerful disposition to situate oneself so as to be able to attend to facial activity. Mothers who become utterly absorbed in their babies' facial expressions provide excellent examples. This fascination facilitates providing care to an infant and permits substantial social interaction. But infants are equally attentive to their caretakers' facial expressions, with the propensity to attend to and use facial activity persisting throughout life. In extreme situations, the facial display may prove very useful when attending to others who have been hurt, or another person's facial grimace of pain may signal danger and allow one to avoid looming personal threat. The functional value of this information argues for ancient bioevolutionary origins of dispositions both to attend to others' facial expressions and to provide information via this communication modality (Fridlund, 1994).

The ability to decipher diverse psychological states through facial activity implies consistencies across individuals in how they behave when experiencing subjective states. These associations between subjective states and overt behavior have both phylogenetic and socialization determinants. Powerful genetic roots are reflected in the physiological regulation, anatomical structure, and behavioral organization of facial displays (Fridlund, 1991) throughout the course of ontogenetic development. Notwithstanding prominent biological bases, children also become acculturated to social standards and normative patterns consistent with the social environments in which they grow up. Through observational learning, direct instruction, and social reinforcement, children and adults come to display patterns of pain and illness behavior that conform to familial and cultural expectations (Craig, 1987). The relatively global, reflexive reactions of very young infants to tissue damage are shaped and transformed during the course of development into differentiated and socially responsive patterns of behavior (Craig, McMahon, Morison, & Zaskow, 1984). Facial displays develop as part of this transformation (Craig, 1998).

Our understanding of the development of facial expressions associated with pain can be enhanced by accounts of the emergence of facial expressions of emotion and their usefulness as social signals (Camras, Malastesta, & Izard, 1991; Ekman, 1993; Huebner & Izard, 1988; Oster, Hegley, & Nagel, 1992; Russell, 1994). Substantial evidence indicates that by the end of the first year of life infants consistently associate specific facial behaviors with affective states, both in terms of producing them and appreciating their significance in others (Reilly & Bellugi, 1996). Theories of the association of specific facial displays with emotional experiences are usually based in the bioevolutionary proposition that there are favorable adaptive consequences for species whose members can signal subjective states and behavioral intentions to conspecifics (Darwin, 1872/1965). The action may have reflected internal homeostatic processes in the first instance, but it often also becomes a social signal because it fulfills a communication function (Adelmann & Zajonc, 1989; Fridlund, 1991). Hypotheses about the adaptive functions of features of facial expression are not difficult to generate. For example, the physical threat usually associated with pain should provoke protective actions. The most prominent action fea-

tures associated with pain—lowering of the brows and narrowing of the eye opening—could reflect efforts to protect these vital organs at the same time as vision is maintained to engage in protective behavior.

Facial activity may also contribute to the experience of pain. Facial feedback models of emotion argue that physiological feedback from the face permits subjective differentiation of emotional states (Adelmann & Zajonc, 1989), with the vigor of the display influencing the intensity of the subjective experience. The position could be extended to pain. Experimentally induced attenuation of facial expression has been associated with diminished autonomic activity, reduced subjective distress, and increased pain tolerance (Colby, Lanzetta, & Kleck, 1977; Lanzetta, Cartwright-Smith, & Kleck, 1976). This seems intuitively acknowledged when people are told to "grin and bear it" or "keep a stiff upper lip." These findings must be interpreted cautiously, as they have been obtained in a limited number of studies, and the mechanisms associated with the effects remain unclear.

SPECIFIC FACIAL ACTIONS ASSOCIATED WITH PAIN

Although a facial grimace of pain tends to be generally recognized, the speed and complexity of facial actions make objective description difficult. Attempts to characterize facial expressions of pain without the benefit of objective, comprehensive coding systems have led to errors in descriptive accounts of the facial display. Darwin (1872/1965), for example, suggested that in pain "the mouth may be closely compressed, or more commonly the lips are retracted, with the teeth clenched or ground together" and "the eyes stare wildly as in horrified astonishment" (pp. 69–70). Recent systematic studies do not confirm this account. Rather, a dropped jaw or open lips are probable, and the eyes are likely to be narrowed or closed.

Decoding facial expressions requires a comprehensive method that objectively identifies all possible actions, their intensity, and their temporal relationships. At present, the Facial Action Coding System (FACS; Ekman & Friesen, 1978) provides the most satisfactory approach, because it is comprehensive, is entirely descriptive, and avoids inference as to underlying subjective states (see Cohn, Zlochower, Lien, & Kanade, 1999, for a review of alternative systems). This fine-grained, anatomically based system identifies 44 discrete facial actions. Each action unit represents the movement of a single facial muscle, or, in a few cases, a group of muscle strands that move as a unit. The typical application uses videotaped, slow-motion, or stop-frame feedback. Coders are trained to apply specific operational criteria to determine which actions have taken place and to identify their onset, offset, and (when possible) intensity over specified time intervals. Table 9.1 illustrates the criteria and rules for identifying one action, "lid tightening," that has consistently been associated with pain in systematic studies. Facial "expressions" (as opposed to specific movements) generally can be defined by two or more specific facial actions that have a common onset or clear overlap in time.

Intercoder reliability for identifying pain-related action units has been consistently high in published investigations (e.g., Craig, Hyde, & Patrick, 1991). When a second trained coder has recoded a randomly selected set of videotaped reactions to pain, reliabilities—calculated as the proportion of agreements relative to the total number of action units identified as occurring by either of the two coders—have consistently exceeded .75 (LeResche & Dworkin, 1988; Prkachin & Mercer, 1989).

With some variation, a relatively distinct subset of facial actions has been recognizable as a facial expression of pain in studies to date. Most investigations have focused upon the short, sharp, acute pain associated with invasive procedures (e.g., Craig et al., 1991; LeResche & Dworkin, 1988) or exacerbation of clinical pain, such as temporomandibular joint (TMJ) disorder (LeResche & Dworkin, 1984), shoulder pathology (Prkachin & Mercer, 1989), chronic low back pain (Hadji-

stavropoulos & Craig, 1994), and surgical repair (Hadjistavropoulos, LaChapelle, MacLeod, Snider, & Craig, 2000). The pattern has also been observed with the tonic discomfort provoked by induced pressure or ischemic pain (Prkachin, 1992a), and with persistent pain arising from surgical incisions (Gilbert et al., 2000). Similar characteristics have been described for people suffering from muscle contraction headaches (Iezzi, Adams, Bugg, & Stokes, 1991), although patients with lung cancer engaging in physical movements displayed minimal facial evidence of distress (Wilkie, 1995). There is also evidence that specific facial expressions exhibited by patients complaining of chest pain can differentiate between adults with heart muscle pathology and those without (Dalton, Brown, Carlson, McNutt, & Greer, 1999). Thus the facial display has the possibility of being indicative of myocardial infarction. In summary, a prototypical pattern of pain display is observed not only when external pain is applied, but also when internal somatic stress instigates increased levels of persistent or phasic pain.

Whereas patients suffering from chronic pain often complain of substantial, unremitting pain, their facial displays more often indicate depressed mood, with facial grimaces occurring only intermittently, apparently when the discomfort is exacerbated (Hadjistavropoulos et al., 2000). For this reason, patients in chronic pain are unlikely to display distress in situations other than those in which the pain has been provoked or intensified. Patients who are asleep or steadfastly inactive to avoid pain would not be expected to display the facial expression.

The key facial actions associated with pain that are consistent across different modalities of pain instigation (Prkachin, 1992a) are as follows (Craig et al., 1991). All studies of adults have identified lowering of the brows and narrowing of the eyes, as a result of tightening the eyelids, as basic to the expression. The majority of studies also have found raising the cheeks (again narrowing the eyes), eyes closed or blinking, raising the upper lip, and parting of lips or dropping of the jaw to be pain-related actions. Individual studies have also identified the following: horizontally stretching the lips, oblique pulling at the corner of the lips, vertically stretching the mouth open, wrinkling the nose, deepening the nasolabial fold, and drooping of the eyelids. Figure 9.1 illustrates facial muscles controlling the FACS action units that have been associated with pain. Figure 9.2 on page 158 provides an artist's drawing of how a patient with low back pain

---

TABLE 9.1. Minimum Requirements for Coding the Occurrence of Action Unit 7 (Lid Tightening) in the Facial Action Coding System (FACS)

1. *Slight* narrowing of the eye opening (due primarily to lower lid raise), or
2. The lower lid is raised and the skin below the eye is drawn up and/or medially towards the inner corner of the eye *slightly*; or
3. *Slight* bulge or pouch of the lower eyelid skin as it is pushed up.

If you did not see the lower lid *move* up, then requirement 1 must be *marked* not slight and requirement 3 must be met.

Note. From Ekman and Friesen (1978). Copyright 1978 by Dr. Paul Ekman, Human Interaction Laboratory, University of California–San Francisco. Reprinted by permission.

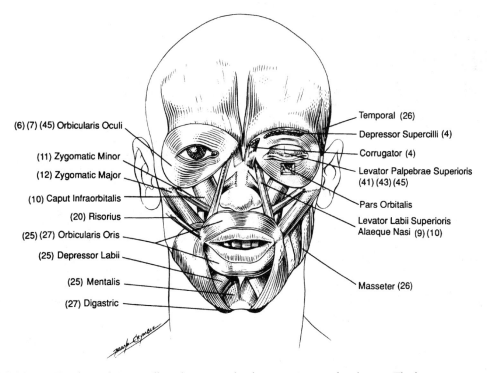

(6) (7) (45) Orbicularis Oculi
(11) Zygomatic Minor
(12) Zygomatic Major
(10) Caput Infraorbitalis
(20) Risorius
(25) (27) Orbicularis Oris
(25) Depressor Labii
(25) Mentalis
(27) Digastric

Temporal (26)
Depressor Supercilli (4)
Corrugator (4)
Levator Palpebrae Superioris (41) (43) (45)
Pars Orbitalis
Levator Labii Superioris Alaeque Nasi (9) (10)
Masseter (26)

FIGURE 9.1. Facial muscles controlling the various facial actions associated with pain. The key action units are identified numerically and have been labeled according to the Facial Action Coding System (FACS; Ekman & Friesen, 1978) as follows: (4) brow lower, (6) cheek raise, (7) lids tight, (9) nose wrinkle, (11) nasolabial deepen, (10) upper lip raise, (12) lip corner pull, (20) lip stretch, (25) lips part, (26) jaw drop, (41) lids droop, (43) eyes closed, (45) blink.

reacted to a painful straight-leg-raising, range-of-motion exercise. This patient's reaction was selected because it provides a composite of many of the facial actions commonly observed. The pattern observed here comprised the brows slightly lowered, the nose wrinkled, the infraorbital triangle (the cheek area) raised, the lower eyelid raised and tightened, a slightly elevated upper lip, eyes closed with a marked tightening, and the lips slightly parted. Patients usually display subsets of these facial actions.

The inconsistencies across studies in the less frequently noted actions identified as pain-related are attributable to a definable set of variables. Other psychological states with expressive markers, such as startle or amused embarrassment, often co-occur with pain and lead to expressions that reflect confounded states. This provides plausible explanations of the not infrequent association between pain and blinking and raising of the lip corner. Other actions—for example, upper-lip raising or horizontal pulling of the lip corners—are probably pain-related but less sensitive indicators. Observers should

understand that there is a core of pain-related actions, as well as associated actions reflecting psychological states that are often, but not always, associated with pain.

Clinicians and others judging a person's pain can be expected to use the configuration of observed actions, including their temporal relationships and intensity. Temporal overlap in pain-related facial movements has been described as a key determinant in the attribution of pain (LeResche & Dworkin, 1988), and it has proven necessary for judgments of more severe pain (Lee & Craig, 1991). Hadjistavropoulos, LaChapelle, and colleagues (1998) have observed that the intensity or vigor of facial actions tends to be the prime determinant of judgments of pain in elderly persons. In some cases, an observer may be dependent upon very brief instances of "microexpressions" of this integrated pattern to appreciate an individual's distress.

Can one be confident that facial activity represents pain? Several strategies have been used to validate the proposition empirically. As noted, facial

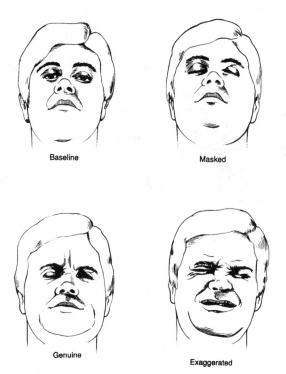

Baseline

Masked

Genuine

Exaggerated

FIGURE 9.2. Facial expressions of a patient with chronic low back pain during (top left) a neutral baseline period prior to onset of motor exercises, (bottom left) straight-leg raising, provoking sharp exacerbation of clinical pain; (top right) repetition of the straight-leg raising, accompanied by instructions to mask the facial display; and (bottom right) repetition of this exercise, along with instructions to exaggerate the response. The video camera was placed above the patient's feet. See Hadjistavropoulos and Craig (1994) for details on the procedure.

activity changes systematically when physical insults known to be painful are applied, and one can readily discriminate between noxious and non-aversive events. Some studies have demonstrated a moderate relationship between facial activity and the intensity of reported painful distress (Craig et al., 1991; Prkachin & Mercer, 1989), but others report nonsignificant associations (LeResche & Dworkin, 1988; Prkachin, 1992a). Prkachin (1992a) concluded that a correlation was not necessarily expected, given that participants were all assessed when their pain was at intolerable levels. It is possible that facial expression might provide the better index of pain experience, given the vulnerability of self-report to bias and situational demand.

A review (Sweet & McGrath, 1998) of the validity of facial measures of infant pain provides

positive correlations of a facial measure of pain with physiological measures ($r = .30$ to .60 in Johnston, Stevens, Yang, & Horton, 1995), cry duration ($r = .44$ in Grunau, Johnston, & Craig, 1990), and adult ratings of discomfort ($r = .65$ in Craig, Grunau, & Aquan-Assee, 1988) and a negative correlation with latency to cry ($r = -.52$ in Grunau & Craig, 1987; $r = -.67$ in Grunau et al., 1990). The facial display diminished when analgesics were applied in randomized controlled trials (Guinsburg, Kopelman, et al., 1998; Taddio, Stevens, et al., 1997) or assessing efficacy of analgesia (Scott et al., 1999), using facial indices of pain as the outcome measure.

Content validity has been observed in studies finding that untrained observers identify the facial display as indicative of pain and are able to discriminate facial displays of pain from aversive, but non-noxious, affective displays (Boucher, 1969). Thus the facial display conveys specific meaning. Judgments of pain severity tend to be correlated with both the severity of the noxious insult applied (Patrick, Craig, & Prkachin, 1986; Prkachin & Mercer, 1989) and the objectively coded vigor of the facial display (Prkachin, Berzins, & Mercer, 1994). LeResche and Dworkin (1988) found that the severity of affective distress during pain, as measured with the McGill Pain Questionnaire, was related to the duration of the pain expression ($r = .69$). LeResche (1982) found that the facial expression of pain shared components with emotional states such as fear, anger, and sadness, but that the overlap with the configuration associated with pain was minimal. LeResche and Dworkin (1988) found no relationship between facial displays of pain and a variety of measures of emotional states the patients were suffering. They concluded that the facial expression of pain taps relatively specific qualities of the pain experience rather than other elements of psychological distress. Thus facial expression displays both sensitivity and specificity as an index of pain.

INDIVIDUAL DIFFERENCES

Although a distinctive pattern of facial activity is observable during pain, there is also substantial variation across situations and individuals. Prkachin (1992a) found significant but modest correlations among facial responses to four types of noxious stimuli (r's ranging from .32 to .39). Interindividual and cross-situational variability appear to be a consequence of the severity and nature of the physical trauma; of psychosocial factors, including cognitive and affective factors, as well as culture-specific social conventions and situational influences; and of long-term personal trait-like dispositions.

Severity and Nature of Physical Distress

The overall magnitude of facial involvement tends to encode pain in a manner graded proportionally to the severity of pain being experienced. Patrick and colleagues (1986) reported moderate correlations between facial activity and the severity of pain provoked by electric shock (multiple mean $r = .43$). The facial display would appear to echo primarily new or renewed pain, in that acute phasic pain and exacerbations of chronic pain are most clearly reflected in the facial display. In a study of facial activity during the persistent pain of the cold pressor test, the facial display was most vigorous at onset, but diminished thereafter, even though pain ratings increased (Craig & Patrick, 1985). In contrast, Feuerstein, Barr, Francoeur, Houle, and Rafman (1982) reported observing an increased incidence of facial grimaces over time in children aged 9 to 14 years during the cold pressor test. It is conceivable that children are more spontaneous in depicting painful experiences in their facial displays. Consistent with the proposition that acute exacerbations in pain are what are reflected in facial activity, Hadjistavropoulos and colleagues (2000) found facial activity to be most vigorous in elderly adults suffering persistent pain when they were engaged in physical activities putting substantial stress on muscles and joints.

Facial actions are differentially sensitive in the extent to which they encode pain severity. Prkachin and Mercer (1989) found cheek raising to have the strongest relationship to subjective pain. Brow lowering, nose wrinkling, lip corner pulling, increasing degrees of mouth opening, and eye closing also correlated with pain in various circumstances, but to varying degrees. Correlations ranged between $r = .44$ and $r = .71$. It is worth emphasizing that the intensity dimension of facial movements is a critical component. In the aforementioned study, in many cases a relationship between pain and facial action was not observed when the actions were coded in a binary format (i.e., present or absent).

It seems probable that all experiences of pain will elicit "primary" facial movements. Prkachin and Mercer (1989) propose brow lowering and eye closing or narrowing as primary movements. Leventhal and Sharp (1965) made the complementary observation that during childbirth heavy knitting and furrowing of the brow were elicited only when distress exceeded a minimum level or threshold. Thereafter, other actions would be recruited, depending upon the specific source of pain and the individual's experience with the condition. Increasing severity and duration of distress would also provoke greater facial involvement. Brow lowering and eye closing would be followed in sequence by the midface actions of upper lip raising, then nose wrinkling. The final phase would include mouth opening, followed, in the extreme, by horizontal stretching of the lips.

LeResche and Dworkin (1988) described the most prominent patterns of facial expression occurring in patients with TMJ disorder who were undergoing painful palpation of the muscles of mastication. The pattern that occurred most frequently during pain consisted of tightening the skin around the eye, lowering the brow, and/or closing the eyes (including blinking). These actions were proposed to be the defining features of pain. A range of lower-face movements also accompanied these actions in the area of the eyes, including raising the upper lip, wrinkling the nose, stretching the lips horizontally, or opening the mouth, but these latter actions were observed to occur no more than 5% of the time. Various facial actions defining specific emotional states (e.g., lip corner pull representing a smile or an expression of happiness) were designated as exclusionary criteria for expressions of pain. Given the complexities of emotional states interacting with pain (Craig, 1999), one could question the assumption that the presence of specific emotional states should preclude the experience of pain.

Cognitive Functioning

The use of facial measures of pain in cognitively impaired people is described by Hadjistavropoulos and colleagues in Chapter 8. Because little is known about the experience of pain in these populations and there is evidence of undermanagement, the development of nonverbal measures and investigation strategies is welcomed.

Affective Correlates

Painful experiences are invariably associated with differing severities and qualities of emotional distress, primarily fear, anxiety, anger, and depression

(Craig, 1999). Patients' faces often disclose forbearance, dismay, panic, anger, or resignation. Again, self-report and nonverbal measures complement each other in providing information about emotional states that accompany the pain experience. Deciphering the range of emotions in facial expressions is made easier by the presence of well-differentiated displays strongly associated with the emotions of sadness, surprise, fear, anger, disgust, contempt, and happiness (Ekman & Friesen, 1986). LeResche and Dworkin (1988) found that patients' emotional reactions during pain were quite variable and included all of disgust, contempt, fear, anger, and sadness. Pain report and pain facial expressions were greater for persons displaying a greater number of different negative affective states. Hale and Hadjistavropoulos (1997) applied the FACS to videotaped facial responses of adults undergoing routine blood tests and found that distinctive emotional displays of disgust, anger, and fear accompanied the pain. Thus attention to emotional correlates of pain can be accomplished through fine-grained analysis of the facial display.

Situational Influences

While less likely to be subjected to voluntary control than self-report, facial displays, along with other nonverbal actions, can be purposefully exaggerated or suppressed on demand by elder children and adults (Craig et al., 1999; Hadjistavropoulos & Craig, 1994, in press). A desire to convince others of the gravity of one's distress or to withhold information that one is in pain often provides a motive for doing so. Differentiated neurophysiological systems for the control of voluntary and involuntary facial muscular systems provide the requisite biological mechanisms (Rinn, 1984). Numerous interventions have a demonstrable immediate impact on the self-report of pain, including hypnosis, instruction in cognitive coping strategies, relaxation training, and social modeling. Limited investigation has been undertaken of the impact of these procedures on nonverbal expression, although tolerance level or willingness to endure painful stimulation tends to covary with self-report.

Exposure to social models who display intolerant or tolerant patterns of response to noxious stimulation has been shown to have an effect on both reports of pain experience and behavior (cf. Craig, 1986). Prkachin, Currie, and Craig (1983) and Prkachin and Craig (1985) demonstrated that exposure to tolerant pain models diminished non-verbal displays of pain, but that the impact appeared minimal relative to the effects of the models on self-report of pain. Patrick and colleagues (1986) found the impact of social models to be substantially greater on self-report than on facial activity. This desynchrony in the impact of a form of situational influence on self-report and facial expression of pain suggests that social influences may be relatively slow to change stylistic patterns of nonverbal pain expression. Nevertheless, socialization in particular familial and cultural contexts may provide the long-term, persistent pressure that can shape both verbal and nonverbal reaction patterns during painful events.

Culture-Specific Differences

Tendencies to be highly reactive or impassive in response to injury are often attributed to a person's ethnic or racial background. However, no studies systematically examining cross-cultural variations in nonverbal displays of pain have been undertaken, despite their potential importance. Evidence for cross-cultural consistency in facial expressions of emotion (Ekman et al., 1987; Russell & Fehr, 1987) suggests that the facial expression of pain should be relatively invariant, although some systematic differences may be expected. Certain "display rules" (Ekman & Friesen, 1969) govern the manner in which emotion will be expressed. For example, people often conform to a social convention that dictates that relatively few emotions should be displayed (Ekman & Friesen, 1969). Socialization within specific familial and cultural contexts is responsible for some cross-cultural variation in the display of emotion (Darwin, 1872/1965; Ekman, Sorensen, & Friesen, 1969), as well as in the display of pain and illness behavior (Craig, 1986; Craig & Patrick, 1985; Craig & Wyckoff, 1987; Sargent, 1984; Weisenberg, 1982).

Personal Dispositions

Some of the variation in the facial display of pain can be attributed to long-term trait-like dispositions that represent the outcome of an interaction between genetic and environmental determinants of personality. Within any distinct ethnic group, some people can be expected to remain nonreactive to pain, whereas others will be highly reactive. Age as a determinant of nonverbal reaction patterns to date has received minimal attention, other than in infants (Johnston, Stevens, Craig, & Grunau, 1993; Lilley, Craig, & Grunau, 1997), although nonverbal pain displays are recognized as crucial to understanding pain in the very young and the very old, given limits in the capacity for verbal communication (see Hadjistavropoulos et al., Chapter 8). Despite evidence of differences between men and women in pain and illness behavior (Feine, Bushnell, Miron, & Duncan, 1991; Unruh, 1996), detailed accounts of behavior during painful events have not been provided. Grunau and Craig (1987) reported that latencies to facial pain activity in neonates were reduced in term-born boys compared to girls, during heel lance for blood collection, but found no differences in amount of facial display between genders. In contrast, Guinsberg and colleagues (2000) recently reported girls showed greater facial display to pain (also to heel lance) in preterm and term-born infants. Craig and colleagues (1991) observed no differences in facial activity in men and women with chronic low back pain when they were reacting to movement-induced exacerbations of their persistent pain. Traditional personality variables have also received limited attention. Prkachin and Mercer (1989) found that intensity and duration of pain-related facial movements were related to the psychological and physical impact of patients' pain problems. Those patients who were more greatly affected by their problems displayed the greater facial activity.

THE FACIAL EXPRESSION OF PAIN IN INFANTS AND YOUNG CHILDREN

Assessing pain in preverbal infants or young children for whom language is unreliable or idiosyncratic is a particular challenge. The younger the child, the greater the dependency of adults on nonverbal assessment. A broad range of cues for pain—including crying (Craig, Gilbert, & Lilley, 2000), facial expression, body movement, and autonomic activity—is usually available for a given child (Pigeon, McGrath, Lawrence, & MacMurray, 1989). However, parents, clinicians, and other concerned observers often find the cues ambiguous, as many of them are not specific to pain and are elicited by diverse need states and events (McGrath, 1996).

A number of investigations have indicated that the most specific behavioral evidence for pain in the infant appears in the facial response to pain

(Craig, 1998; Johnston et al., 1995). Johnston and Strada (1986) reported that the facial response to needle injection pain was more consistent across infants than were cry patterns, heart rate, or body movement. Stevens and Johnston (1991) found that physiological measures of infant response to heel sticks were less satisfactory than facial activity as indicators of pain. Other studies demonstrate that facial activity contributes more to adult judgments of the severity of infant pain than cry and other contextual variables do (Craig et al., 1988; Hadjistavropoulos, Craig, Grunau, & Whitfield, 1994, 1997), although cry is of considerable value in commanding attention to the infant's distress and indicates the severity of distress (Craig et al., 2000; Drummond, Wiebe, & Elliott, 1994).

A specific measure devoted to assessing pain in infants has been developed, based upon facial actions associated with pain in research using the FACS system. The Neonatal Facial Coding System (NFCS) provides an objective, anatomically based, reliable, and detailed approach for studying the infant's facial reaction to painful events (Grunau & Craig, 1987, 1990). In studies using this measure, a relatively stereotyped pattern of facial display has emerged that is consistent through infancy, whether one is characterizing preterm neonates (Craig, Whitfield, Grunau, Linton, & Hadjistavropoulos, 1993) or older infants (Lilley et al., 1997; Oberlander et al., 2000). The facial display comprises lowered brow, eyes squeezed shut, deepened nasolabial furrow (a fold that extends down and out beyond the lip corners), and opened mouth. It is accompanied by a taut cupped tongue in many infants. As well, a protruding tongue appears to indicate states other than pain in term-born infants (Grunau et al., 1990), but it is associated with invasive procedures in preterm infants at 32 weeks gestational age (Grunau, Oberlander, Holsti, & Whitfield, 1998). This description was inclusive of all facial actions displayed by infants experiencing pain (Craig et al., 1994; Lilley et al., 1997) when the faces were also coded with the Baby FACS, the adaptation of the adult FACS system that accommodates anatomical differences between babies and older children or adults (Oster & Rosenstein, 1993). There appears to be greater consistency in the facial expression of infant pain than in adults' facial response. Figure 9.3 illustrates two infants' reactions to heel lancing, and the finding of Grunau and Craig (1987) that the severity of the infants' reaction is related to their asleep–awake behavioral state at the time of the lance. The pattern of the

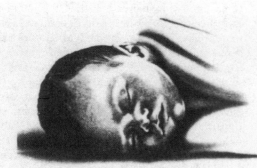
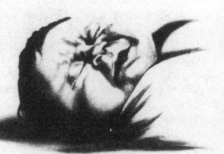

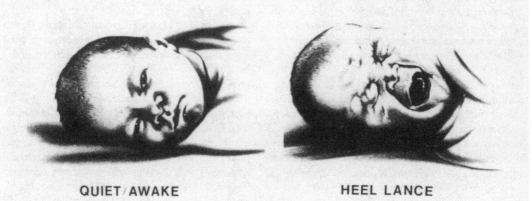

FIGURE 9.3. Infants' facial responses to the heel lance procedure vary with their behavioral state at the time of the lance. Reprinted from *Pain, 28,* R. V. E. Grunau and K. D. Craig, Pain expression in neonates: Facial action and cry, 395–410. Copyright 1987, with permission from Elsevier Science.

display has striking similarities to the facial displays of pain in older children and adults.

The evidence supports the position that newborns have a capacity to experience and communicate pain when subjected to invasive procedures (Anand & Craig, 1996). However, newborns' and infants' experiences of pain are not comparable to those of adults, because they do not have, or are gradually acquiring, older persons' capacity for cognizing the significance of the experience (Craig & Badali, 1999). An infant's experience is dominated by sensory qualities and affective distress, which are perhaps all the more vivid because the adult capacities for anticipating an end or exercising control are not available. Minor facial differences between infant and adult expressions suggest unique features of the infant experience. Most significant is the tendency for young infants to

squeeze their eyes shut, while adults usually keep theirs open but narrowed, only closing them to the most severe pain. Adults are able to use information to terminate or avoid further pain; hence monitoring the situation may be of considerable adaptive value. Because infants do not have this capacity, keeping the eyes shut may have merit in protecting them.

Another prominent age-related variation in facial activity is the correlation between gestational age at birth and the vigor of a neonate's reaction to invasive procedures. Facial reactions become stronger as the infant approaches term (Craig et al., 1993; Johnston et al., 1995; Korol, Goodman, Merchant, & Lawrence, 2000; Scott et al., 1999). The diminished reaction of preterm neonates to invasive procedures may partially account for undermanagement of pain in this population. Shapiro

(1991) found that nurses judged premature neonates to be suffering less than full-term newborns, even though both groups had undergone the same noxious procedure. She concluded, "Lack of recognition of pain in premature neonates may result in unnecessary suffering, increased morbidity and mortality for this vulnerable group" (p. 148).

The lesser reaction of preterm newborns to invasive procedures cannot be interpreted as signifying reduced pain. The work of Fitzgerald and colleagues (Fitzgerald, 1991; Fitzgerald, Millard, & Macintosh, 1989) suggests that "the preterm infant is if anything, supersensitive to painful stimuli when compared with the full term infant" (Fitzgerald & Macintosh, 1989, p. 442). The attenuated reactions of preterms probably reflect limited energy resources available for vigorous and sustained responses. Alternatively, facial neuromuscular systems may not be sufficiently mature to allow these infants to express subjective distress. This cannot be a wholly generalized deficit, because leg withdrawal to stimulation of damaged tissue with von Frey hairs is more vigorous in preterm than in full-term neonates (Fitzgerald & Macintosh, 1989). The deficit would appear to be in the capacity to communicate rather than to experience pain.

Other investigations have demonstrated the sensitivity of infant facial expression during painful events to various interventions. In a number of studies, facial expression has provided an outcome index of pharmacological analgesia, including the impact of EMLA (a topical analgesic) during circumcision (Taddio, Stevens, et al., 1997) and venipuncture (Larsson, Tannfeldt, Lagercrantz, & Olsson, 1998b), fentanyl during mechanical ventilation of preterm infants (Guinsberg et al., 1998), and morphine during invasive procedures (Scott et al., 1999). Nonpharmacological interventions have also been effectively evaluated. A combined auditory and proprioceptive/tactile stimulation procedure was effective in reducing the pain of heel lancing (McCrory, 1990). The food substance, sucrose, and rocking, as a simulation of the vestibular effects of carrying an infant, diminished the facial display of preterm neonates undergoing the routine heelstick procedure (Johnston, Stremler, Stevens, & Horton, 1997). Furthermore, both suckling and sucrose were demonstrably analgesic with newborns when facial expression was used as an index of analgesia (Blass & Watt, 1999). The NFCS is sufficiently sensitive to demonstrate that venipuncture is a more effective and less painful blood-drawing procedure than heel lancing (Larsson, Tannfeldt, Lagercrantz, & Olsson, 1998a). Thus

facial activity provides a useful and valid measure with considerable sensitivity for evaluating a range of pain-reducing procedures for infants.

Perinatal factors, in the form of obstetrical medication and the mode of delivery, were related to the magnitude of the newborn's response to heel lancing (Grunau, Craig, & Drummond, 1989). Facial activity was more vigorous in infants experiencing more stressful deliveries, suggesting the more demanding birth led to greater irritability and a reduced capacity to modulate the response to noxious stimulation.

An enduring impact of early exposure to pain was demonstrated by Taddio, Katz, Ilersich, and Koren (1997). They found that healthy 4- to 6-month-old boys who had been circumcised as neonates displayed a greater facial response, cried longer, and were judged as experiencing more pain to vaccination injections than noncircumcised boys. As well, if premedication with the topical anesthetic EMLA had been done prior to the circumcision, there was a trend for the EMLA-treated infants to have an intermediate pain response across all three measures of pain. There thus appeared to be a long-lasting effect of neonatal pain on subsequent infant pain behavior instigated by alterations in the infants' central neural processing of painful stimuli, with an analgesic capable of diminishing this sensitization to pain. The facial responses of preterm infants to invasive procedures has also been shown to be contingent upon the number of prior invasive procedures to which they had been exposed, suggesting acquired insensitivity to pain (Grunau et al., 2001; Johnston & Stevens, 1996).

Barr, Rotman, Yaremko, Ledur, and Francoeur (1991) have elucidated characteristics of infant colic, demonstrating that infants who satisfied criteria for particularly severe and prolonged bouts of crying and fussing displayed a greater incidence of the facial actions associated with pain before they were fed. A study of the impact of the social context on infant pain behavior (Sweet & McGrath, 1998) demonstrated that mothers engaged in behavior (e.g., reassurance) that, perhaps counterintuitively, enhanced their infants' distress during a painful procedure, and that staff members could decrease the pain behavior by using coping-promoting interactions (e.g., distraction). The impact of social factors appears evident very early in life. Rosmus, Johnston, Chan-Yip, and Yang (in press) reported that Canadian-born Chinese babies, relative to Canadian infants of European descent, displayed greater facial response to routine immunization injections at 2 months of age. Thus a systematic measure of facial activity appears capable of isolating a variety of subtle variations in factors influencing infant procedural pain.

Because the facial displays of toddlers and preschool children during pain have received minimal attention, and there are changes in facial anatomy during the transition from infancy to the toddler years (Oster & Rosenstein, 1993), the NFCS was modified to study this age range. The Child Facial Coding System (CFCS; Chambers, Cassidy, McGrath, Gilbert, & Craig, 1996) was developed to focus on discrete facial actions that account for both gross and subtle movements observed in preschoolers' facial displays of pain. Studies have disclosed that a constellation of actions similar to those observed in neonates and infants occurs consistently during invasive events (e.g., immunization injections, venipuncture, and finger lance; Cassidy et al., 1996; Chambers et al., 1996). Gilbert and colleagues (2000) found that persistent pain during initial postoperative recovery in the postanesthetic recovery unit comprised covarying patterns of brow lowering, deepening of the nasolabial furrow, cheek raising, open mouth, pulling upward of the lip corners, and stretching of the mouth in horizontal and vertical directions. It was noted that there were individual differences in expression and that simultaneous display of all these actions was unusual. The variability in any child's display appears to reflect variations in pain severity. One would not expect a continuous display of pain; vigorous activity is best seen as indicative of exacerbations of discomfort (cf. Hadjistavropoulos et al., 2000). In this sense, the facial display is like self-report. One would not expect either vocalizations or nonverbal behavior to be continuously displayed.

Facial activity has been incorporated as a primary or major component of other scales. The Premature Infant Pain Profile (PIPP; Stevens, Johnston, Petryshen, & Taddio, 1996) is a composite measure, including facial actions (brow bulge, eye squeeze, and nasolabial furrow) and physiological activity (heart rate and blood oxygen saturation), qualified by the gestational age of the infant. The PIPP has been examined for content and discriminant validity, interrater reliability, and internal consistency.

Other coding systems requiring more global judgments of an infant's face also have been productive in understanding emotion and pain. Izard's (1979) Maximally Discriminative Facial Movement Coding System (MAX) requires coders to scan three regions of the face (brow, eyes, and mouth) for particular combinations of activity representing discrete emotional expressions of anger, fear, surprise, and joy, as well as pain. Several studies (Izard, Hembree, Dougherty, & Spizirri, 1983; Izard, Huebner, Risser, McGinness, & Dougherty, 1980) reported that during infancy the early pattern of facial response to immunization injections predominantly suggests pain, but that around 6 to 8 months the pattern becomes one of anticipatory fear prior to the injection, pain following the needle stick, and anger thereafter. The pain response decreases with age, whereas the anger response increases, and the latter is the dominant pattern by 19 months. The anger response is differentiated from the pain response primarily because a child's eyes are open and staring in anger. Individual differences have also been observed, with infants who are slow to be soothed showing significantly more anger, while those who are soothed more readily show less physical distress (Izard, Hembree, & Huebner, 1987). Interesting findings using the MAX also indicate that the capacity to self-regulate negative affect during pain is related to attentional control (Axia, Bonichini, & Benini, 1999). Thus studies of facial activity contribute to a better understanding of infant development.

A COMMUNICATION MODEL OF HUMAN PAIN

The foregoing discussion has emphasized how the subjective experience of pain is encoded in facial expression and how measures of facial activity permit accurate inferences about the subjective state of pain. From a broader communications perspective (Craig, Lilley, & Gilbert, 1996; Prkachin & Craig, 1995), one must understand not only how pain experience becomes manifested in behavior, but also how others attend to, interpret, and respond to specific cues or the configuration of distress presented by the person in pain. Differences are often observed between objective features of the expression of pain and that which is salient and meaningful to the observer.

The specific facial cues attended to by judges when identifying pain have been identified in several studies of adults and children. Brow lowering, eye blinking and narrowing, cheek raising, and upper-lip raising predicted 55% of the variance in ratings of adult pain (mean multiple $r = .74$) (Patrick et al., 1986). Prominent predictor variables for children tended to be taut tongue, open lips, latency to facial activity, vertically stretched mouth, and deepened nasolabial furrow (Craig et al., 1988). These accounted for 43% of adult ratings of affective discomfort displayed by the children. Thus there is agreement in the pain cues that are salient to adult judges. However, the unaccounted-for variance indicates that other factors contribute to the judgments.

Moreover, there is evidence that naïve judges make less than optimal use of the information available in facial expressions when drawing inferences about the pain of others. Prkachin and colleagues (1994) found that although measures of facial activity were significantly and consistently related to patients' reports of pain across a series of tests, observers' ratings were less consistently so. Indeed, on tests that produced relatively low levels of pain, measurements of facial behavior were highly related to pain report, although untrained observers were not able to rate patients' pain reliably at all. These findings imply that it is necessary to receive some systematic training in order to decode pain expressions effectively.

Some evidence exists confirming that decisions about pain reflect more than the objectively identified evidence for pain. Hadjistavropoulos, Ross, and von Baeyer (1990) observed that the physical attractiveness of persons in pain heavily influenced physicians' judgments about the severity of pain expressed in facial displays and biased the judges toward being prepared to provide more care to the less attractive people.

The potential for the individual consciously controlling both verbal and nonverbal behavior to misrepresent more pain or less pain also often concerns observers (Craig et al., 1999). It is possible to manipulate others' impressions by purposefully controlling displays. Certain features are seen as trustworthy and others less so. In terms of facial activity, judges attach primary importance to the upper face and eyes (Lee & Craig, 1991). The observation is consistent with our understanding of the neurophysiological systems that regulate facial activity. The neuromuscular systems for deliberate and spontaneous facial activity differ (Rinn, 1984), with the upper face less amenable to voluntary control. Just as there are differences between felt and false smiles (Ekman, Friesen, & O'Sullivan, 1988) and startle (Ekman, Friesen, & Simons, 1985), genuine and faked pain can be discriminated (Hadjistavropoulos & Craig, 1994; Hadjistavropoulos, Craig, Hadjistavropoulos, & Poole, 1996; Prkachin, 1992b).

Differences between spontaneous and faked facial expressions of pain have been identified in

volunteers, both patients with chronic pain and healthy students. People engaged in faking primarily display the same facial actions, but the display tends to be more severe or intense, and subtle topographic and temporal variations can also be observed (Craig et al., 1991; Hadjistavropoulos & Craig, 1994; Prkachin, 1992a). Patients trying to withhold evidence of pain tend to "leak" signs of distress in the region of the eyes, with cheeks raised, eyes narrowed, and blinks appearing less frequently. The differences are inconspicuous, so it is not surprising that people can be readily fooled into believing another is experiencing genuine pain or not experiencing pain (Hadjistavropoulos et al., 1996; Poole & Craig, 1992).

Figure 9.2, as noted earlier, provides an artist's drawing of the facial behavior of a patient suppressing a pain reaction and exaggerating a pain reaction. In the masked expression, the eyes are closed, and although there is some tension in the lids, there is no marked squeezing or tightening. In the exaggerated expression, the inner and central portion of the brow is lowered, pushing down and reducing visibility of the medial portion of the eyelid; there are marked wrinkles and muscle bulges between the eyebrows; the central portion of the brow and the skin above the brow are pulled together; there are marked crows' feet; the infraorbital triangle (cheek area) is raised, producing bags and wrinkles under the eyes; the nose is wrinkled; the eyes are squeezed shut; there is elongation of the mouth, along with a slight flattening of skin beyond the lip corners; and the lips are parted.

MEASURES OF FACIAL ACTIVITY AS DIAGNOSTIC TOOLS

The focus of the majority of studies using fine-grained methods for capturing the facial display of pain has been on the development of a better understanding. This evidence that facial activity provides for relatively sensitive and specific measurement of pain has led to development of clinical applications. Reflecting the tremendous demands on clinicians, attention to facial displays is usually limited to global judgments of a "facial grimace." When behavioral descriptions of the grimace are provided, they tend to be at variance with what systematic studies have revealed about facial expressions that encode pain (Craig, 1992). The FACS system, described above, is clearly too labor-intensive and complex for clinical application and for many research applications. In consequence, abbreviated methods have been developed that focus upon specific facial actions associated with pain (e.g., the NFCS–Grunau & Craig, 1990; Grunau et al., 1998; the CFCS–Chambers et al., 1996; the PIPP–Stevens et al., 1996). Grunau and colleagues (1998) and Guinsburg and colleagues (1997) demonstrated that the NFCS can be reliably carried out in real time at bedside. Prkachin (1992a) has provided some general proposals for the development of abbreviated pain-coding systems. Alternative proposals using computer vision to develop an automated method of facial display analysis have also been proposed (Cohn et al., 1999). Solomon, Prkachin, and Farewell (1997) have described the development of a program for training people to be able to detect the four facial actions that have been most reliably associated with pain. The program involves descriptions of the key features of each movement, and exposure to simple and then complex examples of the movements in slide and video formats. Exposure of physiotherapy and occupational therapy students to this training program resulted in improved estimations of patients' pain (as evaluated by the difference between the participants' and the patients' pain ratings), compared to the estimations of untrained participants. This provides evidence for the clinical applicability of facial measurement; however, more research is needed to optimize observers' sensitivity.

ACKNOWLEDGMENT

Preparation of this chapter was supported in part by research grants from the Social Sciences and Humanities Research Council of Canada to Kenneth D. Craig.

REFERENCES

Adelmann, P. K., & Zajonc, R. B. (1989). Facial efference and the experience of emotion. *Annual Review of Psychology, 40,* 249–280.

Anand, K. J. S., & Craig, K. D. (1996). New perspectives on the definition of pain [Editorial]. *Pain, 67,* 3–6.

Axia, G., Bonichini, S., & Benini, F. (1999). Attention and reaction to distress in infancy: A longitudinal study. *Developmental Psychology, 35,* 500–504.

Barr, R. G., Rotman, A., Yaremko, S., Ledur, D., & Francoeur, T. E. (1991). The crying of infants with colic. *Pediatrics, 90,* 14–21.

Blass, E. M., & Watt, L. (1999). Suckling and sucrose-induced analgesia in human newborns. *Pain, 83,* 611–623.

Boucher, J. D. (1969). Facial displays of fear, sadness and pain. *Perceptual and Motor Skills, 28,* 239–242.

Camras, L. A., Malatesta, C., & Izard, C. E. (1991). The development of facial expressions in infancy. In R. Feldman & B. Rime (Eds.), *Fundamentals of nonverbal behavior* (pp. 73–105). Cambridge, England: Cambridge University Press.

Cassidy, K. L., McGrath, P. J., Reid, G. J., Chambers, C. T., Gilbert, C. A., Finley, G. A., Brown, T. L., Smith, D. L., Szudek, E., Morley, C., & Morton, B. (1996). *Watch needle watch TV: Audiovisual distraction in preschool immunization.* Poster presented at the 8th World Congress on Pain, Vancouver, British Columbia, Canada.

Chambers, C. T., Cassidy, K. L., McGrath, P. J., Gilbert, C. A., & Craig, K. D. (1996). *Child Facial Coding System: A manual.* Halifax, Nova Scotia, Canada/Vancouver, British Columbia, Canada. Dalhousie University/University of British Columbia.

Cohn, J. F., Zlochower, A. J., Lien, J., & Kanade, T. (1999). Automated face analysis by feature point tracking has high concurrent validity with manual FACS coding. *Psychophysiology, 36,* 35–43.

Colby, C., Lanzetta, J., & Kleck, R. (1977). Effects of the expression of pain on autonomic and pain tolerance responses to subject-controlled pain. *Psychophysiology, 14,* 537–540.

Collier, G. (1985). *Emotional expression.* Hillsdale, NJ: Erlbaum.

Craig, K. D. (1986). Social modeling influences: Pain in context. In R.A. Sternbach (Ed.), *The psychology of pain* (2nd ed., pp. 67–96). New York: Raven Press.

Craig, K. D. (1987). Consequences of caring: Pain in the human context. *Canadian Psychology, 28,* 311–321.

Craig, K. D. (1992). The facial expression of pain: Better than a thousand words? *American Pain Society Journal, 1,* 153–162.

Craig, K. D. (1998). The facial display of pain. In G. A. Finley & P. J. McGrath (Eds.), *Measurement of pain in infants and children* (pp. 103–121). Seattle, WA: International Association for the Study of Pain Press.

Craig, K. D. (1999). Emotions and psychobiology. In P. D. Wall & R. Melzack (Eds.), *Textbook of pain* (4th ed., pp. 293–309). Edinburgh: Churchill Livingstone.

Craig, K. D., & Badali, M. A. (1999). On knowing an infant's pain. *Pain Forum, 8,* 74–77.

Craig, K. D., Gilbert, C. A., & Lilley, C. M. (2000). Cry as an indicator of pain in infants. In R. G. Barr, B. Hopkins, & J. Green (Eds.), *Crying as a signal, a sign, and a symptom* (pp. 23–40). London: Mac Keith Press.

Craig, K. D., Grunau, R. V. E., & Aquan-Assee, J. (1988). Judgment of pain in newborns: Facial activity and cry as determinants. *Canadian Journal of Behavioural Science, 20,* 442–451.

Craig, K. D., Hadjistavropoulos, H. D., Grunau, R.V.E., & Whitfield, M. F. (1994). A comparison of two measures of facial activity during pain in the newborn child. *Journal of Pediatric Psychology, 19,* 305–318.

Craig, K. D., Hill, M. L., & McMurtry, B. (1999). Detecting deception and malingering. In A.R. Block, E. F. Kramer, & E. Fernandez (Eds.), *Handbook of chronic pain syndromes: Biopsychosocial perspectives* (pp. 41–58). Mahwah, NJ: Erlbaum.

Craig, K. D., Hyde, S. A., & Patrick, C. J. (1991). Genuine, suppressed, and faked facial behavior during exacerbation of chronic low back pain. *Pain, 46,* 161–172.

Craig, K. D., Lilley, C. M., & Gilbert, C. A. (1996). Social barriers to optimal pain management in infants and children. *Clinical Journal of Pain, 17,* 247–259.

Craig, K. D., McMahon, R. J., Morison, J. D., & Zaskow, C. (1984). Developmental changes in infant pain expression during immunization injections. *Social Science and Medicine, 19,* 1331–1332.

Craig, K. D., & Patrick, C. J. (1985). Facial expression during induced pain. *Journal of Personality and Social Psychology, 44,* 1080–1091.

Craig, K. D., & Prkachin, K. M. (1980). Social influences on public and private components of pain. In I. G. Sarason & C. Spielberger (Eds.), *Stress and anxiety* (Vol. 7, pp. 57–72). New York: Hemisphere.

Craig, K. D., Whitfield, M. F., Grunau, R. V. E., Linton, J., & Hadjistavropoulos, H. D. (1993). Pain in the preterm neonate: Behavioral and physiological indices. *Pain, 52,* 287–299.

Craig, K. D., & Wyckoff, M. (1987). Cultural factors in chronic pain management. In G. D. Burrows, D. Elton, & G. Stanley (Eds.), *Handbook of chronic pain management* (pp. 99–108). Amsterdam: Elsevier.

Custrini, R. J., & Feldman, R. (1989). Children's social competence and nonverbal encoding and decoding of emotions. *Journal of Clinical Child Psychology, 18,* 336–342.

Dalton, J. A., Brown, L., Carlson, J., McNutt, R., & Greer, S. M. (1999). An evaluation of facial expression displayed by patients with chest pain. *Heart and Lung, 28,* 168–174.

Darwin, C. R. (1965). *The expression of emotions in man and animals.* Chicago: University of Chicago Press. (Original work published 1872)

De Paulo, B. M., Rosenthal, R., Eisenstat, R. A., Rogers, P. L., & Finkelstein, S. (1978). Decoding discrepant nonverbal cues. *Journal of Personality and Social Psychology, 36,* 313–323.

Drummond, J. E., Wiebe, C. F., & Elliott, M. R. (1994). Maternal understanding of infant crying: What does a negative case tell us? *Qualitative Health Research, 4,* 208–223.

Ekman, P. (1993). Facial expression and emotion. *American Psychologist, 48,* 384–392.

Ekman, P., & Friesen, W. V. (1969). The repertoire of nonverbal behavior: Categories, origins, usage and coding. *Semiotica, 1,* 49–98.

Ekman, P., & Friesen, W. V. (1978). *Facial Action Coding System: A technique for the measurement of facial movement.* Palo Alto, CA: Consulting Psychologists Press.

Ekman, P., & Friesen, W. V. (1986). A new pan-cultural facial expression of emotion. *Motivation and Emotion, 10,* 159–168.

Ekman, P., Friesen, W. V., & O'Sullivan, M. (1988). Smiles when lying. *Journal of Personality and Social Psychology, 54,* 414–420.

Ekman, P., Friesen, W. V., O'Sullivan, M., Chan, A., Diacoyanni-Tarlatzis, I., Heider, K., Krause, R., LeCompte, W. A., Pitcairn, R., Ricci-Bitti, P. E., Scherer, K., Tornita, M., & Tzavaras, A. (1987). Universals and cultural differences in the judgments of facial expression of emotion. *Journal of Personality and Social Psychology, 53,* 712–717.

Ekman, P., Friesen, W. V., & Simons, R. (1985). Is the startle reaction an emotion? *Journal of Personality and Social Psychology, 49,* 1416–1426.

Ekman, P., & Rosenberg, E. L. (Eds.). (1997). *What the face reveals: Basic and applied studies of spontaneous expression using the Facial Action Coding System (FACS).* New York: Oxford University Press.

Ekman, P., Sorensen, E. R., & Friesen, W. V. (1969). Pan cultural elements in facial displays of emotion. *Science, 164,* 86–88.

Feine, J. S., Bushnell, M. C., Miron, D., & Duncan, G. H. (1991). Sex differences in the perception of noxious heat stimuli. *Pain, 44,* 255–262.

Feuerstein, M., Barr, R. G., Francoeur, T. E., Houle, M., & Rafman, S. (1982). Potential biobehavioral mechanisms of recurrent abdominal pain in children. *Pain, 13,* 287–298.

Fitzgerald, M. (1991). Development of pain mechanisms. *British Medical Bulletin, 47,* 667–675.

Fitzgerald, M., & Macintosh, N. (1989). Pain and analgesia in the newborn. *Archives of Disease in Childhood, 64,* 441–443.

Fitzgerald, M., Millard, C., & Macintosh, N. (1989). Cutaneous hypersensitivity following peripheral tissue damage in newborn infants and its reversal with topical anaesthesia. *Pain, 39,* 31–36.

Fridlund, A. J. (1991). Evolution and facial action in reflex, social motive, and paralanguage. *Biological Psychology, 32,* 3–100.

Fridlund, A. J. (1994). *Human facial expression: An evolutionary view.* San Diego, CA: Academic Press.

Gilbert, C. A., Lilley, C. M., Craig, K. D., McGrath, P. J., Court, C., Bennett, S. M., & Montgomery, C. (2000). Postoperative pain expression in preschool children: Validation of the Child Facial Coding System. *Clinical Journal of Pain, 15,* 192–200.

Grunau, R. V. E., & Craig, K. D. (1987). Pain expression in neonates: Facial action and cry. *Pain, 28,* 395–410.

Grunau, R. V. E., & Craig, K. D. (1990). Facial activity as a measure of neonatal pain expression. In D. C. Tyler & E. J. Krane (Eds.), *Advances in pain research and therapy* (Vol. 15 pp. 147–155). New York: Raven Press.

Grunau, R. V. E., Craig, K. D., & Drummond, J. E. (1989). Neonatal pain behavior and perinatal events: Implications for research observations. *Canadian Journal of Nursing Research, 21,* 7–17.

Grunau, R. V. E., Johnston, C. C., & Craig, K. D. (1990). Neonatal facial and cry responses to invasive and noninvasive procedures. *Pain, 42,* 295–305.

Grunau, R. E., Oberlander, T., Holsti, L., & Whitfield, M. F. (1998). Bedside application of the Neonatal Facial Coding System in pain assessment of premature neonates. *Pain, 76,* 277–286.

Grunau, R. E., Oberlander, T. F., Whitfield, M. F., Fitzgerald, C., & Lee, S. K. (2001). Demographic and therapeutic determinants of pain reactivity in very low birth weight neonates at 32 weeks' postconceptional age. *Pediatrics, 107,* 105–112.

Guinsburg, R., Berenguel, R. C., de Cassia Xavier, R., de Almeida, M. F. B., & Kopelman, B. I. (1997). Are behavioral scales suitable for preterm and term neonatal pain assessment? In T. S. Jensen, J. A. Turner, & Z. Wiesenfeld-Hallin (Eds.), *Proceedings of the 8th World Congress on Pain: Progress in pain research and management* (Vol. 8, pp. 893–902). Seattle, WA: International Association for the Study of Pain Press.

Guinsburg, R., Kopelman, B. I., Anand, K. J. S., de Almeida, M. F. B., Peres, C. A., & Miyoshi, M. H. (1998). Physiological, hormonal, and behavioral responses to a single fentynal does in intubated and ventilated preterm neonates. *Journal of Pediatrics, 132,* 954–959.

Guinsburg, R., Peres, C., Branco de Almeida, M. F., Balda, R., Berenguel, R. C., Tonelotto, J., & Kopelman, B. I. (2000). Differences in pain expression between male and female newborn infants. *Pain, 85,* 127–133.

Hadjistavropoulos, H. D., & Craig, K. D. (1994). Acute and chronic low back pain: Cognitive, affective and behavioral dimensions. *Journal of Consulting and Clinical Psychology, 62,* 341–349.

Hadjistavropoulos, T., & Craig, K. D. (in press). A theoretical framework for understanding self-report and observational measures of pain: A communications model. *Behaviour Research and Therapy.*

Hadjistavropoulos, H. D., Craig, K. D., Grunau, R. V. E., & Whitfield, M. F. (1994). Judging pain in newborns: Facial and cry determinants. *Journal of Pediatric Psychology, 19,* 485–491.

Hadjistavropoulos, H. D., Craig, K. D., Grunau, R. V. E, & Whitfield, M. F. (1997). Judging pain in infants: Behavioral, contextual, and developmental determinants. *Pain, 73,* 319–324.

Hadjistavropoulos, H. D., Craig, K. D., & Hadjistavropoulos, T. (1998). Cognitive and behavioural responses to illness information: The role of health anxiety. *Behaviour Research and Therapy, 36,* 149–164.

Hadjistavropoulos, H. D., Craig, K. D., Hadjistavropoulos, T., & Poole, G. D. (1996). Subjective judgments of deception in pain expression: Accuracy and errors. *Pain, 65,* 247–254.

Hadjistavropoulos, H. D., Ross, M. A., & von Baeyer, C. (1990). Are physicians' ratings of pain affected by patients' physical attractiveness? *Social Science and Medicine, 31,* 69–72.

Hadjistavropoulos, T., LaChapelle, D., MacLeod, F., Hale, C., O'Rourke, N., & Craig, K. D. (1998). Cognitive functioning and pain reactions in hospitalized elders. *Pain Research and Management, 3,* 145–151.

Hadjistavropoulos, T., LaChapelle, D. L., MacLeod, F. K., Snider, B., & Craig, K. D. (2000). Measuring movement exacerbated pain in cognitively impaired frail elders. *Clinical Journal of Pain, 16,* 54–63.

Hale, C., & Hadjistavropoulos, T. (1997). Emotional components of pain. *Pain Research and Management, 2,* 217–225.

Huebner, R. R., & Izard, C. E. (1988). Mothers' responses to infants' facial expressions of sadness, anger, and physical distress. *Motivation and Emotion, 12,* 185–197.

Iezzi, A., Adams, H. E., Bugg, F., & Stokes, G. S (1991). Facial expressions of pain in muscle-contraction headache patients. *Journal of Psychopathology and Behavioral Assessment, 13,* 269–283.

Izard, C. E. (1979). *The Maximally Discriminative Facial Movement Coding System* (MAX). Newark: University of Delaware Instructional Resources Center.

Izard, C. E., Hembree, E. A., Dougherty, L. M., & Spizirri, C. C. (1983). Changes in facial expressions of 2 to 19-month-old infants following acute pain. *Developmental Psychology, 19,* 418–426.

Izard, C. E., Hembree, E.A., & Huebner, R.R. (1987). Infants' emotion expressions to acute pain: Developmental changes and stability of individual differences. *Developmental Psychology, 23,* 105–113.

Izard, C. E., Huebner, R. R., Risser, D., McGinness, G. C., & Dougherty, L. M. (1980). The young infant's ability to produce discrete emotion expressions. *Developmental Psychology, 16,* 132–140.

Jacox, A. K. (1980). The assessment of pain. In W. L. Smith, H. Merskey, & S. C. Gross (Eds.), *Pain: Meaning and management* (pp. 75–88). New York: SP Medical & Scientific Books.

Johnston, C. C., & Stevens, B. J. (1996). Experience in a neonatal intensive care unit affects pain response. *Pediatrics, 98,* 925–930.

Johnston, C. C., Stevens, B. J., Craig, K. D., & Grunau, R. V. E. (1993). Developmental changes in pain expression in premature, fullterm, two, and four month old infants. *Pain, 52,* 201–208.

Johnston, C. C., Stevens, B. J., Yang, F., & Horton, L. (1995). Differential response to pain by very premature neonates. *Pain, 61,* 471–479.

Johnston, C. C., & Strada, M. E. (1986). Acute pain response in infants: A multidimensional description. *Pain, 24,* 373–382.

Johnston, C. C., Stremler, R. L., Stevens, B. J., & Horton, L. J. (1997). Effectiveness of oral sucrose and simulated rocking on pain response in preterm neonates. *Pain, 72,* 193–199.

Korol, C. T., Goodman, J. T., Merchant, P., & Lawrence, J. (2000). *Contextual influences on the facial expression of pain in the neonatal intensive care unit.* Manuscript submitted for publication.

Kraut, R. E. (1978). Verbal and nonverbal cues in the perception of lying. *Journal of Personality and Social Psychology, 36,* 380–391.

Lanzetta, J. T., Cartwright-Smith, J., & Kleck, R. E. (1976). Effects of nonverbal dissimulation on emotional experience and autonomic arousal. *Journal of Personality and Social Psychology, 33,* 354–370.

Larsson, B. A., Tannfeldt, G., Lagercrantz, H., & Olsson, G. L. (1998a). Venipuncture is more effective and less painful than heel lancing for blood tests in neonates. *Pediatrics, 101,* 882–886.

Larsson, B. A., Tannfeldt, G., Lagercrantz, H., & Olsson, G. L. (1998b). Alleviation of the pain of venipuncture in neonates. *Acta Pediatrica, 87,* 774–779.

Lee, D. E., & Craig, K. D. (1991). *Facial action determinants of observer judgment of subjective states: Complexity and configuration.* Unpublished manuscript.

LeResche, L. (1982). Facial expression in pain: A study of candid photographs. *Journal of Nonverbal Behavior, 7,* 46–56.

LeResche, L., & Dworkin, S. F. (1984). Facial expression accompanying pain. *Social Science and Medicine, 19,* 1325–1330.

LeResche, L, & Dworkin, S. F. (1988). Facial expressions of pain and emotions in chronic TMD patients. *Pain, 35,* 71–78.

Leventhal, H., & Sharp, E. (1965). Facial expressions as indicators of distress. In S.S. Tomkins & C. E. Izard (Eds.), *Affect, cognition and personality* (pp. 296–318). New York: Springer.

Lilley, C. M., Craig, K. D., & Grunau, R. E. (1997). The expression of pain in infants and toddlers: Developmental changes in facial action. *Pain, 72,* 161–170.

McCrory, L. (1990). *The use of continuous sensory stimulation: Proprioceptive–tactile and auditory stimulation to reduce newborns' response to pain.* Unpublished master's thesis, University of Florida.

McGrath, P. J. (1996). There is more to pain measurement in children than "ouch." *Canadian Psychology, 37,* 63–75.

Oberlander, T. F., Grunau, R. E., Whitfield, M. F., Fitzgerald, C., Pitfield, S., & Saul, J. P. (2000). Biobehavioral pain responses in former extremely low birth weight infants at four months' corrected age. *Pediatrics, 105,* 6.

Oster, H., Hegley, D., & Nagel, L. (1992). Adult judgments and fine-grained analysis of infant facial expressions: Testing the validity of a priori coding formulas. *Developmental Psychology, 28,* 1115–1131.

Oster, H., & Rosenstein, D. (1993). *Baby FACS: Analyzing facial movement in infants.* Unpublished manuscript, New York University.

Patrick, C. J., Craig, K. D., & Prkachin, K. M. (1986). Observer judgments of acute pain: Facial action determinants. *Journal of Personality and Social Psychology, 50,* 1291–1298.

Pigeon, H. M., McGrath, P. J., Lawrence, J., & MacMurray, S. B. (1989). Nurses' perceptions of pain in the neonatal intensive care unit. *Journal of Pain and Symptom Management, 4,* 179–183.

Poole, G. D., & Craig, K. D. (1992). Judgments of genuine, expressed, and faked facial expressions of pain. *Journal of Personality and Social Psychology, 63,* 797–805.

Prkachin, K. M. (1992a). The consistency of facial expressions of pain: A comparison across modalities. *Pain, 51,* 297–306.

Prkachin, K. M. (1992b). Dissociating spontaneous and deliberate expressions of pain: Signal detection analyses. *Pain, 51,* 57–65.

Prkachin, K. M., Berzins, S., & Mercer, S. R. (1994). Encoding and decoding of pain expressions: A judgement study. *Pain, 58,* 253–259.

Prkachin, K. M., & Craig, K. D. (1985). Influencing nonverbal expressions of pain: Signal detection analyses. *Pain, 21,* 399–409.

Prkachin, K. M., & Craig, K. D. (1995). Expressing pain: The communication and interpretation of facial pain signals. *Journal of Nonverbal Behavior, 19,* 191–205.

Prkachin, K. M., Currie, A. N., & Craig, K. D. (1983). Judging nonverbal expression of pain. *Canadian Journal of Behavioural Science, 15,* 408–420.

Prkachin, K. M., & Mercer, S. R. (1989). Pain expression in patients with shoulder pathology: Validity, properties and relationship to sickness impact. *Pain, 39,* 257–265.

Reilly, J. S., & Bellugi, U. (1996). Competition on the face: Affect and language in ASL motherese. *Journal of Child Language, 23,* 219–239.

Rinn, W. E. (1984). The neuropsychology of facial expression: A review of the neurological and psychological mechanisms for producing facial expressions. *Psychological Bulletin, 95,* 52–77.

Rosmus, C., Johnston, C. C., Chan-Yip, A., & Yang, F. (2000). Response to pain by Chinese infants. *Social Science and Medicine, 51,* 175–184.

Russell, J. A. (1994). Is there universal recognition of emotion from facial expression? *Psychological Bulletin, 115,* 102–141.

Russell, J. A., & Fehr, B. (1987). Relativity in the perception of emotion in facial expressions. *Journal of Experimental Psychology: General, 116,* 233–237.

Russell, J. A., & Fernandez-Dols, J.-M. (Eds.). (1997). *The psychology of facial expression.* New York: Cambridge University Press.

Sargent, C. (1984). Between death and shame: Dimensions of pain in Bariba culture. *Social Science and Medicine, 19,* 1299–1304.

Scott, C. S., Riggs, K. W., Ling, E. W., Fitzgerald, C. F., Hill, M. L., Grunau, R. V. E., Solimano, A., & Craig, K. D. (1999). Morphine pharmacokinetics and pain assessment in premature newborns. *Journal of Pediatrics, 135,* 423–429.

Shapiro, C. R. (1991). Nurses judgments of pain intensity in term and preterm newborns [Abstract]. *Journal of Pain and Symptom Management, 6,* 148.

Solomon, P. E., Prkachin, K. M., & Farewell, V. (1997). Enhancing sensitivity to facial expression of pain. *Pain, 71,* 297–306.

Stevens, B., & Johnston, C. C. (1991). Premature infant responses to heelstick [Abstract]. *Journal of Pain and Symptom Management, 6,* 206.

Stevens, B., Johnston, C., Petrysen, P., & Taddio, A. (1996). Premature infant pain profile: Development and initial validation. *Clinical Journal of Pain, 12,* 13–22.

Sweet, S. D., & McGrath, P. J. (1998). Relative importance of mothers' versus medical staff's behavior in the prediction of infant immunization pain behavior. *Journal of Pediatric Psychology, 23,* 249–256.

Taddio, A., Katz, J., Ilershich, A. L., & Koren, G. (1997). Effect of neonatal circumcision on pain response during subsequent routine vaccination. *Lancet, 349,* 599–603.

Taddio, A., Stevens, B., Craig, K. D., Rastogi, P., Ben David, S., Hennan, A., Mulligan, P., & Koren, G. (1997). Efficacy and safety of lidocaine-prilocaine cream for pain during circumcision. *New England Journal of Medicine, 336,* 1197–1201.

Unruh, A. M. (1996). Gender variations in clinical pain experience. *Pain, 65,* 123–167.

von Baeyer, C. L., Johnson, M. E., & McMillan, M. J. (1984). Consequences of nonverbal expression of pain: Patient distress and observer concern. *Social Science and Medicine, 19,* 1319–1324.

Weisenberg, M. (1982). Cultural and ethnic factors in reaction to pain. In I. Al-Issa (Ed.), *Culture and psychopathology* (pp. 187–198). Baltimore: University Park Press.

Wilkie, D. J. (1995). Facial expressions of pain in lung cancer. *Analgesia, 1,* 91–99.

Chapter 10

Assessment of Pain Behaviors

FRANCIS J. KEEFE
DAVID A. WILLIAMS
SUZANNE J. SMITH

Although pain is a personal and subjective experience, the fact that someone is experiencing pain is often apparent to others. People who have pain may vocalize their distress by moaning, crying, or complaining, or may exhibit pain-related body postures or facial expressions. These verbal and nonverbal behaviors have been called *pain behaviors* because they serve to communicate the fact that pain is being experienced (Fordyce, 1976). The construct of pain behaviors has emerged as a key component of behavioral formulations of chronic pain (Keefe & Gil, 1986). These formulations emphasize the role that social learning influences can play in the development and maintenance of pain behaviors (Fordyce, 1976; Keefe & Gil, 1986; Turk, Meichenbaum, & Genest, 1983). A patient who has had a low back injury, for example, may exhibit pain behavior long after the normal healing time if his or her spouse or partner responds to pain behavior in an overly solicitous fashion.

The concept of pain behavior is particularly salient in the evaluation of patients with chronic pain who are seen in pain clinics and pain management programs (Keefe, 1989). Many of these patients exhibit a maladaptive pattern of pain behavior that is characterized by an overly sedentary and restricted lifestyle and by excessive dependence on pain medications or family members. Behavioral interventions designed to modify this pain behavior pattern (e.g., activation programs; social reinforcement for engaging in adaptive, well behav-

iors; and time-contingent delivery of pain medications) have been shown to reduce disability and improve psychological functioning of patients with chronic pain (Keefe & Gil, 1986; Turk et al., 1983).

Over the past 20 to 25 years, behavioral and cognitive-behavioral therapists have developed a number of strategies for assessing pain behavior (Keefe, Crisson, & Trainor, 1987). One of the major gaps in the emerging literature on pain behavior observation, however, has been the lack of practical information on how one develops and carries out such behavioral assessments. The purpose of this chapter is to provide clinicians and researchers with detailed information on pain behavior observation methods (see also Hadjistavropoulos, von Baeyer, & Craig, Chapter 8, and Craig, Prkachin, & Grunau, Chapter 9, this volume). The chapter guides the reader through the steps involved in developing an observation method and evaluating its reliability and validity. Although examples drawn from our own research on low back pain and arthritic pain are provided throughout, our intent is to provide guidelines for pain behavior assessment that are applicable to many chronic pain conditions.

The chapter is divided into four major sections. The first section discusses basic elements of pain behavior observation, such as methods of sampling pain behavior, coding category definitions, and observer training. The second section uses an observation method we developed for patients with osteoarthritis (OA) to illustrate practical aspects of each of the basic elements of observation. In the third section, we consider important issues related to the application of pain behavior observation in clinical settings. And in the final section, some future directions are presented for studying the behavioral observation of pain.

BASIC ELEMENTS OF PAIN BEHAVIOR OBSERVATION SYSTEMS

Although a variety of observational strategies can be used to record pain behavior, these strategies share certain basic elements. Five elements common to most observation methods are (1) a rationale for observation, (2) a method for sampling pain behavior, (3) definitions of behavior codes, (4) a method for observer training, and (5) reliability and validity assessments.

Rationale for Observing Pain Behavior

Mr. Smith was having great difficulty tolerating the physical examination. Despite the fact that he had few physical findings, Mr. Smith complained bitterly of chronic back pain. He flinched visibly when the examiner palpated his back. His movements were slow, and he limped in an exaggerated fashion when asked to walk. He gave very detailed descriptions of his back pain and stated that he was not sure that he could cope with the pain much longer.

Most clinicians working in the pain management area have met patients like Mr. Smith. In a medical setting, the behavior of such a patient may influence decisions about the need for further assessment or treatment (Cailliet, 1968). Patients who show exaggerated or inconsistent pain behavior are often considered to be poor candidates for invasive diagnostic testing (e.g., electroymyography) or for medical or surgical interventions (Waddell, McCulloch, Kummel, & Venner, 1980). For a behavioral clinician, the behavior of a patient like Mr. Smith is interesting and important in and of itself.

One of the most common reasons for conducting observations of a patient is to provide a detailed description of the patient's pain behavior. Descriptive data, for example, can be used to document the amount of time that a patient spends up and out of a reclining position (termed *uptime*), to provide a record of medication intake, or to describe the verbal or nonverbal behaviors the patient displays during a physical examination. In behavioral assessment, such descriptive data are used for several purposes. First, descriptive data can be used to pinpoint problem behaviors that may serve as targets for treatment efforts. Careful observations may reveal problem behaviors that patients are reluctant to report. A patient with cancer, for example, may initially deny that pain is a problem, but when asked to swallow or cough may exhibit pain-related facial expressions suggesting that considerable pain is being experienced (Keefe, Brantley, Manuel, & Crisson, 1985). Second, descriptive data can be used to establish an initial baseline measure against which the effects of treatment can be compared. By carrying out observations before treatment, after treatment, and at follow-up intervals, the clinician or investigator can evaluate the degree to which behavioral interventions can modify pain behavior. Finally, descriptive data on pain behavior may be used to predict a patient's response to treatment. Connally and Sanders (1991), for example, found that overt pain behavior recorded prior to a lumbar sympathetic block predicted the amount of pain relief patients reported following initial and subsequent blocks.

The second reason for conducting observations of pain behavior is to analyze the variables controlling that behavior. This application of behavioral observation has been called *functional analysis* (Ferster, 1965), to contrast it with more descriptive static analysis procedures. Functional analysis is designed to identify specific variables that seem to control pain behavior. Social and environmental variables often play an important role in eliciting pain behavior. A patient with an overly solicitous spouse or partner, for example, may report a much higher level of pain when in the presence of that spouse or partner than when in the presence of a neutral observer such as a ward clerk (Block, Kremer, & Gaylor, 1980). Pain behavior may also be affected by its consequences. White and Sanders (1986), for example, found that when an experimenter attended to patients' discussions about their chronic pain, the patients' ratings of pain routinely increased.

The rationale for observing pain behavior is important in determining the specific methods to be used. If the goal is to provide descriptive data, the focus of observation is on specific behaviors exhibited by the patient. Most of the current observation systems for recording pain behavior provide data only on patient behavior. They are thus suitable for a static analysis of behavior. If the goal is to perform a functional analysis, however, the scope of observation must be expanded to include not only patient behavior, but also social or environmental variables (e.g., spouse/partner behavior) that may be controlling that behavior. Although observation systems for performing functional analysis have been used in behavior therapy research for the past 25 to 30 years, these methods have only recently been extended to the chronic pain area (Romano et al., 1991, 1992, 1995).

Sampling and Recording Pain Behavior

One of the major decisions facing anyone who develops an observation system is how the behavior is to be sampled and recorded. There are four common options for sampling and coding behavior: (1) *continuous observation*, (2) *duration recording*, (3) *frequency recording*, and (4) *interval recording*.

In continuous observation, the observer records any behaviors that occurred during the observation session. This approach provides rich detail on behavior and often yields important clues as to environmental variables controlling a particular behavior. For example, a continuous observation of a man with back pain in his home setting may suggest that *downtime* (i.e., reclining) and verbal pain behaviors (e.g., complaining of pain, requests for medications) are strongly influenced by the presence of the patient's spouse. Based on these findings, one could structure a behavioral treatment program so that it focuses not only on modifying the patient's behavior, but also on modifying the spouse's response to that behavior. The major advantages of continuous observation are that they can capture the full complexity of behavior and require minimal training. The major disadvantages are the time and expense involved and the difficulty of coding and reducing the enormous amount of information gathered. Because of these limitations, continuous observation is used sparingly, typically early in the course of assessment when the evaluator is developing ideas about key target behaviors and controlling variables.

A second option for sampling and recording pain behavior is to take a duration measure. This involves simply recording the length of time that the patient takes to perform a specific behavior. For example, when working with a patient who has become dependent on a back brace, one might

record how much time the patient wears the brace each day. Alternatively, one could focus on measuring the duration of well behaviors (e.g., time spent walking or standing) that are incompatible with certain pain behaviors (e.g., time spent reclining) (Fordyce, 1976).

Duration measures provide a simple and practical means for directly observing pain behavior in naturalistic settings. Patients with chronic pain, for example, are often asked to complete diary records of their daily activities so that the duration of time they spend sitting, standing, or walking (uptime) can be recorded. Staff members also may keep duration measures of the amount of time a patient takes to complete a physically demanding task, such as walking a series of laps around a track or climbing a set of stairs. The major disadvantage of duration measures is that someone must be physically present throughout the entire observation period to record behavior in a reliable and valid fashion. Although this is not a problem for behaviors that have a short duration (e.g., time taken to complete a set of 20 sit-ups), it is a serious disadvantage when recording behaviors that can have a long duration (e.g., time spent reclining each day). Although a patient can be asked to observe and record his or her own behavior, the records provided may not be as reliable as those provided by independent observers.

Another option for observing pain behavior is to make frequency counts. In a frequency count, one simply observes and records the number of instances of each of the target behaviors. An observer might keep a frequency count of important pain behaviors, such as the number of times a patient requested medications or the number of times he or she complained of pain. The major limitation of frequency counts is that the observer may need to carry out observations over long time periods to gather reliable and valid data.

A fourth option for sampling and recording pain behavior is interval recording. In interval recording the observation period (e.g., 10 minutes or several hours) is broken down into equal intervals (e.g., 30 seconds or 1 minute long). The observer's task is to watch the patient throughout the interval and simply to note at the end of the interval whether specific behaviors were or were not observed. Interval recording is often used in coding videotaped samples of behavior gathered during standardized or simulated tasks. For example, we have used interval recording methods to observe pain behaviors that occur in patients with chronic low back pain during videotaped sessions in which they are asked to sit, stand, walk, and recline (Keefe & Block, 1982). Using videotaped behavior samples for observation has many advantages. First, videotape provides a permanent record of the patient's behavior, enabling one to carry out repeated observations, check reliability, and refine or develop new coding systems. Second, one can structure a videotaped behavior sample to elicit pain behaviors. Patients can be observed as they engage in simple daily tasks that they tend to avoid doing—for example, walking or transferring from a reclining to a standing position. Third, by applying interval recording methods to videotaped behavior samples, one can obtain data that are easily quantified.

There are several disadvantages of combining videotaped behavior sampling with interval recording methods. First, whenever a patient is being videotaped, there is the potential for reactivity (Keefe, 1989). *Reactivity* refers to the change in behavior that occurs when someone is aware of being observed. Some patients with chronic pain may inhibit their display of pain behavior during a videotaped observation session, whereas others may exaggerate their behavior. Although there is no way to predict how much reactivity will occur, two steps can be taken to minimize the effects of reactivity (Hartmann & Wood, 1982). These include (1) providing patients with minimal information on the categories of behavior being observed, and (2) avoiding interaction with the patient during the observation. It should be noted that reactivity is a problem whenever a patient is observed. The degree of reactivity during a videotaped observation may not be very different from the reactivity that occurs when a physician asks a patient to carry out functional tasks during a physical examination session (Keefe & Block, 1982).

Definitions of Pain Behavior

A visitor to a pain management program was surprised that the patients failed to exhibit many observable signs that they were experiencing pain. The patients were talkative, spending most of their time in the unit's day room in recliners. They rarely displayed pain-related facial expressions or guarded movements indicative of pain.

One of the most important factors in observing pain behavior is how one defines pain behavior. In the example above, the visitor implicitly defined pain behavior on the basis of facial expressions or guarded movements, and failed to note the fact that patients had very low levels of activity and reclined most of the time. Thus implicit assumptions about what constitutes pain behavior can determine whether an individual actually notices the presence of that pain behavior.

Implicit definitions of pain behavior can vary from one individual to another. Some base their judgments of pain behavior on a patient's medication intake, while others focus mainly on verbal complaints or motor behaviors indicative of pain. Fordyce (1976) originally defined *pain behaviors* as those behaviors that communicate to others the fact that pain is being experienced. This definition is a general one that encompasses behaviors ranging from verbal reports of pain to measures of the frequency of doctor visits. To develop a reliable and valid observation system, a more specific operational definition is required. An operational definition indicates precisely what the patient must do and what the observer must record. Thus a good operational definition describes behavior in observable and measurable terms. It also specifies what aspect of the behavior is to be recorded—namely, frequency, duration, or intensity.

Several guidelines can be offered for developing operational definitions for pain behaviors. First, the behavior should occur with sufficient frequency that it can be observed. Behaviors that occur with very low frequency or that cannot be directly observed are generally not suitable for observation. Second, the definitions of the behavior should be written in simple, descriptive language that minimizes inference on the part of observers. This ensures that observers with different backgrounds can use the observation methodology. It also avoids the major problems that occur when observers are attempting to judge why a patient engaged in a particular behavior. Finally, the definition should be written down in a table or manual. Written definitions are particularly useful when multiple categories of behavior are being observed. In such a case, the written definitions provide the basis for initial training of observers.

Observer Training

There is growing recognition that observer training is important in the development of a psychometrically sound observation method (Hartmann & Wood, 1982). The amount of observer training generally varies with the complexity of the observation system. Observation methods that rely on duration measures or frequency counts rarely necessitate intensive observer training. Continuous and interval recording methods that require the coding of multiple categories of behavior, however, typically require a structured observer training program.

Hartmann and Wood (1982) have provided an extensive set of recommendations for training observers. The recommendations include initially giving observers an opportunity to carry out observations on an informal basis, and then following this up with written materials detailing the procedures and coding categories the observers are expected to master. They also recommend having observers carry out practice coding sessions with an experienced observer. Hartmann and Wood suggest that observers reach a criterion level of reliability before starting data collection, and that periodic retraining sessions be conducted to check reliability (see also Dworkin & Sherman, Chapter 32). Finally, they suggest that observers be debriefed after they finish collecting observational data, to identify any problems that had occurred in coding behavior.

Assessing Reliability and Validity

If an observation method is to be truly useful in clinical or research settings it must be both reliable and valid. Reliability can be evaluated in new ways. First, one can determine *interobserver reliability* by examining the degree to which independent observers agree on the behaviors observed. A statistic that provides a good measure of interobserver reliability for dichotomous classification (e.g., presence–absence) is percentage agreement (Hartmann, 1977). The formula for calculating percentage agreement is as follows:

No. agreements/
(No. agreements + No. disagreements)

Agreements are simply the number of instances in which two observers agreed in their coding of specific categories of behavior, and disagreements are the number of instances in which the observers did not agree (for a detailed discussion of several alternative methods of calculating interobserver reliability, see Dworkin & Sherman, Chapter 32). Percentage agreement over 80% is usually considered acceptable. If reliability falls below this level, it usually means that there are problems with the definitions of the coding categories, that the cod-

ing scheme is too complex, or that observer training was not sufficient.

Another statistic used to determine interobserver agreement is kappa, often referred to as Cohen's kappa (Cohen, 1960). The kappa statistic provides a more conservative measure of reliability, since it is chance-corrected. This means that kappa takes into account the number of agreements between observers that one would expect simply by chance. A general formula for calculating kappa is the following:

(No. agreements – No. expected) /
(No. of observations – No. expected)

The number expected is the hypothetical number of agreements one would expect taking into account baseline constraints, such as the independence of observers (Landis & Koch, 1977). Generally, a kappa above .60 is considered an acceptable strength of agreement, and a kappa above .80 is considered nearly perfect agreement (Landis & Koch, 1977).

A second way to assess the reliability of an observation method is to determine the consistency of observed behaviors across time. *Test–retest reliability* refers to the degree to which pain behavior data collected from a patient at one time are correlated with pain behavior data collected at another time. One might, for example, obtain a videotaped behavior sample from a group of patients with chronic low back pain on two occasions separated by a 2-week interval. Correlational analyses could then be carried out to reveal how consistent the levels of behavior were over this time period. Given the varying nature of pain symptoms in chronic pain patients, one might expect the test–retest reliability of pain behavior observations to be in the moderate range ($r = .50–.70$). When test–retest correlations are at the lower end of this range ($r = .50$), it suggests that there is some variability in pain behavior over time. When this occurs, there is the possibility that changes in pain behavior occurring over treatment may reflect variability in the behavior rather than actual treatment effects. One way to deal with this problem is to incorporate control groups (e.g., waiting-list or no-treatment control groups) in behavioral treatment studies that use pain behavior as an outcome variable. This enables one to determine whether the changes in pain behavior that occur following behavioral treatment are significantly greater than the changes in pain behavior that simply occur over time with no treatment.

Several types of validity assessments are relevant in developing or evaluating pain behavior observation methods. First, one needs to examine *concurrent validity*. Concurrent validity is assessed by comparing the results of the observation method to another measure designed to measure a similar construct. For example, one might compare observation data on pain behavior to patients' scores on a self-report measure of pain behavior (Romano et al., 1988). Second, it is important to demonstrate that an observation method has adequate *construct validity*. This term is used to refer to the extent to which a test actually measures what it is intended to measure. One way to assess the construct validity of pain behavior observation systems is to compare trained observers' recordings of pain behavior with naive observers' estimates of the patient's pain. If the behaviors coded by trained observers truly are pain behaviors, then patients having high levels of these behaviors should be rated by naive observers as having higher levels of pain. A third type of validity is *discriminant validity*. This term refers to the extent to which observed pain behaviors discriminate patients having pain from patients who do not. Discriminant validity of an observation system for recording pain behavior in patients having episodic facial pain, for example, could be evaluated by comparing the pain behavior of patients having facial pain at the time of observation with the pain behavior of patients who are pain-free.

Data on the reliability and validity of direct observation methods have primarily come from studies that used trained observers to record pain behavior during videotaped behavior samples. In the early 1980s, we carried out a series of studies evaluating the reliability and validity of an observation method for recording pain behavior in patients with low back pain (Keefe & Block, 1982). The observation method was designed to measure motor pain behaviors occurring during simple daily activities. Patients were asked to engage in a series of standardized tasks (walking, sitting, standing, and reclining). The patients were videotaped as they performed these tasks, and the videotapes were subsequently scored by trained observers using an internal recording method. The categories of pain behavior recorded included guarding (stiff, interrupted, or rigid movement), bracing (pain-avoidant static posturing), rubbing of the painful area, facial grimacing, and sighing. A composite score, total pain behavior, was computed for each patient based on the sum of the number of occurrences of each pain behavior category.

Our research revealed that trained observers were highly reliable in coding the pain behavior categories. Interobserver reliability, determined using the percentage agreement formula, ranged from 93% to 99%. Although we did not assess test–retest reliability, the observation method was sensitive enough to detect changes in pain behavior that occurred following a treatment intervention (Keefe & Block, 1982). The observation method also showed evidence of good concurrent validity; patients' ratings of pain correlated significantly with total pain behavior ($r = .71$, $p < .01$). The construct validity of the observation method was examined by having observers with no knowledge of the pain behavior observation system independently rate patients' pain. The naive observers' ratings correlated significantly with total pain behavior ($r = .67$–$.69$, $p < .05$). Finally, the observation method had adequate discriminant validity, in that the behaviors considered to be pain behaviors were much more frequently observed in pain patients than in pain-free depressed and normal subjects.

Over the past 20 years, numerous studies have provided strong support for the reliability and validity of behavioral observation methods for assessing pain behavior. These include pain behavior observation studies of patients with low back pain (Ohlund et al., 1994; Weiner, Peiper, McConnell, Martinez, & Keefe, 1996), patients with rheumatoid arthritis (Anderson, Bradley, McDaniel, Young, Turner, Agudelo, Gaby, et al., 1987; Anderson, Bradley, McDaniel, Young, Turner, Agudelo, Keefe, et al., 1987; Jawarski, Bradley, Heck, Roca, & Alarcon, 1995; McDaniel et al., 1986), and terminally ill patients with cancer (Ahles et al., 1990). Observation protocols that have shown especially good reliability and validity are those that sample pain behavior during standardized tasks. For a more general and in-depth discussion of psychometric features of any assessment method, see Dworkin and Sherman (Chapter 32).

DEVELOPMENT OF A PAIN BEHAVIOR OBSERVATION SYSTEM FOR RESEARCH

In this section, we present general considerations as well as practical details for developing a standardized method for observing pain behavior. Although the topics presented apply generally to any type of behavioral observation system, as an example we will describe a research system developed for observing pain behavior in patients having OA of the knees.

Determining the Categories of Pain Behavior

Before categories of pain behavior can be selected, researchers must clarify their purpose in using such a system. For example, different behaviors might be selected if the intent is to differentiate the expression of pain from the expression of frustration or depression. Similarly, different behaviors might be selected if the intent is to study high-frequency pain behaviors versus low-frequency behaviors. Once the intent of the system is established, target behaviors can be identified. Ideally, these will be behaviors that (1) occur when pain is present but do not occur when pain is absent, (2) occur with sufficient frequency that the behaviors can be counted during the observation period, (3) can be easily elicited by routine daily tasks, and (4) can be reliably observed.

Since each patient population differs in how pain is expressed, focus groups can help identify potential behaviors for observation. Focus groups should consist of health care providers familiar with patients with pain, patients who suffer from pain themselves, and spouses/partners of patients with pain. These focus groups work best when these parties meet separately, develop a list of potential behaviors indicative of pain, and then meet as an aggregate so as to refine the list of behaviors to those behaviors that all parties agree should be considered in the observation system. Although it may be tempting to retain all behaviors that could indicate pain, systems that use more than five to seven behaviors become cumbersome to raters, and reliability becomes difficult to maintain. It is usually best to retain only those behaviors that occur with high frequency and that clearly differentiate between pain and the expression of other affect. Once the focus groups develop a potential list of behaviors, pilot observations and videotapes should be made of patients displaying the targeted pain behaviors. The videotapes are used to empirically verify the opinions of the focus group members regarding the frequency, observability, and validity of certain behaviors as being indicative of pain expression.

Determining the Categories of Pain Behaviors for OA Pain

In the mid-1980s, we developed an observation method to provide descriptive data on pain behavior in patients having OA of the knees (Keefe, Caldwell, et al., 1987). In this system, coding categories are separated into three major groups:

(1) position codes, (2) movement codes, and (3) pain behavior. The position codes include three common but mutually exclusive body postures: sitting, standing, and reclining. The movement codes include pacing (walking) and shifting (moving from one position to another in the vertical plane). The position and movement codes are included in the observation system so that the relationship of pain behavior to body posture and to dynamic movement can be studied.

The pain behavior categories used with OA patients were identified by means of clinical observations and preliminary analysis of videotaped behavior samples. Five pain behaviors were exhibited by many patients and occurred with reasonable frequency: guarding, active rubbing of the knee, unloading the joint, rigidity, and joint flexing. Table 10.1 provides the operational definition for each of the pain behavior categories, as well as for the position and movement categories included in the scoring system.

Instructions

Some observation systems guide patients through a standardized set of tasks so that each patient performs exactly the same set of tasks. This approach to observation is particularly helpful in research settings where patients will be compared to one another, where patients will be examined as a group, or where data will be collected and compared from multiple sites. When standardized tasks are used, it is essential that both patients and researchers adhere closely to a well-detailed protocol.

Instructions for the OA Behavioral Observation System

In order to elicit pain behavior, patients are asked to perform a sequence of sitting, standing, walking, and reclining tasks. The tasks include a 1- and a 2-minute standing period, a 1- and a 2-minute sitting period, two 1-minute reclining periods, and two 1-minute walking periods. These tasks are appropriate for patients with OA for several reasons. First, the tasks are common daily activities. Second, a number of these tasks tend to increase arthritic pain mildly and thus provide a means of sampling pain behavior. Finally, the tasks are not so demanding that patients would be unable to perform them.

The order of the tasks is randomized for each patient by using a set of cue cards that are shuffled after each observation session. This randomization

TABLE 10.1. Behavioral Categories of the Osteoarthritis (OA) Pain Behavior Observation System

Position codes	
Standing (std)	Patient is in an upright position with one or both feet on the floor for at least 3 sec.
Sitting (sit)	Patient is resting upon buttocks for at least 3 sec. If the patient is in the process of moving to or from a reclining position, do not score as a sit. Rather, this would be included in the shift (see below).
Reclining (rec)	Patient is resting in a horizontal position for at least 3 sec.
Movement codes	
Pacing (pce)	Moving two or more steps in any direction within the interval of 3 sec.
Shifting (sft)	Change in position upward or downward. (Example: Changing from a sitting to a reclining position or a reclining to a standing position.) A shift does not include the transition from standing to walking or walking to standing, since no upward or downward shift is involved.
Pain behavior codes	
Guarding (gd)	Abnormally slow, stiff, interrupted, or rigid movement while shifting from one position to another or while walking.
Active rubbing (ar)	Hands moving over or grabbing the affected knee (knees) and the legs; hands must be palms down, and rubbing must last 3 sec.
Unloading joint (unj)	Shifting of weight from one leg to the other during a stand.
Rigidity (rgd)	Excessive stiffness of the affected knee or knees during activities other than walking (during walking, this would be scored as guarding).
Joint flexing (jf)	Flexing of the affected knee or knees while in a static position (i.e., during standing or sitting). This may take place in conjunction with unloading of a joint.

of standardized tasks is used to prevent order effects. For example, without randomization, reclining might erroneously be shown to elicit greater pain behavior than sitting if reclining always followed 2 minutes of walking.

Before the observation session begins, the individual recording the session explains to the patient the tasks to be performed. The patient is then instructed to perform the task (i.e. sitting, standing, walking, or reclining) that appears on the first cue card for the specified length of time (1 or 2 minutes). Once the time allotted to the task has expired, the patient is asked to perform the second task for the specified time period, then the third, and so on. In order to standardize the length of the observation session, patients are given only the allotted period of time to complete a given task. If they have not completed the task before the time period expires, they are instructed to move on to the next task. For example, if a reclining patient is instructed to sit for 1 minute, but it takes a whole minute to rise from the reclining position, the subject will be instructed to move on to the next task (e.g., walking) once the allotted time for the 1-minute sitting has expired.

Throughout the observation session, attempts are made to minimize conversation and contact with the patient. Conversation with the observer can be distracting to the patient and can thus diminish the desire to express pain if it is present. Similarly, conversation can impede expression of sighing, grimacing, or verbal expressions of pain that are often categories in observation systems. Thus the observer should simply verify that the patient is within the viewfinder of the camera and spend the remainder of the interval watching the stopwatch or ensuring that part of the subject's body is not cropped out of the picture when the task involves movement. More modern systems using remote-controlled video equipment can eliminate the presence of the researcher altogether and simply deliver instructions to the patient via speakers.

Standardizing the Setting

One can gather observational data on pain behavior in almost any setting where there is sufficient room. We have collected observational data in an examination room, a patient's hospital room, or a physical therapy area. When observational measures are being used for research studies, the specific setting for observation is probably less important than making sure the same setting is used within and across the patients being compared. Standardizing the setting for observation helps to reduce variability in behavior that may relate to differences in the physical environment.

The Standardized Setting Used with the OA System

The room in which observation sessions are conducted should have several features. First, it needs to have an examination table, stool for stepping up onto the table, and chair without arms. Patients are asked to recline on the examination table and to use the stool to help them get into the reclining position. This task is somewhat difficult for most patients with OA who have knee pain, and it tends to elicit pain behavior. Transferring in and out of a chair that does not have arms can also be somewhat physically demanding for these patients and thus provides a good opportunity for observing pain behavior.

Second, the room should have adequate space, so that patients can be asked to engage in walking during the observation. A room that is at least 8–10 feet wide is required. Third, approximately 15 feet of space is needed in front of the patient so that the camera can be positioned. This camera placement enables one to keep most of the patient's body in the field of view of the camera. Finally, it is important that the room have adequate lighting and privacy. When remote or mounted minicameras are being used in small rooms, it is important *not* to use the highly distorted fish-eye lenses. Such distortion makes coding more difficult, and subtle shifts in weight can be missed by raters when these distorted lenses are used.

Videotape Equipment

Videotaping is necessary for research purposes. Videotaping facilitates the assessment of interrater agreement, and allows for the reviewing of pain behavior in cases where raters disagree. Advances in video technology have made the taping of pain behaviors much easier over the years. Below, we describe some considerations in purchasing videotaping equipment for behavioral observation.

Videotape Equipment Used in the OA System

In gathering data on pain behavior in patients with OA, we have used a standard-size video camera and VHS-formatted standard-size videocassettes. If re-

cording is done at the slowest speed, a total of 15 observation sessions (10 minutes each) can fit onto one cassette. The newer minicameras are probably less intrusive, but use smaller cassettes that have less recording space on them. We used a tripod to hold the video camera. Although most video cameras can be easily hand-held, a tripod helps to steady the camera and enables the person conducting the observation to attend to other tasks, such as delivering instructions and timing the session.

In our experience, four video camera features have been particularly useful. First, a camera that has a built-in stereo audio microphone is preferred. Stereo is desirable because it enables one to record on two audio tracks. One of these tracks can be dubbed with scoring instructions, and the other can provide an audio record of the session. Second, it is best to use a camera that has the lowest lux level possible. The lower the lux level, the better the quality of picture in dark rooms. A camera that can take good pictures even in a poorly illuminated room enables one to have more flexibility in choosing a room in which to carry out observation sessions. Third, a zoom lens and a wide-angle lens are helpful in situations when the camera must be placed either nearer than 15 feet or farther away than 15 feet from the patient. Fourth, video cameras having graphics capabilities are particularly useful, because they enable one to enter identifying information about the patient directly onto the videotape.

Preparing Videotaped Records for Scoring

After the taping session is completed, the videotape must be prepared for scoring by trained raters. We describe a low-tech method of preparing a videotape for scoring. However, there now exist video-editing software packages for computers equipped with DVD and analog-to-digital conversion hardware that facilitate this step of the scoring processing.

Preparing the Videotape Records for the OA System

The videotaped records are scored using an interval recording system. Each 10-minute record of an observation session is divided into 30-second intervals consisting of a series of 20-second "observe" segments (i.e., raters are instructed to watch the video for pain behavior) and 10-second "record" segments (i.e., raters are instructed to record on the rating sheets any pain behavior that was observed). So as to standardize the timing of the "observe" and "record" segments, verbal instructions to "observe" and "record" can be dubbed onto one of the two stereo tracks of the videotape. A prerecorded master dubbing tape having a voice prompt indicating 20 "observe" intervals (each 20 seconds in length) and 20 "record" intervals (each 10 seconds in length), can be used as a standardized tool for preparing videotapes for coding.

As mentioned previously, video-editing computer software is also now available that can facilitate this type of research. Videotapes can be made and then edited and dubbed through the video-editing programs. These programs also permit raters to enter behavioral codes identifying specific pain behaviors in graphical and quantifiable form directly onto the digital copy of the video. These edited videos can then be transferred to a compact disc (CD) with a CD burner. Large numbers of subjects can be stored on a single CD if this technology is used.

Observer Training

Critical to any behavioral observation system is the training of the observers who will be making the behavioral ratings. If all previously described components (e.g., carefully selected coding categories,

high-quality videotaping and dubbing, etc.) have been developed with care, then the initial training of raters should not be difficult. What is difficult is the maintenance of observer skills. Once trained, observers must continually reestablish their accuracy (see also Dworkin & Sherman, Chapter 32). This is time-consuming and is a facet of using this type of observational system that must be allotted sufficient time and personnel.

Observer Training for the OA System

Observers can be research assistants or college undergraduates. Observers go through a systematic training program that involves several steps. The first step involves learning the definitions of each the coding categories listed in Table 10.1. Observers study the definitions and are tested to ensure that they understand the definitions. Second, the observers are instructed in the use of the scoring form. Table 10.2 displays a sample scoring form. As can be seen, the scoring form provides space for each of 20 recording intervals and groups the individual coding categories into the three major groups (position, movement, and pain behaviors). During each scoring interval, observers simply circle the specific coding categories observed. We use an interval recording method in which the observer simply notes the occurrence of a behavior;

TABLE 10.2. Pain Behavior Scoring Sheet for the Osteoarthritis Pain Behavior Observation System

Patient: _____ Observer: _____ Date: _____ Pain Location: _____

	Position			Movement		Pain behavior				
1.	std	sit	rec	pce	sft	gd	ar	unj	rgd	jf
2.	std	sit	rec	pce	sft	gd	ar	unj	rgd	jf
3.	std	sit	rec	pce	sft	gd	ar	unj	rgd	jf
4.	std	sit	rec	pce	sft	gd	ar	unj	rgd	jf
5.	std	sit	rec	pce	sft	gd	ar	unj	rgd	jf
6.	std	sit	rec	pce	sft	gd	ar	unj	rgd	jf
7.	std	sit	rec	pce	sft	gd	ar	unj	rgd	jf
8.	std	sit	rec	pce	sft	gd	ar	unj	rgd	jf
9.	std	sit	rec	pce	sft	gd	ar	unj	rgd	jf
10.	std	sit	rec	pce	sft	gd	ar	unj	rgd	jf
11.	std	sit	rec	pce	sft	gd	ar	unj	rgd	jf
12.	std	sit	rec	pce	sft	gd	ar	unj	rgd	jf
13.	std	sit	rec	pce	sft	gd	ar	unj	rgd	jf
14.	std	sit	rec	pce	sft	gd	ar	unj	rgd	jf
15.	std	sit	rec	pce	sft	gd	ar	unj	rgd	jf
16.	std	sit	rec	pce	sft	gd	ar	unj	rgd	jf
17.	std	sit	rec	pce	sft	gd	ar	unj	rgd	jf
18.	std	sit	rec	pce	sft	gd	ar	unj	rgd	jf
19.	std	sit	rec	pce	sft	gd	ar	unj	rgd	jf
20.	std	sit	rec	pce	sft	gd	ar	unj	rgd	jf

thus each behavior code is circled only once during any interval. Similar coding sheets can be created for online coding of digitally edited videotape.

The third phase of training involves practice scoring of videotapes. A previously trained observer (the master observer) conducts these practice sessions. The novice observers are shown several 30-second segments of a videotape and are asked to score the patient behaviors they observe. The novices then compare their scoring with that of the master observer. After each practice session, problem areas are addressed, and feedback is provided on the accuracy of coding. As the novices begin to develop their observation skills, the master observer gradually increases the number of intervals being scored. Practice sessions typically begin with a single interval, and then progress to 5, 10, and 15 intervals. Eventually observers should be able to score an entire 20-interval session. Each observer is required to score a practice series of 10-minute videotaped observation sessions and show acceptable reliability with the master observer (over 85% agreement) before he or she is considered fully trained.

The final step of training is to conduct periodic retraining sessions. These sessions are especially important in research applications in which the goal is to obtain reliable and accurate data. Retraining sessions help to prevent the phenomenon known as *observer drift*. Observer drift occurs when observers unwittingly begin to modify coding category definitions after carrying out a series of observations on their own. The retraining sessions should be scheduled periodically (e.g., every 2 weeks or after scoring data from every 10 patients). In the retraining sessions, the master observer reviews coding category definitions and scoring methods, and leads the observers in practice scoring of videotapes. When pain behavior is being scored in a research study, it is important to keep a written log of retraining sessions to document data on interobserver reliability.

Reliability and Validity Data

Examples from the OA System

In our research on patients with OA, we carried out assessments of both the reliability and validity of the pain behavior observation method (Keefe, Caldwell, et al., 1987). In this study, reliability was assessed in two ways. First, we calculated interobserver reliability by having observers independently and simultaneously score the same videotaped behavior sample. Interobserver reliability was

evaluated using the percentage agreement formula for 30 of the first 87 patients with OA knee pain we studied. Our findings revealed a very high degree of interobserver reliability (percentage agreement = 93.7%). Second, in unpublished research, we evaluated the test–retest reliability of our observation method. Pain behavior observations were carried out on a group of 36 patients who, as part of a treatment outcome study (Keefe et al., 1990), were assigned to a routine medical treatment control condition. A 10-minute videotaped behavior sample was obtained prior to entry into the study (time 1), 10 weeks later (time 2), and 6 months after time 2 (time 3). Test-retest reliability was found to be acceptable. Patients' total pain behavior at time 1 correlated significantly with total pain behavior at time 2 ($r = .53$, $p < .005$) and at time 3 ($r = .53$, $p < .005$).

We have also assessed the concurrent, discriminant, and construct validity of this observation method (Keefe, Caldwell, et al., 1987). The concurrent validity of the observation method was supported by the finding that patients' ratings of pain on a 0–10 scale were significantly correlated with their total pain behavior scores ($r = .46$, $p < .0001$). The observation method also showed adequate discriminant validity, in that we found that patients who were having pain at the time of observation ($n = 37$) exhibited significantly more pain behavior ($t = 2.82$, $p < .007$) than those who were pain-free ($n = 14$). To assess the construct validity of the observation method, we showed a series of videotaped segments collected from 20 patients with OA to a group of 13 rheumatologists. The rheumatologists were asked to rate each patient's pain level on a 0–10 rating scale and a 100-millimeter Visual Analogue Scale (VAS). The rheumatologists' ratings were found to be significantly correlated with patients total pain behavior (0–10 ratings, $r = .65$, $p < .002$; VAS ratings, $r = .64$, $p < .003$). Thus patients for whom trained observers scored as having higher levels of pain behavior were similarly viewed by rheumatologists as having more pain, while patients who were scored as having lower levels of pain behavior were viewed by rheumatologists as having less pain.

CLINICAL APPLICATIONS OF BEHAVIORAL OBSERVATION

Issues and Recommendations

Although the research protocol just described offers rigor and control over tasks by giving subjects specific instructions, this method can be criticized for being vulnerable to the effects of patient reactivity to the observation procedure. Reactivity is likely to be high, given the presence of videotaping equipment and the demand by the experimenter to adhere to a fixed activity protocol (Turk & Flor, 1987). When behavioral observation is conducted in the context of a clinical practice, naturalistic observation is generally preferred over the highly controlled standardized methods just described for research.

A number of important issues arise when one tries to incorporate behavioral observation methods into clinical practice settings. First is the issue of time. A commitment to gathering observational data usually means that a clinician will need to make adjustments in workload or shift priorities. Carrying out observations may mean that the practicing clinician has less time available for gathering information via other assessment methods (e.g., interviews) or for carrying out treatment procedures. One of the best ways to reduce the time demands of observation is to carry out preliminary observations before implementing data collection. These observations can help to pinpoint behaviors that can serve as the targets for behavioral observation. A patient, for example, may show one or two pain behaviors (e.g., excessive guarding or pain-avoidant posturing) that are particularly important targets for assessment and treatment efforts. Preliminary observations also can help to identify time periods during the day when pain behaviors are most likely to occur. Observations in a day treatment program, for example, may reveal that there are two times each day when patients are especially likely to exhibit pain behavior. These might be mealtime and the time when patients receive medications. By restricting observation to key periods of the day, one can significantly reduce the costs of observation while still obtaining an adequate sample of pain behavior.

A second issue in applying observation systems in clinical settings is the need for videotape equipment. Most of the sophisticated behavioral observation systems reviewed in this chapter have utilized video cameras and recording equipment. Although this equipment is useful in training observers and providing permanent records of observation sessions, it can be expensive and labor intensive. The goals of behavioral observation can help clarify whether videotaping is needed. For example, if permanent records are needed for research purposes or for training purposes, then videotape can be helpful. On the other hand, if

the data are being used for making clinical decisions about a specific patient and will not be compared to others, then the utility of the videotape is negligible. In summary, we believe that videotape equipment is a helpful tool, but not a necessity, in performing observations. Research has shown that reliable and valid behavioral data can be collected without the assistance of videotape equipment (Hartmann & Wood, 1982). Live observations carried out in naturalistic settings can serve as a basis for defining pain behaviors, developing behavior-sampling strategies, and training observers. Naturalistic observations are not only less expensive; they are probably less intrusive than videotaped observations. People new to the field of behavioral observation should be aware that most practicing behaviorally oriented clinicians rely on live, rather than videotaped, observation methods.

A third important issue for applying observation methods in clinical practice is the need for observer training. The complex and sophisticated behavioral observation methods used in research studies require extensive observer training. Individuals who use these methods to gather data are recruited and trained specifically to serve as observers. In practice settings, one must usually rely on clinical staff to perform the functions of observers. Staff members usually do not have the time for intensive observer training, but they do have considerable clinical expertise, understand the concept of pain behavior, and are capable of providing high-quality observational data if adequately motivated. Brief periods of training can be used to teach staff members to use simple observation methods such as duration measures or frequency counts. With periodic reliability checks and review of recording methods, reliable and valid data on pain behavior can be obtained for clinical use.

Clinical staff members are sometimes resistant to carrying out behavioral observations. They may view observation as a burden that is imposed on their already busy work schedules. Although they may agree to collect data, the quality of the data may not be high. To avoid this problem, the individual staff members who are to serve as observers need to be involved in the focus groups, the development, and the implementation of any pain behavior observation system. We think it is important to involve staffers in writing definitions, setting schedules for observation, and checking reliability. Observation data that are gathered should also be shared with the observers on a regular basis, so that they can be used in evaluating treatment outcome. If observation methods are to be effectively integrated into a pain unit or program, they must be viewed by all as contributing to the clinical management of the patients.

A Clinical Example

In 1990, Shutty, Cundiff, and DeGood developed a pain behavior observation system that could be used unobtrusively in an outpatient setting. Although lacking some of the rigor necessary for a research protocol, this system offered the clinician a time-efficient method of obtaining a rating of pain behavior that could be used to help form his or her clinical impression of the patient. This system is described here in modified form so as to be applicable to patients with low back pain (a naturalistic low back pain system, or NLBPS).

Coding for the NLBPS

Unlike the OA system, the NLBPS capitalizes upon naturalistic observation in a standard clinic setting. The coding categories used for clinical presentation of low back pain, are again separated into three major groups: (l) position codes, (2) movement codes, and (3) pain behavior. The position codes include sitting, standing, and reclining. The movement codes include pacing (walking) and shifting (moving from one position to another in the vertical plane). Again, the position and movement codes are included in the observation system so that the relationship of pain behavior to body posture and dynamic movement can be studied. The pain behaviors that are used with this system are similar to those used in the previously published low back pain behavior observation system (Keefe & Block, 1982) and include guarding, bracing, rubbing, grimacing, and sighing. A sixth behavior, reliance on others, was added to this system. Table 10.3 provides the operational definition for each of the pain behavior categories for the NLBPS.

Instructions and Standardizing the Setting for the NLBPS

Whereas the OA system has observers give instructions to patients to perform certain tasks in order to elicit pain behavior, the NLBPS must rely on naturally occurring behaviors of the patient in the clinical setting. With the naturalistic approach, therefore, it is possible that patients will not perform the tasks that elicit pain in the clinic. Clini-cians, however, can capitalize on features of their own clinic that hold a higher than average likelihood of eliciting pain behavior in their patients. For example, staff members can be instructed to watch for pain behavior when patients sit down in the waiting room. Given this approach, any norms that are established will of course apply only to other patients of the same clinic.

Most clinics offer an opportunity to observe pain behavior during the following common tasks: entering the waiting room (walking), checking in with the receptionist (standing), waiting for the doctor (transition from standing to sitting, and sitting), being called for the appointment (transition from sitting to standing), and leaving the waiting room with the doctor (walking). Nurses and/or receptionists can be trained to observe pain behavior during these naturalistic events.

As mentioned earlier, videotaping is probably not necessary for this type of system. Although small cameras can be installed in clinical settings such as waiting rooms, patients may become suspicious of the cameras if no explanation for their presence is given. This could introduce the unwanted reactive effects that naturalistic observation seeks to reduce. Table 10.4 on page 184 provides a sample coding sheet that can be used in the clinic setting.

Scoring the NLBP

As with the OA system, the occurrence of a pain behavior in the NLBPS is simply identified as present or absent during a specific episode. Thus, for example, there is no need to tally the number of guardings that occur in each episode; rather, the observer simply notes that guarding occurred during that interval. A total pain behavior score can be summed across the four episodes. Clinicians may wish to establish norms for their individual offices and modify the observation episodes to fit their particular office environment.

FUTURE RESEARCH DIRECTIONS

There is a wide variety of important directions for future research on pain behavior observation. In this section we highlight four of these: applying pain behavior observation to new clinical populations, the use of novel palmtop computer approaches, observational studies of patients and their spouses/partners, and studies examining the ability of individuals to detect pain in others.

TABLE 10.3. Behavioral Categories of the Naturalistic Low Back Pain Behavior System (NLBPS)

Position codes	
Standing (std)	Patient is in an upright position with one or both feet on the floor for at least 3 sec.
Sitting (sit)	Patient is resting upon buttocks for at least 3 sec. If the patient is in the process of moving to or from a reclining position, do not score as a sit. Rather, this would be included in the shift (see below).
Reclining (rec)	Patient is resting in a horizontal position for at least 3 sec.
Movement codes	
Pacing (pce)	Moving two or more steps in any direction within the interval of 3 sec.
Shifting (sft)	Change in position upward or downward. (Example: Changing from a sitting to a reclining position or a reclining to a standing position.) A shift does not include the transition from standing to walking or walking to standing since no upward or downward shift is involved.
Pain behavior codes	
Guarding (gd)	Abnormally stiff, interrupted, or rigid movement while shifting from one position to another or during pacing. It includes patients using canes or walkers, and cannot occur during a stationary position (i.e., sit, std, rec). The movement must be hesitant or interrupted, not merely slow.
Bracing (brc)	Position in which an almost fully extended limb supports and maintains an abnormal distribution of weight. It cannot occur during movement (i.e., pce, sft), and must be held for at least 3 sec. It is most frequently the gripping of the edge of a piece of furniture while sitting, but can also be grasping a table, cane, or walker while standing. What appears to be bracing during movement is termed guarding. It can occur with a leg if the patient leans against a wall using no other support, but is not simply the shifting of weight while standing.
Rubbing (rb)	Touching, rubbing, or holding the affected area, which includes low back, hips, and legs, for a minimum of 3 sec. It includes patients' hands in pockets or behind the back, but not the hands folded in a lap. It can occur during an interval of movement or nonmovement. Patients' palm(s) must be touching the affected area to be considered rubbing during a sit. If a clear view is not available, a rub is recorded if touching can be reasonably inferred from the patient's position.
Grimacing (gr)	Obvious facial expression of pain, which may include furrowed brow, narrowed eyes, tightened lips, corners of mouth pulled back, and clenched teeth. It often resembles wincing. Observer must be alert to catch this behavior. It often occurs during a shift.
Sigh (si)	Obvious exaggerated exhalation of air, usually accompanied by shoulders first rising and then falling. Cheeks may be expanded.
Reliance on others (otr)	Obvious reliance on a companion or other person for performing tasks or carrying objects. Examples include using others to check in, carry canes and walkers, get magazines, and find objects in purses or bags. If the patient is leaning on or using others for ambulating, then guarding or bracing should be used.

Applying Behavioral Observation to New Clinical Populations

Can behavioral observation methods be adapted to new clinical populations? Most of the observational methods discussed in this paper have been used to record pain behavior in patients suffering from persistent pain conditions such as low back pain or OA. These methods, however, need not be restricted to these populations. Jay and Elliott (1984), for example, have demonstrated that observational methods can be used to record behavior in children who are experiencing acute pain due to medical procedures. We have recently demonstrated the utility of pain behavior observation in assessing back pain in community-dwelling older adults with OA (Weiner et al., 1996). We are currently extending this observation approach to analyze pain behavior in cognitively impaired nursing home residents (see also Hadjistavropoulos

TABLE 10.4. Sample Pain Behavior Scoring Sheet for the NLBPS

Patient: _____ Observer: _____ Date: _____ Pain Location: _____

1. Observation episode 1: Observe the behavior that occurs from the time the patient enters the waiting room to the time the patient checks in at the reception desk. (If the patient has a companion check in, score using the otr category.)

        std   sit   rec   pce sft   gd brc rb si gr otr

2. Observation episode 2: Observe the behavior that occurs while the patient is standing at the reception desk to check in. (If the patient has a companion check in, score using the otr category.)

        std   sit   rec   pce sft   gd brc rb si gr otr

3. Observation episode 3: Observe the behavior that occurs as the patient walks from the reception desk to a chair, sits down, and sits for 1 minute as he or she waits to be called for the doctor visit.

        std   sit   rec   pce sft   gd brc rb si gr otr

4. Observation episode 4: Observe the behavior that occurs after the patient is called for the doctor visit. This includes rising from the chair, and walking out of the waiting room with the doctor or nurse.

        std   sit   rec   pce sft   gd brc rb si gr otr

et al., Chapter 8). Observational methods are particularly likely to be helpful in evaluating demented patients who have difficulty describing their pain to others. Finally, observational methods have also been used to record pain behavior in very ill patients, such as patients with terminal lung cancer (Ahles et al., 1990).

When one is adapting existent observational systems to new pain populations, there are two important considerations. First, the tasks used to elicit pain behavior during a structured observation session must be relevant to the pain condition being studied. Walking or transferring from one position to another may elicit pain behavior in patients with low back pain, but may be of little value in eliciting pain behavior in a patient having facial pain. Preliminary observations may be needed to determine the best strategies for eliciting and sampling pain behavior. Second, new coding categories may need to be developed. The topography of pain behaviors can vary from one clinical condition to another. Reviewing videotapes of patient behavior can be particularly useful in identifying coding categories for specific pain conditions.

Palmtop Computer Technologies

Palmtop computers can help observers use pain behavior observation systems in the field where videotaping is not an option or where paper-and-pencil recording sheets would be cumbersome. These hand-held computers offer a high-tech method of recording pain behavior coding categories in digital form that can be tallied within the computer or quickly uploaded to a database. Such computers can be programmed to prompt the observer for "observe" and "record" intervals, thus eliminating the need for a stopwatch, and can facilitate the quantification of pain behavior data within the time frame of a patient visit. Thus the clinician can have a measure of pain behavior immediately after the visit that can be a part of his or her dictated report. The disadvantages of this technology are obviously the cost and the need for a programmer to customize the software to capture the nuances of each behavioral observation system.

Observational Studies of Patients and Spouses/Partners

Another emerging area of research incorporates spouses or partners into the observation system. Pain behaviors provide a means of communicating the experience of pain to others and are influenced by social and environmental consequences (Fordyce, 1976). Spouses and partners play an especially significant role in this system, due to their frequency of interaction with patients. An operant behavioral perspective on interaction between a patient and a spouse/partner asserts that if pain behaviors are followed by reinforcing consequences, the rate of pain behaviors will increase over time (Romano et al., 1992). For example, when a spouse/partner responds to pain behaviors in a solicitous manner, such as expressing concern or providing assistance related to the patient's pain or disability, pain behavior is positively reinforced and will increase. Conversely, when a spouse/partner responds to the patient's pain behaviors in a more neutral and less reinforcing fashion—for example, by attending to them but not being overly solicitous—pain behavior may be less likely to occur. Several studies have shown that there are significant associations between spouse/partner responses and patients' reports of pain and activity (Block et al., 1980; Flor, Kerns, & Turk, 1987; Kerns, Haythornthwaite, Southwick, & Giller, 1990; see also Romano & Schmaling, Chapter 18, and Jacob & Kerns, Chapter 19).

An analysis of spouse/partner responses to pain behavior displays may have important clinical implications (see also Romano & Schmaling, Chapter 18, and Jacob & Kerns, Chapter 19). First, by carefully assessing spouse/partner response style, one may be able to distinguish between adaptive and maladaptive interactions between patients and their significant others. This information could be used by clinicians in advising patients and their spouses/partners about interaction patterns that may have beneficial or deleterious effects on the pain experience. Second, early identification of maladaptive interactions may be useful in pinpointing couples who are likely to benefit from couple-based approaches to pain management (e.g. spouse- or partner-assisted pain coping skills training). When the spouse or partner is directly involved in pain management efforts, he or she not only may be able to learn more about the patient's pain, but also can learn how to help prompt and reinforce adaptive behaviors such as exercising and pacing activities.

Romano and colleagues (1991) were the first to develop a structured system for observing and recording the interactions of patients having chronic pain and their spouses (this research thus far has been limited to married couples). This system involves videotaping each couple engaging in a series of household activities: sweeping a floor, changing bed sheets, bundling newspapers, and carrying logs across a room. These activities were chosen because they both elicit pain behaviors from patients and provide a context in which a patient and spouse can interact while working on a task together. The total time to complete these tasks

averages 20 minutes. Each couple is instructed to perform the tasks together, with the patient taking the lead. The videotapes are then coded by trained observers using a modified version of the Living in Family Environments (Hops et al., 1990) computer coding system. This system codes specified behaviors in a continuous, sequential stream in real time. Observers code verbal and nonverbal pain behaviors (e.g., comments referring to physical limitations, limping, stretching) as well as spouse response styles (e.g., facilitative, solicitous, aggressive).

Romano and her colleagues used this observation method to code the behaviors of patients with chronic low back pain and their spouses (Romano et al., 1991, 1992, 1995; see also Romano & Schmaling, Chapter 18). Two interesting findings were obtained in this research. First, spouse solicitous behaviors have been shown both to precede and to follow patient nonverbal pain behaviors (Romano et al., 1992). Second, spouse solicitous responses have been found to be associated with greater frequency of reported pain and higher levels of disability (Romano et al., 1995). Both of these findings are consistent with operant behavioral theory and support the utility of this observational methodology as a research tool.

Assessing the Ability of People to Detect Pain in Others

Clinical observations suggest that people vary substantially in their ability to detect pain in another person. Some individuals seem to be aware of another person's pain and able to track its variations from one moment to another. Other people seem to be unaware of the extent of another person's pain or how it varies.

Beaupre and colleagues (1997) have developed an innovative computer-based methodology to capture these individual differences in people's awareness of another person's pain. They tested this methodology in a study involving patients having pain due to OA of the knees and their spouses. Each patient was videotaped engaging in a series of activities—standing, sitting, walking, and reclining—according to the protocol developed by Keefe and Block (1982) and described previously. The patient then watched this 10-minute videotape of him- or herself while simultaneously providing continuous ratings of the pain intensity. The patient's spouse then viewed the same videotape while making continuous ratings of the patient's pain intensity. The pain intensity ratings were made with a mouse-controlled pointer that could be moved back and forth to indicate pain intensity on a computer-controlled VAS. These ratings were sampled by the computer on a second-by-second basis and averaged over 10-second periods. Statistical analyses were then conducted on the data collected from each couple. Using time series analysis, Beaupre and colleagues found that among some couples, there was a high level of temporal synchrony between a patient's and spouse's ratings of pain over time. In other couples, however, there was very low synchrony between these ratings.

Beaupre and colleagues (1997) also examined factors that might differentiate couples in which a patient and spouse were synchronous in their ratings of the patient's pain from those couples in which there was no synchrony. The level of synchrony tended to be higher among couples in which the spouse was female, the patient had pain for a shorter duration, and the patient had lower levels of disability. These preliminary findings support the notion that there are substantial individual differences in the ability to detect pain in one's spouse, and that women in particular are better at this task than men.

CLOSING COMMENT: THE ROLE OF PAIN BEHAVIOR OBSERVATION IN CLINICAL PRACTICE

Before we complete our discussion of pain behavior observation, it is important to discuss the role that pain behavior plays in the overall assessment of the pain experience. Observations of pain behavior are meant to provide one measure of the pain experience. They are designed to complement, not replace, other forms of pain assessment. Chronic pain is a complex, multidimensional phenomenon (Melzack & Wall, 1965). Thus pain behavior observation should be one component of a comprehensive assessment that includes the use of pain perception measures, standardized psychological tests, and a variety of medical evaluations. That is, to analyze pain behavior, observational data need to be combined with information on the underlying tissue pathology, the perception of pain, and the degree of pain-related suffering (Fordyce, 1979). It is only by viewing pain behavior in its biopsychosocial context that we are likely to achieve significant advances in our ability to assess and treat chronic pain.

REFERENCES

Ahles, T. A., Coombs, D. W., Jensen, L., Stukel, T., Maurer, L. H., & Keefe, F. J. (1990). Development of a behavioral observation technique for the assessment of pain behaviors in cancer patients. *Behavior Therapy, 21,* 449–460.

Anderson, K. O., Bradley, L. A., McDaniel, L. K., Young, L. D., Turner, R. A., Agudelo, C. A., Gaby, N. S., Keefe, F. J., Pisko, E. J., Snyder, R. M., & Semble, E. L. (1987). The assessment of pain in rheumatoid arthritis: Disease differentiation and temporal stability of a behavioral observation method. *Journal of Rheumatology, 14,* 700–704.

Anderson, K. O., Bradley, L. A., McDaniel, L. K., Young, L. D., Turner, R. A., Agudelo, C. A., Keefe, F. J., Pisko, E. J., Snyder, R. M., & Semble, E. L. (1987). The assessment of pain in rheumatoid arthritis: Vaility of a behavioral observation method. *Arthritis and Rheumatism, 30,* 36–43.

Beaupre, P., Keefe, F. J., Lester, N., Affleck, G., Frederickson, B., & Caldwell, D. S. (1997). A computer-assisted observational method for assessing spouses' ratings of osteoarthritis patients' pain. *Psychology, Health and Medicine, 2,* 99–108.

Block, A. R., Kremer, E. F., & Gaylor, M. (1980). Behavioral treatment of chronic pain: Variables affecting treatment efficacy. *Pain, 8,* 367–371.

Cailliet, R. (1968). *Low back pain syndrome.* Philadelphia: Davis.

Cohen, J. (1960). A coefficient of agreement for nominal scales. *Educational and Psychological Measurement, 20,* 37–46.

Connally, G. H., & Sanders, S. H. (1991). Predicting low back pain patients' response to lumbar sympathetic nerve blocks and interdisciplinary rehabilitation: The role of pretreatment overt pain behavior and cognitive coping strategies. *Pain, 44,* 139–146.

Ferster, C. B. (1965). Classification of behavioral pathology. In L. Krasner & L. P. Ullman (Eds.), *Research in behavior modification* (pp. 6–26). New York: Holt, Rinehart & Winston.

Flor, H., Kerns, R. D., & Turk, D. C. (1987). The role of spouse reinforcement, perceived pain, and activity levels of chronic pain patients. *Journal of Psychosomatic Research, 31,* 251–259.

Fordyce, W. E. (1976). *Behavioral methods for chronic pain and illness.* St. Louis, MO: Mosby.

Fordyce, W. E. (1979). Environmental factors in the genesis of low back pain. In J. J. Bonica, J. E. Liebeskind, & D. G. Albe-Fessard (Eds.), *Advances in pain research and therapy* (Vol. 3, pp. 659–666). New York: Raven Press.

Hartmann, D. P. (1977). Considerations in the choice of interobserver reliability estimates. *Journal of Applied Behavior Analysis, 10,* 103–110.

Hartmann, D. P., & Wood, D. D. (1982). Observational methods. In A. S. Bellack, M. Hersen, & A. E. Kazdin (Eds.), *International handbook of behavior modification and therapy* (pp. 109–138). New York: Plenum Press.

Hops, H., Biglan, A., Tolman, A., Arthur, J., Sherman, L., Warner, P., Romano, J., Turner, J., Friedman, L., Bulcroft, R., Holcomb, C., Oosternick, N., & Osteen, V. (1990). *Living in Family Environments*

(*LIFE*) *Coding System*. Eugene, OR: Oregon Research Institute.

Jawarski, T. M., Bradley, L. A., Heck, L. W., Roca, A., & Alarcon, G. S. (1995). Development of an observation method for assessing pain behaviors in children with juvenile rheumatoid arthritis. *Arthritis and Rheumatism, 38,* 1142–1151.

Jay, S. M., & Elliott, C. (1984). Behavioral observation scales for measuring children's distress: The effects of increased methodological rigor. *Journal of Consulting and Clinical Psychology, 52,* 1100–1107.

Keefe, F. J. (1989). Behavioral measurement of pain. In C. R. Chapman & J. D. Loeser (Eds.), *Issues in pain measurement* (pp. 405–424). New York: Raven Press.

Keefe, F. J., & Block, A. R. (1982). Development of an observation method for assessing pain behavior in chronic low back pain patients. *Behavior Therapy, 13,* 363–375.

Keefe, F. J., Brantley, A., Manuel, G., & Crisson, J. E. (1985). Behavioral assessment of head and neck cancer pain. *Pain, 23,* 327–336.

Keefe, F. J., Caldwell, D. S., Queen, R. T., Gil, K. M., Martinez, S., Crisson, S., Crisson, J. E., Ogden, W., & Nunley, J. (1987). Osteoarthritic knee pain: A behavioral analysis. *Pain, 28,* 309–321.

Keefe, F. J., Caldwell, D. S., Williams, D. A., Gil, K. M., Mitchell, D., Robertson, C., Martinez, S., Nunley, J., Beckham, J. C., Crisson, J. E., & Helms, M. (1990). Pain coping skills training in the management of osteoarthritic knee pain: A comparative study. *Behavior Therapy, 21,* 49–62.

Keefe, F. J., Crisson, J. E., & Trainor, M. (1987). Observational methods for assessing pain: A practical guide. In J. A. Blumenthal & D. C. McKee (Eds.), *Applications in behavioral medicine and health psychology: A clinician's source book* (pp. 67–94). Sarasota, FL: Professional Resource Exchange.

Keefe, F. J., & Gil, K. M. (1986). Behavioral concepts in the analysis of chronic pain. *Journal of Consulting and Clinical Psychology, 54,* 776–783.

Kerns, R. D., Haythornthwaite, J., Southwick, S., & Giller, E. L. (1990). The role of marital interaction in chronic pain and depressive symptom severity. *Journal of Psychosomatic Research, 34,* 401–408.

Landis, J. R., & Koch, G. G. (1977). The measurement of observer agreement for categorical data. *Biometrics, 33,* 159–174.

McDaniel, L. K., Anderson, K. O., Bradley, L. A., Young, L. D., Turner, R. A., Agudelo, C. A., & Keefe, F. J.

(1986). Development of an observation method for assessing pain behavior in rheumatoid arthritis patients. *Pain, 24,* 165–184.

Melzack, R., & Wall, P. D. (1965). Pain mechanisms: A new theory. *Science, 150,* 971–979.

Ohlund, C., Lindstrom, I., Areskoug, B., Eek, C., Peterson, L. E., & Nachemson, A. (1994). Pain behavior in industrial subacute low back pain: Part I. Reliability: Concurrent and predictive validity of pain behavior assessments. *Pain, 58,* 201–209.

Romano, J. M., Syrjala, K. L., Levy, R. L., Turner, J. A., Evans, P., & Keefe, F. J. (1988). Observational assessment of pain behaviors: Relationship to patient functioning and treatment outcome. *Behavior Therapy, 19,* 191–202.

Romano, J. M., Turner, J. A., Friedman, L. S., Bulcroft, R. A., Jensen, M. P., & Hops, H. (1991). Observational assessment of chronic pain patient–spouse behavioral interactions. *Behavior Therapy, 22,* 549–567.

Romano, J. M., Turner, J. A., Friedman, L. S., Bulcroft, R. A., Jensen, M. P., Hops, H., & Wright, S. F. (1992). Sequential analysis of chronic pain behaviors and spouse responses. *Journal of Consulting and Clinical Psychology, 60,* 77–782.

Romano, J. M., Turner, J. A., Jensen, M. P., Friedman, L. S., Bulcroft, R. A., Hops, H., & Wright, S. F. (1995). Chronic pain patient–spouse behavioral interactions predict patient disability. *Pain, 63,* 353–360.

Shutty, M. S., Cundiff, G., & DeGood, D. E. (1990). *Development and validation of a brief pain behavior rating scale*. Unpublished manuscript.

Turk, D. C., & Flor, H. (1987). Pain behaviors: The utility and limitations of the pain behavior construct. *Pain, 31,* 277–295.

Turk, D. C., Meichenbaum, D., & Genest, M. (1983). *Pain and behavioral medicine: A cognitive-behavioral perspective*. New York: Guilford Press.

Waddell, G., McCulloch, J. A., Kummel, E., & Venner, R. M. (1980). Nonorganic physical signs in low-back pain. *Spine, 5,* 117–125.

Weiner, D., Peiper, C., McConnell, E., Martinez, S., & Keefe, F. J. (1996). Pain measurement in elders with chronic low back pain: Traditional and alternative approaches. *Pain, 67,* 461–467.

White, B., & Sanders, S. H. (1986). The influence of patients' pain intensity ratings of antecedent reinforcement of pain talk or well talk. *Journal of Behavior Therapy and Experimental Psychiatry, 17,* 155–159.

Part III

MEDICAL AND PHYSICAL EVALUATION OF PATIENTS WITH PAIN

Chapter 11
___

Quantification of Function in Chronic Low Back Pain

___

PETER B. POLATIN
TOM G. MAYER

Chronic low back pain is the "most expensive benign condition in America" (Mayer et al., 1987). Approximately 80% of Americans will suffer a serious episode of low back pain during their lives, and 4% of the population will undergo such an episode each year (Andersson, 1981). In certain occupations, the risk of back injury is as high as 15% per year (Andersson, 1981). Although more than 50% of such episodes resolve within 2 weeks, and 90% resolve within 3 months, those patients who remain symptomatic after that period of time have the poorest prognosis and cost the most in health care dollars (Mayer & Gatchel, 1988). Surgery may be of benefit for only 1% or 2% of patients with a low back pain episode (Mayer et al., 1987). It therefore falls within the province of conservative care to manage the majority of these patients.

In the interest of establishing objective guidelines for assessment, treatment, and therapeutic goal setting, the utilization of measures to quantify lumbar function has been found to be useful (Mayer et al., 1987; Mayer, Barnes, Kishino, et al., 1988; Mayer, Barnes, Nichols, et al., 1988; Mayer & Gatchel, 1988, 1989; Mayer et al., 1986; Mayer, Gatchel, Barnes, Mayer, & Mooney, 1990; Mayer, Kishino, Keeley, Mayer & Mooney, 1985; Mayer & Polatin, 1994; Mayer, Smith, et al., 1985; Mayer, Tencer, Kristoferson, & Mooney,

1984). Functional deficits have also been found to be predictive of and associated with disability (Biering-Sørensen, 1984; Cady, Bischoff, O'Connell, Thomas, & Allen, 1979; Chaffin, 1978; Nachemson, 1983).

WHY QUANTIFY FUNCTION?

Pain perception has been one of the primary indices used in the documentation of human suffering. However, it is a subjective phenomenon influenced by multiple factors (Beals, 1984; Fordyce, Roberts, & Sternbach, 1985; Turk, Meichenbaum, & Genest, 1983; White & Gordon, 1982). Furthermore, similar lesions may produce very different pain reports in different individuals (Gatchel, Mayer, Capra, Diamond, & Barnett, 1986; Mooney, Cairns, & Robertson, 1976). Therefore, although standardized measures of pain are clinically useful, their primary benefit is for intraindividual comparison.

Disability, a direct outcome of chronic pain, is more easily defined objectively in a behavioral context. Within the socioeconomic sphere, it is measured by decreased productivity and represents a major loss for society (Gatchel et al., 1986). Physically, it presents as impaired performance of functional tasks and is frequently accompanied by

191

psychological symptoms, such as depression, anxiety, somatization, and alcohol and drug abuse (Kinney, Polatin, & Gatchel, 1990; Lillo, Gatchel, Polatin, & Mayer, 1991); these symptoms are all well-established concomitants of chronic pain, but are themselves also significant causes of disability. Legally, it is associated with claims for financial compensation based on alleged inability to work, suffering as a result of injury, and the defining of fault with others.

Defining disability within the context of physical function has advantages. It is far less subjective than self-report, as long as certain criteria are met (see also Robinson, Chapter 14, this volume). Initial measures provide a baseline that may define the disabled state as an existing physical entity—the *deconditioning syndrome* (Kondraske, 1986; Mayer & Gatchel, 1989; Mayer & Polatin, 1994)—which the patient can more easily accept than traditional concepts of "dysfunctional" pain. This makes him or her more accessible not only to corrective functional restoration, but to educational and psychotherapeutic interventions as well. Agencies involved in the definition and treatment of disability may be more responsive to human performance measures that directly address the disabled state within the context of the workplace. And, finally, outcome may be more objectively defined by posttreatment functional capacity measures, whereas modification of self-report of pain alone does not necessarily lead to elimination of low back disability (Sturgess, Schaefer, & Sikora, 1984).

The term *deconditioning syndrome* refers to the cumulative physical changes found in chronically disabled patients suffering from spinal dysfunction—changes that have occurred as a result of disuse (Mayer, 2000; Mayer & Gatchel, 1989). Repetitive microtrauma, spinal soft tissue disruption, and perhaps surgery have precipitated scarring, and this has been accompanied by immobilization and inactivity. Muscle atrophy is not as easily discernible in the low back as it is in a dysfunctional extremity, which is readily compared to the unimpaired side. Nevertheless, atrophy of the abdominal flexor and trunk extensor muscle groups has been identified even at a relatively early stage of immobilization (Deyo, Diehl, & Rosenthal, 1986; Hadler, 1986; Mayer & Gatchel, 1988) and almost invariably after posterior lumbar surgery (Rantanen, Hurme, Falck, & Alaranta, 1993; Scapinelli & Candiotto, 1994). The lumbar facet joints typically involved in back extension become immobilized with inactivity, causing progressive loss of joint function and range of motion. With disuse, car-

diovascular fitness and neuromuscular coordination deteriorate. These physical changes result in a patient who is actually exercise-intolerant, with true muscular weakness, lumbar stiffness, poor endurance, and impaired fine motor coordination (Polatin, 1990). Pain sensitivity invariable accompanies this dysfunctional state (Clauw et al., 1999). Prolonged inactivity has therefore exacerbated and perpetuated a state of physical disability that may be individually defined through functional quantification measures. Subsequent efforts at correction through functional restoration represent a valid alternative treatment approach for this patient group.

CRITERIA FOR QUANTIFICATION TESTING

Physical measures of human performance must adhere to certain basic requirements to be useful (Mayer & Gatchel, 1988, 1989; Polatin, 1990). First, a test must be physiologically relevant (i.e., it must measure a specific and defined capacity and not reflect extraneous information). For example, strength of a specific muscle group such as trunk extensors is not accurately measured by a whole body task such as lifting (Gracovetsky & Farfan, 1986). The test must also be valid; in other words, the measurement device must be accurate in its measurement. There must be reproducibility, such that repeatable and precise measurements of a clinical variable are possible—both by the same tester (intertest reliability) and by different testers (interrater reliability). A valid test may not be reproducible, and vice versa. Although an invalid test is useless, problems of reproducibility may be corrected by altering the test protocol (see Dworkin & Sherman, Chapter 32).

A relevant, valid, reproducible, and reliable functional test of human performance will have no clinical value unless it can identify suboptimal effort. Otherwise, invalid low readings may be interpreted as true functional deficits when actually they may be more reflective of poor motivation, pain sensitivity, emotional distress, or malingering. Therefore, each individual test of function must have a built-in mechanism to assess effort.

A relevant, large normative database is required for a test of human performance in order for any meaningful clinical interpretive statement to be made. The larger the database, the more specific the interpretation may be. With very large databases, one is able to extract meaningful information with regard to such variables as age, gender, occupation, structural lesion, or postsurgical status (Mayer, Gatchel, Keeley, Mayer, & Richland, 1991). Because of the proliferation of different test protocols and testing devices in recent years, the size of the normative database must be carefully assessed. Newer devices may have relatively smaller databases than ones that have been in use for an extended period of time, although they may have proven themselves in terms of other criteria for utility and applicability.

TESTS OF FUNCTIONAL CAPACITY IN THE LUMBAR SPINE

There is no single test that can adequately assess lumbar function, but evaluation of separate physical capabilities may be combined to give a statement of functional capacity. Range of motion, particularly in the sagittal plane, provides important information about the functioning of the intervertebral disc and facet joints. Trunk strength is controlled by a number of specific muscle groups moving the lumbar spine in flexion and extension, as well as in rotation, abduction, and adduction. These include the intrinsic muscles (erector spinae, multifidum, quadratus lumborum, psoas, and deep interspinalis and intertransversalis) as well as the extrinsic muscles (abdominal, glutealis, latissimus dorsi, and posterior thigh muscles). When the lumbopelvic unit is isolated by some sort of restraint, the strength of the intrinsic extensors and extrinsic flexors is being measured without the contribution of other extrinsic groups, to give information about isolated trunk strength. Tests of task performance involving the lumbar spine are typically lifting tests, in which the trunk is not isolated. Some give information about maximum weight lifted under defined conditions, whereas others address frequent, repetitive capability to lift over time. The former may address occasional lifting capacity, while the latter delineate lifting endurance. Other tests of work capacity may address other functional tasks less directly related to the low back, such as sitting tolerance, crawling, stooping, bending, or shifting. Assessment of cardiovascular endurance provides important information about overall physical conditioning, as delineated by the work capacity of the body's most important muscle, the heart.

To measure strength and lifting capacity, different technologies may be utilized (Mayer & Gatchel, 1988). *Isometric* testing measures the maximum force a muscle or group of muscles can generate in contraction. It is the most well-established technique, particularly for lifting capacity, but lacks dynamic measurement capability. There is also greater risk for muscle strain with truly maximal exertions. *Isokinetic* testing has the advantage of providing a measurement of dynamic performance with methodology that "locks in" the speed and acceleration variables so that they become known quantities. Torque or force then becomes the only independent variable, making calculation of both interindividual and intraindividual differences relatively easy. Other dependent variables, such as work and power, can be derived from computer-generated curves. *Isodynamic* testing measures torques and position changes occurring around multiple centers. No motion is permitted until a preselected minimum torque is produced, after which the acceleration and velocity increase in proportion to the degree to which a torque exceeds the preset minimum. Therefore, as torque varies, acceleration and velocity also vary without control. Finally, *isotonic* or *isoinertial* testing holds the mass constant or progresses it while the subject does a whole-body motion (lifting) sequentially, and velocity is not controlled. We have found the isokinetic and isotonic testing most helpful in assessing the strength and lifting capacity aspects of lumbar function, although less accurate isometric testing of trunk extensor endurance can still yield useful data with less expensive testing equipment.

Techniques for Measuring Range of Motion

Many of the techniques currently used to measure range of motion in the lumbar spine fail to fulfill necessary criteria of validity, relevance, reproducibility, and effort assessment. Gross lumbar flexion and extension actually consist of motion at the hips as well as at the five lumbar motion segments. Conventional "fingertip-to-floor" and goniometric techniques fail to separate out this compound motion and are therefore invalid. In addition, they have intertest and interrater variability difficulties and include no effort assessment. Three-dimensional digitizers, computerized inclinometers, optical scanners, video combined with light-emitting diodes, and multiposition X-ray imaging are all of research interest, but far too expensive and complicated for general utility in the clinical environment (Brown, Burstein, Nash, & Schock, 1976; Dopf, Mandel, Geiger, & Mayer, 1994; Pearcy, Portek, & Sheperd,

1985; Salisbury & Porter, 1987; Stokes, Wilder, Frymoyer, & Pope, 1980; Whittle, 1982).

The two inclinometer technique has proven to be the most useful method of measuring spinal mobility, and it has been accepted as the preferred test in the third and fourth editions of the *American Medical Association Guides to the Evaluation of Permanent Impairment* (Engelberg, 1988, 1993). An *inclinometer* is a circular fluid-filled disc with a weighted gravity pendulum that remains oriented in the vertical direction; it is readily obtainable in hardware stores, but is also now marketed specifically for mobility testing (see Figure 11.1, top). There is also a more expensive computerized version, the EDI-320 (see Figure 11.1, bottom).

With the patient standing erect, the T12–L1 interspace is identified, as is a point over the convex surface of the sacrum. The first inclinometer is applied over the sacrum, parallel to the spine. The second inclinometer is aligned in the sagittal plane, bridging the T12–L1 spinous processes. The trunk must be in the neutral position while the inclinometers are "zeroed out." The patient is then asked to flex forward maximally while maintaining the knees in extension, and at full flexion the two inclinometers are read. The upper (T12–L1) inclinometer gives the "gross flexion" reading, whereas the lower (sacral) inclinometer gives hip flexion. True lumbar flexion is obtained by subtracting hip flexion from gross flexion and represents motion at the five lumbar segments.

After the patient is returned to the neutral position, he or she is asked to extend maximally, and similar readings are taken, thereby deriving gross lumbar extension, hip extension, and true lumbar extension.

This technique has demonstrated relevance and validity. Sagittal measurements correlate accurately with true lumbar flexion and extension readings obtained on lumbar flexion and extension X-rays (Mayer, Kishino, et al., 1985). Intratester and intertester reliability have been established, as well as a normative database (Keeley et al., 1986). The assessment of effort is provided by measuring maximal supine straight-leg raising (SLR) bilaterally. The inclinometer is placed on each tibial spine with both knees extended. In supine SLR, hamstrings are initially stretched to maximal extensibility, and then the pelvis starts to flex until it is restrained by maximum hyperextension of the contralateral hip. Therefore, SLR should be very close to hip motion, and if the tightest SLR exceeds total sacral (hip) motion by more than 10 degrees, effort has been suboptimal.

In the two-inclinometer technique, a compound motion is being measured, and values are being derived for each component of that motion (i.e., hip and true lumbar flexion and extension). A linear relationship between true lumbar flexion and hip flexion has been demonstrated through the gross lumbar flexion arc for normal subjects (see Figure 11.2) (Mayer et al., 1984). Therefore,

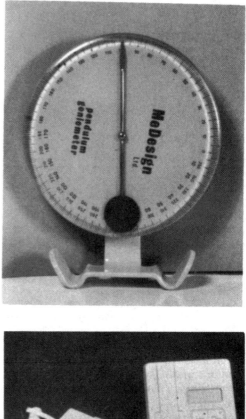

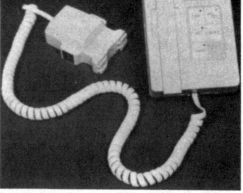

FIGURE 11.1. *Top*: Inclinometer to measure range of motion. *Bottom*: The EDI-320. Reprinted by permission of PRIDE, Dallas, TX.

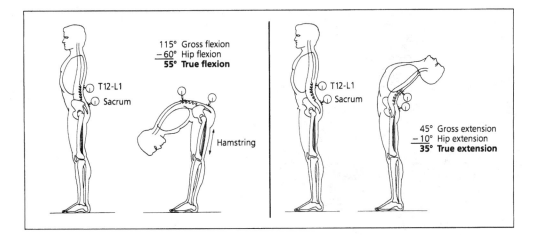

FIGURE 11.2. Two-inclinometer technique to measure spinal range of motion (flexion and extension). From Mayer, Kishino, Keeley, Mayer, and Mooney (1985). Copyright 1985 by PRIDE. Reprinted by permission.

even with identified suboptimal effort and limited gross lumbar flexion, it is still possible to identify structural abnormality by comparing the ratio of true lumbar flexion to hip flexion.

For example, one patient gives the following readings on measurement of lumbar mobility by the two-inclinometer method: gross lumbar flexion, 50 degrees; gross lumbar extension, 15 degrees; sacral (hip) flexion, 20 degrees; sacral (hip) extension, 5 degrees; true lumbar flexion, 30 degrees; true lumbar extension, 10 degrees; and bilateral SLR, 70 degrees. In this case, the SLR exceeds hip mobility by 45 degrees, thereby indicating suboptimal effort. However, the ratio of true lumbar to hip flexion is within normal limits, even if the gross flexion was "held back," thereby indicating that there is no disruption of the normal spine–hip ratio during this flexion movement.

This technique also allows accurate measurement of lateral bend in the lumbar spine. Maintaining the same positions for the first and second inclinometers, the patient is next asked to bend the trunk maximally to the right after "zeroing out" the inclinometers, then to resume neutral position and bend maximally to the left.

The measurement of compound lumbar motion may be adopted for the use of a single inclinometer by conducting each measurement separately, or similarly for the use of the computerized EDI-320 (Figure 11.3). There are some clinicians who find the measurement of total lumbosacral motion at the T12–L1 interspace alone to be adequate, at least to define initial deficits and gauge treatment progress (Rainville, Sobel, & Hartigan, 1994).

Trunk Strength Testing

The various devices for measuring trunk strength are tools with proven research and clinical utility (Flores, Gatchel, & Polatin, 1997). However, they are expensive and require training to be used properly to generate meaningful data. The lumbopelvic unit must be isolated in either the standing, sitting, side-lying, prone, or supine position, thus offering a variety of physiologically induced motion restriction and gravity effects (Mayer & Gatchel, 1989). The isokinetic devices, although not "true to life," do allow accurate measurement of torque, with proven validity and repeatability (Langrana & Lee, 1984; Smith, Mayer, Gatchel, & Becker, 1985).

Trunk flexion, trunk extension, and right and left torso rotation–peak torque can be generated, as well as specific curve shape, from which average-points curve, maximum-points curve, best work repetition curve, and power numbers may be derived (see Figure 11.4). By analyzing the discrepancy between the same points on three separate test curves produced under identical testing conditions, the computer may also generate the "average-points variance" (APV), which has proven to be an assessment of effort on the testing equipment we use, which are the Cybex Isokinetic TEF (torso extension–flexion) and TR (torso rotation) devices (see Figure 11.5 on page 197). This equipment also has the capability to measure isometrically. Other isokinetic/isometric options include the Lido Back System (Loredan, Davis, CA) , Kin-Com (Chatteck, Knoxville, TN), and Biodex Back Attachment (Biodex, New York, NY). The Med-X

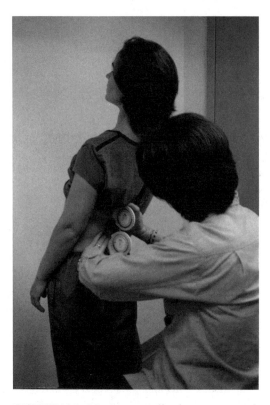

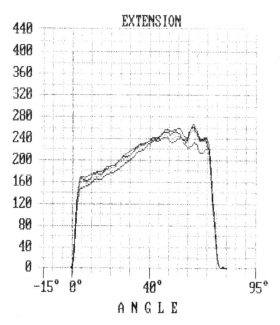

FIGURE 11.4. Cybex isokinetic trunk extensor strength graph for three separate efforts. Reprinted by permission of PRIDE, Dallas, TX.

FIGURE 11.3. Measurement of lumbar extension with two inclinometers. From Mayer and Gatchel (1988). Copyright 1988 by PRIDE. Reprinted by permission.

lumbar extension device testing and rehabilitation device (Med-X, Ocala, FL) measures only isometrically. The Isostation B-200 (Isotechnologies, Raleigh, NC) uses isodynamic technology. It is unusual in that it can measure strength across three axes of rotation, either separately or in combination. Different testing devices have been on the market for different periods of time, with varying normative databases and sometimes differing clinical applications.

There are also several "low-tech" ways of assessing trunk extensor endurance without expensive equipment. The Sorenson test is performed by timing a subject's sustained prone lumbar extension on a table with appropriate restraining straps or on a Roman chair (Biering-Sørenson, 1984). Timing prone static positioning while holding the sternum off the floor, with a pillow under the abdomen to decrease lumbar lordosis, has also been described (Ito, Osamu, Suzuki, & Takahashi, 1996). Rainville and colleagues employ a protocol utilizing the Cybex Eagle back extension machine (Lumex, Ronkonkoma, NY), which is based on

the maximum amount of weight that a patient can lift in four repetitions, beginning with one plate (9.1 kg) and progressing in a standardized manner depending on performance to a specific endpoint (Rainville, Sobel, Hartigan, & Wright, 1997).

Tests of Lifting Capacity

Unlike the isolated trunk strength tests, devices for testing lifting capacity do not stabilize the body above and below the lumbopelvic musculoskeletal unit. Isometric and isokinetic lift tests are not "natural" or "whole-body" tests, in that they impose some restrictions on lifting that remove certain variables present in actual lifting tasks, such as speed and acceleration or position, to allow more precise and reproducible measurements. For instance, the isometric devices used in industry by the National Institute of Occupational Safety and Health standardize a lift by having the patient pull at a bar at a predetermined height above the ground in a straight-back, bent-knee position (leg lift), or a straight-knee, bent-back position (torso lift). Isokinetic devices allow lifting in a more dynamic way, substituting a lifting hand on a cable attached to a dynamometer and thereby permitting a wider selection of body positions and lifting styles during

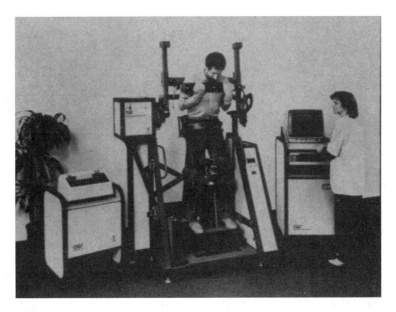

FIGURE 11.5. The Cybex TEF device for the measurement of trunk strength. Reprinted by permission of PRIDE, Dallas, TX.

a test protocol. As in the isokinetic trunk strength testing, with acceleration and speed controlled, the force exerted along the cable and in line with the dynamometer is what is recorded; this allows the derivation of peak force, curve shape, work performed, power consumed, and APV as an effort assessment (see Figures 11.6 and 11.7).

Again, normative databases are essential in using these devices, with previously defined standardized protocols. Our clinical experience has been with the Cybex Liftask (see Figure 11.8), utilizing a three-speed (18 inches/second, 30 inches/second, and 376 inches/second) testing protocol (Kishino et al., 1985). The database has been expanded to include workers in different job categories, as well as comparative norms (Mayer et al., 1991). Other isometric and isokinetic devices include the Lido Lift (Loredan, Davis, CA) and the Ergometrics Strength Testing Unit (Ergometrics, Ann Arbor, MI) (Flores et al., 1997). Whereas the Cybex and Lido devices

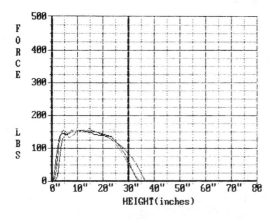

FIGURE 11.6. Isokinetic lifting capacity as measured on Cybex Liftask with three repetitions. Reprinted by permission of PRIDE, Dallas, TX.

```
cybex
PATIENT NAME:
LIFTASK - EXT KNEES/EXT BACK
CYBEX TEST DATE(S)        1/16/1993

SPEED (in/sec)        R 18    30    36
REPETITIONS              3     3     3
START HEIGHT (in.)      00    00    00
END HEIGHT (in.)        29    29    29
BODY WEIGHT (lbs)           (171)

PEAK FORCE (lbs)        125   107    98
PEAK FORCE % BW         73%   62%   57%
HEIGHT OF PEAK FORCE    20    20    17
FORCE @     INCHES
FORCE @     INCHES


TOTAL WORK (BWR,ftlbs)  238   188   148
TOTAL WORK (BWR) %BW   139%  109%   86%
AVG.POWER (BWR,WATTS)   202   266   259
AVG.POWER (BWR) %BW    118%  155%  151%
AVG.FORCE (BWR,lbs)     98    77    61
AVG.FORCE (BWR) %BW     57%   45%   35%
AVG.POINTS VARIANCE     18%   20%   18%
```

FIGURE 11.7. Cybex Liftask data sheet. Reprinted by permission of PRIDE, Dallas, TX.

are limited to vertical lifting, the Ergometrics machine has attachments that enable it also to assess multiplanar lifting capabilities.

However, dynamic psychophysical tests, in which no restriction of activity occurs, are also useful, and more directly address such aspects of performance as task endurance and neuromuscular coordination. The Progressive Isoinertial Lifting Evaluation is one such test (Mayer, Barnes, Kishino, et al., 1988; Mayer et al., 1990) (see Figure 11.9). The protocol involves the lifting of weights in a plastic box from floor to waist (0–30 inches) and waist to shoulder height (30–54 inches). Women begin with a 5-pound load, while men begin with a 10-pound load, and weight is increased by an amount equal to the initial weight every 20 seconds, with a rate of eight lifting movements (four lifting cycles) in each 20-second period. A lifting cycle consists of two lifting movements to return to the starting point (i.e., from floor to waist to floor).

The patient is unaware of the actual amount of weight in the box. The test is terminated when the first of the following endpoints is achieved: (1) fatigue or pain (psychophysical endpoint); (2) achievement of 85% of age-determined "maximum heart rate," unless cardiac precautions are in force (aerobic endpoint); or (3) predetermined safe limits of 45%–55% of body weight (safety endpoint). Results are expressed as (1) maximum weight lifted at the lumbar and cervical levels (floor to waist and waist to overhead), (2) the endurance time to discontinuation for each test, and (3) the final heart rate. Because distance and repetitions are also known, calculations of work and power

consumption are possible and may be normalized to body weight. A normative database exists for this test. An assessment of effort is provided by comparing the final heart rate with the target. With the endurance factor incorporated in the test, it gives a repeatable and objective measure of frequent lifting capacity, which can be translated to job requirements or utilized in training protocols.

Test of Aerobic Capacity (Cardiovascular Endurance)

The most commonly used measure to define aerobic fitness is maximum aerobic capacity (VO_2 max), usually estimated indirectly by means of a step test, bicycle ergometer, or treadmill protocol. Because heart rate increases with increasing oxygen uptake or workload (Astrand & Rodahl, 1977), heart rate may be paired with workloads to predict VO_2 max. Because maximum tests have more intrinsic risks and require more careful monitoring, submaximal tests are more applicable. Both bicycle ergometer and treadmill protocols have demonstrated reliability and validity. Although the treadmill is preferable for maximum tests, the advantage of one over the other for submaximal tests is minimal (Battié, 1991). Patients with back pain have been found to tolerate the bicycle ergometer better, however, and so we use this type of protocol (Mayer & Gatchel, 1988). Testing begins at a predetermined work rate and progresses at regular intervals until the target heart rate (85% of age-related maximum) is reached. The result is expressed as final work rate, the time for the test, and

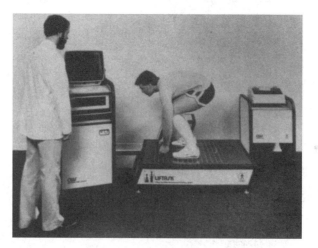

FIGURE 11.8. Cybex Liftask. Reprinted by permission of PRIDE, Dallas, TX.

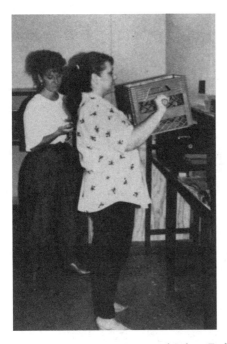

FIGURE 11.9. Progressive Isoinertial Lifting Evaluation. Reprinted by permission of PRIDE, Dallas, TX.

rate of final heart rate to target (as a measurement of effort).

An identical test has been devised, with similarly established normative database, utilizing repetitive cycling motion of the arms instead of the legs. This is the upper-body ergometer, but it is less a test of cardiovascular capacity than of upper-extremity strength and endurance, because the blood vessels supplying the upper extremities are of significantly smaller diameter than those supplying the lower extremities, and thus the cardiovascular demand is less. Nevertheless, in an individual with impaired lower-extremity function, it may provide the only useful endurance test obtainable, with similarly built-in validity, reliability, and some effort assessment. As an upper-extremity endurance test, it also has intrinsic value, particularly in the context of rehabilitation (Mayer & Gatchel, 1988).

Task-Specific Testing

Although human performance evaluation can be very sophisticated, its clinical applicability to functional assessment is still somewhat limited. Ease of administration and cost of the testing are the major problems for the most valid, reliable, and accurate protocols. However, functional task per-

formance is an essential element of occupational therapy and is generally used in *work hardening*, a rehabilitation treatment that focuses on repetitive task training for specific job activities to develop stamina, neuromuscular coordination, and appropriate vocational behaviors.

In the assessment of spinal function, no specific task performance devices stand out as universally applicable at the present time. The multiple-task obstacle course is currently being used in several spine centers (Mayer & Gatchel, 1988). Task performance measured on a structured progression of physical activities that simulate job demands at the workplace delineated on form CA-17 of the U.S. Department of Labor Duty Status Report. There are other devices, in various states of development, that serve a similar function.

USES OF QUANTIFICATION

For tests of lumbar function to be useful, the results must be expressed in relation to deviation from normal, with a medical interpretive summary that integrates the results of the various tests previously described. Such a report, which in our facility is termed a Quantitative Functional Evaluation (QFE), is shown in Figure 11.10.

As an initial evaluation, functional quantification defines the current physical capabilities of the patient's lumbar spine, assuming good effort on testing. The overall level of effort can be accurately determined by reviewing the effort factor for each individual test. But even with suboptimal or poor effort, an initial QFE is a clinical statement of how functional this patient will allow him- or herself to be. Consistently poor effort has meaning in itself, as does inconsistent effort (Kaplan, Wurtele, & Gillis, 1996). Therefore, an initial QFE allows an identification of functional level and raises the issue of psychosocial barriers to functional recovery that may subsequently be identified by further information gathering.

As a statement of disability, only the range-of-motion test of the QFE has recognized validity as defined by the revised *American Medical Association Guides to the Evaluation of Permanent Impairment* (Engelberg, 1988, 1993). In this context, validity has to be strictly controlled. The measurements must be repeated three times and must be consistent with 10% or 5 degrees, whichever is greater. The difference between the tightest SLR and hip flexion plus extension must be less than 10 degrees on each of these repetitions. If valid,

```
Patient Name:
SS#            :
DOI            : 03/06/1990
PT/OT Test     : 06/27/1991   06/27/1991 PRE
```

THORACOLUMBAR QUANTITATIVE FUNCTIONAL EVALUATION

This individual underwent a Quantitative Functional Evaluation which
is a battery of tests of spinal physical capacity. This information
may be used to determine medical impairment of function. % Normal
ratings are based on a limited clinical sample; a large standardized
normative database is being assembled and constantly updated.

```
SELF-REPORT SCORES                PHYSICAL CAPACITY
  Beck Depression        0          Physical Status         R / L
  Pain Drawing                      Neurological Deficit    - / -
    Intensity Score      1/10       FABER                   - / -
    Trunk                2/72     DEFORMITY/POSTURE
    Extremities          0/136      Surgical Scar:          Yes
  Disability Analog      24/150
```

```
LUMBAR RANGE OF MOTION        SAGITTAL                 CORONAL
                              DEGREES                  DEGREES
                     FLEX(% norm)/ EXT(% norm)   RIGHT(% norm)/LEFT(% norm)
  Gross Motion       92 ( 76%) /  26 ( 57%)      40 (114%) / 34 ( 97%)
  True Lumbar        57 ( 87%) /  22 ( 73%)      22 ( 88%) / 22 ( 88%)
  Hip Motion         35 ( 63%) /   4 ( 26%)      20 (200%) / 12 (120%)
  Str.Leg Raise R/L  57 ( 76%) /  59 ( 78%)
  True Spine/Hip Flex Ratio: 162%: Normal ratio probably normal
                                    spine flexibility
  Effort Factor               Fair
```

```
TRUNK STRENGTH (CYBEX)
  Isokinetic Sagittal    PEAK TORQUE (ft-lb)          WORK (lb-ft)
                      FLEX(% norm)/ EXT(% norm)   FLEX(% norm)/ EXT(% norm)
    60/second         199 ( 75%) / 180 ( 52%)     223 ( 77%) / 185 ( 48%)
    120/second        120 ( 45%) / 149 ( 46%)     108 ( 40%) / 149 ( 44%)
    150/second        180 ( 69%) / 161 ( 54%)     163 ( 64%) / 146 ( 50%)
    HSD (Work)             (150/60)               73% (abn) / 79% (nor)
    F/E Ratios (Work) (60/120/150)  120%(abn) /   72% (NL ) / 111% (abn)
    Avg. Pts. Variance  (F/E) at 60/sec.          24         / 25
```

```
CARDIOVASCULAR ENDURANCE        BICYCLE ERGOMETRY      UPPER BODY ERGOMETRY
  Work Rate(Watts)/End. Time     125 / 9:00           131 / 5:15
  Heart Rate/Target              124 / 161             96 / 161
  mVO2(ml/kg/min)/Mets [Calories] 61 / 17             [ 50]
  Fitness Level/Effort Factor    High                 Poor
```

OCCUPATIONAL CAPACITY

```
Working ?                                        No
Job Demand Category (Previous / Anticipated)     4 / N.A.
```

```
Patient Name:                          Test Date: 06/27/1991

Job Lifting Requirements            FLOOR-WAIST       WAIST-OVERHEAD
  Frequent  (lbs)                       50                50
  Occasional (lbs)                    100-120           100-120

Frequent Lifting Capacity           FLOOR-WAIST       WAIST-OVERHEAD
  Final Force (lbs) (% norm)         33 ( 35%)         33 ( 43%)
  Total Work (lb-ft) (% norm)        1380 ( 16%)       1104 ( 20%)
  End.Time (sec) / Power (watts)     60 / 31.3         60 / 25.0
  Final HR / Effort                  88 / Poor         84 / Poor

Isometric Lifting Capacity          MAX-FORCE
  Leg Lift Capacity  (lbs) (% norm)  275( 91%)
  Torso Lift Capacity (lbs) (% norm) 217( 72%)
  Arm Lift Capacity  (lbs) (% norm)  N.A.

Dynamic Isokinetic Lift              PEAK FORCE / POWER
       Lbs.(%n)/WATTS(%n)    Lbs.(%n)/WATTS(%n)    Lbs.(%n)/WATTS(%n)
       18 in/sec.            30 in/sec.            36 in/sec.
Lumbar 240( 71%)/ 370( 70%) 199( 61%)/ 516( 65%)  185( 58%)/ 566( 63%)
Avg. Pts. Variance (Lumbar/Cervical) at 18 in/sec.  28        /
```

```
GLOBAL SCORES
  CUMULATIVE SCORE:      THIS TEST
    Average Test (%)       66
  TEST VALIDITY/EFFORT   Physical Therapy     Occupational Therapy
                            GOOD                   GOOD
```

SUMMARY
Mild pain/disability self-report in a patient with mild true lumbar mobility
deficits associated with severe extensor trunk strength deficits with a reversed
extensor/flexor ratio and high aerobic capacity. The patient's lifting capacity
is at moderately deficient range with drop-off particularly where endurance is
required, but with good effort indicating a patient who should be a good
candidate for functional restoration.

```
Test Interpretation By:
Tom G. Mayer, M.D.

TGM:ptb
```

FIGURE 11.10. Full Quantitative Functional Evaluation (QFE) report.
Reprinted by permission of PRIDE, Dallas, TX.

this measurement may be used in correlating a whole-body medical impairment rating.

An initial QFE has additional usefulness in defining treatment goals for functional restoration to correct the previously delineated deconditioning syndrome and to educate the patient about the existence of these initial functional deficits. Having completed testing, he or she is far more ready to understand the results, and may even be surprised at how poorly he or she has done.

Serial quantification, however, has additional uses. For the patient and the treatment team, retests after a period of rehabilitation provide objective feedback of progress. For the team, serial QFEs help to identify compliance problems and psychosocial barriers in patients who may be giving only lip service to functional recovery. Lack of progress is primarily a result of lack of optimal effort. Mobility, strength, endurance, and neuromuscular coordination *always* improve if the appropriate physical training is taking place. These objective data then allow the treatment team to confront a resistant patient in spite of his or her denial, and then to help him or her overcome whatever barrier may be interfering with the training effort.

A patient who has progressed in functional restoration always shows an improved effort on testing at the end of rehabilitation. This posttreatment QFE is then a valid statement of functional capacity and will allow the treatment team to delineate functional capability to return to a particular job or to "fine-tune" a patient's functional profile for a particular job.

Finally, tracking during a 2-year period after functional restoration, with QFEs repeated at intervals after treatment, allows the physician and the treatment team to follow these patients in a meaningful way and to identify functional deficits if they recur as a result of "slacking off" on prescribed home exercise programs. A normal functional profile is the best defense against recurrent injury for a patient with low back pain, and serial testing allows preventive screening to be enforced (Mayer & Gatchel, 1989).

SUMMARY

Quantification of function in chronic low back pain introduces a degree of objectivity into the clinical assessment and treatment of a problematic patient group. In so doing, it may enhance the effectiveness of more traditional pain modulation techniques. Quantification serves to define the initial

deconditioning state, to document functional improvements in rehabilitation, and to delineate an endpoint from which a patient can resume a normal life. Thereafter, serial testing of previously attained functional gains may delineate recurrent risk factors for reinjury, so that preventive measures may be taken. Therefore, quantification of function is a tool to define disability in physical and ergonomic terms, to guide rehabilitation, to correct functional deficits, to establish a therapeutic endpoint for such disability, and to utilize for relapse prevention. When these techniques of measurement are employed, traditional pain management therapies and physical rehabilitation techniques may be integrated into an interdisciplinary program with enhanced effectiveness.

REFERENCES

Andersson, G. (1981). Epidemiologic aspects on low-back pain in industry. *Spine, 6,* 53–60.

Astrand, P.-O., & Rodahl, K. (1977). *Textbook of work physiology: Physiological bases for exercise* (2nd ed.). New York: McGraw-Hill.

Battié, M. (1991). Aerobic fitness and its measurement. *Spine, 16,* 677–678.

Beals, R. (1984). Compensation and recovery from injury. *Western Journal of Medicine, 140,* 233–237.

Biering-Sørenson, F. (1984). Physical measurements as risk indicators for low back trouble over a one-year period. *Spine, 9,* 106–118.

Brown, R., Burstein, A., Nash, C., & Schock, C. (1976). Spinal analysis using a three-dimensional radiographic technique. *Journal of Biomechanics, 9,* 355–365.

Cady, L., Bischoff, D., O'Connell, E., Thomas, P., & Allen, J. (1979). Strength and fitness and subsequent back injuries in firefighters. *Journal of Occupational Medicine, 21,* 269–272.

Chaffin, D. (1978). Pre-employment strength testing: An updated position. *Journal of Occupational Medicine, 10,* 105–110.

Clauw, D., Williams, D., Lauerman, W., Dahlman, M., Aslami, A., Nachemson, A., Kobrine, A., & Wiesel, S. (1999). Pain sensitivity as a correlate of clinical status in individuals with chronic low back pain. *Spine, 24,* 2035–2041.

Deyo, R., Diehl, A., Rosenthal, M. (1986). How many days of bedrest for acute low back pain? *New England Journal of Medicine, 315,* 1064–1070.

Dopf, C., Mandel, S., Geiger, D., & Mayer, P. (1994). Analysis of spine motion variability using a computerized goniometer compared to physical examination: A prospective clinical study. *Spine, 19,* 586–595.

Engelberg, A. (Ed.). (1988). *American Medical Association guides to the evaluation of permanent impairment* (3rd ed.). Chicago: American Medical Association.

Engelberg, A. (Ed.). (1993). *American Medical Association guides to the evaluation of permanent impairment* (4th ed.). Chicago: American Medical Association.

Flores, L., Gatchel, R., & Polatin, P. (1997). Objectification of functional improvement after nonoperative care. *Spine, 22,* 1622-1633.

Fordyce, W., Roberts, A., & Sternbach, R. (1985). The behavioral management of chronic pain: A response to critics. *Pain, 22,* 113-125.

Gatchel, R., Mayer, T., Capra, P., Diamond, P., & Barnett, J. (1986). Quantification of lumbar function: Part 6. The use of psychological measures in guiding physical functional restoration. *Spine, 11,* 36-42.

Gracovetsky, S., & Farfan, H. (1986). The optimum spine. *Spine, 11,* 543-573.

Hadler, N. (1986). Regional back pain. *New England Journal of Medicine, 315,* 1090-1092.

Ito, T., Osamu, S., Suzuki, H., & Takahashi, M. (1996). Lumbar trunk muscle endurance testing: An inexpensive alternative to a machine for evaluation. *Archives of Physical Medicine and Rehabilitation, 77,* 75-79.

Kaplan, G., Wurtele, S., & Gillis, D. (1996). Maximum effort during functional capacity evaluations: An examination of psychological factors. *Archives of Physical Medicine and Rehabilitation, 77,* 161-164.

Keeley, J., Mayer, T., Cox, R., Gatchel, R., Smith, J., & Mooney, V. (1986). Quantification of lumbar function: Part 5. Reliability of range of motion measures in the sagittal plane and an in vivo torso rotation measurement technique. *Spine, 11,* 31-35.

Kinney, R., Polatin, P., & Gatchel, R. (1990). *The high incidence of psychiatric disorder in chronic low back pain patients.* Paper presented at the annual meeting of the International Society for the Study of the Lumbar Spine, Boston.

Kishino, N., Mayer, T., Gatchel, R., Parrish, M., Anderson, C., Gustin, L., & Mooney, V. (1985). Quantification of lumbar function: Part 4. Isometric and isokinetic lifting simulation in normal subjects and low back dysfunction patients. *Spine, 10,* 921-927.

Kondraske, G. (1986). Towards a standard clinical measure of postural stability. *Proceedings of the 8th Annual Conference of the IEEE Engineering in Medicine and Biology Society, 3,* 1579-1582.

Langrana, N., & Lee, C. (1984). Isokinetic evaluation of trunk muscles. *Spine, 9,* 171-175.

Lillo, E., Gatchel, R., Polatin, P., & Mayer, T. (1991). *The prevalence of major psychiatric disorders in chronic low back pain patients: A replication study.* Paper presented at the annual meeting of the North American Spine Society, Keystone, CO.

Mayer, T. (2000). Quantitative physical and functional capacity assessment. In T. G. Mayer, R. J. Gatchel, & P. B. Polatin (Eds.), *Occupational musculoskeletal disorders: Function, outcomes and evidence* (pp. 36-50). Philadelphia: Lippincott Williams & Wilkins.

Mayer, T., Barnes, D., Kishino, N., Nichols, G., Gatchel, R., Mayer, H., & Mooney, V. (1988). Progressive isoinertial lifting evaluation: I. A standardized protocol and normative database. *Spine, 13,* 993-997.

Mayer, T., Barnes, D., Nichols, G., Kishino, N. D., Coval, K., Piel, B., Hoshino, D., & Gatchel, R. J. (1988). Progressive isoinertial lifting evaluation: Part II. A comparison with isokinetic lifting in a disabled chronic low-back pain industrial population. *Spine, 13,* 998-1002.

Mayer, T., & Gatchel, R. (1988). *Functional restoration for spinal disorders: The sports medicine approach.* Philadelphia: Lea & Febiger.

Mayer, T., & Gatchel, R. (1989). Functional restoration for chronic low back pain: Part I. Quantifying physical function. *Pain Management, 3,* 67-73.

Mayer, T., Gatchel, R., Barnes, D., Mayer, H., & Mooney, V. (1990). Progressive isoinertial lifting evaluation: An erratum notice. *Spine, 15,* 5.

Mayer, T., Gatchel, R., Keeley, J., Mayer, H., & Richland, D. (1991, June). *Building industrial databases: Physical capacity measurements specific to major job categories in U.S. railroads.* Paper presented at the annual meeting of the International Society for the Study of the Lumbar Spine, Heidelberg, Germany.

Mayer, T., Gatchel, R., Kishino, N., Keeley, J., Mayer, H., Capra, P., & Mooney, V. (1986). A prospective short-term study of chronic low back pain patients utilizing novel objective functional measurement. *Pain, 25,* 53-68.

Mayer, T., Gatchel, R., Mayer, H., Kishino, N., Keeley, J., & Mooney V. (1987). A prospective two-year study of functional restoration in industrial low back injury: An objective assessment procedure. *Journal of the American Medical Association, 258,* 1763-1767.

Mayer, T., Kishino, N., Keeley, J., Mayer, S., & Mooney, V. (1985). Using physical measurements to assess low back pain. *Journal of Musculoskeletal Medicine, 2,* 44-59.

Mayer, T., & Polatin, P. (1994). Spinal rehabilitation. In S. Haldeman (Ed.), *Modern developments in the principles and practice of chiropractic* (2nd ed.). Norwalk, CT: Appleton & Lange.

Mayer, T., Smith, S., Kondraske, G., Gatchel, R., Carmichael, T., & Mooney, V. (1985). Quantification of lumbar function: Part 3. Preliminary data on isokinetic torso rotation testing with myoelectric spectral analysis in normal and low back pain subjects. *Spine, 10,* 912-920.

Mayer, T., Tencer, A., Kristoferson, S., & Mooney, V. (1984). Use of noninvasive techniques for quantification of spinal range-of-motion in normal subjects and chronic low-back dysfunction patients. *Spine, 9,* 588-595.

Mooney, V., Cairns, D., & Robertson, J. (1976). A system for evaluating and treating chronic back disability. *Western Journal of Medicine, 124,* 370-376.

Nachemson, A. (1983). Work for all: For those with low back pain as well. *Clinical Orthopedics and Related Research, 179,* 77-85.

Pearcy, M., Portek, I., & Sheperd, J. (1985). The effect of low back pain on lumbar spine movements measured by three dimensional x-ray analysis. *Spine, 10,* 150-153.

Polatin, P. (1990). The functional restoration approach to chronic low back pain. *Journal of Musculoskeletal Medicine, 7,* 17-30.

Rainville, J., Sobel, J., & Hartigan, C. (1994). Comparison of total lumbosacral flexion and true lumbar flexion measured by a dual inclinometer technique. *Spine, 19,* 2698-2701.

Rainville, J., Sobel, J., Hartigan, C., & Wright, A. (1997). The effect of compensation involvement on the reporting of pain and disability by patients referred for rehabilitation of chronic low back pain. *Spine, 22,* 2016-2024.

Rantanen, J., Hurme, M., Falck, B., & Alaranta, H. (1993). The lumbar multifidus muscle five years after surgery for a lumbar intervertebral disc herniation. *Spine, 18,* 568-574.

Salisbury, P., & Porter, R. (1987). Measurement of lumbar sagittal mobility: A comparison of methods. *Spine*, *12*, 190–193.

Scapinelli, R., & Candiotto, S. (1994). Changes in the paravertebral musculature following a traditional herniated lumbar discectomy: A computed tomographic and magnetic resonance study. *Radiological Medicine (Torino)*, *88*, 209–215.

Smith, S., Mayer, T., Gatchel, R., & Becker, T. (1985). Quantification of lumbar function: Part 1. Isometric and multispeed isokinetic trunk strength measures in sagittal and axial planes in normal subjects. *Spine*, *10*, 757–764.

Stokes, I., Wilder, D., Frymoyer, J., & Pope, M. (1980). Assessment of patients with low back pain by biplanar radiogrphic measurements of intervertebral motion. *Spine*, *6*, 233–240.

Sturgess, E., Schaefer, C., & Sikora, T. (1984). Pain center follow-up study of treated and untreated patients. *Archives of Physical Medicine and Rehabilitation*, *65*, 301–303.

Turk, D., Meichenbaum, D., & Genest, M. (1983). *Pain and behavioral medicine: A cognitive-behavioral perspective*. New York: Guilford Press.

White, A., & Gordon, S. (1982). Synopsis: Workshop on idiopathic low-back pain. *Spine*, *7*, 141–149.

Whittle, M. (1982). Calibration and performance of a three-dimensional television system for kinematic analysis. *Journal of Biomechanics*, *15*, 185–196.

Chapter 12

Physical and Occupational Therapy Assessment Approaches

MICHELE CRITES BATTIÉ
LAURA MAY

Theory has been used to guide and advance practice and research in rehabilitation, as well as to aid in communication. Fundamental to theory development are clarity and consistency in defining important concepts, which can guide the choice and design of relevant outcome measures (Minaire, 1992). The global term of *disablement* reflects all the diverse consequences that disease, injury, or congenital abnormalities may have for human functioning (Jette, 1994). The theory of disablement has been a useful tool in guiding initial patient assessment and measurement of subsequent rehabilitation outcomes for physical and occupational therapy (Law et al., 1999; Mayo et al., 1999; Townsend, Ryan, & Law, 1990; Wagstaff, 1982). This chapter briefly discusses the dominant models of disablement used as foundations for establishing the domains of assessment that are routinely given attention in physical and occupational therapy. Other, more general considerations in selecting measures are reviewed as well. Finally, the selection of generic versus condition-specific assessment tools is discussed, as well as examples of assessment approaches for several conditions commonly seen in physical and occupational therapy.

MODELS OF DISABLEMENT: A THEORETICAL BASIS FOR REHABILITATION PERSPECTIVES

Several conceptual schemes or models have been developed to guide disablement research and the development and selection of appropriate assessment or outcome measures. Although no single conceptual model has been adopted universally, two schemes have garnered the most acceptance. The first is a model developed by a sociologist, Saad Nagi (Nagi, 1965); the second is the model set forth in the *International Classification of Impairments, Disabilities, and Handicaps* (ICIDH), a publication of the World Health Organization (WHO, 1980). The four components of each of these models resemble one another, as demonstrated by Figure 12.1. The basic goal of both schemes is to delineate the major pathways from disease to the variety of consequences that may result. One of the key applications of the models is the ability to identify and measure the consequences. It is important to note that, particularly in the case of pain, these pathways are not always unidirectional.

There is general agreement between the two schemes in regard to the first two components of

Nagi Scheme

Active pathology → Impairment → Functional → Disability
Limitation

ICIDH

Disease → Impairment → Disability → Handicap

FIGURE 12.1. Two conceptual schemes for the disablement process.

the models. Both *active pathology* and *disease* refer to the disruption of normal physiological, biochemical, or anatomical processes and the simultaneous attempts by the body to regain homeostasis. In each model, *impairment* refers to abnormality at the body systems level resulting from any cause, which may involve psychological, physiological, or anatomical structure or function. An impairment represents deviation from some norm in the individual's biomedical status (WHO, 1980). Within both models, pain is considered at the level of impairment.

It is at the level of the individual that these two schemes diverge in their use of terminology. Nagi (1965) uses the term *functional limitations* to represent restrictions in performance at the level of the whole person. This concept of attributes involves indicators that are reflected in the characteristics of the person (Nagi, 1991). It is important to note that a limitation in function at the person level may result from differing impairments at lower levels. For example, the inability to lift heavy objects may be related to mechanical problems in the shoulder joint, or it may be a result of diminished cardiac or pulmonary function. The next level in the Nagi scheme, *disability*, represents a relational concept that cannot be solely accounted for in the attributes of the individual (Nagi, 1965). This term is used to assess the individual's capacities to perform socially defined roles expected within a given sociocultural and physical environment. These roles are organized into spheres of life activities such as family, other interpersonal relations, employment, education, recreation, and self-care. In addition, disability includes subjective aspects as defined by the individual and others and the effect of environmental barriers. An example of the application of these terms would include gait restrictions as a functional limitation and the inability to perform personal care or occupational activities as a disability.

Conversely, in the ICIDH model, the term *disability* is defined as the lack of ability to perform an activity that would be considered normal for that person (WHO, 1980). Within this framework, functional limitations, as defined by Nagi, are regarded as an aspect of impairment concerned with individual functions of the body (WHO, 1980). Thus functional limitations are conceptualized at the organ level rather than the level of the whole body. Disability in the ICIDH scheme is concerned with activity restriction of the person; some indicators include locomotion, personal care, family, and occupational roles. These indicators are noted at the level of the person and are measurable in that the functional limitation expresses itself as a reality in everyday life, without reference to others. Some of the indicators here are said to be referential within the concept of disability in the Nagi model. For example, personal care is viewed as a component of a role or multiple roles, and limitations in performing such tasks often result in reciprocal role relationships of dependence (Nagi, 1991).

The final element of the disablement process in the ICIDH scheme is *handicap*. This term represents the disadvantage for a given individual resulting from the presence of impairments or disabilities that limit the fulfillment of normal roles (WHO, 1980). As opposed to the assessment of the individual's abilities in relation to relevant aspects of his or her situation, handicap is a consequence based on the circumstances of the disabled individual that place him or her at a disadvantage relative to other people. It thus reflects the value society attaches to the disability (Wagstaff, 1982). Categories of handicap include orientation (to surroundings), physical independence, mobility (in the individual's surroundings), occupation (ability to occupy time—work and recreation), social integration (participation in customary social relationships), and economic self-sufficiency (WHO, 1980).

Within rehabilitation, the ICIDH model of disablement has been widely accepted as a basis on which to develop and select assessment and outcome measures (Minaire, 1992; Whiteneck, 1994). The model has been criticized, however, for a lack of emphasis on the role of the environment, failure to identify the causes of the limitations in social performance, and difficulty distinguishing some consequences that may be classified under both the disability and the handicap concepts (Jette, 1994; Minaire, 1992). Fuhrer (1994) sites the need to elaborate on subjective and personal value aspects of impairment, disability and handicap in order to link these concepts to other rehabilitation outcomes that are subjective in nature, such as quality of life (QOL). In order to address the limitations and criticisms, WHO has recently published revisions to the ICIDH model, which has been renamed the *International Classification of Functioning and Disability* (ICIDH-2; WHO, 1999). Within the modified model, the dimensions of the main pathway are now renamed *body functions and structure, activities,* and *participation.* Also included are *contextual factors,* which are denoted by environmental and personal factors and have become an integral component of the model.

Among the other models of the disablement process is the framework described by Verbrugge and Jette (1994), which is primarily based on the Nagi scheme, but also includes some of the ideas and elements of the WHO ICIDH model. They have introduced the concepts of *risk, buffer,* and *exacerbating factors,* which can act to modify the main pathway at any level. This model has been applied in the work of Batterham, Dunt, and Disler (1996) in the development of indicators to assess long-term outcomes for people with disabilities. The U.S. Institute of Medicine model (Pope & Tarlov, 1991), which is also based on the Nagi and ICIDH frameworks, has been proposed to identify and evaluate strategic interventions aimed at disability prevention. The disablement model adopted by the U.S. National Center for Medical Rehabilitation Research (NCMRR) is described by Butler and colleagues (1999) as the model chosen to facilitate the evaluation of treatment outcomes in persons with developmental disabilities. This model is conceptually similar to the model proposed by Nagi (1965), with the addition of another level reflecting the *societal limitations* that impose disablement on a person with a disability. To facilitate a smooth transition, should the ICIDH-2 be universally accepted, it was important that the NCMRR model be comparable to the ICIDH-2. Therefore, the additional level of societal limitation corresponded to the contextual factors level proposed in the ICIDH-2. Occupational therapy practice in Canada is guided by the model of occupational performance, which, although not a model of disablement, has been shown to have comple-

mentary components to those of the ICIDH model (Townsend et al., 1990). With this model as a framework, the Canadian Occupational Performance Measure was developed, and this measure has received much attention on an international level (Law et al., 1990).

PAIN MEASUREMENT AND DISABLEMENT

Pain measurement, according to McDowell and Newell (1996), is "the most challenging and difficult area of subjective health measurement" (p. 335). Regardless of underlying pathology, pain is one of the most frequent complaints of clients seen by physical and occupational therapists. In congruence with models of disablement, both professions incorporate a philosophical framework that includes the concept of *holistic health,* such that practice and evaluation are directed by the physical, psychological, social, and cultural realms of an individual's life. Consequently, the evaluation of pain rarely focuses only on the level of impairment of body function, in which pain is viewed as the exteriorization of the pathological state or a reflection of the disturbance at the organ level. For the rehabilitation professional, this is only a starting point. The effects of painful conditions on other aspects of disablement are also of interest in physical and occupational therapy practice. Thus assessment and outcome measurement often include the levels of disability/activity and handicap/participation, allowing the therapist to consider the consequences of pain. It is also recognized that pain not only can lead to functional, social, or environmental consequences, but can also be influenced by them. Measures of such domains are therefore often used in assessments to establish a baseline for the patient's condition at the time of the initial visit, to determine progress toward therapeutic goals at follow-up, or to determine outcomes at discharge. Deciding on whether to assess some or all of the domains of disablement and the specific selection of measurement tools depends on a variety of factors.

GENERAL CONSIDERATIONS IN SELECTING ASSESSMENT APPROACHES/MEASURES

A number of general considerations must be taken into account when one is planning assessments and selecting appropriate tools, most of which are not unique to physical and occupational therapy. These include the importance of the particular attribute (e.g., pain intensity, walking distance, work loss) to the therapeutic goals of the patient and therapist; the reliability, validity, and responsiveness of available assessment tools; and the practicality of the tools for use in the clinical setting. Additional considerations may include whether to select a generic or condition-specific measure, and whether the measure will allow comparisons to relevant reports of similar patients in the professional and scientific literature.

Decisions about the focus of assessment and outcome measures will depend primarily on what factors are of greatest interest and relevance to the condition and goals of therapy established by the patient and therapist. Reducing or controlling pain is a goal of most treatment approaches for patients seeking care for painful conditions. Regaining or maximizing physical functioning and returning to "normal" activities and societal roles, particularly occupational activities, are also goals of importance to both individuals and society. In planning outcome evaluation, the therapist needs to consider how the intervention may change these attributes of disablement within the individual's social context. Those factors that the treatment is specifically designed to influence should be measured. For example, if a treatment is expected to diminish pain, it would seem logical to include a measure assessing pain intensity. If the treatment is intended to improve muscle strength, then a measure of such should be included. For reasons discussed previously, however, it is seldom sufficient to confine the overall goals of either treatment or assessment to the level of impairment or body functions and structure.

There was a time when much treatment and evaluation in physical therapy, in particular, was focused on the level of impairment. This is becoming increasingly less common. Although pain in itself is of significant importance to the patient, many other attributes at the impairment level, such as range of motion and strength, are of importance primarily as they relate to self-care, leisure, and occupational activities that are essential or desirable. Because it cannot be assumed that changes in impairments will necessarily lead to changes in other levels of disablement, treatment goals and outcome measures in rehabilitation usually also target factors at the levels of disability/activity and handicap/participation.

Reliability and validity are essential properties to consider when one is selecting useful measurement tools. In other words, the evaluation tool must yield reproducible results and measure that quality or characteristic which it intends to measure. Evaluating the latter can be complicated, since there is no "gold standard" of measurement for some constructs, such as pain. Thus validity is often established through construct validity, which demonstrates that a measure is associated with other measures of related constructs as would be expected. Self-report measures, which were once thought to be less objective and therefore less valuable than direct measures of physical capacity or performance, are now recognized as providing reliable, valid information on functional status (Deyo, 1988; Myers, Holliday, Harvey, & Hutchinson, 1993).

Responsiveness generally refers to the ability of a measure to detect clinically meaningful changes in a condition (Guyatt, Walter, & Norman, 1987). The differences found in repeat measures of any kind are due to random variation or measurement error and to true changes in the factor being measured. A responsive tool will be capable of detecting and measuring the latter. The minimum amount of change needed in a measure to represent a clinically significant change, however, is not always established even for measurement instruments that have demonstrated reliability and validity.

High measurement reliability and responsiveness are particularly important when one is conducting repeat measures within individuals to gage response to treatment. For example, although measures with reliability coefficients above .75 are viewed as having good reliability, it has been suggested that reliability coefficients should exceed .90 for measures used to evaluate individual patients longitudinally (Portney & Watkins, 1993).

Timing is also an issue when one is using outcome measures to detect changes in disablement, such as when treatment effects are of interest. The timing of follow-up measurements must be consistent with the time that would be expected for a particular treatment approach to have an effect, and must take into account the expected natural history. With respect to pain, earlier, more frequent pain assessment may be indicated in acute conditions, whereas less frequent assessments with longer follow-up may be more appropriate in chronic pain problems.

Another critical issue for an assessment tool to be of value in the clinical environment is its practicality. Among the most important considerations here are the time required of the patient and therapist and the ease of interpretation of results, as well as equipment requirements, space needs, and costs. Whether the patient is required to attend the clinic or whether the assessment can be conducted over the phone may also be a consideration in selecting outcome measures for follow-up.

A study conducted several years ago of Canadian physical therapists examined barriers to the use of standardized outcome measures (Cole, Finch, Gowland, & Mayo, 1994). The three most commonly cited barriers were limited knowledge of instruments, time, and a sense that available instruments did not meet patients' needs. As a response to these perceived barriers, a publication was issued by the Canadian Physiotherapy Association in cooperation with Health and Welfare Canada on outcome measures in physical rehabilitation; this document provides an excellent, pragmatic resource for practitioners (Cole et al., 1994). The development and awareness of rehabilitation-relevant outcome measures continues to increase as the importance of such measures becomes more widely recognized by clinicians, health care administrators, and third-party payers, as well as clinical researchers.

Selecting assessment and outcome measures that have gained wide usage and acceptability has the added benefit of allowing comparisons to other patient data sets reported in the professional and scientific literature. It is becoming increasingly common for professional organizations and research groups to endorse the use of standardized batteries of tests for various conditions. It is hoped that use of common outcome measures will assist in communication and study comparisons (Daltroy, Cats-Baril, Katz, Fossel, & Liang, 1996; Deyo et al., 1998). It is also recognized that these batteries are likely to undergo revision in future years as assessment and outcome measures evolve and as improved methods become available.

GENERIC VERSUS CONDITION-SPECIFIC ASSESSMENT TOOLS

As discussed, the WHO ICIDH model has been helpful in rehabilitation in identifying those attributes that rehabilitation patients and providers view as important. Whereas some attributes are specific to a particular condition or state, others are not. Thus one of the decisions in selecting assessment and outcome measures is whether to use a generic or condition-specific measure. In general, generic measures are more likely to reflect overall physical or psychosocial health and may reflect or identify other problems affecting these, in addition to the specific condition for which care is being sought. Because of their general nature and applicability to a variety of conditions, use of generic measures allows for comparisons across conditions and populations. On the other hand, condition-specific measures address special issues surrounding diagnostic groups and are typically more responsive and better at detecting treatment effects (Patrick & Deyo, 1989). Following are some examples of generic and condition-specific measures of attributes under the broad domains of the WHO model.

Generic Measures to Assess Impairment/Body Functions and Structure

Pain is viewed at the level of impairment in the WHO classification of disablement, although it is recognized that this complex construct is not simply influenced by abnormalities at the body systems level. Therapists usually gain information about the patient's subjective experience of his or her pain, which takes into consideration the duration of the current episode of symptoms; the quality, intensity, and frequency of the pain; and activities or agents that exacerbate or diminish it. In addition, possible consequences of the painful condition for other aspects of impairment, disability, and handicap are explored.

Two commonly used generic measures of pain intensity are the Visual Analogue Scale (VAS) and the Numerical Rating Scale (NRS). The VAS aims to measure pain intensity along a continuous scale represented by a 100-mm line that is anchored by the extremes of "no pain" and "the worst possible pain." It has been validated in populations with various painful conditions, including back pain, cancer, rheumatoid arthritis, and chronic pain (Cole et al., 1994). Test–retest reliability is reportedly high ($r = .99$) (Scott & Huskisson, 1979). With respect to responsiveness, Langley and Sheppeard (1985) found that 21 levels of pain were discernable between minimally detectable to intolerable pain. The NRS involves asking the patient to rate pain on a scale anchored by numbers (usually 0 and 10) representing the extremes of "no pain" and "worst pain imaginable," and can be administered orally or in writing. The VAS and NRS are reported to have a correlation of $r = .80$ (Cole et al., 1994), and both have the appeal of being quick and simple to use in the clinical setting.

The McGill Pain Questionnaire is also in common use in rehabilitation and has the advantage of acknowledging the multidimensional nature of pain and provides information on the sensory and affective qualities of pain, in addition to intensity. Its development, psychometric properties, and usage have been fully discussed by Melzack and Katz in Chapter 3 of this volume.

Range of motion, strength, aerobic capacity, motor control, and other such physical capacities are also viewed at the level of impairment and are frequently targets of therapy and assessment. The limiting factor in physical capacities in painful conditions is often pain rather than physiological restrictions or deficits in the structures themselves. Limitations can also occur through inactivity-induced deconditioning, which is often associated with chronic pain, or directly through underlying pathology. The specific physical capacities of interest depend on the patient's condition and the importance of the activities for which they are needed.

Generic Measures to Assess Disability/Activity

Physical and occupational therapists spend much of their treatment efforts in attempts to facilitate performance of activities in a manner considered normal for particular individuals. It is possible that pain can mediate or be mediated by a patient's performance of these activities. The association between pain and functional disability is often asserted in clinical experiences in which patients report willingness to return to premorbid status "if only their pain wasn't so bad." Unfortunately, research has not been able to substantiate a strong relationship between pain and disability, and it is clear that disability is not an inevitable consequence of impairment (Fuhrer, 1987; Nilges, 1987). From a theoretical viewpoint, impairment and disability are together reflected in the occupational performance components of a model that depicts occupational therapy's understanding of individual performance in daily life (Townsend et al., 1990). Therefore, a comprehensive assessment of a client's condition and response to treatment will include measurement of both impairment and disability.

The measurement of disability to document the impact of pain sometimes involves therapist ratings of observed activity. Functional disability instruments can include measurement of typical activities of daily living (ADLs) such as walking, bathing, or dressing, and/or instrumental activities of daily living (IADLs), which focus on community activities such as cooking, cleaning, or shopping. The area of functional disability assessment

has improved in terms of psychometric evidence; however, there are still problems regarding lack of a theoretical framework for item selection, scoring, and the methodology of reliability and validity studies (Fuhrer, 1987; Keith, 1984; McDowell & Newell, 1996). Although beyond the scope of this chapter, issues to consider in choosing an instrument to document disability also include what the environment or context is, and whether the tool assesses performance or capability (Darragh, Sample, & Fisher, 1998; Haley, Coster, & Binda-Sundberg, 1994; Young, Williams, Yoshida, Bombardier, & Wright, 1996).

When investigating the domain of disability/activity, therapists commonly use measures that focus specifically on those attributes or activities most often affected by a patient's particular condition. However, a few well-known general measures of disability/activity currently used in rehabilitation are noteworthy.

The FIM™

The FIM, originally known as the Functional Independence Measure, is an instrument to measure physical and cognitive ability that has been frequently used in clinical and research settings with various patient groups (Keith, Granger, Hamilton, & Sherwins, 1987). The goal in developing the FIM was to devise a tool useful in evaluating treatments and programs, maintaining quality, determining cost-effectiveness, and making policy decisions (Heinemann et al., 1991). The conceptual basis of the FIM is the estimation of burden of care through the evaluation of 18 items covering independence in self-care, sphincter control, mobility, locomotion, communication, and social cognition (Hamilton, Granger, Sherwin, Zielezny, & Tashman, 1987). Each participant's degree of functional independence is assessed on a 7-point Likert scale, where 1 indicates "total assistance" required and 7 represents "complete independence" (see Appendix 12.A). A total score is derived from the sum of ratings across all items, with possible scores ranging from 18 to 126; higher scores indicate greater independence. Although the FIM will give a basic indication of disability, the rating of assistance required is not done with respect to cause—for example, whether assistance is required due to physical incapability or the effects of pain.

Evaluation of the seven-level FIM has revealed consistently good interrater reliability results for each of the items of assessment, with intraclass correlation coefficients ranging from .88 to .93

(Hamilton, Laughlin, Granger, & Kayton, 1991). Predictive validity has been examined in patients with stroke (Oczkowski & Barreca, 1993; Wilson, Houle, & Keith, 1991), for whom both admission and discharge FIM scores were found to be strong predictors of the likelihood of return home. In both neurological and orthopedic patients, examination of the overall FIM and the Motor and Cognitive subscales using Cronbach's alpha has produced results ranging from .86 to .97, indicating high internal consistency (Dodds, Martin, Stolov, & Deyo, 1993; Stineman et al., 1996). The FIM has also been shown to be responsive to changes in function and to possess adequate discriminant validity in general rehabilitation inpatients (Dodds et al., 1993). Although this tool was originally developed as an observational measure, it has been shown to be similarly effective when completed via questioning patients, which requires substantially less time (Karamehmetoglu et al., 1997).

The Barthel Index

The predecessor of the FIM, the Barthel Index (Mahoney & Barthel, 1965), has also been widely used in rehabilitation, although mostly for neurological and geriatric patients. This scale was originally developed to evaluate long-term care clients with respect to the level of nursing care required. There are 10 weighted items in the original version, which cover function in feeding, bed transfer, personal grooming, toilet transfer, bathing, walking, stairs, dressing, bowel control, and bladder control. One difficulty in the application of the Barthel Index is that alternative versions of the original 10-item scale have been developed (Collin, Wade, Davis, & Horne, 1988; Granger, Albrecht, & Hamilton, 1979; Shah, Vanclay, & Cooper, 1989), and different scoring applies to each. It is difficult to find comprehensive evidence of the psychometric properties for any given version; comparison of results across studies is more difficult as well. Despite this, there have been some good results for reliability and validity for the different versions, although the responsiveness varies depending on the version used (Collin et al., 1989; Granger, Hamilton, Gresham, & Kramer, 1989; Shah et al., 1989; van Bennekom, Jelles, Lankhorst, & Bouter, 1996; Wade & Hewer, 1987).

The Sickness Impact Profile

The Sickness Impact Profile (SIP) is worthy of mention in relation to the level of disability. The SIP is a self-report measure of disability in which the patient assesses his or her behaviors in various activities as they are affected by illness (Bergner, Bobbitt, Carter, & Gilson, 1981). It includes 136 weighted behavior statements in 12 categories, such as "I sit during much of the day" and "I walk shorter distances or stop to rest often." Only the items that describe the client's behavior on that given day are selected. Subscores for Physical and Psychosocial dimensions can be obtained by grouping the category scores for certain items, although there are five categories that are always scored separately (Bergner et al., 1981). One of the main disadvantages is the time required to complete the instrument (usually 30 minutes), although shorter versions have been created for various specific conditions (Post, de Bruin, de Witte, & Schrijvers, 1996; Roland & Morris, 1983; van Straten et al., 1997). The SIP has been used in numerous rehabilitation and medical studies and is widely used in the field of chronic pain (Follick, Smith, & Ahern, 1985; Gill & Feinstein, 1994; Nilges, 1998). It has been extensively tested with positive results in regard to reliability and validity, and has been suggested to be the criterion against which other scales measuring client perception of disability are evaluated (McDowell & Newell, 1996). On a less positive note, the SIP does not fare as well with respect to responsiveness when compared to some other instruments (Beaton, Hogg-Johnson, & Bombardier, 1997; Katz, Larson, Phillips, Fossel, & Liang, 1992).

Functional Capacity Evaluations

Functional capacity evaluations (FCEs) are controversial measures that aim to measure a patient's safe maximum physical abilities for job-related tasks. They are most commonly conducted by physical and occupational therapists and are used to assist in a variety of determinations, including fitness for work following injury and physical capability of performing certain work tasks (King, Tuckwell, & Barrett, 1998; Smith, 1994). Tasks assessed during FCEs vary depending on prospective occupational demands; they usually include dynamic lifting and carrying, positional work, and activities requiring ambulation and hand coordination. Various types of FCE systems exist, and commonly involve psychophysical or kinesiophysical approaches (Alpert, Matheson, Beam, & Mooney, 1991; Isernhagen, 1992; King et al., 1998). The patient is responsible for determining limits in a psychophysical FCE and for stopping performance when he or she believes maximum capacity has been reached. Conversely, with the kinesiophysical approach, the therapist administering the assessment is responsible for stopping tasks when signs of maximum effort are observed; to decide when to do this, the therapist uses standardized criteria, usually related to the quality of the patient's movement patterns. These evaluations are often viewed as objective measures because they involve direct observation of performance, but it is important to recognize that valid test results depend on the cooperation of the patient in performing volitional acts, which can be influenced by motivation and a variety of other factors.

When one is determining whether an injured worker can safely return to work, the results of a FCE are compared to the actual physical demands of the job. If the worker demonstrates functioning at or above job demand levels, it is concluded that the worker can safely return to employment. If the worker does not have a job to return to, the FCE can be used in vocational planning by comparing test results to physical requirements of other occupations (Fishbain et al., 1994). Thus the determinations of safe maximum performance levels can have far-reaching implications with respect to return to work and employability. The reliability and validity of these determinations, therefore, are critical.

Only limited aspects of FCE reliability have been studied. There is some evidence that interrater reliability is acceptable for differentiating light and heavy exertions via kinesiophysical definitions (Isernhagen, Hart, & Matheson, 1999) and for judging whether a lift was performed in a safe manner (Smith, 1994). However, there have been mixed findings related to agreement on the specific level that would constitute safe, maximal lifting, one of the most crucial determinations of FCEs (Lechner, Jackson, Roth, & Straaton, 1994; Smith, 1994). One study exploring interrater reliability of determinations of maximum dynamic strength testing, using kinesiophysical methods in patients with a variety of musculoskeletal disorders, reported fairly good reliability for lifting and carrying tasks (κ = .75–.88) and somewhat lesser reliability for pushing and pulling (κ =.62–.68) (Lechner et al., 1994). Intra- and interrater reliability for most FCE methodologies are not available from peer-reviewed research publications (King et al., 1998).

Sound, prospective cohort studies have yet to be conducted to determine the predictive validity of FCEs. In fact, with few exceptions (Lechner et al., 1994), there is a notable dearth of validity studies of FCEs. Although using observations of maximal abilities as the basis for establishing physical restrictions may appear to be a reasonable approach, it is unknown whether placing such restrictions on individuals truly enhances successful return to work or diminishes the risk of reinjury.

Generic Measures to Assess Handicap/Participation

When one is assessing the level of participation, measurement focuses on the area of health-related quality of life (HRQL). In order to select an outcome measure for HRQL, it is necessary to determine the dimensions of quality of life that would be affected by the condition—and, more importantly, dimensions that would be altered by the rehabilitation intervention (Jette, 1993). With painful conditions where interventions are directed to alleviating pain, the pain dimension will need to be included in an HRQL outcome measure. Many of the generic HRQL measures do include this dimension, but the emphasis varies. A few HRQL measures that are common in rehabilitation include the pain dimension with reference to general and specific functional activities.

The Medical Outcome Study 36-Item Short-Form Health Survey

The Medical Outcome Study 36-Item Short-Form Health Survey (SF-36) is an eight-scale health survey encompassing physical and mental health that was developed for use in clinical practice, research, health policy evaluations, and general population surveys (Ware & Sherbourne, 1992). The eight health concepts, which are assessed by 36 questions, are Physical Functioning; Role Limitations due to Physical Problems; Social Functioning; Bodily Pain; General Mental Health; Role Limitations due to Emotional Problems; Vitality; and General Health Perceptions. With respect to pain, two questions encompass the Bodily Pain scale and refer specifically to pain magnitude during the past 4 weeks and how pain interfered with normal work activity during the same time period. This is a self-report measure that takes approximately 10 minutes to complete. The response set for each question varies and requires some computation to produce the scale scores (higher is better); these scores can then be compared to normative data for the U.S. adult population, which are available in the user's manual (Ware, Kosinski, & Keller, 1994). Software is also available to compute the scores, and comprehensive information regarding the scoring and interpretation of the SF-36 is available online at www.sf-36.com.

Much of the information examining psychometric properties of the SF-36 has been compiled by the test developers and has revealed good to excellent results, which are reviewed in the test manual and other publications (McDowell & Newell, 1996; Ware & Gandek, 1998; Ware et al., 1994). In the assessment of responsiveness, internal consistency, construct validity, and discriminative ability, the SF-36 has performed as well as or better than other measures of HRQL, such as the SIP, the Nottingham Health Profile (NHP), the Duke Health Profile, the Functional Status Questionnaire, the EuroQol, and the Arthritis Impact Measurement Scales (Beaton et al., 1997; Chetter, Spark, Dolan, Scott, & Kester, 1997; Essink-Bot, Krabbe, Bonsel, & Aaronsen, 1997; Katz et al., 1992). However, recent research with specific populations has identified some problems with the SF-36 in relation to sensitivity to change and the usefulness of some of the scale scores, specifically those dealing with role limitations and social functioning (Anderson, Laubscher, & Burns, 1996; O'Mahoney, Rodgers, Thomson, Dobson, & James, 1998; Ruta, Hurst, Kind, Hunter, & Stubbings, 1998; Stadnyk, Calder, & Rockwood, 1998). The widespread use of this instrument and its international acceptance, as demonstrated by an extensive project involving translation and evaluation of the SF-36, suggests that it will become a standard measure in many rehabilitation programs (Bullinger et al., 1998).

Other HRQL Measures

A few other HRQL measures that also include a component directed to pain assessment are worthy of mention. The NHP, mentioned just above, was developed in the United Kingdom and is designed to measure subjective health status in six areas of functioning: Physical Mobility, Energy, Pain, Emotional Reactions, Sleep, and Social Isolation (Hunt et al., 1980). The respondents are asked to indicate their feelings or emotional reactions to 38 weighted questions, using a yes–no format. Test–retest reliability has been shown to be good in patients with musculoskeletal disorders, peripheral vascular disease, and osteoarthritis, with correlations ranging from .75 to .95 (Hunt, McEwen, & McKenna, 1985; Beaton et al., 1997). The dis-

criminative abilities of the NHP appear to be good for multiple patient populations, and there is some evidence that it is responsive to change (Beaton et al., 1997; Essink-Bot et al., 1997; Hunt et al., 1980; O'Brien, Buxton, & Patterson, 1993). Criticism of the NHP has been directed at the low internal consistency of the measure, although the evidence is controversial (Essink-Bot et al., 1997; Kind & Carr-Hill, 1987). In addition, there has been some critical examination of the inappropriate use of the weighted scores with the NHP (Jenkinson, 1991). With respect to pain, it appears that the NHP and the SF-36 are not measuring the same aspects of pain, as demonstrated by a comparison of the dimensions of the two instruments via factor analysis (Essink-Bot et al., 1997; Stansfeld, Roberts, & Foot, 1997). The NHP appears to address the issue of frequency of pain, whereas the SF-36 pain scale is more closely related to the severity of pain.

Unlike the SF-36 and NHP, another HRQL measure mentioned above, the EuroQol, uses a single index score to express health status covering five dimensions: Mobility, Self-Care, Usual Activity, Pain, and Mood (McDowell & Newell, 1996). Using a checklist format, the respondent chooses one of three items in each dimension that best describes his or her health. This instrument was developed to define a core set of generic HRQL items that would then be used in combination with condition-specific measures (EuroQol Group, 1990). The EuroQol generally has shown good to excellent results for test–retest reliability in patients with a variety of specific health conditions and in the general population (Brazier, Walters, Nicholl, & Kohler, 1996; Chetter et al., 1997; Dorman, Slattery, Farrell, Dennis, & Sandercock, 1998; van Agt, Essink-Bot, Krabbe, & Bonsel, 1994). Some evidence has been published indicating that the EuroQol has good concurrent, construct, and discriminant validity, but the results evaluating its responsiveness to change have not been very encouraging (Brazier et al., 1996; Brazier, Jones, & Kind, 1993; Chetter et al., 1997; Dorman et al., 1998; Essink-Bot et al., 1997). Since the EuroQol is intended for use in conjunction with condition-specific tools, the lack of responsiveness may not be of significant concern. With respect to pain assessment, the EuroQol appears to measure the same aspect of pain as the SF-36, as demonstrated by factor analysis (Essink-Bot et al., 1997). Because the SF-36 scores the pain scale separately, as compared to the single index of the EuroQol, it may be preferable to use the SF-36, especially if the intent of measurement is to evaluate change. On the other hand, when formal decision or cost-effectiveness analyses are being considered, the EuroQoL has the advantage of providing a preference-weighted score or measurement of the patient's status on various health factors in a manner required by these forms of analyses (Deyo et al., 1998).

Examples of Condition-Specific Assessment Approaches

Low back pain is the single most common condition seen by physical therapists (Jette, Smith, Haley, & Davis, 1994), and it may top the list for occupational therapists as well. Although the underlying pathology of this common malady is seldom conclusively identified, theories abound in rehabilitation medicine, as they do in other areas of traditional and complimentary medicine. Assessment approaches are in part driven by these theories, particularly for measures at the disease level and the body functions and structure/impairment level. Treatment approaches are also affected.

In studies of beliefs, attitudes, and treatment preferences of family medicine physicians, chiropractors, and physical therapists in Washington State, the effects of different low back pain paradigms were apparent (Battié, Cherkin, Dunn, & Wheeler, 1994; Cherkin, MacCornack, & Berg, 1988). For example, at the times of these studies, the family medicine physicians most commonly believed that the underlying pathology involved the back muscles; the chiropractors cited vertebral subluxation; and the physical therapists cited the intervertebral disc. Not surprisingly, the physicians most commonly prescribed muscle relaxants; the chiropractors manipulated; and the therapists favored the McKenzie approach to evaluation and treatment, focusing on the disc. Many of the current theories held by therapists, and their associated assessment and treatment approaches, relate to mechanical theories such as spinal instability, disc derangement, and adaptive responses of tissues to poor posture or injury that adversely affect spinal mechanics. Most of the assessment methods (particularly at the disease/body function and structure and impairment levels) that are specific to these theories have yet to demonstrate reliability and validity through adequate testing. Other therapists follow a pragmatic approach to patient assessment, and after ruling out known spinal pathology in the initial assessment, accept a diagnosis of nonspecific low back pain and focus on measures of disable-

ment that are of importance to particular patients with this general diagnosis.

Low back pain intensity is frequently assessed via VASs and NRSs. Recently, an international panel of researchers on low back pain proposed several outcome measures for standardized use (Deyo et al., 1998). As an alternative to the VAS for measuring pain severity (which also was advocated), use of the following question was recommended: "During the past week, how bothersome have each of the following symptoms been?" The patient is asked to respond for low back pain and leg pain (sciatica) separately, using a 5-point Likert scale with these descriptors: "not at all" (1), "slightly" (2), "moderately" (3), "very" (4), and "extremely" (5) bothersome. This question has demonstrated construct validity in patients with sciatica through significant associations with use of opioid analgesics, reflex changes, straight-leg raising, functional status and absence from work (Atlas et al., 1996; Patrick et al., 1995). It also has been included in standard batteries of outcome measures advocated by such organizations as the North American Spine Society and the American Academy of Orthopedic Surgeons (Daltroy et al., 1996).

A pain-related measure in common use for back pain problems is the pain drawing. The measure was developed by Ransford, Cairns, and Mooney (1976) as a screening tool for psychological issues surrounding pain and was found to correlate well with Minnesota Multiphasic Personality Inventory findings. Reports of its predictive value for psychological involvement, however, have varied widely, with sensitivity ranging from 42% to 93% (von Baeyer, Bergstrom, Brodwin, & Brodwin, 1983). Pain drawing scoring has been studied by others following the introduction of the tool, and the surface area method of scoring has been found to yield high test–retest reliability ($r = .85$) (Margolis, Chibnall, & Tait, 1988). Pain drawings are also used to document the location of pain and other symptoms.

The physical capacities of strength, endurance, and trunk range of motion are also of frequent interest and are measured with a wide variety of techniques, with varying degrees of documentation regarding reliability and validity.

The domain of back-pain-related disability/activity is most commonly assessed via the Roland and Morris Disability Survey or the Oswestry Low-Back Pain Disability Questionnaire (Fairbank, Davies, Couper, & O'Brien, 1980; Roland & Morris, 1983). Both are widely used and have demonstrated acceptable reliability, validity, and responsiveness (Deyo, 1986, 1988; Fairbank et al., 1980; Roland & Morris, 1983). The Roland and Morris Disability Survey consists of 24 items describing specific behaviors that may be affected by back pain. The survey takes less than 5 minutes to complete, and scoring simply involves summing the positive responses, with a possible range of 0–24. The Oswestry Low-Back Pain Disability Questionnaire addresses 10 areas of ADLs and the degree that they are affected by back pain. Each of the 10 items allows the patient to select one of six responses indicating various levels of pain-related disability. The questionnaire takes less than 5 minutes to complete, and scoring involves summing the scores for each item (0–5); this leads to a score from 0 to 50, which is then multiplied by 2 to yield a percent score (see Appendix 12.B).

Although either instrument is quite acceptable, if telephone follow-up is being considered, the Roland and Morris Disability Survey is better suited for this type of administration. It has also been suggested that this survey may be most useful in primary care settings or other settings where little disability is expected at the end of follow-up (Deyo et al., 1998). Conversely, the Oswestry Low-Back Pain Disability Questionnaire may be most useful in patient groups where the level of disability is expected to remain high, such as in patients with severe chronic low back pain (Baker, Pynsent, & Fairbank, 1989).

Use of either the SF-36 (or SF-12) or the EuroQoL, discussed earlier, is advocated for assessing HRQL in patients with low back pain problems. A simple measure of this construct, which has been advocated as part of a minimum or core of outcome measures for patients with low back pain problems, is provided by the following question: "If you had to spend the rest of your life with the symptoms you have right now, how would you feel about it?" The patient is asked to respond on a 5-point Likert scale ranging from "very dissatisfied" to "very satisfied" (Deyo et al., 1998). Information about days absent from work and days spent on modified work activities due to low back problems are also of frequent interest in assessing the impact of the condition on this important social role. The following two questions have been validated in patients with low back problems, discriminating between surgical and nonsurgical outcomes (Atlas et al., 1996; Patrick et al., 1995) and have been advocated for standard use (Deyo et al., 1998). The questions are "During the past 4 weeks, about how many days did you cut down on the things you usually do for more than half the day because

of back pain or leg pain (sciatica)?" and "During the past 4 weeks, how many days did low back pain or leg pain (sciatica) keep you from going to work or school?"

As mentioned earlier, condition-specific measures of disability are typically preferred to generic measures when treatment effects are of interest. With such interests in mind, self-report instruments measuring disability have been developed for a variety of musculoskeletal conditions, in addition to low back pain. For example, the Western Ontario and McMaster Universities Osteoarthritis Index was designed to measure disability related to osteoarthritis of the knee and hip (Bellamy, Buchanan, Goldsmith, Campbell, & Stitt, 1988). The index includes questions assessing the dimensions of pain, stiffness, and physical functioning. The tool has shown reliability and validity (Bellamy et al., 1988; Bellamy, 1989; Bombardier et al., 1995), and each of the subscale dimensions has demonstrated responsiveness (Bellamy et al., 1988). The questionnaire takes less than 10 minutes to complete; scoring involves summing the item scores for each of the dimensions, and then converting the scores to a range from 0 to 100. This tool has also been used in the study of adults with rheumatoid arthritis affecting the hip and knee, although separate validation studies on this population have not been performed (Jones, 1999).

Lateral epicondylitis provides another example of a common musculoskeletal problem that has been the subject of the development of condition-specific disability assessment tools. A self-report instrument developed by Stratford, Levy, Gauldie, and Miseferi (1987), the Painfree Function Index, includes eight items of activities of daily living for which the patient indicates the presence or absence of associated pain. Test–retest reliability of the index was found to be good (Intraclass Correlation [ICC] = .93), and construct validity was supported through moderate correlations with measures of pain, pain-free grip strength, and overall function (Stratford et al., 1987). More recently a revised measure, the Tennis Elbow Function Scale, was developed and found to have high test–retest reliability (ICC = .92) and construct validity. It also appears to be a more responsive measure than the original Painfree Function Index (Lowe, 1999), but is not yet commonly known or in widespread use. The test includes 10 items of ADLs, and the patient is given five options to respond to each, using a Likert scale ranging from "no discomfort" (0) to "extreme discomfort" (4). The test takes less than 5 minutes to complete and is scored by simply summing the scores for each item, yielding a final score of 0–40 (see Appendix 12.C). Impairment in the form of pain and strength are also commonly assessed in patients with lateral epicondylitis by means of a VAS and maximum or pain-free grip strength measurements. However, pain-free grip strength may be preferred to maximum grip strength when the effects of treatment are of interest, since it has been found to be a more responsive measure (Stratford, Levy, Gauldie, Miseferi, & Levy, 1989; Stratford, Levy, & Gowland, 1993).

The outcome measures primarily used to document pain in clinical practice and research for neurological conditions, such as stroke, brain injury, multiple sclerosis, and Guillain–Barré syndrome, are not condition-specific. The instruments that are most common include the VAS, the McGill Pain Questionnaire, and investigator-generated questionnaires (Chantraine, Baribeault, Uebelhart, & Gremion, 1999; Lahz & Bryant, 1996; Moulin, Hagen, Feasby, Amireh, & Hahn, 1997; Vermote, Ketelaer, & Carton, 1986; Wanklyn, Forster, & Young, 1996). An exception to this trend is in the area of spinal cord injury.

Shoulder pain after spinal cord injury has been documented in persons with quadriplegia or paraplegia, and particularly in wheelchair athletes, with the prevalence rates ranging from 26% to 72% (Burnham, May, Nelson, Steadward, & Reid, 1993; Curtis & Black, 1999; Curtis, Drysdale, et al., 1999; Sie, Waters, Adkins, & Gellman, 1992). Until recently, the prevalence of shoulder pain was primarily measured through a subjective report indicating presence–absence, or through clinical diagnosis of a specific etiology. Most research documenting pain has focused on pain intensity as measured by a simple VAS without reference to specific activity (Kennedy, Frankel, Gardner, & Nuseibeh, 1997; New, Lim, Hill, & Brown, 1997; Störmer et al., 1997). In response to the lack of indices to detect difficulties in the performance of daily activities due to shoulder pain in persons who use wheelchairs, the Wheelchair User's Shoulder Pain Index (WUSPI) was developed (Curtis et al., 1995a). There are 15 items representing performance in functional activities such as transfers, wheelchair mobility, self-care, driving, household chores, and sleeping (see Appendix 12.D). The clients respond to each item on a VAS anchored by the phrases "no pain" at one end and "worst pain ever experienced" at the other, such that the total score ranges from 0 to 150. In addition to these 15 items, a self-administered questionnaire is used to collect demographic and medical history information to identify factors relevant to lifestyle and shoulder pain etiology.

The WUSPI has been shown to have good internal consistency, excellent same-day test–retest reliability ($r = .99$), and concurrent validity with loss of shoulder range of motion (Curtis et al., 1995a, 1995b). Despite excellent results, these studies are limited in that the subjects were mostly male wheelchair athletes, and individuals with lesions above C7 were not included. Preliminary evidence of the responsiveness of this measure is evident by the ability of the WUSPI to document change in pain associated with wheelchair activity after a 6-month exercise program (Curtis, Tyner, et al., 1999). The exercise treatment study and an additional prevalence study (Curtis, Drysdale, et al., 1999; Curtis, Tyner, et al., 1999) included participants with varied functional levels. It was found that the WUSPI was adequate for measuring shoulder pain in subjects with high-level quadriplegia, provided that scores were adjusted for nonperformance items. This tool shows promise; however, the published research to date involves the test developer, and widespread acceptance of this tool would be contingent upon examinations by different authors in different settings.

SUMMARY

To summarize, theories of disablement have played a significant role in directing the attentions of therapists and guiding their approaches to assessment and outcome measurement. In particular, the WHO ICIDH model has been widely used, emphasizing the dimensions of *impairment* or *body structure and function*, *disability* or *activities*, and *handicap* or *participation*. Although pain is viewed at the impairment level, it is recognized that pain is a complex construct that can influence and be influenced by other dimensions of disablement. Given that multiple physical and psychosocial factors can be associated with pain for any given condition, measurement cannot focus solely on pain alone. Functional status, perceived health status, and the ability to fulfill normal roles are important outcome variables as well. Both generic and condition-specific measures are used to assess all dimensions of disablement, and each has its strengths and weaknesses, with selection depending on the purpose of the evaluation and the expected effects of treatment. Condition-specific measures generally have greater responsiveness to clinically meaningful changes and thus are often preferred when one is evaluating the effects of treatment, particularly when influences on functional activities are of interest. Although the combination of measures chosen to produce a meaningful interpretation of outcome may vary, all outcome measures used in clinical trials and practice need to be valid, reliable, and responsive to change. The value of standardized use of psychometrically sound evaluation and outcome measures is becoming increasingly recognized among clinical researchers and therapists. Consequently, measurement instrument development and testing are currently very active areas of clinical research, and outcome measure use among therapists in routine clinical practice continues to grow.

REFERENCES

Anderson, C., Laubscher, S., & Burns, R. (1996). Validation of the Short Form 36 (SF-36) health survey questionnaire among stroke patients. *Stroke, 27*, 1812–1816.

Alpert, J., Matheson, L., Beam, W., & Mooney, V. (1991). The reliability and validity of two new tests of maximum lifting capacity. *Journal of Occupational Rehabilitation, 1*, 13–29.

Atlas, S. J., Deyo, R. A., Keller, R. B., Chapin, A. M., Patrick D. L., Long, J. M., & Singer, D. E. (1996). The Maine Lumbar Spine Study: II: One-year outcomes of surgical and non-surgical management of sciatica. *Spine, 21*, 1777–1786.

Baker, C. D., Pynsent, P. B., & Fairbank, J. C. T. (1989). The Oswestry Disability Index revisited: Its reliability, repeatability, and validity, and a comparison with the St. Thomas's Disability Index. In M. O. Roland & J. R. Jenner (Eds.), *Back pain: New approaches to education and rehabilitation* (pp. 174–186). Manchester, England: Manchester University Press.

Beaton, D. E., Hogg-Johnson, S., & Bombardier, C. (1997). Evaluating changes in health status: Reliability and responsiveness of five generic health status measures in workers with musculoskeletal disorders. *Journal of Clinical Epidemiology, 50*(1), 79–93.

Batterham, R. W., Dunt, D. R., & Disler, P. B. (1996). Can we achieve accountability for long-term outcomes? *Archives of Physical Medicine and Rehabilitation, 77*, 1219–1225.

Battié, M. C., Cherkin, D. C., Dunn, R., & Wheeler, K. (1994). Managing low back pain: Attitudes and treatment preferences of physical therapists. *Physical Therapy 74*(3), 219–226.

Bellamy, N. (1989). Pain assessment in osteoarthritis: Experience with the WOMAC Osteoarthritis Index. *Seminars in Arthritis and Rheumatism, 18*(4, Suppl. 2), 14–17.

Bellamy, N., Buchanan, W. W., Goldsmith, C. H., Campbell, J., & Stitt, L. W. (1988). Validation study of WOMAC: A health status instrument for measuring clinically important patient relevant outcomes to antirheumatic drug therapy in patients with osteoarthritis of the hip or knee. *Journal of Rheumatology, 15*, 1833–1840.

Bergner, M., Bobbitt, R. A., Carter, W. B., & Gilson, B. S. (1981). The Sickness Impact Profile: Development and final revision of a health status measure. *Medical Care, 8*, 787–805.

Brazier, J. E., Jones, N., & Kind, P. (1993). Testing the validity of the EuroQol and comparing it with the SF-36 health status survey questionnaire. *Quality of Life Research, 2*(3), 169–180.

Brazier, J. E., Walters, S. J., Nicholl, J. P., & Kohler, B. (1996). Using the SF-36 and EuroQol on an elderly population. *Quality of Life Research, 5*(2), 195–204.

Bullinger, M., Alonso, J., Apolone, G., Leplège, A., Sullivan, M., Wood-Dauphinee, S., Gandek, B., Wagner, A., Aaronson, N. K., Bech, P., Fukuhara, S., Kaasa, S., & Ware, J. E. (1998). Translating health status questionnaires and evaluating their quality: The IQOLA project approach. *Journal of Clinical Epidemiology, 51*(11), 913–923.

Burnham, R. S., May, L., Nelson, E., Steadward, R., & Reid, D. C. (1993). Shoulder pain in wheelchair athletes: The role of muscle imbalance. *American Journal of Sports Medicine, 21*(2), 238–242.

Butler, C., Chambers, H., Goldstein, M., Harris, S., Leach, J., Campbell, S., Adams, R., & Darrah, J. (1999). Evaluating research in developmental disabilities: A conceptual framework for reviewing treatment outcomes. *Developmental Medicine and Child Neurology, 41*, 55–59.

Chantraine, A., Baribeault, A., Uebelhart, D., & Gremion, G. (1999). Shoulder pain and dysfunction in hemiplegia: Effects of functional electrical stimulation. *Archives of Physical Medicine and Rehabilitation, 80*, 328–331.

Cherkin, D. C., MacCornack, F. A., & Berg, A. O. (1988). Managing low back pain: A comparison of the beliefs and behaviors of family medicine physicians and chiropractors. *Western Journal of Medicine, 149*, 475–480.

Chetter, I. C., Spark, J. I., Dolan, P., Scott, D. J. A., & Kester, R. C. (1997). Quality of life analysis in patients with lower limb ischaemia: Suggestions for European standardisation. *European Journal of Vascular and Endovascular Surgery, 13*, 597–604.

Cole, B., Finch, E., Gowland, C., & Mayo, N. (1994). *Physical rehabilitation outcome measures* (J. Basmajian, Ed.). Toronto: Canadian Physiotherapy Association in cooperation with Health Welfare Canada and the Canada Communications Group—Publishing, Supply, & Services Canada.

Collin, C., Wade, D. T., Davis, S., & Horne, V. (1988). The Barthel ADL Index: A reliability study. *International Disability Studies, 10*, 61–63.

Curtis, K. A., & Black, K. (1999). Shoulder pain in female wheelchair basketball players. *Journal of Orthopaedic and Sports Physical Therapy, 29*(4), 225–231.

Curtis, K. A., Drysdale, G. A., Lanza, R. D., Kolber, M., Vitolo, R. S., & West, R. (1999). Shoulder pain in wheelchair users with tetraplegia and paraplegia. *Archives of Physical Medicine and Rehabilitation, 80*, 453–457.

Curtis, K. A., Roach, K. E., Applegate, E. B., Amar, T., Benbow, C. S., Genecco, T. D., & Gualano, J. (1995a). Development of the Wheelchair User's Shoulder Pain Index (WUSPI). *Paraplegia, 33*, 290–293.

Curtis, K. A., Roach, K. E., Applegate, E. B., Amar, T., Benbow, C. S., Genecco, T. D., & Gualano, J. (1995b). Reliability and validity of the Wheelchair

User's Shoulder Pain Index (WUSPI). *Paraplegia, 33,* 595–601.

Curtis, K. A., Tyner, T. M., Zachary, L., Lentell, G., Brink, D., Didyk, T., Gean, K., Hall, J., Hooper, M., Klos, J., Lesina, S., & Pacillas, B. (1999). Effect of a standard exercise protocol on shoulder pain in long-term wheelchair users. *Spinal Cord, 37*(6), 421–429.

Daltroy, L. H., Cats-Baril, W. L., Katz, J. N., Fossel, A. H., & Liang, M. H. (1996). The North American Spine Society Lumbar Spine Outcome Assessment Instrument: Reliability and validity tests. *Spine, 21,* 741–749.

Darragh, A. R., Sample, P. L., & Fisher, A. G. (1998). Environment effect on functional task performance in adults with acquired brain injuries: Use of the assessment of motor and process skills. *Archives of Physical Medicine and Rehabilitation, 78,* 418–423.

Deyo, R. A. (1986). Comparative validity of the Sickness Impact Profile and shorter scales for functional assessment on low-back pain. *Spine, 11,* 951–954.

Deyo, R. A. (1988). Measuring the functional status of patients with low back pain. *Archives of Physical Medicine and Rehabilitation, 69,* 1044–1053.

Deyo, R. A., Battié, M., Beurskens, A. J. H. M., Bombardier, C., Croft, P., Koes, B., Malmivaara, A., Roland, M., Von Korff, M., & Waddell, G. (1998). Outcome measures for low back pain research: A proposal for standardized use. *Spine, 23,* 2003–2013.

Dodds, T. A., Martin, D. P., Stolov, W. C., & Deyo, R. A. (1993). A validation of the Functional Independence Measure and its performance among rehabilitation inpatients. *Archives of Physical Medicine and Rehabilitation, 74,* 531–36.

Dorman, P., Slattery, J., Farrell, B., Dennis, M., & Sandercock, P. (1998). Qualitative comparison of the reliability of health status assessments with the EuroQol and SF-36 questionnaires after stroke. *Stroke, 29*(1), 63–68.

Essink-Bot, M., Krabbe, P. F. M., Bonsel, G. J., & Aaronson, N. K. (1997). An empirical comparison of four generic health status measures. *Medical Care, 35*(5), 522–537.

EuroQol Group. (1990). EuroQol: A new facility for measurement of health related quality of life. *Health Policy, 16,* 199–208.

Fairbank, J. C. T., Davies, J. B., Couper, J., & O'Brien, J. P. (1980). The Oswestry Low-Back Pain Disability Questionnaire. *Physiotherapy, 66*(8), 271–273.

Fishbain, D. A., Abdel-Moty, E., Cutler, R. K., Khalil, T. M., Sadek, S., Rosomoff, R. S., & Rosomoff, H. L. (1994). Measuring residual functional capacity in chronic back pain patients based on the Dictionary of Occupational Titles. *Spine, 19,* 872–880.

Follick, M. J., Smith, T. W., & Ahern, D. K. (1985). The Sickness Impact Profile: A global measure of disability in chronic low back pain. *Pain, 21,* 67–76.

Fuhrer, M. J. (1987). Overview of outcome analysis in rehabilitation. In M. J. Fuhrer (Ed.), *Rehabilitation outcomes analysis and measurement* (pp. 1–28). Baltimore: Paul H. Brookes.

Fuhrer, M. J. (1994). Subjective well-being: Implications for medical rehabilitation outcomes and models of disablement. *American Journal of Physical Medicine and Rehabilitation, 73,* 358–364.

Gill, T. M., & Feinstein, A. R. (1994). A critical appraisal of the quality of quality of life measurements. *Journal of the American Medical Association, 272*(8), 619–626.

Granger, C. V., Albrecht, G. L., & Hamilton, B. B. (1979). Outcome of comprehensive medical rehabilitation: Measurement by PULSES Profile and the Barthel Index. *Archives of Physical Medicine and Rehabilitation, 60,* 145–154.

Granger, C. V., Hamilton, B. B., Gresham, G. E., & Kramer, A. A. (1989). The stroke rehabilitation outcome study: Part II. Relative merits of the total Barthel Index score and a four-item subscore in predicting patient outcomes. *Archives of Physical Medicine and Rehabilitation, 70,* 100–103.

Guyatt, G. H., Walter, S., & Norman G. (1987). Measuring change over time: Assessing the usefulness of evaluative instruments. *Journal of Chronic Disability, 40,* 171–178.

Haley, S. M., Coster, W. J., & Binda-Sundberg, K. (1994). Measuring physical disablement: The contextual challenge. *Physical Therapy, 74*(5), 443–451.

Hamilton, B. B., Granger, C. V., Sherwin, F. S., Zielezny, M., & Tashman, J. S. (1987). A uniform national data system for medical rehabilitation. In M. J. Fuhrer (Ed.), *Rehabilitation outcomes analysis and measurement* (pp. 137–147). Baltimore: Paul H. Brookes.

Hamilton, B. B., Laughlin, J. A., Granger, C. V., & Kayton, R. M. (1991). Interrater agreement of the seven level Functional Independence Measure (FIM) [Abstract]. *Archives of Physical Medicine and Rehabilitation, 72,* 790.

Heinemann, A. W., Hamilton, B. B., Granger, C. V., Wright, B. D., Linacre, J. M., Betts, H. B., Aguda, B., & Mamott, B. D. (1991). *Rating scale analysis of functional assessment measures.* Chicago: Rehabilitation Institute of Chicago.

Hunt, S. M., McEwen, J., & McKenna, S. P. (1985). Measuring health status: A new tool for clinicians and epidemiologists. *Journal of the Royal College of General Practitioners, 35,* 185–188.

Hunt, S. M., McKenna, S. P., McEwen, J., Backett, E. M., Williams, J., & Papp, E. (1980). A quantitative approach to perceived health status: A validation study. *Journal of Epidemiology and Community Health, 34,* 281–286.

Isernhagen, S. J. (1992). Functional capacity evaluation: Rationale, procedure, and the utility of the kinesiophysical approach. *Journal of Occupational Rehabilitation, 2,* 157–164.

Isernhagen, S. J., Hart, D. L., & Matheson, L. M. (1999). Reliability of independent observer judgements of level of lift in kinesiophysical functional capacity evaluation. *Work, 12,* 145–150.

Jette, A. M. (1993). Using health-related quality of life measures in physical therapy outcomes research. *Physical Therapy, 73*(8), 528–537.

Jette, A. M. (1994). Physical disablement concepts for physical therapy research and practice. *Physical Therapy, 74,* 380–386.

Jette, A. M., Smith, K., Haley, S. M., & Davis, K. D. (1994). Physical therapy episodes of care for patients with low back pain. *Physical Therapy, 74*(2), 101–110.

Jenkinson, C. (1991). Why are we weighting?: A critical examination of the use of time weights in a health status measure. *Social Science and Medicine, 32*(12), 1413–1416.

Jones, C. A. (1999). *Pain and functional outcomes after total hip and knee arthroplasties: A prospective study of a community-based cohort.* Unpublished doctoral dissertation, University of Alberta.

Katz, J. N., Larson, M. G., Phillips, C. B., Fossel, A.H., & Liang, M. H. (1992). Comparative measurement sensitivity of short and longer health status instruments. *Medical Care, 30*(10), 917–925.

Karamehmetoglu, S. S., Karacan, I., Elbasi, N., Demirel, G., Koyuncu, H., & Dosoglu, M. (1997). The Functional Independence Measure in spinal cord injured patients: Comparison of questioning with observational rating. *Spinal Cord, 35*, 22–25.

Keith, R. A. (1984). Functional assessment measures in medical rehabilitation: Current status. *Archives of Physical Medicine and Rehabilitation, 65*, 74–78.

Keith, R. A., Granger, C. V., Hamilton, B. B., & Sherwin, F. S. (1987). The Functional Independence Measure: A new tool for rehabilitation. In M. G. Eisenberg (Ed.), *Advances in clinical rehabilitation* (pp. 6–18). New York: Springer.

Kennedy, P., Frankel, H., Gardner, B., & Nuseibeh, I. (1997). Factors associated with acute and chronic pain following traumatic spinal cord injuries. *Spinal Cord, 35*, 814–817.

Kind, P., & Carr-Hill, R. (1987). The Nottingham Health Profile: A useful tool for epidemiologists? *Social Science and Medicine, 25*(8), 905–910.

King, P. M., Tuckwell, N., & Barrett T. E. (1998). A critical review of functional capacity evaluations. *Physical Therapy, 78*, 852–865.

Lahz, S., & Bryant, R. A. (1996). Incidence of chronic pain following traumatic brain injury. *Archives of Physical Medicine and Rehabilitation, 77*, 889–891.

Langley, G. B., & Sheppeard, H. (1985). The visual analogue scale: Its use in pain measurement. *Rheumatology International, 5*, 145–148.

Law, M., Baptiste, S., McColl, M., Opzoomer, A., Polatajko, H., & Pollack, N. (1990). The Canadian Occupational Performance Measure: An outcome measure for occupational therapy. *Canadian Journal of Occupational Therapy, 57*(2), 82–87.

Law, M., King, G., Russell, D., MacKinnon, E., Hurley, P., & Murphy, C. (1999). Measuring outcomes in children's rehabilitation: A decision protocol. *Archives of Physical Medicine and Rehabilitation, 80*, 629–636.

Lechner, D. E., Jackson, J. R., Roth, D. L., & Straaton, K. V. (1994). Reliability and validity of a newly developed test of physical work performance. *Journal of Occupational Medicine, 36*, 997–1004.

Lowe, K. A. (1999). *The test retest reliability, construct validity, and responsiveness of the Tennis Elbow Function Scale.* Unpublished master's thesis, University of Alberta.

Mahoney, F. I., & Barthel, D. W. (1965). Functional evaluation: The Barthel Index. *Maryland State Medical Journal, 14*, 61–65.

Margolis, R. B., Chibnall, J. T., & Tait, R. C. (1988). Test-retest reliability of the pain drawing instrument. *Pain, 33*, 49–51.

Mayo, N. E., Wood-Dauphinee, S., Ahmed, S., Gordon, C., Higgins, J., McEwen, S., & Salbach, N. (1999). Disablement following stroke. *Disability and Rehabilitation, 21*(5/6), 258–268.

McDowell, I., & Newell, C. (1996). *Measuring health: A guide to rating scales and questionnaires.* New York: Oxford University Press.

Minaire, P. (1992). Disease, illness and health: Theoretical models of the disablement process. *Bulletin of the World Health Organization, 70*, 373–379.

Moulin, D. E., Hagen, N., Feasby, T. E., Amireh, R., & Hahn, A. (1997). Pain in Guillain–Barré syndrome. *Neurology, 48*, 328–331.

Myers, A. M., Holliday, P. J., Harvey, K. A., & Hutchinson, K. S. (1993). Functional performance measures: Are they superior to self-assessments? *Journal of Gerontology, 48*(5), M196–M206.

Nagi, S. (1965). Some conceptual issues in disability and rehabilitation. In M. Sussman (Ed.), *Sociology and rehabilitation* (pp. 100–113). Washington, DC: American Sociological Association.

Nagi, S. (1991). Disability concepts revisited: Implications for prevention. In A. Pope & A. Tarlov (Eds.), *Disability in America: Toward a national agenda for prevention* (pp. 309–327). Washington, DC: National Academy Press.

New, P. W., Lim, T. C., Hill, S. T., & Brown, D. J. (1997). A survey of pain during rehabilitation after acute spinal cord injury. *Spinal Cord, 35*, 658–663.

Nilges, P. (1998). Outcome measures in pain therapy. *Baillière's Clinical Anaesthesiology, 12*(1), 1–18.

O'Brien, B. J., Buxton, M. J., & Patterson, D. L. (1993). Relationship between functional status and health-related quality of life after myocardial infarction. *Medical Care, 31*(10), 950–955.

Oczkowski, W. J., & Barreca, S. (1993). The Functional Independence Measure: Its use to identify rehabilitation needs in stroke survivors. *Archives of Physical Medicine and Rehabilitation, 74*, 1291–1294.

O'Mahoney, P. G., Rodgers, H., Thomson, R. G., Dobson, R., & James, O. F. W. (1998). Is the SF-36 suitable for assessing health status of older stroke patients? *Age and Aging, 27*, 19–22.

Patrick, D. L., & Deyo, R.A. (1989). Generic and disease-specific measures in assessing health status and quality of life. *Medical Care, 27*, S217–S232.

Patrick, D. L., Deyo, R. A., Atlas, S. J., Singer, D. E., Chapin, A., & Keller, R. B. (1995). Assessing health related quality of life in patients with sciatica. *Spine, 20*, 1899–1909.

Pope, A., & Tarlov A. (Eds.). (1991). *Disability in America: Toward a national agenda for prevention.* Washington, DC: National Academy Press.

Portney, L., & Watkins, M. (1993). *Foundations of clinical research: Applications to practice.* Norwalk, CT: Appleton & Lange.

Post, M. W. M., de Bruin, A., de Witte, L., & Schrijvers, A. (1996). The SIP68: A measure of health-related functional status in rehabilitation medicine. *Archives of Physical Medicine and Rehabilitation, 77*, 440–445.

Ransford, A. O., Cairns, D., & Mooney, V. (1976). The pain drawing as an aid to the psychological evaluation of patients with low back pain. *Spine, 1*(2), 127–134.

Roland, M., & Morris, R. (1983). A study of the natural history of back pain: Part I. Development of a reliable and sensitive measure of disability in low back pain. *Spine, 8*, 141–144.

Ruta, D. A., Hurst, N. P., Kind, P., Hunter, M., & Stubbings, A. (1998). Measuring health status in British patients with rheumatoid arthritis: Reliability, validity and responsiveness of the Short Form 36-Item Health Survey (SF-36). *British Journal of Rheumatology, 37*, 425–436.

Scott, J., & Huskinsson E. C. (1979). Vertical or horizontal visual analogue scales. *Annals of the Rheumatic Diseases, 38,* 560.

Sie, I. H., Waters, R. L., Adkins, R. H., & Gellman, H. (1992). Upper extremity pain in the postrehabilitation spinal cord injured patient. *Archives of Physical Medicine and Rehabilitation, 73,* 44–48.

Shah, S., Vanclay, F., & Cooper, B. (1989). Improving the sensitivity of the Barthel Index for stroke rehabilitation. *Journal of Clinical Epidemiology, 42,* 703–709.

Smith, R. L. (1994). Therapists' ability to identify safe maximum lifting in low back pain patients during functional capacity evaluation. *Journal of Orthopaedic and Sports Physical Therapy, 19,* 277–281.

Stadnyk, K., Calder, J., & Rockwood, K. (1998). Testing the measurement properties of the Short Form-36 Health Survey in a frail elderly population. *Journal of Clinical Epidemiology, 51*(10), 827–835.

Stansfeld, S. A., Roberts, R., & Foot, S. P. (1997). Assessing the validity of the SF-36 General Health Survey. *Quality of Life Research, 6,* 217–224.

Stineman, M. G., Shea, J. A., Jette, A., Tassoni, C. J., Ottenbacher, K. J., Fiedler, R., & Granger, C. V. (1996). The Functional Independence Measure: Tests of scaling assumptions, structure, and reliability across 20 diverse impairment categories. *Archives of Physical Medicine and Rehabilitation, 77,* 1101–1108.

Störmer, S., Gerner, H. J., Grüninger, W., Metzmacher, K., Föllinger, S., Wienke, S., Aldinger, W., Walker, N., Zimmerman, M., & Paeslack, V. (1997). Chronic pain/dysaesthesia in spinal cord injury patients: Results of a multicentre study. *Spinal Cord, 35,* 446–455.

Stratford, P., Levy D. R., Gauldie, S., Levy, K., & Miseferi, D. (1987). Extensor carpi radialis tendonitis: A validation of selected outcome measures. *Physiotherapy Canada, 39,* 250–255.

Stratford, P., Levy, D. R., Gauldie, S., Miseferi, D., & Levy, K. (1989). The evaluation of phonophoresis and friction massage as treatments for extensor carpi radialis tendonitis: A randomized controlled trial. *Physiotherapy Canada, 41,* 93–99.

Stratford, P., Levy, D., & Gowland, C. (1993). Evaluative properties used to assess patients with lateral epicondylitis at the elbow. *Physiotherapy Canada, 45,* 160–164.

Townsend, E., Ryan, B., & Law, M. (1990). Using the World Health Organization's *International Classification of Impairments, Disabilities, and Handicaps* in occupational therapy. *Canadian Journal of Occupational Therapy, 57*(1), 16–25.

van Agt, H. M., Essink-Bot, M. L., Krabbe, P.F., & Bonsel, G. J. (1994). Test–retest reliability of health state valuations collected with the EuroQol questionnaire. *Social Science and Medicine, 39*(11), 1537–1544.

van Bennekom, C. A. M., Jelles, F., Lankhorst, G. J., & Bouter, L. M. (1996). Responsiveness of the Rehabilitation Activities Profile and the Barthel Index. *Journal of Clinical Epidemiology, 49*(1), 39–44.

van Straten, A., de Haan, R. J., Limburg, M., Schuling, J., Bossuyt, P. M., & van den Bos, G. A. (1997). The stroke-adapted 30-item version of the Sickness Impact Profile to assess quality of life (SA-SIP30). *Stroke, 28*(11), 2155–2161.

Verbrugge, L. M., & Jette, A. M. (1994). The disablement process. *Social Science and Medicine, 38*(1), 1–14.

Vermote, R., Ketelaer, P., & Carton, H. (1986). Pain in multiple sclerosis patients: A prospective study using the McGill Pain Questionnaire. *Clinical Neurology and Neurosurgery, 88,* 87–93.

Von Baeyer, C. L., Bergstrom, K. J., Brodwin, M. G., & Brodwin, S. K. (1983). Invalid use of pain drawings in psychological screening of back pain patients. *Pain, 16,* 103–110.

Wade, D. T., & Hewer, R. L. (1987). Functional abilities after stroke: Measurement, natural history and prognosis. *Journal of Neurology, Neurosurgery and Psychiatry, 50,* 177–182.

Wagstaff, S. (1982). The use of the *International Classification of Impairments, Disabilities and Handicaps* in rehabilitation. *Physiotherapy, 68,* 233–234.

Wanklyn, P., Forster, A., & Young, J. (1996). Hemiplegic shoulder pain (HSP): Natural history and investigation of associated features. *Disability and Rehabilitation, 18*(10), 497–501.

Ware, J. E., & Gandek, B. (1998). Overview of the SF-36 Health Survey and the International Quality of Life Assessment (IQOLA) project. *Journal of Clinical Epidemiology, 51*(11), 903–912.

Ware, J. E., Kosinski, M., & Keller, S. D. (1994). *SF-36 Physical and Mental Health Summary Scales: A user's manual.* Boston: The Health Insititute.

Ware, J. E., & Sherbourne, C. D. (1992). The MOS 36-Item Short-Form Health Survey (SF-36). *Medical Care, 30*(6), 473–481.

Whiteneck, G. G. (1994). Measuring what matters: Key rehabilitation outcomes. *Archives of Physical Medicine and Rehabilitation, 75,* 1073–1076.

Wilson, D. B., Houle, D. M., & Keith, R. A. (1991). Stroke rehabilitation: A model predicting return home. *Western Journal of Medicine, 154*(5), 587–590.

World Health Organization (WHO). (1980). *International classification of impairments, disabilities, and handicaps.* Geneva: Author.

World Health Organization (WHO). (1999). *International classification of functioning and disability* (Beta-2 draft, short version). Geneva: Author.

Young, N. L., Williams, J. I., Yoshida, K. K., Bombardier, C., & Wright, J. G. (1996). The context of measuring disability: Does it matter whether capability or performance is measured? *Journal of Clinical Epidemiology, 49*(10), 1097–1101.

APPENDIX 12.A. FIM™ INSTRUMENT

L **E** **V** **E** **L** **S**	7 Complete Independence (Timely, Safely) 6 Modified Independence (Device)	**NO HELPER**
	Modified Dependence 5 Supervision (Subject = 100%+) 4 Minimal Assist (Subject = 75%+) 3 Moderate Assist (Subject = 50%+) **Complete Dependence** 2 Maximal Assist (Subject = 25%+) 1 Total Assist (Subject = less than 25%)	**HELPER**

	ADMISSION	DISCHARGE	FOLLOW-UP
Self-Care A. Eating B. Grooming C. Bathing D. Dressing - Upper Body E. Dressing - Lower Body F. Toileting	☐ ☐ ☐ ☐ ☐ ☐	☐ ☐ ☐ ☐ ☐ ☐	☐ ☐ ☐ ☐ ☐ ☐
Sphincter Control G. Bladder Management H. Bowel Management	☐ ☐	☐ ☐	☐ ☐
Transfers I. Bed, Chair, Wheelchair J. Toilet K. Tub, Shower	☐ ☐ ☐	☐ ☐ ☐	☐ ☐ ☐

Locomotion
L.   Walk/Wheelchair
M.   Stairs
	☐ W Walk
	     C Wheelchair
	     B Both
	☐
		☐ W Walk
		     C Wheelchair
		     B Both
		☐
			☐ W Walk
			     C Wheelchair
			     B Both
			☐

Motor Subtotal Score	☐	☐	☐

Communication
N.   Comprehension
O.   Expression
	☐ A Auditory
	     V Visual
	     B Both
	☐ V Vocal
	     N Nonvocal
	     B Both
		☐ A Auditory
		     V Visual
		     B Both
		☐ V Vocal
		     N Nonvocal
		     B Both
			☐ A Auditory
			     V Visual
			     B Both
			☐ V Vocal
			     N Nonvocal
			     B Both

Social Cognition P. Social Interaction Q. Problem Solving R. Memory	☐ ☐ ☐	☐ ☐ ☐	☐ ☐ ☐
Cognitive Subtotal Score	☐	☐	☐
TOTAL FIM Score	☐	☐	☐

NOTE: Leave no blanks. Enter 1 if patient not testable due to risk

APPENDIX 12.B. OSWESTRY LOW-BACK PAIN DISABILITY QUESTIONNAIRE

Please read:

This questionnaire has been designed to give the doctor information as to how your back pain has affected your ability to manage in everyday life. Please answer every section, and mark in each section only the *one box* which applies to you. We realise you may consider that two of the statements in any one section relate to you, but please just *mark the box which most closely describes your problem.*

Section 1—Pain Intensity
- ☐ I can tolerate the pain I have without having to use pain killers.
- ☐ The pain is bad but I manage without taking pain killers.
- ☐ Pain killers give complete relief from pain.
- ☐ Pain killers give moderate relief from pain.
- ☐ Pain killers give very little relief from pain.
- ☐ Pain killers have no effect on the pain and I do not use them.

Section 2—Personal Care (Washing, Dressing, etc.)
- ☐ I can look after myself normally without causing extra pain.
- ☐ I can look after myself normally but it causes extra pain.
- ☐ It is painful to look after myself and I am slow and careful.
- ☐ I need some help but manage most of my personal care.
- ☐ I need help every day in most aspects of self-care.
- ☐ I do not get dressed, wash with difficulty and stay in bed.

Section 3—Lifting
- ☐ I can lift heavy weights without extra pain.
- ☐ I can lift heavy weights but it gives extra pain.
- ☐ Pain prevents me from lifting heavy weights off the floor, but I can manage if they are conveniently positioned, e.g., on a table.
- ☐ Pain prevents me from lifting heavy weights but I can manage light to medium weights if they are conveniently positioned.
- ☐ I can lift only very light weights.
- ☐ I cannot lift or carry anything at all.

Section 4—Walking
- ☐ Pain does not prevent me walking any distance.
- ☐ Pain prevents me walking more than 1 mile.
- ☐ Pain prevents me walking more than ½ mile.
- ☐ Pain prevents me walking more than ¼ mile.
- ☐ I can only walk using a stick or crutches.
- ☐ I am in bed most of the time and have to crawl to the toilet.

Section 5—Sitting
- ☐ I can sit in any chair as long as I like.
- ☐ I can only sit in my favourite chair as long as I like.
- ☐ Pain prevents me from sitting more than 1 hour.
- ☐ Pain prevents me from sitting more than ½ hour.
- ☐ Pain prevents me from sitting more than 10 mins.
- ☐ Pain prevents me from sitting at all.

Section 6—Standing
- ☐ I can stand as long as I want without extra pain.
- ☐ I can stand as long as I want but it gives me extra pain.
- ☐ Pain prevents me from standing for more than 1 hour.
- ☐ Pain prevents me from standing for more than 30 mins.
- ☐ Pain prevents me from standing for more than 10 mins.
- ☐ Pain prevents me from standing at all.

Section 7—Sleeping
- ☐ Pain does not prevent me from sleeping well.
- ☐ I can sleep well only by using tablets.
- ☐ Even when I take tablets I have less than 6 hours sleep.
- ☐ Even when I take tablets I have less than 4 hours sleep.
- ☐ Even when I take tablets I have less than 2 hours sleep.
- ☐ Pain prevents me from sleeping at all.

Section 8—Sex Life
- ☐ My sex life is normal and causes no extra pain.
- ☐ My sex life is normal but causes some extra pain.
- ☐ My sex life is nearly normal but is very painful.
- ☐ My sex life is severely restricted by pain.
- ☐ My sex life is nearly absent because of pain.
- ☐ Pain prevents any sex life at all.

Section 9—Social Life
- ☐ My social life is normal and gives me no extra pain.
- ☐ My social life is normal but increases the degree of pain.
- ☐ Pain has no significant effect on my social life apart from limiting my more energetic interests, e.g., dancing, etc.
- ☐ Pain has restricted my social life and I do not go out as often.
- ☐ Pain has restricted my social life to my home.
- ☐ I have no social life because of pain.

Section 10—Travelling
- ☐ I can travel anywhere without extra pain.
- ☐ I can travel anywhere but it gives me extra pain.
- ☐ Pain is bad but I manage journeys over 2 hours.
- ☐ Pain restricts me to journeys of less than 1 hour.
- ☐ Pain restricts me to short necessary journeys under 30 minutes.
- ☐ Pain prevents me from travelling except to the doctor or hospital.

(cont.)

— —

Scoring (not seen by patients)
For each section the total possible score is 5; if the first statement is marked the section score = 0, if the last statement is marked it = 5. If all ten sections are completed the score is calculated as follows:

Example: $\dfrac{16 \text{ (total scored)}}{50 \text{ (total possible score)}} \times 100 = 32\%$ Example: $\dfrac{16 \text{ (total scored)}}{45 \text{ (total possible score)}} \times 100 = 35.5\%$

Note. From Fairbank, J. C. T., Davies, J. B., Couper, J., and O'Brien, J. P. (1980). The Oswestry Low-Back Pain Disability Questionnaire. *Physiotherapy, 66*(8) 271-273. Copyright 1980 by the Chartered Society of Physiotherapy. Reprinted by permission.

APPENDIX 12.C. TENNIS ELBOW FUNCTION SCALE

Name: _____   Date: _____

Today, do you or *would you have* any elbow discomfort at all with the following activities?

ACTIVITIES	No Discomfort	Slight Discomfort	Moderate Discomfort	Quite a Bit of Discomfort	Extreme Discomfort
a. Your usual work, housework, or school activities	0	1	2	3	4
b. Your usual hobbies, sporting, or recreational activities	0	1	2	3	4
c. Activities like sweeping or raking	0	1	2	3	4
d. Using tools or appliances	0	1	2	3	4
e. Dressing yourself or pulling up your pants/tights	0	1	2	3	4
f. Squeezing or gripping an object	0	1	2	3	4
g. Opening doors with your involved limb	0	1	2	3	4
h. Carrying a small suitcase with your involved limb	0	1	2	3	4
i. Opening a jar or can	0	1	2	3	4
j. Writing or using a keyboard	0	1	2	3	4

Note. Copyright 1995 by Paul Stratford and Jill Binkley. Reprinted by permission.

APPENDIX 12.D. A WHEELCHAIR USER'S SHOULDER PAIN INDEX (WUSPI)

Place an "**X**" on the scale to estimate your level of pain with the following activities. Check box at right if the activity was not performed **in the past week. Based on your experiences in the past week, how much shoulder pain do you experience when:**

Not
Peformed

1. transferring from a bed to a wheelchair?   No Pain [ ] _____ Worst Pain Ever Experienced   [ ]
2. transferring from a wheelchair to a car?   No Pain [ ] _____ Worst Pain Ever Experienced   [ ]
3. transferring from a wheelchair to the tub or shower?   No Pain [ ] _____ Worst Pain Ever Experienced   [ ]
4. loading your wheelchair into a car?   No Pain [ ] _____ Worst Pain Ever Experienced   [ ]
5. pushing your chair for 10 minutes or more?   No Pain [ ] _____ Worst Pain Ever Experienced   [ ]
6. pushing up ramps or inclines outdoors?   No Pain [ ] _____ Worst Pain Ever Experienced   [ ]
7. lifting objects down from an overhead shelf?   No Pain [ ] _____ Worst Pain Ever Experienced   [ ]
8. putting on pants?   No Pain [ ] _____ Worst Pain Ever Experienced   [ ]
9. putting on a t-shirt or pullover?   No Pain [ ] _____ Worst Pain Ever Experienced   [ ]
10. putting on a button-down shirt?   No Pain [ ] _____ Worst Pain Ever Experienced   [ ]
11. washing your back?   No Pain [ ] _____ Worst Pain Ever Experienced   [ ]
12. usual daily activities at work or school?   No Pain [ ] _____ Worst Pain Ever Experienced   [ ]
13. driving?   No Pain [ ] _____ Worst Pain Ever Experienced   [ ]
14. performing household chores?   No Pain [ ] _____ Worst Pain Ever Experienced   [ ]
15. sleeping?   No Pain [ ] _____ Worst Pain Ever Experienced   [ ]

Please answer the following questions to the best of your ability.

1. Age:

2. Sex (circle):   1. Male
                    2. Female

3. Marital status (circle):   1. Single
                              2. Married
                              3. Divorced
                              4. Separated
                              5. Widowed

4. A. How many years have you used a wheelchair? _____ years

   B. Type of wheelchair (circle):   1. Manual
                                      2. Power
                                      3. Both

5. A. What is your disability?   B. Level of spinal cord injury   (write in if applicable)
      (circle one)
      1. Spinal cord injury   1. Cervical _____   1. Complete
      2. Polio   2. Thoracic _____   2. Incomplete
      3. Amputation   3. Lumbar   _____   3. Don't know
      4. Spina bifida   4. Sacral   _____
      5. Other _____

6. Average number of wheelchair transfers per day: _____
   (including transfers to/from bathroom, car, bed, and other)

(cont.)

7. Are you: (circle)   1. Left-handed   2. Right-handed

8. A. Primary occupation: (circle activity in which you spend the *most* time)
   1. Employed
   2. Student
   3. Volunteer
   4. Retired
   5. Other: _____

   B. Total number of work/school hours per week: _____ hours

   C. Total number of hours spent participating in
      sports/leisure activities per week: _____ hours

9. A. Do you drive?   1. Yes   B. If yes, number of hours spent driving per week: _____ hours
                      2. No

   C. If yes, what type of vehicle?   1. Car
                                      2. Van with lift
                                      3. Van without lift
                                      4. Truck/utility vehicle
                                      5. Other _____

MEDICAL HISTORY: (circle the appropriate responses below)

1. Did you have shoulder pain   1. Yes   If yes, which shoulder(s)?   1. Left
   prior to wheelchair use?   2. No   2. Right
                                                                             3. Both

2. Have you had shoulder pain   1. Yes   If yes, which shoulder(s)?   1. Left
   during the time you have used   2. No   2. Right
   a wheelchair?   3. Both

3. Have you had shoulder surgery?   1. Yes   If yes, which shoulder(s)?   1. Left
                                     2. No   2. Right
                                                                             3. Both

4. Do you currently have shoulder   1. Yes   If yes, which shoulder(s)?   1. Left
   pain?   2. No   2. Right
                                                                             3. Both

5. Have you sought medical attention for a shoulder problem?   1. Yes
                                                                2. No

   If yes, who did you see?   1. Physician
                               2. Physical Therapist
                               3. Chiropractor
                               4. Other: _____

6. Circle all of the following   1. Ice
   you have used to relieve   2. Heat
   shoulder pain: 3. Exercise
                                  4. Medication
                                  5. Rest
                                  6. None
                                  7. Other _____

7. Has shoulder pain limited you from performing your usual activities during the past week?   1. Yes
                                                                                                2. No

8. Have you experienced hand or elbow pain or injuries during the time you have used a   1. Yes
   wheelchair?   2. No

Chapter 13

Diagnostic Injection

QUINN HOGAN

A central challenge in caring for patients with chronic pain is discerning the pathophysiological mechanism leading to their condition. Because of the complexity of pain processes and the inherently subjective nature of pain, there is a strong incentive to obtain hard data to identify sites of nociception and pathways signaling pain. Armed with such information, therapeutic efforts may be more accurately aimed at the target provoking pain.

This chapter reviews the use of injections for the diagnosis of pain. Before addressing the use of particular methods, I focus on aspects of anatomy and physiology that create challenges in the application and interpretation of diagnostic neural blockade. My goal is not to discourage use of these techniques, but rather to alert the reader to limitations that could lead to mistakes in diagnosis. I have provided references to published data for topics about which persuasive studies are available, although there are many gaps in our knowledge of the reliability of diagnostic blocks. A more inclusive list of citations can be found in a recent review (Hogan & Abram, 1997). Further research is needed to test the validity of most of these techniques. It is not my intention in this chapter to teach the practical aspects of needle insertion, which are best obtained from hands-on instruction. Standard anesthesia texts may be consulted regarding details of technical methods.

LIMITATIONS OF DIAGNOSTIC INJECTION

With a few exceptions, the goal of neural blockade for diagnosis is selective interruption of a sensory or motor pathway. If relief ensues, the tissues innervated by that pathway are judged to be a contributing pain source. The validity of this model rests on certain assumptions. First, pathology causing pain is located in an exact peripheral location, and impulses from this site travel via a unique and consistent neural route. Second, injection of local anesthetic totally abolishes sensory function of intended nerves and does not affect other nerves. Third, relief of pain following local anesthetic block is attributable solely to block of the target neural pathway.

Peripheral Neural Events

Acute pain fits the simple model of a single pain origin and path, as demonstrated by the ability of specific nerve blocks to provide surgical anesthesia. This experience may lead to similar expectations in chronic pain. However, persistent nociceptive stimulation or injury to a nerve may result in a distributed process in which pain is due to neural events at multiple sites. For instance, it is well demonstrated that spontaneous afferent signals originate in the dorsal root ganglion proximal to axonal injury (Wall & Devor, 1983). Under these conditions, blockade of the peripheral nerve proximal to the injury site can be expected to fail to produce relief, creating the misimpression that the wrong pathway has been blocked. In an opposite fashion, it is possible that blockade of a nerve distal to the site of injury may produce relief (Kibler & Nathan, 1960; Xavier, McDanal, & Kissin, 1988), thereby incorrectly indicating the origin of the pain. This may be due to the block's interruption of the release of neuropeptides into the peripheral tissues by antidromically conducted neural activity (Abram, 1988). Since sympathetic fibers in peripheral nerves are blocked whenever sensory nerves are blocked, local anesthetic techniques at the level of the peripheral nerve cannot distinguish relief due to interruption of a sensory path from relief due to discontinuation of sympathetic motor activity, which may modulate sensory receptor responses (Roberts, 1986), activate injured neurons (Blumberg & Janig, 1984; Devor & Janig, 1981), or facilitate inflammatory processes (Kidd, Cruwys, Mapp, & Blake, 1992).

Spinal Processing

Modulation of the afferent pain signal is due to descending cerebral influences, which may obscure findings during a diagnostic test by producing analgesia in response to stress, regardless of the specific nature of the block. Intense pain from the procedure may diminish the perceived severity of the original pain by stimulating descending inhibition of nociceptive transmission (noxious counterirritation; Sigurdsson & Maixner, 1994), creating the illusion that neural blockade has directly relieved the pain. Conversely, descending modulation may be stimulatory and produce pain that is independent of sensory input (Dubner, Hoffman, & Hayes, 1981). Nonpainful signals can be associated with nociceptive stimuli by conditioning with simultaneous presentation. Diagnostic blocks that produce no relief may suggest a diagnosis of malingering or psychiatric disease, when descending influences are in fact generating sensory activity.

Second-order neurons in the dorsal horn of the spinal cord typically respond to input from primary afferent neurons that innervate a variety of tissues and sites. This is particularly so for those dorsal horn cells that are in the sensory chain for visceral and deep somatic pain (Gillette, Kramis, & Roberts, 1993). Because of this convergence of sensory input, the perception of pain may be dependent on a level of combined neuronal activity from various sites. Interruption of one path of convergent inputs may be sufficient to provide complete pain relief, leading to false assumptions about the source of the pain. Infiltration of a painful trigger point in an abdominal muscle of a patient with pancreatic cancer and coexisting visceral pain may reduce the combined input to a level below the pain threshold, and the interpretation would be that the pain is entirely somatic.

The relationship between stimulus and sensation is not static, but is dependent on the history of preceding neural activity. Plasticity in nociceptive sensory processing is evident when prolonged and intense conditioning stimuli produce hyperalgesia and allodynia. This creates uncertainty in the interpretation of diagnostic blockade. It is possible that interruption of the conditioning stimuli will produce prolonged analgesia, as is often observed following local anesthetic neural blockade (Arner, Lindblom, Meyerson, & Molander, 1990). Alternatively, spinal sensitization may persist independent of afferent activity, with little or no change in pain.

Local Anesthetics

The ideal local anesthetic action for diagnostic blockade would be complete and uniform neural interruption. It is clear that this is usually not the case. Even during successful surgical anesthesia, sensations from the operative site produce somatosensory evoked potentials (Lund, Selmer, Hansen, Hjortso, & Kehlet, 1987). If pain continues after a diagnostic sensory block, one cannot be certain that the injected pathway is not involved, since some neural traffic continues despite neural blockade. Similarly, local anesthetic block of sympathetic pathways does not typically result in total elimination of sympathetic motor activity (Hopf, Weissbach, & Peters, 1990; Malmqvist, Tryggvason, & Bengtsson, 1989). The earliest perturbation of nerve function at very low anesthetic concentrations is the prolongation of the latent interval for refiring (Raymond, 1992). Therefore, information encoded with bursts will be transformed into a more uniform signal. By this means, incomplete local anesthetic block may cause sensations to change without any actual termination of transmission. Because of these features of anesthetic action, an accurate view is of a much more complex and nonuniform neural interruption.

Local anesthetics are absorbed from the injection site into the circulation and then distributed to other tissues. Following injections that require substantial doses of local anesthetic (e.g., greater than 15 ml), it is possible that circulating local anesthetic can have analgesic effects. In the highly vascular area of the stellate ganglion even small injections produce substantial circulating local anesthetic levels (Yokoyama, Mizobuchi, Nakatsuka, & Hirakawa, 1998). It is well proven that typical circulating concentrations of local anesthetics inhibit signal generation originating in injured peripheral nerves (Chabal, Russell, & Burchiel, 1989; Devor, Wall, & Catalan, 1992; Tanelian & MacIver, 1991) and diminish nociceptive signal transmission in the dorsal horn (Bach, Jensen, Dastrup, Stigsby, & Dejgard, 1990). As with nerve block, analgesia from systemic local anesthetic may be prolonged (Edwards, Habib, Burney, & Begin, 1985; Kastrup, Peterson, Dejgard, Angel, & Hilsted, 1987). These actions may produce the mistaken impression that analgesia following diagnostic local anesthetic injection is due to nerve block when in fact it is due to circulating anesthetic.

Psychosocial Issues

A diagnostic injection is a complex social interaction. Pain is an inherently difficult experience to report, and limitations in communication may diminish the yield of information from a procedure. It is also difficult to assure that the patient and doctor have the same agenda. Whereas the doctor may be seeking pathophysiological information, the patient may be looking for reassurance, confirmation of suspicions, proof to persuade doubting family members, and/or certification of disability for legal and financial reasons—or may simply wish to please the doctor. These purposes may enter into the patient's reporting.

Placebo responses must be expected in all diagnostic injections. Patients obtain relief from placebos administered during acute pain about one-third of the time (Beecher, 1955), but obtain relief from chronic pain in about two-thirds of cases after administration of a placebo (Sidel & Abrams, 1940; Traut & Passarelli, 1956), and the probability of analgesia from a placebo is proportionate to the intensity of pain (Levine, Gordon, Bornstein, & Fields, 1979). No personality features predict a placebo response (Liberman, 1964); individuals are not consistent in being responders or nonresponders; and most individuals will eventually respond to a placebo if it is administered repeatedly (Houde, Wallenstein, & Rogers, 1966). Placebo responses may develop over as prolonged an inter-

val as 60 minutes (Fine, Roberts, Gillette, & Child, 1994; Verdugo & Ochoa, 1994), and injections are especially potent placebos (Evans, 1974). The potency and frequency of the placebo effect is underestimated by the majority of physicians and nurses (Goodwin, Goodwin, & Vogel, 1979). It is evident that the physician's convictions play a large role in generating placebo responses, and that even in carefully designed and controlled protocols, unintended communication from the examiner to the subject takes place (Gracely, Dubner, Deeter, & Wolskee, 1985). The ambiguity created by these responses is a major impediment to the valid use of neural blockade for diagnosis.

Anatomy

In most cases, a purpose of diagnostic injection is to distinguish the anatomical site of nociceptive signal generation or the specific path along which they are passed. This assumes that neural structures are found in predictable places and have predictable connections. However, most anatomic parameters show variability around a norm (Hogan, 1993b), and surface and palpation landmarks are unreliable indicators of deep structures. Even determination of vertebral segmental level is usually inaccurate without imaging (Gielen, Slappendel, & Merx, 1991; VanGessel, Forster, & Gamulin, 1993). Variability appears in the segmentation of vertebrae (Willis, 1929) and in the distribution of nerve roots to the intervertebral foramina (Kikuchi, Hasue, Nishiyama, & Ito, 1984; Neidre & MacNab, 1983; Nitta, Tajima, Sugiyama, & Moriyama, 1993), possibly causing correctly performed blocks to produce aberrant results. Even dermatome diagrams are highly inconsistent, dependent on how segmental innervation was determined, so cutaneous pain cannot be attributed to a particular segmental level with certainty. Since visceral and some deep somatic nociception is conveyed to the spinal cord through the same nerves carrying sympathetic efferent fibers, sympathetic block by injection will produce a component of sensory block as well, clouding the diagnostic interpretation (Schott, 1994).

DIAGNOSTIC INJECTION PROCEDURES

Most injections used to diagnose pain processes and pathways have been incompletely studied. Specifically, the validity of the methods have in most cases not been confirmed. The usual limitation is the lack of a "gold standard" against which to compare the injection tests, since for most of these conditions there is no credible standard for proving the diagnosis. Faced with this problem, studies examining injection for diagnosis may enter into circular logic through defining the disease condition by the response to blockade. Numerical values for false-negative rates can rarely be determined, since surgical confirmation is not typically pursued when tests are negative.

Tissue Infiltration

Simple injection into a cutaneous scar, inflamed joint, bursa, or tendon sheath can be used to identify the locus of pain. Failure to relieve tenderness by infiltration of superficial tissues such as skin or muscle focuses attention on a deeper site (bone, joint, nerve root). In general, solutions distribute much more extensively than is intended (Partington & Broome, 1998), so false-positive responses may arise in which relief is due to the anesthetic's acting on tissues other than the target. This method has not been proved by studies, but diagnosis by tissue infiltration with low injectate volumes is direct, simple, and low-risk.

Trigger Point Injection

Myofascial pain syndrome is characterized by discomfort associated with use of affected muscles and reproduction of pain with palpation of localized trigger points in the affected muscle. Since this is commonly found in association with other painful disorders, such as facet arthropathy or radiculopathy, it is often helpful to determine whether a patient's pain is predominantly myofascial, in order to provide specific therapy. Other means of documenting myofascial pain, such as electromyography (EMG), have not been proved reliable (Hatch et al., 1992; Hubbard & Berkoff, 1993).

A small amount of local anesthetic (e.g., 2–5 ml of 1% lidocaine) is injected into the trigger point through a thin (e.g., 25-gauge) needle. Reproduction of pain during injection and relief of pain after injection for the expected duration of local anesthetic, or longer, are used to indicate that myofascial pain is at least partially responsible for the patient's pain. Undesired spread to adjacent nerves needs to be considered in interpreting trigger point injections. For instance, injection of the piriformis muscle, which is deeply situated and not reliably identified by surface landmarks or palpation, is likely to have some effect on the adjacent sciatic nerve. For suspected pain in more superficial muscles or fascia, the simplicity of the procedure for superficial muscles is persuasive.

Somatic Nerve Block

Diagnostic peripheral nerve block is commonly used to predict the likelihood of success after surgical decompression or neurolysis of a peripheral nerve. Diagnostic blocks may also be performed prior to a planned peripheral nerve section, neurolytic block, or cryoanalgesia lesion. Typical settings in which blockade should precede surgery include entrapment neuropathies such as digital nerve entrapment (Morton's neuroma), carpal tunnel entrapment of the median nerve, tarsal tunnel entrapment of the tibial nerve, and neuropathy of the ilioinguinal and iliohypogastric nerves following herniorrhaphy.

The block should be performed at the site of the future surgical or neurolytic procedure to duplicate the response optimally. Small local anesthetic volumes should be used to limit spread to the target nerve, and careful neurological exam should confirm thorough blockade of the intended nerve and normal function of other nerves. In general, a positive response to a block will have greater diagnostic importance than a negative response. For example, in a comparison of median nerve block and subsequently surgery (Green, 1984), a test injection identified 85% of patients with the disease, but identified only 38% of the surgically negative subjects.

Relief of pain following blockade of an injured nerve does not completely confirm the diagnosis of neuropathy at the injection site, since there may be a nociceptive source more distally within the distribution of the blocked nerve. Even pain from a neuropathic source more proximal than the site of block (e.g., radiculopathy or plexopathy) may be relieved by a distal injection procedure (Kibler & Nathan, 1960; Xavier et al., 1988). Even when peripheral local anesthetic nerve block produces profound relief, long term relief after neuroablative procedures is not certain (Noordenbos & Wall, 1981; Younger & Claridge, 1998).

Visceral Nerve Block

Confusing conditions may arise in which it is necessary to distinguish whether thoracic, abdominal, or pelvic pain is due to pathology of visceral elements or somatic structures. Blocking the celiac plexus or the splanchnic nerves proximal to their joining the celiac plexus is carried out to distinguish abdominal pain of visceral origin (such as occurs with pancreatitis, distension of the hepatic capsule, or cholecystitis) from pain arising from a somatic origin (as in the case of entrapment of an intercostal nerve or pain of muscular origin) (Abram & Boas, 1992; Plancarte, Velazquea, & Patt, 1993). In such cases, it is helpful to compare the response of celiac or splanchnic block to that of intercostal block or local infiltration of the abdominal wall.

Prior to neurolysis for the treatment of pancreatic cancer pain, a prognostic celiac or splanchnic block should be performed. This will indicate cases in which blocks may be relatively ineffective due to extensive local tumor spread and resultant inflammation. In the same fashion, blockade of the afferent innervation of the pelvic viscera by superior hypogastric plexus block has been used to predict the response to subsequent neurolytic blockade at this level. The injection should closely duplicate the neurolytic block with regard to needle location and volume of injection. In order to guarantee that the needle position of a successful local anesthetic block is the same as the subsequent neurolytic block, it may be desirable to do both at the same occasion without removing the needle.

Systemic local anesthetic effects may be especially important for these procedures, as relatively large volumes are used. Also, spread of anesthetic to somatic nerves, especially via passage posteriorly to the segmental nerves at the intervertebral foramina and passage into the epidural space, may compromise diagnostic validity.

Sacroiliac Joint Injection

The sacroiliac joint is a probable source of acute and chronic pain, since the joint is well innervated (Solonen, 1957); stimulation by injection of radiographic contrast into the joint in subjects without complaints of back pain produces pain in the immediate area, often also in the surrounding gluteal area, and occasionally into the posterior thigh and knee (Fortin, Dwyer, West, & Pier, 1994). Diagnostic criteria for determining a sacroiliac ori-

gin of low back pain are uncertain. The specificity of physical exam maneuvers, such as Gaenslen's test, are unknown, but often indicate disease in asymptomatic individuals (Dreyfuss, Dryer, Griffin, Hoffman, & Walsh, 1994). Computed tomographic (CT) scans of the joint may show erosions, narrowing of the cartilaginous portion of the joint, and bony sclerosis of the adjacent ilium. However, irregularities and joint asymmetry are typical of healthy joints (Vleeming, Stoeckart, Volkers, & Snijders, 1990), with progressive age-related changes in subjects without complaints (Bowen & Cassidy, 1981). Thus it is often difficult to identify the extent of the sacroiliac contribution to back pain, and relief with anesthetic injection may indicate a role.

Most of the actual joint space is inaccessible due to overhanging iliac bone, so it is probable that needles inserted without X-ray assistance usually fail to enter the joint and are in fact injections into the fibrous structures well outside the joint. If the procedure is done under fluoroscopic or CT control, the inferior extent of the joint line can be identified where iliac bone does not occlude access, and the joint space itself may be entered (Fortin et al., 1994; Hendrix, Lin, & Kane, 1982). It is not clear, however, whether intra-articular spread is necessary to achieve efficacy. Pain relief after injection could also be related to infiltration of anesthetic into the sacrospinalis muscle and give the incorrect impression that the joint is the pain source.

Although there are no well-controlled evaluations of the validity of this technique, it is probable that analgesia after sacroiliac injection with local anesthetic does differentiate sacroiliac arthropathy from facet disease, myofascial pain, or disc disease; however, this remains unproved.

Intervertebral Facet Joint Blockade

The zygapophyseal (facet) joints are paired diarthrodial articulations between the posterior elements of adjacent vertebrae that guide the relative motions of the adjacent vertebrae. The medial branch of the dorsal primary ramus of each spinal nerve supplies portions of the facet joint as well as the supraspinous and interspinous ligaments. Of these, only the facet joint capsule is consistently found to be well innervated by nociceptive fibers, which also penetrate the capsule and supply the synovial folds inside the joint (Giles & Taylor, 1987; McLain, 1994). Each facet joint receives branches from the spinal nerves exiting the vertebral canal through the adjacent intervertebral foramen and from the foramen one segment above (Bogduk, 1982; Bogduk & Long, 1979).

The facet joints clearly can produce pain. Facet menisci and capsule are innervated by small myelinated nerves with substance P, indicative of pain-sensing fibers (El-Bohy et al., 1988; Giles & Harvey, 1987; Giles, Taylor, & Cockson, 1986). Injection of hypertonic saline into or around the lumbar facet joint capsule produces pain in the back, buttocks and proximal thigh (McCall, Park, & O'Brien, 1979; Mooney & Robertson, 1976). Distension of normal cervical facet joint capsules produces unilateral pain referred to occipital and upper neck regions for the atlanto-occipital, atlanto-axial, and C2-C3 joints and scapular pain from joint C6-C7 (Dreyfuss, Michaelsen, & Fletcher, 1994; Dwyer, April, & Bogduk, 1990). Also, physiological recordings in laboratory animals document mechanoreceptive sensory fields in facet joints (Cavanaugh et al., 1989; Yamashita, Cavanaugh, El-Bohy, Getchell, & King, 1990). Rotation and extension between two adjacent vertebrae increases facet stress as does loss of disc height (Dunlop, Adams, & Hutton, 1984), all of which may be stimuli for facet pain.

A controversy remains, however, as to whether the signals originating in the facet joint are a critical component of common clinical conditions. Disc degeneration is a common feature of cases of lumbar and cervical facet disease (Bogduk & April, 1993; Butler, Trafimow, Andersson, McNeill, & Hackman, 1990). Also, changes in facets are a common cause of injury to nerve roots (Epstein et al., 1973). These other disease processes could therefore be the cause of pain in patients with incidental abnormalities of the facet, or at least could contribute to a condition more complex than purely a facet origin of pain. Since there is no histopathological or imaging standard (Murphy, 1984), the frequency of pain from the facet per se has been estimated only by relief in response to injections. This inevitably involves circular logic, but gives a positive indication of cervical facet etiology in 63%–100% of unselected patients with posttraumatic neck pain (April & Bogduk, 1992; Barnsley & Bogduk, 1993; Barnsley, Lord, & Bogduk, 1993; Bogduk & Marsland, 1988; Hove & Gyldensted, 1990; Roy, Fleury, Fontaine, & Dussault, 1988), and in 16%–94% of subjects clinically suspected of having lumbar facet pain (Carette et al., 1991; Carrera, 1980; Destouet, Gilula, Murphey, & Monsees, 1982; Fairbank, McCall, & O'Brian, 1981; Helbig & Lee, 1988; Mooney & Robertson, 1976; Moran, O'Connell, & Walsh, 1988; Mur-

tagh, 1988; Raymond & Dumas, 1984). A random choice of injection level may have no better response than injection into the suspected joint (Marks, Houston, & Thulbourne, 1992), and total absence of pain after injection of local anesthetic into the lumbar facets is uncommon (Carette et al., 1991; Jackson, Jacobs, & Montesano, 1988). These findings indicate that the facets are an origin of at least part of the patients' pain, but rarely the unique or major source.

The site of origin of nonradicular back and neck pain almost always poses a diagnostic dilemma. Many structures in the vertebral column in addition to the facet joints are richly innervated, such as the posterior and anterior longitudinal ligaments, the annular ligament of the intervertebral disc, the anterior dura mater, and the costovertebral joints (Bogduk, 1983; Bogduk, Tynan, & Wilson, 1981; Edgar & Ghadially, 1976; Forsythe & Ghoshal, 1984; Groen, Baljet, & Drukker, 1988, 1990; Stilwell, 1956). Stimulation of these other vertebral elements by injection or during surgery in awake patients with local anesthesia evokes pain in the back, hip, and buttock indistinguishable from pain produced by facet irritation (Edgar & Ghadially, 1976; Fernstrom, 1960; Hirsch, Ingelmark, & Miller, 1963; Kellgren, 1939; Kuslich & Ulstrom, 1991; Murphey, 1968; Smyth & Wright, 1958; Wiberg, 1949), probably due to convergence of sensory input in the dorsal horn of the spinal cord.

Alternative means of diagnosing a facet source of pain have limitations. CT imaging is sensitive, but degenerative facet arthritis is also seen in 10% of asymptomatic patients (Wiesel, Tsourmas, Feffer, Citrin, & Patronas, 1984), making the utility of imaging uncertain. Although the value of bone scan is unproved, a positive finding may support the diagnosis of facet arthropathy and may direct attention to a particular joint. Because there is no specific pathognomonic finding (Helbig & Lee, 1988) or test, the clinical criteria for making the diagnosis of facet pain remain undefined. Therefore, diagnostic injections are often performed to help indicate the contribution of the facet.

Local anesthetic can be injected either into the joint space or around the nerves innervating the joint. Imaging with fluoroscopy is essential, and with advanced disease and joint changes, CT imaging (Murtagh, 1988) or MR imaging (Jerosch, Tappiser, & Asslieuer, 1998) may be helpful. A response is positive if the pain produced by needling is similar to the usual pain, if pain relief is noted in response to local anesthetic injection, and if sensory exam shows no evidence of segmental spinal nerve block. A limitation of this test is that there is no physiological means (such as sensory testing) to confirm the adequacy of the block, although obtaining a proper arthrogram with contrast injection assures delivery of the agent to the intended site.

One must be aware of sources of error in evaluating the response to injection of the facet. Although mechanical irritation of the joint capsule may reproduce the patient's typical pain, cervical (Dwyer et al., 1990; Lora & Long, 1976) and lumbar (Marks, 1989; McCall et al., 1979; Mooney & Robertson 1976) facet stimulation produces broadly overlapping areas of pain distribution even into the distal extremity, so this is not a strong indicator of pain origin. In addition, there is a poor correlation between pain provocation and relief from local anesthetic injection (Fairbank et al., 1981; Moran et al., 1988; Schwarzer, Derby, et al., 1994).

As an alternative to injection within the joint space, some authors advocate interruption of afferent traffic by blocking the medial branch of the posterior primary rami of the spinal nerves innervating the suspected facet joint (Bogduk & Long, 1980). Since there is no cutaneous innervation by these branches, adequacy of this block also cannot be confirmed by sensory testing.

The specificity of facet denervation depends upon limiting anesthetic spread to the target site—either the joint space or nerves to the joint. The facet joints are not capacious, and rupture during intra-articular injection has been identified after injection of more than 1 ml into cervical facets (Dory, 1983) and after most lumbar injections (Destouet et al., 1982; Dory, 1981). Since joint capsule rupture spills local anesthetic into neighboring tissues, including the epidural space (Destouet et al., 1982; Dory, 1981), pain relieved by facet injection could in fact originate in other structures—such as muscle; periosteum and ligaments; and pain-sensitive structures in the vertebral canal, such as anterior dura and posterior longitudinal ligament. In patients with spondylolysis, intra-articular facet injection is consistently followed by spread of solution into the epidural space and to adjacent and contralateral facets, and even laterally along a spinal nerve (Ghelman & Doherty, 1978; Maldague, Mathurin, & Malghem, 1981), limiting the specificity of the test.

Blockade of medial branches may lack specificity, since it not only denervates the joints they supply, but also muscles, ligaments and periosteum into which they also ramify. Therefore, sources of

pain in these alternative sites will be relieved by medial branch block. Fluid distribution during cervical medial branch block is variable, with the area of consistent coverage being a small subset of the area into which spread may be observed. Injectate, however, does not travel to anterior primary rami or to medial branches of adjacent posterior rami (Barnsley & Bogduk, 1993). Since each medial branch supplies parts of two facets, complete denervation of one facet requires partial blockade of the facet above and below. Inevitably, relief from the blocks cannot distinguish pain originating at any of the three. Since medial nerve blockade more accurately simulates the effect of radiofrequency denervation than does intra-articular injection, it should be used on a prognostic basis prior to producing a permanent lesion.

In addition to theoretical limitations of facet blocks, the physician employing them should be aware of technical limitations. Evidence shows that the test results are not readily reproducible. For instance, repeat injection may be positive in only 31% of subjects in whom a first block is positive (Schwarzer, Aprill, Derby, Kine, & Bogduk, 1994). This probably indicates either technical differences between injections (e.g., variable injectate distribution) or random occurrence of positive reports due to placebo response. Even when relief is found during repeated diagnostic injections, there is no feature of the patients' histories or physical exams that correlates with a positive diagnosis by this more demanding criterion (Schwarzer, Aprill, Derby, Fortin, et al., 1994).

As with any technical exercise, proper performance does not guarantee successful neural interruption. Overall success rates for facet blocks have not been determined. Failure to enter the joint during attempted intra-articular injection has been reported in 16%–38% of lumbar injections (Carette et al., 1991; Lynch & Taylor, 1986) and in 44% of cervical facet injections (Roy et al., 1988). Medial branch block has been demonstrated to block pain from subsequent intra-articular injection (with joint capsule distension) in 8 of 9 cases (Kaplan, Dreyfuss, Holbrook, & Bogduk, 1998). The combination of substantial rates of block failure and inability to confirm directly that a particular injection has denervated the joint weakens the diagnostic utility of facet and medial nerve injections.

Since no standard to confirm a facet origin of pain is available for correlation with block findings, the validity of facet block as a diagnostic tool has not been established. The only studies with controls show that response rates are comparable in subjects receiving either actual joint anesthesia or control injections (Fairbank et al., 1981; Jackson, 1992; Lilius, Laasonen, Myllynen, Harilainen, & Gronlund, 1989). Local anesthetic responses are a poor indicator of therapeutic success with steroid (Carette et al., 1991; Hove & Gyldensted, 1990). Facet block by injection has also been shown to be an inconsistent predictor of therapy by radiofrequency lesions (Lora & Long, 1976; McDonald, Lord, & Bogduk, 1999; North, Han, Zahurak, & Kidd, 1994) or fusion surgery (Jackson, 1992).

In conclusion, facet injections have been found useful by a number of authors, but the inability to confirm success of a block and the lack of evidence of diagnostic specificity of these techniques dictate that findings should be interpreted cautiously.

Intervertebral Disc Injection

The annular ligament of the intervertebral disc and the midline posterior longitudinal ligament are well innervated by sensory fibers and may provoke pain (Edgar & Ghadially, 1976; Hirsch et al., 1963; Murphey, 1968; Smyth & Wright, 1958; Wiberg, 1949). Several methods are available for identifying pathological changes in order to identify the source of pain in subjects with back pain. Discography allows examination of the internal structure of the disc by injection of radiopaque contrast into the nucleus pulposus of the disc. Although magnetic resonance imaging (MRI) and CT are sensitive means of identifying changes in disc anatomy, they suffer from inadequate specificity. Asymptomatic discs appear abnormal by these techniques in approximately 20%–50% of subjects under 40 years old and in 90% over the age of 60 years (Boden, Davis, Dina, Patronas, & Wiesel, 1990; Jensen et al., 1994; Powel, Wilson, Szypryt, Symonds, & Worthington, 1986; Weinreb, Wolbarsht, Cohen, Brown, & Maravilla, 1989; Wiesel et al., 1984).

A discogram, ideally made using CT imaging, is positive for disc degeneration if the image reveals altered texture of the nucleus, clefts in the nucleus and annulus, fissures leading to the perimeter of the annulus, or a radial tear that allows contrast to escape (Adams, Dolan, & Hutton, 1986). The validity of discography has been established in studies of cadavers in which imaging is followed by comparison with the dissected specimens (Adams et al., 1986; Videman, Malmivaara, & Mooney, 1987; Yu, Haughton, Sether, & Wagner, 1989).

By imaging alone, however, there is no way to tell which of several abnormal-appearing discs is the source of pain, or indeed whether any are producing pain. Discography allows an additional dynamic component in the test by examining the ability of a disc to produce pain during the injection. Discomfort during contrast injection that duplicates a patient's typical pain is also considered necessary for a completely positive test response. Although there is considerable controversy on these issues (Bogduk & Modic, 1996; Guyer & Ohnmeiss, 1995; Ohnmeiss, Guyer, & Mason, 2000), it is likely that normal discs do not produce pain during discography injection (Walsh et al., 1990). The most stringent criteria for identifying a particular disc as the source of pain are not only visible disruption and concordant pain production, but also normal responses at adjacent discs. Multiple positive discs may be the result of nonspecific reporting by the patient.

There are limitations to discography testing. Some subjects find the pain of needle insertion intolerable, and it is found impossible to enter the nucleus pulposus in about 4%–14% of discs, most often at the L5–S1 level (Colhoun, McCall, Williams, & Cassar Pullicino, 1988; Friedman & Goldner, 1955; Gibson, Buckley, Mulholland, & Worthington, 1986). False-positive lumbar discograms are observed in 17% of asymptomatic subjects, but these false-positive responses are eliminated if pain during injection is required (Walsh et al., 1990). Evidently subjects with pain during injection are a subset of those with abnormal disc anatomy (Grubb, Lipscomb, & Guilford, 1987; Vanharanta et al., 1987). It is less clear how to interpret the results in 2%–24% of patients with back pain who have pain during discography but normal disc anatomy (Grubb et al., 1987; Vanharanta et al., 1987; Zucherman et al., 1988). Complications of discography include discitis (about 0.15% incidence) and dural puncture, as well as the frequent occurrence of increased pain (Guyer & Ohnmeiss, 1995).

The evolution of noninvasive imaging by MRI has in part supplanted discography. In clinical comparison, MRI and discography may differ in up to 45% of patients with back pain (Simmons, Emery, McMillin, Landa, & Kimmich, 1991), due to both normal MRI with abnormal discography and the reverse. MRI that provides clear evidence of either present or absent disc pathology usually agrees with disc injection testing if provoked pain is included in the evaluation (Horton & Daftari, 1992), so discography can safely be reserved for determination of the disease state of discs with in-determinate MRI patterns.

Although discography with evaluation of induced pain can discern structurally abnormal and sensitive discs, this does not establish whether the test necessarily identifies the source of the patient's pain. Using local anesthetic injection to stop disc pain is a natural extension of the test, but has not been evaluated. Successful relief with surgery, typically vertebral fusion, may be considered an indication of correct diagnosis and choice of appropriate surgical level. By this criterion, discography is accurate in 80%–90% of subjects, which is approximately twice the reported accuracy of clinical exam or myelography (Simmons & Segil, 1975). However, false positives are frequent, and a negative test is not a reliable indicator of unsuccessful surgery (Colhoun et al., 1988). Ultimately, the utility of this procedure awaits proof in large, carefully designed and controlled studies, but it is likely that noninvasive imaging will be more desirable in most cases.

Selective Spinal Nerve Injection

In complicated patients with radiating pain, the contribution of root inflammation to pain may not be certain or the level of the pathology may be unclear. Imaging by CT or MRI and electrophysiological evaluation by EMG may be inconsistent or may not fit with clinical findings, or there may be multiple possible sources of pain. A further cause of confusion is the presence of pathology at multiple levels, since the origin of pain may be any one or a combination of sites, as is also true when upper lumbar pathology coexists with hip joint disease. Finally, evaluation is especially difficult after spinal surgery, since imaging is impeded by metallic instrumentation and scar tissue in the epidural space.

Injection of individual spinal nerves by a paravertebral approach (also termed *foraminal injection*, and mistakenly referred to as *nerve root injection*) has been used to elucidate the mechanism and source of pain in these unclear situations. Often this method is used for surgical planning, such as determining the site of foraminotomy. Diagnostic accuracy requires imaging to select the proper level and confirm needle placement in the intervertebral foramen. A paresthesia by gentle contact with the nerve is the final indicator of accurate needle placement in most studies. A test is considered positive for a given nerve if needle contact produces pain similar to the patient's usual pain, and if relief follows local anesthetic injection (including lack of

pain during maneuvers that produced pain prior to the block, such as straight-leg lift or walking). Some authors recommend testing two or three adjacent nerves on separate occasions (Schutz, Lougheed, Wortzman, & Awerbuck, 1973).

Duplication of the typical quality of the pain as a criterion is supported by the demonstration that inflamed nerves are more sensitive to manipulation than normal nerves (Fernstrom, 1960; Smyth & Wright, 1958). However, the distribution of the evoked sensation is less certain to be reliable. As with the stimulation of deep somatic structures, pain radiation with the stimulation of different roots produces overlapping areas of radiation (Smyth & Wright, 1958); these patterns may not distinguish the involved root from adjacent ones. Also, sensations provoked by mechanical stimulation of a nerve root are often more extensive than the area of the expected classical dermatome (Slipman, Pastaras, Palmitier, Huston, & Sterenfeld, 1998). Confirmation of successful blockade by identifying cutaneous anesthesia is desirable for confirming successful block. However, it is not clear that anesthetizing a single spinal nerve should produce discernible peripheral sensory changes, since surgical division of a single root produces no loss of cutaneous sensation (Foerster, 1933).

Because spinal nerve blockade will relieve pain from either pathology of the proximal nerve in the intervertebral foramen or pain transmitted from distal sites by that nerve, interpretation may not be simple. For instance, it is likely that pain due to a nociceptive focus in peripheral tissues innervated by the nerve will be relieved, as well as pain from a neuropathic process in the peripheral nerve. Furthermore, the specificity of spinal nerve block depends critically upon limiting spread of anesthetic to the selected nerve alone. Flow into the intervertebral foramen and epidural space is commonly observed and definitely compromises this assumption (Derby et al., 1992; Dooley, McBroom, Taguchi, & MacNab, 1988; Haueisen, Smith, Myers, & Pryce, 1985; Stanley, McLaren, Euinton, & Getty, 1990; Tajima, Furukawa, & Kuramochi, 1980). Not only will this block pain transmission by the sinuvertebral nerve from the dura, posterior longitudinal ligament, and annular ligament of the disc, but spread via the epidural space to other segmental levels could produce misleading results. To limit undesired spread, the injected volume of local anesthetic should be less than 2 ml, and ideally only 1 ml. The use of a concentrated solution, such as 2% lidocaine, improves the likelihood of adequate block despite small volumes. Because of these various limitations, the test should only be used in the context of thorough overall evaluation.

The frequency with which spinal nerve blockade successfully interrupts nerve conduction has not been determined. Oddly, cutaneous sensory changes have not been examined in any studies using spinal nerve block for diagnosis. In up to 30% of subjects, proper needle placement is not possible because of patient discomfort or anatomical challenges, especially at the S1 level (Haueisen et al., 1985; Schutz et al., 1973).

Several retrospective studies have investigated the ability of selective spinal nerve blocks to diagnose disease and predict surgical outcome. The fraction of patients with injections indicating radiculopathy in whom surgery confirms radicular pathology at the level indicated by the test ranges from 87% to 100% (Dooley et al., 1988; Haueisen et al., 1985; Krempen, Smith, & DeFreest, 1975; Schutz et al., 1973; Stanley et al., 1990). The proportion of patients with a negative injection test who then are found to have normal roots at surgery is approximately 30%–40% (Dooley et al., 1988; Haueisen et al., 1985) but few patients have been studied because surgery is rarely performed following negative injection test. In general, the accuracy of nerve blocks is better than that of imaging or EMG (Haueisen et al., 1985; Stanley et al., 1990). The utility of cervical diagnostic spinal nerve injections has not been formally examined.

In general, a broad group of authorities have found benefits in the use of spinal nerve injection for planning decompressive surgery on complicated patients, although such injection is not precise in its predictions or supported by conclusive studies. Controlled, carefully designed studies are needed to refute or support these beliefs. Studies have repeatedly demonstrated that pain relief by paravertebral spinal nerve injection does not predict success for neuroablative surgery, either dorsal rhizotomy (Loeser, 1972; Onofrio & Campa, 1972) or dorsal root ganglionectomy (North, Kidd, Campbell, & Long, 1991). If steroid is included, spinal nerve injection has been shown to have therapeutic efficacy (Riew et al., 2000).

Greater Occipital Nerve Block

The greater occipital nerve is the continuation of the medial branch of the posterior primary ramus of the C2 spinal nerve, which distributes cutaneous sensory fibers to the scalp as far rostral as the vertex. Several theories implicate this nerve in the production of headache. It has been proposed that the origin of the spinal nerve or the posterior root ganglion may be pinched between the atlas and axis by extension and rotation (Hunter & Mayfield, 1949). Further research proved that this is mechanically unlikely (Bogduk, 1981; Weinberger, 1968). Alternatively, irritation of the greater occipital nerve as it penetrates through the trapezius muscle may be the origin of nerve irritation, which initiates neuralgic pain (Vital, Dautheribes, Baspeyre, Lavignolle, & Senegas, 1989). Finally, irritation of suboccipital muscles and periosteum in the field innervated by the greater occipital nerve has been shown to produce ascending headache (Campbell & Parsons, 1944; Cyriax, 1938; Feinstein, Langton, Jameson, & Schiller, 1954).

Transient elimination of pain by greater occipital nerve block is used as a key criterion in the evaluation of cervicogenic headache (Bovim, Berg, & Dale, 1992; Sjaastad, Fredricksen, & Pfaffenrath, 1990). It should be recognized that cervicogenic headache is a poorly documented entity (Edmeads, 1988) with no consistent histopathological or radiological findings (Pfaffenrath, Dandekar, & Pollmann, 1987) and unpredictable response to surgery (Bovim, Fredriksen, Stolt-Nielsen, & Sjaastad, 1992; Mayfield, 1955).

Selective blockade of the nerve is performed at the site where it penetrates through the trapezius muscle, which shows marked interindividual variability (Bovim et al., 1991; Vital et al., 1989). Anesthesia is confirmed by sensory examination of the scalp ipsilateral and rostral to the injection. The success rate of injection in producing occipital nerve blockade is not determined.

The ability of occipital nerve blockade to identify patients with disease is hampered by inexact definition of cervicogenic headache and no means of confirmation. Most studies, as well as the definition of the condition, come from a single group of authors. In one report (Bovim & Sand, 1992), patients clinically categorized as having either migraine, cervicogenic, or tension-type headaches were tested with greater occipital and supraorbital nerve blocks, the latter as a control. Patients with cervicogenic headaches were most responsive to occipital injection, but supraorbital block also produced relief, and the areas of relief did not always match the distribution of the nerve that was blocked. Ultimately, the diagnostic meaning of a favorable response to cervical nerve block remains ambiguous because of an incomplete understanding of the role of this nerve in producing painful conditions.

Selective Sympathetic Blockade

Sympathetic efferent activity may contribute to a number of pathological conditions, such as sudden sensory–neural hearing loss, peripheral vascular disease, dysrhythmia from long-QT syndrome, central pain (Loh & Nathan, 1978), pain following plexus injury, and trigeminal or postherpetic neuralgia (Hogan, 1993a). Often the role of sympathetic activity is uncertain and controversial. In a large category of poorly defined pain states that are grouped under the terms *reflex sympathetic dystrophy, causalgia,* or *complex regional pain syndrome,* a sympathetic contribution is suspected because blood flow and trophic changes may be evident, but the pathophysiology is largely obscure. In these settings, selective interruption of sympathetic neural traffic to the involved area may provide diagnostic insight and guidance for future therapy.

It is imperative to confirm desired blockade, but practical measurement of sympathetic activity is challenging. Many measures have been used to judge the efficacy of sympathetic blockade, although no single measure has become an accepted standard. Horner's syndrome is easily observed, but documents only blockade of sympathetic fibers to the head. The cervical trunk may be blocked independently of the stellate ganglion or fibers to the brachial plexus, so occurrence of ptosis, meiosis, facial anhydrosis, conjunctival hyperemia, or nasal stuffiness does not assure sympathetic block of fibers to the arm. Skin resistance (sympathogalvanic) response (Bengtsson, Löfström, & Malmqvist, 1985; Lindberg & Wallin, 1981) and pulse amplitude changes (Kim, Arakawa, & Von Lintel, 1975; Meijer, deLange, & Ros, 1988) are difficult to quantify. Microneurography (Lindberg & Wallin, 1981) is direct but invasive and requires elaborate equipment and expertise, as does laser skin blood flow measurement (Bengtsson, Nilsson, & Löfström, 1983). Sweat testing (Benzon, Cheng, Avram, & Molloy, 1985) is cumbersome, time-consuming, and not well accepted by patients, and therefore is not widely used. Most common is the measurement of skin temperature by thermography or contact thermometry. A temperature increase of $1.0°–3.0°C$ is typically used (Carron & Litwiller, 1975; Hardy, 1989; Hogan, Taylor, Goldstein, Stevens, & Kettler, 1994) as a threshold for confirming the onset of sympathetic blockade, but the method is ineffective if the skin is warm at the outset of a block. Stellate, thoracic, or lumbar sympathetic injections that produce no measurable evidence of sympathetic blockade cannot reveal disease pathophysiology, regardless of the response of pain.

Rates of success in actually interrupting sympathetic activity following injections intended for that purpose are incompletely known. Stellate ganglion block predictably produces sympathetic interruption to the head, as demonstrated by Horner's syndrome following approximately 85% of blocks (Hogan, Taylor, et al., 1994; Malmqvist, Bengtsson, & Sorensen, 1992; Ready, Kozody, Barsa, & Murphy, 1982). Blockade of fibers to the hand is much less frequent, with studies showing success in 12%–36% of injections when multiple criteria are applied (Hogan, Dotson, Erickson, Kettler, & Hogan, 1994; Malmqvist et al., 1992; Stevens et al., 1998). There is little difference in the adequacy of sympathetic blockade by paravertebral injection at C7 level compared with C6 (Hogan, Erickson, Haddox, & Abram, 1992; Malmqvist et al., 1992; Matsumoto, 1991; Yamamuro & Kaneko, 1978). Injection through a needle placed at the head of the first rib requires CT guidance but assures successful blockade (Erickson & Hogan, 1993). There are few studies of the success rates for lumbar sympathetic block. Using phenol, approximately 65% of patients show ipsilateral warming (Hatangdi & Boas, 1985). While local anesthetic was shown on average to produce more foot warming on the block side than the contralateral side (Tran et al., 2000), no frequency data was provided.

Stellate ganglion injection may fail to produce sympathetic denervation for several reasons. Multiple alternative routes allow sympathetic fibers to reach peripheral sites without transit through the stellate ganglion (Alexander, Kuntz, Henderson, & Ehrlich, 1949; Groen, Baljet, Boekelaar, & Drukker, 1987; Kirgis & Kuntz, 1942; van Buskirk, 1941). However, the principal reason for failure of injection to produce stellate ganglion blockade is lack of delivery of anesthetic to the ganglion. Whereas the ganglion resides at the lower edge of the head of the first rib (Hogan & Erickson, 1992), solution injected at cervical levels passes anterior into the mediastinum (Guntamukkala & Hardy, 1991; Hogan et al., 1992). In addition to incomplete block, there is evidence of unintended block of somatic elements. Blocks that produced the greatest pain relief were found by careful sensory testing to have a subtle component of somatic afferent anesthesia (Dellemijn, Fields, Allen, McKay, & Rowbotham, 1994).

At lumbar levels, alternative pathways may also allow persistent sympathetic innervation to reach the lower extremities, despite a properly performed lumbar sympathetic block (Cowley & Yeager, 1949). Even crossover of fibers from the contralateral chain has been documented (Kleiman, 1954; Weber, 1957; Yeager & Cowley, 1948). Local anesthetic solution passing to the epidural space along the vertebral body (Evans, Dobben, & Gay, 1967) may result in undesired somatic blockade, thereby producing analgesia that is then attributed to a sympathetic mechanism. All blocks of the paravertebral sympathetic chain inevitably interrupt visceral afferent signals that travel in sympathetic trunks (Schott, 1994). As an example of the confusion that could result from neglecting this fact, a stellate ganglion block might stop arm pain from myocardial ischemia, but could be credited with identifying a sympathetically dependent pain process.

Published reports examining the diagnostic use of sympathetic blockade present findings that raise doubt regarding the relevance of sympathetic testing. The degree of sympathetic dysfunction does not correlate with the response of pain to sympathetic blockade (Loh & Nathan, 1978; Tahmoush, Malley, & Jennings, 1983), and the timing of changes in pain does not necessarily match the onset of manifestations of sympathetic block. Signs of sympathetic blockade do not predict magnitude of pain relief following stellate ganglion block (Price, Long, Wilsey, & Rafii, 1998). When sympathetic activity is measured with microelectrode neurography in limbs with pain relieved by local anesthetic sympathetic block, sympathetic efferent traffic is normal (Torebjork, 1990). Response of pain to sympathetic blockade does not predict levels of norepinephrine and its metabolite in the venous effluent from limbs with features of reflex sympathetic dystrophy (Drummond, Fincj, & Smythe, 1991). In fact, venous plasma catecholamine levels are consistently lower on the painful side than on the unaffected side. These findings make less plausible the belief that sympathetic block analgesia identifies regional sympathetic hyperactivity. The important question of whether the response to sympathetic blockade guides therapy toward a better outcome has not been addressed in any formal way.

The role of sympathetic motor activity in the generation of painful conditions is unresolved and controversial. Although neural blockade holds out hope that solid pathophysiological evidence may be obtained, I believe that the diagnostic value of sympathetic blockade has been overestimated. Appropriate use calls for care in documenting the desired physiological response and for restraint in interpretation of the results. There should be caution to avoid the circular logic of defining sympathetically maintained pain as conditions improved by sympathetic blocks, and defining the blocks as successful if they relieve a pain assumed to be sympathetically maintained.

Intravenous Regional Sympathetic Block

Both guanethidine (Hannington-Kiff, 1974) and bretylium (Hannington-Kiff, 1990) have been delivered into the isolated venous system of the distal extremities for treatment of patients with sympathetically maintained pain. Both drugs inhibit release of norepinephrine from nerve terminals, and guanethidine depletes tissues of norepinephrine. This explains prolonged relief following intravenous regional (IVR) guanethidine in patients who had only brief relief of pain following local anesthetic IVR blockade (Loh, Nathan, Schott, & Wilson, 1980). Therefore, the patients' sustained response to blockade can be interpreted as an indicator of the contribution of sympathetic activity to the generation of the patients' pain. There are theoretical limitations to the use of these injections for diagnosis, since ischemic block produced by the tourniquet may have a profound effect on certain types of pain (see below), and guanethidine has anticholinergic effects and alters central nervous system (CNS) levels of serotonin (Furst, 1967). There have been no comparisons between block with guanethidine or bretylium and block with saline alone.

Studies to date have shown that IVR guanethidine predictably eliminates allodynia but has no effects on other sensory function (Glynn, Basedow, & Walsh, 1981; Loh et al., 1980). Increased peripheral temperature and blood flow follow IVR guanethidine but not IVR saline. Vasodilatation may be delayed by hours after cuff deflation, and complete blockade of vascular control is rare (Loh et al., 1980). There is no temporal relationship between pain relief and manifestations of sympathetic blockade. This may be due to a vasodilatory action of guanethidine that is independent of effects on norepinephrine release (Abboud & Eckstein, 1962). IVR guanethidine is more effective in patients who exhibit dystrophic changes associated with reflex sympathetic dystrophy (Bonelli et al., 1983). Loh and Nathan (1978) found that pain and sensory response were congruent in 9 of 10 painful limbs when IVR guanethidine was compared with local anesthetic sympathetic chain injections. There is a high correlation between relief of pain from intravenous phentolamine and from IVR guanethidine (Arner, 1991). These cross-comparisons support the notion that each is producing analgesia by a common sympatholytic mechanism.

No studies have specifically examined the diagnostic value of IVR sympathetic block in identifying patients who will have long-term therapeutic benefit from systemic or regional sympatholytic measures. The response to IVR guanethidine or bretylium should be evaluated together with clinical findings and response to other diagnostic interventions, such as paravertebral sympathetic blocks or the phentolamine test.

Differential Block by Pressure and Ischemia

Different fiber types convey a variety of painful sensations, each of which is to a great degree unique to each neuronal category. First pain, produced by impulses in small myelinated $A\delta$ fibers, is prompt, is well localized, and has a pricking and sharp character. Second pain, characteristic of nonmyelinated C fibers, is poorly somatotopic, has gradual onset and offset, and has an aching quality. Pain invoked by soft touch of the skin (mechanical allodynia) is probably due to stimulation of fast-conducting $A\beta$ fibers with subsequent aberrant central processing (Torebjork, Lundberg, & LaMotte, 1992). Advances in the neuropharmacology of pain may produce therapies suitable only for certain pathophysiological conditions, making distinctions of fiber types important. As an example, it is likely that capsaicin, which depletes substance P from the skin and central terminals of C fibers, is only effective in treating pain due to unmyelinated fibers.

Local anesthetics block peripheral nerve C fibers prior to $A\delta$ and $A\beta$ fibers, but the reverse is achieved either by direct focal pressure to the nerve or by a tourniquet that produces compression of the nerve and ischemia of the limb. Microneurographic recording of neuronal impulses document that susceptibility to compression and ischemia is greatest for $A\beta$ and $A\delta$ fibers, while C fibers are resistant (Cline, Ochoa, & Torebjork, 1989; Mackenzie, Burke, Skuse, & Lethlean, 1975; Torebjork & Hallin, 1973). Direct compression of the nerve is limited to sites in which the nerve can be pressed against bone, such as the superficial radial nerve at the wrist (Mackenzie et al., 1975;

Torebjork & Hallin, 1973). The psychophysical response to direct compression of a nerve is the same as tourniquet compression and ischemia (Cline et al., 1989), which is more generally applicable.

Compression and ischemia are achieved simply by inflating a tourniquet proximal to the site of extremity pain to a pressure 100 mm Hg above systolic arterial pressure after exsanguination of the limb by elevation. Standard neurological testing is adequate to detect deactivation of the various fibers. The initial sensory event during compression and ischemia of a nerve is intense paresthesia (Merington & Nathan, 1949). Muscle fasciculations representing spontaneous activity in motor axons accompany only prolonged periods of nerve compression (Bostock, Baker, Grafe, & Reid, 1991). After about 5 minutes, conduction in ischemic nerves begins to fail in a decremental fashion, in which impulses travel progressively more slowly and more limited distances before failing (Nielson & Kardel, 1974). Perception of soft touch fails after 5 to 20 minutes, soon followed by loss of sense of cold and first (sharp) pain. These three sensations may be difficult to reliably separate by compression and ischemia (Yarnitsky & Ochoa, 1989). Sense of warmth is inhibited next. Second (aching) pain remains intact after the loss of warmth and may not be completely abolished by compression and ischemia (Mackenzie et al., 1975; Sinclair & Hinshaw, 1950; Yarnitsky & Ochoa, 1991). Findings are usually complete within 30–45 minutes. Efferent sympathetic impulses persist unimpeded (Casale, Glynn, & Buonocore, 1992).

Although compression–ischemic blockade has been used to determine fiber type of transmission in painful conditions (Campbell, Raja, Meyer, & Mackinnon, 1988; Cline et al., 1989; Gracely, Lynch, & Bennett, 1992; Ochoa & Yarnitsky, 1993), practical clinical utility awaits further developments in the taxonomy and neuropharmacology of pain.

Differential Neuraxial Blockade

Spinal or epidural anesthesia, modulated to produce selective block of particular neural pathways, has been used for diagnostic neural block for a substantial period (Ahlgren, Stephen, Lloyd, & McCollum, 1966; McCollum & Stephen, 1964; Ramamurthy & Winnie, 1983). Responses to placebo and local anesthetic solution is employed at different concentrations to determine contribution of sympathetic efferents, sensory fibers, and even motor fibers. The intention is to observe changes in pain during the different phases of the block, and thereby to distinguish the pain origin as psychogenic, sympathetic, nociceptive (sensory-based), or central. A subarachnoid site of injection has been used most extensively, although a long time is required to perform and assess the individual steps. In a modified technique (Akkiineni & Ramamurthy, 1977), a placebo (saline) injection is followed by 100 mg of procaine injected intrathecally. Pain relief following these injections and relief during gradual resolution of neural blockade are noted. An epidural technique has also been used in a fashion similar to the subarachnoid method (Cherry, Gourlay, McLachlan, & Cousins, 1985). Following a placebo injection of saline, 0.25% lidocaine is injected to block sympathetic fibers, then 0.5% lidocaine to block sensation as well, and finally 1% lidocaine to produce surgical anesthesia. Opioid has also been used as the analgesic agent (Cherry et al., 1985), since analgesia is a specific response and there are minimal sensory cues to trigger a placebo response. In this technique, following placebo injections, fentanyl (1 μg/kg in 5 ml normal saline) is injected through an epidural catheter. Analgesia indicates a predominantly nociceptive mechanism of pain instead of a predominantly psychological one, as does reversal of the analgesia by intravenous injection of naloxone (0.4 mg) unobserved by the subject. There has been no formal comparison of these methods to the classical approach.

The validity of differential spinal block has not been established, and there are a number of drawbacks to the technique. It is not clear whether pain fibers or sympathetic fibers are blocked first (Sarnoff & Arrowood, 1946), and the injected solutions may fail to provide the desired block (Ahlgren et al., 1966; McCollum & Stephen, 1964). The entire premise of the ability to achieve a steady state—complete block of certain fiber types while sparing others in the desired order—is flawed. Lack of obvious sensory changes does not assure that neural processing has not been altered, and even a dense block adequate for surgery does not indicate an absence of afferent sensory traffic or efferent sympathetic impulses. Neuraxial opioid block may be ineffective in relieving pain that is nonetheless nonpsychogenic, especially neuropathic and visceral pain or incident pain with movement (Arner & Arner, 1985; Hogan et al., 1991).

There have been no studies to support claims that differential spinal block leads to selection of more effective treatment. One study that examined the relationship between the presence of psychopathology and the incidence of inappropriate responses to differential spinal block concluded that psychopathology was no more likely among those responding inappropriately (Sanders, McKeel, & Hare, 1984). Overall, the ability of differential neuraxial blocks to diagnose various categories of pain generation is unproved. Basic considerations make it probably an unachievable goal.

Systemic Local Anesthetics

Intravenous lidocaine is often effective in providing temporary relief of neuropathic pain, but is generally thought to be ineffective for nociceptive pain. Therefore, it could be used as a means of distinguishing the pathophysiology of a painful condition. Doses range from 1.5 mg/kg in a single bolus with no infusion (Marchettini et al., 1992) to as much as 5 mg/kg over 30 minutes (Bach et al., 1990; Edwards et al., 1985; Kastrup et al., 1987). There have been no comparisons of these techniques. A careful sensory exam and a determination of pain levels are made before drug delivery and at peak effect. Dizziness and lightheaded feelings may accompany the drug injection.

Studies of clinical and experimentally induced pain indicate there is a mild general systemic analgesic effect with high blood concentrations of lidocaine, but selective analgesia of central and peripheral neuropathic pain can be expected with lower lidocaine concentrations (Boas, Covino, & Shahnarian, 1982; Rowlingson, DiFazio, Foster, & Carron, 1980). This selective effect, however, has not been seen in all studies (Marchettini et al., 1992). Although some papers report relief from oral mexiletine in patients who previously responded to intravenous lidocaine (Peterson & Kastrup, 1987; Scott, 1981; Tanelian & Brose, 1991), randomized and controlled studies have not been done to test the ability of systemic lidocaine to predict the response to mexiletine. In general, intravenous lidocaine may be of some diagnostic value in distinguishing between neuropathic and nociceptive pain, although the therapeutic implications of such a distinction may currently be limited.

Systemic Phentolamine

Phentolamine is an alpha-adrenergic blocking agent that may be administered intravenously to determine the degree to which a patient's pain is sympathetically mediated. It has the diagnostic advantage over local anesthetic sympathetic blocks that it does not interrupt afferent traffic from visceral or somatic structures. It would seem logical that analgesia in response to intravenous phentolamine would predict a beneficial response to intermittent or continuous local anesthetic sympathetic blocks or to oral or transdermal sympatholytic drugs. When phentolamine is given in doses adequate to produce evidence of sympathetic block, such as nasal congestion, hypotension, or skin warming, observing an absence of concurrent pain relief is thought to disprove a sympathetic contribution. If placebo produces no analgesia but phentolamine does, pain relief coincident with an increase in skin temperature indicates a sympathetic contribution. Doses of about 0.5 mg/kg are used, and whenever substantial relief of pain is obtained or significant hypotension occurs, the test is terminated (Arner, 1991; Raja, Treede, Davis, & Campbell, 1991). Rather than administration of phentolamine to a predetermined dose, a more thorough method would involve dosing to a physiological endpoint, such as nasal congestion, hypotension, or skin warming, to assure an adequate phentolamine dose. Clearly, careful monitoring and the availability of resuscitation equipment and personnel are required.

Complications include predictable nasal stuffiness and occasional sinus tachycardia, premature ventricular contractions, dizziness, or wheezing (Shir, Cameron, Raja, & Bourke, 1993). The safety of reduced doses of phentolamine has been confirmed in children (Arner, 1991). Subjects with advanced cardiovascular disease, such as heart block, unstable angina, or congestive heart failure, are unsuitable for the test.

As do most diagnostic injections, this test has limitations. Phentolamine has local anesthetic properties (Northover, 1983; Ramirez & French, 1990), which raises the question of whether relief could be resulting from pharmacological mechanisms other than sympathetic interruption. Also, the degree of sympathetic blockade by phentolamine infusion is unclear, since larger doses and more rapid administration produce greater increase in extremity blood flow and temperature, and sympathetic responses persist even after the largest doses examined (Raja, Turnquist, Meleka, & Campbell, 1996). As with other tests of sympathetic function, a fundamental limitation is the ambiguous role of sympathetic function in pain. Even though a patient experiences relief from intravenous phentolamine, oral sympathetic blocking drugs may be ineffective, since side effects (particularly ortho-

static hypotension) may preclude intense blockade comparable to the potent effect of intravenous phentolamine.

Data have been published that support the use of phentolamine infusion for diagnosis. A strong correlation is found between analgesia in response to intravenous phentolamine and analgesia in response to local anesthetic sympathetic blocks in patients with suspected sympathetically maintained pain (Raja et al., 1991). Surprisingly, patients generally experience relief of both spontaneous and evoked pain (allodynia). Another study of patients (Arner, 1991) shows a good concordance of relief with phentolamine and to IVR guanethidine, although a third of the responders to IVR guanethidine failed to have analgesia with intravenous phentolamine. Others (Shir et al., 1993) have found infrequent response to phentolamine infusion in patients with pain despite clinical evidence of a sympathetic contribution, and placebo response is hard to eliminate or recognize (Fine et al., 1994; Verdugo & Ochoa, 1994), making the phentolamine test impossible to interpret. No studies have been carried out to determine whether the response to intravenous phentolamine predicts the therapeutic efficacy of local anesthetic sympathetic blocks or systemic sympathetic blocking agents.

The diagnostic role for intravenous phentolamine appears promising but still unconfirmed. Although responses correlate well with local anesthetic paravertebral sympathetic blocks and guanethidine IVR sympathetic blocks, it is not clear that either of these is a true standard of pure and complete sympathetic interruption. Results of a phentolamine test should be considered in conjunction with clinical findings and other diagnostic tests. As an alternative, a trial of sympatholytic therapy should be considered. The ability of the phentolamine response to predict outcome of therapy with sympatholytic treatments has not been tested.

Systemic Barbiturates

Small intravenous doses of rapidly acting barbiturates have been used in psychiatric practice to promote a state of relaxation to facilitate communication of thoughts (Kaplan & Sadock, 1985). In the diagnosis of pain, a light hypnotic state may be used in combination with physical exam to discern the contribution of cognitive and emotional issues in pain behavior. Because of the complex involvement of cerebral activity and the conscious mind in the production and manifestation of pain and the resulting behavior, changes during barbiturate administration are very difficult to interpret. The physician should be prepared for the occasional exposure of a distressing and disruptive previously unrecognized psychosis during barbiturate administration.

On a neurophysiological level, the response of pain to barbiturates is not simple. Small doses of intravenous barbiturates cause an increase in pain that has a nociceptive basis (Bonica & Loeser, 1990). This antanalgesic effect has been demonstrated in pressure algometry studies (Briggs, Dundee, Bahar, & Clarke, 1982) and may be related to the ability of these drugs to interfere with descending inhibitory mechanisms through a medullary gamma-aminobutyric acid receptor mechanism (Drower & Hammond, 1988). More problematic from a diagnostic point of view, nonnociceptive pain, such as pain related to CNS injury, is often relieved by subanesthetic barbiturate doses (Tasker, 1990). In fact, relief of central pain by barbiturate and lack of analgesia from morphine have been used to predict success of brain stimulation for pain control (89% positive predictive value) (Tsubokawa, Katayama, Yamamoto, Hirayama, & Koyama, 1991).

No controlled studies attesting to the diagnostic utility of this technique are available. Given its purely empirical basis, great caution should accompany the interpretation of data from such tests. It certainly cannot be used to determine whether pain complaints are genuine.

SUMMARY

Unlike any other field in medicine, the pursuit of diagnosis in chronic pain is a uniquely frustrating endeavor, exemplified by ambiguity, subjectivity, and incomplete understanding of pathophysiology. Diagnostic injection may provide insights into these complex situations, but only if its limitations are well understood. The key elements in proper use of these tests is confirmation of a desired physiological effect (i.e., block of the intended pathways and none other), and awareness of alternative mechanisms of relief that may confound interpretation. These techniques are only suitable as supplements to overall patient evaluation.

ACKNOWLEDGMENT

Portions of this chapter are adapted from Hogan, Q., and Abram, S. (1997). Neural blockade for diagnosis and prognosis: A review. Anesthesiology, 86, 216-241.

REFERENCES

Abboud, F. M., & Eckstein, J. W. (1962). Vasodilator action of guanethidine. Circulation Research, 11, 788-796.

Abram, S. E. (1988). Pain mechanisms in lumbar radiculopathy. Anesthesia and Analgesia, 67, 1135-1137.

Abram, S. E., & Boas, R. A. (1992). Sympathetic and visceral nerve blocks. In J. L. Benumof (Ed.), Clinical procedures in anesthesia and intensive care (pp. 796-805). Philadelphia: Lippincott.

Adams, M. A., Dolan, P., & Hutton, W. C. (1986). The stages of disc degeneration as revealed by discograms. Journal of Bone and Joint Surgery, 68(B), 36-41.

Ahlgren, E. W., Stephen, C. R., Lloyd, E. A. C., & McCollum, D. E. (1966). Diagnosis of pain with a graduated spinal block technique. Journal of the American Medical Association, 195, 125-128.

Akkineni, S. R., & Ramamurthy, S. (1977). Simplified differential spinal block. American Society of Anesthesiology Annual Management Abstracts, 765-766.

Alexander, W., Kuntz, A., Henderson, W., & Ehrlich, E. (1949). Sympathetic ganglion cells in ventral nerve roots: Their relation to sympathectomy. Science, 109, 484.

Aprill, C., & Bogduk, N. (1992). The prevalence of cervical zygapophyseal joint pain: A first approximation. Spine, 17, 744-747.

Arner, S. (1991). Intravenous phentolamine test: Diagnostic and prognostic use in reflex sympathetic dystrophy. Pain, 46, 17-22.

Arner, S., & Arner, B. (1985). Differential effects of epidural morphine in the treatment of cancer-related pain. Acta Anaesthesiologica Scandinavica, 29, 32-36.

Arner, S., Lindblom, U., Meyerson, B. A., & Molander, C. (1990). Prolonged relief of neuralgia after regional anesthetic blocks: A call for further experimental and systematic clinical studies. Pain, 43, 287-297.

Bach, F. W., Jensen, T. S., Kastrup, J., Stigsby, B., & Dejgard, A. (1990). The effects of intravenous lidocaine on nociceptive processing in diabetic neuropathy. Pain, 40, 29-34.

Barnsley, L., & Bogduk, N. (1993). Medial branch blocks are specific for the diagnosis of cervical zygapophyseal joint pain. Regional Anesthesia, 18, 242-250.

Barnsley, L., Lord, S., & Bogduk, N. (1993). Comparative local anaesthetic blocks in the diagnosis of cervical zygapophyseal joint pain. Pain, 55, 99-106.

Beecher, H. K. (1955). The powerful placebo. Journal of the American Medical Association, 159, 1602-1606.

Bengtsson, M., Löfström, J. B., & Malmqvist, L.-Å. (1985). Skin conduction changes during spinal analgesia. Acta Anaesthesiologica Scandinavica, 29, 67-71.

Bengtsson, M., Nilsson, G. E., & Löfström, J. B. (1983). The effect of spinal analgesia on skin blood flow, evaluated by laser Doppler flowmetry. Acta Anaesthesiologica Scandinavica, 17, 206.

Benzon, H. T., Cheng, S., Avram, M., & Molloy, R. (1985). Sign of complete sympathetic blockade: Sweat test or sympathogalvanic response. *Anesthesia and Analgesia, 64,* 415-419.

Blumberg, H., & Janig, W. (1984). Discharge pattern of afferent fibers from a neuroma. *Pain, 20,* 335-353.

Boas, R. A., Covino, B. G., & Shahnarian, A. (1982). Analgesic responses to IV lidocaine. *British Journal of Anaesthesia, 54,* 501-505.

Boden, S. D., Davis, D. O., Dina, T. S., Patronas, N. J., & Wiesel, S. W. (1990). Abnormal magnetic-resonance scans of the lumbar spine in asymptomatic subjects. *Journal of Bone and Joint Surgery, 72*(A), 403-408.

Bogduk, N. (1981). The anatomy of occipital neuralgia. *Clinical and Experimental Neurology, 17,* 167-184.

Bogduk, N. (1982). The clinical anatomy of cervical dorsal rami. *Spine, 4,* 319-330.

Bogduk, N. (1983). The innervation of the lumbar spine. *Spine, 8,* 286-293.

Bogduk, N., & Aprill, C. (1993). On the nature of neck pain, discography and cervical zygapophyseal joint blocks. *Pain, 54,* 213-217.

Bogduk, N., & Long, D. M. (1980). Percutaneous lumbar medial branch neurotomy: A modification of facet denervation. *Spine, 5,* 193-200.

Bogduk, N., & Long, D. M. (1979). The anatomy of the so-called "articular nerves" and their relationship to facet denervation in the treatment of low-back pain. *Journal of Neurosurgery, 51,* 172-177.

Bogduk, N., & Marsland, A. (1988). The cervical zygapophyseal joints as a source of neck pain. *Spine, 13,* 610-617.

Bogduk, N., & Modic, M. T. (1996). Lumbar discography. *Spine, 21,* 402-404.

Bogduk, N., Tynan, W., & Wilson, A. S. (1981). The nerve supply to the human lumbar intervertebral discs. *Acta Anatomica, 132,* 9-56.

Bonelli, S., Conoscente, F., Movilia, B.G., Restelli, L., Francucci, B., & Grossi, E. (1983). Regional intravenous guanethidine vs. stellate ganglion block in reflex sympathetic dystrophies: A randomized trial. *Pain, 16,* 297-307.

Bonica, J. J., & Loeser, J. D. (1990). Medical evaluation of the patient with pain. In J. J. Bonica (Ed.), *The management of pain* (2nd ed., pp. 563-579). Philadelphia: Lea & Febiger.

Bostock, H., Baker, M., Grafe, P., & Reid, G. (1991). Changes in excitability and accommodation of human motor axons following brief periods of ischemia. *Journal of Physiology (London), 441,* 537-557.

Bovim, G., Berg, R., & Dale, L. G. (1992). Cervicogenic headache: Anesthetic blockades of cervical nerves (C2-C5) and facet joint (C2/C3). *Pain, 49,* 315-320.

Bovim, G., Bonamico, L., Fredriksen, T. A., Lindboe, C. F., Stolt-Nielsen, A., & Sjaastad, O. (1991). Topographic variations in the peripheral course of the greater occipital nerve. *Spine, 16,* 475-478.

Bovim, G., Fredriksen, T. A., Stolt-Nielsen, A., & Sjaastad, O. (1992). Neurolysis of the greater occipital nerve in cervicogenic headache: A follow up study. *Headache, 32,* 175-179.

Bovim, G., & Sand, T. (1992). Cervicogenic headache, migraine without aura and tension-type headache: Diagnostic blockade of greater occipital and supraorbital nerves. *Pain, 51,* 43-48.

Bowen, V., & Cassidy, J. D. (1981). Macroscopic and microscopic anatomy of the sacroiliac joint from embryonic life until the eighth decade. *Spine, 6,* 620-628.

Briggs, L. P., Dundee, J. W., Bahar, M., & Clarke, R. S. J. (1982). Comparison of the effect of diisopropyl phenol (ICI 35868) and thiopentone on response to somatic pain. *British Journal of Anaesthesia, 54,* 307-311.

Butler, D., Trafimow, J. H., Andersson, G. B. J., McNeill, T. W., & Hackman, M. S. (1990). Discs degenerate before facets. *Spine, 15,* 111-113.

Campbell, J. N., Raja, S. N., Meyer, R. A., & Mackinnon, S. E. (1988). Myelinated afferents signal the hyperalgesia associated with nerve injury. *Pain, 32,* 89-94.

Campbell, D. G., & Parsons, C. M. (1944). Referred head pain and its concomitants. *Journal of Nervous and Mental Disease, 99,* 544-551.

Carette, S., Marcoux, S., Truchon, R., Grondin, C., Gagnon, J., Allard, Y., & Latulippe, M. (1991). A controlled trial of corticosteroid injection into facet joints for chronic low back pain. *New England Journal of Medicine, 325,* 1002-1007.

Carrera, G. F. (1980). Lumbar facet joint injection in low back pain and sciatica: Preliminary results. *Radiology, 137,* 665-557.

Carron, H., & Litwiller, R. (1975). Stellate ganglion block. *Anesthesia and Analgesia, 54,* 567-570.

Casale, R., Glynn, C., & Buonocore, M. (1992). The role of ischaemia in the analgesia which follows Bier's block technique. *Pain, 50,* 169-175.

Cavanaugh, J. M., El-Bohy, A., Hardy, W. N., Getchell, T. V., Getchell, M. L., & King, A. I. (1989). Sensory innervation of soft tissues of the lumbar spine in the rat. *Journal of Orthopedic Research, 7,* 378-388.

Chabal, C., Russell, L. C., & Burchiel, K. J. (1989). The effect of intravenous lidocaine, tocainide, and mexiletene on spontaneously active fibers originating in rat sciatic neuromas. *Pain, 38,* 333-338.

Cherry, D. A., Gourlay, G. K., McLachlan, M., & Cousins, M. J. (1985). Diagnostic epidural opioid blockade and chronic pain: Preliminary report. *Pain, 21,* 143-152.

Cline, M. A., Ochoa, J., & Torebjork, H. E. (1989). Chronic hyperalgesia and skin warming caused by sensitized C nociceptors. *Brain, 112,* 621-647.

Colhoun, E., McCall, I. W., Williams, L., & Cassar Pullicino, V. N. (1988). Provocation discography as a guide to planning operations on the spine. *Journal of Bone and Joint Surgery, 70*(B), 267-271.

Cowley, R. A., & Yeager, G. H. (1949). Anatomic observations on the lumbar sympathetic nervous system. *Surgery, 25,* 880-890.

Cyriax, J. (1938). Rheumatic headache. *British Medical Journal, ii,* 1367-1368.

Dellemijn, P. L. I., Fields, H. L., Allen, R. R., McKay, W. R., & Rowbotham, M. C. (1994). The interpretation of pain relief and sensory changes following sympathetic blockade. *Brain, 117,* 1475-1487.

Derby, R., Kine, G., Saal, J. A., Reynolds, J., Goldthwaite, N., White, A. H., Hsu, K., & Zucherman, J. (1992). Response to steroid and duration of radicular pain as predictors of surgical outcome. *Spine, 17,* S176-S183.

Destouet, J. M., Gilula, L. A., Murphey, W. A., & Monsees, B. (1982). Lumbar facet joint injection: Indication, technique, clinical correlation, and preliminary results. *Radiology, 145,* 321-325.

Devor, M., & Janig, W. (1981). Activation of myelinated afferents ending in neuroma by stimulation of the sympathetic supply in the rat. *Neuroscience Letters, 24*, 43-47.

Devor, M., Wall, P. D., & Catalan, N. (1992). Systemic lidocaine silences neuroma and DRG discharge without blocking nerve conduction. *Pain, 48*, 261-268.

Dooley, J. F., McBroom, R. J., Taguchi, T., & MacNab, I. (1988). Nerve root infiltration in the diagnosis of radicular pain. *Spine, 13*, 79-83.

Dory, M. A. (1981). Arthrography of the lumbar facet joints. *Radiology, 140*, 23-27.

Dory, M. A. (1983). Arthrography of the cervical facet joints. *Radiology, 148*, 379-382.

Dreyfuss, P., Dryer, S., Griffin, J., Hoffman, J., & Walsh, N. (1994). Positive sacroiliac screening tests in asymptomatic adults. *Spine, 19*, 1138-1143.

Dreyfuss, P., Michaelsen, M., & Fletcher, D. (1994). Atlanto-occipital and lateral atlanto-axial joint pain patterns. *Spine, 19*, 1125-1131.

Drower, E. J., & Hammond, D. L. (1988). GABAergic modulation of nociceptive threshold: Effects of THIP and bicuculline microinjected in the ventral medulla of the rat. *Brain Research, 450*, 316-324.

Drummond, P. D., Fincj, P. M., & Smythe, G. A. (1991). Reflex sympathetic dystrophy: The significance of differing plasma catecholamine concentrations in affected and unaffected limbs. *Brain, 114*, 2025-2036.

Dubner, R., Hoffman, D., & Hayes, R. (1981). Neuronal activity in medullary dorsal horn of awake monkeys trained in a thermal discrimination task: III. Task-related responses and their functional role. *Journal of Neurophysiology, 46*, 444-464.

Dunlop, R. B., Adams, M. A., & Hutton, W. C. (1984). Disc space narrowing and the lumbar facet joints. *Journal of Bone and Joint Surgery, 66*(B), 706-710.

Dwyer, A., Aprill, C., & Bogduk, N. (1990). Cervical zygapophyseal joint pain patterns: I. A study in normal volunteers. *Spine, 15*, 453-457.

Edgar, M. A., & Ghadially, J. A. (1976). Innervation of the lumbar spine. *Clinical Orthopedics and Related Research, 115*, 35-41.

Edmeads, J. (1988). The cervical spine and headache. *Neurology, 38*, 1874-1878.

Edwards, W. T., Habib, F., Burney, R. G., & Begin, G. (1985). Intravenous lidocaine in the management of various chronic pain states. *Regional Anesthesia, 10*, 1-6.

El-Bohy, A., Cavanaugh, J. M., Getchell, M. L., Bulas, T., Getchell, T. V., & King, A. I. (1988). Localization of substance P and neurofilament immunoreactive fibers in the lumbar facet joint capsule and supraspinous ligament of the rabbit. *Brain Research, 460*, 379-382.

Epstein, J. A., Epstein, B. S., Lavine, L. S., Carras, R., Rosenthal, A. D., & Sumner, P. (1973). Lumbar nerve root compression at the intervertebral foramina caused by arthritis of the posterior facets. *Journal of Neurosurgery, 39*, 362-369.

Erickson, S. J., & Hogan, Q. (1993). CT guided stellate ganglion injection: Description of technique and efficacy of sympathetic blockade. *Radiology, 188*, 707-709.

Evans, F. J. (1974). The placebo response in pain reduction. *Advances in Neurology, 4*, 289-300.

Evans, J., Dobben, G., & Gay, G. (1967). Peridural effusion of drugs following sympathetic blockade. *Journal of the American Medical Association, 200*, 573-578.

Fairbank, J. C. T., McCall, I. W., & O'Brian, J. P. (1981). Apophyseal injection of local anesthetic as a diagnos-

tic aid in primary low-back pain syndromes. *Spine, 6*, 598-605.

Feinstein, B., Langton, J. N. K., Jameson, R. M., & Schiller, F. (1954). Experiments on pain referred from deep somatic tissues. *Journal of Bone and Joint Surgery, 36*(A), 981-997.

Fernstrom, U. (1960). A discographical study of ruptured lumbar intervertebral discs. *Acta Chirurgica Scandinavica, S258*, 10-60.

Fine, P. G., Roberts, W. J., Gillette, R. G., & Child, T. R. (1994). Slowly developing placebo responses confound tests of intravenous phentolamine to determine mechanisms underlying idiopathic chronic low back pain. *Pain, 56*, 235-242.

Foerster, O. (1933). The dermatomes in man. *Brain, 56*, 1-39.

Forsythe, W. B., & Ghoshal, N. G. (1984). Innervation of the canine thoracolumbar vertebral column. *Anatomical Record, 208*, 57-63.

Fortin, J. D., Dwyer, A. P., West, S., & Pier, J. (1994). Sacroiliac joint: Pain referral maps upon applying a new injection/arthrography technique: Part I. Asymptomatic volunteers. *Spine, 19*, 1475-1482.

Friedman, J., & Goldner, M. Z. (1955). Discography in evaluation of lumbar disk lesions. *Radiology, 65*, 653-662.

Furst, C. I. (1967). The biochemistry of guanethidine. *Advances in Drug Research, 4*, 133-161.

Ghelman, B., & Doherty, J. H. (1978). Demonstration of spondylolysis by arthrography of the apophyseal joint. *American Journal of Roentgenography, 130*, 986-987.

Gibson, M. J., Buckley, J., Mulholland, R. C., & Worthington, B. S. (1986). Magnetic resonance imaging and discography in the diagnosis of disc degeneration. *Journal of Bone and Joint Surgery, 68*(B), 369-373.

Gielen, M. J., Slappendel, R., & Merx, J. L. (1991). Asymmetric onset of sympathetic blockade in epidural anesthesia shows no relation to epidural catheter position. *Acta Anaesthesiologica Scandinavica, 35*, 81-84.

Giles, L. G. F., & Harvey, A. R. (1987). Immunohistochemical demonstration of nociceptors in the capsule and synovial folds of human zygapophyseal joints. *British Journal of Rheumatology, 26*, 362-364.

Giles, L. G. F., & Taylor, J. R. (1987). Human zygapophyseal joint capsule and synovial fold innervation. *British Journal of Rheumatology, 26*, 93-98.

Giles, L. G. F., Taylor, J. R., & Cockson, A. (1986). Human zygapophyseal joint synovial folds. *Acta Anatomica, 126*, 110-114.

Gillette, R. G., Kramis, R. C., & Roberts, W. J. (1993). Characterization of spinal somatosensory neurons having receptive fields in lumbar tissues of cats. *Pain, 54*, 85-98.

Glynn, C. J., Basedow, R. W., & Walsh, J. A. (1981). Pain relief following post-ganglionic sympathetic blockade with I.V. guanethidine. *British Journal of Anaesthesia, 53*, 1297-1301.

Goodwin, J. S., Goodwin, J. M., & Vogel, A. V. (1979). Knowledge and use of placebos by house officers and nurses. *Annals of Internal Medicine, 91*, 106-110.

Gracely, R. H., Dubner, R., Deeter, W. R., & Wolskee, P. J. (1985). Clinical expectations influence placebo analgesia. *Lancet, i*, 43.

Gracely, R. H., Lynch, S. A., & Bennett, G. J. (1992). Painful neuropathy: Altered central processing maintained dynamically by peripheral input. *Pain, 51*, 175–194.

Green, D. P. (1984). Diagnostic and therapeutic value of carpal tunnel injection. *Journal of Hand Surgery, 9A*, 850–854.

Groen, G. J., Baljet, B., Boekelaar, A. B., & Drukker, J. (1987). Branches of the thoracic sympathetic trunk in the human fetus. *Anatomy and Embryology, 176*, 401–411.

Groen, G. J., Baljet, B., & Drukker, J. (1988). The innervation of the spinal dura mater: Anatomy and clinical implications. *Acta Neurochirgerie, 92*, 39–46.

Groen, G. J., Baljet, B., & Drukker, J. (1990). Nerves and nerve plexuses of the human vertebral column. *American Journal of Anatomy, 188*, 282–296.

Grubb, S. A., Lipscomb, H. J., & Guilford, W. B. (1987). The relative value of lumbar roentgenograms, metrizamide myelography, and discography in the assessment of patients with chronic low-back syndrome. *Spine, 12*, 282–286.

Guntamukkala, M., & Hardy, P. A. J. (1991). Spread of injectate after stellate ganglion block in man: An anatomical study. *British Journal of Anaesthesia, 66*, 643–644.

Guyer, D., & Ohnmeiss, D. D. (1995). Lumbar discography: Position statement from the North American Spine Society Diagnostic and Therapeutic Committee. *Spine, 18*, 2048–2059.

Hannington-Kiff, J. G. (1974). Intravenous regional sympathetic block with guanethidine. *Lancet, i*, 1019–1020.

Hannington-Kiff, J. G. (1990). Retrograde intravenous sympathetic target blocks in limbs. In M. Stanton-Hicks (Ed.), *Pain and the sympathetic nervous system* (pp. 191–126). Boston: Kluwer.

Hardy, P. (1989). Stellate ganglion block with bupivacaine: Minimum effective concentration of bupivacaine and the effect of added potassium. *Anaesthesia, 44*, 398–399.

Hatangdi, V., & Boas, R. (1985). Lumbar sympathectomy: A single needle technique. *British Journal of Anaesthesia, 57*, 285–289.

Hatch, J. P., Moore, P. J., Cyr-Provost, M., Boutros, N. N., Seleshi, E., & Borcherding, S. (1992). The use of electromyography and muscle palpation in the diagnosis of tension-type headache with and without pericranial muscle involvement. *Pain, 49*, 175–178.

Haueisen, D. C., Smith, B. S., Myers, S. R., & Pryce, M. L. (1985). The diagnostic accuracy of spinal nerve injection studies. *Clinical Orthopaedics and Related Research, 198*, 179–183.

Helbig, T., & Lee, C. K. (1988). The lumbar facet syndrome. *Spine, 13*, 61–64.

Hendrix, R. W., Lin, P. P., & Kane, W. J. (1982). Simplified aspiration or injection technique for the sacroiliac joint. *Journal of Bone and Joint Surgery, 64(A)*, 1249–1252.

Hirsch, C., Ingelmark, B., & Miller, M. (1963). The anatomical basis for low back pain. *Acta Orthopaedica Scandinavica, 33*, 1–17.

Hogan, Q. (1993a). The sympathetic nervous system in post-herpetic neuralgia. *Regional Anesthesia, 18*, 271–273.

Hogan, Q. (1993b). Tuffier's line: The normal distribution of anatomic parameters. *Anesthesia and Analgesia, 78*, 194–195.

Hogan, Q., & Abram, S. (1997). Neural blockade for diagnosis and prognosis: A review. *Anesthesiology, 86*, 216–241.

Hogan, Q., Dotson, R., Erickson S., Kettler, R., & Hogan, K. (1994). Local anesthetic myotoxicity: A case and review. *Anesthesiology, 80*, 942–947.

Hogan, Q., & Erickson, S. (1992). MR imaging of the stellate ganglion: Normal appearance. *American Journal of Roentgenography, 158*, 655–659.

Hogan, Q., Erickson, S., Haddox, J. D., & Abram, S. (1992). The spread of solutions during "stellate ganglion" blockade. *Regional Anesthesia, 17*, 78–83.

Hogan, Q., Haddox, J. D., Abram, S., Weissman, D., Taylor, M. L., & Janjan, N. (1991). Epidural opiates and local anesthetics for the management of cancer pain. *Pain, 46*, 271–279.

Hogan, Q., Taylor, M. L., Goldstein, M., Stevens, R., & Kettler, R. (1994). Success rates in producing sympathetic blockade by paratracheal injection. *Clinical Journal of Pain, 10*, 139–145.

Hopf, H., Weissbach, B., & Peters, J. (1990). High thoracic segmental epidural anesthesia diminishes sympathetic outflow to the legs, despite restriction of sensory blockade to the upper thorax. *Anesthesiology, 73*, 882–889.

Horton, W. C., & Daftari, T. (1992). Which disc as visualized by magnetic resonance imaging is actually a source of pain? *Spine, 17*, S164–S171.

Houde, R. W., Wallenstein, M. S., & Rogers, A. (1966). Clinical pharmacology of analgesics: A method of assaying analgesic effect. *Clinical Pharmacology and Therapeutics, 1*, 163–174.

Hove, B., & Gyldensted, C. (1990). Cervical analgesic facet joint arthrography. *Neuroradiology, 32*, 456–459.

Hubbard, D. R., & Berkoff, G. M. (1993). Myofascial trigger points show spontaneous needle EMG activity. *Spine, 18*, 1803–1807.

Hunter, C. R., & Mayfield, F. H. (1949). Role of the upper cervical roots in the production of pain in the head. *American Journal of Surgery, 78*, 743–749.

Jackson, R. P., Jacobs, R. R., & Montesano, P. X. (1988). Facet joint injection in low-back pain: A prospective statistical study. *Spine, 13*, 966–971.

Jackson, R. P. (1992). The facet syndrome. *Clinical Orthopaedics and Related Research, 279*, 110–121.

Jensen, M. C., Brant-Zawadzki, M. N., Obuchowski, N., Modic, M., Malkasian, D., & Ross, J. S. (1994). Magnetic resonance imaging of the lumbar spine in people without back pain. *New England Journal of Medicine, 331*, 69–73.

Jerosch, J., Tappiser, R., & Asslieuer, J. (1998). MRI-controlled facet block—technique and initial results. *Biomedizinische Technik, 43*, 249–252.

Kaplan, M., Dreyfuss, P., Holbrook, B., Bogduk, N. (1998). The ability of lumbar medial branch blocks to anesthetize the zygapophysial joint. *Spine, 23*, 847–852.

Kaplan, H. I., & Sadock, B. J. (Eds.). (1985). *Comprehensive textbook of psychiatry* (4th ed.). Baltimore: Williams & Wilkins.

Kastrup, J., Peterson, P., Dejgard, A., Angel, H. R., & Hilsted, J. (1987). Intravenous lidocaine infusion: A new treatment for chronic painful diabetic neuropathy? *Pain, 28*, 69–75.

Kellgren, J. H. (1939). On the distribution of pain arising from deep somatic structures with charts of segmental pain areas. *Clinical Science, 4*, 35–46.

Kibler, R. F., & Nathan, P. W. (1960). Relief of pain and paresthesiae by nerve block distal to a lesion. *Journal of Neurology, Neurosurgery and Psychiatry, 23,* 91–98.

Kidd, B. L., Cruwys, S., Mapp, P. I., & Blake, D. R. (1992). Role of the sympathetic nervous system in chronic joint pain and inflammation. *Annals of Rheumatic Disease, 51,* 1188–1191.

Kikuchi, S., Hasue, M., Nishiyama, K., & Ito, T. (1984). Anatomic and clinical studies of radicular symptoms. *Spine, 9,* 23–30.

Kim, J. M., Arakawa, K., & Von Lintel, T. (1975). Use of pulse-wave monitor as a measurement of diagnostic sympathetic block and of surgical sympathectomy. *Anesthesia and Analgesia, 54,* 289–296.

Kirgis, H., & Kuntz, A. (1942). Inconstant sympathetic neural pathways. *Archives of Surgery, 44,* 95–102.

Kleiman, A. (1954). Evidence of the existence of crossed sensory sympathetic fibers. *American Journal of Surgery, 87,* 839–841.

Krempen, J. S., Smith, B., & DeFreest, L. J. (1975). Selective nerve root infiltration for the evaluation of sciatica. *Orthopedic Clinics of North America, 6,* 311–315.

Kuslich, S. D., & Ulstrom, C.L. (1991). The tissue origin of low back pain and sciatica: A report of pain response to tissue stimulation during operations on the lumbar spine using local anesthesia. *Orthopedic Clinics of North America, 22,* 181–187.

Levine, J. D., Gordon, N. C., Bornstein, J. C., & Fields, H. L. (1979). Role of pain in placebo analgesia. *Proceedings of the National Academy of Sciences USA, 76,* 3528–3531.

Liberman, R. (1964). An experimental study of the placebo response under three different situations of pain. *Journal of Psychiatric Research, 2,* 233–246.

Lilius, G., Laasonen, E. M., Myllynen, P., Harilainen, A., & Gronlund, G. (1989). Lumbar facet joint syndrome: A randomized clinical trial. *Journal of Bone and Joint Surgery, 71*(B), 681–684.

Lindberg, L., & Wallin, B. G. (1981). Sympathetic skin nerve discharges in relation to amplitude of skin resistance responses. *Psychophysiology, 18,* 268–270.

Loeser, J. D. (1972). Dorsal rhizotomy for the relief of chronic pain. *Journal of Neurosurgery, 36,* 745–750.

Loh, L., & Nathan, P. W. (1978). Painful peripheral states and sympathetic block. *Journal of Neurology, Neurosurgery and Psychiatry, 41,* 664–671.

Loh, L., Nathan, P. W., Schott, G. D., & Wilson, P. G. (1980). Effects of regional guanethidine in certain painful states. *Journal of Neurology, Neurosurgery and Psychiatry, 43,* 446–451.

Lora, J., & Long, D. (1976). So-called facet denervation in the management of intractable back pain. *Spine, 2,* 121–126.

Lund, C., Selmer, P., Hansen, D. B., Hjortso, N.-C., & Kehlet, H. (1987). Effects of epidural bupivacaine on somatosensory evoked potentials after dermatomal stimulation. *Anesthesia and Analgesia, 66,* 34–38.

Lynch, M. C., & Taylor, J. F. (1986). Facet joint injection for low back pain. *Journal of Bone and Joint Surgery, 68*(B), 138–141.

Mackenzie, R. A., Burke, D., Skuse, N. F., & Lethlean, A. K. (1975). Fiber function and perception during cutaneous nerve block. *Journal of Neurology, Neurosurgery and Psychiatry, 38,* 865–873.

Maldague, B., Mathurin, P., & Malghem, J. (1981). Facet joint arthrography in lumbar spondylosis. *Radiology, 140,* 29–36.

Malmqvist, E. L., Bengtsson, M., & Sorensen, J. (1992). Efficacy of stellate ganglion block: A clinical study with bupivacaine. *Regional Anesthesia, 17,* 340–347.

Malmqvist, L., Tryggvason, B., & Bengtsson, M. (1989). Sympathetic blockade during extradural analgesia with mepivacaine or bupivacaine. *Acta Anaesthesiologica Scandinavica, 33,* 444–449.

Marchettini, P., Lacerenza, M., Marangoni, C., Pellegata, G., Sotgiu, M. L., & Smirne, S. (1992). Lidocaine test in neuralgia. *Pain, 48,* 377–382.

Marks, R. (1989). Distribution of pain provoked from lumbar facet joints and related structures during diagnostic spinal infiltration. *Pain, 39,* 37–40.

Marks, R. C., Houston, T., & Thulbourne, T. (1992). Facet joint injection and facet nerve block: A randomised comparison in 86 patients with chronic low back pain. *Pain, 49,* 325–328.

Matsumoto, S. (1991). Thermographic assessments of the sympathetic blockade by stellate ganglion block: Comparison between C7-SGB and C6-SGB in 40 patients. *Masui: Japanese Journal of Anesthesiology, 40,* 562–569.

Mayfield, F. H. (1955). Neurosurgical aspects: Symposium on cervical trauma. *Clinical Neurosurgery, 2,* 83–99.

McCall, I. W., Park, W. M., & O'Brien, J. P. (1979). Induced pain referral from posterior lumbar elements in normal subjects. *Spine, 4,* 441–446.

McCollum, D. E., & Stephen, C. R. (1964). The use of graduated spinal anesthesia in the differential diagnosis of pain of the back and lower extremities. *Southern Medical Journal, 57,* 410–416.

McDonald, G. J., Lord, S. M., & Bogduk, N. (1999). Long term follow-up of patients treated with cervical radio frequency neurotomy for chronic neck pain. *Neurosurgery, 45,* 61–67.

McLain, R. F. (1994). Mechanicoreceptor endings in human cervical facet joints. *Spine, 19,* 195–201.

Meijer, J., deLange, J., & Ros, H. (1988). Skin pulse wave monitoring during lumbar epidural and spinal anesthesia. *Anesthesia and Analgesia, 67,* 356–359.

Merington, W. R., & Nathan, P. W. (1949). A study of post-ischemic paresthesiae. *Journal of Neurology, Neurosurgery and Psychiatry, 12,* 1–18.

Mooney, V., & Robertson, J. (1976). The facet syndrome. *Clinical Orthopaedics and Related Research, 115,* 149–156.

Moran, R., O'Connell, D., & Walsh, M. G. (1988). The diagnostic value of facet joint injections. *Spine, 13,* 1407–1410.

Murphey, F. (1968). Sources and patterns of pain in disc disease. *Clinical Neurosurgery, 15,* 343–351.

Murphy, W. A. (1984). The facet syndrome. *Radiology, 151,* 533.

Murtagh, F. R. (1988). Computed tomography and fluoroscopy guided anesthesia and steroid injection in facet syndrome. *Spine, 13,* 686–689.

Neidre, A., & MacNab, I. (1983). Anomalies of the lumbosacral nerve roots: Review of 16 cases and classification. *Spine, 8,* 294–299.

Nielson, V. K., & Kardel, T. (1974). Decremental conduction in normal human nerves subjected to ischemia? *Acta Physiologica Scandinavica, 92,* 249–262.

Nitta, H., Tajima, T., Sugiyama, H., & Moriyama, A. (1993). Study of dermatomes by means of selective lumbar spinal nerve block. *Spine, 13,* 1782-1786.

Noordenbos, W., & Wall, P. D. (1981). Implications of the failure of nerve resection and graft to cure chronic pain produced by nerve lesions. *Journal of Neurology, Neurosurgery and Psychiatry, 44,* 1068-1073.

North, R. B., Han, M., Zahurak, M., & Kidd, D. H. (1994). Radiofrequency lumbar facet denervation: Analysis of prognostic factors. *Pain, 57,* 77-83.

North, R. B., Kidd, D. H., Campbell, J. N., & Long, D. M. (1991). Dorsal root ganglionectomy for failed back surgery syndrome: A 5-year follow-up study. *Journal of Neurosurgery, 74,* 236-242.

Northover, B.J. (1983). A comparison of the electrophysiological actions of phentolamine with those of some other antiarrhythmic drugs on tissues isolated from the rat heart. *British Journal of Pharmacology, 80,* 85-93.

Ochoa, J. L., & Yarnitsky, D. (1993). Mechanical hyperalgesias in neuropathic pain patients: Dynamic and static subtypes. *Annals of Neurology, 33,* 465-472.

Ohnmeiss, D. D., Guyer, R. D., & Mason, S. L. (2000). The relation between cervical discographic pain responses and radiographic images. *Clinical Journal of Pain, 16,* 1-5.

Onofrio, B. M., & Campa, H. K. (1972). Evaluation of rhizotomy: Review of 12 years' experience. *Journal of Neurosurgery, 36,* 751-755.

Partington, P. F., & Broome, G. H. (1998). Diagnostic injection around the shoulder: Hit and miss? *Journal of Shoulder and Elbow Surgery, 7,* 147-150.

Peterson, P., & Kastrup, J. (1987). Dercum's disease (adiposa dolorosa): Treatment of the severe pain with intravenous lidocaine. *Pain, 28,* 77-80.

Pfaffenrath, V., Dandekar, R., & Pollmann, W. (1987). Cervicogenic headache: The clinical picture, radiologic findings and hypotheses of its pathophysiology. *Headache, 27,* 495-499.

Plancarte, R., Velazquez, R., & Patt, R. B. (1993). Neurolytic blocks of the sympathetic axis. In R. B. Patt (Ed.), *Cancer pain* (pp. 377-435). Philadelphia: Lippincott.

Powel, M. C., Wilson, M., Szypryt, P., Symonds, E. M., & Worthington, B. S. (1986). Prevalence of lumbar disc degeneration observed by magnetic resonance in symptomless women. *Lancet, ii,* 1366-1367.

Price, D. D., Long, S., Wilsey, B., & Rafii, A. (1998). Analysis of peak magnitude and duration of analgesia produced by local anesthetics injected into sympathetic ganglia of complex regional pain syndrome patients. *Clinical Journal of Pain, 14,* 216-226.

Raja, S. N., Treede, R.-D., Davis, K. D., & Campbell, J. N. (1991). Systemic alpha-adrenergic blockade with phentolamine: A diagnostic test for sympathetically maintained pain. *Anesthesiology, 74,* 691-698.

Raja, S. N., Turnquist, J. L., Melcka, S. M., & Campbell, J. N. (1996). Monitoring adequacy of α-adrenoreceptor blockade following systemic phentolamine administration. *Pain, 64,* 197-204.

Ramamurthy, S., & Winnie, A. P. (1993). Diagnostic maneuvers in painful syndromes. *International Anesthesiology Clinics, 83,* 47-59.

Ramirez, J. M., & French, A. S. (1990). Phentolamine selectively affects the fast sodium component of sensory adaptation in an insect mechanoreceptor. *Journal of Neurobiology, 21,* 893-899.

Raymond, J., & Dumas, J.-M. (1984). Intraarticular facet block: diagnostic test or therapeutic procedure? *Radiology, 151,* 333-336.

Raymond. S. A. (1992). Subblocking concentrations of local anesthetics: Effects on impulse generation and conduction in single myelinated sciatic nerve axons in frog. *Anesthesia and Analgesia, 75,* 906-921.

Ready, L. B., Kozody, R., Barsa, J. E., & Murphy, T. M. (1982). Side-port needles for stellate ganglion block. *Regional Anesthesia, 7,* 160-163.

Riew, K. D., Yin, Y., Gilula, L., Bridwell, K. H., Lenke, L. G., Lauryssen, C., & Goette, K. (2000). The effect of nerve-root injections on the need for operative treatment of lumbar radicular pain. *Journal of Bone Joint Surgery, 82*(A), 1589-1593.

Roberts, W. J. (1986). A hypothesis on the physiological basis for causalgia and related pains. *Pain, 24,* 297-311.

Rowlinson, J. C., DiFazio, C. A., Foster, J., & Carron, H. (1980). Lidocaine as an analgesic for experimental pain. *Anesthesiology, 52,* 20-22.

Roy, D. F., Fleury, J., Fontaine, S. B., & Dussault, R. (1988). Clinical evaluation of cervical facet joint infiltration. *Journal of the Canadian Association of Radiologists, 39,* 118-120.

Sanders, S. H., McKeel, N. L., & Hare, B. D. (1984). Relationship between psychopathology and graduated spinal block findings in chronic pain patients. *Pain, 19,* 367-372.

Sarnoff, S. J., & Arrowood, J. G. (1946). Differential spinal block. *Surgery, 20,* 150-159.

Schott, G. D. (1994). Visceral afferents: Their contribution to 'sympathetic dependent' pain. *Brain, 117,* 397-413.

Schutz, H., Lougheed, W. M., Wortzman, G., & Awerbuck, B. G. (1973). Intervertebral nerve-root in the investigation of chronic lumbar disc disease. *Canadian Journal of Surgery, 16,* 217-221.

Schwarzer, A. C., Aprill, C. N., Derby, R., Fortin, J., Kine, G., & Bogduk, N. (1994). Clinical features of patients with pain stemming from the lumbar zygapophyseal joints. *Spine, 19,* 1132-1137.

Schwarzer, A. C., Aprill, C. N., Derby, R., Kine, G., & Bogduk, N. (1994) The false-positive rate of uncontrolled diagnostic blocks of the lumbar zygapophyseal joints. *Pain, 58,* 195-200.

Schwarzer, A. C., Derby, R., Aprill, C. N., Fortin, J., Kine, G., & Bogduk, N. (1994). The value of the provocation response in lumbar zygapophyseal joint injections. *Clinical Journal of Pain, 10,* 309-313.

Scott, R. M. (1981). Mexilitine and vascular headaches. *New Zealand Medical Journal, 93,* 92-93.

Shir, Y., Cameron, L. B., Raja, S., & Bourke, D. L. (1993). The safety of intravenous phentolamine administration in patients with neuropathic pain. *Anesthesia and Analgesia, 76,* 1008-1011.

Sidel, N., & Abrams, M. I. (1940). Treatment of chronic arthritis: Results of vaccine therapy with saline injections as controls. *Journal of the American Medical Association, 114,* 1740-1742.

Sigurdsson, A., & Maixner, W. (1994). Effects of experimental and clinical noxious counterirritants on pain perception. *Pain, 57,* 265-275.

Simmons, E. H., & Segil, C. (1975). An evaluation of discography in the localization of symptomatic levels in discogenic disease of the spine. *Clinical Orthopaedics and Related Research, 108,* 57-69.

Simmons, J. W., Emery, S. F., McMillin, J. N., Landa, D., & Kimmich, S. J. (1991). Awake discography: A comparison with magnetic resonance imaging. *Spine, 16,* S216-S221.

Sinclair, D. C., & Hinshaw, J. R. (1950). A comparison of the sensory dissociation produced by procaine and by limb compression. *Brain, 73,* 480-498.

Sjaastad, O., Fredricksen, T. A., & Pfaffenrath, V. (1990). Cervicogenic headache: diagnostic criteria. *Headache, 30,* 725-726.

Slipman, C. W., Plastaras, C. T., Palmitier, R. A., Huston, C. W., & Sterenfeld, E. B. (1998). Symptom provocation of fluoroscopically guided cervical nerve root stimulation. *Spine, 20,* 2235-2242

Smyth, M. J., & Wright, V. (1958). Sciatica and the intervertebral disc. *Journal of Bone and Joint Surgery, 40*(A), 1401-1418.

Solonen, K. A. (1957). The sacroiliac joint in light of anatomical, roentgenological and clinical studies. *Acta Orthopaedica Scandinavica, 27*(S), 1-27.

Stanley, D., McLaren, M. I., Euinton, H. A., & Getty, C. J. M. (1990). A prospective study of nerve root infiltration in the diagnosis of sciatica. *Spine, 15,* 540-543.

Stevens, R. A., Stotz, A., Kao, T. C., Powar, M., Burgess, S., & Kleinman, B. (1998). The relative increase in skin temperature after stellate ganglion block is predictive of a complete sympathectomy of the hand. *Regional Anesthesia and Pain Medicine, 23,* 266-270.

Stilwell, D. L. (1956). The nerve supply of the vertebral column and its associated structures in the monkey. *Anatomical Record, 125,* 139-162.

Tahmoush, A. J., Malley, J., & Jennings, J. R. (1983). Skin conductance, temperature, and blood flow in causalgia. *Neurology, 33,* 1483-1486.

Tajima, T., Furukawa, K., & Kuramochi, E. (1980). Selective lumbosacral radiculography and block. *Spine, 5,* 68-77.

Tanelian, D. L., & Brose, W. G. (1991). Neuropathic pain can be relieved by drugs that are use-dependent sodium channel blockers: Lidocaine, carbamazepine, and mexiletine. *Anesthesiology, 74,* 949-951.

Tanelian, D. L., & MacIver, M. B. (1991). Analgesic concentrations of lidocaine suppress tonic A-delta and C fiber discharges produced by acute injury. *Anesthesiology, 74,* 934-936.

Tasker, R. R. (1990). Pain resulting from central nervous system pathology (central pain). In J. J. Bonica (Ed.), *The management of pain* (pp. 271-272). Philadelphia: Lea & Febiger.

Torebjork, E. (1990). Clinical and neurophysiological observations relating to pathophysiological mechanisms in reflex sympathetic dystrophy. In M. Stanton-Hicks, W. Janig, & R. A. Boas (Eds.), *Reflex sympathetic dystrophy* (pp. 71-80). Boston: Kluwer.

Torebjork, H. E., & Hallin, R. G. (1973). Perceptual changes accompanying controlled preferential blocking of A and C fibre responses in intact human skin nerves. *Experimental Brain Research, 16,* 321-332.

Torebjork, H. E., Lundberg, L. E. R., & LaMotte, R. H. (1992). Central changes in processing mechanoreceptive input in capsaicin-induced secondary hyperalgesia in humans. *Journal of Physiology, 448,* 765-780.

Tran, K. M., Frank, S. M., Raja, S. N., El-Rahmany, H. K., Kim, L. J., & Vu, B. (2000). Lumbar sympathetic block for sympathetically maintained pain: Changes in cutaneous temperatures and pain perception. *Anesthesia and Analgesia, 90,* 1396-1401.

Traut, F. F., & Passarelli, E. W. (1956). Study in the controlled therapy of degenerative arthritis. *Archives of Internal Medicine, 98,* 181-186.

Tsubokawa, T., Katayama, Y., Yamamoto, T., Hirayama, T., & Koyama, S. (1991). Chronic motor cortex stimulation for the treatment of central pain. *Acta Neurochirurgica,* Suppl. 52, 137-139.

van Buskirk, C. (1941). Nerves in the vertebral canal: Their relation to the sympathetic innervation of the upper extremities. *Archives of Surgery, 43,* 427-432.

Van Gessel, E. F., Forster, A., & Gamulin, Z. (1993). Continuous spinal anesthesia: Where do spinal catheters go? *Anesthesia and Analgesia, 76,* 1004-1007.

Vanharanta, H., Sachs, B. L., Spivey, M. A., Guyer, R. D., Hochschuler, S. H., Rashbaum, R. F., Johnson, R. G., Ohnmeiss, D., & Mooney, V. (1987). The relationship of pain provocation to lumbar disc deterioration as seen by CT/discography. *Spine, 12,* 295-298.

Verdugo, R., & Ochoa, J. L. (1994). 'Sympathetically maintained pain': Phentolamine block questions the concept. *Neurology, 44,* 1003-1010.

Videman, T., Malmivaara, A., & Mooney, V. (1987). The value of the axial view in assessing discograms: An experimental study with cadavers. *Spine, 12,* 299-304.

Vital, J. M., Dautheribes, M., Baspeyre, H., Lavignolle, B., & Senegas, J. (1989). An anatomic and dynamic study of the greater occipital nerve (n. of Arnold). *Surgical and Radiologic Anatomy, 11,* 205-210.

Vleeming, A., Stoeckart, R., Volkers, A. C. W., & Snijders, C. J. (1990). Relation between form and function in the sacroiliac joint: Part I. Clinical anatomic aspects. *Spine, 15,* 130-132.

Wall, P. D., & Devor, M. (1983). Sensory afferent impulses originate from dorsal root ganglia as well as from the periphery in normal and nerve injured rats. *Pain, 17,* 321-339.

Walsh, T. R., Weinstein, J. N., Spratt, K. F., Lehmann, T. R., Aprill, C., & Sayre, H. (1990). Lumbar discography in normal subjects. *Journal of Bone and Joint Surgery, 72*(A), 1081-1088.

Weber, R. (1957). An analysis of the cross communications between the sympathetic trunks in the lumbar region in man. *Annals of Surgery, 145,* 365-370.

Weinberger, L. M. (1968). Cervico-occipital pain and its surgical treatment: The myth of the bony millstones. *American Journal of Surgery, 135,* 243-247.

Weinreb, J. C., Wolbarsht, L. B., Cohen, J. M., Brown, C. E. L., & Maravilla, K. R. (1989). Prevalence of lumbosacral intervertebral disk abnormalities on MR images in pregnant and aymptomatic nonpregnant women. *Radiology, 170,* 125-128.

Wiberg, G. (1949). Back pain in relation to the nerve supply of the intervertebral disc. *Acta Orthopaedica Scandinavica, 19,* 211-221.

Wiesel, S. W., Tsourmas, N., Feffer, H. L., Citrin, C. M., & Patronas, N. (1984). A study of computer-assisted tomography. I. The incidence of positive CAT scans in an asymptomatic group of patients. *Spine, 9,* 549-551.

Willis, T. A. (1929). An analysis of vertebral anomalies. *American Journal of Surgery, 6,* 163-168.

Xavier, A. V., McDanal, J., & Kissin, I. (1988). Relief of sciatic radicular pain by sciatic nerve block. *Anesthesia and Analgesia, 67,* 1177-1180.

Yamamuro, M., & Kaneko, T. (1978). The comparison

of stellate ganglion block at the transverse process of the 7th and the 6th cervical vertebra. *Masui: Japanese Journal of Anesthesiology, 27,* 376–389.

Yamashita, T., Cavanaugh, J. M., El-Bohy, A. A., Getchell, T. V., & King, A. I. (1990). Mechanosensitive afferent units in the lumbar facet joint. *Journal of Bone and Joint Surgery, 72*(A), 865–870.

Yarnitsky, D., & Ochoa, J. L. (1989). Sensations conducted by large and small myelinated fibers are lost simultaneously under compression–ischemia block. *Acta Physiologica Scandinavica, 137,* 319.

Yarnitsky, D., & Ochoa, J. L. (1991). Differential effect of compression-ischemia block on warm sensation and heat induced pain. *Brain, 114,* 907–913.

Yeager, G. H., & Cowley, R. A. (1948). Anatomical observations on the lumbar sympathetics with evaluation of sympathectomies in organic vascular disease. *Annals of Surgery, 127,* 953–967.

Yokoyama, M., Mizobuchi, S., Nakatsuka, H., & Hirakawa, M. (1998). Comparison of plasma lidocaine concentrations after injection of a fixed small volume in the stellate ganglion, the lumbar, epidural space, or a single intercostal nerve. *Anesthesia and Analgesia, 87,* 112–115.

Younger, A. S., & Claridge, R. J. (1998). The role of diagnostic block in the management of Morton's neuroma. *Canadian Journal of Surgery, 41,* 127–130.

Yu, S., Haughton, V. M., Sether, L. A., & Wagner, M. (1989). Comparison of MR and diskography in detecting radial tears of the anulus: A postmortem study. *American Journal of Neuroradiology, 10,* 1077–1081.

Zucherman, J., Derby, R., Hsu, K., Picetti, G., Kaiser, J., Schofferman, J., Goldthwaite, N., & White, A. (1988). Normal magnetic resonance imaging with abnormal discography. *Spine, 13,* 1355–1359.

Chapter 14

Disability Evaluation in Painful Conditions

JAMES P. ROBINSON

Patients with painful conditions often receive work disability benefits as well as medical or surgical care for their problems. Typically, a physician must assert that they are disabled from work in order for them to receive disability benefits. The information and opinions provided by physicians are used by adjudicators in disability agencies to determine whether the patients are eligible for benefits under various work disability programs.

Physicians perform disability evaluations on patients in two different contexts. Sometimes they interact with patients solely for the purpose of performing disability evaluations. For example, insurance companies and disability agencies often retain independent medical examiners to do the evaluations. However, most disability evaluations are performed by treating physicians; that is, a physician who is treating a patient also evaluates the patient's ability to work and communicates this information to a disability agency or insurance company.

The judgments a physician must make during a disability evaluation are the same, regardless of whether he or she is a treating physician or an independent medical examiner. However, there are significant differences between the challenges faced by treating physicians and those faced by independent medical examiners. First, independent medical examiners have no ongoing contact with the patients whom they evaluate, and no responsibility to provide treatment. In contrast, treating physicians have the challenge of blending the adjudica-

tive role they play when they perform disability evaluations with the clinical role they play in their other interactions with patients (Robinson, in press). Second, physicians who choose to become independent medical examiners do so only because they are willing to perform disability evaluations. They often make disability evaluations an important part of their professional activities, and take courses to enhance their ability to perform these evaluations. In contrast, treating physicians often have a distaste for performing disability evaluations, and have only minimal knowledge about how the evaluations should be performed.

In this chapter I focus on practical strategies that treating physicians can use when they perform disability evaluations. It is important to note at the outset that it is impossible to write a step-by-step "cookbook" for conducting disability evaluations. The question "How do you evaluate disability in a patient with chronic pain?" is just as complex as the question "How do you provide medical or surgical care for a patient with chronic pain?" In both instances a chapter can describe general principles, but the application of these principles to specific patients requires a good deal of clinical judgment.

One factor that contributes greatly to the complexity of disability evaluation is the diversity of the insurance companies and governmental agencies that administer disability programs. For example, in the United States, there are 50 state workers' compensation systems, three federal workers' compensation systems, two disability programs operated by the Social Security Administration (SSA), a Department of Veterans Affairs disability program, and several disability programs offered by private insurance companies. Also, many public assistance (welfare) programs provide disability benefits, and miscellaneous other programs (such as Medicare and Medicaid) deal to some extent with disability (Demeter, Andersson, & Smith, 1996; Rondinelli & Katz, 2000; Williams, 1991; Wolfe & Potter, 1996). Because of the multitude of disability programs, virtually any statement about disability is likely to have exceptions, and it is difficult even to define concepts unambiguously.

BASIC CONCEPTS

Disability

The two fundamental concepts in the area of disability are *impairment* and *disability*. These terms do not have unique definitions, because different disability agencies define them in slightly different ways.

In its broadest meaning, *disability* refers to an inability to carry out necessary tasks in any important domain of life because of a medical condition. For example, a person with C5 quadriplegia is disabled in the sense of being unable to carry out many basic activities of daily living. This chapter focuses on the more restricted concept of work disability, which can be informally defined as the inability to work because of a medical condition.

Work disability can be subcategorized in several ways. The most important distinctions are between total and partial disability, and between temporary and permanent (or long term) disability. Various disability agencies have programs tailored to these different categories of work disability. For example, the SSA programs are designed for people who are permanently and totally disabled; workers' compensation time loss benefits are paid to individuals who are totally, temporarily disabled; many private disability insurance policies provide benefits when an individual is disabled from performing his or her usual work, even if he or she is not totally disabled.

Impairment

In the United States, the most widely used system for assessing impairment is the one developed by the American Medical Association (AMA) and described in the fourth edition of its publication

Guides to the Evaluation of Permanent Impairment (American Medical Asociation, 1993).[1] The discussion of impairment in this chapter is based on concepts described in this volume (hereafter referred to as the *Guides*).

The *Guides* defines impairment as "a deviation from normal in a body part or organ system and its functioning" (American Medical Asociation, 1993, p. 1). Impairment is important because it permits disability agencies to distinguish between medical and nonmedical causes of workplace failure. Disability programs provide benefits to people who fail in the workplace because of a medical condition (i.e., who have an impairment), but not to ones who fail in the workplace because of poor job skills or other nonmedical factors.

The *Guides* attempts to quantify impairment. Impairments associated with a wide range of medical conditions are construed as being measurable on a scale ranging from 0% (when there is no impairment) to 100% (when a person is completely incapacitated). The *Guides* assumes that impairment measures the medical component of work disability, and that the magnitude of an individual's impairment correlates with the severity of his or her disadvantage in the workplace. Thus a physician who uses the *Guides* attempts to determine not only whether a patient has an impairment, but also how severe the impairment is.

A few practical points need to be made about impairment and disability. First, despite rhetoric that can be found in various monographs (e.g., American Medical Association, 1993), the distinction between impairment and disability is often unclear (Robinson, in press). Second, when a person seeking disability benefits is evaluated, the "bottom line" of the evaluation is the decision about whether or not he or she is actually disabled. The assessment of impairment is important because it is an intervening step in the broader task of assessing disability. Finally, physicians are typically asked questions about both impairment and disability when they perform evaluations on patients. The discussion below focuses on disability evaluations; it assumes that when a physician performs a disability evaluation, the evaluation includes an impairment assessment.

ISSUES ADDRESSED IN DISABILITY EVALUATIONS

Physicians are typically asked to address the following when they conduct disability evaluations:

1. Diagnosis
2. Causation
3. Need for further treatment
4. Impairment
5. Ability to work

Examples of the questions posed by disability agencies are listed in Table 14.1. The second column of the table presents questions that were addressed to an independent medical examiner by a workers' compensation board. The patient was a woman who had sustained a noncatastrophic neck injury in the course of her work. The third column lists questions that were addressed to a physician who

was treating a man for a non-work-related median neuropathy. The patient had a disability policy through a private insurance company, and the questions were written by the company. The table is organized to show how questions were worded by the two agencies, and which of the key issues the questions addressed. Note that the questions from the workers' compensation board addressed all five of the issues listed above, whereas the questions from the private insurance company addressed only three of them. This reflects the different mandates of the two agencies; for example, workers' compensation programs are responsible only for injuries that occur at work, whereas many

TABLE 14.1. Typical Issues Addressed and Specific Questions Asked in Disability Evaluations

	Specific questions asked	
Issue addressed	Workers' compensation system: Questions to independent medical examiner	Private insurance company: Questions to treating physician
Diagnosis	What are the diagnoses based on objective findings?	Diagnoses _____ Subjective symptoms _____ Objective findings _____
Causation	Please state which, if any, of the diagnosed conditions are work related?	
Maximal medical improvement	Is Ms. X medically stable or has she reached preinjury status? What treatment would you recommend?	Has patient reached maximal medical improvement? Would any further therapy be reasonably expected to result in full or partial recovery?
Impairment rating	If Ms. X is medically stable, does she have a ratable permanent partial impairment according to the *Guides*, fourth edition?	
Ability to work	Can Ms. X return to her job of injury? (Her job description is attached.)	1. Rate patient's physical impairment Class 1—no limitation Class 2—capable of medium work Class 3—capable of light work Class 4—capable of sedentary work Class 5—incapable of minimal activity or sedentary work 2. Please describe fully how patient's symptoms/limitations affect ability to work. 3. Would job modification enable patient to work with impairment? 4. Would vocational counseling and/ or retraining be recommended?

private disability programs provide benefits regardless of how a policy holder became disabled.

A fundamental goal of the disability evaluation process is to determine whether a patient can work. From this perspective, items 1–4 in the list above can be viewed as preliminary items that set the stage for addressing the crucial question of item 5. For example, Figure 14.1 displays the type of algorithm that many disability agencies follow, at least when a patient is being evaluated for long-term or permanent disability.

PROBLEMS ASSOCIATED WITH DISABILITY EVALUATION IN PAINFUL CONDITIONS

Disability evaluation is a complex area for many reasons. These have been discussed in other publications (Robinson, 2001, in press) and are only briefly mentioned here.

1. Disability agencies have to a large extent defined the concepts and procedures to be used in disability evaluations. However sensible these concepts may be from an administrative standpoint, they are often difficult for physicians to apply.

2. One central tenet of disability agencies is that impairment should be public and objectively measurable—that is, that a skilled physician should be able to determine the nature and severity of a patient's impairment.

3. As a corollary of item 2 above, disability agencies focus on what might be called a *mechanical failure* model of impairment (Osterweis, Kleinman, & Mechanic, 1987). The assumption is that activity limitations of people are (or should be) closely linked to measurable evidence of failure or dysfunction in certain organs or body parts, rather than to self-reported subjective barriers such as anxiety or pain.

4. Disability is particularly difficult to evaluate in painful conditions, precisely because they violate the assumption that impairment is objectively measurable and closely linked to mechanical failure of an organ or body part. Patients with chronic pain routinely complain of activity restrictions that cannot be fully understood in terms of

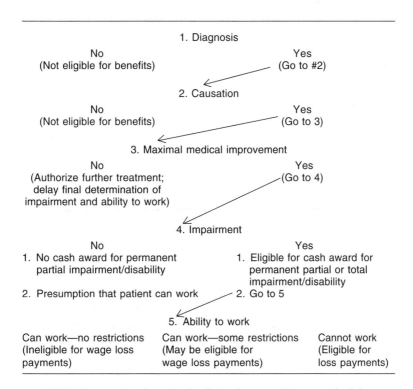

FIGURE 14.1. An algorithm for the evaluation of long-term disability.

mechanical failure of some body part or organ. The mismatch between the subjective reports of patients with chronic pain and the objective evidence for mechanical failure of their organs creates a fundamental dilemma for a disability evaluator. At one extreme, the disability evaluator may ignore a patient's subjective appraisals and rely strictly on objective evidence of organ dysfunction. At the opposite extreme, the evaluator may rely strictly on the subjective appraisals and apparent activity restrictions of the patient, regardless of whether they can be objectified in terms of measurable failure or dysfunction of an organ. Finally, the evaluator may rate impairment on the basis of some composite of objective and subjective factors. No disability agency or disability evaluation system has offered an acceptable resolution to this dilemma.

PAIN AND IMPAIRMENT IN THE *GUIDES*

The "mechanical failure" model of disability evaluation described above is somewhat oversimplified. For example, the *Guides* (American Medical Association, 1993) provides concepts that go beyond this model when impairment associated with pain is being assessed. Although the *Guides* focuses on objective evidence of organ dysfunction as the basis for impairment ratings, it attempts to incorporate what might be called *expected pain* or *typical pain* (Robinson, 2001) into impairment ratings.

As an example, consider the rating of impairment for a person with a chronic lumbar radiculopathy. A disability evaluator could use the *diagnosis-related estimates* (DRE) model (American Medical Association, 1993) to make a rating. The patient would probably receive a DRE category III rating, which translates to 10% impairment. Ostensibly, this rating would be based strictly on objective factors, such as the patient's imaging studies and neurological examination. However, the *Guides* makes it clear that the rating also takes into account the pain that would typically be part of a chronic radiculopathy. At the beginning of the volume is this statement: "In general, the impairment percents shown in the chapters that consider the various organ systems make allowance for the pain that may accompany the impairing conditions" (American Medical Association, 1993, p. 9).

Thus the *Guides* acknowledges that pain contributes to impairment, and attempts to factor pain into impairment ratings. In most of its chapters,

however, it deals only with *expected pain* or *typical pain*. Except in Chapter 15, it does not incorporate what has been called *magnified pain* or *unverifiable pain* (Robinson, 2001).

The *Guides* elaborates additional concepts related to impairment assessment in painful conditions in its Chapter 15, which is devoted exclusively to this subject. Concepts described in this chapter appear to be inconsistent with ones outlined in the rest of the book. For example, the authors of the chapter state:

(1) Pain evaluation does not lend itself to strict laboratory standards of sensitivity, specificity, and other scientific criteria; (2) chronic pain is not measurable or detectable on the basis of the classic, tissue-oriented model; (3) pain evaluation requires acknowledging and understanding a multifaceted, biopsychosocial model that transcends the usual, more limited disease model. (American Medical Association, 1993, p. 304)

In essence, Chapter 15 of the *Guides* asserts that factors other than objectively measurable organ dysfunction and expected pain need to be considered when impairment associated with painful conditions is being rated. But the chapter does not give any specific information about what these other factors are, or how a disability evaluator can incorporate them into an impairment rating. Also, it does not provide information about how an evaluator might blend information in Chapter 15 with information in the other chapters of the book. As a practical matter, informal observation suggests that the concepts outlined in Chapter 15 are rarely used by disability evaluators.

In summary, although the *Guides* goes beyond the mechanical failure model of disability evaluation, it still does not answer this crucial question: How does an evaluator integrate subjective data and objective data into the evaluation of disability in a patient with chronic pain?

PRACTICAL STRATEGIES FOR DISABILITY EVALUATION

Preliminaries: A Word of Caution

The discussion below is largely based on my experiences as a private practitioner, an attending physician at a university-based pain center, an independent medical examiner, and a consultant to the Washington State Department of Labor and Industries. It is *not* based on scientific data, because such data do not exist. For example, data on the reliability of disability evaluations are scanty (Clark et al., 1988; Clark & Haldeman, 1993), and there are virtually no credible scientific data on the predictive or concurrent validity of the evaluations. In the absence of scientific data, it is impossible to say what decision-making strategies are appropriate when one performs disability evaluations. In this ambiguous situation, it is easy for practitioners (and authors of chapters) to fall into the trap of believing they are making valid judgments when in fact their judgments are based on a variety of biases (Gilovich, 1991; Robinson, 2001).

Philosophical Issues: The Ethics of Disability Evaluation

It is beyond the scope of this chapter to discuss ethical dilemmas in disability evaluation in any detail. Suffice it to say that such dilemmas abound, and that they are particularly acute when a physician evaluates a patient whom he or she is treating. Many of these dilemmas are discussed in a thoughtful paper by Sullivan and Loeser (1992).

Some of the most difficult dilemmas involve trust. Patients put their trust in treating physicians because they expect their physicians to be advocates for them. Although physicians are often forced to balance the needs of patients against other factors (such as the cost of medical care), most of them perceive themselves as putting the needs of their patients first. Thus a kind of symmetry exists: Patients place their trust in physicians, and physicians reciprocate by acting as agents for patients.

When physicians perform disability evaluations on patients whom they are treating, there is a potential for them to abuse the trust that patients have placed in them. Sullivan and Loeser (1992) describe the dilemma as follows:

> Encounters between physician and patient for the purposes of treating and rating disability create fundamentally different relationships. When the aim of medical diagnosis is the selection of effective treatment for the patient's pain, the physician acts as agent for the patient. When the aim of diagnosis is rating the patient's disability, the physician acts as agent for the state. The purpose of the former encounter is to reduce suffering; the purpose of the latter encounter is to assign compensation as mandated by law or regulation. If two different physicians perform these tasks, there is little chance for confusion about the nature of the relationship on the part of the patient. If one individual is performing both functions, the potential for confusion and exploitation of trust is higher. (p. 1830)

Sullivan and Loeser conclude that physicians should refuse to perform disability evaluations on patients whom they are treating. Unfortunately, this option is frequently not available to a treating physician. If a physician refuses to complete a disability form, several adverse consequences ensue. Sometimes the patient's disability benefits are summarily halted. In other situations, the disability agency refuses to pay the physician for his or her clinical services. Some disability agencies have the legal right to impose fines on physicians who do not submit disability forms. In essence, physicians frequently have no choice other than to fill out a disability form on patients they are treating. When physicians do this, however, they need to be aware that they are treading on morally ambiguous terrain. They need to ask themselves the following questions:

1. *What are your attitudes toward disability?* Some physicians empathize with patients who are applying for disability. They believe that the patients are likely to experience severe emotional and physical stress if economic circumstances compel them to remain in the work force. At the opposite extreme, some physicians perceive disability applicants as con artists who are trying to manipulate "the system" and get benefits that they do not deserve. The available evidence suggests that both of these perspectives are oversimplified.

For most workers, the workplace provides many benefits. In addition to financial rewards, work provides people with social contacts and binds them to the community. The psychosocial benefits of work can best be appreciated by the extensive research on unemployment among people who are not disabled. The general thrust of this research is that when people are separated from the workplace—for example, by being laid off during an economic recession—they and their families are at increased risk for a number of adverse outcomes, including depression, anxiety, substance abuse, social isolation, family dissolution, and suicide (Atkinson, Liem, & Liem, 1986; Hammarstrom & Janlert, 1997; Kaplan et al., 1987; Mrazek & Haggerty, 1994; Rahmqvist & Carstensen, 1998). The implication of this research is clear: The mental health of most people—even those with significant medical problems—is better served by remaining in the work force than by leaving it.

In addition to the psychological losses associated with separation from the work environment, injured workers suffer severe economic losses when they go on disability (Reno, Mashaw, & Gradison,

1997). Thus, the notion that disabled people are "milking the system" is almost certainly wrong. In fact, one of the tragedies of disability is that everyone seems to lose: the injured workers, their families, the people who pay disability insurance premiums, and society at large.

Third, many observers of disability systems have speculated that the process of interacting with disability agencies has detrimental effects on patients (Robinson, Rondinelli, & Scheer, 1997). For example, Hadler (1996) has argued that as patients try to prove their incapacitation to disability adjudicators, they become more and more convinced that they really are disabled. Some observers have suggested the term *disability syndrome* to describe the set of dysfunctional attitudes and beliefs that develops over time as a person adapts to the role of being a disabled person. Thus patients who seem straightforward and highly motivated soon after injuries often become more resistant to rehabilitation later on (Krause & Ragland, 1994; Robinson et al., 1997).

Disability syndrome is an inferred construct that is difficult to validate. But it is at least consistent with studies demonstrating that significant numbers of people seem to get "stuck" in disability systems. For example, research indicates that after a person has been awarded disability benefits by the SSA, the probability is only about 3% that he or she will ever return to the work force (Muller, 1992). Also, numerous studies on disabled workers with industrial compensation claims have shown that whereas the vast majority of them return to work within a few weeks after injury, ones who are still disabled at 6 months after injury have a high probability of protracted disability (Cheadle et. al., 1994; Robinson, 1998).

2. *How much do you know about the disability agencies with which you interact?* When physicians perform disability evaluations on their patients, they act as intermediaries between the patients and various agencies that provide benefits for people who are disabled from work. In order to understand disability evaluation, physicians need to have some understanding of these disability agencies, since they typically define the issues that must be addressed in a disability evaluation.

Unfortunately, this understanding is difficult to achieve, in part because of the enormous heterogeneity of disability agencies and the programs they administer. Also, the policies and practices that a disability agency follows when it determines eligibility for benefits are generally not available to physicians. In this ambiguous situation, physicians can increase their understanding substantially by reviewing monographs that deal with disability agencies and disability evaluation (Demeter et al., 1996; Osterweis et al., 1987; Rondinelli & Katz, 2000). Also, physicians who are observant as they perform disability evaluations on patients can learn a lot about the disability agencies with which they interact.

3. *How do you integrate disability evaluation into an overall strategy of disability management?* I focus on disability evaluation in this chapter. In practical situations, however, treating physicians do not do disability evaluations in isolation. Broadly speaking, a treating physician needs to develop strategies for *disability management* for patients he or she is treating. Disability management encompasses at least four areas: assessment of disability risk, establishment of a treatment contract with a patient, prevention of disability, and evaluation of disability. These areas are linked. Thus, if a physician fails to assess disability risk adequately or to develop reasonable disability prevention strategies, he or she will probably find disability evaluation particularly difficult.

4. *How much importance do you give to the subjective appraisals that patients make regarding their ability to work?* At one extreme, a physician might accept what patients say about their physical capacities more or less at face value. Such a physician would run the risk of being duped by patients with chronic pain and/or greatly underestimating the capacities of the patients. At the opposite extreme, a physician might try to make decisions about the disability status of patients strictly on the basis of objective findings, and react skeptically to reports of incapacitation that are not closely linked to objective findings.

A position somewhere between these two extremes is probably most appropriate. The perceptions that patients have about their abilities certainly should not be ignored or automatically discounted. As a practical matter, research demonstrates that these self-appraisals are important predictors of whether or not patients with pain problems will perform well on physical tests or succeed in getting off disability (Fishbain et al., 1997, 1999; Hazard, Bendix, & Fenwick, 1991; Hidding et al., 1994; Hildebrandt et al., 1997; Kaplan, Wurtele, & Gillis, 1996). Thus a physician who makes disability decisions without considering patients' appraisals is discarding valuable data. As a result, his or her decisions can go awry in two ways. First, they can pressure patients to return to work in jobs that the patients are realistically not capable of performing. Second, they may be completely in-effective in resolving disability issues. Consider, for example, a man with chronic pain who is released to work by his physician, even though he is convinced that he is unable to work. Such a patient (or his attorney) is likely to seek out a different physician who will provide a different opinion regarding his disability. In this setting, the physician who released the patient for work may believe that he or she has successfully got-ten the patient off disability, but the belief is illusory.

But the fact that patients' perceptions are im-portant does not mean that they are valid, or that they are immutable. In fact, research suggests just the opposite; that is, it suggests that patients with chronic pain often have distorted views of their capabilities, and that these views are modifiable (Alaranta et al., 1994; Estlander et al., 1991; Jensen, Turner, & Romano, 1994; Lipchik, Milles, & Covington, 1993). These results have implications for both the evaluation and the management of disability by a treating physician. When perform-ing a disability evaluation, the physician needs to consider the validity of a patient's stated activity limitations in light of the biomedical information available and his or her assessment of the patient's credibility. He or she should reserve the right to challenge the patient's self-assessments and to make decisions that are discordant with these assessments. In the course of treatment, the treat-ing physician needs to promote changes in per-ceptions that are unduly self-defeating and medi-cally unsubstantiated.

It is worth noting that such challenges are likely to be met with resistance. Patients with chronic pain generally do not welcome suggestions by physicians that their perceptions are inaccurate. They often give a message something like this: "I am the only one who really knows about my pain. You outsiders can only guess." A treating physi-cian thus needs to approach the issue of inaccu-rate perceptions with a good deal of tact.

In summary, the treating physician should carefully assess patients' perceptions regarding their ability to perform various tasks, and, whenever feasible, should render disability judgments that are consistent with these perceptions. But this does not mean that the physician should let patients with chronic pain control the terms of discussion about disability or the outcomes of disability evaluations. Instead, the physician should be ready to challenge the appraisals of patients when he or she believes that they are inaccurate.

Mechanics

Overview

Table 14.2 provides an algorithm that can help you as a physician approach disability evaluations syste-matically. The major sections are as follows:

1. Before the disability form arrives
2. Initial review of the disability form
3. Getting additional data
4. Addressing the main questions
5. Objective findings
6. Psychogenic pain
7. Filling out the form
8. Follow-up

Before the Disability Form Arrives

Initial Assessment of Risk for Protracted Dis-ability. You will do a better job of responding to disability requests if you have thought about the disability issues that might arise for a particular pa-tient, and have done some preliminary work to resolve or mitigate these. You should do at least a preliminary analysis of several issues at the time of initial evaluation of patients. You may well re-vise your assessment of these issues as you learn more about a patient.

TABLE 14.2. Overview of Steps during Disability Evaluation

1. Before the disability form arrives
   a. Initial assessment of risk for protracted disability
   b. Contracting
2. Initial review of the disability form
   a. Who should fill out the form?
   b. What disability agency is requesting the form?
   c. What issues are you asked to address?
   d. Overall assessment of the patient
   e. Assessment of patient credibility
   f. Discussion of the form with the patient
3. Getting additional data
4. Addressing the main questions
   a. Diagnosis
   b. Causation
   c. Need for further treatment
   d. Impairment
   e. Physical capacities
   f. Ability to work
5. Objective findings
6. Psychogenic pain
7. Filling out the disability form
8. Follow-up

1. A key issue is that you should assess the current disability status of every patient with pain when you first evaluate him or her. Is the patient currently working? If so, is he or she struggling on the job because of pain, or missing a lot of time from work? If the patient is not working, is this because of his or her health or for some other reason? If the patient is disabled from work, how long has he or she been disabled? Is there any history of disability or work instability prior to the index injury for which the patient is seeing you?

2. In addition to obtaining factual information about the disability status of patients, you should assess their perceptions regarding disability. What barriers to return to work do they identify? Are they optimistic or pessimistic about the probability of returning to work? Do they believe that their employers and the workers' compensation system have treated them fairly? Remember that patients' perceptions are important predictors of the actual outcomes of claims.

3. You should look for disability "red flags" as you carry out the history and physical examination. There is no single list of red flags that has been demonstrated in published research to predict risk of long-term disability, but experts in the field of musculoskeletal medicine and disability have developed lists by consensus (Frymoyer & Cats-Baril, 1987; Washington State Department of Labor and Industries, 1999). Table 14.3 lists a set of risk factors that were identified on the basis of input from physicians in the Washington State Medical Association and senior claims adjudicators at the Washington State Department of Labor and Industries. Note that the list includes factors in the environment around the patient, rather than just personal attributes of the patient. This reflects the opinion of experts that factors external to an individual patient have a substantial bearing on the likelihood that the patient will become chronically disabled. Some of these "systems issues" are difficult for a clinician to assess, especially when parties to a claim have a hidden agenda of some kind.

4. Without being unduly cynical, you need to be aware of the possibility that any of the participants in a disability claim can have a hidden agenda. Opportunities for deception are particularly rich in workers' compensation claims.

a. An extensive medical literature on secondary gain, compensation neurosis, and malingering has dealt with hidden agendas of patients (Bellamy, 1997; Fishbain et al., 1995; Loeser, Henderlite, &

TABLE 14.3. Proposed List of Risk Factors for Prolonged Disability

Group 1: Catastrophic—*Cases with catastrophic injuries are very likely to benefit from medical case management.*
☐ 1. Catastrophic

Group 2A: High Risk—*Cases with any of these factors are likely to benefit from medical case management, unless there is clear evidence the worker is about to return to work.*
☐ 1. Hospitalized within 28 days of injury, for reasons related to industrial injury
☐ 2. Worker who is 45 years old or older with carpal tunnel syndrome
☐ 3. 90 or more days of time-loss

Group 2B: High Risk—*The presence of one or more of the following may indicate an increased likelihood of long-term disability and, therefore, some potential benefit from case management or other intensive services.*

A. Medical Factors
☐ 1. Presence of secondary medical condition
☐ 2. Injury to dominant hand
☐ 3. Hospitalized within 28 days of injury for reasons unrelated to industrial injury
☐ 4. Pre-existing psychiatric conditions

B. Injury Descriptions
☐ 1. Non-overt injury—injury occurring in course of usual work activities
☐ 2. No objective findings on examinations
☐ 3. Diagnosis not consistent with injury description
☐ 4. Time gap in report of injury
☐ 5. Unwitnessed accident

C. Provider/Patient Factors
☐ 1. No identifiable treatment plan or goals
☐ 2. Over-utilization of health care delivery systems and services by either patient or provider, or over-referral by physician. May include frequent changes of attending physician
☐ 3. Misuse of scheduled medications by patient
☐ 4. Physician fostering illness beliefs
☐ 5. Number of surgeries both related and unrelated to work-related problem. May include a number of unsuccessful surgeries in the same area
☐ 6. Spread of diagnosis over time; newly contended diagnosis
☐ 7. No documented medical progress

D. Psychosocial Factors
☐ 1. Exaggerated illness behavior: Presence of non-organic signs (Waddell signs); no objective findings
☐ 2. Evidence of abuse of alcohol, illicit drug or prescription medication
☐ 3. Presence of depression or avoidance anxiety, post-traumatic disorder or other dysphoric affects (for example, anger at employer or supervisor or L&I [the Washington State Department of Labor and Industries])
☐ 4. History of childhood abuse, physical or sexual abuse, substance abuse in caretaker or family instability
☐ 5. Presence of personality traits or disorders. For example, presence of specific somatization traits or problematic interpersonal relationships; arrests

(cont.)

TABLE 14.3. (cont.)

E. Demographic Factors
☐ 1. Low educational level, including illiteracy
☐ 2. English not primary language
☐ 3. Age greater than 50 and employed in heavy industry
☐ 4. Back or lower extremity injury with medium or heavy labor employment
☐ 5. Nearing retirement age

F. Job Factors
☐ 1. Anger at employer
☐ 2. Employer anger at worker
☐ 3. Miscellaneous employer factors: seasonal work, strike, plant closure, job becoming obsolete, etc.
☐ 4. Loss of job in which the injury occurred
☐ 5. Singular work history in heavy industry
☐ 6. Complaints of inability to function
☐ 7. History of poor job performance, frequent job change, short duration of employment, job dissatisfaction or job termination prior to claims filing
☐ 8. Employer or worker not active in return-to-work efforts
☐ 9. Worker is not clearly headed back to work
☐ 10. Perception of the worker that he or she will be retrained "for a better job" or other misperceptions of L&I vocational entitlement

G. Administrative Factors
☐ 1. Third-party involvement
☐ 2. Recent claim closures; application for reopening
☐ 3. Employer protest
☐ 4. Current income, including time-loss, compares favorably to net income prior to injury
☐ 5. Multiple L&I claims (may include a number of previous claims)
☐ 6. Loss of driver's license or other credentials
☐ 7. Loss of medical insurance
☐ 8. Originally non-time-loss claim that has become time-loss
☐ 9. Non-compliance with medical or vocational treatment
☐ 10. Worker or physician perception that L&I is unresponsive or adversarial

Note. From Washington State Department of Labor and Industries (1999).

Conrad, 1995; Mendelson, 1988; Voiss, 1995). Most experts in disability believe that frank malingering or deception is uncommon among patients who seem to report excessive disability, but you should be alert to the following:

1. Is there any evidence that a patient who claims to be disabled is "double-dipping" (i.e., working at the same time he or she is getting disability benefits)?

2. Is there evidence from surveillance tapes or other collateral sources that a patient's physical capabilities are far greater than he or she claims?

b. Other parties to a workers' compensation claim—including employers and adjudicators for disability agencies—can have hidden agendas. Their agendas have been ignored almost completely in research on disability, so you need to use clinical judgment in deciding whether participants in a disability claim are behaving in a deceptive manner. You should consider the following:

1. Is there evidence that the disability system is "playing hardball" with the patient? For example, does it appear that the patient has had his or her claim closed arbitrarily? Has the compensation carrier refused to authorize services requested by the attending physician? Does it appear that the patient's claims manager is requesting multiple evaluations in order to maneuver the patient out of the disability system on the basis of "preponderance of evidence"?

2. Is there any indication that the patient's former employer has created misleading job descriptions? Has put pressure on the patient not to file a workers' compensation claim? Has fired the patient in apparent response to the patient's report of injury?

5. Based on items 1–4 above, you should formulate some preliminary assessment of the patient's risk for protracted disability.

Contracting. Your ability to respond to disability forms will also be enhanced if you establish ground rules with your patient at the beginning of treatment. At the very least, it is advisable to describe your approach to disability management and disability evaluation to the patient. You should also indicate what you expect from the patient in the arena of disability. For example, some physicians will treat disabled patients only if the patients express a commitment to return to work.

Initial Review of the Disability Form

1. You should first consider whether you are the most appropriate person to fill out the form. For example, suppose you are acting as a pain

consultant for a general physician who has been treating a patient for an extended period of time. In such a scenario, it might well be most appropriate for the general physician to fill out disability forms.

2. You should review the form and identify the disability agency that has sent it. Do you know anything about that agency? (If not, you may end up filling out the form in a way that leads to problems for you or your patient later.) Also, you should see which of the five key issues—diagnosis, causation, need for further treatment, impairment, and ability to work—you are being asked to assess. You should try to formulate tentative answers and, in the process, to identify important information gaps.

3. As you consider your answers, you should formulate an overall assessment of the patient with respect to disability issues. It is often best to think of a narrative that you might write to describe the patient. This (imaginary) narrative should address the five basic issues to the extent that they are relevant to the patient you are evaluating.

4. Your overall assessment should include a consideration of the credibility of the patient whom you have been asked to evaluate. The rationale for this is simple but compelling. As noted earlier, disability assessment of patients with chronic pain is difficult primarily because their statements about their activity limitations often cannot be easily rationalized in terms of objectively measurable organ pathology. As a practical matter, if you consider a patient's statements about his or her incapacitation to be valid, you will be more likely to judge him or her disabled than if you make a judgment based strictly on organ pathology. The question then become this: Should your patient's statements be accepted as valid? To answer this, you must decide whether or not the statements are credible.

The importance of patient credibility has been acknowledged by the SSA, the administrative body that administers the largest disability programs in the United States (Social Security Ruling, 1996). However, neither the SSA nor any other disability agency (as far as I am aware) gives any specific guidelines about how to assess patient credibility. Table 14.4 lists factors that are thought to be relevant to patient credibility. Be aware, though, that the list has not been validated, and that research on deception by medical patients suggests that physicians are not particularly good at assessing patient credibility (Faust, 1995; Hall & Pritchard, 1996).

It is important to note that treating physicians have an advantage over independent medical examiners in the assessment of patient credibility. A

TABLE 14.4. Characteristics Associated with High Patient Credibility

1. No preexisting condition
2. No medical comorbidities
3. Definite stimulus (e.g., crushed by a tree)
4. Definite tissue damage (e.g., fracture)
5. Symptoms, signs, activity limitations fit expectations for the medical problem
6. Consistent findings over repeated examinations
7. No exaggerated pain behavior
8. No inconsistencies between symptoms/signs noted in MD's office and behavior outside the office
9. No chronic psychiatric disorders or long-term psychosocial risk factors
10. No reactive psychiatric problems (e.g., anxiety disorder, depression)
11. Patient motivated to return to productivity
12. Job opportunities exist
13. No incentives for disability

Note. Adapted from Robinson (1997).

major reason for this is that treating physicians have the opportunity to observe their patients over extended periods of time. As they observe the consistency of physical findings over repeated examinations and patients' responses to various therapies, physicians gradually gain a sense about the credibility of their patients.

5. Discuss the form with the patient. At the very least, you should let the patient know that you have received a request for information about his or her disability status. To the extent feasible, you should find out how your patient believes you should answer questions on the disability form. In particular, it is helpful to the get the patient's view of his or her physical limitations. Also, it is important to see whether the patient challenges any of the factual information provided along with the disability form. For example, it is not uncommon for patients to object strenuously to the information provided in job analyses.

Obtaining Additional Data

You will sometimes find that you need additional information in order to fill out a disability form responsibly. For example, additional past medical records are sometimes crucial. These might include a report of the initial injury, or records from physicians who treated the patient soon after the injury. Sometimes medical records covering the period prior to the index injury are extremely informative.

Sometimes a disability form will prompt you to do an overall clinical reassessment of your patient. This could consist of a thorough reexamination in your office, or updated radiological or laboratory tests.

You may also need objective data regarding the physical capacities of a patient. Objective performance data can be obtained from a functional capacities evaluation, or from a work hardening program or a pain center. (See below.)

Finally, you may need input from a patient's employer. This is particularly important when the patient alleges that the employer has provided distorted information about the demands of his or her job. One way to clarify the demands of a job is to meet with both the patient and a representative of the company for which he or she has worked.

Addressing the Main Questions

Diagnosis. You will generally not have difficulty providing a diagnosis for a patient. You should be aware, though, that adjudicators will sometimes make inferences about causation on the basis of a diagnosis. For example, if you diagnose a patient as having lumbar degenerative disc disease, an adjudicator might take the position that the patient's back pain was not caused by a specific accident.

Causation. Concepts that are helpful in the assessment of causation are given in Table 14.5. Causation is important when a patient is seeking disability benefits from an agency that is responsible only for medical conditions that arise in certain circumstances. For example, workers' compensation carriers are responsible only for conditions that arise out of employment; automobile insurance carriers are responsible only for injuries that occur in motor vehicle accidents. The assessment of causation is difficult both conceptually (Kramer & Lane, 1992) and practically. This is particularly true for patients who have cumulative trauma disorders and/or disorders without clear-cut biological markers. Another difficult situation arises when a patient sustains an injury to a body part that has previously been injured. For example, a patient who has undergone a lumbar discectomy in the remote past may report a return of radicular symptoms after falling down. In this kind of setting, a disability agency may ask you to apportion causation of the patient's impairment between the index injury and his or her preexisting lumbar disc condition.

TABLE 14.5. Factors to Consider in Assessing Causation

1. Did patient have similar problem prior to index event?
2. Was the nature of the accident consistent with patient's present problem?
3. Is there any biological marker that clearly and specifically ties patient's problems to the accident (e.g., complete quadriplegia)?
   a. Alternatives:
      1. Biological marker with uncertain relation to exposure (e.g., carpal tunnel syndrome)
      2. No biological marker (e.g., headaches)
4. Is patient's problem mentioned in initial medical evaluation following injury?
5. Is there a paper trail (i.e., a record of ongoing treatment, and consistency of symptoms and findings)?
6. Did patient have any other injuries after the index injury?
7. Are symptoms/signs on your initial exam interpretable? Credible?
8. Are findings consistent over time on repeated examination?
9. Are there any reinforcers that might give patient an incentive to manipulate you?
10. Overall, how credible do you find the patient?

It is worth noting that disability agencies differ significantly in the standard they set for establishing causation. Some agencies follow the principle that in order for an index injury to be accepted as the cause of a patient's impairment, the injury must be the major factor contributing to the impairment. Others adopt a much lower standard of causation that has been described as "lighting up." When this standard applies, an index injury may be viewed as the cause of an impairment even when the injury is minor and impairment is severe. For example, consider a man with a multiply operated knee who falls at work, develops an effusion in the knee, and is told by an orthopedist that he needs a total knee replacement. If this man's workers' compensation carrier operated under the "lighting up" standard of causation, his knee symptoms and need for a total knee replacement would be viewed as caused by his slip and fall.

Physicians should indicate the factors they consider when they make a causation assessment, and should indicate when their statements about causation are based on their medical training, as opposed to being based on common sense that a nonphysician could use. For example, suppose a woman has alleged that she injured her low back in an automobile accident, and that review of records reveals that she was already receiving treatment for low back pain when the accident occurred. The historical information would cast ambiguity on the causal role of the motor vehicle accident in her current back pain. However, the ambiguity would be equally apparent to a nonphysician and a physician.

Need for Further Treatment. Table 14.6 lists factors to consider in determining whether a patient needs further treatment. It is important to be aware, though, that the determination of whether a patient needs additional treatment is fraught with ambiguity.

Disability agencies generally adopt an idealized model of the course of recovery following an injury. The model is shown in Figure 14.2. It embodies the assumption that people show rapid improvement following injury, but then level off and reach a plateau. Before patients reach this hypothetical plateau, they presumably can benefit from further treatment. When they reach the plateau, they are considered to have achieved *maximal medical improvement* (MMI). When a patient

has reached MMI, insurance companies and/or disability agencies typically refuse to pay for additional medical care, and attempt to make a final determination regarding a patient's impairment and work capacity. From an administrative perspective, the model is convenient because it provides guidelines for intervention and decision making. For example, when a patient has reached point X on the graph, curative treatment should be abandoned, and a permanent partial impairment rating should be made.

Unfortunately, patients frequently present with clinical problems that are hard to conceptualize in terms of the idealized recovery shown in Figure 14.2. The difficulties in this area are myriad. For example, it is not at all clear that patients with repetitive strain injuries should be expected to follow the trajectory shown in Figure 14.2. Another problem is that patients may have comorbidities that complicate recovery and make it difficult to determine when they have reached MMI. An example is a patient with diabetes who has a work-related carpal tunnel syndrome in addition to a peripheral polyneuropathy.

A final complication of the MMI concept is that a patient who has reached maximal benefit from a particular kind of treatment may not have reached maximal benefit from treatment in general. For example, consider a woman who is examined 6 months after a low back injury. Assume that her treatment has consisted entirely of chiropractic care during the 6-month interval, and that she has not shown any measurable improvement during the past two months. This patient might be judged to have reached maximal medical benefit *from chiropractic care,* but an examining physician would understandably be uncertain about whether she could benefit from physical therapy, epidural steroids, lumbar surgery, aggressive use of various medications, or other therapies not provided by her chiropractor. This problem is not just a hypothetical one, since examiners routinely find that even patients with very chronic pain have not had exposure to all the plausible treatment approaches for their condition.

One other consideration is extremely important for a treating physician. It does not bear on the process of determining MMI, but does bear on the consequences that follow the determination that a patient has reached MMI. Disability and health insurance companies typically take the position that no more medical treatment should be authorized after a patient has reached MMI. This administrative perspective frequently does not match the clinical needs of patients. For example,

TABLE 14.6. Issues to Consider in Determining Maximal Medical Improvement (MMI)

1. Is patient's condition best construed as:
   a. A distinct injury?
   b. A repetitive strain (overuse) syndrome?
   c. A disease?
2. How long does it usually take for people with this condition to recover, or to reach a stable plateau?
   a. Is there a predictable course?
   b. Is patient's condition likely to get worse in the future?
3. How much time has elapsed since the index condition began?
4. What has been the trend over time with respect to function of the affected organ or body part?
   a. Steady improvement?
   b. Very little change over time?
   c. Deterioration?
   d. Widely fluctuating?
5. What has been the trend of time with respect to patient's symptoms?
   a. Steady improvement?
   b. Very little change over time?
   c. Deterioration?
   d. Widely fluctuating?
6. Does patient have concurrent medical conditions that obscure recovery curve from the index condition?
7. Has patient had access to treatment approaches that are appropriate for his or her condition?

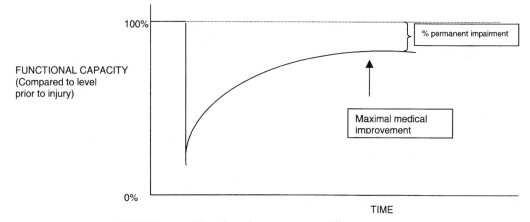

FUNCTIONAL CAPACITY
(Compared to level
prior to injury)

100%

% permanent impairment

Maximal medical
improvement

0%

TIME

FIGURE 14.2. Hypothetical recovery curve following an injury.

a man may have reached MMI from a low back injury in the sense that a significant period of time has elapsed since injury, and no further curative treatment is available. But the individual might still need *maintenance* treatment for his condition—for example, ongoing medication. This issue is often ignored by agencies that administer benefits.

Impairment. Disability systems typically specify the system that physicians are required to use when they rate patients' impairments. Table 14.7 shows steps that should be followed if you rate impairment according to the *Guides*. The *Guides* usually allows more than one way to rate the impairment associated with a medical condition. At the very least, virtually any chronic pain condition can be rated either according to rules set out for the affected body part or organ, or according to the principles set out in Chapter 15 of the volume, which deals exclusively with pain. As a practical matter, most physicians use ratings for the affected organ or body part, rather than ratings based on concepts given in Chapter 15. For example, if you were rating impairment in a patient with low back pain, you should use the concepts outlined in Chapter 3 of the *Guides* ("The Musculoskeletal System"), rather than the ones outlined in Chapter 15.

It is important to remember that the *Guides* recognizes that impairment rating involves clinical judgment, rather than simply the mechanical application of formulas. At one point, the volume suggests that an examiner can reduce an impairment rating on the basis of clinical judgment:

The physician must utilize the entire gamut of clinical skill and judgment in assessing whether or not the results of measurements or tests are plausible and

relate to the impairment being evaluated. If in spite of an observation or test result the medical evidence appears not to be of sufficient weight to verify that an impairment of a certain magnitude exists, the physician should modify the impairment estimate accordingly, describing the modification and explaining the reason for it in writing. (American Medical Association, 1993, p. 8)

TABLE 14.7. Issues to Consider in Using the *Guides* to Determine Impairment

1. Select section of the *Guides* that is devoted to the patient's condition (e.g., lumbosacral spine).
2. Follow rules given in the *Guides* for determining percent impairment.
3. Decide whether, in your clinical judgment, the impairment rating accurately reflects the burden that the patient bears as a result of his or her condition.
   a. Modify the rating *downward* if you believe that pain behaviors are excessive, and invalidate measurements used in the *Guides* to determine impairment. (Example: A patient with low back pain demonstrates severely restricted range of motion of the lumbar spine.)
   b. Modify the rating *upward* if you believe that the patient's pain limits him or her more than the evaluation procedures described in the *Guides* suggest. You may rationalize this upward adjustment on the basis of concepts given in Chapter 15 ("Pain") or Chapter 14 ("Mental and Behavioral Disorders") of the *Guides*.
   c. Note: The *Guides* volume recognizes that its formal rules for evaluating impairment may not lead to an impairment rating that adequately captures the burden imposed by a medical condition. It indicates that if that situation arises, the examining physician should use his or her clinical judgment to modify the rating.

At another point, the volume recognizes the potential need for a physician to award a higher impairment rating than a simple mechanical application of the AMA rating system would imply: "If the examiner determines that the estimate for the anatomic impairment does not sufficiently reflect the severity of the patient's condition, the examiner may increase the impairment percent, explaining the reason for the increase in writing" (p. 64).

As Table 14.7 indicates, after you have rated your patient's impairment according to principles outlined in the chapter of the *Guides* devoted to the organ system to which his or her problem is relevant, you should consider modifying the rating to take into accounts the patient's pain complaints and credibility. In theory, the rating could be either increased or decreased at this point.

Physical Capacities. The assessment of physical capacities is a precursor to the determination of a patient's ability to work. Disability agencies typically request detailed data on physical capacities, and usually provide supplementary forms for this purpose. Figure 14.3 provides an example of a typical physical capacities form.

Table 14.8 outlines issues you should consider in assessing the physical capacities of your patient. In general, a clinical evaluation in your office will not provide the detailed physical capacities information that you will need to fill out a physical capacities form. You can supplement information gleaned from your clinical evaluation in a variety of ways.

The simplest way is to ask the patient to estimate his or her capacities. You should consider filling out a physical capacities form on the basis of a patient's reports only if you judge the patient to be highly credible, or if you do not have access to objective data regarding the patient's capacities. (If you follow this approach, you should indicate this on the form.)

Another way to obtain physical capacities data is to refer a patient for a functional capacities evaluation (FCE) (King, Tuckwell, & Barrett, 1998; Lechner, 1998; Rondinelli & Katz, 2000). FCEs are formal, standardized assessments typically performed by physical therapists. They typically last from 2 to 5 hours. The therapist gathers information about a patient's strength, mobility, and endurance in tasks related to the work that the patient is expected to do. As noted by King and colleagues (1998), FCEs are popular with insurance carriers and attorneys because they provide objective performance data. However, in their compre-

TABLE 14.8. Issues to Consider in Determining Physical Capacities

1. What physical capacities issues need to be addressed in order to determine the patient's eligibility for disability benefits? (Example: Most jobs do not require employees to run. Therefore, the ability of a patient to run is usually irrelevant to an evaluation of his or her disability.)
2. Does the patient have a clear diagnosis?
3. Does this diagnosis provide clear information about the nature and severity of the activity restrictions the patient is likely to have?
4. Are the patient's symptoms and physical findings consistent over time, and consistent with his or her diagnosis?
5. Does the patient describe activity limitations that are plausible, given the medical information you have on him or her?
6. Do you have reports or behavioral data on the patient's activities outside your medical office?
   a. Data from day-to-day life (e.g., reports from spouse/partner or employer; surveillance tapes)?
   b. Data from a functional capacity evaluation?
   c. Data from a rehabilitation program, such as a work hardening program or a pain center?
7. What is your overall assessment of the patient's credibility?

hensive review, King and colleagues note that there are virtually no data that validate FCEs against actual job performance.

Finally, you can get physical capacities data on a patient by referring him or her to a functional restoration program, a pain center, or a work hardening program (Hildebrandt et al., 1997; Mayer & Gatchel, 1988; Niemeyer et al., 1994). A common feature of these programs is that they both assess physical capacities and provide treatment designed to improve those capacities. The performance data from one of these programs have more face validity than performance data from a FCE, because functional restoration programs, work hardening programs, and pain centers typically observe performance over a few weeks and indicate what patients can do after they have completed rehabilitative treatment.

Ability to Work. As noted above, the ability of a patient to work is in many respects the key issue in a disability evaluation. In essence, disability agencies are required to make wage compensation payments to patients if and only if the patients are judged not to be employable because of a medical condition. Unfortunately, assessing employ-

1. In an 8-hour workday, this patient can:

	TOTAL AT ONE TIME (hours)	TOTAL DURING 8-HR DAY (hours)
A. Sit	0 ½ 1 2 3 4 5 6 7 8	0 ½ 1 2 3 4 5 6 7 8
B. Stand	0 ½ 1 2 3 4 5 6 7 8	0 ½ 1 2 3 4 5 6 7 8
C. Walk	0 ½ 1 2 3 4 5 6 7 8	0 ½ 1 2 3 4 5 6 7 8

2. Patient can lift:

	Never	Occasionally	Frequently	Continuously
Up to 5 lbs				
5–10 lbs				
11–20 lbs				
21–25 lbs				
26–50 lbs				
51–100 lbs				

3. Patient can carry:

	Never	Occasionally	Frequently	Continuously
Up to 5 lbs				
5–10 lbs				
11–20 lbs				
21–25 lbs				
26–50 lbs				
51–100 lbs				

4. Patient is able to:

	Never	Occasionally	Frequently	Continuously
Bend				
Squat				
Crawl				
Climb				
Crouch				
Kneel				
Stoop				
Reach overhead				

5. Patient can use hands for repetitive actions such as:

	Simple Grasp	Push/Pull	Fine Manipulation
Right:	__Yes __No	__Yes __No	__Yes __No
Left:	__Yes __No	__Yes __No	__Yes __No

6. Patient can use feet for repetitive movements, as in operating foot controls:

Right	Left	Both
__Yes __No	__Yes __No	__Yes __No

KEY: "Occasionally" = 1%–33% of an 8-hour workday
"Frequently" = 34%–66% of an 8-hour workday
"Continuously" = 67%–100% of an 8-hour workday

FIGURE 14.3. A physical capacities form.

263

ability is difficult, and there is no simple set of techniques to apply when a decision about employability is requested. Table 14.9 outlines issues that you should consider when you judge a patient's employability.

As Figure 14.4 suggests, a physician makes a judgment about a patient's employability by balancing the patient's capacities (or limitations) against the demands of jobs for which the patient is being considered. Both sides of the balance involve difficult measurements. Issues related to assessing physical capacities are discussed above.

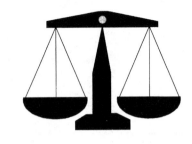

Capacities (Impairments)   Work Demands

FIGURE 14.4. Balancing capacity against work demands.

TABLE 14.9. Issues to Consider in Determining Employability

1. What specific questions about employability are you being asked to address?
   a. Can patient work at a specified job?
   b. What general category of work can the patient perform (sedentary, light, medium, heavy, very heavy)?
   c. Is the patient employable in any capacity?
2. For work in a specific job:
   a. Is there a job analysis?
   b. Does the patient agree with the demands stated on the job analysis?
   c. Are there any collateral sources of information about the job (e.g., information from the employer)?
   d. Do you believe the patient can perform the job with modifications?
   e. Do you believe the patient needs assistance in transitioning to the job (e.g., a graduated reentry, or a work hardening program)?
3. Do you have reliable physical capacities data that permit you to determine the appropriateness of a specific job, or the appropriateness of a general work category?
4. Are there any "trick questions"?
   a. Description of a job with minimal physical requirements (e.g., phone solicitor)?
   b. Description of a job that seems inappropriate for the patient from an economic and career standpoint (e.g., description of a cashiering job for a person who has spent the last 20 years working as an electrician)?
5. Based on the questions addressed to you, does it seem that the disability agency is making a sincere attempt to find a place in the work force for the patient, as opposed to trying to "set the patient up" (i.e., contrive vocational options that will maneuver him or her out of the disability system)?
6. Does it appear that the patient is making a sincere effort to return to work, or is he or she exaggerating pain complaints and/or maneuvering in some way to get long-term disability?

As far as the demands of jobs are concerned, the physician usually has to rely on information provided by vocational rehabilitation counselors (VRCs) or employers. In workers' compensation claims, VRCs often prepare formal job analyses. Figure 14.5 gives a sample job analysis. Note that the job analysis form includes a section in which the evaluating physician is asked to give his or her opinion about whether or not the worker can perform the job.

A detailed job analysis can be extremely helpful in the assessment of the work demands that a patient is likely to face. However, you need to check with the patient to see whether he or she agrees with the physical requirements listed in a job analysis. If the patient vigorously disputes the job analysis, you should make an attempt to reconcile the discrepancy.

Several problems involving employability determinations occur frequently enough to warrant further discussion.

1. Sometimes you will be asked whether your patient can do a specific job, and you will be provided with a job analysis. In other situations, you will be asked much broader questions. For example, you might be asked to rate the general category of work for which the patient is suited. Broad work categories are defined in the *Dictionary of Occupational Titles* (U.S. Department of Labor, Employment and Training Administration, 1977) and a supplementary publication by Field and Field (1992; see also Lechner, 1998); they are "sedentary," "light," "medium," "heavy," and "very heavy." The problem with these work categories is that they may not capture specific activity limitations of your patient. When you are asked to place your patient in a general work category, probably the best approach is to get physical capacities data and use them to assign the patient.

Job Title: Taxi Dispatcher
DOT: 913.367-010
GOE: 07.04.05
SVP: 3

Job Description: Dispatches taxicabs in response to telephone requests for service by entering client name and pick-up and drop-off locations into the computer. Directs calls to dispatch supervisor if needed.

Job Qualifications: Good customer service skills; ability to type and learn computer program.

Types of Machines, Tools, Special Equipment Used: Telephone with headset, computer.

Materials, Products, Subject Matter, Services: Local and suburban transit and interurban buses.

Work Schedule: Full time, 8-hour shifts.

Physical Demands:
1. Stand: Occasionally. Daily total 0.5 hours.
2. Walk: Occasionally. Daily total 0.5 hours.
3. Sit: Constantly with option to stand. Daily total 7 hours.
4. Lift/carry: Occasionally lift/carry ounces.
5. Push/pull: Occasionally with minimum force to open file drawers and keyboard trays.
6. Controls: Frequently use controls on telephone. Most calls are incoming.
7. Climb: Not required.
8. Balance: Not required.
9. Bend/stoop: Rarely to occasionally.
10. Crouch: Not required.
11. Twist: Occasionally at the neck while answering the phones.
12. Kneel: Not required.
13. Crawl: Not required.
14. Handle/grasp: Occasionally handle/grasp office supplies and handset.
15. Fine manipulation/fingering: Frequent to constant typing is involved during workday. Fingering to dial telephone.
16. Feeling: Not required.
17. Reach: Occasionally at mid-waist level, three-quarters to full arm extension.
18. Vision: Correctable vision is desirable.
19. Talk/hear: Speech and hearing are mandatory.
20. Taste/smell: Not required.
21. Environmental factors: Office environment. Floors are carpeted.
22. Work environment access: On-site parking available.

Physician's Judgment:
__ The injured worker can perform this job without restrictions and can return to work on _____.
__ The injured worker can perform this job without restrictions, but only on a part-time basis for __ hours per day, __ days per week. The worker can be expected to return to full-time work in __ days/weeks.
__ The injured worker can perform this job, but only with the following modifications: _____
_____
   Modifications are needed on a __ permanent __ temporary basis.
__ The injured worker temporarily cannot perform this job, based on the following physical limitations: _____
_____
   Anticipated release date: _____
__ The injured worker permanently cannot perform this job, based on the following physical limitations:
_____

Comments:

_____   _____
Signature of Physician   Date

FIGURE 14.5. A job analysis.

2. Sometimes you will be presented with "trick questions" dealing with employability. As an example, imagine that you are treating a man with chronic low back pain who has failed multiple spine surgeries, and continues to complain of relentless pain despite the implantation of an intrathecal opiate delivery system. Imagine that you do not believe it is realistic for this patient to return to competitive employment. Suppose that a disability agency asks you whether your patient can work as a telephone solicitor. This question poses a dilemma. If you indicate "Yes," your patient will probably have his disability benefits terminated. If you say "No," you are implicitly saying that the patient's low back pain prevents him from doing a job that has essentially no physical demands. The "trick" in this type of situation is that disability adjudicators or VRCs sometimes concoct jobs specifically because they demand essentially nothing in the way of physical capacities. When you see a trick question like this one, you have good reason to be suspicious that the disability system is maneuvering to terminate the patient's benefits. In this situation, it is appropriate to be protective of your patient and to demand details regarding the proposed job. For example, you should ask the adjudicator whether there is a market for the phone solicitor job, and whether the patient would have to commute to an office in order to perform the job.

3. Some patients drag their feet and emphasize the severity of their incapacitation. These behaviors should make you suspicious of their agendas. In such a situation, it is reasonable to stick closely to objective data regarding the patient's capacities, rather than to be influenced strongly by the patient's subjective assessments.

It is important to make an employability determination that is acceptable to your patient whenever this is possible. As noted earlier, physicians sometimes feel that they have resolved a difficult disability claim when they say a patient is capable of employment. If the patient strongly disagrees with this conclusion, he or she may simply go to another physician or retain an attorney. In many instances, the anticipated resolution of the claim turns out to be ephemeral. The recommendation here is *not* to let the patient dictate what you say on a disability form. But it is important to listen carefully to your patient's concerns about employment, and to look for an employment plan that is both medically sensible and acceptable to the patient and the disability system.

It is worth noting that you can sometimes use disability evaluations as springboards to mobilize patients to take an active role in their vocational rehabilitation. Some patients with chronic disabilities passively wait for "the system" to solve their vocational dilemmas. When they see the jobs that are proposed during disability evaluations, they are often appalled. In this setting, a treating physician can encourage a patient to become more active in seeking vocational options on his or her own. Some patients will take this advice and find jobs that fit their physical limitations and their economic needs. Thus a disability evaluation can provide the stimulus for patients to become more actively involved in their own rehabilitation.

Objective Findings

It is routine for disability agencies to ask physicians to base their opinions on objective findings. This request may seem innocuous, but it has profound implications. As noted above, disability agencies attempt to make decisions based on objectively measurable evidence of incapacitation. But patients with painful conditions typically report incapacitation that goes beyond measurable damage to their organs. Even if you find a patient's pain complaints very credible, you will invariably have difficulty stating objective findings that make his or her activity limitations inevitable. For example, consider a patient with low back pain who reports that he or she can sit for only 20 minutes at a time. There is no objective measure that would make this limitation inevitable.

The request for objective findings can create at least two kinds of problems for you as an examining physician. First, some patients—for example, ones with fibromyalgia or chronic headaches—may not have any unequivocally objective findings. Second (and far more important), even when patients have objective findings, the findings rarely explain the extent of the incapacitation that the patients report.

As a step toward a strategy for dealing with requests for objective findings, it is important to note that the term *objective findings* is not precisely defined. In general, it refers to laboratory or physical findings that are objectively measurable and are not subject to voluntary control or manipulation by a patient. Objective findings can be contrasted with *subjective findings*, such as patients' reports of pain intensity or activity restrictions caused by pain. However, as shown in Table 14.10, a lot of clinically important examination findings are *semi-*

objective. They are objective in the sense that they can be observed and measured. But they are not completely objective, since patients can to some extent voluntarily modify them. Most of the adjudicators who request objective findings are not aware of these subtleties.

There is a fairly simple way to finesse the objective findings issue. If you do not find your patient credible, it would be perfectly reasonable to indicate that there are no objective findings to support his or her claimed incapacitation. But if your patient has consistent physical findings that you find credible, you can simply list them in the space where you are requested to give objective findings. In most instances, the findings you list will be accepted by the disability system, even if they are only semiobjective or do not necessarily explain the activity restrictions your patient reports. If your findings are challenged, you can indicate that in your clinical judgment they represent valid indices of the patient's condition.

Psychogenic Pain

A physician who does disability evaluations on patients with chronic pain needs to have at least a

---

TABLE 14.10. "Objective Findings" and "Subjective Findings" in Low Back Pain

Objective findings

1. X-ray abnormalities (e.g., fracture, scoliosis, spondylolisthesis, disc space narrowing, osteophytes)
2. MRI abnormalities (e.g., spinal stenosis, disc herniation)
3. Electromyographic abnormalities (e.g., positive waves and fibrillations, absent H-reflex)

Subjective findings

1. Patient-reported pain intensity
2. Activity restrictions reported by patient

Semiobjective findings

1. Abnormal posture (e.g., loss of lumbar lordosis, list)
2. Abnormal gait
3. Muscle spasms
4. Soft tissue hypersensitivity (myofascial pain)
5. Reduced range of motion
6. Abnormal straight-leg raising
7. Some lower-extremity deep tendon reflex findings (e.g., reflexes difficult to elicit in patient who is tense)
8. Reduced sensory function in lower extremities
9. Reduced lower-extremity strength

---

rudimentary familiarity with psychogenic pain. Unfortunately, the concepts surrounding psychogenic pain are generally ambiguous, and there is significant disagreement among experts regarding how to apply them (Fishbain, 1996; Hiller, Rief & Fichter, 1997; Jackson, 1992; King, 1995; Sullivan, in press; Sullivan & Katon, 1993; Sullivan & Turk, 2001). (See also Sullivan, Chapter 15, this volume.)

A terminological issue needs to be addressed at the outset. *Psychogenic pain* can be used in a broad sense to refer to pain complaints that are best understood in psychological terms rather than biomedical terms (i.e., complaints in which psychological factors appear to play a major role in onset or maintenance). It can also be used in a more restricted sense to refer to two diagnoses given in the American Psychiatric Association's (1994) *Diagnostic and Statistical Manual of Mental Disorders*, fourth edition (DSM-IV): pain disorder associated with psychological factors (307.80), and pain disorder associated with both psychological factors and a general medical disorder (307.89). The DSM-IV indicates that these diagnoses should be considered when two conditions are met: (1) A patient's pain complaints can best be understood in psychological terms, and (2) the complaints *cannot* be better explained in terms of a psychotic, mood, or anxiety disorder. Thus pain disorder has the quality of a "wastebasket diagnosis"—it is given only when a patient's pain complaints seem to be affected by psychological factors and no specific Axis I diagnosis can be made. For nonpsychiatrists, the broader concept of psychogenic pain is more useful.

It is appropriate for physicians to consider the possibility of psychogenic pain in patients with chronic pain for at least two reasons. First, as indicated above, patients with chronic pain routinely report symptoms and activity restrictions that cannot be rationalized in terms of objectively measurable biological deficits. There are multiple reasons for the mismatch between the restrictions that a patient reports and the biomedical abnormalities that a physician can observe, but one possibility is that psychological factors may be leading the patient to amplify his or her reports of incapacitation. Second, there is abundant research demonstrating high levels of psychopathology (Fishbain et al., 1988; Robinson, Robinson, & Shelton, 1999) and psychological distress (Turk & Okifuji, 1997; Turk, Okifuji, Sinclair, & Starz, 1996, 1998; Wells, 1994) in patients with chronic pain.

However, it is important to avoid the simplistic dichotomy of concluding something like this: "I'll find the source of my patient's pain either on the

MRI [magnetic resonance imaging] or on the MMPI [Minnesota Multiphasic Personality Inventory]." Chronic pain is a dilemma for patients and physicians precisely because it often cannot be neatly compartmentalized into "biogenic" and "psychogenic" subgroups. In attempting to understand a patient's pain complaints, it is important to consider a variety of possible explanations, and to avoid premature closure. No one has developed a widely accepted framework in terms of which to conceptualize pain complaints that are not easily explained in terms of biological dysfunction, but as a prudent physician, you should consider the following general categories:

1. The patient's pain may be a manifestation of a pathophysiological process that is obscure enough to have eluded detection.

2. The patient's pain may reflect central sensitization.

3. The pain may best be construed in psychological terms—either as a manifestation of a pain disorder, or as a manifestation of an anxiety, mood, or psychotic disorder.

4. The pain may best be construed in terms of "systems issues" (Robinson et al., 1997) such as financial disincentives or poor employment opportunities.

If you are a nonpsychiatric physician, your best strategy is to ask for help with the assessment of patients who appear to have psychological or systems issues that may be influencing their pain complaints. In order to implement this strategy, you would need to do at least a preliminary assessment of these factors. But if you maintain a high index of suspicion and a low threshold for seeking psychiatric or psychological consultation, you should be able to get the help you need. If you follow this strategy, do not be surprised if you get some puzzling reports back. As noted above, no one has been able to articulate a coherent, widely accepted perspective on psychogenic pain at a clinical level, and the forensic implications of psychogenic pain are even murkier.

Filling Out the Form

Once you have addressed the issues described above, your work in filling out a disability form is largely done. However, there are three other matters that you should consider.

1. When you fill out a disability form, you are acting as an intermediary between the medical system and an administrative or legal system. The manner in which the disability agency responds to the form you submit will be governed by the administrative and legal mandate under which the agency functions. In many instances, the agency's response will depend on specific words that you use in answering questions. For example, if you are writing a report on behalf of an applicant for Social Security disability benefits, your report will probably have a greater impact if you compare your patient's clinical findings to the appropriate listing that the SSA uses when it determines whether an applicant is eligible for disability benefits. (Listings are described in the book *Disability Evaluation under Social Security, 1994*. In contrast, you may use language that is sensible from a medical standpoint when you fill out a disability form, and then find that the disability agency to which it is submitted interprets it in a completely different way. There is no easy way to solve this problem. Ideally, you should be aware that it exists, and you should learn enough about the legal and administrative mandates of disability systems that you do not accidentally use wording that is misinterpreted or misused.

2. It is not unusual for disability forms to ask questions that physicians are simply unable to answer. For example, it is often impossible for a physician to determine causation in problems such as low back pain and cumulative trauma disorders of the upper extremities. When you encounter such an item, you should feel free to withhold judgment. However, it is often effective to indicate the difficulty of the item on the form—for example, to say, "Neither I nor any other physician can answer this question on the basis of the information available."

3. Sometimes the questions asked in a disability form are so specific that they do not give you a chance to communicate an overall perspective on your patient. As a practical matter, you may find that the information you provided on the disability form does not convey the general assessment that you constructed when you first reviewed the form ("Initial Review of the Disability Form," above). In this situation, you should write a cover letter to accompany the disability form. In it, you should communicate your overall perspective on the patient and any critical information that was not given when you answered the specific questions on the form.

Follow-Up

Sometimes your interaction with a disability system will end after you have sent in a single disability form. For example, the SSA generally asks a treating physician to fill out only a single form. Other agencies, such as the workers' compensation companies, will ask you to participate in sequential disability determinations that may extend over months or even years.

In either case, your responses to a disability form may have ongoing consequences for your relationship with your patient. Some patients will object if your statements on a disability form suggest that they are capable of working. They will usually look for another physician if you give the "wrong" answers. In other situations, you and your patient may agree about the information you put on a disability form, but the disability agency to which the form is submitted may reach a decision that is adverse to the patient's interests. The patient may then feel that you have sold him or her out. The best way to avoid such recriminations is to tell your patient at the outset that disability decisions are made by adjudicators rather by physicians, and that you cannot provide information that will guarantee a favorable outcome.

Another consequence of a disability evaluation is that the patient's medical and wage replacement payments may change dramatically. It is helpful to discuss this openly with a patient before a final decision has been made by the disability agency. For example, if you have been treating a patient under a workers' compensation claim, you should discuss whether the patient wants to continue treatment after the claim has been closed, and, if so, how he or she will pay for the treatment.

INTEGRATING DISABILITY EVALUATION INTO CLINICAL PRACTICE

The discussion above demonstrates that disability evaluations are difficult for treating physicians to perform. A physician who tries to incorporate disability evaluation into his or her practice must deal with several challenges:

1. Disability evaluations require information and skills that physicians typically do not acquire in their training. For example, they require a physician to know about the policies of various disability agencies.

2. Agencies that request disability evaluations typically challenge assumptions that are fundamental to clinical medicine. The clearest example of this is the demand for objective findings. This

demand challenges the view that an essential task of a physician is to combine objective findings, semiobjective findings, and symptoms into a coherent picture of a patient. In essence, disability evaluation procedures embody skepticism about the clinical judgments that are fundamental to the practice of medicine.

3. Even for physicians who have spent the time necessary to gain expertise in the art of disability evaluation, the evaluations are time-consuming and tedious. They frequently require extensive record reviews, efforts to reconcile conflicting opinions, and a lot of paperwork.

4. Disability evaluations can have significant effects on the doctor–patient relationship. In particular, patients frequently become hostile when they perceive that their treating physicians are understating the severity of their incapacitation.

5. Disability evaluations raise significant ethical challenges for a treating physician. Many physicians worry that in the course of performing the evaluations, they may misuse the trust that patients place in them. They may also be concerned about the outcomes of their disability evaluations. At one extreme, they are likely to feel angst if patients whom they perceive as severely incapacitated are denied disability benefits. At the opposite extreme, when patients with very minimal incapacitation receive disability benefits, treating physicians may feel that they have failed to represent the legitimate need of society to refuse disability benefits to individuals who do not have incapacitating medical problems.

6. The ethical concerns above are aggravated by the lack of validation of disability evaluation procedures. Thoughtful physicians realize that their judgments about the ability of their patients to work have important consequences, but they have no way to determine whether their judgments are well founded.

Given all these difficulties, some physicians are understandably tempted to avoid making judgments about whether or not their patients are disabled. Unfortunately, this is not a viable option. As noted above, society requires physicians to make disability determinations on patients whom they are treating. Physicians may do disability evaluations thoughtfully or thoughtlessly, but they do not have the option of simply not doing them.

Another option is for a physician to develop expertise in the area of disability evaluation. For example, a physician might gain familiarity with major disability agencies, and attend courses on independent medical examinations (e.g., ones conducted by the American Board of Independent Medical Examiners).

There is a third option that is probably the most appropriate one for the majority of physicians. It is to get help from consultants. Clinicians are used to requesting consultation regarding medical care of their patients. Medical specialists have an important role to play because they have more expertise than nonspecialists in certain areas of clinical medicine. In the same way, some physicians—especially ones trained in physical medicine and rehabilitation or occupational medicine—have enough expertise in disability evaluation to provide consultation to other physicians. If you decide that it is infeasible to acquire expertise in disability evaluation, you should identify physicians in your community who can assist you in making disability determinations on your patients.

NOTE

1. This chapter makes several references to the American Medical Association's *Guides to the Evaluation of Permanent Impairment*. These all refer to the 4th edition of the *Guides*. Recently, the 5th edition of the *Guides* has been published. Some of the statements made in this chapter apply to both editions. However, the 5th edition's chapter on rating pain-related impairment (Chapter 18) is completely different from the corresponding chapter (Chapter 15) in the 4th edition of the *Guides*. In particular, the new chapter describes a detailed protocol for an examiner to follow when rating pain-related impairment. Also, it discusses in detail the many complex conceptual issues an evaluator needs to consider when reaching conclusions about impairment secondary to pain.

As one of the authors of Chapter 18 of the 5th edition of the *Guides*, I believe that it represents a significant improvement over the corresponding chapter in the 4th edition. At this point, however, the new edition of the *Guides* has not been available long enough for anyone to know whether it will play a bigger role in impairment evaluations than did Chapter 15 of the 4th edition.

REFERENCES

Alaranta, H., Rytokoski, U., Rissanen, A., Talo, S., Ronnemaa, T., Puukka, M. A., Karppi, S.-L., Videman, T., Kallio, V., & Slatis, P. (1994). Intensive physical and psychosocial training program for patients with chronic low back pain. *Spine, 19,* 1339–1349.

American Medical Association. (1993). *Guides to the evaluation of permanent impairment* (4th ed.). Chicago: Author.

American Psychiatric Association. (1994). *Diagnostic and statistical manual of mental disorders* (4th ed.). Washington, DC: Author.

Atkinson, T., Liem, R., & Liem, J. (1986). The social cost of unemployment: Implications for social support. *Journal of Health and Social Behavior, 54,* 454–460.

Bellamy, R. (1997). Compensation neurosis. *Clinical Orthopaedics and Related Research, 336,* 94–106.

Cheadle, A., Franklin, G., Wolfhagen, C., Savarino, J., Liu, P. Y., Salley, C., & Weaver, M. (1994). Factors influencing the duration of work-related disability: A population-based study of Washington State workers' compensation. *American Journal of Public Health, 84,* 190–196.

Clark, W. L., & Haldeman, S. (1993). The development of guideline factors for the evaluation of disability in neck. *Spine, 18,* 1736–1745.

Clark, W. L., Haldeman, S., Johnson, P., Morris, J., Schulenberger, C., Trauner, D., & White, A. (1988). Back impairment and disability determination: Another attempt at objective, reliable rating. *Spine, 13,* 332–341.

Demeter, S. L., Andersson, G. B. J., & Smith, G. M. (1996). *Disability evaluation.* Chicago: American Medical Association.

Estlander, A., Mellin, G., Vanharanta, H., & Hupli, M. (1991). Effects and follow-up of a multimodel treatment program including intensive physical training for low back pain patients. *Scandinavian Journal of Rehabilitation Medicine, 23,* 97–102.

Faust, D. (1995). The detection of deception. *Neurologic Clinics of North America, 13,* 255–265.

Field, J. E., & Field, T. F. (1992). *Classification of jobs.* Athens, G A: Elliott & Fitzpatrick.

Fishbain, D. A. (1996). Where have two DSM revisions taken us for the diagnosis of pain disorder in chronic pain patients? *American Journal of Psychiatry, 153,* 137–138.

Fishbain, D. A., Cutler, R. B., Rosomoff, H. L., Khalil, T., & Steele-Rosomoff, R. (1997). Impact of chronic pain patients' job perception variables on actual return to work. *Clinical Journal of Pain, 13,* 197–206.

Fishbain, D. A., Cutler, R. B., Rosomoff, H. L., Khalil, T., & Steele-Rosomoff, R. (1999). Prediction of "intent," "discrepancy with intent," and "discrepancy with nonintent" for the patient with chronic pain to return to work after treatment at a pain facility. *Clinical Journal of Pain, 15,* 141–150.

Fishbain, D. A., Goldberg, M., Labbe, E., Steele, R., & Rosomoff, H. (1988). Compensation and noncompensation chronic pain patients compared for DSM-III operational diagnoses. *Pain, 32,* 197–206.

Fishbain, D. A., Rosomoff, H. L., Cutler, R. B., & Rosomoff, R. S. (1995). Secondary gain concept: A review of the scientific evidence. *Clinical Journal of Pain, 11,* 6–21.

Frymoyer, J. W., & Cats-Baril, W. (1987). Predictors of low back pain disability. *Clinical Orthopaedics and Related Research, 221,* 89–98.

Gilovich, T. (1991). *How we know what isn't so.* New York: Free Press.

Hadler, N. M. (1996). If you have to prove you are ill, you

can't get well: The object lesson of fibromyalgia. *Spine, 21*, 2397–2400.

Hall, H. V., & Pritchard, D. A. (1996). *Detecting malingering and deception.* Delray Beach, FL: St. Lucie Press.

Hammarstrom, A., & Janlert, U. (1997). Nervous and depressive symptoms in a longitudinal study of youth unemployment—selection or exposure? *Journal of Adolescence, 20*, 293–305.

Hazard, R. G., Bendix, A., & Fenwick, J. W. (1991) Disability exaggeration as a predictor of functional restoration outcomes for patients with chronic low-back pain. *Spine, 16*, 1062–1067.

Hidding, A., Van Santen, M., De Klerk, E., Gielen, X., Boers, M., Geenen, R., Vlaeyen, J., Kester, A., & van der Linden, S. (1994). Comparison between self-report measures and clinical observations of functional disability in ankylosing spondylitis, rheumatoid arthritis, and fibromyalgia. *Journal of Rheumatology, 21*, 818–823.

Hildebrandt, J., Pfingsten, M., Saur, P., & Jansen, J. (1997). Prediction of success from a multidisciplinary treatment program for chronic low back pain. *Spine, 22*, 990–1001.

Hiller, W., Rief, W., & Fichter, M. M. (1997). How disabled are patients with somatoform disorders? *General Hospital Psychiatry, 19*, 432–438.

Jackson, J. E. (1992). After a while, no one believes you: Real and unreal pain. In M. D. Good, P. E. Brodwin, B. J. Good, et al. (Eds.), *Pain as human experience: An anthropological perspective* (pp. 138–168). Berkeley: University of California Press.

Jensen, M. P., Turner, J. A., & Romano, J. M. (1994). Correlates of improvement in multidisciplinary treatment of chronic pain. *Journal of Consulting and Clinical Psychology, 62*, 172–179.

Kaplan, G. A., Roberts, R. E., Camacho, T. C., & Coyne, J. C. (1987). Psychosocial predictors of depression. *American Journal of Epidemiology, 125*, 206–220.

Kaplan, G. M., Wurtele, S. K., & Gillis, D. (1996). Maximal effort during functional capacity evaluations: An examination of psychological factors. *Archives of Physical Medicine and Rehabilitation, 77*, 161–164.

King, P. M., Tuckwell, N., & Barrett, T. E. (1998). A critical review of functional capacity evaluations. *Physical Therapy, 78*, 852–866.

King, S. A. (1995). Review: DSM-IV and pain. *Clinical Journal of Pain, 11*, 171–176.

Kramer, M. S., & Lane, D. A. (1992). Causal propositions in clinical research and practice. *Journal of Clinical Epidemiology, 45*, 639–649.

Krause, N., & Ragland, D. R. (1994). Occupational disability due to low back pain: A new interdisciplinary classification based on a phase model of disability. *Spine, 19*, 1011–1020.

Lechner, D. E. (1998). Functional capacity evaluation. In P. M. King (Ed.), *Sourcebook of occupational rehabilitation* (pp. 209–227). New York: Plenum Press.

Lipchik, G. L., Milles, K., & Covington, E. C. (1993). The effects of multidisciplinary pain management treatment on locus of control and pain beliefs in chronic non-terminal pain. *Clinical Journal of Pain, 9*, 49–57.

Loeser, J. D., Henderlite, S. E., & Conrad, D. E. (1995). Incentive effects of workers' compensation benefits: A literature synthesis. *Medical Care Research, 52*, 34–59.

Mayer, T. G., & Gatchel, R. J. (1988). *Functional restoration for spinal disorders: The sports medicine approach.* Philadelphia: Lea & Febiger.

Mendelson, G. (1988). *Psychiatric aspects of personal injury claims.* Springfield, IL: Charles C Thomas.

Muller, L. S. (1992). Disability beneficiaries who work and their experience under program work incentives. *Social Security Bulletin, 55*, 2–19.

Mrazek, P. J., & Haggerty, R. J. (Eds.). (1994). *Reducing risks for mental disorder.* Washington, DC: National Academy Press.

Niemeyer, L. O., Jacobs, K., Reynolds-Lynch, K., Bettencourt, C., & Lang, S. (1994). Work hardening: Past, present and future—the Work Programs Special Interest Section national work hardening outcome study. *American Journal of Occupational Therapy, 48*, 327–339.

Osterweis, M., Kleinman, A., & Mechanic, D. (Eds.). (1987). *Pain and disability.* Washington, DC: National Academy Press.

Rahmqvist, M., & Carstensen, J. (1998). Trend of psychological distress in a Swedish population from 1989 to 1995. *Scandinavian Journal of Social Medicine, 3*, 214–222.

Reno, V. P., Mashaw, J. L., & Gradison, B. (Eds.). (1997). *Disability.* Washington, DC: National Academy of Social Insurance.

Robinson, J. P. (1997, June). *Psychological aspects of disability.* Paper presented to the Employer Advisory Group, Valley Medical Center, Renton, WA.

Robinson, J. P. (1998). Disability in low back pain: What do the numbers mean? *American Pain Society Bulletin, 8*, 9–13.

Robinson, J. P. (2001). Evaluation of function and disability. In J. D. Loeser, S. D. Butler, C. R. Chapman, & D. C. Turk (Eds.), *Bonica's management of pain* (3rd ed., pp. 342–362). Philadelphia: Lippincott Williams & Wilkins.

Robinson, J. P. (in press). Pain and disability. In P. Wilson & T. Jensen (Eds.), *Clinical pain management.* London: Edward Arnold.

Robinson, J. P., Robinson, K. A., & Shelton, J. L. (1999). *Psychiatric independent medical examinations on injured workers with back pain.* Paper presented at the World Congress of the International Association for the Study of Pain, Vienna.

Robinson, J. P., Rondinelli, R. D., & Scheer, S. J. (1997). Industrial rehabilitation medicine: 1. Why is industrial rehabilitation medicine unique? *Archives of Physical Medicine and Rehabilitation, 78*, S3–S9.

Rondinelli, R. D., & Katz, R. T. (Eds.). (2000). *Impairment rating and disability evaluation.* Philadelphia: Saunders.

Social Security Ruling 96-7, 61 Fed. Reg. 34483–34488 (1996).

Sullivan, M. D. (in press). DSM-IV pain disorder: A case against the diagnosis. *International Review of Psychiatry.*

Sullivan, M. D., & Katon, W. (1993). Somatization: The path between distress and somatic symptoms. *American Pain Society Journal, 2*, 141–149.

Sullivan, M. D., & Loeser, J. D. (1992). The diagnosis of disability. *Archives of Internal Medicine, 152*, 1829–1835.

Sullivan, M. D., & Turk, D. C. (2001). Psychiatric illness, depression, and psychogenic pain. In J. D. Loeser, S. D. Butler, C. R. Chapman, & D. C. Turk (Eds.),

Bonica's management of pain (3rd ed., pp. 483–500). Philadelphia: Lippincott Williams & Wilkins.

Turk, D. C., & Okifuji, A. (1997). Evaluating the role of physical, operant, cognitive, and affective factors in the pain behaviors of chronic pain patients. *Behavior Modification, 21,* 259–280.

Turk, D. C., Okifuji, A., Sinclair, J. D., & Starz, T. W. (1996). Pain, disability, and physical functioning in subgroups of patients with fibromyalgia. *Journal of Rheumatology, 23,* 1255–1262.

Turk, D. C., Okifuji, A., Sinclair, J. D., & Starz, T. W. (1998). Differential responses by psychosocial subgroups of fibromyalgia syndrome patients to an interdisciplinary treatment. *Arthritis Care and Research, 11,* 397–404.

U.S. Department of Labor, Employment and Training Administration. (1977). *Dictionary of occupational titles* (4th ed.). Washington, DC: U.S. Government Printing Office.

Voiss, D. V. (1995). Occupational injury: Fact, fantasy, or fraud? *Neurologic Clinics of North America, 13,* 431–446.

Washington State Department of Labor and Industries. (1999). *Attending doctor's handbook* (Rev. ed.). Olympia, WA: Author.

Wells, N. (1994). Perceived control over pain: Relation to distress and disability. *Research in Nursing and Health, 17,* 295–302.

Williams, C. A. (1991). *An international comparison of workers' compensation.* Boston: Kluwer.

Wolfe, F., & Potter, J. (1996). Fibromyalgia and work disability. *Rheumatic Disease Clinics of North America, 22,* 369–391.

Part IV

PSYCHOLOGICAL EVALUATION OF PATIENTS WITH PAIN

Chapter 15

Assessment of Psychiatric Disorders

MARK D. SULLIVAN

Psychiatric disorders are common in patients with chronic nonmalignant pain, but are still poorly understood. Epidemiological evidence supports the use of inclusive rather than exclusive models of psychiatric diagnosis in medical settings. Patients with medical disorders are more likely than those without to have comorbid psychiatric disorders. But often psychiatric disorders are not considered in the differential diagnosis of physical symptoms such as pain until medical disorders have been "ruled out." This stigma-driven policy can lead to unnecessary testing, iatrogenic injury, and poor clinical management of patients. Any time a pain problem has become chronic and disabling, psychiatric disorders should be considered.

Any discussion of psychiatric disorders in patients with chronic pain is haunted by the concept of *psychogenic pain*. We are drawn to the concept of psychogenic pain because it fills the gaps left when our attempts to explain clinical pain exclusively in terms of tissue pathology fail. Psychogenic pain, however, is an empty concept. Positive criteria for the identification of psychogenic pain, mechanisms for the production of psychogenic pain, and specific therapies for psychogenic pain are lacking. Psychiatric diagnosis of many disorders, such as depression, can be very helpful to clinicians and patients by pointing toward specific effective therapies. But the diagnosis of psychogenic pain too often only serves to stigmatize further the patients who experience chronic pain.

In the discussion that follows, psychiatric disorders as defined in the *Diagnostic and Statisti-*

cal Manual of Mental Disorders, fourth edition (DSM-IV; American Psychiatric Association, 1994), are used as an organizing strategy. It is important to note, however, that the categorical model of mental disorder favored by psychiatrists and used in DSM-IV can imply more discontinuity between those with and those without a mental disorder that is actually the case. For example, it is common for patients with chronic pain to meet criteria for a number of mental disorders partially. It is therefore sometimes useful to think of these disorders as dimensions rather than categories. The DSM-IV nevertheless provides a well-recognized and systematic template for the discussion of psychiatric disorders in patients with chronic pain.

When asked to evaluate patients at our Multidisciplinary Pain Center, I typically consider the following issues: depression, anxiety (panic, posttraumatic stress disorder [PTSD], and history of physical or sexual abuse), substance abuse or dependence, somatization disorder, and personality disorders. Other issues are addressed as indicated, such as obsessive–compulsive disorder (OCD), attention-deficit/hyperactivity disorder (ADHD), dementia, psychosis, and antisocial behavior. I do not usually use a structured interview for psychiatric diagnosis. But for readers who prefer some guidance and structure, the least cumbersome and most useful interview in the general medical setting is the PRIME-MD (Spitzer et al., 1994). This includes a screening questionnaire followed by interview modules. A new self-report instrument, the Patient Health Questionnaire, has recently been reported to yield psychiatric diagnoses similar to those derived from the PRIME-MD structured interview (Spitzer, Kroenke, & Williams, 1999).

DEPRESSIVE DISORDERS

Major Depression

One must begin by distinguishing between depressed mood and the clinical syndrome of major depression. It is important to note, especially when working with patients who have chronic pain, that depressed mood or dysphoria is not necessary for the diagnosis of major depression. Anhedonia, the inability to enjoy activities or experience pleasure,

is an adequate substitute. It is common for patients with chronic pain to deny dysphoria but to acknowledge that enjoyment of all activities has ceased, even those without obvious relation to their pain problem (e.g., watching TV for a patient with low back pain).

The DSM-IV criteria for a major depressive episode are listed in Table 15.1. These include both psychological symptoms such as worthlessness and somatic symptoms such as insomnia. It is important to note that somatic symptoms count toward a diagnosis of major depression unless they are due to "the direct physiological effects of a general medical condition" or medication. The poor sleep, poor concentration, and lack of enjoyment

---

TABLE 15.1. DSM-IV Criteria for Major Depressive Episode

A. Five (or more) of the following symptoms have been present during the same 2-week period and represent a change from previous functioning; at least one of the symptoms is either (1) depressed mood or (2) loss of interest or pleasure.

  Note: Do not include symptoms that are clearly due to a general medical condition, or mood-incongruent delusions or hallucinations.

  (1) depressed mood most of the day, nearly every day, as indicated by either subjective report (e.g., feels sad or empty) or observation made by others (e.g., appears tearful). Note: In children and adolescents, can be irritable mood.
  (2) markedly diminished interest or pleasure in all, or almost all, activities most of the day, nearly every day (as indicated by either subjective account or observation made by others)
  (3) significant weight loss when not dieting or weight gain (e.g., a change of more than 5% of body weight in a month), or a decrease or increase in appetite nearly every day. Note: In children, consider failure to make expected weight gains.
  (4) insomnia or hypersomnia nearly every day
  (5) psychomotor agitation or retardation nearly every day (observable by others, not merely subjective feelings of restlessness or being slowed down)
  (6) fatigue or loss of energy nearly every day
  (7) feelings of worthlessness or excessive or inappropriate guilt (which may be delusional) nearly every day (not merely self-reproach or guilt about being sick)
  (8) diminished ability to think or concentrate, or indecisiveness, nearly every day (either by subjective account or as observed by others)
  (9) recurrent thoughts of death (not just fear of dying), recurrent suicidal ideation without a specific plan, or a suicide attempt or a specific plan for committing suicide

B. The symptoms do not meet criteria for a Mixed Episode.

C. The symptoms cause clinically significant distress or impairment in social, occupational, or other important areas of functioning.

D. The symptoms are not due to the direct physiological effects of a substance (e.g., a drug of abuse, a medication) or a general medical condition (e.g., hypothyroidism).

E. The symptoms are not better accounted for by Bereavement, i.e., after the loss of a loved one, the symptoms persist for longer than 2 months or are characterized by marked functional impairment, morbid preoccupation with worthlessness, suicidal ideation, psychotic symptoms, or psychomotor retardation.

Note. Reprinted by permission from the *Diagnostic and Statistical Manual of Mental Disorders*, Fourth Edition. Copyright 1994 American Psychiatric Association.

often experienced by patients with chronic pain are frequently attributed to pain rather than depression. However, since they are not direct physiological effects of pain, these symptoms should count toward a diagnosis of depression. In fact, studies of depression in medically ill populations have generally found greater sensitivity and reliability with "inclusive models" of depression diagnosis that accept all symptoms as relevant to the diagnosis than with models that try to identify the cause of each symptom (Koenig, George, Peterson, & Pieper, 1997).

Patients with chronic pain will often dismiss a depression diagnosis, stating that their depression is a "direct reaction" to their pain problem. Psychiatry has long debated the value of distinguishing a "reactive" form of depression caused by adverse life events and an endogenous form of depression caused by biological and genetic factors (Frank, Anderson, Reynolds, Ritenour, & Kupfer, 1994). Life events are important in many depressive episodes, though they play a less important role in recurrent and very severe or melancholic or psychotic depressions (Brown, Harris, & Hepworth, 1994). Currently, the only life event that will exclude a person from a depression diagnosis who otherwise qualifies for one is bereavement. Determining whether a depression is a "reasonable response" to life's stress may be very important to patients seeking to decrease the stigma of a depression diagnosis and has been of interest to pain investigators. It is not, however, important in deciding that treatment is necessary and appropriate. Indeed, there is no clarity in assessment to be gained from debating whether the depression caused the pain or the pain caused the depression. If patients meet the criteria outlined in Table 15.1, it is likely that they can benefit from appropriate treatment.

When one is considering the diagnosis of depression in a patient with chronic pain, important alternatives include bipolar disorder, substance-induced mood disorder, and dysthymic disorder. Patients with bipolar disorder have extended periods of abnormally elevated as well as abnormally depressed mood. These periods of elevated mood need to last more than one continuous day and include features such as inflated self-esteem, decreased need for sleep, and racing thoughts. A history of manic or hypomanic episodes predicts an atypical response to antidepressant medication and increases the risk of antidepressant-induced mania. Substance-induced mood disorders can also occur in those with pain. Patients with chronic pain may be taking medications such as steroids, dopamine-blocking agents (including antiemetics), or sedatives (including "muscle relaxants") that produce a depressive syndrome. Patients' current medication lists should be scrutinized before additional medications are prescribed. One patient with pain and other neurological symptoms after pancreas transplant, whom I placed on sertraline for probable depression, had a full remission of all depressive symptoms after a consultant neurologist discontinued his metoclopramide.

Dysthymic Disorder

Dysthymic disorder is a chronic form of depression lasting 2 years or longer. Individuals with dysthymia are at high risk of developing major depression as well. This combined syndrome has often been called *double depression* (Keller, Hirschfeld, & Hanks, 1997). It is important to note dysthymia because it is frequently invisible in medical settings, often being dismissed as "just the way that patient is." Dysthymia has been shown to respond to many antidepressants, including the selective serotonin reuptake inhibitors (Thase et al., 1996). Treatment of double depression can be particularly challenging due to treatment resistance and concurrent personality disorders (Rush & Thase, 1997). Psychiatric consultation may be useful when dysthymia or double depression is suspected.

Relationships between Depressive Disorders and Chronic Pain

Prevalence rates of depression among patients in pain clinics have varied widely, depending on the method of assessment and the population assessed. Rates as low as 10% and as high as 100% have been reported (Romano & Turner, 1985). The reason for the wide variability may be attributable to a number of factors, including the methods used to diagnose depression (e.g., interview, self-report instruments), the criteria used (e.g., DSM-IV, cutoff scores on self-report instruments), the set of disorders included in the diagnosis of depression (e.g., presence of depressive symptoms, major depression), and referral bias (e.g., higher reported prevalence of depression in studies conducted in psychiatry clinics compared to rehabilitation clinics). The majority of studies report depression in over 50% of patients with chronic pain sampled (Fishbain, Goldberg, Meagher, Steele, & Rosomoff,

1986). However, these studies are typically done in pain clinic settings and may be overestimates of the rates of depression in unselected patients with chronic pain.

Studies of primary care populations (where generalization is less problematic) have revealed a number of factors that appear to increase the likelihood of depression in patients with chronic pain. Dworkin, Von Korff, and LaResche (1990) reported that patients with two or more pain complaints were much more likely to be depressed than those with a single pain complaint. Number of pain conditions reported was a better predictor of major depression than was pain severity or pain persistence (Dworkin et al., 1990). Von Korff, Ormel, Keefe, and Dworkin (1992) developed a four-level scale for grading chronic pain severity based on pain disability and pain intensity: (1) low disability and low intensity, (2) low disability and high intensity, (3) high disability–moderately limiting, and (4) high disability–severely limiting. Depression, use of opioid analgesics, and doctor visits all increased as chronic pain grade increased. When dysfunctional primary care patients with back pain are followed for a year, those whose back pain improves also show improvement of depressive symptoms to normal levels (Von Korff, Deyo, Cherkin, & Barlow, 1993).

These epidemiological studies provide solid evidence for a strong association between chronic pain and depression, but do not address whether chronic pain causes depression or depression causes chronic pain. As indicated above, this question has more importance in medicolegal contexts than in clinical contexts. But since it is a perennial question, some attempt to answer it should be made. Prospective studies of patients with chronic musculoskeletal pain have suggested that chronic pain can cause depression (Atkinson et al., 1991), that depression can cause chronic pain (Magni, Moreschi, Rigatti-Luchini, & Merskey, 1994), and that they exist in a mutually reinforcing relationship (Rudy, Kerns, & Turk, 1988).

One fact often raised to support the idea that pain causes depression is that a patient's current depressive episode often began after the onset of the pain problem. The majority of studies appear to support this contention (Brown, 1990). However, it has been documented that many patients with chronic pain (especially those disabled patients seen in pain clinics) have often had past episodes of depression that predated their pain problem by years (Katon, Egan, & Miller, 1985). This has led some investigators to propose that there may exist

a common trait of susceptibility to dysphoric physical symptoms (including pain) and to negative psychological symptoms (including anxiety as well as depression). They conclude that "pain and psychological illness should be viewed as having reciprocal psychological and behavioral effects involving both processes of illness expression and adaptation" (Von Korff & Simon, 1996, p. 107).

Patients with chronic pain often feel they are battling to have their suffering recognized as real. They will resist a depression diagnosis if they see it as a way of dismissing their suffering. Even if clinicians are sensitive to these issues, they must recognize that legal proceedings, insurance companies, and workers' compensation boards can look on a depression diagnosis with prejudice. Traditional and industrial societies appear to hold individuals less responsible for somatic symptoms than for psychological symptoms. This difference may be especially prominent in modern Western biomedicine, where symptom complexes are validated or invalidated through their correspondence with objective disease criteria (Fabrega, 1990). A somatic "idiom of distress" therefore becomes the favored means of communication for communicating distress of any origin that is overwhelming or disabling (Good, 1992). Pain is a more acceptable reason for disability than depression is in many cultures. Therefore, cultural incentives exist for translation of depression into pain. Since depressed patients have many physical symptoms, these can become the focus of clinical communication and concern. Giving patients with chronic pain permission to talk of distress in the clinical setting using nonsomatic terms can facilitate treatment, as long as they do not feel that somatic elements of their problem are not being neglected or discounted. I try to validate depression an understandable response to a chronic pain problem. This can often be accomplished with a statement such as "It is easy to see how you might become depressed with all the pain you have been having."

ANXIETY DISORDERS

It is not unusual for patients with symptoms of pain to be anxious and worried. Anxiety and concern about symptoms, however, are not synonymous with a psychiatric diagnosis of an anxiety disorder. When patients with chronic pain do suffer from an anxiety disorder, it is rare that this is their sole psychiatric diagnosis. Most pain patients with chronic anxiety (i.e., generalized anxiety disorder) will also meet criteria for either major depression or dysthymia. In these cases, treatment should be directed toward the mood disorder. With successful treatment of the mood disorder, the anxiety should be relieved as well. Benzodiazepines should almost always be avoided, because they are associated with tolerance, dependence, and withdrawal. Prolonged use may promote inactivity and cognitive impairment.

Panic Disorder

Panic disorder is a common, disabling psychiatric illness associated with high medical service utilization and multiple medically unexplained symptoms. In the pain clinic setting, panic disorder should be considered especially in patients with chest pain, abdominal pain, or headaches. The diagnosis of panic disorder requires recurrent, unexpected panic attacks (see Table 15.2), followed by at least a month of worry about having another panic attack, about the implications or consequences of the panic attacks, or behavioral changes related to the attacks. These attacks should not be the direct physiological consequence of a substance or other medical condition. The panic attacks

---

TABLE 15.2. DSM-IV Criteria for Panic Attack

Note: A Panic Attack is not a codable disorder. Code the specific diagnosis in which the Panic Attack occurs (e.g., 300.21 Panic Disorder With Agoraphobia).

A discrete period of intense fear or discomfort, in which four (or more) of the following symptoms developed abruptly and reached a peak within 10 minutes:

(1) palpitations, pounding heart, or accelerated heart rate
(2) sweating
(3) trembling or shaking
(4) sensations of shortness of breath or smothering
(5) feeling of choking
(6) chest pain or discomfort
(7) nausea or abdominal distress
(8) feeling dizzy, unsteady, lightheaded, or faint
(9) depersonalization (feelings of unreality) or depersonalization (being detached from oneself)
(10) fear of losing control or going crazy
(11) fear of dying
(12) paresthesias (numbness or tingling sensations)
(13) chills or hot flushes

Note. Reprinted with permission from the *Diagnostic and Statistical Manual of Mental Disorders,* Fourth Edition. Copyright 1994 American Psychiatric Association.

---

should not be better accounted for by another mental disorder such as PTSD (described below) or OCD. At least two unexpected attacks are required for the diagnosis, though most patients have more.

One of the most common problems with panic disorder is fears of undiagnosed, life-threatening illness. Patients with panic disorder can receive extensive medical testing and treatment for their somatic symptoms before the diagnosis of panic disorder is made and appropriate treatment initiated.

Lifetime prevalence of panic disorder throughout the world is estimated to be 1.5% to 3.5%. One-year prevalence rates range from 1% to 2%. Panic disorder is two to three times more common in women than in men. Age of onset is variable, but most typically occurs between late adolescence and the mid-30s. Of all common mental disorders in the primary care setting, panic disorder is most likely to produce moderate to severe occupational dysfunction and physical disability (Ormel et al., 1994). It is also associated with the greatest number of disability days in the past month.

The most common complication of panic disorder is agoraphobia, or fear of public places. Patients with panic disorder learn to fear places where escape might be difficult or help not available in case they have an attack. One-half to two-thirds of patients with panic disorder also suffer from major depression. These patients are the most disabled patients with panic disorder. The differential diagnosis of patients presenting with panic symptoms in the medical setting includes thyroid, parathyroid, adrenal, and vestibular dysfunction; seizure disorders; cardiac arrhythmias; and drug intoxication or withdrawal. Patients with panic disorder typically present in the medical setting with cardiological, gastrointestinal, or neurological complaints (Zaubler & Katon, 1996).

Chest pain is one of the most common complaints presented to primary care physicians, but a specific medical etiology is identified in only 10%–20% of cases. From 43% to 61% of patients who have normal coronary arteries at angiography, and 16%–25% of patients presenting to emergency rooms with chest pain, have panic disorder. A number of these patients will eventually receive the diagnoses of vasospastic angina, costochondritis, esophageal dysmotility, or mitral valve prolapse. High rates of psychiatric disorders have been found in some of these groups as well (Carney, Freedland, Ludbrook, Saunders, & Jaffe, 1990). Many of these patients remain symptomatic and disabled 1 year later, despite reassurance concerning coronary artery disease (Beitman et al., 1991).

Approximately 11% of primary care patients will present the problem of abdominal pain to their physician each year. Fewer than a quarter of these complaints will be associated with a definite physical diagnosis in the following year. Among the most common reasons for abdominal pain is irritable bowel syndrome (IBS). It is estimated that IBS accounts for 20%–52% of all referrals to gastroenterologists. Various studies have found that 54%–74% of these patients with IBS have associated psychiatric disorders. One study determined that patients with IBS had much higher current (28% vs 3%) and lifetime (41% vs. 25%) rates of panic disorder than a comparison group with inflammatory bowel disease (Walker, Gelfand, Gelfand, & Katon, 1995). This suggests that the psychiatric disorder was not simply a reaction to the abdominal distress.

Among 10,000 persons assessed in a community survey who consulted their physicians for headache, 15% of females and 13% of males had a history of panic disorder. Further studies have suggested that migraine headache is the type of headache most strongly associated with panic attacks (Stewart, Breslau, & Keck, 1994). Often anxiety symptoms precede the onset of the headaches, while depressive symptoms often have their onset after the headaches. Some authors have suggested that a common predisposition exists to headaches (especially migraines and chronic daily headache), anxiety disorders, and major depression.

Posttraumatic Stress Disorder

Following direct personal exposure to an extreme psychologically traumatic event, some individuals develop PTSD—a syndrome that includes reexperiencing the event, avoidance of stimuli associated with the event, and persistent heightened arousal. PTSD was originally described following exposure to military combat, but is now recognized to occur following sexual or physical assault, natural disasters, accidents, life-threatening illnesses, and other events that induce feelings of intense fear, hopelessness, or horror. Persons may develop the disorder after experiencing or just witnessing these events. DSM-IV diagnostic criteria for PTSD are provided in Table 15.3. A short screening scale for DSM-IV PTSD has recently been validated (Breslau, Peterson, Kessler, & Schultz, 1999).

Up to 80% of Vietnam veterans with PTSD report chronic pain in limbs, back, torso, or head (Beckham et al., 1997). Increased physical symp-

TABLE 15.3. DSM-IV Diagnostic Criteria for Posttraumatic Stress Disorder (PTSD)

A. The person has been exposed to a traumatic event in which both of the following were present:

  (1) the person experienced, witnessed, or was confronted with an event or events that involved actual or threatened death or serious injury, or a threat to the physical integrity of self or others
  (2) the person's response involved intense fear, helplessness, or horror. Note: In children, this may be expressed instead by disorganized or agitated behavior.

B. The traumatic event is persistently reexperienced in one (or more) of the following ways:

  (1) recurrent and intrusive distressing recollections of the event, including images, thoughts, or perceptions. Note: In young children, repetitive play may occur in which themes or aspects of the trauma are expressed.
  (2) recurrent distressing dreams of the event. Note: In children, there may be frightening dreams without recognizable content.
  (3) acting or feeling as if the traumatic event were recurring (includes a sense of reliving the experience, illusions, hallucinations, and dissociative flashback episodes, including those that occur on awakening or when intoxicated). Note: In young children, trauma-specific reenactment may occur.
  (4) intense psychological distress at exposure to internal or external cues that symbolize or resemble an aspect of the traumatic event
  (5) physiological reactivity on exposure to internal or external cues that symbolize or resemble an aspect of the traumatic event

C. Persistent avoidance of stimuli associated with the trauma and numbing of general responsiveness (not present before the trauma), as indicated by three (or more) of the following:

  (1) efforts to avoid thoughts, feelings, or conversations associated with the trauma
  (2) efforts to avoid activities, places, or people that arouse recollections of the trauma
  (3) inability to recall an important aspect of the trauma
  (4) markedly diminished interest or participation in significant activities
  (5) feeling of detachment or estrangement from others
  (6) restricted range of affect (e.g., unable to have loving feelings)
  (7) sense of foreshortened future (e.g., does not expect to have a career, marriage, children, or a normal life span)

(cont.)

TABLE 15.3. (cont.)

D. Persistent symptoms of increased arousal (not present before the trauma), as indicated by two (or more) of the following:

   (1) difficulty falling or staying asleep
   (2) irritability or outbursts of anger
   (3) difficulty concentrating
   (4) hypervigilance
   (5) exaggerated startle response

E. Duration of the disturbance (symptoms in Criteria B, C, and D) is more than 1 month.

F. The disturbance causes clinically significant distress or impairment in social, occupational, or other important areas of functioning.

Specify if:
   Acute: if duration of symptoms is less than 3 months
   Chronic: if duration of symptoms is 3 months or more

Specify if:
   With Delayed Onset: if onset of symptoms is at least 6 months after the stressor

Note. Reprinted by permission from the *Diagnostic and Statistical Manual of Mental Disorders*, Fourth Edition. Copyright 1994 American Psychiatric Association.

toms, including muscle aches and back pain, are also more common in Gulf War veterans with PTSD than in those without PTSD (Baker, Mendenhall, Simbartl, Magan, & Steinberg, 1997). The prevalence of PTSD in medical populations has been shown to be quite high. Averaging the prevalence rates of PTSD across a number of studies reveals that after motor vehicle accidents causing sufficient injury to require medical attention, 29.5% of patients meet the criteria for PTSD; for over one-half of these patients, the symptoms resolve within 6 months (Blanchard & Hickling, 1997). In one study, 15% of patients with idiopathic facial pain seeking treatment were found to have PTSD (Aghabeigi, Feinmann, & Harris, 1992). In another study, 21% of patients with fibromyalgia were found to have PTSD (Amir et al., 1997). Case reports have associated reflex sympathetic dystrophy (RSD), also known as complex regional pain syndrome (CRPS), with PTSD. Other studies suggest that 50% to 100% of patients presenting at pain treatment centers meet the diagnostic criteria for PTSD (Kulich, Mencher, Bertrand, & Maciewicz, 2000). Pain patients with

PTSD have been shown to have more pain and affective distress than those without PTSD (Geisser, Roth, Bachman, & Eckert, 1996), so it is not surprising that PTSD rates among patients with pain increase as one moves into more specialized treatment settings.

The relationship between pain and PTSD is multifaceted. Pain and PTSD may both result from a traumatic event. Sometimes acute pain can constitute the traumatic event, as described in a case of traumatic eye enucleation (Schreiber & Galai-Gat, 1993). PTSD also appears to permit induction of an opioid-mediated stress-induced analgesia. PTSD-related stimuli can result in a naloxone-reversible decreased sensitivity to noxious stimuli in affected individuals (Pitman, van der Kolk, Orr, & Greenberg, 1990). I often screen for PTSD with a question such as this: "Have you ever been through some severe trauma, such as an assault or a rape, about which you still have nightmares or flashbacks?" It is probably even more important to assess whether the trauma that gave rise to the chronic pain problem has also produced PTSD. Questions such as "Do you still have nightmares or flashbacks about your accident?" or "Do you avoid anything that might remind you of your accident?" will help a clinician determine whether accident-related PTSD needs to be pursued further.

The relation between childhood maltreatment and chronic pain has received a lot of attention in recent years. Multiple studies have demonstrated higher rates of childhood maltreatment in patients with chronic pain than in comparison groups. They have also shown poorer coping among abused patients with pain (Spertus, Burns, Glenn, Lofland, & McCracken, 1999). However, the relationship between childhood psychological trauma and adult somatic symptoms is complex and multifaceted (Walker, Unützer, & Katon, 1998). PTSD, dissociation, somatization, and affect dysregulation represent a spectrum of adaptations to trauma. They may occur together or separately (van der Kolk et al., 1996). The best way to incorporate information about childhood maltreatment into the treatment of the adult patient with chronic pain is as yet unclear. At minimum, it signals caregivers that establishing a therapeutic alliance may be difficult. It may also signal that the "here-and-now" focus of the cognitive-behavioral therapy frequently used for patients with pain will not be adequate. But chronic pain treatment trials have not yet grouped patients by trauma history or attempted treatment matching by trauma history.

SUBSTANCE ABUSE AND DEPENDENCE

Diagnosis

Diagnosis of substance abuse and dependence in patients with chronic pain is controversial, because it is difficult to achieve consensus on what constitutes a *maladaptive* pattern of substance use. DSM-IV distinguishes between substance dependence and substance abuse. The essential feature of substance dependence is continued use of a substance despite a cluster of cognitive, behavioral, and physiological problems. It is characterized by tolerance, withdrawal, and compulsive drug-taking behavior. DSM-IV criteria for substance dependence are presented in Table 15.4.

The essential feature of DSM-IV substance abuse is a maladaptive pattern of substance use characterized by recurrent and significant adverse consequences. These include impaired role function, use in physically hazardous situations, and legal problems. It is distinguished from DSM-IV substance dependence in that it does not require tolerance, dependence, or a compulsive pattern of use.

Opioid Use and Other Issues

Traditionally, opioids have been considered appropriate for terminal cancer pain, where tolerance, dependence, and dose escalation are limited in their importance by the impending death of the patients.

TABLE 15.4. DSM-IV Criteria for Substance Dependence

A maladaptive pattern of substance use, leading to clinically significant impairment or distress, as manifested by three (or more) of the following, occurring at any time in the same 12-month period:

(1) tolerance, as defined by either of the following:

    (a) a need for markedly increased amounts of the substance to achieve intoxication or desired effect
    (b) markedly diminished effect with continued use of the same amount of the substance

(2) withdrawal, as manifested by either of the following:

    (a) the characteristic withdrawal syndrome for the substance (refer to Criteria A and B of the criteria sets for Withdrawal from the specific substances)
    (b) the same (or a closely related) substance is taken to relieve or avoid withdrawal symptoms

(3) the substance is often taken in larger amounts or over a longer period than was intended
(4) there is a persistent desire or unsuccessful efforts to cut down or control substance use
(5) a great deal of time is spent in activities necessary to obtain the substance (e.g., visiting multiple doctors or driving long distances), use the substance (e.g., chain-smoking), or recover from its effects
(6) important social, occupational, or recreational activities are given up or reduced because of substance use
(7) the substance use is continued despite knowledge of having a persistent or recurrent physical or psychological problem that is likely to have been caused or exacerbated by the substance (e.g., current cocaine use despite recognition of cocaine-induced depression, or continued drinking despite recognition that an ulcer was made worse by alcohol consumption)

Specify if:
With Physiological Dependence: evidence of tolerance or withdrawal (i.e., either Item 1 or 2 is present)
Without Physiological Dependence: no evidence of tolerance or withdrawal (i.e., neither Item 1 nor 2 is present)

Course specifiers (see [DSM-IV] text for definitions):
    Early Full Remission
    Early Partial Remission
    Sustained Full Remission
    Sustained Partial Remission
    On Agonist Therapy
    In a Controlled Environment

Note. Reprinted by permission from the *Diagnostic and Statistical Manual of Mental Disorders*, Fourth Edition. Copyright 1994 American Psychiatric Association.

But they have been considered problematic for patients with chronic noncancer pain, where long-term function is an essential issue. A large percentage of patients referred to multidisciplinary pain centers report taking opioids at the time of assessment. Following treatment, the majority of these patients report significantly reduced pain concurrent with elimination of opioid medication (Turk & Okifuji, 1997).

Portenoy (1990) and others have argued forcefully that chronic opioid therapy can be appropriate and beneficial in *some* patients with chronic noncancer pain. One of the current unanswered questions is what factors characterize those patients who are likely to benefit from long-term opioids without problems of addiction, tolerance, or increased disability. To date, there have been no long-term, double-blind studies that help to select the group for whom long-term opioids are beneficial.

Prevalence rates for substance abuse and dependence in patients with chronic pain are variable, due to differences in definitions used and populations assessed. Studies completed to date suggest that substance abuse and dependence occur in a minority of patients with chronic pain on opioids. They do not answer the more difficult question as to whether opioids are, on balance, beneficial treatment for these patients. Future studies involving random assignment of patients with chronic pain to opioid treatment will be necessary to answer the question of what patients, with what characteristics, are able to obtain benefits (pain reduction and improvement of function) from long-term opioids without developing deleterious effects. One useful question to ask to screen for potential substance abuse or dependence is "Do you ever save pain medication to give yourself a 'mental break' at some point during the week?"

Since small amounts of alcohol use can retard response to antidepressant medication, it is important to inquire about alcohol use that may not otherwise meet criteria for abuse or dependence in patients who are candidates for antidepressant medication. I seek zero alcohol use in patients I place on antidepressant medication. Significant others and other third parties are indispensable sources of information about substance abuse or dependence. We routinely include a significant other in the initial evaluation of new patients disabled by chronic pain. I am also quite liberal in my use of urine toxicology screens in any patients with histories of substance abuse or dependence, or with possible current substance use disorders. Often this is the only way to be sure about the cause

of a patient's altered mental status, such as affective lability, cognitive impairment, and treatment nonresponse. Unfortunately, toxicology screens detect highly lipid soluble compounds (such as tetrahydrocannabinol from marijuana) for a much longer time than other compounds (such as cocaine) that are more critical to treatment planning.

SOMATOFORM DISORDERS

Current psychiatric theory dictates diagnoses of somatoform disorders rather than "abnormal illness behavior" or "misuse of the sick role." The essential feature of the somatoform disorders is the presence of physical symptoms that suggest a general medical condition but are not fully explained by a general medical condition. These symptoms must cause impairment in social and occupational functioning. The somatoform disorders are distinguished from factitious disorders and malingering in that the symptoms are not intentionally produced or feigned. The most valuable diagnosis among the somatoform disorders, in my experience, is somatization disorder.

Somatization Disorders

Somatization disorder is a chronic condition characterized by a pattern of multiple and recurrent somatic complaints resulting in medical treatment and impairment in role functioning but not explained by a general medical condition. For this particular somatoform diagnosis, the somatic symptoms must be persistent and pervasive. These complaints must begin before 30 years of age and last for a period of years. Diagnostic criteria for somatization disorder are displayed in Table 15.5.

Somatization disorder must be distinguished from medical disorders producing multiple and scattered symptoms, such as multiple sclerosis or systemic lupus erythematosis. It must also be distinguished from panic disorder. This also produces multiple somatic symptoms, but is a more acute and treatable psychiatric disorder. Panic disorder is an acute, episodic disorder; it does not lead to lifelong symptoms or health care utilization. It also generally has an abrupt onset, unlike somatization disorder, which has a chronic, indolent course.

The prevalence of somatization disorder in the community has been reported to be between 0.13% and 0.4%, with the vast majority of cases being women (Smith, 1991). Prevalence estimates in the

TABLE 15.5. DSM-IV Diagnostic Criteria for Somatization Disorder

A. A history of many physical complaints beginning before age 30 years that occur over a period of several years and result in treatment of being sought or significant impairment in social, occupational, or other important areas of functioning.

B. Each of the following criteria must have been met, with individual symptoms occurring at any time during the course of the disturbance:

   (1) *four pain symptoms:* a history of pain related to at least four different sites or functions (e.g., head, abdomen, back, joints, extremities, chest, rectum, during menstruation, during sexual intercourse, or during urination)

   (2) *two gastrointestinal symptoms:* a history of at least two gastrointestinal symptoms other than pain (e.g., nausea, bloating, vomiting other than during pregnancy, diarrhea, or intolerance of several different foods)

   (3) *one sexual symptom:* a history of at least one sexual or reproductive symptom other than pain (e.g., sexual indifference, erectile or ejaculatory dysfunction, irregular menses, excessive menstrual bleeding, vomiting throughout pregnancy)

   (4) *one pseudoneurological symptom:* a history of at least one symptom or deficit suggesting a neurological condition not limited to pain (conversion symptoms such as impaired coordination or balance, paralysis or localized weakness, difficulty swallowing or lump in throat, aphonia, urinary retention, hallucinations, loss of touch or pain sensation, double vision, blindness, deafness, seizures; dissociative symptoms such as amnesia; or loss of consciousness other than fainting)

C. Either (1) or (2):

   (1) after appropriate investigation, each of the symptoms in Criterion B cannot be fully explained by a known general medical condition or the direct effects of a substance (e.g., a drug of abuse, or medication)

   (2) when there is a related general medical condition, the physical complaints or resulting social or occupational impairment are in excess of what would be expected from the history, physical examination, or laboratory findings

D. The symptoms are not intentionally produced or feigned (as in Factitious Disorder or Malingering).

Note. Reprinted by permission from the *Diagnostic and Statistical Manual of Mental Disorders*, Fourth Edition. Copyright 1994 American Psychiatric Association.

primary care setting have ranged from 0.2% to 5%. Studies of patients referred to pain clinics have produced estimates from 8% to 12% (Kouyanou, Pither, Rebe-Hesketh, & Wessely, 1998). Although prevalence rates clearly increase from community to primary care to tertiary care settings, patients with somatization disorder remain in the clear minority in all settings, including pain clinics.

Unexplained somatic symptoms are common problems in medical settings that extend far beyond the bounds of somatization disorder. Various attempts have been made to assess the prevalence of an abridged version of somatization disorder in primary care, requiring four to six unexplained symptoms (4.4% of patients) or three symptoms persistent over a 2-year period (8.2% of patients) (Kroenke et al., 1997). Even these abridged forms of somatization disorder are associated with increased rates of disability, health care utilization, and mood and anxiety disorders.

Although the initial emphasis with somatization disorder was on a discrete familial, even genetic, disorder, recent evidence suggests that somatization is a process that exists along a spectrum of severity (Liu, Clark, & Easton, 1997). A recent large international study confirms that medically unexplained somatic symptoms are very common, whereas full-fledged somatization disorder is quite rare (Gureje, Simon, Ustun, & Goldberg, 1997). A great deal of confusion exits between somatization as a *process* and somatization as a *disorder*. Somatization as a *process*, meaning the somatic experience of distress, is ubiquitous (Sullivan & Katon, 1993). It accounts for the majority of symptoms presented to primary care physicians. It is most frequently associated with transient stressors (and is therefore time limited) or acute psychiatric disorders (which are very treatable). Somatization *disorder* is a rare, chronic, and treatment-resistant condition that characterizes the most severely and chronically distressed individuals. When clinicians use the term *somatizer* to refer to a patient with unexplained symptoms, it is unclear whether they are implying the process or the disorder. The primary value in diagnosing somatization disorder in the pain clinic setting is that it identifies a treatment-resistant group. This is the only group in which I have seen the "symptom substitution" in response to cognitive-behavioral pain treatment that has been predicted by psychodynamic theorists. Full rehabilitation of patients with somatization disorder is extremely difficult. Often treatment must focus on preventing iatrogenic injury (Kouyanou, Pither, & Wessely, 1997)

Although somatization disorder frequently occurs within families and may have a genetic component, it also appears to have a strong association with childhood physical and sexual abuse (Pribor, Yutzy, Dean, & Wetzel, 1993). A significant percentage of patients who meet criteria for somatization disorder also meet criteria for borderline personality disorder (Hudziak et al., 1996). This has led some investigators to question the independence of these diagnoses and others, and to stress their common origin in severe childhood abuse. Borderline personality disorder is a severe, chronic pattern of chaotic and dysfunctional interpersonal relationships. Patients with these disorders are characterized by pervasive distress and distrust and by recurrent despair. Diagnostic criteria for borderline personality disorder are presented in Table 15.6.

TABLE 15.6. DSM-IV Diagnostic Criteria for Borderline Personality Disorder

A pervasive pattern of instability of interpersonal relationships, self-image, and affects, and marked impulsivity beginning by early adulthood and present in a variety of contexts, as indicated by five (or more) of the following:

(1) frantic efforts to avoid real or imagined abandonment. **Note:** Do not include suicidal or self-mutilating behavior covered in Criterion 5.
(2) a pattern of unstable and intense interpersonal relationships characterized by alternating between extremes of idealization and devaluation
(3) identity disturbance: markedly and persistently unstable self-image or sense of self
(4) impulsivity in at least two areas that are potentially self-damaging (e.g., spending, sex, substance abuse, reckless driving, binge eating). **Note:** Do not include suicidal or self-mutilating behavior covered in Criterion 5.
(5) recurrent suicidal behavior, gestures, or threats, or self-mutilating behavior
(6) affective instability due to a marked reactivity of mood (e.g., intense episodic dysphoria, irritability, or anxiety usually lasting a few hours and only rarely more than a few days)
(7) chronic feelings of emptiness
(8) inappropriate, intense anger or difficulty controlling anger (e.g., frequent displays of temper, constant anger, recurrent physical fights)
(9) transient, stress-related paranoid ideation or severe dissociative symptoms

Note. Reprinted by permission from the *Diagnostic and Statistical Manual of Mental Disorders*, Fourth Edition. Copyright 1994 American Psychiatric Association.

In a recent study of 200 patients with back pain attending a pain clinic, 51% of patients had some personality disorder and 15% had borderline personality disorder by structured psychiatric interview (Polatin, Kinney, Gatchel, Lillo, & Mayer, 1993). This is a strikingly high prevalence of these disorders compared to other clinical populations. Patients with borderline personality disorder are often considered difficult by their primary care physicians and may be referred more frequently to pain clinics. There is some controversy about the validity of these diagnoses, especially as to whether they constitute a cause or an effect of the chronic pain problem (Weisberg & Keefe, 1997).

Pain Disorder

In many common pain syndromes (e.g., low back pain, headache, fibromyalgia), it is difficult to identify the tissue pathology giving rise to symptoms. When a somatic cause for pain cannot be identified, many clinicians begin to seek psychological causes. The identification of *psychogenic pain* is a difficult, and perhaps impossible, task. Pain disorder is the current psychiatric diagnosis that most closely corresponds to the concept of psychogenic pain.

Since *pain disorder* is an important but problematic concept at the interface of pain medicine and psychiatry, it is important to understand some of the history of the concept. In DSM-II (published in 1968), there was no specific diagnosis pertaining to pain. Painful conditions caused by emotional factors were considered part of the "psychophysiological disorders." DSM-III introduced a new diagnostic category for pain problems, *psychogenic pain disorder* (American Psychiatric Association, 1980). To qualify for this diagnosis, a patient needed to have severe and prolonged pain inconsistent with neuroanatomical distribution of pain receptors or without detectable organic etiology or pathophysiological mechanism. Related organic pathology was allowed, but the pain had to be "grossly in excess" of what was expected on the basis of physical exam. Accepted evidence that psychological factors were involved in the production of the pain were (1) a temporal relationship between pain onset and an environmental event producing psychological conflict; (2) the pain's appearing to allow avoidance of some noxious event or responsibility; and/or (3) the pain's promoting emotional support or attention that the individual would not have otherwise received. It is important to note that this kind of evidence never *proves* that psychological factors have caused a pain complaint.

Difficulties in establishing that pain was psychogenic led to changes in the diagnosis for DSM-III-R (American Psychiatric Association, 1987; see Stoudemire & Sandu, 1987). In DSM-III-R, the diagnosis was renamed *somatoform pain disorder*, and three major changes were made in the diagnostic criteria. The requirements for etiological psychological factors and lack of other contributing mental disorders were eliminated, and a requirement for "preoccupation with pain for at least six months" was added. The diagnostic criteria were thus reduced to the following:

(1) Preoccupation with pain for at least six months
(2) Either a or b:
    (a) appropriate evaluation uncovers no organic pathology or pathophysiologic mechanism to account for the pain
    (b) when there is related organic pathology, the complaint of pain or resulting social or occupational impairment is grossly in excess of what would be expected from the findings (American Psychiatric Association, 1987, p. 266)

In DSM-III-R, therefore, somatoform pain disorder became purely a diagnosis of exclusion. The diagnosis was made when medical disorders were excluded in a patient "preoccupied" with pain.

The members of the DSM-IV subcommittee on pain disorder found that despite these changes, somatoform pain disorder was rarely used in research projects or clinical practice. They identified a number of reasons for this: (1) The meaning of "preoccupation with pain" was unclear; (2) whether pain exceeded that expected was difficult to determine; (3) the diagnosis did not apply to many patients disabled by pain where a medical condition was contributory; (4) the term *somatoform pain disorder* implied that this pain was somehow different from organic pain; and (5) acute pain of less than 6 months' duration was excluded (King & Strain, 1992). They therefore proposed the DSM-IV category of pain disorder, described in Table 15.7.

The DSM-IV subcommittee tried to devise a broader diagnostic grouping encompassing both acute and chronic pain problems. They wanted to have all the factors relevant to the onset or maintenance of the pain delineated, *and* also to have a diagnostic category that would not require more training than the majority of DSM-IV users would be expected to have. These two requirements may

TABLE 15.7. DSM-IV Diagnostic Criteria for Pain Disorder

A. Pain in one or more anatomical sites is the predominant focus of the clinical presentation and is of sufficient severity to warrant clinical attention.

B. The pain causes clinically significant distress or impairment in social, occupational, or other important areas of functioning.

C. Psychological factors are judged to have an important role in the onset, severity, exacerbation, or maintenance of the pain.

D. The symptom of deficit is not intentionally produced or feigned (as in Factitious Disorder or Malingering).

E. The pain is not better accounted for by a Mood, Anxiety, or Psychotic Disorder and does not meet criteria for Dyspareunia.

Code as follows:
307.80 Pain Disorder Associated with Psychological Factors: psychological factors are judged to have the major role in the onset, severity, exacerbation, or maintenance of the pain. (If a general medical condition is present, it does not have a major role in the onset, severity, exacerbation, or maintenance of the pain.) This type of Pain Disorder is not diagnosed if criteria are also met for Somatization Disorder.

Specify if:
  Acute: duration of less than 6 months
  Chronic: duration of 6 months or longer

307.89 Pain Disorder Associated with Both Psychological Factors and a General Medical Condition: both psychological factors and a medical condition are judged to have important roles in the onset, severity, exacerbation, or maintenance of the pain. The associated general medical condition or anatomical site of the pain (see below) is coded on Axis III.

Specify if:
  Acute: duration of less than 6 months
  Chronic: duration of 6 months or longer

Note: The following is not considered to be a mental disorder and is included here to facilitate differential diagnosis.

Pain Disorder Associated with a General Medical Condition: a general medical condition has a major role in the onset, severity, exacerbation, or maintenance of the pain. (If psychological factors are present, they are not judged to have a major role

(*cont.*)

TABLE 15.7. (cont.)

in the onset, severity, exacerbation, or maintenance of the pain.) The diagnostic code for the pain is selected based on the associated general medical condition if one has been established (see Appendix G) or on the anatomical location of the pain if the underlying general medical condition is not yet clearly established—for example, low back (724.2), sciatic (724.3), pelvic (625.9), headache (784.0), facial (784.0), chest (786.50), joint (719.4), bone (733.90), abdominal (789.0), breast (611.71), renal (788.0), ear (388.70), eye (379.91), throat (784.1), tooth (525.9), and urinary (788.0).

Note. Reprinted by permission from the *Diagnostic and Statistical Manual of Mental Disorders*, Fourth Edition. Copyright 1994 American Psychiatric Association.

not be compatible. Furthermore, no guidance is given in determining when psychological factors have a major role in pain or are considered important enough in the presence of a painful medical disorder to be coded as a separate mental disorder. Given the high rates of mood and anxiety disorders among disabled patients with chronic pain, many patients most appropriate for the diagnosis might be excluded. Although depression and anxiety diagnoses point toward specific proven therapies, this is not true for pain disorder. The diagnosis thus continues covertly as a diagnosis of exclusion, with neither clear inclusion criteria nor implications for therapy.

Multiple studies have also demonstrated the association between medically unexplained symptoms (pain and nonpain) and psychiatric disorders. A linear relationship has been demonstrated between the lifetime number of medically unexplained physical symptoms and the lifetime number of depressive and anxiety disorders or the degree of neuroticism or harm avoidance the patient demonstrates on psychological testing (Russo, Katon, Sullivan, Clark, & Buchwald, 1994). Increased psychiatric morbidity has been repeatedly demonstrated for levels of unexplained medical symptoms far below the number required for a DSM diagnosis of somatization disorder (Escobar, Burnham, Karno, Forsythe, & Golding, 1987). This suggests that the somatoform disorders may be less distinct than implied by their separate DSM categories, and that they have a strong kinship with the depressive and anxiety disorders (Aigner & Bach, 1999). It may be more accurate and productive to think of somatization as a process present in varying degrees throughout the

population, rather than as a set of disorders affecting a small subset of the population (Sullivan & Katon, 1993).

Conversion Disorder

The essential feature of conversion disorder is an alteration in voluntary motor or sensory function that suggests a neurological or general medical disorder. Classical examples include hysterical paralysis, blindness, or mutism. Psychological factors must be associated with the initiation or exacerbation of this deficit. Diagnostic criteria for conversion disorder are displayed in Table 15.8.

TABLE 15.8. DSM-IV Diagnostic Criteria for Conversion Disorder

A. One or more symptoms or deficits affecting voluntary motor or sensory function that suggest a neurological or other general medical condition.

B. Psychological factors are judged to be associated with the symptom or deficit because the initiation or exacerbation of the symptom or deficit is preceded by conflicts or other stressors.

C. The symptom or deficit is not intentionally produced or feigned (as in Factitious Disorder or Malingering).

D. The symptom or deficit cannot, after appropriate investigation, be fully explained by a general medical condition, or by the direct effects of a substance, or as a culturally sanctioned behavior or experience.

E. The symptom or deficit causes clinically significant distress or impairment in social, occupational, or other important areas of functioning or warrants medical evaluation.

F. The symptom or deficit is not limited to pain or sexual dysfunction, does not occur exclusively during the course of Somatization Disorder, and is not better accounted for by another mental disorder.

Specify type of symptom or deficit:
  With Motor Symptom or Deficit
  With Sensory Symptom or Deficit
  With Seizures or Convulsions
  With Mixed Presentation

Note. Reprinted by permission from the *Diagnostic and Statistical Manual of Mental Disorders*, Fourth Edition. Copyright 1994 American Psychiatric Association.

Great caution must be exercised in making the diagnosis of conversion disorder, because the presence of relevant psychological factors does not exclude the possibility of a concurrent organically caused condition.

In "Psychogenic Pain and the Pain-Prone Patient," George Engel (1959) proposed that psychogenic pain arose from guilt and an intolerance of success. He indicated that it functioned as a substitute for loss or a replacement for aggression. He furthermore stated that "patients with conversion hysteria constitute the largest percentage of the pain-prone population" (p. 910). Others have also contended that pain is probably the most common conversion symptom encountered clinically (Ziegler, Imboden, & Myer, 1960). However, only case reports exist to support this contention. Pain is not a classic conversion disorder symptom, because it is not a neurological deficit or incapacity. Whether chronic pain can ever qualify as a conversion disorder by itself is controversial. Some, for example, have contended that RSD/CRPS can be understood as a conversion reaction; however, this is also highly controversial (Ochoa & Verdugo, 1995). Some elements of conversion disorders appear to be present in patients with RSD/CRPS (e.g., indifference or neglect toward the affected body part), though it is highly unlikely that the condition is entirely psychogenic.

Rather than labeling some chronic pain problems as conversion reactions and not others, it may be more useful to understand what components of conversion reaction may be present in chronic pain problems. Being ill surely creates problems in living for those affected. Being ill, however, can also solve problems in living. For example, being ill provides an excuse for not being at school or not meeting a deadline at work. These interpersonal advantages of illness were originally recognized by Freud and termed *secondary gain*.

The term *secondary gain* has been distorted and misunderstood in the care of chronic pain, probably due to medicolegal pressures. A number of corrections are in order. First, all illnesses are characterized by some secondary gain, not just illnesses considered to be psychogenic. Being sick *always* has advantages as well as disadvantages. Second, secondary gain includes all potential interpersonal benefits of illness, not just monetary advantages. Many of the advantages of illness are quite subtle and individualized. Third, secondary gain must be understood in the context of *primary gain*, the intrapersonal advantages of illness. For example, focusing on pain rather than depression

may allow patients to avoid self-blame and thereby achieve primary gain. This is a common phenomenon in chronic pain. Indeed, blame avoidance has been hypothesized by some to be one of the main functions of somatization (Bridges, Goldberg, Evan, & Sharpe, 1991). Thus some traditional elements of conversion disorder may be present in many chronic pain problems that do not qualify as conversion disorders per se.

Purely psychogenic or conversion models of chronic pain have some questionable implications for diagnosis and therapy of chronic pain disorders. Interview of the patient with a suspected conversion disorder with the aid of an amytal (sodium amobarbital) infusion has been a standard tool in psychiatric diagnosis (Fackler, Anfinson, & Rand, 1997). It is more common that motor and sensory deficits will resolve under amytal sedation than that pain will. Furthermore, some patients have had violent or suicidal reactions to abrupt resolution of their somatic symptoms under amytal, possibly due to the loss of face-saving primary gain aspects of the illness. Psychodynamic theories of the origin of conversion symptoms imply that psychological treatments alone will be effective. Psychodynamic treatments for chronic pain, however, have little documented success. The most effective psychological treatments, such as cognitive-behavioral therapy, include a reactivation component that will address the profound disuse and deconditioning found in many patients with chronic pain.

CONCLUSION

Psychiatric diagnosis and treatment can add an essential and often neglected component to the conceptualization and treatment of chronic pain problems. However, it is absolutely critical to avoid a dualistic model that postulates that pain is *either* physical or mental in origin. This model alienates patients who feel blamed for their pain; it is also inconsistent with modern models of pain causation. Since the gate control theory of pain was introduced, multiple lines of evidence suggest that pain is a product of efferent as well as afferent activity in the nervous system. Tissue damage and nociception are neither necessary nor sufficient for pain. Indeed, it is now widely recognized that the relationship between pain and nociception is highly complex and must be understood in terms of the situation of the organism as a whole.

We are only beginning to understand the complexities of the relationship between pain and suffering. Pain usually, but not always, produces suffering. Suffering can, through somatization, produce pain. We have traditionally understood this suffering, as we have understood nociception, as arising from a form of pathology intrinsic to the sufferer; hence the traditional view that pain is due to either tissue pathology (nociception) or due to psychopathology (suffering). An alternative model that allows us to escape this dualism is to think of pain as a "transdermal process" with causes outside as well as inside the body. For humans, social pathology can be as painful as tissue pathology. Psychological trauma as well as physical trauma appears to contribute to many chronic pain problems. We can investigate the physiology and the psychology of this "sociogenic" pain without losing sight of its origins in relations *between* people.

Psychological care for patients with chronic pain should occur within the medical treatment setting whenever possible. This is the most effective way to reassure patients that the somatic elements of their problems are not neglected. It also allows integration of somatic and psychological treatments in the most effective manner.

REFERENCES

Aghabeigi, B., Feinmann, C., & Harris, M. (1992). Prevalence of post-traumatic stress disorder in patients with chronic idiopathic facial pain. *British Journal of Oral and Maxillofacial Surgery, 30,* 360–364.

Aigner, M., & Bach, M. (1999). Clinical utility of DSM-IV pain disorder. *Comprehensive Psychiatry, 40,* 353–357.

American Academy of Pain Medicine and American Pain Society. (1997).*The use of opioids for the treatment of chronic pain: A consensus statement of the American Academy of Pain Medicine and the American Pain Society.* Glenview, IL: Authors.

American Psychiatric Association. (1980). *Diagnostic and statistical manual of mental disorders* (3rd ed.). Washington, DC: Author.

American Psychiatric Association. (1987). *Diagnostic and statistical manual of mental disorders* (3rd ed., rev.). Washington, DC: Author.

American Psychiatric Association. (1994). *Diagnostic and statistical manual of mental disorders* (4th ed.). Washington, DC: Author.

Amir, M., Kaplan, Z., Neumann, L., Sharabani, R., Shani, N., & Buskila, D. (1997). Posttraumatic stress disorder, tenderness and fibromyalgia. *Journal of Psychosomatic Research, 42,* 607–613.

Atkinson, J. H., Hampton, J., Slater, M. A., Patterson, T. L., Gant, I., & Garfin, S. R. (1991). Prevalence, onset, and risk of psychiatric disorders in men with chronic low back pain: A controlled study. *Pain, 45,* 111–121.

Baker, D. G., Mendenhall, C. L., Simbartl, L. A., Magan, L. K., & Steinberg, J. L. (1997). Relationship between posttraumatic stress disorder and self-reported physical symptoms in Persian Gulf War veterans. *Archives of Internal Medicine, 157,* 2076–2078.

Beckham, J. C., Crawford, A. L., Feldman, M. E., Kirby, A. C., Hertzberg, M. A., Davidson, J. R., & Moore, S. D. (1997). Chronic posttraumatic stress disorder and chronic pain in Vietnam combat veterans. *Journal of Psychosomatic Research, 43,* 379–389.

Beitman, B. D., Kushner, M. G., Basha, I., Lamberti, J., Mukerji, V., & Bartels, K. (1991). Follow-up status of patients with angiographically normal coronary arteries and panic disorder. *Journal of the American Medical Association, 265,* 1545–1549.

Blanchard, E. B., & Hickling, E. J. (1997). *After the crash: Assessment and treatment of motor vehicle accident survivors.* Washington, DC: American Psychological Association.

Breslau, N., Peterson, E. L., Kessler, R. C., & Schultz, L. R. (1999). Short screening scale for DSM-IV posttraumatic stress disorder. *American Journal of Psychiatry, 156,* 908–911.

Bridges, K., Goldberg, D., Evans, B., & Sharpe, T. (1991). Determinants of somatization in primary care. *Psychological Medicine, 21,* 473–483.

Brown, G. K. (1990). A causal analysis of chronic pain and depression. *Journal of Abnormal Psychology, 99,* 127–137.

Brown, G. W., Harris, T. O., & Hepworth, C. (1994). Life events and endogenous depression. *Archives of General Psychiatry, 51,* 525–534.

Carney, R. M., Freedland, K. E., Ludbrook, P. A., Saunders, R. D., & Jaffe, A. S. (1990). Major depression, panic disorder, and mitral valve prolapse in patients who complain of chest pain. *American Journal of Medicine, 89,* 757–760.

Dworkin, S.F., Von Korff, M., & LeResche, L. (1990). Multiple pains and psychiatric disturbance: An epidemiologic investigation. *Archives of General Psychiatry, 47,* 239–244.

Engel, G. L. (1959). Psychogenic pain and the pain-prone patient. *American Journal of Medicine, 26,* 899–918.

Escobar, J. I., Burnham, M. A., Karno, M., Forsythe, A., & Golding, J. M. (1987). Somatization in the community. *Archives of General Psychiatry, 44,* 713–718.

Fabrega, H., Jr. (1990). The concept of somatization as a cultural and historical product of Western medicine. *Psychosomatic Medicine, 52,* 653–672.

Fackler, S. M., Anfinson, T. J., & Rand, J. A. (1997). Serial sodium amytal interviews in the clinical setting. *Psychosomatics, 38,* 558–564.

Fishbain, D. A., Goldberg, M., Meagher, B. R., Steele, R., & Rosomoff, H. (1986). Male and female chronic pain patients categorized by DSM-III psychiatric diagnostic criteria. *Pain, 26,* 181–187.

Frank, E., Anderson, B., Reynolds, C. F., Ritenour, A., & Kupfer, D. J. (1994). Life events and the Research Diagnostic Criteria endogenous subtype. *Archives of General Psychiatry, 51,* 519–524.

Geisser, M. E., Roth, R. S., Bachman, J. E., & Eckert, T. A. (1996). The relationship between symptoms of post-traumatic stress disorder and pain, affective disturbance and disability among patients with accident and non-accident related pain. *Pain, 66,* 207–214.

Good, M.D., Good, B. J., & Kleinman, A. (Eds.). (1992). *Pain as human experience: An anthropological perspective.* Berkeley: University of California Press.

Gureje, O., Simon, G. E., Ustun, T. B., & Goldberg, D. P. (1997). Somatization in a cross-cultural perspective: A WHO study in primary care. *American Journal of Psychiatry, 154,* 989-995.

Hudziak, J. J., Bofffeli, T. J., Kreisman, J. J., Battaglia, M. M., Stanger, C., & Guze, S. B. (1996). Clinical study of the relation of borderline personality disorder to Briquet's syndrome (hysteria), somatization disorder, antisocial personality disorder, and substance abuse disorders, *American Journal of Psychiatry, 153,* 1598-1606.

Katon, W., Egan, K., & Miller, D. (1985). Chronic pain: Lifetime psychiatric diagnoses and family history. *American Journal of Psychiatry, 142,* 1156-1160.

Keller, M. B., Hirschfeld, R. M., & Hanks, D. (1997). Double depression: A distinctive subtype of unipolar depression. *Journal of Affective Disorders, 45,* 65-73.

King, S. A., & Strain, J. J. (1992). Revising the category of somatoform pain disorder. *Hospital and Community Psychiatry, 43,* 217-219.

Koenig, H. G., George, L. K., Peterson, B. L., & Pieper, C. F. (1997). Depression in medically ill hospitalized older adults: Prevalence, characteristics, and course of symptoms according to six diagnostic schemes. *American Journal of Psychiatry, 154,* 1376-1383.

Kouyanou, K., Pither, C. E., Rabe-Hesketh, S., & Wessely, S. (1998). A comparative study of iatrogenesis, medication abuse, and psychiatric morbidity in chronic pain patients with and without medically explained symptoms. *Pain, 76,* 417-426.

Kouyanou, K., Pither, C. E., & Wessely, S. (1997). Iatrogenic factors and chronic pain. *Psychosomatic Medicine, 59,* 597-604.

Kroenke, K., Spitzer, R. L., deGruy, F. V., III, Hahn, S. R., Linzer, M., Williams, J. B., Brody, D., & Davies, M. (1997). Multisomatoform disorder: An alternative to undifferentiated somatoform disorder for the somatizing patient in primary care. *Archives of General Psychiatry, 54,* 352-358.

Kulich, R. J., Mencher, P., Bertrand, C., & Maciewicz, R. (2000). Comorbidity of post-traumatic stress disorder and pain: Implications for clinical and forensic assessment. *Current Review of Pain, 4,* 36-48.

Liu, G., Clark, M. R., & Eaton, W. W. (1997). Structural factor analyses for medically unexplained somatic symptoms of somatization disorder in the Epidemiologic Catchment Area study. *Psychological Medicine, 27,* 617-626.

Magni, G., Moreschi, C., Rigatti-Luchini, S., & Merskey, H. (1994). Prospective study on the relationship between depressive symptoms and chronic musculoskeletal pain. *Pain, 56,* 289-297.

Ochoa, J. L., & Verdugo, R. J. (1995). Reflex sympathetic dystrophy: A common clinical avenue for somatoform expression. *Neurology Clinics of North America, 13,* 351-363.

Ormel, J., Von Korff, M., Ustun, T. B., Pini, S., Korten, A., & Oldehinkel, T. (1994). Common mental disorders and disability across cultures. *Journal of the American Medical Association, 272,* 1741-1748.

Pitman, R. K., van der Kolk, B. A., Orr, S. P., & Greenberg, M. S. (1990). Naloxone-reversible analgesic response to combat-related stimuli in posttraumatic stress disorder: A pilot study. *Archives of General Psychiatry, 47,* 541-544.

Polatin, P. B., Kinney, R. K., Gatchel, R. J., Lillo, E., & Mayer, T. G. (1993). Psychiatric illness and chronic low back pain. *Spine, 18,* 66-71.

Portenoy, R. K. (1990). Chronic opioid therapy in nonmalignant pain. *Journal of Pain and Symptom Management, 5*(1, Suppl), S46-S62.

Pribor, E. F., Yutzy, S. H., Dean, J. T., & Wetzel, R. D. (1993). Briquet's syndrome, dissociation, and abuse. *American Journal of Psychiatry, 150,* 1507-1511.

Romano, J. M., & Turner, J. A. (1985). Chronic pain and depression: Does the evidence support a relationship? *Psychological Bulletin, 97,* 18-34.

Rudy, T. E., Kerns, R. D., & Turk, D. C. (1988). Chronic pain and depression: Toward a cognitive behavioral mediation model. *Pain, 35,* 129-140.

Rush, A. J., & Thase, M. E. (1997). Strategies and tactics in the treatment of chronic depression. *Journal of Clinical Psychiatry, 58*(Suppl. 13), 14-22.

Russo, J., Katon, W., Sullivan, M., Clark, M., & Buchwald, D. (1994). Severity of somatization and its relationship to psychiatric disorders and personality. *Psychosomatics, 35,* 546-556.

Schreiber, S., & Galai-Gat, T. (1993). Uncontrolled pain following physical injury as the core trauma in posttraumatic stress disorder. *Pain, 54,* 107-110.

Smith, G. R. (1991). *Somatization disorder in the medical setting.* Washington, DC: American Psychiatric Press.

Spertus, I. L., Burns, J., Glenn, B., Lofland, K., & McCracken, L. (1999). Gender differences in associations between trauma history and adjustment among chronic pain patients. *Pain, 82,* 97-102.

Spitzer, R. L., Kroenke, K., & Williams, J. B. (1999). Validation of a self-report version of the PRIME-MD: The PRIME-MD PHQ 3000 study. *Journal of the American Medical Association, 282,* 1737-1744.

Spitzer, R. L., Williams, J. B., Kroenke, K., Linzer, M., deGry, F. V., III, Hahn, S. R., Brody, D., & Johnson, J. G. (1994). Utility of a new procedure for diagnosing mental disorders in primary care: The PRIME-MD 1000 study. *Journal of the American Medical Association, 272,* 1749-1756.

Stewart, W., Breslau, N., & Keck, P. E., Jr. (1994). Comorbidity of migraine and panic disorder. *Neurology, 44*(10, Suppl. 7), S23-S27.

Stoudemire, A., & Sandu, J. (1987). Psychogenic/Idiopathic pain syndromes. *General Hospital Psychiatry, 9,* 79-86.

Sullivan, M. D., & Katon, W. J. (1993). Somatization: The path from distress to somatic symptoms. *American Pain Society Journal, 2,* 141-149.

Thase, M. E., Fava, M., Halbreich, U., Kocsis, J. H., Koran, L., Davidson, J., Rosenbaum, J., & Harrison, W. (1996). A placebo-controlled, randomized clinical trial comparing sertraline and imipramine for the treatment of dysthymia. *Archives of General Psychiatry, 53,* 777-784.

Turk, D. C., & Okifuji, A. (1997). What factors affect physicians' decisions to prescribe opioids for chronic non-cancer pain patients? *Clinical Journal of Pain, 13,* 330-336.

van der Kolk, B. A., Pelcovitz, D., Roth, S., Mandel, F. S., McFarlane, A., & Herman, J. L. (1996). Dissociation, somatization, and affect dysregulation: The complexity of adaptation of trauma. *American Journal of Psychiatry, 153*(7, Suppl.), 83-93.

Von Korff, M., Deyo, R. A., Cherkin, D., & Barlow, W. (1993). Back pain in primary care: Outcomes at 1 year. *Spine, 18,* 855–862.

Von Korff, M., Ormel, J., Keefe, F. J., & Dworkin, S. F. (1992). Grading the severity of chronic pain. *Pain, 50,* 133–149.

Von Korff, M., & Simon, G. (1996). The relationship between pain and depression. *British Journal of Psychiatry, 168*(Suppl. 30), 101–108.

Walker, E. A., Gelfand, A. N., Gelfand, M. D., & Katon, W. J. (1995). Psychiatric diagnoses, sexual and physical victimization, and disability in patients with irritable bowel syndrome or inflammatory bowel disease. *Psychological Medicine, 25,* 1259–1267.

Walker, E. A., Unützer, J., & Katon, W. J. (1998). Understanding and caring for the patient with multiple unexplained medical symptoms. *Journal of the American Board of Family Practice, 11,* 347–356.

Weisberg, J. N., & Keefe, F. J. (1997). Personality disorders in the chronic pain population. *Pain Forum, 6,* 1–9.

Zaubler, T. S., & Katon, W. (1996). Panic disorder and medical comorbidity: A review of the medical and psychiatric literature. *Bulletin of the Menninger Clinic, 60*(2, Suppl. A), A12–A38.

Ziegler, F. J., Imboden, J. B., & Myer, E. (1960). Contemporary conversion reaction: A clinical study. *American Journal of Psychiatry, 116,* 901–903.

Chapter 16

Assessment of Psychological Status Using Interviews and Self-Report Instruments

LAURENCE A. BRADLEY
NANCY L. McKENDREE-SMITH

A thorough evaluation of individuals with chronic pain must include an assessment of the psychological and social factors associated with their subjective experiences and pain behaviors. Studies of persons with a wide variety of pain syndromes over the past 20 years have shown that psychological distress and environmental stressors are associated with reports of pain and related symptoms (Bradley et al., 1993; Haythornthwaite, Sieber, & Kerns, 1991), functional impairment (Aaron, Bradley, Alarcón, et al., 1997; Haley, Turner, & Romano, 1985; Lorish, Abraham, Austin, Bradley, & Alarcón, 1991), health-care-seeking behavior (Aaron et al., 1996; Kersh et al., in press), and resumption of work (Gallagher et al., 1989).

Thus the goals of psychological assessment are to identify (1) psychosocial factors that may affect pain perception and behavior as well as functional impairment, (2) specific treatment goals for each patient, and (3) intervention strategies that may produce maximum patient improvement (Romano, Turner, & Moore, 1989). In this chapter we focus on the use of interviews and self-report measures of affective distress, psychiatric morbidity, and functional disability in psychological assessment. We first review several strategies for selecting patients for psychological evaluation. We then describe both structured and semistructured interviews for assessing the psychosocial dimensions of

chronic pain and for making reliable and valid psychiatric diagnoses. Finally, we examine a large number of self-report instruments that are used to evaluate patients' psychological status, environmental stressors, pain-related disability, fear of pain, and readiness to adopt self-management strategies. Other selected psychological evaluation procedures, such as the measurement of pain beliefs and perceptions as well as pain behavior, may be found in other chapters of this volume. (See Jensen & Karoly, Chapter 2; Melzack & Katz, Chapter 3; Craig, Prkachin, & Grunau, Chapter 9; Keefe, Williams, & Smith, Chapter 10; and DeGood & Tait, Chapter 17.)

SELECTING PATIENTS FOR PSYCHOLOGICAL EVALUATION

Patients with chronic pain often undergo psychological evaluation only when physical findings that may underlie their symptoms cannot be identified. However, psychological assessment is useful for any patient who (1) displays high levels of pain behavior or functional impairment, despite receiving appropriate medical treatment; (2) exhibits substantial psychological distress; or (3) excessively uses health care services, medications, or alcohol (Romano et al., 1989).

Other patient selection strategies may be used for patients seen in tertiary care centers. For example, university-based clinics for patients with rheumatic disease are usually staffed by multidisciplinary teams composed of rheumatologists, orthopedic surgeons, psychologists, nurses, physical and occupational therapists, and social workers. The treatment teams often perform brief psychosocial assessments on all patients at their initial visits, in order to identify individuals who require more intensive psychological evaluation and treatment. As a result, appropriate behavioral and pharmacological interventions may be initiated during the early phases of treatment, with the goals of reducing morbidity and excessive health care resource utilization.

Another strategy, which we use in our university-based gastroenterology clinic, is to perform a complete psychological assessment on all patients who are referred for evaluation of symptoms of functional disease, such as irritable bowel syndrome (IBS) or chest pain of unknown etiology (CPUE). Patients are advised before their arrival that a psychological evaluation will be performed as part of the medical diagnostic process. In order to reduce patients' concerns that their symptoms will not be viewed as legitimate, they are informed that the psychological assessment is mandatory for all patients.

Regardless of the procedure that is used to identify patients for psychological evaluation, physicians and psychologists must educate and prepare patients before the evaluation occurs. Specifically, it is necessary to reassure patients that their pains are not considered to be imaginary or the result of mental illness. Rather, the psychological evaluation is required to identify interactions between pathophysiological and psychological processes that affect patients' physical symptoms, disabilities, and social and family activities. The evaluation may also suggest interventions that might help to reduce pain or improve other dimensions of health status. Finally, information should be given regarding the specific assessment procedures that will be administered, the professionals who will perform the assessment, the time required to complete the assessment, and the manner in which feedback will be given to the patients and their physicians (Romano et al., 1989).

In addition, the psychological assessments are performed on the second day of the 3-day evaluation, prior to completion of the medical diagnostic procedures. The physicians and psychologists then meet with the patients to provide feedback regarding the results of the entire evaluation and to discuss their treatment plans, which often involve both medical and psychological regimens. These professionals also convey the same information in a joint written report and by telephone to the referring physicians.

INTERVIEWS

Psychological assessment of patients with persistent pain requires at least one interview and the administration of one or more self-report measures. Interviews may be used to evaluate behavioral or personality factors that might influence patients' pain and health status as well as to make specific diagnoses based on the criteria of the *Diagnostic and Statistical Manual of Mental Disorders*, fourth edition (DSM-IV; American Psychiatric Association, 1994; see Sullivan, Chapter 15, this volume). The self-report measures described later in this chapter are used for many of the same purposes, as well as to evaluate patients' affective states, pain-related cognitions, and other factors that may influence their health status and responses to treatment.

Behavioral Interviews

A behavioral interview should involve both the patient and spouse/partner or some other family member. Because the interview is usually the first procedure performed in the psychological assessment, it is helpful to begin by explaining that its purpose is to determine how pain has affected the patient's life and what factors may influence the pain. It is also helpful to encourage the spouse/partner or other family member to contribute information and his or her opinion during the interview, even if a question is not directed specifically to this family member. This allows the interviewer to compare the responses and assess the interactions of the patient and family member.

Structured Interviews

Few structured behavioral interviews have been developed for use with chronic pain patients. However, one of the most well-known structured interviews is the Psychosocial Pain Inventory (PSPI; Getto, Heaton, & Lehman, 1983; Heaton et al., 1982). This measure is used to gather information from the patient and family member about 25 psychosocial aspects of chronic pain, such as stressful life events, social reinforcement of pain behavior, medication usage, health-care-seeking behavior, and familial models for chronic pain. Table 16.1 summarizes the 25 PSPI items, each of which is scored on a 3-point or 4-point scale using a standardized system. A high score on a PSPI item indicates a greater contribution of that item to the patient's pain problem. It should be noted that administration of the protocol requires 1½ to 2 hours.

An initial study involving 169 consecutive patients with chronic pain attending a multidisciplinary pain clinic found evidence of high interrater reliability ($r = .98$) and a mean item–total correlation coefficient of .30 (Heaton et al., 1982). No other reliability data have been reported. Heaton and colleagues (1982) also provided evidence regarding the convergent validity of the instrument. This was established by modest but significant correlations (r's = .26) between total PSPI scores and the Total and Sensory Pain Rating Indices of the McGill Pain Questionnaire (MPQ). The authors

TABLE 16.1. Summary of Psychosocial Pain Inventory (PSPI) Items

1. Pain duration
2. Disability income and litigation
3. Major stressful life events prior to pain onset
4. Major stressful life events prior to pain worsening
5. Major stressful life events prior to pain assessment
6. Pain-related stressors avoided by patient
7. Number of pain-related surgeries
8. Duration (months) of pain-related hospitalizations
9. Number of primary physicians for pain
10. Amount of previous relief from pain
11. Current pain-related medications
12. Pain behavior at home
13. Social reinforcement of pain behavior
14. Pain-reducing behaviors
15. Daytime hours spent reclining due to pain
16. Decrease in home/family responsibilities
17. Employment history prior to pain
18. Change in work status after pain onset
19. Plans for activities if pain is decreased
20. Previous painful or disabling medical problems of at least 1-month duration
21. Physician visits prior to pain onset
22. Maximum number of medications (any kind) used daily for at least 6 months prior to pain onset
23. Exposure to models for chronic pain or illness in family
24. History of alcohol abuse
25. Pain behavior observed in interview

Note. From Getto, Heaton, and Lehman (1983). Copyright 1983 by Raven Press, Ltd. Adapted by permission.

found that total PSPI scores were significantly associated with only 1 of the 10 clinical scales of the Minnesota Multiphasic Personality Inventory (MMPI), Hypochondriasis ($r = .21$); this finding supported its divergent validity. Finally, Getto and colleagues (1983) provided evidence regarding the predictive validity of the PSPI. They reported a study of 32 patients with acute pain who were treated by neurosurgeons with either surgical or conservative interventions. Getto et al. reported that pretreatment PSPI scores accurately differentiated patients who were classified by the neurosurgeons as either treatment successes or failures. When a cutoff score of 30 was used, the PSPI identified 72% of the successes and 79% of the failures. Thus it appears that high PSPI scores are associated with high subjective ratings of pain and with physicians' judgments of treatment response, independently of patients' psychopathology levels.

The Interactive Microcomputer Patient Assessment Tool for Health (IMPATH; Monsein, 1990; Nelson, 1986) represents another structured interview that is noteworthy for its computerized format. The instrument consists of 400 dichotomous, multiple-choice, and visual analogue questions that are presented to patients on a computer screen. The patient responds to each question by pressing the appropriate computer key. These responses are stored and analyzed, and a printout is provided for the health care provider. This printout provides (1) the patient's medical history data; (2) a list of psychological, behavioral, cognitive, and social factors that may contribute to the patient's current pain problems; and (3) a series of scales regarding symptom severity and the degree to which pain has negatively affected the patient's daily activities. The printout also includes the patient's scores on four validity scales that are designed to detect positive and negative response biases, random answering, and low accuracy in the patient's IMPATH responses. These scales are similar to the validity scales constructed for the MMPI.

The IMPATH manual (Nelson, 1986) presents reliability and validity data regarding the responses of 128 patients with head and neck pain of myofascial origin and 95 healthy volunteers. The internal reliability of each IMPATH scale was reported to be at least .80, and the minimum test–retest reliability coefficient over a 2-week period for these scales was .87. Evidence regarding the construct validity of the instrument was provided by the finding that each IMPATH item differentiated the patient sample from the healthy controls. In addition, correlational analyses revealed that the

IMPATH scales measure relatively independent constructs. It should be stressed, however, that it has not been shown that the instrument represents a reliable and valid measure for patients with pain syndromes other than myofascial head and neck pain.

Neither the PSPI nor the IMPATH has received a great deal of attention in the research literature. No investigators, other than the instrument developers, have published reports of the psychometric properties of these two measures. Thus, at present, we recommend usage of both instruments primarily for research purposes.

Semistructured Interviews

Due to the limited research on structured interviews, most practitioners have chosen to perform their behavioral interviews using a semistructured format. For example, we have adopted a modified version of the interview that was originally appended to the MPQ (Melzack, 1975). Other useful interview formats may be found in Karoly and Jensen (1989), Phillips (1988), and Gatchel (2000). Table 16.2 shows a summary of items included in the Phillips interview.

Regardless of the specific format that is chosen, the behavioral interview has several objectives (Bradley, 1989; Romano et al., 1989). The first objective is to obtain a "pain history." This should include a description of the events that may have precipitated the onset of pain and the course of the patient's pain over time with regard to intensity, frequency, sensory, and affective qualities, as well as location. Collection of this information may be aided by the use of the MPQ and of a pain drawing (Ransford, Cairns, & Mooney, 1976). The history should also include questions regarding prior pain treatments and the patient's responses to these treatments. This information is critical so that the practitioner may avoid duplication of "failed" interventions or determine whether these unsuccessful treatments may be attributed to problems such as inadequate dosages of pharmacological agents, use of "passive" (e.g., massage, heat) rather than "active" (e.g., exercise program) physical therapy, or patient nonadherence with the treatment regimen.

The second objective of the interview is to identify the events that precede exacerbations in the patient's pain perceptions or pain behavior, as well as the events that follow these exacerbations. For example, suppose a female patient with IBS reports that she dislikes attending business-related

TABLE 16.2. Summary of Items Included in Semistructured Interview

Is there evidence of:

1. Depression: _____
2. Anxiety: _____
3. Avoidance/confrontation activity patterns: _____
4. Inactivity/unfit: _____
5. Lack of evolved pain coping strategies: _____
6. Drug dependency: _____
7. Poor inadequate understanding of chronic pain/physical mechanisms: _____
8. Work disruption: _____
9. Marital problems: _____
10. Other: _____
11. Motivation for treatment: _____
12. Sources of reinforcement for pain:
    (a) financial
    (b) sympathy, attention, support from significant others and health-care providers
    (c) provision of time to engage in pleasurable activities
    (d) avoidance of work, school, unpleasant activities (e.g., home or family related), social events
    (e) other

Note. From Philips (1988, p. 198). Copyright 1988 by Springer Publishing Company. Adapted by permission.

dinners with her spouse and that she always experiences increases in her symptoms a few hours prior to these dinners. The patient also states that she takes analgesic or antispasmodic medication in response to the increases in her pain. In addition, she has recently had to increase the medication dosage in order to control her pain. Based on this information, the interviewer may generate several hypotheses that can be evaluated with additional questions and review of other assessment measures. First, it may be speculated that, due to several chance pairings of increased pain during previous business dinners, the events associated with preparing for these dinners now serve as conditioned stimuli that automatically elicit severe pain and other IBS symptoms. We may also speculate that the patient's medication usage is reinforced by the sedating side effects of the medication. Indeed, the increased dosages required by the patient suggest that she may be developing a physiological tolerance for or dependence on the medication (cf. Fordyce, 1976).

During this portion of the interview, it also should be noted how persons in the patient's environment respond to the patient's use of medication and other pain behaviors (see Romano & Schmaling, Chapter 18). With regard to the patient with IBS described above, it should be determined whether family members bring medication to the patient or provide reinforcement to her after medication usage. One example of positive reinforcement (i.e., positive consequences) would be increased attention or nurturance from the patient's spouse or children when they see her use medication. Several investigators have found that patients' reports of pain and pain behaviors are greatest when patients perceive that their spouses/partners provide supportive or solicitous responses to expressions of pain (Block, Kremer, & Gaylor, 1980; Flor, Kerns, & Turk, 1987; Gil, Keefe, Crisson, & Van Dalfsen, 1987; Kerns et al., 1991). This relationship may be especially strong when couple satisfaction is high (Flor et al., 1987). Negative reinforcement for pain behavior (i.e., avoidance of unpleasant events) might occur if the patient is encouraged by her spouse to remain at home rather than attend his business dinners. Another example of negative reinforcement might occur if the patient's family is characterized by interpersonal conflict. In this case, reduced interactions with the spouse or children following medication intake might reward the patient with IBS for frequent usage of her medication or for increasing the dosage.

The results of this portion of the interview might suggest that an appropriate treatment plan must attend to the reinforcement contingencies associated with this patient's medication usage and her avoidance of business-related dinners. For example, treatment might include teaching the patient's family to withdraw positive reinforcement for medication usage and to reward relatively healthy behavior (such as discussing her concerns with her spouse about attending these dinners).

The third objective of the interview is to evaluate the patient's daily activities. It is necessary to determine (1) how the patient usually spends his or her time during the day and evening, (2) which activities have been performed more often or less often since the onset of pain, and (3) whether any activities have been modified or eliminated since pain onset. The information that is gathered during this portion of the interview may be supplemented by direct observations of the patient's behavior or responses to activity diaries (see Keefe et al., Chapter 10) and functional capacity evaluations (see Polatin & Mayer, Chapter 11, and Battié & May, Chapter 12).

Information regarding changes in the patient's daily activities may allow an evaluator to generate hypotheses regarding reinforcement contingencies related to the patient's pain behavior, in addition to those described earlier in this section. For example, if the performance of physically demanding, pleasurable activities has not decreased greatly, but the performance of similarly demanding, aversive responsibilities has been substantially reduced, we might hypothesize that the patient's behavior has been influenced by negative reinforcement (Romano et al., 1989). This discordance in behavior would be exemplified by a man with chronic back pain who reports that he is unable to perform factory work that requires standing and repetitive movement of the upper extremities, but is able to serve as an umpire for his daughter's softball games. Although the physical requirements of the two activities are not entirely equal, we would have to consider the possibility that the patient's work-related pain behavior has been reinforced by the avoidance of monotonous activity in an unpleasant environment. This hypothesis would gain support if we also learned that the patient had experienced interpersonal conflicts with his job supervisor or coworkers (Bigos et al., 1991). Indeed, this information would suggest that the outcome of any vocational rehabilitation services offered to the patient might be poor if the patient were placed in another work environment that he considered aversive (Linton & Bradley, 1992).

Information about the patient's daily activities also may allow us to determine the extent to which the patient exacerbates his or her suffering. For example, the restriction or elimination of activities due to the expectation of increased pain may lead to excessive disability or pain behavior resulting from distorted gait or physical deconditioning (Bradley, 1989). Intensive physical reconditioning or anxiety management may be necessary for the patient to successfully perform the activities that have been avoided (Vlaeyen et al., 1999). Conversely, a patient may describe behavior characterized by constant activity that is not reduced until the intensity of pain becomes severe. This individual will require instruction in appropriately modulating his or her activity level so that pain does not become a signal that automatically elicits rest, medication intake, or reinforcement from others in the environment.

The fourth objective of the interview is to determine whether the patient has any relatives or friends who suffer from chronic pain or disabilities similar to those of the patient. Careful questioning may reveal that the patient spends a considerable amount of time with individuals who also have chronic pain problems (Gamsa & Vikis-Freibergs, 1991; Keefe & Bradley, 1984). Similarly, the interview may show that the patient's childhood was characterized by parental reinforcement for or modeling of maladaptive illness behaviors (e.g., school or work absenteeism in response to minor symptoms). These childhood experiences may have important implications for the patient's current pain behavior or psychological adjustment (Schanberg, Keefe, Lefebvre, Kredrich, & Gil, 1998; Spirito, DeLawyer, & Stark, 1991). Thus experiences during childhood and as an adult may provide the patient with a great deal of opportunity to learn complex, maladaptive, chronic pain behaviors (e.g., inappropriate use of medication or health care services). This may occur particularly often among patients with chronic pain syndromes such as IBS and fibromyalgia (FM) that tend to be found among multiple family members (Neumann & Buskila, 1997; Pellegrino, Waylonis, & Sommer, 1989; Whitehead, Winget, Fedoravicius, Wooley, & Blackwell, 1982). Indeed, several investigators have reported that a history of chronic pain among one's relatives is a significant premorbid risk factor for suffering from a chronic pain syndrome (e.g., Buskila, Neumann, Hazanov, & Carmi, 1996; Gamsa & Vikis-Freibergs, 1991; Mikhail & von Baeyer, 1990).

Another family-related issue that has recently received a great deal of attention is whether the patient has suffered physical or sexual abuse. Haber and Roos (1985) were the first investigators to study histories of abuse among patients with chronic pain. They reported that of 151 consecutive female patients who presented to a university-based chronic pain center, 53% reported histories of physical or sexual abuse during childhood or as adults. Of all women reporting abuse, 16% reported sexual abuse, 43% reported physical abuse, and 41% reported experiencing both types of abuse. Ninety percent of the women reported abuse during their adult years (over 18 years of age). The mean duration of

abuse among the adults was 12 years; spouses were involved in 71% of these incidents. In addition, 17% of the victims reported abuse during childhood or adolescence, with 10% of those incidents involving incestuous relationships with a parent. Moreover, the abused patients, relative to those who had not been abused, were twice as likely to have suffered pain without a specific precipitating injury or identified cause and to have a significantly greater number of previous medical problems for which they had sought treatment.

Drossman and colleagues (1990) reported that physical and sexual abuse were also common among female patients in a university-based specialty clinic for patients with gastrointestinal (GI) disorders. These investigators reported that of 206 consecutive females referred to the gastroenterology clinic, 30% reported histories of childhood sexual abuse, and 4% reported frequent childhood physical abuse. The proportions of these women who reported sexual and physical abuse during adulthood were 40% and 4%, respectively. It should be noted that the greater frequency of sexual than of physical abuse among these patients is not consistent with the rates reported by Haber and Roos (1985) and other early investigators (e.g., Domino & Haber, 1987). However, using Drossman and colleagues' interview-based assessment instrument, we also have found higher rates of sexual abuse, compared to physical abuse, among patients at specialty clinics for GI disorders and FM (Alexander et al., 1998; Scarinci, McDonald-Haile, Bradley, & Richter, 1994). In addition, our investigations as well as that of Drossman and colleagues have shown that patients who report a history of abuse are characterized by higher levels of pain, disability, psychiatric morbidity, and affective distress, as well as by more frequent use of pain medications and outpatient health care visits (Table 16.3). Similar associations between abuse history and pain and other dimensions of health status have been reported in samples drawn from the general population (Linton, 1997) and primary care medical settings (Dickinson, deGruy, Dickinson, & Candib, 1999; Walker et al., 1999). There is also evidence that severity of abuse is associated with greater deficits in health status (Leserman et al., 1996).

Relatively few data are available concerning male patients who have been physically or sexually abused. However, Wurtele, Kaplan, and Keairnes (1990) found that 7% of 45 consecutive male patients attending a chronic pain rehabilitation program reported a history of sexual abuse.

TABLE 16.3. Associations between Abuse History and Measures of Health Status in Patients with Fibromyalgia (FM)

| Variable | FM patient group ($n = 75$) | | t | p |
	Abused ($n = 43$)	Nonabused ($n = 32$)		
Total outpatient visits	13.8 ± 2.0	9.0 ± 1.2	1.91	.030
Medication for pain	3.5 ± 0.2	2.8 ± 0.3	1.99	.025
MPQ	38.1 ± 2.4	31.1 ± 2.3	-2.05	.022
SIP–Total	21.7 ± 2.0	16.9 ± 1.8	-1.77	.038
Number of lifetime psychiatric diagnoses	4.0 ± 0.4	1.4 ± 0.3	-5.16	.001

Note: MPQ, McGill Pain Questionnaire; SIP–Total, Sickness Impact Profile Total Disability.

Karol, Micka, and Kuskowski (1992) also studied 100 consecutive male patients attending outpatient clinics for chronic back pain. Six percent reported a history of sexual abuse, and 16% reported that they had been physically abused.

Based on the evidence cited above, we suggest that assessments of all patients with chronic pain should include a careful evaluation of possible sexual and physical abuse. Table 16.4 shows the interview questions that we used to assess abuse among patients with GI disorders and FM (Alexander et al., 1998; Scarinci et al., 1994). These questions were originally used in a Canadian national postal survey and were later used in two U.S. research studies (Briere & Runtz, 1988; Drossman et al., 1990). With regard to the treatment of patients who report histories of abuse, merely giving such a patient an opportunity to discuss these experiences with an empathic health professional often provides some emotional relief (Cahill, Llewelyn, & Pearson, 1991). Nevertheless, many patients must be referred to experienced therapists, who may help them to resolve issues such as poor self-image, self-blame for the abuse, sexual dysfunction, and suppressed anger and rage.

A further objective of the behavioral interview is to evaluate the degree to which the patient is experiencing affective disturbance. Depression is commonly found among patients with chronic pain (Romano & Turner, 1985). A few investigators have suggested that chronic pain is usually a manifestation of an underlying affective disorder (e.g., Blumer & Heilbronn, 1982; Hudson & Pope, 1996). However, most investigators acknowledge that although psychological distress may contribute to the development of chronic pain in some predisposed individuals, depression and other mood disorders generally interact with chronic pain. That is, these disorders are frequently consequences of chronic pain and they also tend to

enhance pain perception (Ahles, Yunus, & Masi, 1987; Atkinson, Slater, Patterson, Grant, & Garfin, 1991; Brown, 1990; Gamsa, 1990; Magni, Moreschi, Rigatti-Luchini, & Merskey, 1994). Thus, it should be determined whether the patient has experienced any change in mood or outlook on life since the onset of pain, and whether the patient has experienced vegetative signs of depression such as sleep disturbance, change in food intake, or decreased desire for sexual intercourse. It is also important to evaluate patients' level of satisfaction with their relationships with spouses or significant others. Several investigators have

TABLE 16.4. Interview Items Used to Assess Sexual and Physical Abuse

Sexual Abuse[a]

During your childhood (<14 years) or adulthood, has anyone ever:
    A. exposed the sex organs of their body to you?
    B. threatened to have sex with you?
    C. touched the sex organs of your body?
    D. made you touch the sex organs of their body?
    E. tried forcefully or succeeded to have sex when you didn't want this?

Physical Abuse[b]

When you were a child (now that you are an adult), did an older person (does any other adult):
    Hit, kick, or beat you?
    (1 = never, 2 = seldom, 3 = occasionally, 4 = often)

Note. Adapted from Drossman et al. (1990, p. 829). Copyright 1990 by the American College of Physicians. Adapted by permission.

[a]Patients are considered to be sexually abused if they answer "yes" to any sexual abuse question, except for category A during adulthood.

[b]Patients are considered to be physically abused if they answer "often" to the physical abuse question.

demonstrated that patient depression is inversely related to couple satisfaction (e.g., Kerns, Haythornthwaite, Southwick, & Giller, 1990; Kerns & Turk, 1984; see Romano & Schmaling, Chapter 18). Kerns and colleagues (1990) also have shown that patient depression tends to be greatest when couple satisfaction is low and the patient perceives that his or her spouse/partner responds punitively to expressions of pain.

Finally, it is important to determine the degree to which patients may be experiencing difficulty in sexual functioning. Difficulty in sexual functioning may be associated with depression and decreased couple satisfaction, as patients often report during the interview that they have experienced difficulty in achieving or maintaining erections, decreased vaginal lubrication, or dyspareunia. Decreased lubrication, dyspareunia, and restricted movement may be especially pronounced among patients with rheumatic diseases (Anderson, Bradley, Young, McDaniel, & Wise, 1985).

Psychiatric Interviews

Although questions regarding affective distress should be included in the behavioral interview, structured psychiatric interviews should also be used to evaluate patients with chronic pain (Clouse, 1991). For example, Beitman and colleagues (1991) have reported that between 34% and 59% of patients with CPUE also meet the DSM-III-R criteria for panic disorder. Independent investigators have reported similar prevalence rates for panic disorder among these patients (Cormier et al., 1988; Katon et al., 1988). These prevalence rates are substantially higher than those found among patients with other chronic pain syndromes (16.2%; Katon, Egan, & Miller, 1985). Panic disorder may cause CPUE in some patients, because anxiety disorders may alter the thresholds of visceral afferent mechanisms and thereby cause people to perceive low intensity esophageal stimuli as painful (Bradley, Scarinci, & Richter, 1991). Furthermore, psychiatric disorders (such as panic disorder) among patients with CPUE have been shown to be associated with the use of negative coping strategies such as wishful thinking, which may exacerbate pain (Vitaliano, Katon, Maiuro, & Russo, 1989).

Both pharmacological and cognitive-behavioral interventions may be used to reduce panic disorder symptoms as well as pain episodes among patients with CPUE (Beitman et al., 1989; Cannon et al.,

1994; Klimes, Mayou, Pearce, Coles, & Fagg, 1990; Mayou, Bass, & Bryant, 1999). Thus it appears that the use of a reliable and valid psychiatric interview may enable an evaluator to identify a specific target associated with episodes of CPUE that may respond well to appropriate treatment. The psychiatric interview may also allow identifiction of patients who have mixed symptoms of anxiety and depression that do not meet diagnostic criteria for specific psychiatric disorders, but that nevertheless place them at risk for more severe somatic complaints as well as mood and anxiety disorders when they are exposed to substantial life stresses (Katon & Roy-Byrne, 1991).

Two structured psychiatric interviews have been used extensively in studies of patients with chronic pain. The first is the Diagnostic Interview Schedule (DIS; Helzer & Robins, 1988; Robins, Helzer, Croughan, & Ratcliff, 1981). The DIS was originally developed to provide reliable and valid diagnoses based on DSM-III or DSM-III-R criteria (American Psychiatric Association, 1987); however, an updated version is now available that is in accord with DSM-IV criteria (American Psychiatric Association, 1994). The DIS is a highly structured interview that requires specialized training. Training courses are offered twice a year at Washington University (DIS Training/Department of Psychiatry, 4940 Audubon Avenue, St. Louis, MO 63110). A computerized version of the DIS (CDIS-IV) is also available from Washington University. Nevertheless, we recommend that potential users of the CDIS-IV undergo training in order to understand the structure of the DIS and to learn to respond appropriately to patients' questions regarding interview items.

Test–retest reliability studies of the original DIS reported median kappa coefficients for lifetime psychiatric diagnoses over 1-year intervals ranging from .37 to .59 (Helzer, Spitznagel, & McEvoy, 1987; Vandiver & Sher, 1991). The validity of the DIS was established by examining the lifetime diagnoses assigned to large samples of psychiatric patients and controls by groups of psychiatrists and lay interviewers, both of whom used the DIS. Kappa coefficients ranged between .47 and 1.00; these indicate a high level of concordance between the diagnoses assigned by the psychiatrists and those assigned by the lay interviewers, even after chance agreements were controlled for (Robins et al., 1981). Recent epidemiological studies, however, suggest that the DIS may underdetect diagnoses made by psychiatrists especially in respondents who are older, are male, and have low levels of impairment (Eaton, Neufeld, Chen, & Cai, 2000).

The second psychiatric interview is the Structured Clinical Interview for DSM (SCID; Spitzer, Williams, Gibbon, & First, 1990). This instrument was also developed originally to make diagnoses according to the DSM-III-R criteria, but has been updated for use with the DSM-IV (First, Spitzer, William, & Gibbon, 1997). The SCID was designed for use by experienced clinicians, who may supplement the structured interview with (1) additional questions to clarify differential diagnosis, (2) challenges to inconsistencies in subjects' self-reports, or (3) ancillary information drawn from hospital records, family members, or other clinical staff (Spitzer, Williams, Gibbons, & First, 1992). A detailed training manual and training videotapes are available (First et al., 1997; Spitzer et al., 1990). In addition, a computerized version of the screening version of the SCID for Axis I and Axis II disorders has been developed by the American Psychiatric Association (First, Gibbon, Williams, & Spitzer, 2000). The reliability of the original SCID was evaluated by examining the consistency with which trained clinicians assigned lifetime diagnoses to a large sample of psychiatric patients and controls. Williams and colleagues (1992) found that the mean kappa for patient diagnosis was .68; the mean kappa for the controls, however, was .51. The lower reliability coefficients for the diagnoses assigned to the healthy controls were attributed primarily to the low base rates of psychiatric disorders within this subject sample.

In summary, it appears that the interrater reliabilities for the DIS and the SCID are approximately equal. However, few data concerning the other psychometric properties of the SCID have been published, whereas the reliability and validity of the DIS have been examined in several published studies. We agree with Spitzer and colleagues (1992) that the DIS decision tree procedure occasionally produces diagnoses that do not appear to be consistent with clinical impressions. At these times, supplementary source material that can be used in making diagnoses with the SCID appears to be desirable. We recommend that relatively inexperienced clinicians obtain training in and use the DIS. Relatively experienced clinicians may wish to obtain training in the use of both the DIS and the SCID. These individuals then may choose whichever instrument best meets the needs of their clinical settings or research efforts.

SELF-REPORT INSTRUMENTS

We have described the important psychosocial factors that may influence pain perception and behavior that may be evaluated by structured and semistructured interviews in the preceding section. Most health care professionals also administer self-report measures of affective disturbance and related constructs to patients with chronic pain. These instruments are very important for clinical and research purposes because they provide standardized, reliable, and valid assessments of psychosocial variables. The other advantage is that they require little professional time and cost for administration and scoring. Moreover, the self-report instruments tend to be more sensitive to treatment-related changes than are psychiatric diagnoses or other interview data.

In this portion of this chapter, we first review the literature concerning two measures of depression that have been widely used with patients who have chronic pain: the Beck Depression Inventory (BDI) and the Center for Epidemiologic Studies–Depression scale (CES-D). We then examine four comprehensive measures of psychological status that are frequently used with patients who have chronic pain. These are the MMPI, the Symptom Checklist-90 Revised (SCL-90R), the Millon Behavioral Health Inventory (MBHI), and the Illness Behavior Questionnaire (IBQ). This is followed by a discussion of several measures of environmental stressors that may influence pain. The chapter then examines three measures designed to provide assessments of disability and adaptation to chronic pain. Finally, measures of pain-related anxiety/fear and pain stages of change are reviewed.

Measures of Depression: The BDI and the CES-D

Both the BDI and the CES-D are brief and easy to score. The BDI (Beck & Steer, 1993) has 21 items in which the patient circles the statement that best describes how he or she has felt during the past week. Alpha coefficients for the BDI range from .73 to .95 in both psychiatric and nonpsychiatric populations (Beck, Steer, & Garbin, 1988). The CES-D has 20 items reflecting depressive symptomatology that are rated on a 0–3 scale. Alpha coefficients for the CES-D range from .85 for a general population to .90 for a psychiatric population (Radloff, 1977).

The BDI was originally developed by Aaron Beck to assess the cognitive components of depression. Nevertheless, it contains a large number of items concerning somatic disturbances, such as sleep disturbance and weight change. These items, therefore, may artificially inflate the scores of patients with chronic pain (Wesley, Gatchel, Polatin, Kinney, & Mayer, 1991; Williams & Richardson, 1993). This problem may be especially important in evaluations of patients with diseases that produce fatigue and other symptoms of depression, such as rheumatoid arthritis (RA) and systemic lupus erythematosus (Bradley, 1994). In contrast, the CES-D has relatively fewer items with somatic content. Therefore, we suggest that the CES-D is more appropriate than the BDI for the evaluation of patients with rheumatological disorders (Bradley, 1994).

Several authors (Geisser, Roth, & Robinson, 1997; Turner & Romano, 1984) reported good sensitivity and specificity for the BDI in identifying depression in patients with chronic pain. Geisser and colleagues (1997) also found that both the BDI and CES-D significantly discriminated between patients with chronic pain who did and did not have major depression. Diagnoses obtained via self-report measures were compared to those obtained via clinical interview. Using statistically derived cutoff scores of 21 rather than the usual 14 on the BDI and 27 rather than 14 on the CES-D, these authors found that although the overall hit rates were similar, there were some differences in sensitivity and specificity for the two measures. The CES-D had better sensitivity (81.8% vs. 68.2%), while the BDI demonstrated greater specificity (78.4% vs. 72.7%). The investigators noted that removing the somatic items from each scale did not result in improvements in the measures' abilities to detect depression accurately. However, an independent study reported that the CES-D was more sensitive to changes in depression severity than the BDI (Santor, Zuroff, Ramsey, Cervantes, & Palacios, 1995). This increased sensitivity may be due in part to its relatively low somatic content.

In summary, then, both the CES-D and the BDI appear to be adequate tools for assessing depression in the population with chronic pain, although relatively higher than usual cutoff scores must be used to obtain the best results in terms of sensitivity and specificity. Use of lower cutoff scores may lead to excessive numbers of false positives. The finding that the CES-D is more sensitive to change may make it the measure of choice for researchers or clinicians interested in measuring outcomes of pharmacological and cognitive-behavioral inteventions, especially in populations with rheumatological disorders.

Comprehensive Measures of Psychological Status

Minnesota Multiphasic Personality Inventory

The MMPI is the most commonly used instrument in clinical settings for evaluating the psychological status of patients with chronic pain. The original MMPI was a 566-item questionnaire made up of 10 scales designed to assess psychological disturbance and three additional validity scales. The revised version of this instrument, the MMPI-2 (Hathaway et al., 1989), includes 567 items and the same clinical and validity scales as those found in the original instrument. In addition, 15 new content scales have been developed to enhance the understanding of patients in the clinical setting and to help predict their behavior during treatment (Ben-Porath & Sherwood, 1993). Both MMPI forms require patients' raw scores on each scale to be converted to standard T-scores, so that they may be compared with the responses produced by a large normative sample.

The primary differences between the original and revised versions of the MMPI are that (1) the normative sample used for the MMPI-2 is more representative of the U.S. population with regard to ethnic group membership, religious preference, and education; and (2) 90 of the MMPI items have been eliminated and 68 items have been modified for the MMPI-2 (Levitt, 1990). However, only 12 items from the MMPI's 13 basic validity and clinical scales were eliminated from the MMPI-2, in an attempt to maximize consistency between profiles produced by patients on the two instruments. Finally, the method for transforming subjects' raw scores into T-scores on the MMPI-2 has been modified so that direct comparisons can be made of T-scores on the clinical and supplemental content scales (Ben-Porath & Graham, 1991). As a result, between 10% and 33% of the 2-point code types (e.g., elevations on the Hypochondriasis [Hs] and Hysteria [Hy] scales) produced by psychiatric patients on the original MMPI will not be replicated with the MMPI-2 (Ben-Porath & Graham, 1991).

The standardization samples utilized for profile interpretation with both versions of the MMPI are not appropriate for the assessment of patients with chronic pain (Bradley, Prokop, Gentry, Van der Heide, & Prieto, 1981). For example, one study (Pincus, Callahan, Bradley, Vaughn, & Wolfe, 1986) identified five items from the MMPI Hs, Depression (D), and Hy scales that reliably differentiated a sample of patients with RA from healthy controls. The patients' responses to these items reflected disease activity (as measured by grip strength and self-report of disability) rather than psychological status (see Table 16.5). Similar findings have been reported by independent investigators (Moore, McFall, Kivlahan, & Capestany, 1988; Naliboff, Cohen, & Yellin, 1982; Prokop, 1986).

In response to the problem of MMPI interpretation, several groups of investigators have used hierarchical clustering methods to identify the MMPI and MMPI-2 profile patterns that are produced most frequently by patients with chronic pain and the behaviors that are associated with each of these patterns. For example, we (Bradley, Prokop, Magolis, & Gentry, 1978; Bradley & Van der Heide, 1984) identified and replicated three MMPI profile patterns across four samples of patients with low back pain. We found that MMPI profiles characterized by elevations on the Hs, D, and Hy scales were associated with perceptions of severe pain; affective disturbance; and large disruptions in vocational, social, marital/sexual, and family endeavors. Profiles with elevations on the scales noted above, as well as on the Psychopathic Deviate and Schizophrenia scales, tended to be associated with difficulty giving up positive reinforcements for pain behavior; high levels of psychopathology; and relatively moderate disruptions in vocational, social, marital/sexual, and family endeavors.

An independent study of patients with the elevated scales described above showed that they were also characterized by high levels of depression, anxiety, vulnerability, and hostility (Wade, Dougherty, Hart, & Cook, 1992). Profiles without elevations on the clinical scales were associated with relatively few pain-related disabilities in daily functioning. Similar MMPI and MMPI-2 profile patterns and behavioral correlates have

been identified among independent samples of patients with back pain (McGill, Lawlis, Selby, Mooney, & McCoy, 1983) and patients with diverse chronic pain syndromes presenting to university-based pain treatment centers (Costello, Hulsey, Schoenfeld, & Ramamurthy, 1987; Guck, Meilman, Skultety, & Poloni, 1988; Riley & Robinson, 1998). Costello and colleagues (1987) have also identified a profile pattern characterized by elevations only on the Hs and Hy scales. However, no unique correlates for this profile pattern have been identified.

It was originally anticipated that the identification of distinct MMPI profile patterns would help clinicians tailor treatments for patient subgroups with similar MMPI profiles and pain-related behaviors (Bradley et al., 1978). Although this goal has not been achieved, several investigators have attempted to determine whether specific MMPI profile patterns are associated with different responses to various treatment packages. Two studies have shown that MMPI profile patterns do not reliably predict outcome following interdisciplinary pain clinic treatment (Guck et al., 1988; Moore, Armentrout, Parker, & Kivlahan, 1986). However, McCreary (1985) demonstrated that the responses of patients with chronic pain to conservative orthopedic management were accurately predicted by their MMPI profile patterns. The proportion of accurate predictions ranged from 61% to 99% among the male patients and from 65% to 89% among the females. Moreover, a study of work-disabled patients' responses to the MMPI-2 (Moore, McCallum, Holman, & O'Brien, 1991) found that among the males, profiles characterized by elevations on the Hs, D, Hy, Psychopathic Deviante, and Schizophrenia scales were associated with a significantly poorer return-to-work rate (33%) than the remaining profile patterns (83%

TABLE 16.5. Responses of Patients with Rheumatoid Arthritis to "Disease-Related" MMPI Items and Their Relation to Mean Health Assessment Questionnaire (HAQ) Scores and Grip Strength

	Mean HAQ scores		Mean grip strength values	
MMPI item	True	False	True	False
9. I am about as able to work as I ever was.	0.63	1.70[a]	126	95
51. I am in just as good physical health as most of my friends.	0.73	1.62[b]	124	97
153. During the past few years I have been well.	0.92	1.79[a]	124	87[c]
163. I do not tire quickly.	0.79	1.47	153	98[c]
243. I have few or no pains.	0.88	1.51	149	92[d]

Note. From Pincus, Callahan, Bradley, Vaughn, and Wolfe (1986, p. 1463). Copyright 1986 by the American Rheumatism Association. Adapted by permission.

[a]p < .001; [b]p = .006; [c]p < .03; [d]p = .002.

and 91%) at a 12-month follow-up assessment. This finding is consistent with the behavioral correlates identified for the same profile pattern derived from the MMPI (Bradley & Van der Heide, 1984). Profile patterns did not predict return to work among the female patients, due to the high rates of work return associated with each pattern (78%–88%).

One investigation has examined the predictive validity of the MMPI-2 Negative Treatment Indicators (*TRT*) content scale in a group of male patients with chronic pain treated at a Department of Veterans Affairs hospital (Clark, 1996). After demographic factors and duration of pain were controlled for, *TRT* scores were a significant predictor of patients' BDI scores and performance on a physical capacity evaluation. The *TRT* scale's power to predict posttreatment physical capacity remained significant even after pretreatment physical capacity was controlled for. In contrast, a study of Dutch patients with chronic back pain revealed that several MMPI-2 clinical and content scales involving emotional distress and somatic complaints predicted treatment-related change in self-reports of pain intensity and disability. These scales, however, did not predict change in trunk muscle performance (Vendrig, Derksen, & de Mey, 1999).

We find it very encouraging that the profile patterns derived from the MMPI responses of patients with chronic pain have been replicated in studies using the MMPI-2. We remain concerned, however, that MMPI profile patterns have not been shown consistently to predict treatment outcome. It appears that the profile patterns are better predictors of responses to surgical and nonsurgical treatment when stringent criteria are used to evaluate pattern homogeneity (Henrichs, 1987). Therefore, we suggest that clinicians and investigators studying the profile patterns associated with the MMPI-2 continue to use conservative methods for defining these patterns (Sines, 1964). Moreover, since statistical algorithms used to derive MMPI profile patterns in one setting may not generalize to other locales (Robinson, Swimmer, & Rallof, 1989), clinicians and investigators should continue to derive profile patterns and behavioral correlates based on the responses of patients at their respective institutions ("local norms"). This will allow for comparisons between local findings and the MMPI profile patterns and correlates already identified in the literature. Finally, we encourage further evaluation of the predictive validity of the *TRT* and other MMPI-2 content scales in both women and men with chronic pain (see, e.g., Clark, 1996).

Since there are problems associated with the MMPI, such as its length, the contamination of items with physical symptoms, and the uncertain predictive validity of profile patterns for patients with chronic pain, health care professionals have examined the utility of several alternative multiscale instruments in assessing the psychological status of such patients. These instruments include the SCL-90R (Derogatis, 1983), the MBHI (Millon, Green, & Meagher, 1982), and the IBQ (Pilowsky & Spence, 1975).

Symptom Checklist-90 Revised

The SCL-90R is a 90-item self-report measure of nine major psychological disturbances (Somatization, Obsessive–Compulsive, Interpersonal Sensitivity, Depression, Anxiety, Hostility, Phobic Anxiety, Paranoid Ideation, and Psychoticism). Three global measures of psychological distress also may be derived. The Global Severity Index is the measure that is most frequently reported in the literature. The SCL-90R requires patients to rate on a 6-point scale the extent to which each of the 90 physical or psychiatric symptoms has bothered them in the past 7 days. The patients' raw scores on each scale are transformed to standard *T*-scores and are interpreted in a manner similar to that used with the MMPI.

The reliability and validity of the SCL-90R with psychiatric patients have been demonstrated in a large number of studies summarized by Derogatis (1983). The SCL-90R is much briefer than the MMPI. Thus it often produces less patient resistance to psychological assessment than does the latter instrument. In addition, Parker and colleagues (1990) have reported that among a sample of patients with RA, only the Depression and Hostility scales are associated with disease severity or activity as measured by rheumatologists' judgments and anatomical stage comparisons.

Despite the advantages of the SCL-90R noted above, several studies have raised questions regarding its utility for patients with chronic pain. For example, although Derogatis originally derived 10 factors from the responses of psychiatric patients, Shutty, DeGood, and Schwartz (1986) extracted only five factors from the SCL-90R responses of a sample of patients with chronic pain. Similarly, Buckelew, DeGood, Schwartz, and Kerler (1986) found different item response patterns among samples of psychiatric inpatients and patients with chronic pain. The former patients tended to endorse equivalent levels of somatic and cognitive distress items on the SCL-90R, whereas the latter patients' reports of psychological distress were generally restricted to somatic signs of anxiety and depression. Therefore, it appears that different dimensions of distress underlie the SCL-90R responses of psychiatric inpatients and patients with chronic pain. It is not valid, then, to interpret the latter patients' responses on the basis of norms produced by the former patients.

Several groups of investigators have derived SCL-90R scoring methods for use with chronic pain patients. Jamison, Rock, and Parris (1988) have adopted a strategy for interpreting SCL-90R scores similar to one used with the MMPI (Bradley & Van der Heide, 1984). These investigators have empirically derived three subgroups of patients with chronic pain based on their SCL-90R responses. They found that patients with elevated scores on the majority of the scales, relative to those with scale scores within normal limits, reported the highest levels of (1) functional disability, (2) sleep disturbance, (3) usage of sleep medication, (4) family conflict, and (5) emotional distress. Butterworth and Deardorff (1987) identified three subgroups of patients with craniomandibular pain identical to those derived by Jamison and his colleagues based on SCL-90R responses. Using a revised scoring method based on their derived factors, Shutty and DeGood (1987) conducted a cluster-analytic study and found three replicable subgroups of male patients with back pain: (1) one subgroup reporting symptoms across almost all dimensions, (2) a second subgroup reporting a variety somatic complaints, and (3) a third subgroup reporting only back pain related somatic symptoms. Finally, Williams, Urban, Keefe, Shutty, and France (1995) attempted to replicate these findings in an outpatient pain clinic population consisting of men and women with heterogeneous pain complaints. These investigators derived three subgroups of patients that resembled those identified by Shutty and DeGood (1987). They also found the factor scoring method to be superior to standard scoring for these patients, as the former method produced patient clusters that were more distinct in reports of pain and pain behavior. However, no information has been published regarding the predictive validity of any of these SCL-90R subgroups with regard to treatment outcome.

A shortened version of the SCL-90R, the Brief Symptom Inventory (BSI; Derogatis & Spencer, 1983), is also available. This 53-item instrument also provides scores on nine subscales and three global scales. The BSI has not been used as extensively with pain patients as the SCL-90R; thus its reliability and validity with these patients are not well established.

Millon Behavioral Health Inventory

The MBHI is a 150-item self-report measure that was designed to evaluate the psychological functioning of medical patients. It includes: (1) eight scales that assess various dimensions of patients' styles of relating to health care providers (e.g., Cooperative, Forceful); (2) six scales that assess major psychosocial stressors (e.g., Future Despair, Social Alienation); and (3) six scales that assess probable response to illness (e.g., GI Susceptibility) and treatment interventions (e.g., Pain Treatment Responsivity). Patients respond to each item with "true" or "false," and their raw scores on each scale are transformed into "base rate" scores. Thus, for example, an elevated base rate score on GI Susceptibility indicates that the score is significantly greater than that expected, given the base rate of this variable within a normative sample of medical patients.

The MBHI has several advantages relative to the MMPI. First, it contains fewer items than the MMPI. Moreover, the items are not contaminated by symptoms of physical illness, and the norms are based on the responses of patients with a variety of medical (rather than psychiatric) disorders. The reliability and construct validity of the MBHI scales have been established in a series of studies summarized by Millon and colleagues (1983).

We have found the Somatic Anxiety and GI Susceptibility scales to be quite useful in our studies of patients with GI tract pain. For example, we have shown that these scales reliably differentiate patients with CPUE or IBS from patients with benign esophageal diseases and two groups of healthy control subjects (Richter et al., 1986). Among the patients with CPUE, the prevalence rates of significant psychological disturbance identified by the MBHI and the DIS were nearly equivalent. In addition, we have found excellent agreement between the MBHI scales and the SCL-90R Somatization and Global Severity Index scales in the assessment of patients with CPUE and hypertensive lower esophageal sphincter pressures (Waterman et al., 1989). Finally, we have demonstrated that the frequently reported association between stress and gastroesophageal reflux symptoms (heartburn) may be attributed to a tendency of persons with high levels of chronic anxiety to report intense reflux symptoms during stress in the absence of changes in esophageal acid exposure (Bradley et al., 1993).

The MBHI would be of exceptional value to clinicians and research investigators if it were confirmed that the instrument accurately predicted outcomes of treatment programs for patients with a variety of chronic pain syndromes. Unfortunately, two investigations have failed to show reliable relationships between the MBHI Pain Treatment Responsivity scale and patients' changes on subjective and objective outcome measures following treatment in a multidisciplinary pain clinic (Gatchel, Mayer, Capra, Barnett, & Diamond, 1986; Sweet, Breuer, Hazlewood, Toye, & Pawl, 1985). Negative results also have been reported for patients who participated in a behavioral program for chronic headaches (Gatchel, Deckel, Weinberg, & Smith, 1985), and for patients undergoing surgery for low back pain (Herron, Turner, Ersek, & Weiner, 1992). Nevertheless, Gatchel and colleagues (1986) did demonstrate that patients with chronic back pain who scored low on the Cooperative Style scale and high on the Sensitive Style scale showed poor treatment outcome.

Illness Behavior Questionnaire

The IBQ is a 62-item self-report measure that evaluates seven dimensions of abnormal illness behavior. Abnormal illness behavior is defined as "symptom complaints in the absence of somatic pathology, or the adoption by the patient of a sick role which the physician considers logically inconsistent with medical findings" (Hoon, Feuerstein, & Papciak, 1985, p. 385). The seven dimensions of abnormal illness behavior assessed by the IBQ are (1) General Hypochondriasis, (2) Disease Conviction, (3) Psychological versus Somatic Focus of Disease, (4) Affective Inhibition, (5) Affective Disturbance, (6) Denial of Life Problems Unrelated to Pain, and (7) Irritability. Patients respond to each IBQ item with "true" or "false." Although three relatively normal and three abnormal patterns have been identified by Pilowsky and Spence (1976), there are no norms against which patients' IBQ scale scores can be compared. The instrument also has been criticized for the lack of information regarding internal and test–retest reliability, as well as the use of inappropriate factor procedures in the derivation of the IBQ scales (Bradley et al., 1981). However, an interview form of the IBQ has been shown to be associated with adequate interrater reliability (mean percentage agreement of 88%) (Pilowsky, Bassett, Barrett, Petrovic, & Minniti, 1983).

With respect to construct validity, several investigations have shown that patients with diverse chronic pain syndromes or pain symptoms without organic pathology produce higher IBQ scores than controls (Drossman et al., 1988; Pilowsky, Chapman, & Bonica, 1977; Speculand, Goss, Spence, & Pilowsky, 1981). It has also been shown that the IBQ is associated with observational measures of abnormal illness behavior (Waddell, Pilowsky, & Bond, 1989) and pain behavior (Keefe, Crison, Maltbie, Bradley, & Gil, 1986).

Finally, a factor analytic study of the IBQ (Zonderman, Heft, & Costa, 1985) produced six factors that closely resembled those originally derived by Pilowsky and Spence (1975). These were (1) Health Worry, (2) Illness Disruption, (3) Affective Inhibition, (4) Affective Disturbance, (5) Avowed Absence of Life Problems, and (6) Irritability. Zonderman et al. found, however, that each of the factor scales was correlated significantly with Eysenck's Neuroticism scale (Eysenck & Eysenck, 1968). Thus it appears that the IBQ may primarily measure anxiety or other neurotic features, rather than specific patterns of abnormal illness behavior. This probably accounts for the IBQ's low predictive validity with regard to outcome of low back surgery after psychological stress was controlled for (Waddell et al., 1989). Moreover, in a study of the Disease Conviction subscale, Dworkin, Cooper, and Siegfried (1996) suggested that scores may reflect the consequences of chronic pain rather than an inappropriate belief in the presence of disease. We believe that future investigators must provide evidence for the reliability of the IBQ and demonstrate that the IBQ scales are associated with relevant criterion variables (e.g., pain behavior, return to work following surgery) independently of neuroticism before they can be used with confidence to assess abnormal illness behavior.

Summary

All of the psychological status measures described above have strengths and weaknesses. We recommend use of the MMPI and MBHI, however, since these instruments appear to possess the greatest strengths and fewest weaknesses. The MMPI has been used in numerous studies of populations with pain patient. The development of reliable MMPI and MMPI-2 profile patterns has helped to resolve some of the difficulties associated with the interpretation of profiles based on a psychiatric reference sample and with the instrument's predictive validity. Nevertheless, the length of the MMPI continues to reduce cooperation with psychological assessment among some patients with chronic pain.

The MBHI's greatest strengths are that it is relatively brief and that its norms are based on the responses of medical patients. Several of the scales regarding psychosocial stressors (e.g., GI Susceptibility) have been shown to differentiate patients with chronic pain from those with other chronic illnesses and from healthy controls. Greater attention, however, should be devoted to the utility of the remaining MBHI scales and to improving the predictive validity of the Pain Treatment Responsivity scale.

Both the SCL-90R and IBQ are brief measures that may be easily administered to patients with chronic pain. However, the value of both of these instruments in chronic pain assessment has been reduced by important questions that have been raised regarding their factor structures and predictive validity.

Measures of Major Stressful Life Events and Daily Hassles

Several investigators have begun to examine the extent to which self-reports of environmental stressors are associated with psychological distress and pain behavior. This interest in environmental stressors stems from the associations that have been established within "healthy" populations among stress, psychosocial variables, and physical as well as psychiatric symptoms (see, e.g., Kohn, Lafreniere, & Gurevich, 1991). Investigators typically have chosen to examine major life stressors (such as divorce, unemployment, and financial problems), as well as "hassles" or everyday events that are perceived as annoying or irritating (such as lack of sleep or rest, exposure to noise, or difficulty in relaxing). These investigators have most frequently assessed major life stressors with the Life Experiences Survey (Sarason, Johnson, & Siegel, 1978) and the Life Events and Difficulties Schedule (Brown & Harris, 1978). They have used the Daily Stress Inventory (Brantley, Waggoner, Jones, & Rappaport, 1987), the Schedule of Recent Life Events (Kohn & Macdonald, 1992), and the Hassles Scale (Kanner, Coyne, Schafer, & Lazarus, 1981) to evaluate the influence of everyday stressors on pain and other symptoms. All of these methods have been shown to be reliable and valid measures of different dimensions of environmental stress.

With regard to major life stressors, patients with back pain of unknown etiology appear significantly more likely to report adverse life events prior to pain onset than are patients whose back pain is due to a specific cause such as a herniated disc (Crauford, Creed, & Jayson, 1990). Major life events also differentiate patients with nonulcerative dyspepsia (upper abdominal pain that persists in the absence of an organic cause) from healthy control persons (Bennett, Beaurepaire, Langeluddecke, Kellow, & Tennant, 1991). However, patients with FM and IBS have tended to show levels of major life stress equal to or lower than those found in control groups composed of healthy persons or individuals with other chronic illnesses (Dailey, Bishop, Russell, & Fletcher, 1990; Drossman et al., 1988; Wolfe et al., 1984). Nevertheless, one prospective study of community residents with FM revealed that major stressors, such as beginning a new job or a change in residence, were significantly associated with seeking initial treatment for painful symptoms (Aaron, Bradley, Alexander, et al., 1997).

Several investigators have reported that the accuracy of patients' retrospective reports of major life events tends to decrease sharply as the time periods between those events and the assessments increase (e.g., Raphael, Cloitre, & Dohrenwend, 1991). There are methods for improving the accuracy of patients' recall of stressful events, such as the use of interviewer-administered checklists and structured probes (Dohrenwend, Link, Kern, Shrout, & Markowitz, 1987). However, these methods may be too time-consuming for use in a busy clinic setting or in research studies in which patient response burden must be considered.

Many investigators have directed their attention to measures of everyday stressors or hassles. Daily hassles have been shown to be positively associated with self-reports of psychological stress and health-care-seeking behavior among persons with FM (Dailey et al., 1990), negatively associated with use of adaptive coping strategies and overall well-being among patients with RA (Beckham, Keefe, Caldwell, & Roodman, 1991; Dwyer, 1997), and positively associated with reports of disease activity among patients with Crohn's disease (Garrett, Brantley, Jones, & McKnight, 1991). Several studies have examined the possible link between daily hassles and the experience of painful symptoms. Volinn, Lai, McKinney, and Loeser (1988) demonstrated that socioeconomic factors that can produce both major life events and everyday stressors are associated with pain behavior displayed by residents of large communities. These investigators examined differences in industrial insurance claim rates for back pain as a function of county in the state of Washington. They found that after they controlled for variables likely to predict back pain compensation claims, socioeconomic factors such as unemployment rate, per capita income, and percentage of individuals receiving food stamps accounted for approximately one-third of the variance in the rate of claims. Put another way, claims for disabling back pain increased in conjunction with greater economic hardship and job insecurity.

Several groups of investigators have studied the differential effects of major life events and daily hassles on patients with headache. Holm and colleagues (1986) found that hassles, but not major life events, were more prevalent in patients with tension headache than in healthy controls. Similarly, DeBenedittis and Lorenzetti (1992) found no significant differences between healthy controls and patients with chronic headache in the incidence or valence of major life events. However, the patients with headache reported greater frequency and intensity of daily hassles, even when potential headache-related items were excluded. Furthermore, patients with tension-type headache and mixed headache reported greater frequency and intensity of daily hassles than patients with migraine headaches. Fernandez and Sheffield (1996) examined the relationship between frequency and intensity of headaches and life stress. The average severity of daily hassles made a significant, albeit modest (5%–6% of the variance), contribution to the prediction of both the frequency and intensity of headaches.

Johnson, Gunning, and Lewis (1996) reported a possible link between daily hassles and health care seeking in patients suffering from heartburn. These investigators compared the hassles scores of patients seeking treatment for heartburn, community residents with heartburn who had not sought medical treatment for their condition (i.e., nonpatients), and healthy individuals. Patients reported a significantly greater number of daily hassles than nonpatients with heartburn, even when heartburn intensity was included as a covariate. Interestingly, the patients' average intensity rating of the hassles was significantly lower than that for either healthy individuals or nonpatients. Thus the patients may have shown high sensitivity to negative events, and thus may have regarded even low-intensity events as hassles. This propensity could have contributed to the decision to seek health care. In contrast, we recently reported that after demographic factors, psychiatric history, and other psychosocial factors,

were controlled for, severity of daily hassles (as measured by the Schedule of Recent Life Events) was a significant predictor of status as a patient or nonpatient with FM (Kersh et al., in press).

In summary, the growing literature regarding the association between environmental stressors and chronic pain is characterized by findings that differ as a function of type of pain syndrome and stressor. We recommend that all patient assessments devote attention to this issue, using either interview questions or one of the self-report methods discussed above.

Measures of Disability

The Sickness Impact Profile

The Sickness Impact Profile (SIP; Bergner, Bobbitt, Carter, & Gilson, 1981) is a 136-item measure of functional disability that may be administered as an interview or as a self-report questionnaire. The SIP provides a profile of patient disability on 12 dimensions of functioning: ambulation, mobility, body care and movement, social interaction, communication, alertness, emotional behavior, sleep and rest, eating, work, home management, and recreation. These dimensions may also be combined to form Physical, Psychosocial, and Total Disability scales. Each SIP item describes a specific dysfunctional behavior, and patients indicate whether or not each item applies to them. Scores are calculated for the Physical and Psychosocial Scales as well as for the Total Disability Scale by using predetermined weights that reflect the relative severity of each item. The test–retest reliabilities of these SIP scores over a 3-week interval have been shown to vary from .69 to .87 (Deyo, 1986; for a review, see DeBruin, DeWitte, Stevens, & Diederiks, 1992). The validity of the SIP was originally established by comparing patients' SIP responses with direct home observations of the patients' behavior. However, it has also been shown that SIP scores are significantly associated with self-reports of pain; with results of physical examination measures such as spinal flexion and straight-leg raising; and with scores on several other functional disability measures, such as the Functional Status Index (Jette, 1980) and the Index of Well-Being (Liang, Larson, Cullen, & Schwartz, 1985).

Studies of patients with arthritis have shown the efficiency and sensitivity of the SIP to be equal or superior to that of several other instruments with regard to changes in patient mobility, global functioning, and social functioning (Liang et al., 1985).

Follick, Smith, and Ahern (1985) have also produced positive evidence regarding the concurrent validity and sensitivity to change of SIP scores produced by patients with chronic back pain. As a result, numerous investigators have used the SIP as an outcome measure (e.g., Sanders & Brena, 1993; Turner & Clancy, 1988; Turner, Clancy, McQuade, & Cardenas, 1990) and a criterion measure (e.g., Hopman-Rock, Kraaimaat, Odding, & Bijlsma, 1998; Romano et al., 1995) in studies of patients with chronic pain.

The major drawback of the SIP is its length. Patients who are highly disabled often have difficulty in responding to 136 items without assistance. Therefore, Roland and Morris (1983) developed a 24-item version of the SIP. Although Deyo (1986) has presented positive evidence regarding the reliability and validity of this short SIP form, it should be noted that its items focus almost exclusively on the physical dimension of disability. The correlations between the short form of the SIP and the Physical and Psychosocial dimensions of the full SIP are .89 and .59, respectively (Deyo, 1986).

A 68-item short-form version of the SIP (SIP-68) has been developed that covers a wider range of areas of functioning (DeBruin, Diederiks, DeWitte, Stevens, & Philipsen, 1994). Item selection was based on a principal-components analysis that did not replicate the original 12-factor structure of the SIP. The 68 items constituting the short form loaded on six factors: Somatic Autonomy, Mobility Control, Psychic Autonomy and Communication, Social Behavior, Emotional Stability, and Mobility Range. The total score of the SIP-68 was highly correlated with the original version, and internal consistency was adequate, with alphas ranging from .72 to .85 (DeBruin, Diederiks, et al., 1994). Test–retest reliability of the SIP-68 has been assessed over four administrations in a 19-day period (day 1, day 3, day 17, and day 19). This revealed reliability coefficients of .97 for the total SIP-68 scores. Coefficients for the six category scores ranged from .90 to .97. Internal consistency, assessed by Cronbach's alpha, ranged from .90 to .92 for the total score and .49 to .87 for the category scores. Internal consistency did not substantially differ, regardless of whether the SIP-68 was administered as an independent instrument or as part of the full-length SIP (DeBruin, Buys, DeWitte, & Diederiks, 1994). Further analysis indicated that the SIP-68 does not differ from the original version in sensitivity to change in functional status (DeBruin, Diederiks, DeWitte, Stevens, & Philipsen, 1997). The strong psychometric properties of the SIP-68

suggest that it may prove to be a more useful measure of disability in patients with chronic pain than other brief instruments with important psychometric limitations, such as the Medical Outcome Study 36-Item Short-Form Health Survey (Gatchel, Polatin, Mayer, Robinson, & Dersh, 1998; Ware & Sherbourne, 1992).

The Chronic Illness Problem Inventory

Despite the strengths of the SIP described above, several investigators have devised alternative measures of disability (Bradley, 1989). One of the most promising of these alternatives is the Chronic Illness Problem Inventory (CIPI; Kames, Naliboff, Heinrich, & Schag, 1984). The CIPI is a 65–item self-report measure that assesses behavioral problems associated with a variety of chronic illnesses. Similar to the SIP, each CIPI item describes a problem in functioning; patients rate the extent to which each item applies to them on a 5-point scale. The advantages of the CIPI relative to the SIP are that it is brief and that it evaluates several behavioral dimensions that are not included in the SIP. The 18 CIPI scales consist of Activities of Daily Living, Inactivity, Social Activity, Family/Friends Contact, Employment, Sleep, Eating, Finances, Medication, Cognition, Physical Appearance, Body Deterioration, Sex, Assertion, Medical Interaction, Marital Overprotection, Marital Difficulty, and Nonmarital Relationships.

The initial CIPI reliability studies revealed that the internal consistencies (alpha coefficients) for the 18 scales ranged from .78 to .98. The test–retest reliability coefficients over a 1-week interval ranged from .69 to .97. The validity of the CIPI was established by demonstrating an agreement rate of 80% between problems identified by patients on the instrument and those noted on their evaluations by a clinical psychologist (Kames et al., 1984). In addition, the CIPI was shown to reliably differentiate patients with chronic pain from those with chronic respiratory disease or obesity Kames et al., 1984). Romano, Turner, and Jensen (1992) showed that the CIPI scores produced by patients with chronic pain are significantly correlated with their SIP scores (r's = .72 before treatment and .62 following treatment). These correlation coefficients also indicate that a substantial amount of variance is not shared by the two instruments, despite their strong association with each other (Romano et al., 1992). Thus the CIPI and SIP appear to be complementary measures of dysfunction among patients with chronic low back pain.

The West Haven–Yale Multidimensional Pain Inventory

Only one group of investigators has devoted effort to developing a comprehensive self-report instrument that evaluates the impact of diverse chronic pain syndromes on multiple dimensions of patients' lives. The West Haven–Yale Multidimensional Pain Inventory (WHYMPI; Kerns, Turk, & Rudy, 1985) is a 56-item measure with three sections. The first section includes items regarding (1) interference of pain with daily activities, work, family relationships, and social activities; (2) support from spouse or significant other; (3) pain severity and suffering; (4) perceived life control; and (5) negative mood. The second section assesses patients' perceptions of the degree to which spouses or significant others display solicitous, distracting, or punishing responses to pain or suffering behavior. The final WHYMPI section assesses the frequency with which patients engage in household chores, outdoor work, activities away from home, and social activities. Patients respond to the WHYMPI items on 7-point scales. These responses may be compared to a large normative database (see Jacob & Kerns, Chapter 19). Kerns and colleagues (1985) have demonstrated that the internal reliability coefficients of all WHYMPI scales range from .70 to .90; the test–retest reliabilities of these scales over a 2-week interval range from .62 to .91.

The validity of the WHYMPI was originally supported by the results of exploratory and confirmatory and exploratory factor-analytic investigations. These studies also revealed that the WHYMPI scales derived by factor analysis were significantly correlated with several criterion measures of anxiety, depression, marital satisfaction, pain severity, and health locus of control. Subsequent factor-analytic studies of the WHYMPI (Bernstein, Jaremko, & Hinkley, 1995; Riley, Zawacki, Robinson, & Geissner, 1999) have generally confirmed the original structure of the instrument. However, they also have identified some anomalies, such as items with loadings on more than one factor and associations among some of the subscales that are meant to be orthogonal.

Other validity studies (Turk, Okifuji, Sinclair, & Starz, 1996; Turk & Rudy, 1990; Walter & Brannon, 1991) have shown that three WHYMPI profile patterns may be reliably identified within samples of patients with chronic low back pain, temporomandibular disorders, FM, and headaches. These patterns have been labeled Dysfunctional, Interpersonally Distressed, and Adaptive Coper profiles. Dysfunctional profile patterns are characterized by relatively high levels of pain severity, life interference, and affective distress, as well as relatively low levels of life control and activity. Interpersonally Distressed profile patterns are characterized by relatively low levels of support from significant others in the environment. The Adaptive Coper profile patterns are the converse of the Dysfunctional patterns. That is, they are characterized by relatively low levels of pain severity, activity interference, and affective distress, as well as by relatively high levels of life control. Dysfunction, as measured by the WHYMPI, is related to psychopathology on the MMPI (Etscheidt, Steger, & Braverman, 1995). Dysfunctional patterns are also associated with relatively high levels of pain-related fear, anxiety, and avoidance behaviors (Asmundson, Norton, & Allerdings, 1997; McCracken, Spertus, Janeck, Sinclair, & Wetzel, 1999). Additionally, in a study of patients with FM, those with the Dysfunctional and Interpersonally Distressed patterns reported higher levels of pain, disability, and depression than those with the Adaptive Copers pattern (Turk et al., 1996). Notably, this tripartite classification scheme for patients with chronic pain has been replicated with alternate measures of the WHYMPI constructs (Jamison, Rudy, Penzien, & Mosley, 1994). This suggests that the three WHYMPI subgroup classifications are quite robust. These studies also indicate that it usually is not possible to classify between 20% and 30% of patients with chronic pain in one of the three WHYMPI subgroups. A recent study, however, showed that a minor supplement to the instructions explaining the phrase *significant other* significantly reduces the number of patients who cannot be classified due to missing data (Okifuji, Turk, & Everleigh, 1999; see Jacob & Kerns, Chapter 19, to view the new instructions).

Several studies (Dahlstrom, Widmark, & Carlsson, 1997; Turk, Okifuji, Sinclair & Starz, 1998; Turk, Rudy, Kubinski, Zaki, & Greco, 1996) have demonstrated the WHYMPI's utility in predicting treatment response. Turk and colleagues (1998) examined the outcomes of patients with FM in an outpatient pain treatment program as a function of WHYMPI classification. Those with the Dysfunctional pattern showed significant reductions in pain, affective distress, perceived disability, and perceived interference of pain. Those with the Adaptive Copers pattern showed significant reductions in pain, but showed no change in affective distress or disability as their pretreatment scores on these were quite low. Those with the Interpersonally Distressed pattern, however, had a generally poor response to treatment. Similarly, Turk, Rudy, Kubinski, and colleagues (1996) reported that patients with Dysfunctional patterns and temporomandibular disorders showed significantly greater improvements in pain, depression, and medication use when they received cognitive therapy in addition to stress management and use of an intraoral appliance, compared to stress management and the appliance alone. In contrast, Dahlstrom and colleagues (1997) found a significant association between Dysfunctional WHYMPI profiles and treatment failure among patients with temporomandibular disorders.

Summary

In summary, there are three self-report measures that may be used to assess disability and suffering among patients with diverse chronic pain syndromes. One of these measures, the SIP, measures disability in both the physical and psychosocial domains of functioning. This instrument is the most extensively studied disability measure in the chronic pain literature; it is especially useful in treatment outcome studies, due to its high levels of sensitivity and measurement efficiency. There is a large response burden associated with the SIP because of its length. However, the SIP-68 is a promising alternative to the original instrument, due to its relative brevity and strong psychometric properties. Investigators also may wish to use the CIPI as a complementary instrument, given that it assesses several areas of suffering (e.g., finances, sex, medical interaction) that are not evaluated by the SIP. The WHYMPI is a measure of disability and response to chronic pain that is noteworthy for its assessment of a large number of behavioral and psychosocial dimensions with only 56 items. Recent studies have also suggested that the WHYMPI may be useful for predicting treatment response. The WHYMPI represents a highly valuable assessment tool for clinicians or investigators who wish to measure multiple dimensions of adaptation to chronic pain without placing an excessive response burden on patients.

Measures of Pain-Related Anxiety and Fear

Fordyce (1976) first suggested that relationships exist between chronic pain and constructs such as anxiety, fear, and avoidance learning. Investigators devoted little attention to these relationships until the 1990s. However, researchers developed and validated four measures of pain-related anxiety and fear between 1990 and 1999.

The Pain Anxiety Symptoms Scale (PASS; McCracken, Zayfert, & Gross, 1992) is a 53-item scale that assesses fear of pain across cognitive, behavioral, and physiological domains. The PASS items were rationally derived for inclusion in four subscales: Fear of Pain, Cognitive Anxiety, Somatic Anxiety, and Escape and Avoidance. Patients respond to these items on a 6-point scale ranging from 0 ("never") to 6 ("always"). Internal consistency is good, with Cronbach's alpha ranging from .81 to .89 for the subscales and .94 for the total score (McCracken et al., 1992). Evidence for the construct validity of the instrument was established by moderate correlations of PASS scores with other measures of anxiety (McCracken et al., 1992). In addition, the PASS Cognitive Anxiety subscale was more strongly associated with cognitive anxiety than with somatic anxiety as measured by the Cognitive Somatic Anxiety Questionnaire (CSAQ; Schwartz, Davidson, & Goleman, 1978). Similarly, PASS Somatic or Anxiety scores were more strongly related to somatic than cognitive anxiety on the CSAQ. We recently found that patients with FM who produce high total scores on the PASS show significant increases in pain and in blood flow in the right anterior cingulate cortex during anticipation of acute pain (Alberts et al., 2000).

McCracken and colleagues (1992) established the concurrent validity of the PASS by demonstrating significant correlations between the PASS and the interference scale of the WHYMPI, the BDI, and self-reports of disability as measured by the Pain Disability Index (Pollard, 1984). Furthermore, the PASS was a better predictor of disability and interference than measures of general anxiety and emotional distress, as well as the Sensory scale of the MPQ (McCracken et al., 1992). A subsequent study (Burns, Mullen, Higdon, Wei, & Lansky, 2000) found that the PASS accounted for little unique variance in self-reported disability among workers injured on the job, after trait anxiety, depression, and pain severity were controlled for. Nevertheless, these and other investigators also reported that PASS scores are related to behavioral measures of disability. Patients' PASS scores are positively correlated with reports of anxiety on a leg-raising exercise (McCracken et al., 1992) and are negatively associated with measures of lifting and carrying capacity (Burns et al., 2000). Finally, a factor-analytic study of PASS responses produced a five-factor solution that showed moderate correspondence with the four domains of the instrument. The five derived factors were Catastrophic Thoughts, Physiological Anxiety, Escape/Avoidance, Cognitive Interference, and Coping Strategies (Larsen, Taylor, & Asmundson, 1997).

The Tampa Scale (TS; Clark, Kori, & Broeckel, 1996) was developed as a measure of *kinesiophobia*, or the fear of movement/(re)injury (Kori, Miller, & Todd, 1990). The TS is a 13-item scale in which items are rated on a 4-point Likert scale ranging from "strongly disagree" to "strongly agree." Factor analysis has identified two underlying dimensions: Activity Avoidance and Pathological Somatic Focus. Internal consistency for the total scale is adequate, with an alpha coefficient of .86 (Clark et al., 1996). Although the validity of this instrument has not been well studied in North America, investigations in the Netherlands have found that the TS is correlated with patients' reports of catastrophizing and depression and with performance on behavioral tasks such as lifting and trunk extension–flexion (Crombez, Vlaeyen, Heuts, & Lysens, 1999; Vlaeyen, Kole-Snijders, Boeren, & van Eek, 1995), as well as with muscle reactivity in patients high on negative affect (Vlaeyen et al., 1999).

The Fear-Avoidance Beliefs Questionnaire (FABQ; Waddell, Newton, Henderson, Somerville, & Main, 1993) evaluates patients' beliefs about how physical activity and work may affect their back pain. It is a 16-item questionnaire that utilizes a 7-point Likert scale with responses ranging from "strongly disagree" to "strongly agree." A test-retest reliability study over 48 hours revealed that patients showed an exact item agreement of 71% and an average kappa coefficient for the 16 items of .74 (Waddell et al., 1993). Principal-components analysis produced a two-factor structure: (1) fear–avoidance beliefs related to work and (2) fear–avoidance beliefs about physical activity in general. These factor scales are significantly correlated with disability ratings produced by back pain patients (Waddell et al., 1993). In addition, fear-avoidance belief scores regarding general physical activity are negatively correlated with performance on behavioral tasks (Crombez et al., 1999; Vlaeyen et al., 1995).

The Fear of Pain Questionnaire–III (FPQ-III) is the newest measure of pain anxiety. This 30-item questionnaire was designed to measure fear of pain in healthy persons, as well as in patients with painful conditions (McNeil & Rainwater, 1998). Respondents use a 5-point Likert scale ranging from "not at all" to "extreme" to rate the amount of fear they would experience in each of 30 events involving pain. Principal-components analysis identified a three-factor structure: Fear of Severe Pain, Fear of Minor Pain, and Fear of Medical Pain. Test-retest reliability over a 3-week interval was .74 for the total score, with coefficients ranging from .60 to .76 across the three subscales. Internal consistency is good, with alpha coefficients ranging from .87 to .92. The validity of the FPQ-III has been examined in clinical populations, such as patients treated in an inpatient pain program, as well as in patients with chronic headache (Hursey & Jacks, 1992; McNeil & Rainwater, 1998). Hursey and Jacks (1992) found that the FPQ-III scores of patients with headache were positively associated with their reports of life disruptions, depression and anxiety.

In summary, several instruments have been developed to assess anxiety and fear related to pain. Preliminary studies provide support for their use in the research setting. However, no studies have established whether patients' responses to these measures are associated with response to treatment or disability behavior over extended time periods. Thus it is not yet appropriate to use these measures to make clinical predictions about patients' responses to treatment, or to make judgments about patients' eligibility for disability compensation.

The Pain Stages of Change Questionnaire

Although many of the psychological status measures used with patients who have chronic pain are intended to evaluate psychopathology, most clinicians and investigators agree that "normal" psychological factors must also be assessed. Much of the work in this area has been devoted to the evaluation of patients' coping strategies and perceptions of self-efficacy, as these factors tend to be associated with outcomes produced by cognitive-behavioral and other self-management therapies (see DeGood & Tait, Chapter 17).

Recently, however, some investigators have begun to examine factors associated with changes in health behaviors that may also be relevant to pain. One especially promising product of this work is the Pain Stages of Change Questionnaire (PSOCQ; Kerns, Rosenberg, Jamison, Caudill, & Haythornthwaite, 1997). The PSOCQ is based on the transtheoretical model of behavioral change (Prochaska & DiClemente, 1984) and is designed to assess the degree to which patients are ready to adopt a self-management approach to their chronic pain condition. This model suggests that each individual shows variations in his or her readiness to alter different health-related behaviors. Therefore, the PSOCQ includes four scales that correspond to the model's stages of readiness for behavioral change (i.e., Precontemplation, Contemplation, Preparation, and Action/Maintenance). These scales include 30 items to which patients respond on a 6-point Likert scale ranging from "strongly disagree" to "strongly agree." Internal reliability is good, with alpha coefficients ranging from .77 to .86. The PSOCQ is also characterized by short-term stability, as its test–retest reliability coefficients over 1 to 2 weeks range from .74 to .88 (Kerns et al., 1997).

The criterion-related validity of the PSOCQ was established by the finding that the instrument accurately distinguished the completers of a cognitive-behavioral pain treatment program from the noncompleters (Kerns et al., 1997). Baseline Precontemplation and Contemplation scores best discriminated these two groups. In addition, increased scores from baseline to posttreatment on the Action/Maintenance scale and decreases on the Precontemplation scale were associated with improved outcomes (Kerns & Rosenberg, 2000). Although it is necessary to attempt to replicate these results in other treatment settings, the PSOCQ may prove to be a highly accurate predictor of patients' responses to self-management therapies for pain.

CONCLUSIONS

In this chapter, we have reviewed a wide array of psychological assessment procedures that may be used with patients who have chronic pain. We noted that assessment of patients with chronic pain requires the administration of at least one interview with the patient and spouse (or other family member) and one or more patient self-report measures. A semistructured interview (e.g., Gatchel, 2000; Karoly & Jensen, 1989; Phillips, 1988) is usually most appropriate. This interview should include questions regarding (1) the patient's pain history, (2) events that precede or follow exacerbations in the patient's pain perceptions or behavior, (3) the patient's daily activities, (4) social models for pain and disability, (5) occurrence of sexual or physical abuse, and (6) affective disturbance.

The information that is derived from the interview should be compared and integrated with the patient's responses to one or more self-report measures, in order to help support evaluative inferences regarding the patient and to aid in treatment planning. These self-report measures should provide information regarding psychological status, environmental stressors, functional disability, pain-related cognitions, and related aspects of psychosocial adaptation. If the evaluation must be limited to only one instrument, we suggest that the WHYMPI would be the most appropriate and useful assessment measure. However, we usually prefer to use multiple assessment measures. When it is possible to use more than one measure, investigators and clinicians may consider using either the MMPI or the MBHI to evaluate psychological status. These assessment devices also may be supplemented by a structured psychiatric interview such as the DIS or SCID. Environmental stressors may be evaluated with measures such as the Life Experiences Survey, the Schedule of Recent Life Events, or the Daily Stress Inventory. Retrospective reports of major life events over long time periods, however, are often inaccurate. It is also important to evaluate pain-related anxiety or fear that might be related to treatment outcomes. The PASS is probably the instrument of choice in most situations at present because it has been evaluated by a large number of investigators. The PSOCQ is a promising instrument for patient evaluation and tailoring treatment to patients' needs. Finally, the SIP (or SIP-68) and the CIPI may be used either singly or in combination to evaluate disability across a large number of domains of functioning.

ACKNOWLEDGMENTS

Preparation of this chapter was supported by grants from the National Institute of Arthritis and Musculoskeletal and Skin Diseases (No. 1 RO1 AR43136-05, No. P60 AR20164), and the National Institute of Diabetes and Digestive and Kidney Diseases (No. RO1 DK42428). We would also like to thank Brian C. Kersh and Erin S. Straight for their assistance in preparing the manuscript.

REFERENCES

Aaron, L. A., Bradley, L. A., Alarcón, G. S., Alexander, R. W., Triana-Alexander, M., Martin, M. Y., & Alberts, K. R. (1996). Psychiatric diagnoses in patients with fibromyalgia are related to health care-seeking behavior rather than to illness. *Arthritis and Rheumatism, 39*(3), 436–445.

Aaron, L. A., Bradley, L. A., Alarcón, G. S., Triana-Alexander, M., Alexander, R. W., Martin, M. Y., & Alberts, K. R. (1997). Perceived physical and emotional trauma as precipitating events in fibromyalgia: Association with health care seeking and disability status but not pain severity. *Arthritis and Rheumatism, 40,* 453–460.

Aaron, L. A., Bradley, L. A., Alexander, M. T., Alexander, R. W., Alberts, K. R., Martin, M. Y., & Alarcón, G. S. (1997). Work stress, psychiatric history, and medication usage predict initial use of medical treatment for fibromyalgia symptoms: A prospective analysis. In T. S. Jensen, J. A. Turner, & Z. Wiesenfeld-Hallin (Eds.), *Proceedings of the 7th World Congress on Pain: Progress in pain research and management* (pp. 683–691). Seattle, WA: International Association for the Study of Pain Press.

Ahles, T. A., Yunus, M. B., & Masi, A. T. (1987). Is chronic pain a variant of depressive disease?: The case of primary fibromyalgia syndrome. *Pain, 29,* 105–111.

Alberts, K. R., Bradley, L. A., Alarcón, G. S., Mountz, J. M., Sotolongo, A., & Liu, H.-G. (2000). Anticipation of acute pain and high arousal feedback in women with fibromyalgia (FM), high pain anxiety, and high negative affectivity (NA) evokes increased pain and anterior cingulate cortex (ACC) activity without nociception. *Arthritis and Rheumatism, 44,* S637.

Alexander, R. W., Bradley, L. A., Alarcón, G. S., Triana-Alexander, M., Aaron, L. A., Alberts, K. R., Martin, M. Y., & Stewart, K. E. (1998). Sexual and physical abuse in women with fibromyalgia: Association with outpatient health care utilization and pain medication usage. *Arthritis Care and Research, 11,* 102–115.

American Psychiatric Association. (1987). *Diagnostic and statistical manual of mental disorders* (3rd ed., rev.). Washington, DC: Author.

American Psychiatric Association. (1994). *Diagnostic and statistical manual of mental disorders* (4th ed.). Washington, DC: Author.

Anderson, K. O., Bradley, L. A., Young, L. D., McDaniel, L. K., & Wise, C. M. (1985). Rheumatoid arthritis: Review of psychological factors related to etiology, effects, and treatment. *Psychological Bulletin, 98,* 358–387.

Asmundson, G. J., Norton, G. R., & Allerdings, M. D. (1997). Fear and avoidance in dysfunctional chronic back pain patients. *Pain, 69,* 231–236.

Atkinson, J. H., Slater, M. A., Patterson, T. L., Grant, I., & Garfin, S. R. (1991). Prevalence, onset, and risk of psychiatric disorders in men with chronic low back pain: A controlled study. *Pain, 45,* 111–131.

Beck, A. T., & Steer, R. A. (1993). *Beck Depression Inventory.* San Antonio, TX: Psychological Corporation.

Beck, A. T., Steer, R. A., & Garbin, M. G. (1988). Psychometric properties of the Beck Depression Inventory: Twenty-five years of evaluation. *Clinical Psychology Review, 8,* 77–100.

Beckham, J. C., Keefe, F. J., Caldwell, D. S., & Roodman, A. A. (1991). Pain coping strategies in rheumatoid arthritis: Relationship to pain, disability, depression, and daily hassles. *Behavior Therapy, 22,* 113–124.

Beitman, B. D., Basha, I. M., Trombka, L. H., Jayaratna, M. A., Russell, B., Flaker, G., & Anderson, S. (1989). Pharmacotherapeutic treatment of panic disorder in patients presenting with chest pain. *Journal of Family Practice, 28,* 177–180.

Beitman, B. D., Mukerji, V., Kushner, M., Thomas, A. M., Russell, J. L., & Logue, M. B. (1991). Validating studies for panic disorder in patients with angiographically normal coronary arteries. *Medical Clinics of North America, 75,* 1143–1155.

Bennett, E., Beaurepaire, J., Langeluddecke, P., Kellow, J., & Tennant, C. (1991). Life stress and non-ulcer dyspepsia: A case–control study. *Journal of Psychosomatic Research, 35,* 579–590.

Ben-Porath, Y. S., & Graham, J. R. (1991). Resolutions to interpretive dilemmas created by the Minnesota Multiphasic Personality Inventory 2 (MMPI-2): A reply to Strassberg. *Journal of Psychopathology and Behavioral Assessment, 13,* 173–179.

Ben-Porath, Y. S., & Sherwood, N. E. (1993). *The MMPI-2 content component scales: Development, psychometric characteristics, and clinical application.* Minneapolis: University of Minnesota Press.

Bergner, M., Bobbitt, R. A., Carter, W. B., & Gibson, B. S. (1981). The Sickness Impact Profile: Development and final revision of a health status measure. *Medical Care, 19,* 787–805.

Bernstein, I. H., Jaremko, M. E., & Hinckley, B. S. (1995). On the utility of the West Haven–Yale Multidimensional Pain Inventory. *Spine, 20,* 956–963.

Bigos, S. J., Battie, M. C., Spengler, D. M., Fisher, L. D., Fordyce, W. E., Hansson, T. H., Nachemson, A. L., & Wortley, M. D. (1991). A prospective study of work perceptions and psychosocial factors affecting the report of back injury. *Spine, 16,* 1–6.

Block, A. R., Kremer, E. F., & Gaylor, M. (1980). Behavioral treatment of chronic pain: The spouse as a discriminative cue for pain behavior. *Pain, 9,* 243–252.

Blumer, D., & Heilbronn, M. (1982). Chronic pain as a variant of depressive disease: The pain-prone disorder. *Journal of Nervous and Mental Disease, 170,* 381–406.

Bradley, L. A. (1989). Psychological evaluation of the low back pain patient. In C. D. Tollison & M. L. Krieger (Eds.), *Interdisciplinary rehabilitation of low back pain* (pp. 33–50). Baltimore: Williams & Wilkins.

Bradley, L. A. (1994). Psychological dimensions of rheumatoid arthritis. In F. Wolfe & T. Pincus (Eds.), *Rheumatoid arthritis: Pathogenesis, assessment, outcome, and treatment* (pp. 273–295). New York: Marcel Dekker.

Bradley, L. A., Prokop, C. K., Gentry, W. D., Van der Heide, L. H., & Prieto, E. J. (1981). Assessment of chronic pain. In C. K. Prokop & L. A. Bradley (Eds.), *Medical psychology: Contributions to behavioral medicine* (pp. 91–117). New York: Academic Press.

Bradley, L. A., Prokop, C. K., Margolis, R., & Gentry, W. D. (1978). Multivariate analyses of the MMPI profiles of low pack pain patients. *Journal of Behavioral Medicine, 1,* 253–272.

Bradley, L. A., Richter, J. E., Pulliam, T. J., Haile, J. M., Scarinci, I. C., Schan, C. A., Dalton, C. B., & Sally, A. N. (1993). The relationship between stress and symptoms of gastroesophageal reflux: The influence of psychological factors. *American Journal of Gastroenterology, 88,* 11–19.

Bradley, L. A., Scarinci, I. C., & Richter, J. E. (1991). Pain threshold levels and coping strategies among patients who have chest pain and normal coronary arteries. *Medical Clinics of North America, 75,* 1189–1202.

Bradley, L. A., & Van der Heide, L. H. (1984). Pain-related correlates of MMPI profile subgroups among back pain patients. *Health Psychology, 3,* 157–174.

Brantley, P. J., Waggoner, C. D., Jones, G. N., & Rappaport, N. B. (1987). A Daily Stress Inventory: Development, reliability, and validity. *Journal of Behavioral Medicine, 10,* 61–74.

Briere, J., & Runtz, M. (1988). Multivariate correlates of childhood psychological and physical maltreatment among university women. *Child Abuse and Neglect, 12,* 331–341.

Brown, G. K. (1990). A causal analysis of chronic pain and depression. *Journal of Abnormal Psychology, 99,* 127–137.

Brown, G. W., & Harris, T. (1978). *Social origins of depression: A study of psychiatric disorder in women.* New York: Free Press.

Buckelew, S. P., DeGood, D. E., Schwartz, D. P., & Kerler, R. M. (1986). Cognitive and somatic item response patterns of pain patients, psychiatric patients, and hospital employees. *Journal of Clinical Psychology, 42,* 852–860.

Burns, J. W., Mullen, J. T., Higdon, L. J., Wei, J. M., & Lansky, D. (2000). Validity of the Pain Anxiety Symptoms Scale (PASS): Prediction of physical capacity variables. *Pain, 84,* 247–252.

Buskila, D., Neumann, L., Hazanov, I., & Carmi, R. (1996). Familial aggregation in the fibromyalgia syndrome. *Seminars in Arthritis and Rheumatism, 26,* 605–611.

Butterworth, J. C., & Deardoff, W. W. (1987). Psychometric profiles of craniomandibular pain patients: Identifying specific subgroups. *Journal of Craniomandibular Practice, 5,* 225–232.

Cahill, C., Llewelyn, S. P., & Pearson, C. (1991). Treatment of sexual abuse which occurred in childhood: A review. *British Journal of Clinical Psychology, 30,* 1–12.

Cannon, R. O., III, Quyyumi, A. A., Mincemoyer, R., Stine, A. M., Gracely, R. H., Smith, W. B., Geraci, M. F., Black, B. C., Uhde, T. W., Waclawiw, M. A., Maher, K., &, Benjamin, S. B. (1994). Imipramine in patients with chest pain despite normal coronary angiograms. *New England Journal of Medicine, 330,* 1411–1417.

Clark, M. E. (1996). MMPI-2 Negative Treatment Indicators content and content component scales: Clinical correlates and outcome prediction for men with chronic pain. *Psychological Assessment, 8,* 32–38.

Clark, M. E., Kori, S. H., & Broeckel, J. (1996, November). *Kinesiophobia and chronic pain: Psychometric characteristics and factor analysis of the Tampa Scale.* Paper presented at the 15th Annual Scientific Meeting of the American Pain Society, Washington, DC.

Clouse, R. E. (1991). Psychiatric disorders in patients with esophageal disease. *Medical Clinics of North America, 75,* 1081–1096.

Cormier, L. E., Katon, W., Russo, J., Hollifield, M., Hall, M. L., & Vitaliano, P. P. (1988). Chest pain with negative cardiac diagnostic studies: Relationship to psychiatric illness. *Journal of Nervous and Mental Disease, 176,* 351–358.

Costello, R. M., Hulsey, T. L., Schoenfeld, L. S., & Ramamurthy, S. (1987). P-A-I-N: A four-cluster MMPI typology for chronic pain. *Pain, 30,* 199–209.

Crauford, D. I. O., Creed, F., & Jayson, M. I. V. (1990). Life events and psychological disturbance in patients with low-back pain. *Spine, 15,* 490–494.

Crombez, G., Vlaeyen, J. W. S., Heuts, P. H. T. G., & Lysens, R. (1999). Pain-related fear is more disabling than pain itself: Evidence on the role of pain-related fear in chronic back pain disability. *Pain, 80,* 329–339.

Dailey, P. A., Bishop, G. D., Russell, I. J., & Fletcher, E. M. (1990). Psychological stress and the fibrositis fibromyalgia syndrome. *Journal of Rheumatology, 17,* 1380–1385.

Dahlstrom, L., Widmark, G., & Carlsson, S. G. (1997). Cognitive-behavioral profiles among different categories of orofacial pain patients: Diagnostic and treatment implications. *European Journal of the Oral Sciences, 105,* 377–383.

DeBenedittis, G., & Lorenzetti, A. (1992). The role of stressful life events in the persistence of primary headache: Major events vs. daily hassles. *Pain, 51,* 35–42.

DeBruin, A. F., Buys, M., DeWitte, L. P., & Diederiks, J. P. M. (1994). The Sickness Impact Profile: SIP68, a short generic version. First evaluation of the reliability and reproducibility. *Journal of Clinical Epidemiology, 47,* 863–871.

DeBruin, A. F., DeWitte, L. P., Stevens, F., & Diederiks, J. P. M. (1992). Sickness Impact Profile: The state of the art of a generic functional status measure. *Social Science and Medicine, 35,* 1003–1014.

DeBruin, A. F., Diederiks, J. P. M., DeWitte, L. P., Stevens, L. P., & Philipsen, H. (1994). The development of a short generic version of the Sickness Impact Profile. *Journal of Clinical Epidemiology, 47,* 407–418.

DeBruin, A. F., Diederiks, J. P. M., DeWitte, L. P., Stevens, L. P., & Philipsen, H. (1997). Assessing the responsiveness of a functional status measure: The Sickness Impact Profile versus the SIP68. *Journal of Clinical Epidemiology, 50,* 529–540.

Derogatis, L. (1983). *The SCL-90R manual–II: Administration, scoring and procedures.* Towson, MD: Clinical Psychometric Research.

Derogatis, L., & Spencer, P. (1983). *BSI manual I: Administration and procedures.* Baltimore: Johns Hopkins University School of Medicine, Clinical Psychometric Unit.

Deyo, R. A. (1986). Comparative validity of the Sickness Impact Profile and shorter scales for functional assessment in low-back pain. *Spine, 11,* 951–954.

Dickinson, L. M., deGruy, F. V., III, Dickinson, W. P., & Candib, L. M. (1999). Health-related quality of life and symptom profiles of female survivors of sexual abuse. *Archives of Family Medicine, 8,* 35–43.

Dohrenwend, B. P., Link, B. G., Kern, R., Shrout, P. E., & Markowitz, J. (1987). Measuring life events: The problems of variability within event categories. In B. Cooper (Ed.), *Psychiatric epidemiology: Progress and prospects* (pp. 103–119). London: Croom Helm.

Domino, J. V., & Haber, J. D. (1987). Prior physical and sexual abuse in women with chronic headache: Clinical correlates. *Headache, 27,* 310–314.

Drossman, D. A., Leserman, J., Nachman, G., Li, Z., Gluck, H., Toomey, T. C., & Mitchell, M. (1990). Sexual and physical abuse in women with functional or organic gastrointestinal disorders. *Annals of Internal Medicine, 113,* 828–833.

Drossman, D. A., McKee, D. C., Sandler, R. S., Mitchell, C. M., Cramer, E. M., Lowman, B. C., & Burger, A. L. (1988). Psychosocial factors in the irritable bowel syndrome: A multivariate study of patients and nonpatients with irritable bowel syndrome. *Gastroenterology, 95,* 701–708.

Dworkin, R. H., Cooper, E. M., & Siegfried, R. N. (1996). Chronic pain and disease conviction. *Clinical Journal of Pain, 12,* 111–117.

Dwyer, K. A. (1997). Psychosocial factors and health status in women with rheumatoid arthritis: Predictive models. *American Journal of Preventive Medicine, 13,* 66–72.

Eaton, W. W., Neufeld, K., Chen, L. S., & Cai, G. (2000). A comparison of self-report and clinical diagnostic interviews for depression: Diagnostic Interview Schedule and Schedules for Clinical Assessment in Neuropsychiatry in the Baltimore Epidemiologic Catchment Area follow-up. *Archives of General Psychiatry, 57,* 217–222.

Etscheidt, M. A., Steger, H. G., & Braverman, B. (1995). Multidimensional Pain Inventory profile classifications and psychopathology. *Journal of Clinical Psychology, 51,* 29–36.

Eysenck, H. J., & Eysenck, S. B. G. (1968). *The manual of the Eysenck Personality Inventory.* San Diego, CA: Educational and Industrial Testing Service.

Fernandez, E., & Sheffield, J. (1996). Relative contributions of life events versus daily hassles to the frequency and intensity of headaches. *Headache, 36,* 595–602.

First, M. B., Gibbon, M., Williams, J. B. W., & Spitzer, R. L. (2000). *SCID Screen Patient Questionnaire Computer Program.* North Tonawanda, NY: Multi-Health Systems.

First, M. B., Spitzer, R. L., Gibbon, M., & Williams, J. B.W. (1997). *User's guide for the Structured Clinical Interview for DSM-IV Axis I Disorders: SCID-I clinician version.* Washington, DC: American Psychiatric Press.

Flor, H., Kerns, R. D., & Turk, D. C. (1987). The role of the spouse in the maintenance of chronic pain. *Journal of Psychosomatic Research, 31,* 251–259.

Follick, M. J., Smith, T. W., & Ahern, D. K. (1985). The Sickness Impact Profile: A global measure of disability in chronic low back pain. *Pain, 21,* 67–76.

Fordyce, W. E. (1976). *Behavioral methods for chronic pain and illness.* St. Louis, MO: Mosby.

Gallagher, R. M., Rauh, V., Haugh, L. D., Milhous, R., Gallas, P. W., Langelier, R., McClallen, J. M., & Frymoyer, J. (1989). Determinants of return-to-work among low back pain patients. *Pain, 39,* 55–67.

Gamsa, A. (1990). Is emotional disturbance a precipitator or a consequence of chronic pain? *Pain, 42,* 183–195.

Gamsa, A., & Vickis-Freibergs, V. (1991). Psychological events are both risk factors in, and consequences of chronic pain. *Pain, 44,* 271–277.

Garrett, V. D., Brantley, P. J., Jones, G. N., & McKnight, G. T. (1991). The relation between daily stress and Crohn's disease. *Journal of Behavioral Medicine, 14,* 87–96.

Gatchel, R. J. (2000). How practitioners should evaluate personality to help manage patients with chronic pain. In R. J. Gatchell & J. N. Weisberg (Eds.), *Personality characteristics of patients with pain* (pp. 241–257). Washington, DC: American Psychological Association.

Gatchel, R. J., Deckel, A. W., Weinberg, N., & Smith, J. E. (1985). The utility of the Millon Behavioral Health Inventory in the study of chronic headaches. *Headache, 25,* 49–54.

Gatchel, R. J., Mayer, T. G., Capra, P., Barnett, J., & Diamond, P. (1986). Millon Behavioral Health Inventory: Its utility in predicting physical function in patients with low back pain. *Archives of Physical Medicine and Rehabilitation, 67,* 878–882.

Gatchel, R. J., Polatin, P. B., Mayer, T. G., Robinson, R., & Dersh, J. (1998). Use of the SF-36 health status survey with a chronically disabled back pain population: Strengths and limitations. *Journal of Occupational Rehabilitation, 8,* 237–246.

Geisser, M. E., Roth, R. S., & Robinson, M. E. (1997). Assessing depression among persons with chronic pain using the Center for Epidemiological Studies—Depression Scale and the Beck Depression Inventory: A comparative analysis. *Clinical Journal of Pain, 13,* 163–170.

Getto, C. J., Heaton, R. K., & Lehman, R. A. (1983). PSPI: A standardized approach to the evaluation of psychosocial factors in chronic pain. *Advances in Pain Research and Therapy, 5,* 885–889.

Gil, K. M., Keefe, F. J., Crisson, J. E., & Van Dalfsen, P. J. (1987). Social support and pain behavior. *Pain, 29,* 209–217.

Guck, T. P., Meilman, P. W., Skultety, M., & Poloni, I. D. (1988). Pain-patient Minnesota Multiphasic Personality Inventory (MMPI) subgroups: Evaluation of long-term treatment outcome. *Journal of Behavioral Medicine, 11,* 159–169.

Haber, J. D., & Roos, C. (1985). Effects of spouse abuse and/or sexual abuse in the development and maintenance of chronic pain in women. *Advances in Pain Research and Therapy, 9,* 889–895.

Haley, W. E., Turner, J. A., & Romano, J. M. (1985). Depression in chronic pain patients: Relation to pain, activity, and sex differences. *Pain, 23,* 337–343.

Hathaway, S. R., McKinley, J. C., Butcher, J. N., Dahlstrom, W. G., Graham, J. R., Tellegen, A., & Kaemmer, B. (1989). *Minnesota Multiphasic Personality Inventory–2: Manual for administration.* Minneapolis: University of Minnesota Press.

Haythornthwaite, J. A., Sieber, W. J., & Kerns, R. D. (1991). Depression and the chronic pain experience. *Pain, 46,* 177–184.

Heaton, R. K., Getto, C. J., Lehman, R. A. W., Fordyce, W. E., Brauer, E., & Groban, S. E. (1982). A standardized evaluation of psychosocial factors in chronic pain. *Pain, 12,* 165–174.

Helzer, J. E., & Robins, L. N. (1988). The Diagnostic Interview Schedule: Its development, evaluation, and use. *Social Psychiatry and Psychiatric Epidemiology, 23,* 6–16.

Helzer, J. E., Spitznagel, E. L., & McEvoy, L. (1987). The predictive validity of lay Diagnostic Interview Schedule diagnoses in the general population: A comparison with physician examiners. *Archives of General Psychiatry, 44,* 1069–1077.

Henrichs, T. F. (1987). MMPI profiles of chronic pain patients: Some methodological considerations that concern clusters and descriptors. *Journal of Clinical Psychology, 43,* 650–660.

Herron, L., Turner, J. A., Ersek, M., & Weiner, P. (1992). Does the Millon Behavioral Health Inventory (MBHI) predict lumbar laminectomy outcome?: A comparison with the Minnesota Multiphasic Personality Inventory (MMPI). *Journal of Spinal Disorders, 5,* 188–192.

Holm, J. E., Holroyd, K. A., Hursey, K. G., & Penzien, D. B. (1986). The role of stress in recurrent tension headache. *Headache, 26,* 160–167.

Hoon, P. W., Feuerstein, M., & Papciak, A. S. (1985). Evaluation of the chronic low back pain patient: Conceptual and clinical considerations. *Clinical Psychology Review*, 5, 377–401.

Hopman-Rock, M., Kraaimaat, F. W., Odding, E., & Bijlsma, J. W. (1998). Coping with pain in the hip or knee in relation to physical disability in community-living elderly people. *Arthritis Care and Research*, 11, 243–252.

Hudson, J. I., & Pope, H. G., Jr. (1996). The relationship between fibromyalgia and major depressive disorder. *Rheumatic Diseases Clinics of North America*, 22, 385–303.

Hursey, K. G., & Jacks, S. D. (1992). Fear of pain in recurrent headache sufferers. *Headache*, 32, 283–286.

Jamison, R. N., Rock, D. L., & Parris, W. C. V. (1988). Empirically derived Symptom Checklist 90 subgroups of chronic pain patients: A cluster analysis. *Journal of Behavioral Medicine*, 11, 147–158.

Jamison, R. N., Rudy, T. E., Penzien, D. B., & Mosley, T. H. (1994). Cognitive-behavioral classifications of chronic pain: Replication and extension of empirically derived patient profiles. *Pain*, 57, 277–292.

Jette, A. M. (1980). Functional status instrument: Reliability of a chronic disease evaluation instrument. *Archieves of Physical Medicine and Rehabilitation*, 61, 395–401.

Johnson, B. T., Gunning, J., & Lewis, S. A. (1996). Health care seeking by heartburn sufferers is associated with psychosocial factors. *American Journal of Gastroenterology*, 91, 2500–2504.

Kames, L. D., Naliboff, B. D., Heinrich, R. L, & Schag, C. C. (1984). The Chronic Illness Problem Inventory: Problem-oriented psychosocial assessment of patients with chronic illness. *International Journal of Psychiatry in Medicine*, 14, 65–75.

Kanner, A. D., Coyne, J. C., Schaefer, C., & Lazarus, R. S. (1981). Comparison of two modes of stress measurement: Daily hassles and uplifts versus major life events. *Journal of Behavioral Medicine*, 4, 1–39.

Karol, R. L, Micka, R. G., & Kuskowski, M. (1992, March). *Physical, emotional, and sexual abuse among pain patients and health care practitioners.* Poster presented at the meeting of the Society of Behavioral Medicine, New York.

Karoly, P., & Jensen, M. P. (1989). *Multimethod assessment of chronic pain.* New York: Pergamon Press.

Katon, W., Egan, K., & Miller, D. (1985). Chronic pain: Lifetime psychiatric diagnoses and family history. *American Journal of Psychiatry*, 142, 1156–1160.

Katon, W., Hall, M. L., Russo, J., Cormier, L., Hollifield, M., Vitaliano, P. O., & Beitman, B. D. (1988). Chest pain: Relationship of psychiatric illness to coronary arteriographic results. *American Journal of Medicine*, 84, 1–9.

Katon, W., & Roy-Byrne, P. P. (1991). Mixed anxiety and depression. *Journal of Abnormal Psychology*, 100, 337–445.

Keefe, F. J., & Bradley, L. A. (1984). Behavioral and psychological approaches to the assessment and treatment of chronic pain. *General Hospital Psychiatry*, 6, 49–54.

Keefe, F. J., Crisson, J. E., Maltbie, A., Bradley, L., & Gil, K. M. (1986). Illness behavior as a predictor of pain and overt behavior patterns in chronic low back pain patients. *Journal of Psychosomatic Research*, 30, 543–551.

Kerns, R. D., Haythornthwaite, J., Southwick, S., & Giller, E. L. (1990). The role of marital interaction in chronic pain and depressive symptom severity. *Journal of Psychosomatic Research*, 34, 401–408.

Kerns, R. D., & Rosenberg, R. (2000). Predicting responses to self-management treatments for chronic pain: Application of the pain stages of change model. *Pain*, 84, 49–55.

Kerns, R. D., Rosenberg, R., Jamison, R. N., Caudill, M. A., & Haythornthwaite, J. (1997). Readiness to adopt a self-management approach to chronic pain: The Pain Stages of Change Questionnaire (PSOCQ). *Pain*, 72, 227–234.

Kerns, R. D., Southwick, S., Giller, E. L., Haythornthwaite, J. A., Jacob, M. C., & Rosenberg, R. (1991). The relationship between reports of pain-related social interactions and expressions of pain and affective distress. *Behavior Therapy*, 22, 101–111.

Kerns, R. D., & Turk, D. C. (1984). Depression and chronic pain: The mediating role of the spouse. *Journal of Marriage and the Family*, 46, 845–852.

Kerns, R. D., Turk, D. C., & Rudy, T. E. (1985). The West Haven–Yale Multidimensional Pain Inventory (WHYMPI). *Pain*, 23, 345–356.

Kersh, B. C., Bradley, L. A., Alarcon, G. S., Alberts, K. R., Sotolongo, A., Martin, M. Y., Aaron, L. A., Dewaal, D. F., Domino, M. L., Chaplin, W. F., Palardy, N. R., Cianfrini, L. R., Triana-Alexander, M. (in press). *Psychosocial and health status variables independently predict health care seeking in fibromyalgia. Arthritis Care and Research.*

Klimes, I., Mayou, R. A., Pearce, M. J., Coles, L., & Fagg, J. R. (1990). Psychological treatment for atypical noncardiac chest pain: A controlled evaluation. *Psychological Medicine*, 20, 605–611.

Kohn, P. M., Lafreniere, K., & Gurevich, M. (1991). Hassles, health, and personality. *Journal of Personality and Social Psychology*, 61, 478–482.

Kohn, P. M., & Macdonald, J. E. (1992). The survey of Recent Life Experiences: A decontaminated hassles scale for adults. *Journal of Behavioral Medicine*, 15, 221–236.

Kori, S. H., Miller, R. P., & Todd, D. D. (1990). Kinesiophobia: A new view of chronic pain behavior. *Pain Management*, 3, 35–43.

Larsen, D. K., Taylor, S., & Asmundson, G. J. G. (1997). Exploratory factor analysis of the Pain Anxiety Symptoms Scale in patients with chronic pain complaints. *Pain*, 69, 27–34.

Leserman, J., Drossman, D. A., Li, Z., Toomey, T. C., Nachman, G., & Glogan, L. (1996). Sexual and physical abuse history in gastroenterology practice: How types of abuse impact health status. *Psychosomatic Medicine*, 58, 4–15.

Levitt, E. E. (1990). A structural analysis of the impact of MMPI-2 on MMPI-1. *Journal of Personality Assessment*, 55, 572–577.

Liang, M. H., Larson, M. G., Cullen, K. E., & Schwartz, J. A. (1985). Comparative measurement efficiency and sensitivity of five health status instruments for arthritis research. *Arthritis and Rheumatism*, 28, 542–547.

Linton, S. J. (1997). A population-based study of the relationship between sexual abuse and back pain: Establishing a link. *Pain*, 73, 47–53.

Linton, S. J., & Bradley, L. A. (1992). An 18-month follow-up of a secondary prevention program for back pain:

Help and hindrance factors related to outcome maintenance. *Clinical Journal of Pain, 8,* 227–236.

Lorish, C. D., Abraham, N., Austin, J., Bradley, L. A., & Alarcón, G. C. (1991). Disease and psychosocial factors related to physical functioning in rheumatoid arthritis. *Journal of Rheumatology, 8,* 1150–1157.

Magni, G., Moreschi, C., Rigatti-Luchini, S., & Merskey, H. (1994). Prospective study on the relationship between depressive symptoms and chronic musculoskeletal pain. *Pain, 56, 289–297.*

Mayou, R. A., Bass, C. M., & Bryant, B. M. (1999). Management of non-cardiac chest pain: From research to clinical practice. *Heart, 81,* 387–392.

McCracken, L. M., Spertus, I. L., Janeck, A. S., Sinclair, D., & Wetzel, F. T. (1999). Behavioral dimensions of adjustment in persons with chronic pain: Pain-related anxiety and acceptance. *Pain, 80,* 283–289.

McCracken, L. M., Zayfert, C., & Gross, R. T. (1992). The Pain Anxiety Symptoms Scale: Development and validation of a scale to measure fear of pain. *Pain, 50,* 67–73.

McCreary, C. (1985). Empirically derived MMPI profile clusters and characteristics of low back pain patients. *Journal of Consulting and Clinical Psychology, 53,* 558–560.

McGill, J., Lawlis, F., Selby, D., Mooney, V., & McCoy, C. E. (1983). The relationship of Minnesota Multiphasic Personality Inventory (MMPI) profile clusters to pain behaviors. *Journal of Behavioral Medicine, 6,* 677–692.

McNeil, D. W., & Rainwater, A. J., III. (1998). Development of the Fear of Pain Questionnaire–III. *Journal of Behavioral Medicine, 21,* 389–410.

Melzack, R. (1975). The McGill Pain Questionnaire: Major properties and scoring methods. *Pain, 1,* 277–299.

Mikhail, S. F., & von Baeyer, C. L. (1990). Pain, somatic focus, and emotional adjustment in children of chronic headache sufferers and controls. *Social Science and Medicine, 31,* 51–59.

Millon, T., Green, C., & Meagher, R. (1983). *Millon Behavioral Health Inventory manual* (3rd ed.). Minneapolis, MN: National Computer Systems.

Monsein, M. (1990). Soft tissue pain and disability. *Advances in Pain Research and Therapy, 17,* 183–200.

Moore, J. E., Armentrout, D. P., Parker, J. C., & Kivlahan, D. R. (1986). Empirically-derived pain-patient MMPI subgroups: Prediction of treatment outcome. *Journal of Behavioral Medicine, 9,* 51–63.

Moore, J. E., McCallum, S., Holman, C., & O'Brien, S. (1991). *Prediction of return to work after pain clinic treatment by MMPI-2 clusters.* Paper presented at the meeting of the American Pain Society, New Orleans, LA.

Moore, J. E., McFall, M. E., Kivlahan, D. R., & Capestany, F. (1988). Risk of misinterpretation of MMPI Schizophrenia scale elevations in chronic pain patients. *Pain, 32,* 207–213.

Naliboff, B. D., Cohen, M. J., & Yellin, A. N. (1982). Does the MMPI differentiate chronic illness from chronic pain? *Pain, 13,* 333–341.

Nelson, A. F. (1986). *Impath TMJ: User reference manual.* Minneapolis, MN: Chronic Illness Care.

Neumann, L., & Buskila, D. (1997). Quality of life and physical functioning of relatives of fibromyalgia patients. *Seminars in Arthritis and Rheumatism, 26,* 834–839.

Okifuji, A., Turk, D. C., & Everleigh, D. J. (1999). Improving the rate of classification of patients with the Multidimensional Pain Inventory (MPI): Clarifying the meaning of "significant others." *Clinical Journal of Pain, 15,* 290–296.

Parker, J. C., Buckelew, S. P., Smarr, K. L., Buescher, K. L., Beck, N. C., Frank, R. G., Anderson, S. L., & Walker, S. E. (1990). Psychological screening in rheumatoid arthritis. *Journal of Rheumatology, 17,* 1016–1021.

Pellegrino, M. J., Waylonis, G. W., & Sommer, A. (1989). Familial occurrence of primary fibromyalgia. *Archives of Physical Medicine and Rehabilitation, 70,* 61–63.

Phillips, H. C. (1988). *The psychological management of chronic pain: A treatment manual.* New York: Springer.

Pilowsky, I., Bassett, D., Barrett, R., Petrovic, L., & Minniti, R. (1983). The Illness Behavior Assessment Schedule: Reliability and validity. *International Journal of Psychiatry in Medicine, 13,* 11–28.

Pilowsky, I., Chapman, C. R., & Bonica, J. J. (1977). Pain, depression, and illness behavior in a pain clinic population. *Pain, 4,* 183–192.

Pilowsky, I., & Spence, N. D. (1975). Patterns of illness behavior in patients with intractable pain. *Journal of Psychosomatic Research, 19,* 279–287.

Pilowsky, I., & Spence, N. D. (1976). Illness behavior syndromes associated with intractable pain. *Pain, 2,* 61–71.

Pincus, T., Callahan, L. F., Bradley, L. A., Vaughn, W. K., & Wolfe, F. (1986). Elevated MMPI scores for hypochondriasis, depression, and hysteria in patients with rheumatoid arthritis reflect disease rather than psychological status. *Arthritis and Rheumatism, 29,* 1456–1466.

Pollard, C. A. (1984). Preliminary validity study of the pain disability index. *Perceptual and Motor Skills, 59,* 974.

Prochaska, J. O., & DiClemente, C. C. (1984). *The transtheoretical approach: Towards a systematic eclectic framework.* Homewood, IL: Dow Jones Irwin.

Prokop, C. K. (1986). Hysteria scale elevations in low back pain patients: A risk facor for misdiagnosis? *Journal of Consulting and Clinical Psychology, 54,* 558–562.

Ransford, A. O., Cairns, D., & Mooney, V. (1976). The pain drawing as an aid to the psychologic evaluation of patients with low-back pain. *Spine, 1,* 127–134.

Radloff, L. (1977). The CES-D scale: A self-report depression scale for research in the general population. *Journal of Applied Psychological Measurement, 1,* 385–401.

Raphael, K. G., Cloitre, M., & Dohrenwend, B. P. (1991). Problems of recall and misclassification with checklist methods of measuring stressful life events. *Health Psychology, 10,* 62–74.

Richter, J. E., Obrecht, W. F., Bradley, L. A., Young, L. D., Anderson, K. O., & Castell, D. O. (1986). Psychological profiles of patients with the nutcracker esophagus. *Digestive Diseases and Sciences, 31,* 131–138.

Riley, J. L., & Robinson, M. E. (1998). Validity of MMPI-2 profiles in chronic back pain patients: Differences in path models of coping and somatization. *Clinical Journal of Pain, 14,* 324–335.

Riley, J. L., Zawacki, T. M., Robinson, M. E., & Geisser, M. E. (1999). Empirical test of the factor structure of the West Haven–Yale Multidimensional Pain Inventory. *The Clinical Journal of Pain, 15,* 24–30.

Robins, L. N., Helzer, J. E., Croughan, J., & Ratcliff, K. S. (1981). National Institute of Mental Health Diagnostic Interview Schedule. *Archives of General Psychiatry, 38,* 381–389.

Robinson, M. E., Swimmer, G. I., & Rallof, D. (1989). The P-A-I-N MMPI classification system: A critical review. *Pain, 37,* 211–214.

Roland, M., & Morris, R. (1983). A study of the natural history of back pain: Part I. Development of a reliable and sensitive measure of disability in low-back pain. *Spine, 8,* 141–144.

Romano, J. M., & Turner, J. A. (1985). Chronic pain and depression: Does the evidence support a relationship? *Psychological Bulletin, 97,* 18–34.

Romano, J. M., Turner, J. A., & Jensen, M. P. (1992). The Chronic Illness Problem Inventory as a measure of dysfunction in chronic pain patients. *Pain, 49,* 71–75.

Romano, J. M., Turner, J. A., Jensen, M. P., Friedman, L. S., Bulcroft, R. A., Hops, H., & Wright, S. F. (1995). Chronic pain patient–spouse behavioral interactions predict patient disability. *Pain, 63,* 353–360.

Romano, J. M., Turner, J. A., & Moore, J. E. (1989). Psychological evaluation. In C. D. Tollison (Ed.), *Handbook of chronic pain management* (pp. 38–51). Baltimore: Williams & Wilkins.

Sanders, S. H., & Brena, S. F. (1993). Empirically derived chronic pain patient subgroups: The utility of multidimensional clustering to identify differential treatment effects. *Pain, 54,* 51–56.

Santor, D. A., Zuroff, D. C., Ramsey, J. O., Cervantes, P., & Palacios, J. (1995). Examining scale discriminability in the BDI and CES-D as a function of depressive severity. *Psychological Assessment, 7,* 131–139.

Sarason, I. G., Johnson, J. H., & Siegel, J. M. (1978). Assessing the impact of life changes: Development of the Life Experiences Survey. *Journal of Consulting and Clinical Psychology, 46,* 932–946.

Scarinci, I. C., McDonald-Haile, J., Bradley, L. A., & Richter, J. E. (1994). Altered pain perception and psychosocial features among women with gastrointestinal disorders and history of abuse: A preliminary model. *American Journal of Medicine, 97,* 108–118.

Schanberg, L. E., Keefe, F. J., Lefebvre, J. C., Kredich, D. W., & Gil, K. M. (1998). Social context of pain in children with juvenile primary fibromyalgia syndrome: Parental pain history and family environment. *Clinical Journal of Pain, 14,* 107–115.

Schwartz, G. E., Davidson, R. J., & Goleman, D. J. (1978). Patterning of cognitive and somatic processes in the self-regulation of anxiety: Effects of meditation vs. exercise. *Psychosomatic Medicine, 40,* 321–328.

Shutty, M. S., & DeGood, D. E. (1987). Cluster analyses of responses of low-back pain patients to the SCL-90: Comparison of empirical versus rationally derived subscales. *Rehabilitation Psychology, 32,* 133–144.

Shutty, M. S., DeGood, D. E., & Schwartz, D. P. (1986). Psychological dimensions of distress in chronic pain patients: A factor analytic study of Symptom Checklist-90 responses. *Journal of Consulting and Clinical Psychology, 54,* 836–842.

Sines, J. O. (1964). Actuarial methods as an appropriate strategy for the validation of diagnostic tests. *Psychological Review, 71,* 517–523.

Speculand, B., Goss, A. N., Spence, N. D., & Pilowsky, I. (1981). Intractable facial pain and illness behavior. *Pain, 11,* 213–219.

Spirito, A., DeLawyer, D. D., & Stark, L. J. (1991). Peer relations and social adjustment of chronically ill children and adolescents. *Clinical Psychology Review, 11,* 539–564.

Spitzer, R. L, Williams, J. B. W., Gibbon, M., & First, M. B. (1990). *Structured Clinical Interview for DSM-III-R.* Washington, DC: American Psychiatric Press.

Spitzer, R. L, Williams, J. B. W., Gibbon, M., & First, M. B. (1992). The Structured Clinical Interview for DSM-III-R (SCID): I. History, rationale and description. *Archives of General Psychiatry, 49,* 624–629.

Sweet, J. J., Breuer, S. R., Hazlewood, L. A., Toye, R., & Pawl, R. P. (1985). The Millon Behavioral Health Inventory: Concurrent and predictive validity in a pain treatment center. *Journal of Behavioral Medicine, 8,* 215–226.

Turk, D. C., Okifuji, A., Sinclair, J. D., & Starz, T. W. (1996). Pain, disability, and physical functioning in subgroups of patients with fibromyalgia. *Journal of Rheumatology, 23,* 1255–1262.

Turk, D. C., Okifuji, A., Sinclair, J. D., & Starz, T. W. (1998). Differential responses by psychosocial subgroups of fibromyalgia syndrome patients to an interdisciplinary treatment. *Arthritis Care and Research, 11,* 397–404.

Turk, D. C., & Rudy, T. E. (1990). The robustness of an empirically derived taxonomy of chronic pain patients. *Pain, 43,* 27–35.

Turk, D. C., Rudy, T. E., Kubinski, J. A., Zaki, H. S., & Greco, C. M. (1996). Dysfunctional patients with temporomandibular disorders: Evaluating the efficacy of a tailored treatment protocol. *Journal of Consulting and Clinical Psychology, 64,* 139–146.

Turner, J. A., & Clancy, S. (1988). Comparison of operant behavioral and cognitive-behavioral group treatment for chronic low back pain. *Journal of Consulting and Clinical Psychology, 56,* 261–266.

Turner, J. A., Clancy, S., McQuade, K. J., & Cardenas, D. D. (1990). Effectiveness of behavioral therapy for chronic low back pain: A component analysis. *Journal of Consulting and Clinical Psychology, 58,* 573–579.

Turner, J. A., & Romano, J. M. (1984). Self-report screening measures for depression in chronic pain patients. *Journal of Clinical Psychology, 40,* 909–913.

Vandiver, T., & Sher, K. J. (1991). Temporal stability of the Diagnostic Interview Schedule. *Psychological Assessment, 3,* 277–281.

Vendrig, A. A., Derksen, J. L., & deMey, H. R. (1999). Utility of selected MMPI-2 scales in the outcome prediction for patients with chronic back pain. *Psychological Assessment, 11,* 381–385.

Vitaliano, P. P., Katon, W., Maiuro, R. D., & Russo, J. (1989). Coping in chest pain patients with and without psychiatric disorders. *Journal of Consulting and Clinical Psychology, 57,* 338–343.

Vlaeyen, J. W. S., Kole-Snijders, A. M. J., Boeren, R.G.B., & van Eek, H. (1995). Fear of movement/(re)injury in chronic low back pain and its relation to behavioral performance. *Pain, 62,* 363–372.

Vlaeyen, J. W. S., Seleen, H. A. M., Peters, M., de Jong, P., Aretz, E., Beisiegel, E., & Weber, W. E. (1999). Fear of movement/(re)injury and muscular reactivity in chronic low back pain patients: An experimental investigation. *Pain, 82,* 297–304.

Volinn, E., Lai, D., McKinney, S., & Loeser, J. D. (1988). When back pain becomes disabling: A regional analysis. *Pain, 33,* 33–40.

Waddell, G., Newton, M., Henderson, I., Somerville, D., & Main, C. J. (1993). A Fear-Avoidance Beliefs Questionnaire (FABQ) and the role of fear–avoidance beliefs in chronic low back pain and disability. *Pain, 52,* 157–168.

Waddell, G., Pilowsky, I., & Bond, M. R. (1989). Clinical assessment and interpretation of abnormal illness behavior in low back pain. *Pain, 39,* 41–53.

Wade, J. B., Dougherty, L. M., Hart, R. P., & Cook, D. B. (1992). Patterns of normal personality structure among chronic pain patients. *Pain, 48,* 37–43.

Walker, E. A., Gelfand, A., Katon, W. J., Koss, M. P., Von Korff, M., Bernstein, D., & Russo, J. (1999). Adult health status of women with histories of childhood abuse and neglect. *American Journal of Medicine, 107,* 332–339.

Walter, L., & Brannon, L. (1991). A cluster analysis of the Multidimensional Pain Inventory. *Headache, 31,* 476–479.

Ware, J. E., & Sherbourne, C. D. (1992). The MOS 36-item Short Form Health Survey (SF-36). *Medical Care, 30,* 473–483.

Waterman, D. C., Dalton, C. B., Ott, D. J., Castell, J. A, Bradley, L. A., Castell, D. O., & Richter, J. E. (1989). Hypertensive lower esophageal sphincter: What does it mean? *Journal of Clinical Gastroenterology, 11,* 139–146.

Wesley, A. L., Gatchel, R. J., Polatin, P. B., Kinney, R. A., & Mayer, T. G. (1991). Differentiation between somatic and cognitive/affective components in commonly used measures of depression in patients with chronic low back pain: Let's not mix apples and oranges. *Spine, 16,* S213–S215.

Whitehead, W. E., Winget, C., Fedoravicius, A. S., Wooley, S., & Blackwell, B. (1982). Learned illness behavior in patients with irritable bowel syndrome and peptic ulcer. *Digestive Diseases and Sciences, 27,* 202–208.

Williams, A. C., & Richardson, P. H. (1993). What does the BDI measure in chronic pain? *Pain, 55,* 259–266.

Williams, D. A., Urban, B., Keefe, F. J., Shutty, M. S., & France, R. (1995). Cluster analysis of pain patients' responses to the SCL-90R. *Pain, 61,* 81–91.

Williams, J. B., Gibbon, M., First, M. B., Spitzer, R. L, Davies, M., Borus, J., Howes, M. J., Kane, J., Pope, H. G., Rounsaville, B., & Wittchen, H-V. (1992). The Structured Clinical Interview for DSM-III-R (SCID): II. Multi-site test–retest reliability. *Archives of General Psychiatry, 49,* 630–636.

Wolfe, F., Cathey, M. A., Kleinhekel, S. M., Amos, S. P., Hoffman, R. G., Young, D. Y., & Hawley, D. J. (1984). Psychological status in primary fibrositis and fibrositis associated with rheumatoid arthritis. *Journal of Rheumatology, 11,* 500–506.

Wurtele, S. K., Kaplan, G. M., & Keairnes, M. (1990). Childhood sexual abuse among chronic pain patients. *Clinical Journal of Pain, 6,* 110–113.

Zonderman, A. B., Heft, M. W., & Costa, P. T. (1985). Does the Illness Behavior Questionnaire measure abnormal illness behavior? *Health Psychology, 4,* 425–436.

Chapter 17

Assessment of Pain Beliefs and Pain Coping

DOUGLAS E. DeGOOD
RAYMOND C. TAIT

The purpose of this chapter is to describe and evaluate the psychometric assessment tools available to clinicians and researchers to assess both pain beliefs and patients' efforts to cope with chronic pain. Since 1992 (when the first edition of this volume was published), the research on pain beliefs has progressed at a slow, steady pace, while the research on coping with pain has exploded. A recent search of psychological abstracts on the latter topic reveals well over 1,000 coping-related publications since that time. Needless to say, this chapter cannot provide an exhaustive review of the literature that has accumulated on coping with pain. For that, the interested reader is referred to several recent reviews (Boothby, Thorn, Stroud, & Jensen, 1999; DeGood, 2000). Instead, this chapter focuses on key developments relevant to pain beliefs and coping that have occurred over the past decade.

THEORETICAL BACKGROUND

Our interest in the beliefs and attitudes of patients with chronic pain began in the clinic rather than the laboratory. Twenty-five years ago, when we first began to work with patients in pain, we frequently observed the expected mood disturbances, conflicts regarding medications, activity restrictions, employ-ment difficulties, and couple conflicts. Less anticipated but equally prevalent among these patients, however, were persistent maladaptive beliefs about the diagnosis and treatment of pain. Despite multiple diagnostic studies and failed, invasive treatments, it was not uncommon for patients to expect, if not demand, more of the same.

The approach in our settings, usually involving a review of past diagnostics and an emphasis on conservative treatments over surgery, was frequently met with disappointment, skepticism, and anger. Recommendations to increase physical exercise, use less medication, and practice relaxation techniques were not what patients expected from a university medical clinic. Patients often responded negatively to such suggestions: "Yes, but in my case there must be something that has been overlooked," or more dramatically, "You don't seem to understand how much I hurt." In addition, these individuals often complained that no one had ever explained the cause of their pain, so they were compelled to continue their desperate search for a doctor who "will just tell me what is wrong."

These are not isolated examples. Many patients find it inconceivable that self-management therapies (e.g., biofeedback, hypnosis) can improve painful conditions; they believe that this would imply that their condition is nonphysical, and therefore less respectable. Such patients may approach

320

psychological therapy feeling compelled to prove their sanity rather than to consider new treatment options, preferring instead to exaggerate symptoms or pursue high-risk treatments in order to legitimize their pain complaints. With the advantage of hindsight, we now know that such beliefs are only a sample of the dysfunctional beliefs that can contribute to misunderstanding and treatment noncompliance or failure (DeGood, 1983; DeGood & Kiernan, 1997–1998). Thus these observations underscore the need to assess and understand patients' beliefs about pain if we are to maximize response to treatment.

A topic closely aligned with beliefs and attitudes regarding pain is that of pain coping skills. In fact, the psychology of pain management is mostly about how people manage to cope with pain. Coping, whether adaptive or maladaptive, represents an individual's attempts to resolve pain-related problems, and is strongly influenced by beliefs about pain. Adherence with treatment represents an aspect of coping that, in turn, reflects a belief that the treatment is appropriate and likely to be helpful. These beliefs are especially important when adherence is likely to be tested (e.g., the course of treatment is not smooth).

Thus, beliefs about the nature of pain and about coping with pain should not be viewed as artifacts of the chronic pain experience that will disappear once a correct diagnosis is made and corresponding treatment initiated. Rather, maladaptive cognitions can lie at the heart of the chronic pain problem. Recognizing that beliefs compatible with treatment must exist if patients are to cope effectively with pain, in New Zealand the National Advisory Committee on Health and Disability (1997) has identified "maladaptive attitudes and beliefs about back pain" as a significant risk factor for developing long-term disability from low back pain. Likewise, Gatchel and Ecker (1999) list "maladaptive attitudes and beliefs about pain" as among the prime risk factors in identifying patients likely to move from acute pain into chronic pain and disability.

Attention to pain beliefs and pain coping is a critical component of a cognitive-behavioral approach to understanding pain. This perspective views coping with pain as a dynamic process wherein patients' beliefs, attitudes, and thinking styles mediate their emotional and behavioral responses. Stated differently, Turk and Rudy (1986) emphasize that a cognitive-behavioral perspective focuses attention on the "attitudes and beliefs of patients regarding their understanding of their plights, of

the health care system, of appropriate behavioral responses to disease, of their own capabilities and of their responses to stress" (p. 762).

DEFINITIONS AND RELATIONSHIPS AMONG TERMS

Beliefs have been defined as personally formed or culturally shared cognitive configurations (Wrubel, Benner, & Lazarus, 1981). They differ from *attitudes*, defined as our feelings about events, because beliefs refer to our understanding of events (Fishbein & Ajzen, 1975). Thus they are preexisting notions about the nature of reality, which mold our perception of our environment and ourselves and shape its meaning (Lazarus & Folkman, 1984). Beliefs may be so generalized or wide-ranging as to qualify as stable personality dispositions, or they may be highly specific to a particular context (Lazarus & Folkman, 1984).

Although *expectancies* are often considered synonymous with *beliefs*, they refer more specifically to beliefs about the future, especially relationships between a set of events and future consequences. Most relevant to pain management are so-called *self-efficacy expectancies*, which refer to beliefs about one's capacity to execute the behavior required to produce a certain outcome (Bandura, 1977). *Self-efficacy beliefs* differ from *outcome expectancy beliefs*. The latter are beliefs that a behavior will lead to a specific outcome, regardless of whether the person can execute the behavior. By comparison, self-efficacy beliefs are based on behaviors within a person's repertoire, and thus represent appraisals of personal control.

Pain beliefs differ in significant ways from *coping responses*. Whereas pain beliefs are mental appraisals of a situation, coping involves the set of responses an individual produces. Hence a pain belief is always a cognition, while a coping response may be a cognition or an overt behavior. Moreover, patients will readily acknowledge their beliefs about pain and its treatment, whereas self-reports regarding their coping responses to pain may or may not be the ones that are actually employed (DeGood, 2000). Finally, coping responses may be either adaptive or maladaptive, depending upon variables such as the internal and external resources available to the individual and the demands posed by the stressor (Lazarus & Folkman, 1984).

An example may clarify the meaning of the terms presented above and illustrate how beliefs can interact with actual coping behavior. Picture a patient with musculoskeletal back pain who has been instructed that a set of stretching exercises will be helpful for managing pain. The patient may or may not believe this information to be accurate (a treatment outcome expectancy belief). Even if the recommendation is believed to be valid, the patient may doubt his or her own ability to perform the exercises (self-efficacy belief). For either or both of these reasons, the patient may not perform the exercises (coping response). If the patient does perform the exercise and encounters an increase in pain, the patient may or may not continue with the exercise regimen. Therefore, if the exercise routine is to become a stable coping response, four steps must occur: (1) The therapeutic benefit of the prescribed exercise must be believed; (2) the capability to perform the exercise must exist; (3) the exercise must actually be performed; and (4) the outcome must yield a perception of pain mastery. Although exercising may be viewed as the critical (coping) behavior, the beliefs regarding this behavior may be more critical in determining whether the coping response occurs or is maintained. If the coping response were cognitive rather than an overt behavior, a similar analysis would apply.

THE PLACE OF BELIEF AND COPING ASSESSMENT IN THE EVALUATION PROCESS

A single trip to an emergency room readily demonstrates individual differences in response to pain. When pain is of a short-term nature, presumably healing is little affected by individual differences in beliefs and coping. However, when pain moves from an acute to a chronic phase, cognitive and behavioral variables gradually take on increasing significance. With chronic pain, in addition to the stress of the pain itself is the frustration of unobtainable relief (Gatchel & Ecker, 1999). This can only increase feelings of helplessness, hopelessness, and depression. Practical problems regarding career, finances, social functioning, and sexual activity can also tax coping resources.

Not surprisingly, when psychologists first began to work in the pain field, the psychological assessment process centered on evaluation of conventional symptoms of psychopathology, especially disturbances in mood state. But over the past 20 years there has been a shift toward inclusion of constructs related to individual differences in vulnerability and coping. At the time of initial contact, patients with pain will typically discuss

their pain-related experiences, opinions, and expectations more readily than psychosocial factors, which they may view as irrelevant to pain. Finding an entry point is crucial to the change process, because treatment will fail if the patient does not understand the personal relevance of the philosophy, intervention methods, and goals of the treatment program. Gradually, specific measures designed to assess health beliefs and patterns of coping have emerged as useful supplements, if not alternatives, to traditional measures of personality and psychopathology. The sections to follow describe some of the instruments that have been developed for this purpose and identify those that hold the most promise for clinical use.

PAIN BELIEFS ASSESSMENT

Categories of Beliefs

Beliefs relevant to pain can be categorized into three domains: (1) basic philosophical assumptions about the nature of the self and the world; (2) beliefs sufficiently generalized and stable to be considered personality traits; and (3) beliefs specific to the experience of pain. The first category of beliefs has to do with loosely organized, but deep-seated, ethical and philosophical assumptions about such values as justice, fairness, suffering, and personal responsibility. If one believes that life should be free of pain, that belief can intensify suffering associated with the experience of chronic pain. Because beliefs in this category are often highly personalized, inconsistent, and contradictory, they are also difficult to assess.

Beliefs falling into the second category tend to be more organized and rooted in everyday life. Because they are stable across time and situation, such beliefs are often conceptualized as personality traits. Considering beliefs that translate into negative traits, Lazarus (1991) suggests that "people carry around with them private and recurrent personal meanings that lead them to react inappropriately to an encounter with a sense of betrayal, victimization, rejection, abandonment, inadequacy, or whatever" (p. 363). Of course, other such beliefs may contribute to positive adaptation, including popular psychological constructs such as *hardiness* (Kobasa, 1979; Pollock & Duffy, 1990), *locus of control* (Rotter, 1966; Wallston, Wallston, & DeVellis, 1978), *attributional style* (Abramson, Seligman, & Teasdale, 1978), and *self-efficacy* (Bandura, 1977).

Certainly beliefs falling into the second category can be studied in patients with pain (see, e.g.,

Weisburg & Gatchel, 2000); nevertheless, the most productive of the beliefs research has focused on specific patient beliefs about pain. These pain-specific beliefs have to do with the "nuts and bolts" concerning what patients believe should be done to diagnose and control pain. As reflected in the introduction to this chapter, pain-specific beliefs, such as the insistence that further diagnostic procedures are needed, are intimately associated with a patient's response to treatment recommendations. Some beliefs about the etiology of pain and the corresponding expectations about diagnosis and treatment that have particular relevance for subsequent adherence and outcome are listed in Table 17.1.

Early Measures of Pain Beliefs

Some of the pain beliefs measurement tools described in the first edition of this volume (DeGood & Shutty, 1992) are found infrequently in the more recent pain literature. These include the Cognitive Error Questionnaire (Lefebvre, 1981), the Gottlieb Pain Beliefs Questionnaire (Gottlieb, 1984, 1986), the Pain Information and Beliefs Questionnaire

TABLE 17.1. Sample Dimensions of Beliefs about Chronic Pain and Pain Treatment

Etiology of pain
- Somatic only vs. interaction of multiple factors
- External vs. internal (e.g., accident vs. aging)
- Someone is to blame vs. unfortunate natural or chance event
- Pain as symptom of disease vs. pain as a benign condition

Diagnostic expectations regarding:
- History taking
- Clinical medical exam
- Laboratory tests, esp. radiological
- Psychosocial evaluation

Treatment expectations
- Patient active vs. passive (e.g., exercise/self-relaxation vs. surgery/medications)
- Invasive vs. noninvasive procedures
- Fix/repair vs. rehabilitation mindset
- Medical only vs. multidisciplinary
- Somatic/medical vs. psychological/behavioral

Outcome goals
- Complete cure vs. partial relief
- Rapid vs. gradual improvement
- Sensory comfort vs. improved quality of life
- Return to prior full functioning vs. partial functioning

(Schwartz, DeGood, & Shutty, 1985; Shutty & DeGood, 1990), the Pain and Impairment Relationship Scales (Riley, Ahern, & Follick, 1988), and the Pain Cognition Questionnaire (Boston, Pearce, & Richardson, 1990). Even though theses measures can be found in studies that made a seminal contribution to the early evolution of beliefs assessment, continued use of these instruments has been limited by a number of factors. In some cases the instruments are unwieldy to administer, unclear in underlying factor structure, or too restricted in focus. As a result, each has limited potential for becoming part of the repertoire of measures used in routine individual clinical assessment of the patient with chronic pain. However, these measures may still be of value to the researcher with a particular focused interest.

A more recent example of a restricted-focus pain belief measure is the Pain Beliefs Questionnaire (PBQ) of Edwards, Pearce, Turner-Stokes, and Jones (1992). Following factor analysis of the original 20-item scale, the questionnaire was reduced to 12 items with an Organic Beliefs scale (8 items) and a Psychological Beliefs scale (4 items). The construct validity of these two subscales was then explored with 40 additional patients with pain. In this group there were significant associations found between scores on the PBQ Organic Beliefs scale and scores on the Chance and Powerful Others scales of the Multidimensional Health Locus of Control instrument (MHLC; Wallston et al., 1978), and between the PBQ Psychological Beliefs scale and the Internal scale of the MHLC. No relationship, however, emerged between either PBQ scale and pain intensity.

As was the case for several of the older measures, the PBQ appears to be valid and useful for researchers concerned with a highly specific issue—in this case, measurement of beliefs regarding organic versus psychological etiology. But it is too limited in scope to provide the clinician with a comprehensive picture of patient beliefs. The next section covers several measures with broader measurement goals and a more extensive psychometric research base.

Instruments Currently Recommended for Research and Clinical Applications

Survey of Pain Attitudes

The pain beliefs instrument that has been most extensively studied and has gained the widest use is the Survey of Pain Attitudes (SOPA). The initial published version (Jensen, Karoly, & Huger, 1987) had 24 items, each rated on a 5-point scale. These items were designed to assess five dimensions related to patient beliefs about pain: (1) Control, (2) Disability, (3) Medical Cures, (4) Solicitude, and (5) Medication. A sixth dimension, Emotion (i.e., beliefs about the influence of emotions on pain), was added in a subsequent 35-item version (Jensen & Karoly, 1989). Initial psychometric analyses revealed the 35-item SOPA to have high internal consistency within subscales and to be stable over time (Jensen & Karoly, 1989). Subsequent analyses revealed the SOPA to be associated with patient reports of pain behavior and coping responses as well as sensitive to attitudinal changes following conservative pain treatment. (Jensen & Karoly, 1991; Jensen, Turner, & Romano, 1991).

In a third revision of the SOPA (Jensen, Turner, Romano, & Lawler, 1994), the scale was increased to 57 items (see Appendix 17.A). Additional items were added to the Medication and Disability subscales, and a seventh dimension was added, Harm (i.e., beliefs that pain is evidence of physical harm). Subscale scores with this version continued to demonstrate acceptable internal consistency, test–retest reliability, and convergent/discriminant validity (Jensen et al., 1994). Scale scores derived from this version have been related to treatment outcomes; changes in beliefs from pre- to posttreatment were correlated with changes in measures of physical and emotional functioning.

Tait and Chibnall (1997) developed a briefer, 30-item version (SOPA-B) of the SOPA that also demonstrates a seven-dimension factor structure. Correlations between subscales in the brief and standard versions of the SOPA ranged from .79 to .97. The SOPA-B also demonstrated other psychometric properties, including convergent/discriminative validity with other pain variables, that appear similar to the properties of the lengthier version. However, Jensen, Turner, and Romano (2000) have developed a slightly different 35-item short version, which they argue conforms more closely to the content and psychometric properties of the original 57-item SOPA.

The SOPA has now undergone three major revisions and is available in two abbreviated versions. Since its inception, it has consistently demonstrated strong psychometric qualities and good clinical utility involving patient responses to conservative pain management. Its demonstrated relationship to treatment outcome makes it especially appealing to clinicians as well as researchers interested in the assessment of pain cognition. The 57-item version remains somewhat cumbersome to use and presently lacks normative standards against which to compare individual response profiles. Nonetheless, it is currently a useful instrument for both research and clinical applications.

Pain Beliefs and Perceptions Inventory

The Pain Beliefs and Perceptions Inventory (PBAPI; Williams & Thorn, 1989) is a 16-item questionnaire that originally measured three dimensions of patient beliefs derived from factor analysis: (1) Self-Blame, (2) Mystery (i.e., perception of pain as mysterious), and (3) Stability (i.e., beliefs about the stability/permanence of pain over time). The initial study (Williams & Thorn, 1989) showed that these three scales are face-valid and possess high internal consistency. The belief that pain is permanent and likely to persist despite treatment was positively associated with pain intensity ratings and decreased compliance with conservative treatment. In addition, the belief that pain is mysterious (i.e., that pain has no explanation) was inversely associated with posttreatment ratings of psychological distress and somatization. Finally, beliefs in both the stability and the mysterious nature of pain were associated with negative self-perceptions and decreased control over pain. A study by Williams and Keefe (1991) also supported the validity of the PBAPI. They examined the relationship between PBAPI beliefs and coping strategies. A cluster analysis of PBAPI responses revealed three patient subgroups that differed in patterns of coping strategies. For example, patients who believed that their pain was mysterious and permanent reported a greater tendency to catastrophize about pain and employed fewer cognitive coping strategies than did patients who believed their pain was of short duration and understandable.

Recent factor analyses (Herda, Siegeris, & Basler, 1994; Strong, Ashton, & Chant, 1992) have indicated, however, a four-factor structure in which the Stability scale divides into two subscales: beliefs that pain is a constant and enduring experience (Constancy) and beliefs about the chronicity of pain (Acceptance). Constancy showed higher correlations with self-reported symptoms (anxiety, general physical troubles, and pain intensity) than did Acceptance, Self-Blame, or Mystery. Appendix 17.B presents the PBAPI with a four-factor solution in which Permanence replaces Acceptance.

Whether this scale has three or four dimensions is not as critical for the clinician as the question of clinical utility. Clearly this measure has strong psychometric grounding and taps dimensions with proven relevance to patient behavior. These properties are probably behind its increasing acceptance as an instrument both in English-speaking and in other countries (Herda et al., 1994). Several caveats should be noted, however. First, the limited scope of the PBAPI may restrict its clinical appeal. Furthermore, high levels of self-blame are uncommonly reported, potentially reducing the utility of the Self-Blame scale. Finally, the Mystery scale seems to measure something very akin to catastrophizing, so that its added value remains to be seen. Nonetheless, these are empirical questions requiring further attention rather than abandonment of the subscales in question. Other dimensions of the PBAPI (Constancy, Acceptance) seem to have considerable potential for current clinical use.

Cognitive Risk Profile

After abandoning the Pain Information and Beliefs Questionnaire (Shutty & DeGood, 1990) due to inherent limitations in the videotaped format, DeGood and colleagues began development of a wider-ranging pain beliefs instrument. This instrument, the Cognitive Risk Profile (CRP), has now gone through several iterations. The CRP is intended to assess several dimensions identified through prior research as potential roadblocks to treatment success. The most recent version of the CRP (see Appendix 17.C) consists of 68 items, each rated on a 6-point scale. Each item asks the patient to rate his or her level of agreement–disagreement with a statement about pain that has been judged to be either adaptive or maladaptive, and thus potentially related to response to treatment. Both exploratory and confirmatory factor analyses have supported the current scale construction (DeGood et al., 1996; Klocek, DeGood, & Chastain, 1997). These show the CRP to consist of nine scales: (1) Philosophic Beliefs, (2) Denial Mood Affects Pain, (3) Denial Pain Affects Mood, (4) Perception of Blame, (5) Lack of Social Support, (6) Disability Entitlement, (7) (waiting for) Medical Breakthrough, (8) Multidisciplinary Skepticism (i.e., skepticism about a multidisciplinary approach to pain treatment), and (9) Conviction of Hopelessness. Moderate concurrent validity has been established through independent clinical interview (Klocek et al., 1997) and associations with depression and activity level (Cook, DeGood, & Chastain, 1999). Predictive validity based on a small treatment outcome study of 45 patients

(DeGood et al., 1996) has also been reported. Moderate correlations (.35–.55 range) among the scales suggest that they do not represent entirely independent dimensions of risk.

The intent of the CRP, to identify factors that put patients at risk for treatment failure, makes it clinically appealing. In addition, several of the scales reflect factors that are highly familiar to clinicians, and thus have considerable face validity. Although the CRP is built on an extensive amount of psychometric research, the current form is too lengthy for what it purports to measures, the subscales are too highly intercorrelated, and norms have not been established for subgroups of patients with pain. Thus it remains a tool with clinical promise that is still in need of further refinement.

Pain Stages of Change Questionnaire

The Pain Stages of Change Questionnaire (PSOCQ; Kerns, Rosenberg, Jamison, Caudill, & Haythornwaite, 1997; see also Bradley & McKendree-Smith, Chapter 16, this volume) reflects a different approach to pain beliefs assessment. It measures cognitions that are relevant to a patient's *readiness for change*. It is based on a model that examines stages in change processes—a model that has successfully predicted response to treatment for a number of health risk behaviors (Prochaska & DiClemente, 1984). Recently, this model has been adapted to the assessment of patients' readiness to adopt a self-management approach to chronic pain. The PSOCQ, a 30-item self-report instrument, assesses attitudes and beliefs about four stages relevant to self-management: Precontemplation, Contemplation, Action, and Maintenance (see Appendix 17.D).

A study of 241 patients supports the factor structure of the scales, as well as the discriminant and criterion validity for each scale (Kerns et al., 1997). Moreover, each of the four scales was found to be internally consistent and stable over time. In a recent study (Kerns & Rosenberg, 2000) of 109 patients with chronic pain participating in cognitive-behavioral treatment, it was found that, relative to patients that completed treatment, 50 patients who dropped out had significantly higher Precontemplation scores and lower Contemplation scores prior to treatment. Overall, it was found that pre- to posttreatment changes in the PSOCQ scales were associated with improved outcomes.

This new scale is easily administered and has evident face validity. Initial research supports its other psychometric properties as well. It fits nicely within the tradition of cognitive assessment of pain beliefs, especially in relationship to predicting response to treatment. It also adds a conceptual framework that is particularly appealing to clinicians interested in predicting treatment response for often skeptical referral sources and/or insurance carriers. Nonetheless, because of the preliminary nature of its psychometric support, further work is needed to examine its predictive validity.

Concluding Comment on Pain Beliefs

In the nearly 10 years since the first edition of this volume, maladaptive beliefs have increasingly come to be recognized as a major risk factor in poor response to treatment for chronic pain. Also, change in beliefs has become more clearly linked to positive treatment outcomes than was true a decade ago. However, understanding of and beliefs about pain are still most likely to be assessed by interviewing a patient with pain, rather than via psychometric assessment tools. Of the measures that have been described, the SOPA and the shorter SOPA-B have the strongest psychometric base and the most immediate clinical utility. Most of the other measures, including those of historical significance, either require further development or are useful primarily for exploring particular research questions.

Several problems remain to be clarified relevant to pain beliefs. First, there is ongoing conceptual confusion between pain beliefs and pain coping. Similarly, the relationship between pain beliefs and coping behaviors is confusing and difficult to sort out in the literature. Likewise, the process by which pain beliefs translate into attempts at coping is often unclear. Clearer conceptual models, such as an adaptation of the Lazarus and Folkman (1984) transactional model of stress as proposed by Thorn, Rich, and Boothby (1999), may be helpful.

There also are problems associated with research design. In many studies beliefs, coping, and even outcome measures are intertwined in a manner leading to conceptual confusion. One solution to this problem might be to restrict beliefs to the realm of cognition and coping to the realm of overt behavior (Jensen, Turner, Romano, & Strom, 1995). At a less radical level and at the very least, further attention to conceptual issues is needed among researchers as they design studies of these elusive constructs.

Another issue involves measurement. Belief measures have emphasized the assessment of mal-

adaptive beliefs. It is not clear, however, that a low score on a negative belief scale is the equivalent of a positive belief. More research is needed on relations between adaptive and maladaptive pain beliefs, as well as the relative contribution of each to coping and treatment outcome.

Another ongoing question concerns the origin of beliefs relevant to pain. Are pain beliefs the products of misinformation, idiosyncratic medical experiences, or the psychosocial environment? To what degree do they precede or follow the onset of pain? Such information is critical in terms of prevention and modification of maladaptive beliefs. In light of information that mere exposure to new (and presumably correct) information is not always sufficient to change pain beliefs (Shutty, DeGood, & Tuttle, 1990), it would be useful to further explore from whence maladaptive beliefs are derived.

Little research to date has considered the impact of beliefs, particularly on response to treatment, in interaction with moderator variables such as age, gender, employment, and economic circumstances. Similarly, little attention has been paid to the interface of beliefs with recent developments in the field of pain management. The delivery of pain management services may not always be reflected in the content of assessment tools. Although beliefs have been heavily studied in the context of behavioral interventions, they have been less studied as they apply to interventional strategies that are frequently employed in current pain management health care (e.g., implantable spinal cord stimulation).

COPING WITH PAIN

As noted earlier, a voluminous literature on coping has sprung up since 1992. Nonetheless, any discussion of coping should begin with the transactional model of stress (Lazarus & Folkman, 1984), a theory that predates 1992 but continues to guide research on coping with pain. Accordingly, the first subsection below addresses that model and, very briefly, measures directly associated with it. The next subsection surveys research on several established measures of coping: the Vanderbilt Pain Management Inventory (VPMI; Brown & Nicassio, 1987), and especially the Coping Strategies Questionnaire (CSQ; Rosenstiel & Keefe, 1983), the instrument that has driven much of the coping research since 1992. The following subsection examines psychometric developments since 1992, especially longitudinal studies and studies of mediating/moderating variables associated with coping and pain. Psychometric developments since 1992 are then examined, including both modifications of established instruments and newly developed instruments. The final part of this section examines both clinical applications of the present research and directions for further study.

Conceptual Basis of Coping

The transactional model of stress defines *coping* as "constantly changing cognitive and behavioral efforts to manage specific external and/or internal demands that are appraised as taxing, or exceeding the resources of the person" (Lazarus & Folkman, 1984, p. 141). This definition recognizes that coping is a fluid process, subject to change across situations and over time. Similarly, it represents coping as a process composed of appraisals, responses, and reappraisals. Appraisals and responses are both colored by individual differences, including differences in beliefs, expectancies, personality and biological characteristics, and social roles. Faced with similar stressors (e.g., pain), individuals are likely to respond differently; one may appraise pain as a threat, while the other may appraise it as a challenge.

The Ways of Coping Checklist (WCCL; Folkman & Lazarus, 1980) was developed to assess coping responses to a broad range of emotion-focused (internal) and problem-focused (external) demands, dimensions intrinsic to the transactional model. Both the WCCL and a 42-item modified version developed to assess somewhat different dimensions (Vitaliano, Russo, Carr, Maiuro, & Becker, 1985) were used extensively in early research on patients in pain (DeGood & Shutty, 1992; Jensen, Turner, Romano, & Karoly, 1991). Each has seen relatively little recent use, possibly because the factor structure of the WCCL has not held up with medical patients (Wineman, Durand, & McCulloch, 1994), and possibly because neither version was designed for specific health conditions such as chronic pain (Endler, Parker, & Summerfeldt, 1993).

Research on Established Measures

Vanderbilt Pain Management Inventory

The VPMI is a 19-item questionnaire that assesses active and passive coping strategies specifically relevant to chronic pain (Brown & Nicassio, 1987).

The VPMI defines active strategies as attempts by the patient to deal with pain through his or her own resources, and passive strategies as helplessness or relying on others (Nicholas, Wilson, & Goyen, 1992). Correlational studies have shown passive coping to be associated with higher levels of pain, pain-related disability, and psychological distress, while active coping has been associated with more positive affect and higher levels of activity (Snow-Turek, Norris, & Tan, 1996; Zautra et al., 1995). Longitudinal studies have followed a similar pattern. Six months after assessment, patients who coped passively with musculoskeletal pain reported higher levels of pain than did patients who coped actively (Potter & Jones, 1992). Similarly, greater pain-related disability was reported at a 9-month follow-up by patients with temporomandibular dysfunction (Turner, Whitney, Dworkin, Massoth, & Wilson, 1995), and greater psychosocial interference was described at a 4-year follow-up by patients with rheumatoid arthritis (RA) (Smith & Wallston, 1992).

Despite the generally supportive pattern of findings described above, several problems have been identified with the VPMI. Relative to passive coping, VPMI active coping has been less predictive of adjustment to pain. Similarly, psychometric properties of the VPMI appear to be inferior to those of the active and passive coping dimensions derived from the CSQ (Snow-Turek et al., 1996). Finally, the VPMI has been critiqued because its composition does not allow assessment of specific coping strategies that fall within the active and passive coping categories (Smith, Wallston, Dwyer, & Dowdy, 1997).

Coping Strategies Questionnaire

The CSQ (Rosenstiel & Keefe, 1983) has formed the backbone of research on coping and adjustment to pain. Unlike the VPMI, the CSQ assesses relatively specific coping strategies: six cognitive coping strategies and one behavioral coping strategy. Items for each coping strategy subscale are rated as to the frequency with which they are used (0 = "never," 6 = "always"). The subscales for cognitive coping strategies include Diverting Attention, Reinterpreting Pain, Coping Self-Statements, Ignoring Pain, Praying or Hoping, and Catastrophizing. The behavioral coping strategy subscale is Increasing Activity. In addition, there are two self-efficacy items reflecting "perceived control over pain" and "ability to decrease pain." The CSQ has been used in two lines of research: (1) factor-analytic studies aimed at identifying superordinate constructs relevant to coping, and (2) studies of individual scales aimed at identifying specific coping strategies associated with good or poor adjustment.

CSQ Composite Measures. Numerous composites have been derived from the CSQ since 1992. One such composite is Coping Attempts, a construct that subsumes Coping Self-Statements, Reinterpreting Pain, Ignoring Pain, Increasing Activity, and Diverting Attention (all of the cognitive coping strategies except catastrophizing). Although there is evidence that Coping Attempts correlates negatively with disability (Gil et al., 1993; Martin et al., 1996) and with psychosocial dysfunction (Jensen, Turner, & Romano, 1992), the evidence is not unanimous (see, e.g., Nicassio, Schoenfeld-Smith, Radojevic, & Schuman, 1995; Thompson, Gil, Abrams, & Phillips, 1992) and is generally modest in terms of effect sizes. The mixed results and modest effects may result from aggregating disparate coping strategies into a single score, leading to a loss of information (Jensen et al., 1992). Alternatively, the pattern of findings may reflect clinical practice, as most patients with pain employ relatively few active coping strategies (Geisser, Robinson, & Riley, 1999; Haythornthwaite, Menefee, Heinberg, & Clark, 1998; Schmitz, Saile, & Nilges, 1996).

Another composite derived from factor analysis of the CSQ is Pain Control and Rational Thinking. Typically, this composite has included the Catastrophizing subscale (loading negatively) and the two self-efficacy items (loading positively). Studies of the construct have shown higher scores to be linked with less reported pain (Beckham, Keefe, Caldwell, & Roodman, 1991; Keefe et al., 1991; Schanberg, Lefebvre, Keefe, Kredich, & Gil, 1997; Tota-Faucette, Gil, Williams, Keefe, & Goli, 1993), less widespread pain (Schanberg et al., 1997), and less distress and disability (Beckham et al.,1991; Dozois, Dobson, Wong, Hughes, & Long, 1996; Keefe et al., 1991). Although the consistency of these findings is noteworthy, it is difficult to ascertain whether the results reflect coping strategies, self-efficacy beliefs, or some combination of the two.

Another line of composite research has identified Active and Passive Coping dimensions in the CSQ (e.g., Beckham et al., 1991; Nicholas et al., 1992). Active Coping, composed of such items as "I pretend it's not part of me," has correlated with higher levels of activity and lower levels of

psychological distress (see, e.g., Snow-Turek et al., 1996). Longitudinal research has shown Active Coping to predict gains in jaw mobility among patients with temporomandibular dysfunction (Turner et al., 1995) and with increased *uptime* (i.e., time spent in other than a reclining position) at a 3-month follow-up of patients with low back pain (Spinhoven & Linssen, 1991). As with the previous composite, Active Coping is composed of items that reflect multiple coping strategies, making it difficult to determine the contribution of particular coping strategies to pain adjustment.

Yet another CSQ composite that has been studied in regard to adjustment to pain is Coping Flexibility (Haythornthwaite et al., 1998). Unlike previous composites, derived from factor analyses, Coping Flexibility has been defined as simply the number of strategies (excluding Catastrophizing) frequently employed to cope with pain. Patients describing a high number of frequently used coping strategies have reported higher levels of perceived control over pain, suggesting that flexibility contributes to effective coping. Although this finding is in agreement with research showing that coping flexibility is important for effective pain management (Blalock, DeVellis, & Giorgino, 1995), the omission of the Catastrophizing scale from data analysis should be noted. It was omitted because of ongoing disagreement over whether it is an appraisal or a coping strategy, but its omission complicates interpretation of the results, because Catastrophizing has been established as an important predictor of adjustment (Geisser et al., 1999).

Several CSQ composites are associated with poor adjustment to pain and/or poor outcomes. In research using a modified version of the CSQ that was adapted for sickle cell disease (SCD), the construct of Negative Thinking/Passive Adherence (catastrophizing, fear self-statements, anger self-statements, resting, heat/cold/massage, taking fluids, isolation, decreased activity, and control) has been linked with poor adjustment to SCD: lower levels of activity (Thompson et al., 1992), higher levels of hospitalization (Gil, Abrams, Phillips, & Williams, 1992), and more health care contacts (Gil et al., 1993). Pain Avoidance (a composite of Praying or Hoping and Diverting Attention) has been associated with levels of pain-related disability, distress, and pain intensity, with the Praying or Hoping variable accounting for most of the variance in the results (Geisser, Robinson, & Henson, 1994).

Although research on composite measures has identified several constructs of clinical significance, several problems characterize this line of study. Because most composites were empirically derived, their composition typically varies somewhat across samples (Boothby et al., 1999). Furthermore, because the superordinate constructs reflected in the composites include items from multiple CSQ subscales, the subscales within these constructs may be differentially associated with criterion variables (see, e.g., Geisser, Robinson, & Henson, 1994). Thus theoretically and clinically important information can be lost that is clearer in research focusing on individual coping strategies.

Catastrophizing. Catastrophizing, defined as "an exaggerated negative orientation toward pain stimuli and pain experience" (Sullivan, Stanish, Waite, Sullivan, & Tripp, 1998, p. 253), is the single construct from the coping literature that has received the most attention since 1992. Catastrophizing has been associated with many variables reflecting poor adjustment to pain: psychological distress (Geisser, Robinson, Keefe, & Weiner, 1994; Hill, Niven, & Knussen, 1995; Jensen et al., 1992; Ulmer, 1997), disability (Lester, Lefebvre, & Keefe, 1996; Lin & Ward, 1996; Martin et al., 1996; Robinson et al., 1997), and levels of pain intensity (Geisser, Robinson, Keefe, & Weiner, 1994; Harkapaa, 1991; Hill, 1993; Wilkie & Keefe, 1991). Discrepant findings, such as those regarding catastrophizing and disability (see, e.g., Jensen et al., 1992; Pfingsten, Hildebrandt, Leibing, Franz, & Saur, 1997), only underscore the need for further research on the construct.

Several important practical and theoretical questions about catastrophizing have been raised. For example, Sullivan and D'Eon (1990) found that clinical psychologists viewed catastrophizing and depression as virtually synonymous. Evidence shows, however, that they are not synonymous: Catastrophizing has been associated with self-reports of pain intensity independently of depression (Flor, Behle, & Birbaumer, 1993; Geisser, Robinson, Keefe, & Weiner, 1994; Sullivan, Bishop, & Pivik, 1995). Similarly, Geisser and Roth (1998), after controlling for negative affect, still found a significant relationship between catastrophizing and disability.

There is also considerable disagreement regarding the category to which the concept belongs. By dint of its inclusion in the CSQ, it was judged initially to represent a way of coping with pain. Noting that the CSQ Catastrophizing scale reflects automatic, irrational cognitions rather than pur-

poseful responses, Jensen, Turner, and Romano (1991) have suggested that catastrophizing is better considered as an appraisal. Noting that catastrophizing can "increase distress and can mobilize the individual for action" (Keefe, Kashikar-Zuck, et al., 1997, p. 197), others have contended that catastrophizing does represent a coping strategy.

Although most research using the CSQ has continued to include the Catastrophizing scale as a measure of coping, there appears to be increasing agreement that catastrophizing represents a belief, rather than a coping response (Boothby et al., 1999; Geisser et al., 1999; Haythornthwaite et al., 1998). Regardless of its category, the weight of research evidence clearly underscores the importance of catastrophizing in coping research. Geisser and colleagues (1999), in fact, have argued that it should receive increased attention—perhaps as a variable that moderates the likelihood of coping adaptively to pain. This stance has not been universally embraced (Haythornthwaite & Heinberg, 1999; Keefe, Lefebvre, & Smith, 1999; Thorn et al., 1999), but the ongoing debate underscores the need for further research aimed at clarifying its theoretical and clinical role.

Diverting Attention. Research regarding the use of attention diversion (e.g., "I try to think of something pleasant") as a coping strategy has been inconclusive. When diverting attention has been associated with positive adjustment to pain, the association has generally been moderated by another variable, such as low levels of pain intensity (Affleck, Urrows, Tennen, & Higgins, 1992), flexible goal setting (Schmitz et al., 1996), or pain acuity (Stevens, 1992).

Reinterpreting Pain. There is some evidence supporting the efficacy of reinterpretation strategies (e.g., "I tell myself it doesn't hurt") in reducing pain among patients undergoing painful procedures (see, e.g., Buckelew et al., 1992). Research with chronic pain, however, has been mixed. Perhaps, the best support has come from longitudinal studies, although these too have yielded mixed results (Affleck et al., 1992; Keefe, Affleck, et al., 1997). Additional longitudinal research is warranted, if only to clarify reasons for the discrepant results.

Coping Self-Statements. Despite the fact that coping self-statements (e.g., "I tell myself that I can overcome the pain") are often taught in multidisciplinary treatment settings, research regarding their efficacy has been sufficiently mixed that some have argued that further study of this coping strategy may not be warranted (Boothby et al., 1999). It may be, however, that coping self-statements are efficacious only under certain conditions, such as relatively low levels of pain intensity (Jensen et al., 1992). Similarly, coping self-statements may be mediated by beliefs, such as self-efficacy (Haythornthwaite et al., 1998; Keefe, Kashikar-Zuck, et al., 1997; Large & Strong, 1997). Research that provides a better understanding of mediating and moderating variables appears important if the impact of positive self-statements on adjustment to pain is to be appreciated in clinical settings.

Ignoring Pain. The strategy of ignoring pain (e.g., "I don't think about the pain") also has generated mixed results even in studies where its efficacy is likely to be greatest, such as painful procedures (see, e.g., Chaves & Brown, 1987; Kashikar-Zuck et al., 1997). Because the preponderance of studies show no relations between ignoring pain as a coping strategy and adjustment to chronic pain, Boothby and colleagues (1999) have concluded that further research on this strategy does not appear promising.

Praying or Hoping. The use of praying or hoping (e.g., "I have faith in doctors that someday there will be a cure for my pain") as a coping strategy generally has been associated with poor adjustment to pain (see, e.g., Ashby & Lenhart, 1994). Inconsistencies in the research (e.g., Jensen et al., 1992) have been explained several ways. In a factor analysis of the CSQ, Praying or Hoping items loaded on distinct factors (Robinson et al., 1997), suggesting that inconsistencies may have been the product of psychometric properties of the CSQ. From a more clinical perspective, Boothby and colleagues (1999) suggest that the findings may reflect a tendency for people to hope and pray more often when they are doing badly, rather than do badly because of praying/hoping. Although research should clarify reasons for inconsistencies in the literature, the value of this set of coping strategies for clinical practice is not clear.

Increasing Activity. Unlike routine physical exercise, the strategy of increasing activities to distract from pain (e.g., "I do something active, like household chores or projects") has demonstrated little utility as a means of coping with pain (Boothby et al., 1999). It may be, as with other coping strategies, that other variables (e.g., pain intensity, pain acuity) moderate the effects of increased activity on chronic pain adjustment.

Methodological Developments

Longitudinal Studies

A number of longitudinal studies using established measures of coping strategies (e.g., the CSQ, the VPMI) have demonstrated the importance of coping strategies as determinants of long-range adjustment. Because of their pre–post design, however, the studies could not clarify processes that influenced adjustment. Several longitudinal studies have been conducted since 1992 that shed light on such processes.

In a study of 75 patients with RA, Affleck and colleagues (1992) looked at daily fluctuations in coping strategies, levels of joint pain, and mood over a period of 75 days. To assess daily coping functions, participants completed and mailed to the investigators the Daily Coping Inventory (Stone & Neale, 1984), a measure that assesses seven coping categories: (1) direct action to reduce pain; (2) relaxation; (3) distraction; (4) redefinition; (5) emotional expression; (6) spiritual comfort; and (7) emotional support. Regression analyses showed that the most frequently used strategies involved taking direct action to reduce pain and relaxation. Patients who used more relaxation reported lower levels of pain across the study. Whereas those who used more coping strategies reported higher daily levels of pain, those levels declined across the study time period as mood steadily improved. Several interesting interactions between coping and level of pain severity also emerged. At low levels of pain, emotional support and distraction were associated with improved mood; at high levels of pain, those strategies were associated with poorer mood.

A later study of 53 patients with RA over a 30-day time period examined similar data, but used both within-persons (in which the person rather than the day is the unit of analysis) and across-persons analyses (Keefe, Affleck, et al., 1997). Both within- and across-persons results showed more frequent use of coping strategies among patients reporting higher levels of daily pain, a finding consistent with the previous study. Although within-person analyses yielded a host of other associations among pain, coping, and mood, perhaps the most interesting results involved carryover effects found for coping on pain and mood the following day. Next-day improvements in both pain and mood were associated with prior-day pain coping activity. Ratings of coping efficacy also predicted next-day improvements in pain.

Although studies such as those described above are immensely laborious, they provide important information regarding daily processes associated with pain coping. They provide the strongest support to date for coping activity as a positive contributor to adjustment. By use of daily ratings, they also minimize potentially distorting effects of memory on self-reports (Eich, Rachman, & Lopatka, 1990; Salovey, Smith, Turk, Jobe, & Willis, 1993; see also Haythornthwaite & Fauerbach, Chapter 22). Though they are not yet used in outcome studies, such time series designs are likely to clarify processes associated with positive and negative treatment outcomes.

Moderating Variables

Because coping is a fluid phenomenon (Lazarus & Folkman, 1984), it is important that situation-specific, changeable elements of the coping process be better understood. Research on variables that may moderate relations between coping and adjustment is beginning to clarify some of the conditions that influence coping effectiveness. For example, several studies have shown that level of pain intensity moderates relations between coping strategies and adjustment. Affleck and colleagues (1992) found that high levels of coping activity were associated with improved mood for patients reporting low levels of pain, but with worsened mood for patients reporting high levels of pain. Similarly, Jensen and Karoly (1991) found that diverting attention, ignoring pain, and using coping self-statements were positively associated with levels of activity for patients with low levels of pain, but not for patients with high levels of pain. Associations that hold only for high levels of pain have also been found: Frequent use of coping self-statements has been linked to poor adjustment to pain for patients reporting high (but not low) levels of pain intensity (Jensen et al., 1992). These and other studies underscore the importance of pain intensity as a moderating factor that differentially affects relations between coping and adjustment.

Demographic variables also moderate relations between coping and adjustment. A recent study of patients with RA showed that older patients were more likely than younger patients to use maladaptive coping strategies in response to mild pain, but not severe pain (Watkins, Shifren, Park, & Morrell, 1999). On the other hand, the same study reported that adults across the age range used more active coping strategies in response to mild pain and more maladaptive strategies in response to severe pain. Other studies (e.g., Sullivan et al., 1995) have suggested that gender may be another demographic variable that moderates coping and pain.

Whereas pain intensity and demographic variables have been studied as moderator variables, psychological moderators are relatively understudied. One variable that has been examined involves flexibility of goal setting. In a study of expectations regarding goal setting among patients with chronic pain, patients who were flexible in setting goals reported less depression and disability reported less depression and disability than inflexible patients (Schmitz et al., 1996). These data suggest that flexible goal setting may moderate the efficacy of specific coping strategies used with pain—a finding consistent with other studies of patients who have adapted successfully to pain (see, e.g., Large & Strong, 1997; Strong & Large, 1995). It is likely that flexibility in goal setting represents only one of a larger set of beliefs and expectancies that moderate coping efficacy. Other pain-specific beliefs and/or attitudes that deserve attention as potential moderators include acceptance (McCracken, 1998), readiness to accept change (Kerns et al., 1997), and catastrophizing (DeGood, 2000; Geisser et al., 1999).

Psychometric Developments

Revised Instruments

Revisions have been proposed recently for both the VPMI and the CSQ. The Vanderbilt Multidimensional Pain Coping Inventory (VMPCI) represents a significant revision of the VPMI (Smith et al., 1997). Whereas the VPMI uses 19 items to assess two dimensions relevant to coping, the VMPCI has 49 items that assess 11 subscales: Planful Problem-Solving, Positive Reappraisal, Distraction, Confrontative Coping, Distancing/Denial, Stoicism, Use of Religion, Self-Blame, Self-Isolation, Wishful Thinking, and Disengagement. In a study of the relative utility of the two instruments among 378 patients with RA, the VMPCI demonstrated more predictive power in assessing physical and psychological function. Moreover, because of its subscale structure, it provided a richer set of predictors than did the VPMI. These initial results suggest that it is an instrument deserving of further study.

Revisions to the CSQ also have been recently proposed. In a factor analysis of 965 patients with chronic pain, Robinson and colleagues (1997) found five factors that were generally consistent with CSQ subscales (Diverting Attention, Catastrophizing, Ignoring Pain, Reinterpreting Pain, and Coping

Self-Statements). They also found four other factors that differed from those of the CSQ (Hoping, Praying, Increasing Activity, and Distancing from Pain). In another factor analysis of data provided by 472 patients with chronic pain, Riley and Robinson (1997) compared the goodness of fit of several factor solutions. They found that a six-factor solution provided the best fit: Diverting Attention, Catastrophizing, Ignoring Pain, Distancing from Pain, Coping Self-Statements, and Praying. They recommended that the CSQ be revised to include only the 27 items that made up these stable subscales. Although the suggested factor structure has been applied in recent work (Hadjistavropoulos, MacLeod, & Asmundson, 1999), psychometric studies of a revised CSQ are still needed.

New Instruments

Three instruments relevant to coping with pain that have been developed since 1992 are reviewed here: the Pain Catastrophizing Scale (PCS; Sullivan et al., 1995), the Chronic Pain Coping Inventory (CPCI; Jensen et al., 1995), and the Pain Coping Questionnaire (PCQ; Reid, Gilbert, & McGrath, 1998). The PCS (see Appendix 17.E) is a brief, 13-item instrument that examines three components of catastrophizing: Rumination ("I can't stop thinking about how much it hurts"), Magnification ("I worry that something serious may happen"), and Helplessness ("There is nothing I can do to reduce the intensity of the pain"). Initial studies of the PCS with undergraduates showed catastrophizing to predict levels of pain and distress reported in response to pain inductions. In a more applied setting, PCS scores predicted levels of pain and distress among clinical patients undergoing electromyographic procedures (Sullivan et al., 1995). PCS scores have also been associated with thought intrusions among patients awaiting painful dental procedures (Sullivan & Neish, 1997), and with pain, disability, and employment status among patients with intractable musculoskeletal pain (Sullivan et al., 1998). The latter study also showed PCS scores, especially scores on the Rumination subscale, to predict disability even after the researchers controlled for variance associated with levels of pain intensity, depression, and anxiety. Although the PCS is brief, has promising psychometric properties, and measures an important clinical construct, further study in clinical populations is needed.

In contrast to the many instruments that have focused on cognitive strategies, the CPCI (Jensen et al., 1995) was developed in both a self-report

and a significant-other format to assess behavioral coping. Appendix 17.F presents sample items from the self-report version. The item pool for the CPCI was derived from a list of coping responses incorporated into pain treatment programs and/or emphasized in the literature. Factor analysis (based on 176 patients with chronic pain) of 64 total items yielded eight factors, reflecting illness- and wellness-focused strategies. The eight subscales included Guarding, Resting, Asking for Assistance, Relaxation, Task Persistence, Exercising/Stretching, Coping Self-Statements, and Seeking Social Support. Initial results showed that Guarding, Resting, and Asking for Assistance (illness-focused strategies) were associated with poor adjustment to pain. Task Persistence was the only wellness-focused strategy associated with a good adjustment.

A follow-up study of the CPCI (Hadjistavropoulos et al., 1999) examined its psychometric properties in a group of 210 patients with chronic pain, all of whom were involved in workers' compensation. Factor analysis revealed an eight-factor solution, paralleling the factor structure reported above. Regression analyses showed several CPCI subscales discussed in the previous study (Asking for Assistance, Guarding, and Task Persistence) to account for significant variance in a measure of adjustment. These initial studies show the CPCI to be a promising, behaviorally oriented measure of coping.

Unlike the instruments above, developed for adult applications, the PCQ (Reid et al., 1998) was designed for use with children. The PCQ is a 39-item instrument written for subjects who read at approximately a third-grade level. The original psychometric research was conducted on 340 healthy children and 76 children with recurrent pain conditions, ranging from 3rd to 12th grades. The PCQ contains eight subscales, all with good internal reliabilities ($\alpha > .75$), nested within three superordinate constructs: Approach, Distraction, and Emotion-Focused Avoidance. Of these, Approach and Distraction correlated positively with each other and negatively with Emotion-Focused Avoidance. Approach strategies included Information Seeking, Problem Solving, Seeking Social Support, and Positive Self-Statements. Distraction strategies included Behavioral Distraction and Cognitive Distraction. Emotion-Focused Avoidance strategies included Externalizing and Internalizing/Catastrophizing. Correlations computed between PCQ subscales and measures of pain, distress, and disability generally supported the adaptive nature of Approach and Distraction strategies and the maladaptive nature of Emotion-Focused Avoidance strategies. Although further investigation of this instrument is ongoing across a broader age range, it is likely that the PCQ will see increasing use, as it addresses an assessment need for an underserved population.

Concluding Comments on Coping

From this discussion of coping strategies, it is clear that considerable progress has been made since publication of the earlier chapter (DeGood & Shutty, 1992). Extensive study of the CSQ has revealed several overarching coping constructs (e.g., Pain Control and Rational Thinking) that are associated with adjustment to pain. Perhaps more important clinically has been the work on specific coping strategies. Measures such as the CSQ (Rosenstiel & Keefe, 1983), the VMPCI (Smith et al., 1997), and the CPCI (Jensen et al., 1995) assess specific cognitive and behavioral coping strategies associated with adjustment to pain. Although these tools allow assessment of a broader range of coping strategies than was available in 1992, they probably do not exhaust the coping strategies that could be assessed. For example, recent research suggests that problem solving, a construct for which there is no established measure in the pain literature, is a skill relevant to adjustment to pain (Kole-Snijders et al., 1999). Further elaboration of the role of specific coping skills in adjusting to pain is certain to come.

Associated with the shift in attention to specific coping strategies, several established instruments have undergone additional study and proposed revision. As noted above, the VPMI (Brown & Nicassio, 1987) served as a catalyst for the VMPCI (Smith et al., 1997). Because of its focus on specific strategies, the VMPCI is likely to supplant the VPMI in coping research. Until it undergoes further psychometric attention, however, its value in clinical applications is difficult to assess. Revisions have also been proposed for the CSQ (Riley & Robinson, 1997; Robinson et al., 1997). Should further research show that the revised, briefer version of the CSQ provides improved assessment of specific skills, it will see widespread clinical use. Until that time, however, its clinical value remains uncertain. Thus, because the CSQ already focuses on specific coping skills and has substantial support in the clinical literature, it remains the single instrument of most value in clinical settings.

The CSQ has promoted the study of catastrophizing, a construct with clear clinical significance, even if its theoretical role remains in question (Geisser et al., 1999). The recent development of an instrument explicitly designed to measure that construct, the PCS (Sullivan et al., 1995), is likely to promote further clinical and theoretical investigation of this important construct. Because of the clear clinical importance of catastrophizing and in recognition of its psychometric support, the PCS appears to be a tool of considerable value in clinical assessment.

Although considerable progress has occurred, a number of questions remain about coping with pain. Longitudinal studies have just begun to clarify processes relevant to coping and pain adjustment. The daily tracking strategy used in longitudinal research, though laborious, holds considerable promise for a better understanding of causal mechanisms linking coping and adjustment. Clearly, further attention to this area is needed.

Attention is also needed to assessment of coping in outcome research. Outcome instruments keyed to treatment interventions (e.g., the CPCI; Jensen et al., 1995) hold promise for outcome research, especially if treatment interventions are keyed to coping variables. In addition, the daily tracking methodology used in longitudinal research holds promise for tracking the course of treatment-related change in outcome research in a more fine-grained manner.

Additional attention is needed to coping across the life span. The PCQ (Reid et al., 1998) is an instrument that is likely to facilitate attention to this question among children and adolescents. It awaits further psychometric support, but it addresses a clear need in clinical practice and should be considered for use in pediatric settings where pain adjustment is a frequent focus. Although a similar need exists for older adults, especially in light of evidence that they cope differently with pain than do younger adults (Watkins et al., 1999), a comparable instrument does not yet exist. In light of the prevalence of pain in this group and its relative underassessment (Ferrell, 1996), attention to both adaptive and maladaptive coping in this age group is likely to provide considerable benefit.

Finally, a methodological issue clearly deserving more study involves the role of moderating, or interactive variables. Several descriptive variables have been shown to moderate relations between coping and adjustment, including levels of pain intensity, age, gender, and pain duration. Other variables that might influence relations between coping and adjustment have received less attention. There is a particular need for research examining attitudes and beliefs that moderate or mediate coping efficacy, such as readiness for change, flexibility in goal setting, and self-efficacy. In this regard, Turner, Jensen, and Romano (2000) recently determined from a sample of 169 patients that belief scores significantly and independently predicted physical disability and depression, even when the researchers controlled (via multiple regression) for age, sex, pain intensity, catastrophizing, and coping. Coping scores with similar controls significantly predicted physical disability, but not depression. The implication is that even though beliefs and coping may share considerable common variance, individual patients may require treatment strategies targeting individual components of the pain puzzle. More attention to these and other variables is likely to give us a better theoretical understanding of the fluid processes that influence the efficacy of coping efforts. At least as important is a better understanding of moderating and mediating influences, which will help us to identify for whom and under what conditions coping strategies are most likely to help and/or hinder adjustment to pain.

REFERENCES

Abramson, L. Y., Seligman, M. E. P., & Teasdale, J. D. (1978). Learned helplessness in humans: Critique and reformulations. *Journal of Abnormal Psychology, 87,* 49–74.

Affleck, G., Urrows, S., Tennen, H., & Higgins, P. (1992). Daily coping with pain from rheumatoid arthritis: Patterns and correlates. *Pain, 51,* 221–229.

Ashby, J. S., & Lenhart, R. S. (1994). Prayer as a coping strategy for chronic pain patients. *Rehabilitation Psychology, 39,* 205–209.

Bandura, A. (1977). Self-efficacy: Toward a unifying theory of behavioral change. *Psychological Review, 84,* 191–215.

Beckham, J. C., Keefe, F. J., Caldwell, D. S., & Roodman, A. A. (1991). Pain coping strategies in rheumatoid arthritis: Relationships to pain, disability, depression, and daily hassles. *Behavior Therapy, 22,* 113–124.

Blalock, S. J., DeVellis, B. M., & Giorgino, K. B. (1995). The relationship between coping and psychological well-being among people with osteoarthritis: A problem-specific approach. *Annals of Behavioral Medicine, 17,* 107–115.

Boothby, J. L., Thorn, B. E., Stroud, M. W., & Jensen, M. P. (1999). Coping with pain. In R. J. Gatchel & D. C. Turk (Eds.), *Psychosocial factors in pain: Critical perspectives* (pp. 343–359). New York: Guilford Press.

Boston, K., Pearce, S. A., & Richardson, P. H. (1990). The Pain Cognition Questionnaire. *Journal of Psychosomatic Research, 34,* 103–109.

Brown, G. K., & Nicassio, P. M. (1987). Development of a questionnaire for the assessment of active and passive coping strategies in chronic pain patients. *Pain, 31,* 53–63.

Buckelew, S. P., Conway, R. C., Shutty, M. S., Lawrence, J. A., Grafing, M. R., Anderson, S. K., Hewett, J. E., & Keefe, F. J. (1992). Spontaneous coping strategies to manage acute pain and anxiety during electrodiagnostic studies. *Archives of Physical Medicine and Rehabilitation, 73,* 594–598.

Chaves, J. F., & Brown, J. M. (1987). Spontaneous cognitive strategies for the control of clinical pain and stress. *Journal of Behavioral Medicine, 10,* 263–276.

Cook, A. J., DeGood, D. E., & Chastain, D. C. (1999, August). *Age differences in pain beliefs.* Poster presented at the 9th World Congress on Pain, Vienna.

DeGood, D. E. (1983). Reducing medical patients' reluctance to participate in psychological therapies: The initial session. *Professional Psychology, 14,* 491–502.

DeGood, D. E. (2000). The relationship of pain coping strategies to adjustment and functioning. In J. N. Weisburg & R. J. Gatchel (Eds.), *Personality characteristics of pain patients: Recent advances and future directions* (pp. 129–164). Washington, DC: American Psychological Association.

DeGood, D. E., & Kiernan, B. D. (1997–1998). Pain related cognitions as predictors of pain treatment outcome. *Advances in Medical Psychotherapy, 9,* 73–90.

DeGood, D. E., Kiernan, B. D., Cundiff, G., Klocek, J., Adams, L., & Ferguson, J. (1996, August). *Development of a patient self-report inventory for predicting pain treatment response: The Cognitive Risk Profile.* Poster presented at the 8th World Congress on Pain, Vancouver, British Columbia, Canada.

DeGood, D. E., & Shutty, M. S. (1992). Assessment of pain beliefs, coping, and self-efficacy. In D. C. Turk & R. Melzack (Eds.), *Handbook of pain assessment* (pp. 214–234). New York: Guilford Press.

Dozois, D. J. A., Dobson, K. S., Wong, M., Hughes, D., & Long, A. (1996). Predictive utility of the CSQ in low back pain: Individual vs. composite measures. *Pain, 66,* 171–180.

Edwards, L. C., Pearce, S. A., Turner-Stokes, L., & Jones, A. (1992). The Pain Beliefs Questionnaire: An investigation of beliefs in the causes and consequences of pain. *Pain, 51,* 267–272.

Eich, E., Rachman, S., & Lopatka, C. (1990). Affect, pain and autobiographical memory. *Journal of Abnormal Psychology, 99,* 174–178.

Endler, N .S., Parker, J. D. A., & Summerfeldt, L. J. (1993). Coping with health problems: Conceptual and methodological issues. *Canadian Journal of Behavioural Science, 25,* 384–399.

Ferrell, B. A. (1996). Overview of aging and pain. In B. R. Ferrell & B. A. Ferrell (Eds.), *Pain in the elderly* (pp. 1–10). Seattle, WA: International Association for the Study of Pain Press.

Fishbein, M., & Ajzen, I. (1975). *Belief, attitude, intention and behavior: An introduction to theory and research.* Reading, MA: Addison-Wesley.

Flor, H., Behle, D. J., & Birbaumer, N. (1993). Assessment of pain-related cognitions in chronic pain patients. *Behaviour Research and Therapy, 31,* 63–73.

Folkman, S., & Lazarus, R. S. (1980). An analysis of coping in a middle-aged community sample. *Journal of Health and Social Behavior, 21,* 219-239.

Gatchel, R. J., & Ecker, J. (1999). Psychosocial predictors of chronic pain and response to treatment. In R. J. Gatchel & D. C. Turk (Eds.), *Psychosocial factors in pain: Critical perspectives* (pp. 412-434). New York: Guilford Press.

Geisser, M. E., Robinson, M. E., & Henson, C. D. (1994). The Coping Strategies Questionnaire and chronic pain adjustment: A conceptual and empirical reanalysis. *Clinical Journal of Pain, 10,* 98-106.

Geisser, M. E., Robinson, M. E., Keefe, F. J., & Weiner, M. L. (1994). Catastrophizing, depression and the sensory, affective and evaluative aspects of chronic pain. *Pain, 59,* 79-83.

Geisser, M. E., Robinson, M. E., & Riley, J. L. (1999). Pain beliefs, coping, and adjustment to chronic pain: Let's focus more on the negative. *Pain Forum, 8,* 161-168.

Geisser, M. E., & Roth, R. S. (1998). Knowledge of and agreement with pain diagnosis: Relation to pain beliefs, pain severity, disability, and psychological distress. *Journal of Occupational Rehabilitation, 8,* 73-88.

Gil, K. M., Abrams, M. R., Phillips, G., & Williams, D. A. (1992). Sickle cell disease pain: 2. Predicting health care use and activity level at 9-month follow-up. *Journal of Consulting and Clinical Psychology, 60,* 267-273.

Gil, K. M., Thompson, R. J., Keith, B. R., Tota-Faucette, M., Noll, S., & Kinney, T. R. (1993). Sickle cell disease pain in children and adolescents: Change in pain frequency and coping strategies over time. *Journal of Pediatric Psychology, 18,* 621-637.

Gottlieb, B. S. (1984, November). *Development of the Pain Beliefs Questionnaire: A preliminary report.* Paper presented at the annual meeting of the Association for Advancement of Behavior Therapy, Philadelphia.

Gottlieb, B. S. (1986, August). *Predicting outcome in pain programs: A matter of cognition.* Paper presented at the annual meeting of the American Psychological Association, Washington, DC.

Hadjistavropoulos, H. D., MacLeod, F. K., & Asmundson, G. J. G. (1999). Validation of the Chronic Pain Coping Inventory. *Pain, 80,* 471-481.

Harkapaa, K. (1991). Relationships of psychological distress and health locus of control beliefs with the use of cognitive and behavioral coping strategies in low back pain patients. *Clinical Journal of Pain, 7,* 275-282.

Haythornthwaite, J. A., & Heinberg, L. J. (1999). Coping with pain: What works, under what circumstances, and in what ways? *Pain Forum, 8,* 172-175.

Haythornthwaite, J. A., Menefee, L. A., Heinberg, L. J., & Clark, M. R. (1998). Pain coping strategies predict perceived control over pain. *Pain, 77,* 33-39.

Herda, C. A., Siegeris, K., & Basler, H. D. (1994). The Pain Beliefs and Perceptions Inventory: Further evidence for a four-factor structure. *Pain, 57,* 85-90.

Hill, A. (1993). The use of pain coping strategies by patients with phantom limb pain. *Pain, 55,* 347-353.

Hill, A., Niven, C. A., & Knussen, C. (1995). The role of coping in adjustment to phantom limb pain. *Pain, 62,* 79-86.

Jensen, M. P., & Karoly, P. (1989, March). *Revision and cross-validation of the Survey of Pain Attitudes (SOPA).*

Poster presented at the annual meeting of the Society of Behavioral Medicine, San Francisco.

Jensen, M. P., & Karoly, P. (1991). Control beliefs, coping efforts, and adjustment to chronic pain. *Journal of Consulting and Clinical Psychology, 59,* 431-438.

Jensen, M. P., Karoly, P., & Huger, R. (1987). The development and preliminary validation of an instrument to assess patients' attitudes toward pain. *Journal of Psychosomatic Research, 31,* 393-400.

Jensen, M. P., Turner, J. A., & Romano, J. M. (1991). Self-efficacy and outcome expectancies: Relationship to chronic pain coping strategies and adjustment. *Pain, 44,* 263-269.

Jensen, M. P., Turner, J. A., & Romano, J. M. (1992). Chronic pain coping measures: Individual vs. composite scores. *Pain, 51,* 273-280.

Jensen, M. P., Turner, J. A., & Romano, J. M. (2000). Pain belief assessment: A comparison of short and long versions of the Survey of Pain Attitudes. *Journal of Pain, 1,* 138-150.

Jensen, M. P., Turner, J. A., Romano, J. M., & Lawler, B. K. (1994). Relationship of pain-specific beliefs to chronic pain adjustment. *Pain, 57,* 301-309.

Jensen, M. P., Turner, J. A., Romano, J. M., & Karoly, P. (1991). Coping with chronic pain: A critical review of the literature. *Pain, 47,* 249-283.

Jensen, M. P., Turner, J. A., Romano, J. M., & Strom, S. E. (1995). The Chronic Pain Coping Inventory: Development and preliminary validation. *Pain, 60,* 203-216.

Kashikar-Zuck, S., Keefe, F. J., Kornguth, P., Beaupre, P., Holzberg, A., & Delong, D. (1997). Pain coping and the pain experience during mammography: A preliminary study. *Pain, 73,* 165-172.

Keefe, F. J., Affleck, G., Lefebvre, J. C., Starr, K., Caldwell, D. S., & Tennen, H. (1997). Pain coping strategies and coping efficacy in rheumatoid arthritis: A daily process analysis. *Pain, 69,* 35-42.

Keefe, F. J., Caldwell, D. S., Martinez, S., Nunley, J., Beckham, J., & Williams, D. A. (1991). Analyzing pain in rheumatoid arthritis patients: Pain coping strategies in patients who have had knee replacement surgery. *Pain, 46,* 153-160.

Keefe, F. J., Kashikar-Zuck, S., Robinson, E., Salley, A., Beaupre, P., Caldwell, D., Baucom, D., & Haythornthwaite, J. (1997). Pain coping strategies that predict patients' and spouses' ratings of patients' self-efficacy. *Pain, 73,* 191-199.

Keefe, F. J., Lefebvre, J. C., & Smith, S. J. (1999). Catastrophizing research: Avoiding conceptual errors and maintaining a balanced perspective. *Pain Forum, 8,* 176-180.

Kerns, R. D., & Rosenberg, R. (2000). Predicting responses to self-management treatments for chronic pain: Application of the pain stages of change model. *Pain, 84,* 49-55.

Kerns, R. D., Rosenberg, R., Jamison, R. N., Caudill, M. A., & Haythornthwaite, J. (1997). Readiness to adopt a self-management approach to chronic pain: The Pain Stages of Change Questionnaire (PSOCQ). *Pain, 72,* 227-234.

Klocek, J., DeGood, D., & Chastain, D. (1997, October). *Augmenting clinical interview assessment of pain patients with the Cognitive Risk Profile (CRP).* Poster presented at the annual meeting of the American Pain Society, New Orleans, LA.

Kobasa, S. C. (1979). Stressful life events, personality, and health: An inquiry into hardiness. *Journal of Personality and Social Psychology, 37*, 1–11.

Kole-Snijders, A. M. J., Vlaeyen, J. W. S., Goossens, M. E. J. B., Ruten-van Molken, M. P. M. H., Heuts, P. H. T. G., van Breukelen, G., & van Eek, H. (1999). Chronic low-back pain: What does cognitive coping skills training add to operant behavioral treatment? Results of a randomized clinical trial. *Journal of Consulting and Clinical Psychology, 67*, 931–944.

Large, R. G., & Strong, J. (1997). The personal constructs of coping with chronic low back pain: Is coping a necessary evil? *Pain, 73*, 245–252.

Lazarus, R. A. (1991). Cognition and motivation in emotion. *American Psychologist, 46*, 353–367.

Lazarus, R. S., & Folkman, S. (1984). *Stress, appraisal, and coping.* New York: Springer.

Lefebvre, M. F. (1981). Cognitive distortion in depressed psychiatric and low back pain patients. *Journal of Consulting and Clinical Psychology, 49*, 517–525.

Lester, N., Lefebvre, J. C., & Keefe, F. J. (1996). Pain in young adults: III. Relationships of three pain-coping measures to pain and activity interference. *Clinical Journal of Pain, 12*, 291–300.

Lin, C., & Ward, S. E. (1996). Perceived self-efficacy and outcome expectancies in coping with chronic low back pain. *Research in Nursing and Health, 19*, 299–310.

Martin, M. Y., Bradley, L. A., Alexander, R. W., Alarcon, G. S., Triana-Alexander, M., Aaron, L. A., & Alberts, K. R. (1996). Coping strategies predict disability in patients with primary fibromyalgia. *Pain, 68*, 45–53.

McCracken, L. M. (1998). Learning to live with the pain: Acceptance of pain predicts adjustment in persons with chronic pain. *Pain, 74*, 21–27.

National Advisory Committee on Health and Disability. (1997). *Guide to assessing yellow flags in acute low back pain.* Wellington, New Zealand: Ministry of Health.

Nicassio, P. M., Schoenfeld-Smith, K., Radojevic, V., & Schuman, C. (1995). Pain coping mechanisms in fibromyalgia: Relationship to pain and functional outcomes. *Journal of Rheumatology, 22*, 1552–1558.

Nicholas, M. K., Wilson, P. H., & Goyen, J. (1992). Comparison of cognitive-behavioral group treatment and an alternative non-psychological treatment for chronic low back pain. *Pain, 48*, 339–347.

Pfingsten, M., Hildebrandt, J., Leibing, E., Franz, C., & Saur, P. (1997). Effectiveness of a multimodal treatment program for chronic low-back pain. *Pain, 73*, 77–85.

Pollock, S. E., & Duffy, M. E. (1990). The Health-Related Hardiness Scale: Development and psychometric analysis. *Nursing Research, 39*, 218–222.

Potter, R. G., & Jones, J. M. (1992). The evolution of chronic pain among patients with musculoskeletal problems: A pilot study in primary care. *British Journal of General Practice, 42*, 462–464.

Prochaska, J. O., & DiClemente, C. C. (1984). *The transtheoretical approach: Crossing traditional boundaries of change.* Homewood, IL: Dow Jones/Irwin.

Reid, G. J., Gilbert, C. A., & McGrath, P. J. (1998). The Pain Coping Questionnaire: Preliminary validation. *Pain, 76*, 83–96.

Riley, J. F., Ahern, D. K., & Follick, M. J. (1988). Chronic pain and functional impairment: Assessing beliefs about their relationship. *Archives of Physical Medicine and Rehabilitation, 59*, 579–582.

Riley, J. L., & Robinson, M. E. (1997). CSQ: Five factors or fiction? *Clinical Journal of Pain, 13*, 156–162.

Robinson, M. E., Riley, J. L., Myers, C. D., Sadler, I. J., Kvaal, S. A., Geisser, M. E., & Keefe, F. J. (1997). The Coping Strategies Questionnaire: A large sample, item level factor analysis. *Clinical Journal of Pain, 13*, 43–49.

Rosenstiel, A. K., & Keefe, F. J. (1983). The use of coping strategies in chronic low back pain patients: Relationship to patient characteristics and current adjustment. *Pain, 17*, 33–44.

Rotter, J. B. (1966). Generalized expectancies for internal versus external control of reinforcement. *Psychological Monographs: General and Applied, 80*(1, Whole No. 609).

Salovey, P., Smith, A. F., Turk, D. C., Jobe, J. B., & Willis, G. B. (1993). The accuracy of memory for pain: Not so bad most of the time. *American Pain Society Journal, 2*, 184–191.

Schanberg, L. E., Lefebvre, J. C., Keefe, F. J., Kredich, D. W., & Gil, K. M. (1997). Pain coping and the pain experience in children with juvenile chronic arthritis. *Pain, 73*, 181–189.

Schmitz, U., Saile, H., & Nilges, P. (1996). Coping with chronic pain: Flexible goal adjustment as an interactive buffer against pain-related distress. *Pain, 67*, 41–51.

Schwartz, D. P., DeGood, D. E., & Shutty, M. S. (1985). Direct assessment of beliefs and attitudes of chronic pain patients. *Archives of Physical Medicine and Rehabilitation, 66*, 806–809.

Shutty, M. S., & DeGood, D. E. (1990). Patient knowledge and beliefs about pain and its treatment. *Rehabilitation Psychology, 35*, 43–54.

Shutty, M. S., DeGood, D. E., & Tuttle, D. H. (1990). Chronic pain patients' beliefs about their pain and treatment outcomes. *Achives of Physical Medicine and Rehabilitation, 71*, 128–132.

Smith, C. A., & Wallston, K. A. (1992). Adaptation in patients with chronic rheumatoid arthritis: Application of a general model. *Health Psychology, 11*, 151–162.

Smith, C. A., Wallston, K. A., Dwyer, K. A., & Dowdy, S. W. (1997). Beyond good and bad coping: A multidimensional examination of coping with pain in persons with rheumatoid arthritis. *Annals of Behavioral Medicine, 19*, 11–21.

Snow-Turek, A L, Norris, M. P., & Tan, G. (1996). Active and passive coping strategies in chronic pain patients. *Pain, 64*, 455–462.

Spinhoven, P., & Linssen, A. C. G. (1991). Behavioral treatment of chronic low back pain: I. Relation of coping strategy use to outcome. *Pain, 45*, 29–34.

Stevens, J. J. (1992). Interaction of coping style and cognitive strategies in the management of acute pain. *Imagination, Cognition, and Personality, 11*, 225–232.

Stone, A., & Neale, J. (1984). New measure of daily coping: Development and preliminary results. *Journal of Personality and Social Psychology, 46*, 892–906.

Strong, J., Ashton, R., & Chant, D. (1992). The measurement of attitudes towards and beliefs about pain. *Pain, 48*, 227–236.

Strong, J., & Large, R. G. (1995). Coping with chronic pain: An idiographic exploration through focus groups. *International Journal of Psychiatry in Medicine. 25*, 361–377.

Sullivan, M. J. L., & D'Eon, J. (1990). Relation between catastrophizing and depression in chronic pain patients. *Journal of Abnormal Psychology, 99,* 260–263.

Sullivan, M. J. L., & Neish, N. (1997). Psychological predictors of pain during dental hygiene treatment. *Probe, 31,* 123–127.

Sullivan, M. J. L., Bishop, S., & Pivik, J. (1995). The Pain Catastrophizing Scale: Development and validation. *Psychological Assessment, 7,* 524–532.

Sullivan, M. J. L., Stanish, W., Waite, H., Sullivan, M., & Tripp, D. A. (1998). Catastrophizing, pain, and disability in patients with soft-tissue injuries. *Pain, 77,* 253–260.

Tait, R. C., & Chibnall, J. T. (1997). Development of a brief version of the Survey of Pain Attitudes. *Pain, 70,* 229–235.

Thompson, R. J., Gil, K. M., Abrams, M. R., & Phillips, G. (1992). Stress, coping, and psychological adjustment of adults with sickle cell disease. *Journal of Consulting and Clinical Psychology, 60,* 433–440.

Thorn, B. E., Rich, M. A., & Boothby, J. L. (1999). Pain beliefs and coping attempts: Conceptual model building. *Pain Forum, 8,* 169–171.

Tota-Faucette, M. E., Gil, K. M., Williams, D. A., Keefe, F. J., & Goli, V. (1993). Predictors of response to pain management treatment. *Clinical Journal of Pain, 9,* 115–123.

Turk, D. C., & Rudy, T. E. (1986). Assessment of cognitive factors in chronic pain: A worthwhile enterprise? *Journal of Consulting and Clinical Psychology, 54,* 766–768.

Turner, J. A., Jensen, M. P., & Romano, J. M. (2000). Do beliefs, coping, and catastrophizing independently predict functioning in patients with chronic pain? *Pain, 85,* 115–125.

Turner, J. A., Whitney, C., Dworkin, S. F., Massoth, D., & Wilson, L. (1995). Do changes in patient beliefs and coping strategies predict temporomandibular disorder treatment outcomes? *Clinical Journal of Pain, 11,* 177–188.

Ulmer, J. F. (1997). An exploratory study of pain, coping, and depressed mood following burn injury. *Journal of Pain and Symptom Management, 13,* 148–157.

Vitaliano, P. P., Russo, J., Carr, J. E., Maiuro, R. D., & Becker, J. (1985). The Ways of Coping Checklist: Revision and psychometric properties. *Multivariate Behavioral Research, 20,* 3–26.

Wallston, K. A., Wallston, B. S., & DeVellis, R. (1978). Development of the Multidimensional Health Locus of Control (MHLC) scales. *Health Education Monographs, 6,* 160–170.

Watkins, K. W., Shifren, K., Park, D. C., & Morrell, R. W. (1999). Age, pain, and coping with rheumatoid arthritis. *Pain, 82,* 217–228.

Weisberg, J. N., & Gatchel, R. J. (Eds.). (2000). *Personality characteristics of pain patients: Recent advances and future directions.* Washingon, DC: American Psychological Association.

Wilkie, D. J., & Keefe, F. J. (1991). Coping strategies of patients with lung cancer-related pain. *Clinical Journal of Pain, 7,* 292–299.

Williams, D. A., & Keefe, F. J. (1991). Pain beliefs and the use of cognitive-behavioral coping strategies. *Pain, 46,* 185–358.

Williams, D. A., & Thorn, B. E. (1989). An empirical assessment of pain beliefs. *Pain, 36,* 351–358.

Wineman, N. M., Durand, E. J., & McCulloch, B. J. (1994). Examination of the factor structure of the Ways of Coping Questionnaire with clinical populations. *Nursing Research, 43,* 268–273.

Wrubel, J., Benner, P., & Lazarus, R. S. (1981). Social competence from the perspective of stress and coping. In J. Wine & M. Syme (Eds.), *Social competence* (pp. 61–99). New York: Guilford Press.

Zautra, A. J., Burleson, M. H., Smith, C. A., Blalock, S. J., Wallston, K. A., DeVellis, R. F., DeVellis, B. M., & Smith, T. W. (1995). Arthritis and perceptions of quality of life: An examination of positive and negative affect in rheumatoid arthritis patients. *Health Psychology, 14,* 399–408.

APPENDIX 17.A. SURVEY OF PAIN ATTITUDES (SOPA)

Instructions: Please indicate how much you agree with each of the following statements about your pain problem by using the following scale:

    0 = This is very untrue for me.
    1 = This is somewhat untrue for me.
    2 = This is neither true nor untrue for me (or it does not apply to me).
    3 = This is somewhat true for me.
    4 = This is very true for me.

1. There are times when I can influence the amount of pain I feel	0 1 2 3 4
2. The pain I feel is a sign that damage is being done	0 1 2 3 4
3. I do not consider my pain to be a disability	0 1 2 3 4
4. Nothing but my pain really bothers me	0 1 2 3 4
5. Pain is a sign that I have not been exercising enough	0 1 2 3 4
6. My family does not understand how much pain I am in	0 1 2 3 4
7. I count more on my doctors to decrease my pain than I do on myself	0 1 2 3 4
8. I will probably always have to take pain medication	0 1 2 3 4
9. When I hurt, I want my family to treat me better	0 1 2 3 4
10. If my pain continues at its present level, I will be unable to work	0 1 2 3 4
11. The amount of pain I feel is out of my control	0 1 2 3 4
12. I do not expect a medical cure for my pain	0 1 2 3 4
13. Pain does not have to mean that my body is being harmed	0 1 2 3 4
14. I have had the most relief from pain with the use of medications	0 1 2 3 4
15. Anxiety increases the pain I feel	0 1 2 3 4
16. There is little that I can do to ease my pain	0 1 2 3 4
17. When I am hurting, I deserve to be treated with care and concern	0 1 2 3 4
18. I pay doctors so they will cure me of my pain	0 1 2 3 4
19. My pain problem does not need to interfere with my activity level	0 1 2 3 4
20. My pain is physical, not emotional	0 1 2 3 4
21. I have given up my search for the complete elimination of my pain through doctors	0 1 2 3 4
22. It is the responsibility of my family to help me when I feel pain	0 1 2 3 4
23. Stress in my life increases the pain I feel	0 1 2 3 4
24. Exercise and movement are good for my pain problem	0 1 2 3 4
25. Just by concentrating or relaxing, I can "take the edge" off of my pain	0 1 2 3 4
26. I will get a job to earn money regardless of how much pain I feel	0 1 2 3 4
27. Medicine is one of the best treatments for chronic pain	0 1 2 3 4
28. I am unable to control most of my pain	0 1 2 3 4
29. A doctor's job is to find pain treatments that work	0 1 2 3 4
30. My family needs to learn how to take better care of me when I am in pain	0 1 2 3 4
31. Depression increases the pain I feel	0 1 2 3 4
32. If I exercise, I could make my pain problem much worse	0 1 2 3 4
33. I can control my pain by changing my thoughts	0 1 2 3 4
34. I need more tender loving care than I am now getting when I am in pain	0 1 2 3 4
35. I consider myself disabled	0 1 2 3 4
36. I wish my doctor would stop giving me pain medications	0 1 2 3 4

(cont.)

37. My pain is mostly emotional, and not so much a physical problem	0	1	2	3	4
38. My pain gets in the way of movement and exercise	0	1	2	3	4
39. I have learned to control my pain	0	1	2	3	4
40. I trust that doctors can cure my pain	0	1	2	3	4
41. I know for sure I can learn to manage my pain	0	1	2	3	4
42. My pain does not stop me from leading a physically active life	0	1	2	3	4
43. My physical pain will never be cured	0	1	2	3	4
44. There is a connection between my emotions and my pain level	0	1	2	3	4
45. I can do everything as well as I could before I had a pain problem	0	1	2	3	4
46. If I do not exercise regularly, my pain problem will get worse	0	1	2	3	4
47. I am not in control of my pain	0	1	2	3	4
48. No matter how I feel emotionally, my pain stays the same	0	1	2	3	4
49. Pain will never stop me from doing what I really want to do	0	1	2	3	4
50. When I find the right doctor, he or she will know how to reduce my pain	0	1	2	3	4
51. If my doctor prescribed pain medications for me, I would throw them away	0	1	2	3	4
52. Whether or not a person is disabled by pain depends more on attitude than the pain itself	0	1	2	3	4
53. If I can change my emotions, I can influence my pain	0	1	2	3	4
54. I will never take pain medications again	0	1	2	3	4
55. Exercise can decrease the amount of pain I experience	0	1	2	3	4
56. No medical procedure can help my pain	0	1	2	3	4
57. My pain would stop anyone from leading an active life	0	1	2	3	4

SOPA Scoring Key
Control: 1, 11*, 16*, 25, 28*, 33, 39, 41, 47*, 53
Disability: 3*, 10, 19*, 26*, 35, 42*, 45*, 49*, 52*, 57
Harm: 2, 5*, 13*, 24*, 32, 38, 46*, 55*
Emotion: 4*, 15, 20*, 23, 31, 37, 44, 48*
Medication: 8, 14, 27, 36*, 51*, 54*
Solicitude: 6, 9, 17, 22, 30, 34
Medical Cure: 7, 12*, 18, 21*, 29, 40, 43*, 50, 56*

*Reverse-scored items. Transform these items (i.e., 4 minus rating given) before summing with other items.

Note. Copyright 1996 by Mark P. Jensen and Paul Karoly. Reprinted by permission.

APPENDIX 17.B. PAIN BELIEFS AND PERCEPTIONS INVENTORY (PBAPI)

Please indicate the degree to which you agree or disagree with each of the following statements. Simply circle the number that corresponds with your level of agreement.

	Strongly Disagree	Disagree	Agree	Strongly Agree
1. No one's been able to tell me exactly why I'm in pain.	-2	-1	1	2
2. I used to think my pain was curable but now I'm not so sure.	-2	-1	1	2
3. There are times when I am pain-free.	-2	-1	1	2
4. My pain is confusing to me.	-2	-1	1	2
5. My pain is here to stay.	-2	-1	1	2
6. I am continuously in pain.	-2	-1	1	2

(cont.)

	Strongly Disagree	Disagree	Agree	Strongly Agree
7. If I am in pain, it is my own fault.	−2	−1	1	2
8. I don't know enough about my pain.	−2	−1	1	2
9. My pain is a temporary problem in my life.	−2	−1	1	2
10. It seems like I wake up with pain and I go to sleep with pain.	−2	−1	1	2
11. I am the cause of my pain.	−2	−1	1	2
12. There is a cure for my pain.	−2	−1	1	2
13. I blame myself if I am in pain.	−2	−1	1	2
14. I can't figure out why I'm in pain.	−2	−1	1	2
15. Someday I'll be 100% pain-free again.	−2	−1	1	2
16. My pain varies in intensity but is always with me.	−2	−1	1	2

Four-Factor Scoring Solution
    Scales: Mystery $(1 + 4 + 8 + 14)/4$
             Permanence $(2 + 5 + 9R + 12R + 15R)/5$
             Constancy $(3R + 6 + 10 + 16)/4$
             Self-Blame $(7 + 11 + 13)/3$

Note. Copyright 1987 by David A. Williams. Reprinted by permission.

APPENDIX 17.C. COGNITIVE RISK PROFILE (CRP)

Questionnaire instructions: Please fill in the circle next to each statement that best expresses how much you agree or disagree with that statement. Please try to respond to ALL questions, even if you are not sure if the question applies to you. There are no correct answers, we want to understand your own experiences and reactions to pain.

strongly AGREE
    moderately AGREE
        slightly AGREE
            slightly DISAGREE
                moderately DISAGREE
                    strongly DISAGREE

① ② ③ ④ ⑤ ⑥	1. Learning to pace myself can help with my pain.
① ② ③ ④ ⑤ ⑥	2. Pain can give me bad dreams.
① ② ③ ④ ⑤ ⑥	3. It seems that I have never really been thoroughly examined for my pain.
① ② ③ ④ ⑤ ⑥	4. I feel very discouraged about my pain problem.
① ② ③ ④ ⑤ ⑥	5. It seems that taking pain killing medication is about all I can do for my pain.
① ② ③ ④ ⑤ ⑥	6. I'm afraid my pain is here to stay.
① ② ③ ④ ⑤ ⑥	7. I expect to be free of pain at the end of my treatment.
① ② ③ ④ ⑤ ⑥	8. My family is very understanding and helpful with my pain problem.
① ② ③ ④ ⑤ ⑥	9. My pain is not anyone's fault, it's just bad luck.
① ② ③ ④ ⑤ ⑥	10. No matter what I try to do, my pain always stays the same.
① ② ③ ④ ⑤ ⑥	11. Improvement in my pain condition will require an operation.
① ② ③ ④ ⑤ ⑥	12. My church or community will help me if I need help.
① ② ③ ④ ⑤ ⑥	13. Feeling angry can increase my pain.
① ② ③ ④ ⑤ ⑥	14. I am satisfied with the medical care I have received so far.
① ② ③ ④ ⑤ ⑥	15. Pain can put me in a bad mood.

(cont.)

strongly AGREE
　moderately AGREE
　　slightly AGREE
　　　slightly DISAGREE
　　　　moderately DISAGREE
　　　　　strongly DISAGREE

① ② ③ ④ ⑤ ⑥　16. Because others cannot see my pain, they often do not understand how much I hurt.

① ② ③ ④ ⑤ ⑥　17. I may have to sue to get what is due me.

① ② ③ ④ ⑤ ⑥　18. Right now I am unable to do any kind of work, or most other normal activity.

① ② ③ ④ ⑤ ⑥　19. I fear that I could become paralyzed or confined to a wheelchair.

① ② ③ ④ ⑤ ⑥　20. Exercise can help me manage my pain.

① ② ③ ④ ⑤ ⑥　21. My life should be pain free.

① ② ③ ④ ⑤ ⑥　22. There must be some higher purpose for me to have so much pain.

① ② ③ ④ ⑤ ⑥　23. I do not deserve to have all of this pain.

① ② ③ ④ ⑤ ⑥　24. I expect my pain will just get worse and worse.

① ② ③ ④ ⑤ ⑥　25. Worry can increase the pain I feel.

① ② ③ ④ ⑤ ⑥　26. Talking with a counselor might help me to deal with my pain.

① ② ③ ④ ⑤ ⑥　27. My mood on a given day has nothing to do with my level of pain.

① ② ③ ④ ⑤ ⑥　28. People who can accept their pain manage better than those who cannot accept it.

① ② ③ ④ ⑤ ⑥　29. The best thing for me is to stay off my feet as much as I can.

① ② ③ ④ ⑤ ⑥　30. I get bored because pain keeps me from doing what I would like to do.

① ② ③ ④ ⑤ ⑥　31. Maybe I can learn to cope better, even if my pain does not go away.

① ② ③ ④ ⑤ ⑥　32. My pain was caused by someone else's neglect or carelessness.

① ② ③ ④ ⑤ ⑥　33. Doctors should do more to help with my pain.

① ② ③ ④ ⑤ ⑥　34. It really bothers me when others say I look fine.

① ② ③ ④ ⑤ ⑥　35. My attitude and the way I think are an important part of how to manage my pain.

① ② ③ ④ ⑤ ⑥　36. I fear that exercise could make my pain problem worse.

① ② ③ ④ ⑤ ⑥　37. I have no choice but to support myself with a disability pension.

① ② ③ ④ ⑤ ⑥　38. Learning relaxation and stress management skills could help me better manage my pain.

① ② ③ ④ ⑤ ⑥　39. I believe more medical tests are needed to find what is really causing my pain.

① ② ③ ④ ⑤ ⑥　40. No one should have to suffer such lasting pain as mine.

① ② ③ ④ ⑤ ⑥　41. When I see people who are pain free, I resent all of my discomfort.

① ② ③ ④ ⑤ ⑥　42. Stress in my life can make my pain feel worse.

① ② ③ ④ ⑤ ⑥　43. I am afraid pain will keep me from ever returning to work (or other normal activity).

① ② ③ ④ ⑤ ⑥　44. My pain problem puts a lot of pressure on my family.

① ② ③ ④ ⑤ ⑥　45. Pain can make me feel depressed.

① ② ③ ④ ⑤ ⑥　46. A pain problem is worse than any other type of problem.

① ② ③ ④ ⑤ ⑥　47. My pain could be completely cured if only a doctor could find my real problem.

① ② ③ ④ ⑤ ⑥　48. I could use more help than I've been getting from my friends.

(cont.)

strongly AGREE
| moderately AGREE
| | slightly AGREE
| | | slightly DISAGREE
| | | | moderately DISAGREE
| | | | | strongly DISAGREE
| | | | | |

① ② ③ ④ ⑤ ⑥   49. Almost everything I try to do seems to make my pain worse.

① ② ③ ④ ⑤ ⑥   50. The insurance providers I have had to deal with can be very aggravating.

① ② ③ ④ ⑤ ⑥   51. There must be a medicine that can control my pain.

① ② ③ ④ ⑤ ⑥   52. No one seems to understand what I go through in living every day with pain.

① ② ③ ④ ⑤ ⑥   53. I certainly have a right to disability benefits, after all of the pain I have had.

① ② ③ ④ ⑤ ⑥   54. Doctors just don't take my pain seriously enough.

① ② ③ ④ ⑤ ⑥   55. I am in good health except for my pain.

① ② ③ ④ ⑤ ⑥   56. I will gradually have to become more physically active in order to get better.

① ② ③ ④ ⑤ ⑥   57. It is unfair for me to have to suffer so much pain.

① ② ③ ④ ⑤ ⑥   58. I believe someday a cure will be found for my pain condition.

① ② ③ ④ ⑤ ⑥   59. My pain level on a given day has nothing to do with my mood.

① ② ③ ④ ⑤ ⑥   60. I have been treated fairly by the insurance system.

① ② ③ ④ ⑤ ⑥   61. My life is hardly worth living with all of this pain.

① ② ③ ④ ⑤ ⑥   62. I should receive financial compensation for my pain and suffering.

① ② ③ ④ ⑤ ⑥   63. If only certain people had listened to me more carefully, I would not have all of this pain.

① ② ③ ④ ⑤ ⑥   64. This pain often leaves me feeling frustrated and angry.

① ② ③ ④ ⑤ ⑥   65. My pain makes me worry about the future.

① ② ③ ④ ⑤ ⑥   66. I should not have to work with this much pain.

① ② ③ ④ ⑤ ⑥   67. I believe my pain problem is quite rare.

① ② ③ ④ ⑤ ⑥   68. No matter how I feel emotionally, my pain stays the same.

CRP Scoring Key

Philosophic Beliefs	21*, 22, 23*, 28, 34*, 40*, 41*, 46*, 57*, 61*
Denial Mood Affects Pain	13, 25, 35, 42, 59*, 68*
Denial Pain Affects Mood	2, 15, 27*, 30, 44, 45, 64, 65
Perception of Blame	9, 14, 17*, 32*, 33*, 60, 63*
Lack of Social Support	8, 12, 16*, 48*, 50*, 52*, 54*
Disability Entitlement	18*, 37*, 43*, 53*, 62*, 66*
Medical Breakthrough	3*, 7*, 39*, 47*, 51*, 58*, 67*
Multidisciplinary Skepticism	1, 5*, 11*, 20, 26, 29*, 31, 36*, 38, 56
Conviction of Hopelessness	4*, 6*, 10*, 19*, 24*, 49*, 55

*Reverse-scored items.

APPENDIX 17.D. THE PAIN STAGES OF CHANGE QUESTIONNAIRE (PSOCQ)

This questionnaire is to help us better understand the way you view your pain problem. Each statement describes how you *may* feel about this particular problem. Please indicate the extent to which you tend to agree or disagree with each statement. In each example, please make your choice is based on *how you feel right now*, not how you have felt in the past or how you would like to feel.

Circle the response that best describes how much you agree or disagree with each statement.

	Strongly Disagree	Disagree	Undecided or unsure	Agree	Strongly Agree
1. I have been thinking that the way I cope with my pain could improve.	1	2	3	4	5
2. I am developing new ways to cope with my pain.	1	2	3	4	5
3. I have learned some good ways to keep my pain problem from interfering with my life.	1	2	3	4	5
4. When my pain flares up, I find myself automatically using coping strategies that have worked in the past, such as a relaxation exercise or mental distraction technique.	1	2	3	4	5
5. I am using some strategies that help me better deal with my pain problem on a day-to-day basis.	1	2	3	4	5
6. I have started to come up with strategies to help myself control my pain.	1	2	3	4	5
7. I have recently realized that there is no medical cure for my pain condition, so I want to learn some ways to cope with it.	1	2	3	4	5
8. Even if my pain doesn't go away, I am ready to start changing how I deal with it.	1	2	3	4	5
9. I realize now that it's time for me to come up with a better plan to cope with my pain problem.	1	2	3	4	5
10. I use what I have learned to help keep my pain under control.	1	2	3	4	5
11. I have tried everything that people have recommended to manage my pain and nothing helps.	1	2	3	4	5
12. My pain is a medical problem and I should be dealing with physicians about it.	1	2	3	4	5
13. I am currently using some suggestions people have made about how to live with my pain problem.	1	2	3	4	5
14. I am beginning to wonder if I need to get some help to develop skills for dealing with my pain.	1	2	3	4	5
15. I have recently figured out that it's up to me to deal better with my pain.	1	2	3	4	5
16. Everybody I speak with tells me that I have to learn to live with my pain, but I don't see why I should have to.	1	2	3	4	5
17. I have incorporated strategies for dealing with my pain into my everyday life.	1	2	3	4	5
18. I have made a lot of progress in coping with my pain.	1	2	3	4	5
19. I have recently come to the conclusion that it's time for me to change how I cope with my pain.	1	2	3	4	5

(cont.)

	Strongly Disagree	Disagree	Undecided or unsure	Agree	Strongly Agree
20. I'm getting help learning some strategies for coping better with my pain.	1	2	3	4	5
21. I'm starting to wonder whether it's up to me to manage my pain rather than relying on physicians.	1	2	3	4	5
22. I still think despite what doctors tell me, there must be some surgical procedure or medication that would get rid of my pain.	1	2	3	4	5
23. I have been thinking that doctors can only help so much in managing my pain and that the rest is up to me.	1	2	3	4	5
24. The best thing I can do is find a doctor who can figure out how to get rid of my pain once and for all.	1	2	3	4	5
25. Why can't someone just do something to take away my pain?	1	2	3	4	5
26. I am learning to help myself control my pain without doctors.	1	2	3	4	5
27. I am testing out some coping skills to manage my pain better.	1	2	3	4	5
28. I have been wondering if there is something I could do to manage my pain better.	1	2	3	4	5
29. All of this talk about how to cope better is a waste of my time.	1	2	3	4	5
30. I am learning ways to control my pain other than with medications or surgery.	1	2	3	4	5

Scoring of the Pain Stages of Change Questionnaire

Precontemplation: Sum (11, 12, 16, 22, 24, 25, 29)/7
Contemplation: Sum (1, 7, 8, 9, 14, 15, 19, 21, 23, 28)/10
Action: Sum (2, 6, 20, 26, 27, 30)/6
Maintenance: Sum (3, 4, 5, 10, 13, 17, 18)/7

To account for sporadic missing data, sums should be divided by the number of non-missing items. Any scale with more than 25% of its items missing should be considered missing.

Note. From Kerns, R. D., Rosenberg, R., Jamison, R. N., Caudill, M. A., & Haythornthwaite, J. (1997). Readiness to adopt a self-management approach to chronic pain: The Pain Stages of Change Questionnaire (PSOCQ). *Pain*, 72, 227–234. Copyright 1997 by the International Association for the Study of Pain. Reprinted by permission.

APPENDIX 17.E. PAIN CATASTROPHIZING SCALE (PCS)

Name:_____ Age:_____ Gender:_____ Date:_____

Everyone experiences painful situations at some point in their lives. Such experiences may include headaches, tooth pain, joint or muscle pain. People are often exposed to situations that may cause pain such as illness, injury, dental procedures or surgery.

We are interested in the types of thoughts and feelings that you have when you are in pain. Listed below are thirteen statements describing different thoughts and feelings that may be associated with pain. Using the following scale, please indicate the degree to which you have these thoughts and feelings when you are experiencing pain.

0—not at all   1—to a slight degree   2—to a moderate degree   3—to a great degree   4—all the time

(cont.)

When I'm in pain . . .

1. ☐ I worry all the time about whether the pain will end.
2. ☐ I feel I can't go on.
3. ☐ It's terrible and I think it's never going to get any better.
4. ☐ It's awful and I feel that it overwhelms me.
5. ☐ I feel I can't stand it anymore.
6. ☐ I become afraid that the pain will get worse.
7. ☐ I keep thinking of other painful events.
8. ☐ I anxiously want the pain to go away.
9. ☐ I can't seem to keep it out of my mind.
10. ☐ I keep thinking about how much it hurts.
11. ☐ I keep thinking about how badly I want the pain to stop.
12. ☐ There's nothing I can do to reduce the intensity of the pain.
13. ☐ I wonder whether something serious may happen.
   . . . *Total*

APPENDIX 17.F. SAMPLE ITEMS FROM THE CHRONIC PAIN COPING INVENTORY (CPCI), SELF-REPORT VERSION

Illness-focused coping

1. Guarding: Protecting part of the body to avoid pain
   Sample item: Avoided using part of my body (e.g., hand, arm, leg)

2. Resting: Avoiding activity as a way of avoiding pain increases
   Sample item: I rested as much as I could

3. Asking for Assistance: Requesting help from others for customary tasks
   Sample item: Asked someone to do something for me

4. Medication Use (Opioid, Nonsteroidal, Sedative–Hypnotic): Using medications of different types to reduce pain
   Sample item: List each medication that you took for pain during the past week, and indicate the number of days that you took each medication during the past week.

Wellness-focused coping

1. Relaxation: Engaging in a specific relaxation technique to cope with pain
   Sample item: Focussed on relaxing my muscles

2. Task Persistence: Maintaining levels of activity despite pain
   Sample item: I didn't let the pain interfere with my activities

3. Exercise/Stretch: Engaging in therapeutic physical activity specifically designed for pain management
   Sample item: Exercised to improve my overall physical condition for at least 5 minutes

4. Coping Self-Statements: Using self-talk strategies intended to reduce distress
   Sample item: Reminded myself that I had coped with pain before

Other coping

1. Seeking Social Support: Turning to another for distraction or emotional support
   Sample item: Called a friend on the phone to help me feel better

Chapter 18

Assessment of Couples and Families with Chronic Pain

JOAN M. ROMANO
KAREN B. SCHMALING

The assessment of the patient with chronic pain is incomplete without consideration of the social context in which the patient functions (see Jacob & Kerns, Chapter 19, this volume). The family arguably provides the most important social influence on the development of concepts of health and illness and on responses to acute and chronic health care problems (Kerns, 1995). Families provide the context in which early experiences of illness and caretaking occur, and in which beliefs about the meanings of symptoms and the appropriate individual and family response to them are formed.

There has been increasing recognition that couple and family functioning in the context of chronic health problems such as pain are multidimensional and involve a continuing dynamic interplay between the patient and his or her significant others as they appraise, cope, and respond to challenges related to the patient's health, as well as to other life stresses and situations. These processes will both affect and be affected by the patient's chronic pain and dysfunction (Kerns & Weiss, 1994; Patterson & Garwick, 1994).

In this chapter, we focus on the assessment of the family, particularly the couple, when one adult member has a chronic nonmalignant pain problem. We have chosen to focus primarily on the couple, given that most of the research literature pertaining to the families of patients with

chronic pain is based on the study of couples. In addition, it is most often the case that the clinician will have access to the spouse or partner rather than to other family members during assessment and treatment of adults with chronic pain.

We first describe the major theoretical models that have been applied to the study of couples and family systems in which one member has chronic pain, and then describe and review the most commonly used methods and measures for assessing couple and family functioning. Finally, we will discuss areas in need of further research and suggest directions for future studies.

MODELS OF THE ROLE OF THE FAMILY IN CHRONIC PAIN

Behavioral Models

Arguably, the most influential description of the role of the social environment and its impact on chronic pain was provided by Wilbert Fordyce in his seminal work, *Behavioral Methods for Chronic Pain and Illness*, published in 1976. Fordyce made the conceptual breakthrough of considering *pain behaviors* (behaviors that would be commonly construed as indicating pain; see also Keefe, Williams, & Smith, Chapter 10, this volume) not simply as responses elicited by a nociceptive stimulus, but as operant behaviors that could come under the

346

control of social and environmental contingencies of reinforcement. This conceptualization was particularly pertinent to the patient with chronic pain, in that Fordyce hypothesized that the longer pain persisted, the more opportunity existed for pain behaviors to be influenced by the environment. According to this model, if a patient's pain behaviors result in increased positive or decreased negative consequences, such contingencies can contribute to the perpetuation of pain behaviors through operant learning processes. This model does not imply that pain is not "real," nor does it imply a conscious attempt to manipulate the social environment. Rather, it suggests that through learning mechanisms a shaping process may occur, such that pain behavior may be influenced by contingencies such as the social responses of significant others, contributing to the continuation of pain behaviors and to diminished functioning over time. However, operant learning processes may explain only a portion of the variance in patient dysfunction and pain behaviors, with other potential influences including physiological factors (such as deconditioning) and psychological disorders (such as depression).

Despite the important conceptual advance represented by the application of behavioral theory to the assessment and treatment of chronic pain and disability, behavioral models have been criticized for being overly restrictive in their conceptualization of chronic pain and for paying insufficient attention to the role that cognitive factors (such as beliefs and attributions about pain or the responses of others) may play in influencing suffering and functioning in people with chronic pain (Novy, Nelson, Francis, & Turk, 1995; Turk & Flor, 1987).

Cognitive-Behavioral and Cognitive-Behavioral Transactional Models

Cognitive-behavioral approaches to the assessment and treatment of patients with chronic pain have become widely used over the last 15 to 20 years, with a growing body of evidence supporting their efficacy and applicability (Compas, Haaga, Keefe, Leitenberg, & Williams, 1998; National Institutes of Health Technology Assessment Panel, 1996). Cognitive-behavioral therapy is based on a theoretical model in which a patient's affect and behavior are strongly influenced by how the patient views and interprets his or her experiences. One implication of this model is that the patient's be-

liefs and attributions regarding pain will influence how the patient responds emotionally and behaviorally to pain. However, this model also implies that the effect of the social environment on the patient's pain behaviors and dysfunction will be influenced by the patient's cognitions—for example, the beliefs that the patient holds regarding the appropriateness or meaning of others' responses to pain behaviors. In addition, the model implies that the responses of significant others in the patient's environment may be strongly influenced by the beliefs that they hold regarding the nature of the patient's pain and disability and of the appropriateness of different responses to pain behaviors (Turk, Kerns, & Rosenberg, 1992). Thus whether a particular partner response functions to reinforce pain behaviors may depend upon the patient's beliefs and interpretation of that behavior in the context of the relationship with the partner, much as other cognitive-behavioral formulations of interpersonal relationships have incorporated beliefs and attributions into their theoretical models (see, e.g., Bradbury & Fincham, 1990).

Kerns, Turk, and their colleagues have provided an expanded theoretical model of family functioning in chronic pain and illness, which they have termed the *cognitive-behavioral transactional model* (Kerns & Weiss, 1994; Turk & Kerns, 1985). This model draws on cognitive-behavioral and operant behavioral perspectives, models of family adjustment and adaptation, and stress and coping models (Kerns & Weiss, 1994). It also emphasizes the importance of the family as an active system that seeks out and evaluates information and responds to stress and demands based on both individual and shared schemas (relatively stable sets of beliefs regarding the family and its sociocultural context). This model supports assessment at multiple levels (individual, dyadic, and family system) of behavior, cognitions, mood, and global adjustment and functioning (Kerns & Weiss, 1994).

Family Systems and Family Contextual-Interactional Models

Family systems models generally posit that difficulties in interpersonal systems such as the family may be expressed as dysfunction in one person, the identified patient (see, e.g., Bowen, 1978). This dysfunction may take the form of chronic medical symptomatology. Specific family interaction patterns have been postulated to be associated with poorly explained medical symptoms or problems.

These patterns include *enmeshment, overprotectiveness, rigidity,* and *lack of conflict resolution.* An enmeshed, or fused, family would be characterized by a relative lack of differentiation or boundaries between individuals. An overprotective family would be unable to tolerate family members' distress and would avert or negate distress in others. Rigid families may appear quite invested in the maintenance of familial rules and status quo, and of inflexible roles within the family. Finally, families characterized by a lack of conflict resolution avoid acknowledging or addressing conflict and its resolution. Such patterns are posited to interfere with appropriate adaptation, coping with stress, and resolution of individual symptoms and family dysfunction.

Several specific systems models of family functioning have been articulated and have given rise to the development of model-driven family assessment devices. One systems model, the circumplex model (Olson, Sprenkle, & Russell, 1979), is a typology for classifying families on two key dimensions of family behavior: adaptability and cohesion. *Adaptability* refers to the family's ability to reorganize itself in response to stress. *Cohesion* refers to the emotional bonding among family members. The circumplex model posits that a moderate or balanced level of both adaptability and cohesion is necessary for good family functioning.

Another model, the McMaster model of family functioning (Epstein, Bishop, & Levin, 1980), assumes that the purpose of the family is the social, psychological, and biological development of its members through basic, developmental, and hazardous (e.g., crisis management) tasks. The model contains six dimensions of family functioning: problem solving, communication, roles, affective responsiveness, affective involvement, and behavior control. Assessment methods based on the circumplex and McMaster's models have been developed, but as yet relatively few studies have applied them to families with chronic pain (Basolo-Kunzer, Diamond, Maliszewski, Weyermann, & Reed, 1991; Roy, 1989; Roy & Thomas, 1989).

Summary

The family environment of the patient with chronic pain has been the focus of theorists informed by behavioral, cognitive-behavioral, and family systems perspectives. These perspectives share an emphasis on the potent repercussions one person's experience of pain can have in a family, but they differ in their temporal focus and degree of empirical support. Behavioral theory has tended to focus on proximal behavioral transactions and their effects on subsequent behavior and functioning, whereas systems theory focuses on larger shifts in roles and responsibilities over longer periods of time. More empirical support exists for the behavioral perspective, perhaps in part because its focus on smaller, discrete behaviors facilitates investigation. Further refinement of cognitive-behavioral models would be facilitated by the development and validation of measures of patient and partner cognitions (e.g., attributions and appraisals) regarding patient pain behaviors and partner responses to them (Kerns & Weiss, 1994). Few empirical studies have tested family systems theory as applied to chronic pain. However, advances in testing this model in the families of children with chronic abdominal disease (Wood et al., 1989) suggest the possibility that similar methodologies might be applicable to the study of families of patients with chronic pain.

THE IMPACT OF CHRONIC PAIN ON THE PARTNER

Given the enormous impact of chronic pain on a patient's physical and psychosocial functioning, it would be difficult to imagine that partner and family functioning would not also be affected by the experience of living with someone in chronic pain. Such effects are predicted by family systems and cognitive-behavioral transactional models as reviewed above, and research findings are consistent with this view. A number of studies have found evidence of increased psychological distress among partners of patients with chronic pain (Ahern, Adams, & Follick, 1985; Kerns & Turk, 1984; Schwartz, Slater, Birchler, & Atkinson, 1991; Taylor, Lorentzen, & Blank, 1990). Relationship dissatisfaction has also been reported in patients with chronic pain (Flor, Turk, & Rudy, 1989; Kerns & Turk, 1984), as well as partners of such patients (Ahern et al., 1985; Flor, Turk, & Scholz, 1987; Kerns & Turk, 1984; Maruta & Osborne, 1978; Maruta, Osborne, Swanson, & Halling, 1981).

However, not all studies have reported elevated levels of relationship distress, and a number have reported mean levels of relationship satisfaction in the normal range. For example, Flor, Breitenstein, Birbaumer, and Fürst (1995) found that ratings of relationship distress did not differentiate couples with back pain from healthy control couples, and the percentage of "happy" couples was higher in the group with pain (53%) compared to the controls (43%). Basolo-Kunzer and colleagues (1991) also found no difference in relationship satisfaction or adjustment between a sample of patients with headache and their spouses compared to controls. A number of other studies have also reported mean relationship adjustment scores in the nondistressed range for patients with chronic pain and their partners (Block & Boyer, 1984; Flor, Kerns, & Turk, 1987; Hewitt, Flett, & Mikail, 1995; Romano et al., 1995; Stampler, Wall, Cassisi, & Davis, 1997), using well-validated measures of relationship satisfaction and adjustment.

A number of factors may bear on these apparently discrepant findings. There is strong evidence that patients with chronic pain do not form a homogeneous group on measures of physical and psychological functioning, and empirically derived subgroups of patients have been identified (Jamison, Rudy, Penzien, & Mosley, 1994; Turk & Rudy, 1988, 1990; see also Turk & Okifuji, Chapter 21). One such subgroup has been labeled Interpersonally Distressed; it consists of patients reporting significantly lower levels of perceived support and relationship satisfaction (Turk, Okifuji, Sinclair, & Starz, 1996; Turk & Rudy, 1988, 1990). This result suggests that reliance on group mean relationship adjustment or satisfaction scores may obscure the presence of a significant subgroup of distressed couples in a sample. Thus it would be helpful in future studies of relationship satisfaction and adjustment in patients with chronic pain and their partners for researchers to report not only the means and standard deviations of these measures, but also the percentages of patients and partners falling into distressed and nondistressed groups, using generally accepted cutting scores for these purposes.

Another factor potentially affecting reported rates of relationship distress is self-selection bias. Couples in which there is significant relationship distress may not agree to participate in studies involving examination of the relationship; this may result in an underrepresentation of distressed couples in these studies. In addition, patients and partners recruited from specialty pain clinics may not be representative of those seen in primary care settings. Findings based on patients in pain clinics may not generalize to the larger population of patients with chronic pain not seen in such settings.

With these limitations in mind, the research as a whole suggests a pattern for partners to show lower levels of relationship satisfaction than do patients (Ahern et al., 1985; Basolo-Kunzer et al., 1991; Block & Boyer, 1984; Flor, Kerns, & Turk, 1987; Flor, Turk, & Scholz, 1987; Hewitt et al., 1995; Kerns, Haythornthwaite, Southwick, & Giller, 1990; Kerns & Turk, 1984; Romano, Turner, & Clancy, 1989; Romano et al., 1995; Stampler et al., 1997), although not all studies have tested these differences statistically. Significant differences in level of relationship satisfaction have been reported (Ahern et al., 1985; Flor, Turk, & Scholz, 1987) between patients and partners, with partners reporting lower levels of satisfaction. One possible interpretation of this pattern is that living with a partner with chronic pain may be associated with a relative burden, which may dampen the healthy partner's perception of the relationship.

Alternatively, patients and partners may differ in systematic ways other than their pain versus pain-free status that are associated with relationship satisfaction. For example, gender may provide a potential explanation for the trend in patient versus partner differences in relationship satisfaction. One study (Romano, Turner, & Clancy, 1989) found that in couples where the patients with chronic pain were male and the partners were female, partners reported significantly lower relationship satisfaction than did patients. This pattern was not seen in couples in which the patients were female and the partners were male. Such a gender effect has been suggested previously by Flor, Turk, and Scholz (1987), Hafstrom and Schram (1984), and Kerns and Turk (1984). Women have been called the "emotional barometers" in heterosexual relationships (Barry, 1970) and tend to be relatively less satisfied with their relationships than men (Schumm, Webb, & Bollman, 1998). However, the findings of Basolo-Kunzer and colleagues (1991) were not consistent with this pattern, in that couples reported greater relationship satisfaction when the patients were male. This result may reflect differences in the patient population (patients with headache) in the Basolo-Kunzer and colleagues study compared to other patients with chronic pain, or other unknown differences.

In summary, there appears to be good evidence that there is a large subgroup of partners who report significant relationship dissatisfaction and psychological distress. However, distress and dissatisfaction are not universal, and continued research is needed to identify factors associated with good versus poor adjustment to living with a partner who has a chronic pain problem. The clarification of the contributions of patient status, pain severity, pain site, pain-related disability, gender, and other variables awaits future research efforts.

THE ROLE OF COUPLE AND FAMILY ASSESSMENT IN THE CLINICAL EVALUATION OF THE PATIENT WITH CHRONIC PAIN

A thorough evaluation of the psychosocial factors associated with the onset, maintenance, and course of a chronic pain problem is crucial for understanding important influences on a patient's pain. Evaluation of the patient–partner relationship, of how the partner and patient conceptualize and manage the patient's pain and disability, and of how the partner responds to the patient's pain behaviors forms an important part of this assessment process both prior to and during treatment. Such a comprehensive psychosocial evaluation ideally provides information regarding (1) factors that may directly contribute to ongoing pain and disability (e.g., deconditioning, severe fear/avoidance of movement); (2) factors that may have an indirect impact on treatment or outcome (e.g., stresses that are not directly attributable to pain, but that affect function); (3) treatable conditions that may be addressed to improve functioning and reduce suffering (e.g., depression); and (4) targets for treatment and indices of treatment outcome (e.g., physical capacities, functional disability, work status, pain level).

METHODS FOR ASSESSING COUPLE AND FAMILY FUNCTIONING IN THE CONTEXT OF CHRONIC PAIN

In this section, we describe some of the most commonly used methods to assess aspects of couple and family functioning, and review methods of clinical interviewing, questionnaires, and direct observational methods. Excellent reviews of couple and family assessment instruments are available, although not written with a focus on the application to patients with chronic pain and their partners or families. Readers interested in self-report family assessment instruments are referred to Halvorsen (1991) or Tutty (1995). Self-report couple assessment measures are reviewed in Weiss and Heyman (1997). Readers interested in observational coding systems for use with families or couples may want to familiarize themselves with

issues in the choice of an observational system (see, e.g., Schmaling, DeKlyen, & Jacobson, 1989), before considering specific candidate systems (see review by Weiss & Heyman, 1990).

The Clinical Interview

Psychological evaluation of the patient with chronic pain typically includes an interview of the patient and often of the partner or another close family member, usually conducted separately (Romano, Turner, & Moore, 1989). Interviews may be supplemented by questionnaires or psychometric testing. Informal clinical observation of patient and partner behavior usually occurs in the course of interviewing; more formal observational assessment of the patient's pain behaviors or of patient–partner interactions is more likely to be conducted in research than in clinical settings. In this section, we focus on the areas of the clinical interview of the patient and partner that are most pertinent to assessing couple and family functioning, as listed in Table 18.1. For a more complete description of the psychological evaluation of the patient with chronic pain, please see Romano, Turner, and Moore (1989; see also Bradley & McKendree-Smith, Chapter 16).

The clinical interview of the patient and partner is the primary source of information regarding the quality of interpersonal relationships within the family, as well as the patterns of the partner's and family's responses to the patient's pain behaviors. One area of inquiry for both the patient and partner should involve determining how the patient communicates pain (i.e., what pain behaviors the patient demonstrates) and how the partner and other family members respond when this occurs. Frequent solicitous behaviors by the partner and family—coupled with excessive patient disability and a relative absence of pathophysiology, especially in the context of relationship satisfaction—suggest that social contingencies may be playing a significant role in reinforcing pain behavior and dysfunction.

The theoretical rationale for assessing the responses of significant others to a patient's pain behavior has its roots in the concept of conducting a behavioral analysis of factors associated with increased or decreased pain and disability, to discover potential social-environmental reinforcers of pain and illness behavior (Fordyce, 1976). However, the beliefs and assumptions that a patient and partner have about the patient's pain problem also

TABLE 18.1. Couple and Family Issues to Assess in Interviewing Both Patient and Partner

Cognitive-behavioral analysis

1. Changes in the patient's and partner's activity since pain onset, and how these have affected the family.
2. Description of the patient's pain behaviors.
3. Responses of the partner/family to pain behaviors.
4. Responses of the partner/family to the patient's well behaviors and activity.
5. Beliefs of the patient and partner about the cause of the pain. (Does either believe that pain is a signal of potential harm or damage?)
6. Patient's perceptions and interpretations of the partner's responses to his or her pain behaviors.
7. Partner's perceptions and interpretations of the patient's pain behaviors.
8. Changes in roles and functions of the patient and partner since pain onset.
9. Partner's observations concerning the patient's emotional distress and adjustment to chronic pain.

Relationship issues

1. Quality of the patient–partner relationship.
2. Stresses and strains having an impact on the couple and family.
3. Changes in the relationship since pain onset.
4. Sexual adjustment and changes since pain onset; factors other than pain affecting sexual adjustment.
5. Strengths and resources of the couple.

Financial issues

1. Impact of pain on financial status of the couple/family.
2. Patient's and partner's perceptions of compensation/litigation issues.
3. Patient's and partner's views of vocational issues, return to work.

Social history and family of origin issues

1. Family relationships and attachment.
2. History of pain, disability, or chronic illness in family members.
3. Patient history of abuse or neglect.
4. Patient's family psychiatric history: history of psychological disorders, alcohol or other substance abuse/dependence.

should be assessed. Beliefs such as the conviction that pain signals harm or damage may prevent patients from engaging in activity and may lead partners to take over the patient's activities. It is also important to inquire about how a patient and partner interpret each other's behaviors. For example, solicitous behaviors may occur frequently in response to pain behaviors, yet may not be reinforcing if the patient interprets the partner's solici-

tousness as demeaning or as evidence that the patient is incapable. Conversely, behaviors that appear to be negative or punishing, such as the partner's withdrawing from the patient when pain behaviors occur, actually may be positively reinforcing if they allow the patient "time out" from stressful or conflictual interaction with the partner.

It is also crucial to assess the responses of the partner and family to activity and other *well behaviors*—that is, behaviors incompatible with disability. As noted above, a partner may discourage activity for fear of injury to a patient. The partner may fear that the entire family will "pay for" the patient's activity by having to suffer with the patient through increased pain, and perhaps further medical evaluation or treatment. As a result, the partner may need help in overcoming fears of the patient's activity and in learning to support and encourage activity as part of functional restoration.

A transactional or family systems model also stresses the role changes that may occur when one member is disabled and unable to perform normal functions, which are then taken over by the partner or other family members. Such role changes may produce a reapportionment of responsibilities and control within the family, potentially creating initial stress as the family adjusts (Patterson & Garwick, 1994). However, over time, new roles may become the norm, meaning that attempts by the patient to resume former roles and responsibilities may be met with resistance by other family members. Helping family members to identify positive consequences for the patient's functional restoration and strategies for change that will accommodate the needs of both patient and partner is crucial for successful treatment outcome.

In both patient and partner interviews, assessment of the quality of the relationship is important for understanding the context in which pain behaviors and partner responses are occurring, as well as for understanding the extent of cohesiveness and support (or, conversely, stress and discord) in the relationship. It is often informative to ask each individual about the effects of the pain problem on their relationship, and about the quality of the relationship both before and after pain onset. The possibility that pain behaviors and disability may perform maintenance roles in the family must be considered; in some cases, couples may remain together primarily because of pain (e.g., "I couldn't leave him like this"). In other cases, caretaking may enhance feelings of closeness or intimacy, perhaps allowing emotional expression that was not otherwise possible (e.g., "The pain has brought us closer together"). Pain may have the effect of stabilizing or destabilizing relationships, depending on the nature of the patient's and partner's needs.

These processes have important implications for treatment. If a pain problem has stabilized the relationship by providing additional closeness and intimacy, attempts to rehabilitate the patient to work and more normal functioning may threaten this homeostasis and meet with resistance if this pattern is not recognized and dealt with during treatment. Likewise, if the only factor now holding the couple together is the pain problem, the patient may resist treatment for fear of losing the partner. In addition, significant relationship conflict may form a major stressor in the patient's life that can contribute to depression and dysfunction. Conversely, a healthy partnership in which the relationship is not dependent on continuing patient dysfunction and in which the partner can be a supportive ally of improved functioning can bode well for treatment aimed at decreasing disability.

Often chronic pain is associated with reductions in the frequency and quality of a couple's sexual activity (Maruta & Osborne, 1978; Maruta, Osborne, Swanson, & Halling, 1981), and it is important to assess sexual functioning before and after pain onset with both the patient and partner in a sensitive manner to determine how the pain problem has affected this aspect of the relationship. Frequently patients will report that sexual activity provokes increased pain during and after the activity. Increased pain can lead to avoidance of sex by both the patient and partner. However, other factors as well may be responsible for changes in sexual activity. Depression may result in loss of interest in sex. Conflict in the relationship or primary sexual dysfunction may be the underlying reason for avoidance of sex, with pain providing a more acceptable reason for reduced intimacy. Avoidance of sex may also be related to a history of sexual abuse. Some studies have reported an association between such abuse and certain types of pain such as pelvic pain, although a definitive causal relationship has not been established (Walker & Stenchever, 1993).

Finally, it is important to assess the strengths and resources of the couple and family, which can be drawn on to support the process of change during treatment or to maintain gains after treatment. These strengths may include shared humor, mutual interests and activities outside of pain, strong commitments to children and work, capacity for caring and intimacy, and ability to support

each other's problem-solving skills, among others. Perceived partner support has been linked to lower levels of depressive symptoms (Kerns & Turk, 1984). Family cohesion as rated by patients has been associated with lower levels of patient depressive symptoms; partner-rated cohesion has been associated with lower levels of patient disability, as well as fewer overt patient pain behaviors (Romano, Turner, & Jensen, 1997). Family support has also been associated with better outcome of pain treatment (Jamison & Virts, 1990), although differences in demographic and work-related injury status do not appear to have been controlled in this study and may have influenced outcome.

The financial implications of the patient's pain problem for the family constitute a difficult but important topic to address. Although relatively few patients are found to be consciously malingering for financial gain, many patients whose pain problem is the result of an industrial injury or motor vehicle accident may be involved in compensation or litigation proceedings, with significant current or potential impact on their families' financial situation (see review by Main, 1999). Often a patient is not working because of pain, and both patient and partner may worry about the patient's ability ever to sustain work again, as well as about the long-term financial stability of the family. Such stresses can contribute to depression and relationship strain. Although a full review of issues of compensation and litigation and their implications for rehabilitation of patients with chronic pain is beyond the scope of this chapter (see Robinson, Chapter 14), it is important to assess these areas, as a patient's and partner's beliefs and fears may need to be addressed if treatment aimed at improved functioning and work is to be successful.

In addition to the above-noted inquiries regarding current family and couple functioning, it is important to obtain basic information regarding the patient's and partner's families of origin. In particular, it may be useful to obtain information about role models for chronic illness behavior and any experiences the patient and partner may have had earlier in life with extended illness or disability in themselves or in close family members. In addition, a family psychiatric history can provide important data about the presence of depression or other psychological disorders, or alcohol or other substance abuse or dependence, in family members. Information about the patient's early developmental history may be important for treatment planning. Histories of physical or sexual abuse or of neglect may be relevant to coping and adjustment to chronic pain (see Bradley and McKendree-Smith, Chapter 16), and have been linked to higher utilization of health care (Alexander et al., 1998).

Questionnaire Measurement

The use of reliable and valid questionnaire instruments can provide valuable information to complement the clinical interviews of the patient and partner, and serves as a mainstay of research addressing questions of patient and family functioning and response to chronic pain. In this section, we review commonly used instruments for assessing general relationship satisfaction and family environment and their application to patients with chronic pain, and also questionnaire measures of partner responses to patient pain behavior. (Sample items from the questionnaires described below can be found in Table 18.2.)

Questionnaire Measurement of Relationship Satisfaction

Locke–Wallace Marital Adjustment Test. The Marital Adjustment Test (MAT; Locke & Wallace, 1959) is a 15-item scale that is probably the earliest standardized self-report instrument designed to assess intimate relationship quality. Items are scored with different weights, which are indicated on the instrument. The total score ranges between 2 and 158, with higher scores indicative of greater satisfaction.

The MAT has been used in a number of studies of couples with chronic pain to assess relationship satisfaction. Block (1981) and Stampler and

colleagues (1997) noted that partners reporting more relationship satisfaction on the MAT had greater physiological reactivity to patient pain behaviors than partners in unsatisfied relationships did. Block and Boyer (1984) found that better relationship adjustment as assessed by the MAT was associated significantly with more partner optimism about the course of the patient's illness, stronger perceptions that the patient was functionally limited, and stronger perceptions that psychological factors did not contribute to the patient's difficulties. They hypothesized that this pattern of perceptions might increase the likelihood of solicitous discouragement of activity and reinforcement of pain behavior by satisfied partners.

Flor, Kerns, and Turk (1987) found a positive relationship between relationship satisfaction assessed with the MAT and spouse solicitousness. This was replicated by Flor, Turk, and Scholz (1987) in a different sample of males with chronic pain and their partners. In this latter study, they also found a positive relationship between relationship satisfaction and reported pain. Kerns and colleagues (1990) found that among couples with satisfied relationships, greater pain severity was associated with more solicitous partner responses to pain. In summary, the MAT has been a useful instrument to characterize relationship satisfaction and has been a significant predictor of pain-relevant variables, both alone and in its interaction with partner responses to pain (Kerns et al., 1990).

Dyadic Adjustment Scale. The Dyadic Adjustment Scale (DAS; Spanier, 1976) is a widely used relationship questionnaire. The DAS consists of 32 items designed to assess the quality of the rela-

TABLE 18.2. Sample Questionnaire Items

Topic and questionnaire(s)	Sample item
Relationship satisfaction	
Marital Adjustment Test (MAT)	"Do you ever wish you had not married?"
Dyadic Adjustment Scale (DAS)	"Do you and your partner engage in outside interests together?"
Partner responses to patient pain	
West Haven–Yale Multidimensional Pain Inventory (WHYMPI)	"[My partner] takes over my jobs or duties."
Family environment	
Family Environment Scale (FES)	"Family members rarely become openly angry."
Family Adaptability and Cohesion Scale III (FACES III)	"Family members ask each other for help."
McMaster Family Assessment Device (FAD)	"Anything goes in our family."

tionship as perceived by each individual in a couple. Good internal consistency, test–retest reliability, and criterion-related validity have been reported (Spanier, 1976). The total score (range = 0–151) is used to measure global relationship satisfaction and has been shown to be sensitive to change in couple therapy (e.g., Jacobson et al., 1984). Adequate normative data exist, and reference ranges for scores that reflect normal and distressed relationships have been carefully developed (Eddy, Heyman, & Weiss, 1991; Jacobson, Follette, & Revenstorf, 1986; Jacobson & Truax, 1991). In addition to the total score, four component scores can be derived for Dyadic Satisfaction, Cohesion, Consensus, and Affectional Expression. Finally, the DAS also includes items related to the individual's commitment to the relationship and willingness to work on improving the relationship; responses to these items may be useful for clinicians considering initiating couples therapy.

The DAS has been used to assess the level of relationship adjustment in couples in which one partner has chronic pain (cf. Romano, Turner, & Clancy, 1989; Romano et al., 1995), as well as the association of relationship adjustment to pain-related patient and partner functioning. For example, Basolo-Kunzer and colleagues (1991) found that among patients with headaches, patients with relatively greater relationship satisfaction on the DAS were significantly more likely to report continuous headaches than those reporting less relationship satisfaction. Hewitt and colleagues (1995) reported that partner perfectionism was associated with lower patient relationship satisfaction, as well as fewer supportive partner responses to pain.

The DAS appears to be a useful instrument to quantify relationship satisfaction among couples dealing with pain. It has demonstrated reliability and validity, and DAS scores may have potentially important relationships with pain-relevant variables. An advantage of the use of the DAS in couples with pain is the ability to compare DAS scores in a given couple or sample of couples with well-established normative data, and with other patient samples.

*Questionnaire Measurement
of Partner Responses to Patient
Pain Behaviors and Disability*

The most commonly used measure of partner responses to patient pain behaviors is Part II of the West Haven–Yale Multidimensional Pain Inventory (WHYMPI; Kerns, Turk, & Rudy, 1985; see also Jacob & Kerns, Chapter 19). The WHYMPI was developed as an assessment instrument for use with patients with chronic pain that would provide a brief but comprehensive evaluation of salient dimensions of the experience of chronic pain. There are three main parts to this inventory. Part I assesses pain severity and interference with activities and functioning; perceived life control; affective distress; and perceived support from partner, family, and significant others. Part II evaluates patients' perceptions of the range and frequency of responses by significant others to patient pain and suffering behaviors, and is most relevant to the present review. Fourteen specific responses are divided into three subscales: Solicitous, Punishing, and Distracting responses. Part III of the WHYMPI assesses patient engagement in common domestic, household, social, and recreational activities.

The significant-other version of Part II, developed by Kerns and Rosenberg (1995), has the same responses and scales as the patient version described above, but is designed to allow the significant other to provide his or her self-report of responses to the patient's pain behaviors. This measure has been demonstrated to have adequate internal consistency and criterion-related validity (Kerns & Rosenberg, 1998).

Part II of the WHYMPI has frequently been used in studies testing behavioral theory regarding the role that partner behavior may play in contributing to or maintaining chronic pain behavior. In general, studies have supported a positive relationship between solicitous partner responding and increased patient pain and dysfunction, although the correlational nature of these studies does not allow for conclusions about causation to be drawn. Solicitous responses by the partner to patient pain behaviors as measured by the WHYMPI have been found to be significantly related to patient ratings of greater pain severity and lower patient activity (Flor, Kerns, & Turk, 1987; Flor et al., 1989). The Solicitous response scale of the WHYMPI also has shown a significant association to more frequent patient pain behaviors (Kerns et al., 1991), as well as to observed solicitous behaviors in partners of patients with chronic pain (Romano et al., 1991).

The relationship of the Punishing scale of the WHYMPI to patient functioning has yielded less consistent findings. Flor, Kerns, and Turk (1987) found a positive association between punishing responses and patient activity levels. However, other studies have not demonstrated significant relationships between punishing responses on the

WHYMPI and patient disability (Turk et al., 1992), pain intensity (Kerns et al., 1990; Turk et al., 1992), or pain behavior (Turk et al., 1992). A more consistent finding has been that punishing responses are associated with poorer patient mood and psychological adjustment (Kerns et al., 1990; Schwartz, Slater, & Birchler, 1996; Turk et al., 1992).

As noted previously, Turk and Rudy (1988) developed an empirically derived taxonomy of patients with chronic pain, and identified three major profile types based on cluster analysis of WHYMPI profiles: Dysfunctional, Interpersonally Distressed, and Adaptive Coper (see Turk & Okifuji, Chapter 21). Patients in the Interpersonally Distressed group reported lower levels of support from families and significant others and lower levels of relationship satisfaction, compared to patients in the other two groups (Rudy, Turk, Zaki, & Curtin, 1989; Turk & Rudy, 1988). In addition, a recent study demonstrated that patients in the Interpersonally Distressed group may show a poorer response to standard interdisciplinary pain treatment (Turk, Okifuji, Sinclair, & Starz, 1998). These findings suggest the importance of assessment of interpersonal distress as part of the evaluation process prior to treatment, because it may be necessary to provide more intensive intervention targeting the relationship with the significant other or family during pain treatment for a patient experiencing high levels of familial discord or relationship distress.

Questionnaire Measures of Family Environment

Family Environment Scale. The Family Environment Scale (FES; Moos & Moos, 1986) is a 90-item measure consisting of 10 scales that reflect different components of family functioning: relationships, personal growth, and system maintenance. Although the psychometric properties of the FES have typically been reported to be adequate (Moos & Moos, 1986), other studies have led some to question the reliability and validity of the FES (Loveland-Cherry, Youngblut, & Leidy, 1989; Roosa & Beals, 1990).

A number of research studies using the FES have focused on comparing the family environments of patients with pain problems to those of healthy, pain-free persons. Feuerstein, Sult, and Houle (1985) found that patients with low back pain reported greater conflict and control, and less active recreation, than healthy controls. Naidoo and Pillay (1994) found that the family environments

of women with low back pain could be characterized as less cohesive, independent, and organized, but more conflictual, than those of healthy controls. A small sample of seven women with chronic pain reported significantly less cohesion, but more conflict, than the families of seven women without pain or illness (Dura & Beck, 1988). Kopp and colleagues (1995), using the German version of the FES, reported that patients with headache or low back pain reported less active recreation and moral–religious orientation in their families than in those of healthy controls. In addition, the family environments of patients with headache were less expressive, but evidenced greater structure and organization, than those of healthy persons.

Romano and colleagues (1997) compared adults with chronic pain with healthy controls on five FES scales (Cohesion, Expressiveness, Conflict, Organization, and Control) and found that patients with chronic pain reported significantly less cohesion and more control than did healthy persons. More depressive symptoms were associated with more conflict and less cohesion; in addition, conflict and disability were significantly positively related. In a study of patients with chronic headache, patients reported less expressiveness but more structure and organization in their family environments than did headache-free controls (Ehde, Holm, & Metzger, 1991).

Taken together, the studies that have used the FES to characterize the family environments of patients with chronic pain suggest that such families tend to be more controlled and conflictual, and less cohesive and engaged in less active recreation, than healthy control families. These preliminary conclusions must be tempered by the fact that not all studies have yielded this pattern of findings and a number of them have been based on small samples.

The FES has also been found to predict response to treatment. Tota-Faucette, Gil, Williams, Keefe, and Goli (1993) reported data from 119 patients who participated in an inpatient pain management program where family participation was encouraged, but variable. In this study, the FES was scored for its three superordinate factors: Supportiveness, Disorganization, and Control. They found that more family control was predictive of greater pain report and more discomfort with activity at the end of treatment.

Family Adaptability and Cohesion Scale III. The Family Adaptability and Cohesion Scale III (FACES III; Olson, Portner, & Lavee, 1985) is a set of 20 items, each of which is responded to twice on a 5-point Likert-type scale; the two response sets are "Describe your family now" and "Ideally, how would you like your family to be?" The odd-numbered items are summed to obtain the Cohesion score, and the even-numbered items are summed to obtain the Adaptability score. The scores are interpreted so that relatively higher Cohesion scores are indicative of family enmeshment, and higher Adaptability scores are indicative of family chaos. Cohesion, adaptability, and communication are the three key dimensions of family functioning posited by the circumplex model (Olson et al., 1979).

Few studies have used the FACES III to characterize the families of patients with chronic pain. Roy and Thomas (1989) presented data from an uncontrolled study of 52 patients with chronic pain and their partners. Based on the interpretive guidelines for the FACES III provided by Olson and colleagues (1985), the authors concluded that the families were functioning in the chaotic range of adaptation, with "loose" emotional bonding. Basolo-Kunzer and colleagues (1991) reported a study comparing 117 patients with headache and partners to 108 control couples on the FACES III. Contrary to their hypothesis, there was no difference between the couples with headache and the control couples on the Cohesion and Adaptability subscales of the FACES III or on a measure of couple satisfaction. In addition, the scores in both groups on the FACES III were reported as similar to normative data for this measure (Olson et al., 1985). However, they did find that Cohesion and Adaptability scores were significantly positively related to patient pain. Further controlled research will be necessary to determine the utility of this instrument for families in which one person has chronic pain.

McMaster Family Assessment Device. The McMaster Family Assessment Device (FAD; Epstein, Baldwin, & Bishop, 1983) consists of 60 statements (e.g., "We confide in each other") that the respondent endorses on a 4-point Likert-type scale. The questionnaire can be scored for a General Functioning subscale and six subscales designed to reflect dimensions of family functioning posited by the McMaster model: Problem Solving, Communication, Roles, Affective Responsiveness, Affective Involvement, and Behavior Control.

Hewitt and colleagues (1995) administered the FAD to 83 patients with chronic pain and their partners and reported that the patients' General Functioning scores did not differ from their part-

ners' or from those of the normative nonclinical sample reported in the original Epstein and colleagues (1983) article. Further work is need to determine whether the FAD is appropriately sensitive to the dysfunction typically observed in families with chronic pain and detected by other family assessment instruments.

Questionnaire Measures:
Summary and Recommendations

Our review of existing questionnaires that assess relationship and family functioning, and significant others' responses to patients' pain behavior, suggests that well-developed instruments exist to measure these constructs. Choosing from among multiple existing questionnaires requires a balanced consideration of factors such as the length of the questionnaire and respondent burden, reliability and validity information, and extant data applying a questionnaire to samples with chronic pain. In the assessment of couples and families of patients with chronic pain, the DAS (Spanier, 1976) and the FES (Moos & Moos, 1986) are recommended to assess the quality and functioning of intimate relationships and families, based on their psychometric characteristics and available data supporting their utility in this population. The MAT (Locke & Wallace, 1959) also has considerable empirical support in this population. The WHYMPI (Kerns et al., 1985) represents the most empirically supported questionnaire measure of partner responses to patient pain behavior and is recommended when a patient- or partner-reported measure of this construct is needed.

Observation Measures

Relatively few studies have used direct observational methods to examine the interactions of couples or families in which one or more members have a chronic pain problem. Most studies have relied on the self-report of the patient and partner, thus potentially introducing issues of reporting bias and shared method variance when examining relationships among variables. Observational research tends to be more expensive, labor-intensive, and time-consuming than research that involves the administration of questionnaires, but these costs may be offset by strengths such as the potential for increased objectivity of data collection. In addition, the use of observational data allows for more precise measurement of dimensions of couple and family interaction that may have important theoretical and clinical implications.

Observational measures of patient activity or pain behavior have been used as outcome measures in studies examining the role of partner solicitousness in patient pain behavior. Lousberg, Schmidt, and Groenman (1992) demonstrated that patients whose partners described themselves as solicitous reported higher pain levels and walked on a treadmill for a shorter period of time when the partners were present than did patients with nonsolicitous partners. Observed pain behaviors, as measured by an expanded version of the Keefe and Block (1982) observational protocol, were found to vary by partner presence versus absence and by the type of partner support provided (Paulsen & Altmaier, 1995). Schwartz, Slater, and Birchler (1994) reported that patients who had participated in a stress interview condition were significantly more likely to terminate a cycling task prematurely than were those in a neutral interaction condition.

Similarly, partner responses and behavior have been assessed through sources other than self-report or patient report. Block (1981) used physiological recording to assess the responses of partners to patients' pain behavior and noted greater physiological reactivity of satisfied partners to displays of patient distress. Manne and Zautra (1989) interviewed the partners of patients with rheumatoid arthritis about the impact of the patients' illness on the partners. The interviews were taped and later coded for the number of critical remarks. They found that partner criticism and patient perception of partner criticism were associated with poorer patient adjustment.

A more complex coding scheme for measuring interactional patterns, the *Kategoriensystem für Partnerschaftliche Interaktion* (KPI; Hahlweg et al., 1984), was used by Flor and colleagues (1995) in a study involving physiological as well as interactional measures to examine the relationship of partner solicitousness to pain report and behaviors. Partners of patients with chronic back pain used more acceptance and agreement in their discussions than did healthy control partners. Patients with highly solicitous partners also used less self-disclosure.

The KPI, however, does not measure patient pain behavior, nor capture directly the solicitous responses of the partner to patient pain behaviors. A series of studies (Romano et al., 1991, 1992, 1995) was conducted in which a methodology was developed for directly observing and quantifying patient pain behaviors and partner responses. Patients with chronic pain and their partners were videotaped while engaging in a series of standardized activities such as sweeping, folding laundry and making a bed. The tapes were then coded using the Living in Family Environments coding system (LIFE; Hops, Davis, & Longoria, 1995). This is a real-time sequential coding system that provides data not only on the rates of different behavior codes, but also on the probability of sequences of behavior, such as the likelihood that partner solicitous behaviors will precede or follow patient pain behaviors. For this research, the LIFE was modified to specifically include affect and content codes reflecting verbal and nonverbal pain behaviors, as well as solicitous behaviors. (See Romano et al., 1991, for a more detailed description of the methodology and coding system.) The coding of pain behaviors and partner responses was found to be reliable and valid (Romano et al., 1991).

Use of the LIFE coding system revealed that partner solicitous responses were significantly more likely to precede and follow patient pain behaviors in patients with chronic pain than in control couples (Romano et al., 1992). In addition, partner solicitous responses following patient nonverbal behaviors were associated with greater disability in patients who were more depressed, and with more frequent pain behaviors in those with higher self-reported pain (Romano et al., 1995), even when patient age, gender, and pain level were statistically controlled. These findings provide observational corroboration of previous results from studies based on self-reports of patients and partners. However, most studies in this area have been correlational, and conclusions about causation and direction of influence cannot be drawn as yet. In addition, there is likely a reciprocal relationship between a patient's pain behaviors and responses from the partner, such that over time each may shape the other's behavior. Longitudinal studies to examine such learning processes, as well as studies in which partner responses to pain behaviors are systematically altered to determine effects on subsequent pain behaviors, need to be conducted to provide more stringent tests of behavioral theory.

SUMMARY AND FUTURE DIRECTIONS

The assessment of the couple and family context of patients with chronic pain is an essential component of the psychosocial evaluation of such patients. The research literature provides consistent support for the importance of the family to the adjustment of the patient with chronic pain, and for the impact that chronic pain in the patient appears to have on the family, particularly the partner.

However, many unresolved questions and issues remain. Research in this area has tended to be descriptive and correlational, and more systematic tests of theoretical models are needed to refine them further. Development of well-validated instruments to assess cognitive as well as behavioral, contextual, and interactive variables are needed to provide more comprehensive assessment, and to test complex models that posit synergistic effects among these classes of variables, such as the cognitive-behavioral transactional model (Kerns & Weiss, 1994). Longitudinal studies in which the family environment, the beliefs and behavior of the patient and partner, and their transactions in relationship to pain and disability are assessed over time (ideally over the course of the transition from acute to chronic pain) could potentially elucidate processes predictive of long-term functioning and adjustment in patients and family members.

Although this review has focused primarily on assessment of couples, the effects of chronic pain in a parent on children requires additional research and clinical attention. Some studies have suggested that children of patients with chronic pain may be at increased risk for illness behaviors and maladjustment (Chun, Turner, & Romano, 1993; Dura & Beck, 1988; Jamison & Walker, 1992; Rickard, 1988), but the mechanisms by which such increased risk may occur remain unclear. Developmental factors, such as deficits in attachment, that may increase vulnerability to the development of dysfunctional chronic pain also require further investigation (Mikulincer & Florian, 1998).

Another area in need of further research is that of how social support is related to solicitous behavior, and how these classes of partner responses function in relationship to patient pain behaviors and disability. This issue has particular relevance for treatment. As discussed previously, research evidence and behavioral theory suggest that solicitous partner responses may have deleterious effects on patient physical functioning, whereas social support in general appears to be associated with better psychological functioning (Turk et al., 1992). Further research is needed to distinguish these classes of behavior and to identify types of support that are associated with improved mood and psychosocial function, but not with poorer physical functioning.

Factors that might moderate these relationships, such as gender or relationship satisfaction, also require further investigation.

Observational assessment of couples in which one member has chronic pain appears to merit further development and application. The collection of physiological, overt behavioral, and self-report data has greatly enhanced the ability of researchers to test hypotheses regarding couples' interactions and functioning in the field of relationship assessment (Gottman & Levenson, 1992). Although each of these modes of assessment has been used in different studies of patients with chronic pain and/or their partners as reviewed above, the use of concurrent multimodal assessment is in its infancy in this population. The development, refinement, and application of more sophisticated assessment instruments and methodologies to the evaluation of couples and families with chronic pain are needed at this point, to move the field beyond descriptive research to more comprehensive testing of theoretical models and their implications for treatment.

REFERENCES

Ahern, D. K., Adams, A. E., & Follick, M. J. (1985). Emotional and marital disturbance in spouses of chronic low back pain patients. *Clinical Journal of Pain, 1*, 69–74.

Alexander, R. W., Bradley, L. A., Alarcon, G. S., Triana-Alexander, M., Aaron, L. A., Alberts, K. R., Martin, M. Y., & Stewart, K. E. (1998, April). Sexual and physical abuse in women with fibromyalgia: Association with outpatient health care utilization and pain medication usage. *Arthritis Care Research, 11*(2), 102–115.

Barry, W. (1970). Marriage research and conflict: An integrative review. *Psychological Bulletin, 73*, 41–54.

Basolo-Kunzer, M., Diamond, S., Maliszewski, M., Weyermann, L., & Reed, J. (1991). Chronic headache patients' marital and family adjustment. *Issues in Mental Health Nursing, 12*, 133–148.

Block, A. R. (1981). An investigation of the response of the spouse to chronic pain behavior. *Psychosomatic Medicine, 43*, 415–422.

Block, A. R., & Boyer, S. L. (1984). The spouse's adjustment to chronic pain: Cognitive and emotional factors. *Social Science in Medicine, 19*, 1313–1317.

Bowen, M. (1978). *Family therapy in clinical practice.* New York: Aronson.

Bradbury, T. N., & Fincham, F. D. (1990). Attributions in marriage: Review and critique. *Psychological Bulletin, 107*, 3–33.

Chun, D. Y., Turner, J. A., & Romano, J. M. (1993). Children of chronic pain patients: Risk factors for maladjustment. *Pain, 52*, 311–317.

Compas, B. E., Haaga, D. A. F., Keefe, F. J., Leitenberg, H., & Williams, D. A. (1998). Sampling of empirically supported psychological treatments from health psychology: Smoking, chronic pain, cancer, and bulimia nervosa. *Journal of Consulting and Clinical Psychology*, 66, 89-112.

Dura, J. R., & Beck, S. J. (1988). A comparison of family functioning when mothers have chronic pain. *Pain*, 35, 79-89.

Eddy, J. M., Heyman, R. E., & Weiss, R. L. (1991). An empirical investigation of the Dyadic Adjustment Scale: Exploring the differences between marital "satisfaction" and "adjustment." *Behavioral Assessment*, 13, 199-220.

Ehde, D. M., Holm, J. E., & Metzger, D. L. (1991). The role of family structure, functioning, and pain modeling in headache. *Headache*, 31, 35-40.

Epstein, N. B., Baldwin, L. M., & Bishop, D. S. (1983). The McMaster Family Assessment Device. *Journal of Marital and Family Therapy*, 9, 171-180.

Epstein, N. B., Bishop, D. S., & Levin, S. (1980). The McMaster model of family functioning. *Advances in Family Psychiatry*, 2, 73-89.

Feuerstein, M., Sult, S., & Houle, M. (1985). Environmental stressors and chronic low back pain: Life events, family, and work environment. *Pain*, 22, 295-307.

Flor, H., Breitenstein, C., Birbaumer, N., & Fürst, M. (1995). A psychophysiological analysis of spouse solicitousness towards pain behaviors, spouse interaction, and pain perception. *Behavior Therapy*, 26, 255-272.

Flor, H., Kerns, R. D., & Turk, D. C. (1987). The role of spouse reinforcement, perceived pain, and activity levels of chronic pain patients. *Journal of Psychosomatic Research*, 31, 251-259.

Flor, H., Turk, D. C., & Rudy, T. E. (1989). Relationship of pain impact and significant other reinforcement of pain behaviors: The mediating role of gender, marital status, and marital satisfaction. *Pain*, 38, 45-50.

Flor, H., Turk, D. C., & Scholz, O. B. (1987). Impact of chronic pain on the spouse: Marital, emotional, and physical consequences. *Journal of Psychosomatic Research*, 31, 63-71.

Fordyce, W. E. (1976). *Behavioral methods for chronic pain and illness*. St. Louis, MO: Mosby.

Gottman, J. M., & Levenson, R. W. (1992). Toward a typology of marriage based on affective behavior: Preliminary differences in behavior, physiology, health, and risk for dissolution. *Journal of Personality and Social Psychology*, 63, 221-233.

Hafstrom, J. L., & Schram, V. R. (1984). Chronic illness in couples: Selected characteristics, including wives' satisfaction with and perception of marital relationships. *Family Relationships*, 33, 195-203.

Hahlweg, K., Reisner, L., Kohli, G., Vollmer, M., Schindler, L., & Revenstorf, D. (1984). Development and validity of a new system to analyze interpersonal communication (KPI). In K. Hahlweg & N. Jacobson (Eds.), *Marital interaction: Analysis and modification* (pp. 182-198). New York: Guilford Press.

Halvorsen, J. G. (1991). Self-report family assessment instruments: An evaluative review. *Family Practice Research Journal*, 11, 221-255.

Hewitt, P. L., Flett, G. L., & Mikail, S. F. (1995). Perfectionism and relationship adjustment in pain patients and their spouses. *Journal of Family Psychology*, 9, 335-347.

Hops, H., Davis, B., & Longoria, N. (1995). Methodological issues in direct observation: Illustrations with the Living in Familial Environments (LIFE) coding system. *Journal of Clinical Child Psychology*, 24, 193-203.

Jacobson, N. S., Follette, W. C., & Revenstorf, D. (1986). Toward a standard definition of clinically significant change. *Behavior Therapy*, 17, 308-311.

Jacobson, N. S., Follette, W. C., Revenstorf, D., Baucom, D. H., Hahlweg, K., & Margolin, G. (1984). Variability in outcome and clinical significance of behavioral marital therapy: A reanalysis of outcome data. *Journal of Consulting and Clinical Psychology*, 52, 497-504.

Jacobson, N. S., & Truax, P. (1991). Clinical significance: A statistical approach to defining meaningful change in psychotherapy research. *Journal of Consulting and Clinical Psychology*, 59, 12-19.

Jamison, R. N., Rudy, T. E., Penzien, D. B., & Mosley, T. H. (1994). Cognitive-behavioral classification of chronic pain: Replication and extension of empirically derived patient profiles. *Pain*, 57, 277-292.

Jamison, R. N., & Virts, K. L. (1990). The influence of family support on chronic pain. *Behaviour Research and Therapy*, 28, 283-287.

Jamison, R. N., & Walker, L. S. (1992). Illness behavior in children of chronic pain patients. *International Journal of Psychiatry in Medicine*, 22, 329-342.

Keefe, F. J., & Block, A. R. (1982). Development of an observation method of assessing pain behavior in chronic low back pain patients. *Behavior Therapy*, 13, 363-375.

Kerns, R. D. (1995). Family assessment and intervention in chronic illness. In P. M. Nicassio & T. W. Smith (Eds.), *Managing chronic illness: A biopsychosocial perspective* (pp. 207-244). Washington, DC: American Psychological Association.

Kerns, R. D., Haythornthwaite, J., Southwick, S., & Giller, E. L. (1990). The role of marital interaction in chronic pain and depressive symptom severity. *Journal of Psychosomatic Research*, 34, 401-408.

Kerns, R. D., & Rosenberg, R. (1995). Pain-relevant responses from significant others: Development of a significant-other version of the WHYMPI scales. *Pain*, 61, 245-249.

Kerns, R. D., Southwick, S., Giller, E. L., Haythornthwaite, J. A., Jacob, M. C., & Rosenberg, R. (1991). The relationship between reports of pain-related social interactions and expressions of pain and affective distress. *Behavior Therapy*, 22, 101-111.

Kerns, R. D., & Turk, D. C. (1984). Depression and chronic pain: The mediating role of the spouse. *Journal of Marriage and the Family*, 46, 845-852.

Kerns, R. D., Turk, D. C., & Rudy, T. E. (1985). The West Haven-Yale Multidimensional Pain Inventory (WHYMPI). *Pain*, 23, 345-356.

Kerns, R. D., & Weiss, L. H. (1994). Family influences on the course of chronic illness: A cognitive-behavioral transactional model. *Annals of Behavioral Medicine*, 16, 116-121.

Kopp, M., Richter, R., Rainer, J., Lopp-Wilfling, P., Rumpold, G., & Walter, M. H. (1995). Differences in family functioning between patients with chronic headache and patients with chronic low back pain. *Pain*, 63, 219-224.

Locke, H. J., & Wallace, K. M. (1959). Short marital adjustment and prediction tests: Their reliability and validity. *Marriage and Family Living, 21,* 251–255.

Lousberg, R., Schmidt, A. J. M., & Groenman, N. H. (1992). The relationship between spouse solicitousness and pain behavior: Searching for more experimental evidence. *Pain, 51,* 75–79.

Loveland-Cherry, C. J., Youngblut, J. M., & Leidy, N. W. K. (1989). A psychometric analysis of the Family Environment Scale. *Nursing Research, 38,* 262–266.

Main, C. J. (1999). Medicolegal aspects of pain: The nature of psychological opinion in cases of personal injury. In R. J. Gatchel & D. C. Turk (Eds.), *Psychosocial factors in pain: Critical perspectives* (pp. 132–147). New York: Guilford Press.

Manne, S. L., & Zautra, A. J. (1989). Spouse criticism and support: Their associations with coping and psychological adjustment among women with rheumatoid arthritis. *Journal of Personality and Social Psychology, 56,* 608–617.

Maruta, T., & Osborne, D. (1978). Sexual activity in chronic pain patients. *Psychosomatics, 19,* 531–537.

Maruta, T., Osborne, D., Swanson, D. W., & Halling, J. M. (1981). Chronic pain patients and spouses: Marital and sexual adjustment. *Mayo Clinic Proceedings, 56,* 307–310.

Mikulincer, M., & Florian, V. (1998). The relationship between adult attachment styles and emotional and cognitive reactions to stressful events. In J. A. Simpson & W. S. Rholes (Eds.), *Attachment theory and close relationships* (pp. 143–165). New York: Guilford Press.

Moos, R. H., & Moos, B. S. (1986). *Family Environment Scale manual.* Palo Alto, CA: Consulting Psychologists Press.

Naidoo, P., & Pillay, Y. G. (1994). Correlations among general stress, family environment, psychological distress, and pain experience. *Perceptual and Motor Skills, 78,* 1291–1296.

National Institutes of Health Technology Assessment Panel on Integration of Behavioral and Relaxation Approaches into the Treatment of Chronic Pain and Insomnia. (1996). Integration of behavioral and relaxation approaches into the treatment of chronic pain and insomnia. *Journal of the American Medical Association, 276,* 313–318.

Novy, D. M., Nelson, D. V., Francis, D. J., & Turk, D. C. (1995). Perspectives of chronic pain: An evaluative comparison of restrictive and comprehensive models. *Psychological Bulletin, 118,* 238–247.

Olson, D., Portner, J., & Lavee, Y. (1985). *FACES-III.* St. Paul: University of Minnesota, Department of Family Social Science.

Olson, D., Sprenkle, D., & Russell, C. S. (1979). Circumplex model of marital and family systems: I. Cohesion and adaptability dimensions, family types, and clinical applications. *Family Process, 18,* 3–28.

Patterson, J. M., & Garwick, A. W. (1994). The impact of chronic illness on families: A family systems perspective. *Annals of Behavioral Medicine, 16,* 131–142.

Paulsen, J. S., & Altmaier, E. M. (1995). The effects of perceived versus enacted social support on the discriminative cue function of spouses for pain behaviors. *Pain, 60,* 103–110.

Rickard, K. (1988). The occurrence of maladaptive health-related behaviors and teacher-rated conduct problems in children of chronic low back pain patients. *Journal of Behavioral Medicine, 11,* 107–116.

Romano, J. M., Turner, J. A., & Clancy, S. L. (1989). Sex differences in the relationship of pain patient dysfunction to spouse adjustment. *Pain, 39,* 289–295.

Romano, J. M., Turner, J. A., Friedman, L. S., Bulcroft, R. A., Jensen, M. P., & Hops, H. (1991). Observational assessment of chronic pain patient–spouse behavioral interactions. *Behavior Therapy, 11,* 549–567.

Romano, J. M., Turner, J. A., Friedman, L. S., Bulcroft, R. A., Jensen, M. P., Hops, H., & Wright, S. F. (1992). Sequential analysis of chronic pain behaviors and spouse responses. *Journal of Consulting and Clinical Psychology, 60,* 777–782.

Romano, J. M., Turner, J. A., & Jensen, M. P. (1997). The family environment in chronic pain patients: Comparison to controls and relationship to patient functioning. *Journal of Clinical Psychology in Medical Settings, 4,* 383–395.

Romano, J. M., Turner, J. A., Jensen, M. P., Friedman, L. S., Bulcroft, R. A., Hops, H., & Wright, S. F. (1995). Chronic pain patient–spouse behavioral interactions predict patient disability. *Pain, 63,* 353–360.

Romano, J. M., Turner, J. A., & Moore, J. E. (1989). Psychological evaluation. In C. D. Tollison (Ed.), *Handbook of chronic pain management* (pp. 38–51). Baltimore: Williams & Wilkins.

Roosa, M. W., & Beals, J. (1990). Measurement issues in family assessment: The case of the Family Environment Scale. *Family Process, 29,* 191–198.

Roy, R. (1989). Couple therapy and chronic headache: A preliminary outcome study. *Headache, 29,* 455–457.

Roy, R., & Thomas, M. R. (1989). Nature of marital relations among chronic pain patients. *Contemporary Family Therapy, 11,* 277–285.

Rudy, T. E., Turk, D. C., Zaki, H. S., & Curtin, H. D. (1989). An empirical taxometric alternative to traditional classification of temporomandibular disorders. *Pain, 36,* 311–320.

Schmaling, K. B., DeKlyen, M., & Jacobson, N. S. (1989). Direct observational methods for studying family functioning. In C. N. Ramsey, Jr. (Ed.), *Family systems in medicine* (pp. 215–226). New York: Guilford Press.

Schumm, W. R., Webb, F. J., & Bollman, S. R. (1998). Gender and marital satisfaction: Data for the National Survey of Families and Households. *Psychological Reports, 83,* 319–327.

Schwartz, L., Slater, M. A., & Birchler, G. R. (1994). Interpersonal stress and pain behaviors in chronic pain patients. *Journal of Consulting and Clinical Psychology, 62,* 861–864.

Schwartz, L., Slater, M. A., & Birchler, G. R. (1996). The role of pain behaviors in the modulation of marital conflict in chronic pain couples. *Pain, 65,* 227–233.

Schwartz, L., Slater, M. A., Birchler, G. R., & Atkinson, J. H. (1991). Depression in spouses of chronic pain patients: The role of patient pain and anger, and marital satisfaction. *Pain, 44,* 61–67.

Spanier, G. B. (1976). Measuring dyadic adjustment: New scales for assessing the quality of marriage and similar dyads. *Journal of Marriage and the Family, 38,* 15–28.

Stampler, D. B., Wall, J. R., Cassisi, J. E., & Davis, H. (1997). Marital satisfaction and psychophysiological responsiveness in spouses of patients with chronic pain. *International Journal of Rehabilitation and Health, 3,* 159-170.

Taylor, A. G., Lorentzen, L. J., & Blank, M. B. (1990). Psychologic distress of chronic pain sufferers and their spouses. *Journal of Pain and Symptom Management, 5,* 6-10.

Tota-Faucette, M. E., Gil, K. M., Williams, D. A., Keefe, F. J., & Goli, V. (1993). Predictors of response to pain management treatment: The role of family environment and changes in cognitive processes. *Clinical Journal of Pain, 9,* 115-123.

Turk, D. C., & Flor, H. (1987). Pain greater than pain behaviors: The utility and limitations of the pain behavior construct. *Pain, 31,* 277-295.

Turk, D. C., & Kerns, R. D. (1985). The family in health and illness. In D. C. Turk & R. D. Kerns (Eds.), *Health, illness and families: A life span perspective* (pp. 1-22). New York: Wiley.

Turk, D. C., Kerns, R. D., & Rosenberg, R. (1992). Effects of marital interaction on chronic pain and disability: Examining the down side of social support. *Rehabilitation Psychology, 37,* 259-274.

Turk, D. C., Okifuji, A., Sinclair, J. D., & Starz, T. W. (1996). Pain, disability, and physical functioning in subgroups of patients with fibromyalgia. *Journal of Rheumatology, 23,* 1255-1262.

Turk, D. C., Okifuji, A., Sinclair, J. D., & Starz, T. W. (1998). Differential responses by psychosocial sub-

groups of fibromyalgia syndrome patients to an interdisciplinary treatment. *Arthritis Care and Research, 11,* 397-404.

Turk, D. C., & Rudy, T. E. (1988). Toward an empirically derived taxonomy of chronic pain patients: Integration of psychological assessment data. *Journal of Consulting and Clinical Psychology, 56,* 233-238.

Turk, D. C., & Rudy, T. E. (1990). The robustness of an empirically derived taxonomy of chronic pain patients. *Pain, 43,* 27-35.

Tutty, L. M. (1995). Theoretical and practical issues in selecting a measure of family functioning. *Research on Social Work Practice, 5,* 80-106.

Walker, E. A., & Stenchever, M. A. (1993). Sexual victimization and chronic pelvic pain. *Obstetrics and Gynecology Clinics of North America, 20,* 795-807.

Weiss, R. L., & Heyman, R. E. (1990). Observation of marital interaction. In F. D. Fincham & T. N. Bradbury (Eds.), *The psychology of marriage: Basic issues and applications* (pp. 87-117). New York: Guilford Press.

Weiss, R. L., & Heyman, R. E. (1997). A clinical-research overview of couples interactions. In W. K. Halford & H. J. Markman (Eds.), *Clinical handbook of marriage and couples interventions* (pp. 13-41). Chichester, England: Wiley.

Wood, B., Watkins, J. B., Boyle, J. T., Nogueira, J., Zimand, E., & Carroll, L. (1989). The "psychosomatic family" model: An empirical and theoretical analysis. *Family Process, 28,* 399-417.

Chapter 19

Assessment of the Psychosocial Context of the Experience of Chronic Pain

MARY CASEY JACOB
ROBERT D. KERNS

HISTORICAL AND THEORETICAL PERSPECTIVE

Attention to the role of psychological and social factors in the thorough assessment of pain states has long been emphasized in both the clinical and experimental literatures. The influence of mood and cognition on the experience of pain—and, conversely, the effects of pain on one's psychological state and behavior—are universally accepted. In fact, predominant historical perspectives on pain consider the phenomenon to be defined by its psychosocial context. As a function of the rapid pace of clinical research in the last decade, the domain of psychosocial factors relevant to the assessment of the pain experience is rapidly expanding.

Emphasis on the broad domain of psychosocial factors is no more apparent than in the chronic pain area. This state of affairs is largely a function of the development of clinical constructs such as the *chronic pain syndrome* (Black, 1975), *psychogenic pain disorder* (Engel, 1959), and *pain behavior* (Fordyce, 1974)—terms that by their definition encourage a focus on psychosocial factors as cardinal features of the pain experience. Elaboration of traditional psychodynamic models (Blumer & Heilbronn, 1982), and the articulation of operant conditioning (Fordyce, 1976) and cognitive-behavioral (Turk, Meichenbaum, & Genest, 1983) conceptualizations of chronic pain, have encour-

aged consideration of psychological and interpersonal factors in the development and maintenance of the pain problem. The cognitive-behavioral perspective, in particular, has emphasized the importance of a broad domain of potentially relevant variables in defining the often deleterious impact of the chronic pain experience, and in identifying possible psychosocial contributors to the problems of the individual with chronic pain.

Clinical investigators and scholars in the area of chronic pain emphasize thorough assessment of the broad domain of psychosocial factors in order to fully understand the idiosyncrasies of the experience for any given individual, and to identify multiple targets for intervention in a comprehensive pain treatment and rehabilitation program. Indeed, multidimensional and multimodal clinical programs—based in part on a consideration of psychosocial, in addition to biomedical, factors—are rapidly replacing discipline-specific and unidimensional treatment centers as the state of the art in chronic pain management. Research designed to examine interactions of psychological and interpersonal variables with biomechanical and physiological parameters is a burgeoning area of investigation that will likely continue to influence clinical assessment and the development of treatment and rehabilitation alternatives.

The primary historical emphasis in the area of chronic pain has been on describing the often deleterious impact or influence of pain on psychological and social functioning, and the bulk of empirical work in this area has been devoted to this purpose. Psychological distress, particularly clinical depression and anxiety disorders, has been cited as a frequent concomitant of chronic pain (Banks & Kerns, 1996; Romano & Turner, 1985). Additional clinical and social problems commonly noted to occur include unemployment or underemployment, marital and family dysfunction, alcohol and other substance abuse and dependence, and general declines in social and recreational functioning. With ongoing investigation, the list of documented problems or changes in the psychosocial functioning of patients with chronic pain continues to grow.

Conversely, the development and refinement of contemporary models that incorporate or emphasize psychological processes in the experience of pain has led to a search for specific psychological and social variables that contribute to the development, maintenance, or expression of pain and its impact. Most noteworthy is the gate control theory of pain, which emphasizes cognitive-evaluative and motivational-affective processes in addition to sensory-discriminative processes, in the experience of pain (Melzack & Wall, 1965). The viability of this model has been instrumental in opening the door to others who have proposed specific psychological models to explain the development and maintenance of chronic pain (e.g., Fordyce, 1976; Turk et al., 1983).

Central to the assessment of the psychosocial context of the chronic pain experience is attention to the role of the family (Flor, Turk, & Rudy, 1987; Kerns, 1999; Payne & Norfleet, 1986; Turk, Flor, & Rudy, 1987). Strong empirical support for a role of the family in the perpetuation of chronic pain and associated disability and distress has accumulated over the past 15 years. In large part, research in this area is directly attributable to advances in the development of theoretically derived and psychometrically sound methods for the assessment of family functioning. Included among these methods are those developed or refined for assessment of pain-relevant communication among family members. These developments have led to further theoretical refinements as well as to proposals for the application of specific family therapy approaches for improving chronic pain management (Kerns, 1999).

Two historically distinct theories of family functioning have particularly influenced the field of chronic pain and pain management over the past

several years. The integration of family systems and family stress theories has led to the development of a single influential framework for understanding the role of the family with a chronically ill individual, including an individual with persistent pain. This model, termed the *family adjustment and adaptation response model*, is important in that it emphasizes the complexity of family functioning, particularly principles of systems theory, in attempting to explain the family's response to a member's experience of persistent pain (Patterson, 1988; Patterson & Garwick, 1994). The cognitive-behavioral perspective, specifically as it has been informed by operant conditioning theory and to the extent that it emphasizes the central role of pain-relevant communication, has also been heuristically important. Kerns and his colleagues (Kerns, 1995, 1999; Kerns & Payne, 1996; Kerns & Weiss, 1994) have further articulated a cognitive-behavioral transactional model to explain the role of families in the course of chronic illness—a model that shares important features with both of these theoretical perspectives.

It is unfortunate that research and clinical wisdom generally continue to view the relationship between the experience of pain and psychosocial variables in unidirectional terms. That is, it is typically thought either that chronic pain may be caused by psychosocial factors or that it provokes psychosocial sequelae. This apparent divergence in theoretical perspectives and the resultant split of scientific and clinical focus of attention compromises a view of these associations as reciprocal and dynamic. It seems much more reasonable to appreciate that the psychosocial context in which chronic pain develops and continues to exist is inextricably linked with the phenomenon of pain itself. Consistent with this perspective, Karoly (1985) has encouraged a view that the *context* of the pain experience should be viewed as the primary unit of inquiry or investigation in pain assessment. The psychosocial context, then, should be considered as relevant to the understanding of the development as well as impact of the experience of chronic pain. A cross-sectional approach to assessment of psychosocial factors is to be avoided, or at least interpretation of psychosocial data should consider reciprocal and dynamic relationships among variables, including the individual's report of pain.

Thus far we have emphasized the broad domain of psychosocial variables that may be relevant to the assessment of chronic pain, the reciprocal and dynamic relationships among these variables, and the importance of thorough assessment of these variables in order to develop a reasonable understanding of the individual's pain and associated problems, and to develop realistic and comprehensive plans for intervention. Several additional factors should be considered when one is developing an assessment plan and deciding upon specific measures. These choices can clearly influence the quality of the data collected, as well as their interpretation and ultimate utility.

OVERVIEW OF THE ASSESSMENT PROCESS

Regardless of theoretical perspective, clinicians involved in the assessment of the psychosocial context of the chronic pain experience are generally encouraged to adopt a hypothesis-testing approach to evaluation. A broadly based consideration of the full scope of psychological and social functioning typically begins the assessment process. Most commonly, this review is conducted in an interview format that is relatively standardized across individuals, regardless of the specifics of their pain complaints. Two examples are offered later in this chapter: the Pain Assessment Report (Holzman, Kerns, & Turk, 1981) and the Psychosocial Pain Inventory (PSPI; Heaton, Lehman, & Getto, 1985). Questionnaires are frequently used as adjuncts to the interview. Examples of the most commonly used psychosocial questionnaires and critical discussions of their psychometric properties and clinical uses are provided below. The content domains include educational accomplishments and vocational functioning, family and marital or couple status and functioning, and social and recreational functioning. Psychological well-being should be specifically addressed, with particular attention to levels of affective distress, and to alcohol and drug use (illicit and prescription). Consideration should be given to both historical information and present functioning. Emphasis should be placed on changes in functioning over time, especially those that are temporally associated with alterations in the individual's pain complaint, medical condition, or psychosocial concerns.

Based upon this broad screening or review process, specific psychosocial problem areas should be identified, and hypotheses should be developed to explain the link between them and the pain problem. These problem areas then serve as targets for further assessment and investigation. Efforts should be made to specify psychosocial problems in quantifiable terms, to identify important

mediators of their development and maintenance, and to identify potential mediators for change. Various standardized assessment procedures (ranging from standardized depression inventories to the instruments described below), as well as strategies specifically developed by the clinician for this purpose (e.g., a diary to record social and recreational activity level and its relationship to pain intensity), are likely to be used.

Whenever possible, clinicians and researchers should avoid relying on a single measure to assess specific content domains (e.g., marital/couple functioning). Optimally, data are collected via multiple methods (e.g., interviews, questionnaires, and diaries) to avoid the biases or sources of error inherent in any single method or specific instrument. Information from sources other than the patient is also valuable, and in certain situations critical, in making accurate judgments about psychosocial functioning. The inclusion of spouses/partners or other family members or close friends is a routine part of many pain programs' assessment protocols.

Clinicians will do best to consider the assessment process as an ongoing component of intervention for most patients. Initial interactions with a patient and others set the stage for more structured interventions. With this in mind, the concerns that many pain patients have about contact with mental health professionals or the specific focus on psychosocial functioning should be addressed in a straightforward and preemptive fashion. Emphasis during the assessment process should be on engaging the patient and others in a collaborative effort that will maximize treatment participation and outcomes. Goals of the assessment process should be specified, and the importance of assuming a broad view of chronic pain and its impact should be emphasized. Assessment should continue beyond the specification of problems and the development of treatment or rehabilitation goals. Ongoing reevaluation of these goals and outcomes throughout the application of intervention strategies is desirable, in order to permit identification of new problems or concerns, progress toward or modification of treatment goals, and refinement in intervention strategies.

Thus far our discussion has offered a broad framework in which to consider the assessment of the psychosocial context in chronic pain. In the following pages, we describe a number of methods and instruments that are either commonly used, or little known but deserving of attention and evaluation. All are creative efforts to add a psychosocial component to the evaluation of chronic pain.

ASSESSMENT INSTRUMENTS

Interviews

The most commonly used method for the collection of psychosocial information is the clinical interview. The interview is typically the initial contact between the patient and clinician, and often between significant others in the patient's life and the clinician. Because it is the initial contact, the interview has a significant influence on the expectancies of the patient and on the outcome of subsequent assessment and intervention. The interview serves multiple purposes, including the identification of potential problem areas and targets for further assessment; the development of possible intervention strategies; and, importantly, the motivation of patients for further contact with the clinician. Interviews vary with regard to degree of structure, the inclusion (or not) of significant others, the scope of the interview, and the breadth versus depth of information gathered. These variables are likely to be influenced by the theoretical perspective of the clinician. Readers interested in further information about general interview strategies are referred to Gordon (1975) and Haynes (1978). Discussions of the clinical pain interview are also readily available (e.g., Karoly & Jensen, 1987; Turk et al., 1983).

Pain Assessment Report

A specific example of a semistructured pain assessment interview is the Pain Assessment Report (Holzman et al., 1981). This preintervention interview serves to collect a broad range of specific and quantifiable information relevant to the psychosocial assessment of chronic pain. Goals of the interview include those common among clinical interviews, but because of its structure and emphasis on quantification, it also has the advantage of being useful for research.

Clinicians using the Pain Assessment Report follow a specific format for collection of information, referring to a manual that describes methods for coding patient responses in measurable terms. Content domains include a review of the history, site, and presumed diagnosis of the pain complaint; variables perceived by the patient as influencing the pain experience; history and present use of prescribed and over-the-counter pain medications, illicit substances, and alcohol; history of past medical and surgical treatment, physical therapy, and other interventions related to the pain problem; perceived cognitive, behavioral, and physical means of coping with pain; educational, vocational, and avocational history and current status, with an emphasis on changes related to the pain problem; current status, satisfaction, and pain-related changes in family and marital/couple relations and domestic activities; social functioning; and psychological functioning, with an emphasis on mood, sleep, mental status, and current or past psychological treatment. Although the structured nature of the interview and the availability of a detailed coding manual should increase the reliability of the information collected, reliability and validity of the measure have not been reported. The Pain Assessment Report and coding manual may be obtained from one of us (RDK).

Psychosocial Pain Inventory

A slightly different approach to interviewing has been taken by Heaton and his colleagues in their development of the PSPI (Getto, Heaton, & Lehman, 1983; Heaton et al., 1981, 1982, 1985). The PSPI was developed to allow reliable quantification of psychosocial variables hypothesized to influence the experience and the expression of pain. This, in turn, allows testing of hypotheses such as those Fordyce (1976) and Sternbach (1974) have put forth.

The PSPI is a 25-question structured interview developed and tested initially on 169 consecutive patients with pain at the Pain Clinic at the University of Colorado Health Sciences Center. The authors report choosing a structured format because in their experience they get more information this way, and it communicates to patients that many of their experiences are normal for patients with chronic pain. In addition, it can reassure patients who might react to a more traditional psychiatric interview with suspiciousness and concern about what the interviewer is trying to uncover. Patients are encouraged to add anything of significance, and the interviewer is free to pursue other topics as advisable. The PSPI is meant to generate a minimum patient database, and to guide further assessment. Topics addressed include pain-contingent financial gain, rest, solicitous responding by others, medication use, illness behaviors, stressful life events, and the impact of pain behaviors on interpersonal relationships. Uniquely, the PSPI also includes items inquiring about past learning history related to the sick role.

The original item pool contained 31 questions. In development, evaluators conducted the interview with 169 patients and significant others jointly, taking 1–2 hours for each interview (Getto & Heaton, 1985). Originally, each item was scored on a 4-point scale (0–3, with equal weighting) and specific descriptors anchored each point. Seven items, however, turned out to be clearly bimodal, and so now are scored as 0 or 2. Also, 6 of the original 31 items were deleted because of low variability. Total possible scores range from 0 to 68. In the test sample the range was 9–54, with a mean of 30 and a standard deviation of 7.9. Interrater reliability on a sample of 24 patients was .98 for total inventory scores.

During development, PSPI scores were compared to Minnesota Multiphasic Personality Inventory (MMPI) scores, McGill Pain Questionnaire (MPQ; Melzack, 1975) responses, physician impressions of exaggerated reports of pain, and objective physical findings. PSPI scores were largely unrelated to MMPI scores, except that patients with low PSPI scores appeared slightly more defensive and less somatically concerned than patients scoring higher on the PSPI. Patients with higher PSPI scores tended to use more MPQ adjectives and adjectives of greater severity, particularly sensory adjectives.

Almost 27% of the sample had been seen as exaggerating their symptoms by the examining physician. These patients also tended to have higher PSPI scores and elevated MMPI Depression scores. In terms of objective physical findings, patients with objective findings were more likely to score higher on the PSPI. Heaton et al. (1982) argue that this shows that psychosocial influences operate strongly for patients with pain, regardless of physical findings.

In a small study of 32 patients with acute pain who were undergoing neurosurgical evaluations, the hypothesis that patients who score high on the PSPI are unlikely to respond to purely medical intervention or advice was tested (Heaton et al., 1982). Nineteen of the patients received surgery, and the others received rest, traction, medication, and/or physical therapy. At a 6-month follow-up, the 18 patients considered significantly improved had a lower mean PSPI score than those who did not improve or those who got worse. Although this study was small, it did provide tentative support for the hypothesis that the PSPI can predict response to treatment, and it is consistent with the authors' report that total scores above 30 are correlated with a stronger influence of psychosocial factors in the chronic pain problem and with a poorer response to standard medical treatment (Getto & Heaton, 1985).

The PSPI appears useful for clinicians, and provides for uniform assessment by teams with many members and by clinicians of varied backgrounds. The authors point out that it does not obviate the need for standard psychiatric assessment, such as screening with the MMPI or diagnostic interviewing. Although the authors suggest that the PSPI will be sensitive to treatment gains, the evidence remains to be gathered. Since the first edition of this chapter was published (Kerns & Jacob, 1992), no further psychometric data have been published, although the instrument is being used in published studies (Wade, Dougherty, Hart, Rafii, & Price, 1992).

Self-Report Measures

West Haven–Yale Multidimensional Pain Inventory

In assessing the dynamic relationship between psychosocial variables and pain, interviews are generally supplemented by self-report measures. The West Haven–Yale Multidimensional Pain Inventory (WHYMPI; Kerns, Turk, & Rudy, 1985) is a multifactor instrument designed to assess the broad domain of psychosocial variables relevant to the chronic pain experience. The instrument is theoretically linked to a cognitive-behavioral perspective on chronic pain (Turk et al., 1983) and health assessment (Turk & Kerns, 1985). As such, it places an emphasis on patients' idiosyncratic beliefs or appraisals of their pain problems, the impact of pain on their lives, and the responses of others. The instrument is designed to provide a brief, psychometrically sound, and comprehensive assessment of important components of the pain experience. The authors encourage its use in the context of a multimodal and multidimensional assessment regimen.

The WHYMPI is a 52-item, 12-scale inventory divided into three parts. Section 1 consists of five scales designed to evaluate important dimensions of the chronic pain experience: perceived Interference of pain in vocational, social/recreational, and family and marital/couple functioning; Support and concern from significant others; Pain Severity; Life-Control with regard to activities of daily living and daily problems; and Affective Distress. Section 2 assesses patients' perceptions of the responses of others to their demonstrations and complaints of pain. Three scales assess the perceived frequencies of Negative, Solicitous, and Distracting responses. Section 3 assesses patients' reports of their participation in four categories of common daily activities: Household Chores, Outdoor Work, Activities Away from Home, and Social Activities. In addition to the individual scale scores, derivation of a General Activity score (the combination of the four activity scale scores) has been recommended for some purposes (Turk & Rudy, 1990). For the 12 WHYMPI scales, the number of items loading on each scale range from two in the case of the Life-Control scale to nine for the Interference scale. The WHYMPI is presented in Appendix 19.A.

Original development of the WHYMPI was conducted on a sample of 120 patients with chronic pain who were heterogeneous with regard to site and etiology of their pain complaints. The sample was drawn from two Veterans Administration (VA) Medical Centers and therefore was largely male. Otherwise, the sample can generally be viewed as typical of many hospital-based pain treatment centers and included patients who had a long duration of pain (mean > 10 years) and a substantial history of failed treatment efforts.

Twenty-two items for Section 1 of the instrument were developed to assess six a priori domains relevant to the comprehensive assessment of pain severity and the impact of pain on patients' lives. Those domains were identical to the final scales named above, except that the Interference scale was originally conceptualized as two separate domains measuring pain-related Interference and Dissatisfaction with present levels of functioning. Confirmatory factor analysis was used to verify the reliability of the six scales. However, a high correlation between the Interference and Dissatisfaction scales led to combining these scales into a single Interference scale. Two items were dropped because they failed to meet established criteria for convergent and discriminant validity. The resulting five scales were subsequently found to have adequate degrees of internal consistency (alphas ranging from .72 to .90) and stability over a 2-week test–retest period (r's ranging from .69 to .86).

Section 2 was developed to evaluate patients' perceptions of the range and frequency of responses by a significant other (most often a spouse/partner or close family member) to displays of pain and suffering. The original 21 items were derived from interviews with significant others about how they responded to the family member with pain. Exploratory factor analysis was conducted on the data from the 95 patients (out of the sample of 115) who reported living with a spouse/partner or family member. A three-factor solution was selected based on established criteria, and three scales composed of 14 of the original 21 items were identified and named. These scales were each found to have reasonable levels of internal consistency (alphas ranged from .74 to .84) and stability (r's ranging from .62 to .89).

Thirty items for Section 3 of the WHYMPI were derived from published activity lists and lists of activity goals for patients already seen at a pain program at one of the VA Medical Centers. Four reliable factors were identified on the basis of factor analysis. Eighteen of the original items were retained. Each resulting scale demonstrated good levels of reliability (alphas ranging from .70 to .86) and stability (r's ranging from .83 to .91).

Several authors have conducted their own factor analyses on these items, and in general their results support the factor structures reported here. (See, for example, Riley, Zawacki, Robinson, & Geisser, 1999.)

Validity of the scales of the WHYMPI was examined in two ways. Interscale correlations were all lower than each scale's index of internal consistency, suggesting that each scale contains a unique reliable variance or discriminant distinctiveness from the other scales. Factorial validity was also examined by submitting the 12 scales from the WHYMPI along with several other standardized measures of pain-relevant constructs to exploratory factor analysis. The WHYMPI scales loaded significantly and meaningfully on factors that also included conceptually related standardized measures. For example, the Affective Distress and Life-Control scales from the WHYMPI loaded significantly on the first factor, along with standardized measures of depression and anxiety.

Since its publication in 1985, the WHYMPI has been used in research projects that support its heuristic value and clinical utility. Studies have documented its sensitivity to improvements in pain and functioning (Kerns & Haythornthwaite, 1988; Kerns, Turk, Holzman, & Rudy, 1986); the ability of several of its scales to discriminate level of depressive symptom severity (Kerns & Haythornthwaite, 1988); the viability of the Pain Severity and General Activity scales as brief and reliable measures of pain intensity and adaptive functioning, respectively (Holmes & Stevenson, 1990); and the predictive utility of the Section 2 response scales in analyses of the role of social interactions in the maintenance of pain and disability (Faucett & Levine, 1991; Flor, Kerns, & Turk, 1987; Flor, Turk, & Rudy, 1989; Kerns, Haythornthwaite, Southwick, & Giller, 1990;

Kerns et al., 1991). The individual scales have also been found to capture parts of the experience of pain with little overlap with other important and useful tools, such as the Beck Depression Inventory (Beck & Beamesderfer, 1974; Beck, Ward, Mendelson, Mock, & Erbaugh, 1961) and the MPQ (De Gagne, Mikail, & D'Eon, 1995; Melzack, 1975).

Rudy (1989) proposed a revision of the WHYMPI that contains two additional items in both the Life Control and Interference scales. Computer scoring of this version is also available (Rudy, 1989).

The WHYMPI has been translated into a number of other languages, including Spanish, Dutch, French, Italian, Japanese, Chinese, Portuguese, Finnish, Icelandic, and Swedish, and has been found to be reliable and valid in those versions (Linton, Jensen, Bodin, Nygren, & Carlsson, 1998; Lousberg et al., 1997, 1999).

Rudy, Turk, and their colleagues (Rudy, Turk, Zaki, & Curtin, 1989; Turk & Rudy, 1988, 1990) have proposed an empirically derived taxonomy of patients with chronic pain called the Multiaxial Assessment of Pain, based on analyses of the WHYMPI scale scores. In a series of studies these investigators have identified three reliable profiles or categories of patients with chronic pain: Dysfunctional, Interpersonally Distressed, and Adaptive Copers. These profiles have been confirmed as similar in groups of patients suffering from chronic low back pain, headache, and temporomandibular joint pain (Turk & Rudy, 1990, 1992). Together, these findings support the discriminant validity of the WHYMPI and its utility as a clinical assessment tool in the context of a comprehensive evaluation protocol that also assesses medical and physical parameters.

Okifuji, Turk, and Eveleigh (1999) recently demonstrated that a minor modification to the WHYMPI instructions clarifying the definition of a *significant other* can greatly reduce the number of missing responses to Section 2 of the measure and improve the rate of classification of patients into one of the primary subgroups described above. In the first of two studies, these authors found that unmarried individuals and those living alone were more likely than others to fail to complete Section 2, suggesting that difficulty with interpretation of the term *significant other* might be responsible for the problem of missing responses. In a second study of 143 people reporting chronic pain, individuals were administered a modified version of the WHYMPI in which *significant other* was

defined as "the person with whom you feel closest," and were asked to specify who their "significant other" was. The data from this study are compelling and encourage modification of the measure as proposed by these authors. The WHYMPI in Appendix 19.A incorporates this modification.

Robinson and colleagues (1997) have shown that the WHYMPI and other instruments can be manipulated by patients wishing to score as coping poorly. Bruehl, Lofland, Sherman, and Carlson (1999) have developed a scale designed to detect random responding that may be of interest and use to clinicians working with patient populations where there is a question about malingering.

In summary, the WHYMPI has been found to be useful in varied settings as a measure of psychosocial functioning for clinical as well as research purposes. The strengths of the WHYMPI are its brevity, the ease with which it is scored (by hand or computer), its demonstrated reliability and validity, and its demonstrated utility in multiple clinical research investigations.

Family Environment Scale

The Family Environment Scale (FES; Moos & Moos, 1986) is a 90-item questionnaire that measures the social-environmental characteristics of families. Development of the FES was specifically informed by family systems theory and its key constructs. There are 10 subscales that make up three central dimensions of family functioning: a Family Relationship dimension (Cohesion, Expressiveness, and Conflict subscales), a Personal Growth dimension (Independence, Achievement Orientation, Intellectual–Cultural Orientation, Active–Recreational Orientation, and Moral–Religious subscales), and a Family System Maintenance Dimension (Organization and Control subscales). Over the past decade, investigators have employed the FES to examine potential relationships between family functioning and chronic pain conditions. For example, Ehde, Holm, and Metzger (1991) found that FES subscales differentiated between families with individuals experiencing headache and families without a member with headaches. In a more recent study, Schanberg, Keefe, Lefebvre, Kredick, and Gil (1998) administered the FES to both adolescents with juvenile primary fibromyalgia syndrome and their parents, and found that incongruity between parent and child responses to the FES was associated with greater impairment in functioning among the adolescents. In both studies, the authors concluded that their findings suggest a role of the family in helping to determine the individual's coping response to the pain condition, if not some role in the development and perpetuation of the pain condition itself.

Chronic Illness Problem Inventory

The Chronic Illness Problem Inventory (CIPI; Kames, Naliboff, Heinrich, & Schag, 1984) is a 65-item instrument intended to assess patient functioning in the areas of physical limitations, psychosocial functioning, health care behaviors, and marital adjustment. Its form has been influenced by the emphasis Turk and his colleagues (Turk, Sobel, Follick, & Youkilis, 1980) have placed on measures of competency as a way of focusing on patient-environment.

In developing the CIPI, mental health clinicians working in areas of chronic illness generated 74 items in 24 "problem areas" thought to be of concern to people with chronic illness and amenable to treatment. These items were initially administered to 115 patients with pain. Initial analyses included (1) tests of internal consistency using Cronbach's alpha; (2) factor analyses; and (3) frequency distributions (items with extremely low frequencies were discarded unless they were thought to represent significant concerns of patients with chronic illness but not of patients with pain). These analyses resulted in a 65-item inventory with 18 scales. Coefficient alphas ranged from .78 to .98 ($M = .85$). A 1-week test–retest sample of 30 patients resulted in coefficients ranging from .69 to .97 ($M = .87$).

The validity of the 65-item inventory was evaluated by comparing scores on individual scales to the results of a psychological evaluation by a clinical psychologist on the pain team. There was an 80% chance that problems noted by the psychologist were indicated on the CIPI, and a 72% chance that the psychologist and the CIPI agreed on the absence of a specific problem.

A second approach to validity testing involved administering the CIPI to patients with pain (back, head and neck, and multiple sites), people in treatment for obesity, and people with respiratory problems (mostly chronic obstructive pulmonary disease). Sample size for these analyses are unknown. Results indicated that the patients with pain reported more problems and problems of greater severity than other groups.

Furthermore, the specific problem areas endorsed by particular patient groups were as expected (e.g., the patients with pain reported the greatest difficulty with activity). In addition, some problem areas (e.g., sex and marital/couple concerns) were endorsed by all groups, suggesting the existence of problem areas common to chronic illness generally.

In a study by Romano, Turner, and Jensen (1992), the CIPI was found to share a substantial amount of variance with the Sickness Impact Profile (described later in this chapter). However, these authors also acknowledge that there is a significant amount of unshared variance between these measures, suggesting they may be addressing somewhat different aspects of dysfunction.

The CIPI is intended to be used as a screening device that can assist in focusing an assessment, and as an outcome measure that can assist in evaluating progress in treatment (Kames, Rapkin, Naliboff, Afifi, & Ferrer-Brechner, 1990). Romano, Turner, and Jensen (1992) suggest that its ease of administration and scoring, as well as its preliminary psychometric properties make it very attractive, but that its 18 scales make it somewhat unwieldy. Given these continued concerns, the CIPI should be used with some caution and always with additional indices of dysfunction.

Illness Behavior Inventory

A measure with potential usefulness for screening and measuring treatment gains is the Illness Behavior Inventory (IBI; Turkat & Pettegrew, 1983). Developed from a behavioral perspective, the IBI is a 20-item self-report measure of *illness behaviors*; such a behavior is defined as "an overt behavior performed by an individual which indicates that he or she is physically ill or in physical discomfort" (Turkat & Pettegrew, 1983, p. 36). The authors state that the original domain of 46 items was generated clinically after an exhaustive review of the literature proved relatively unhelpful, given that much of the literature purportedly addressing illness behavior actually relies on intrapsychic concepts (see discussion of the Illness Behavior Questionnaire, below).

The original 46 items were administered to 40 graduate nursing students, a population selected for relative healthiness but sensitivity to health and illness. Because of the large number of items relative to the sample size, the data were explored with elementary linkage analysis. Two factors were found, and they have been named

Work-Related Illness Behavior (9 items) and Social Illness Behavior (11 items). Other items were discarded. Cronbach's alphas were .89 and .88, respectively. Test–retest reliabilities on a sample of 32 undergraduate linguistic students at 2-week intervals were .97 for Work-Related Illness Behavior and .93 for Social Illness Behavior; individual item coefficients ranged from .82 to 1.00. A confirmatory structural analysis of the original nursing data set, compared to data from an unreported number of patients with back pain, indicated good stability of IBI items across subject populations.

In a test of discriminant validity, 22 patients with diabetic neuropathy were classified as high or low in illness behavior by medical staff. Scores for the total IBI as well as the two subscales were significantly different, in the expected direction, for the two groups.

The authors also report that the IBI has good concurrent validity, based on data from three studies (Turkat & Pettegrew, 1983). In the first study, the patients with diabetic neuropathy mentioned above also completed a diabetes symptom questionnaire's health interview survey with questions on disability and medical utilization, as well as the MPQ. In the second study, 50 patients with low back pain provided information about their medical utilization and cost, hospitalizations, and days lost from work. In the third study, 152 healthy college students completed the IBI. In all cases, scores were positively and significantly related to medical utilization, to Mechanic and Volkart's (1960) Sick Role Tendency Scale, and to Pilowsky's (1967) Hypochondriasis Scale.

Finally, predictive validity was assessed by administering the IBI and other measures to 63 female undergraduates. Regression analyses predicted outpatient medical utilization, bed disability days, and responses on a scale measuring the tendency to seek and receive medications from physicians (Wolinsky & Wolinsky, 1981).

These early tests of the IBI are promising. It is simple to use, appears psychometrically sound, and seems to have both clinical and research uses. Although individual items are written about "illness," the IBI has been used with low back pain patients without difficulty, and it would be easy to substitute "pain" for "illness" in individual items. The IBI's emphasis on self-observed behaviors can help educate patients about importance of behavioral expressions of pain in the development of a chronic pain mindset and in the maintenance of the pain itself.

Illness Behavior Questionnaire

The concept of *illness behaviors* is also the focus of the Illness Behavior Questionnaire (IBQ; Pilowsky & Spence, 1983). It is based on the sociology of illness as Parsons (1951) and Mechanic and Volkhart (1960) have written about it. Pilowsky (1967, 1970) has worked to integrate these sociological concepts into a clinical understanding of hypochondriasis and abnormal illness behavior.

Scale development took place on 100 unselected patients with pain (Pilowsky & Spence, 1975). The original questionnaire contained 52 items asking about patients' attitudes toward their illnesses, perceived reactions of others to the illness, and psychosocial variables. These 52 items were factor-analyzed in several steps, with seven factors ultimately interpreted; the seven are currently called General Hypochondriasis, Disease Conviction, Psychological versus Somatic Focusing, Affective Disturbance, Affective Inhibition, Denial, and Irritability. In its most recent form, the IBQ has 62 items. Two second-order factors have also been identified: Affective State (a composite of General Hypochondriasis, Affective Disturbance, and Irritability) and Disease Affirmation (a composite of Disease Conviction and Psychological versus Somatic Focusing).

Pilowsky and his colleagues (Pilowsky & Spence, 1975; Waddell, Pilowsky, & Bond, 1989) have used the IBQ in several studies with patients with chronic pain. In these studies it was found that such patients characteristically endorse items contributing to the Disease Affirmation scale. These patients are somatically preoccupied, have a firm belief that their pain is "real," and reject suggestions or implications that psychological factors play a role in their pain. These findings are consistent with clinical practice, where many patients are initially resistant to a rehabilitation approach to pain management, fearing that it implies the pain is "in their heads."

Other studies have used the IBQ to examine the personality and patterns of illness behavior of subgroups of patients with chronic pain (Keefe, Crisson, Maltbie, Bradley, & Gil, 1986; Schnurr, Brooke, & Rollman, 1990) as well as other clinical populations (Byrne, 1982; Joyce, Bushnell, Walshe, & Morton, 1986). The IBQ has also been demonstrated to be sensitive to treatment effects including surgery for pain (Waddell et al., 1989) and comparisons of psychotherapy and amitriptyline in the treatment of chronic pain (Pilowsky & Barrow, 1990).

The IBQ has moderate reliability and good validity (Williams, 1988). We had previously written (Kerns & Jacob, 1992) that its clinical usefulness in a comprehensive pain assessment may be limited because the form in which the information is packaged does not assist the clinician in planning or monitoring interventions. Some clinical applications, however, have been described. Keefe and his colleagues (1986) found that the IBQ scores were quite predictive of a number of indices of pain and pain behavior, and they argue that their findings support the use of the IBQ in a behavioral assessment of patients with chronic pain. Miller and Hafner (1991) have found that Disease Conviction scores predict utilization of both general practitioners and specialists, and that Denial scores predict utilization of specialists. Given its important theoretical foundations, it is clear that in addition to its possible clinical usefulness, the IBQ is a valuable research instrument.

Sickness Impact Profile

Of all the instruments we review in this chapter, the Sickness Impact Profile (SIP; Bergner, Bobbitt, Carter, & Gilson, 1981) is the most comprehensively tested and revised. Boldly stated, the SIP was designed to be a measure of perceived health status so sensitive that it would detect changes within groups and over time, regardless of the medical, demographic, or cultural variables involved. Because many developed countries are beginning to shift attention from cure and rehabilitation to prevention, traditional variables such as morbidity and mortality were considered inadequate outcome measures. Bergner and colleagues (1981) hypothesized that a broad measure of daily activities would be sensitive to changes in health status, and this is the focus of the SIP.

The SIP was developed during multiple field trials over a 6-year period (Bergner, Bobbitt, Kressel, et al., 1976; Bergner, Bobbitt, Pollard, et al., 1976; Bergner et al., 1981; Gilson et al., 1975; Pollard, Bobbitt, Bergner, Martin, & Gilson, 1976). Test populations included a mixed group of 246 inpatients, outpatients, home care patients, patients at a walk-in clinic, and nonpatients; patients treated by rehabilitation medicine; patients seen by speech pathologists; outpatients with chronic problems; prepaid health plan enrollees; a random sample of 696 prepaid health plan patients; and 199 patients from a family medicine clinic who considered themselves sick.

The process of developing the SIP was much too extensive to be reviewed in detail here. The numerous analyses, reported in their final form in Bergner and colleagues (1981), resulted in an instrument with 136 items and 12 categories or scales: Sleep and Rest, Eating, Work, Home Management, Recreation and Pastimes, Ambulation, Mobility, Body Care and Movement, Social Interaction, Alertness Behavior, Emotional Behavior, and Communication. The first five scales are considered Independent categories; the second three are considered Physical categories; and the last four are called Psychosocial categories. The SIP can be self-administered or administered by an interviewer in 20–30 minutes. The overall alpha was .94, and the test–retest on a sample of 53 was .92. Convergent and discriminant validity were evaluated with the multitrait, multimethod technique and were found to be good. In an early and unpublished manual (Anonymous, 1978), it is noted that an investigator can administer only those scales of interest without compromising their reliability or construct validity, but warns against picking and choosing among individual items. It is not clear whether this continues to be the case (Bergner et al., 1981).

Although lengthy and cumbersome to score, the SIP is a psychometrically sound instrument that provides a wealth of information, some of it psychosocial. According to Williams (1988), several investigators have found it to be clinically useful in working with patients with chronic pain. A number of authors have found it to be a sensitive measure of change following psychological treatments for chronic pain (Sanders & Brena, 1993; Turner, 1982; Turner & Clancy, 1988). The SIP has been found to be useful in a variety of cultures (Sanders et al., 1992) and has been translated into at least one foreign language (Chwalow et al., 1992).

Roland and Morris (1983a, 1983b) have developed a short form (24 items) of the SIP worded especially for people with back pain. They report the (same-day) test–retest reliability of the SIP Roland scale to be .94, and Deyo (1986) found the test–retest reliability to be the same as that of the full SIP. The Roland scale has shown to be treatment-sensitive (Hadler, Curtis, Gillings, & Stinnett, 1987; Klein & Eek, 1990), to be sensitive to improvements over time (Deyo, 1986; Roland & Morris, 1983a, 1983b), and to be correlated in the expected directions with other pain-related measures (Deyo & Centor, 1986; Weinstein, Spratt, Lehmann, McNeill, & Hejna, 1986). It does appear that the SIP Roland scale is more representative of the SIP Physical category than of the Independent or Psychosocial categories (Deyo, 1986; Jensen, Strom, Turner, & Romano, 1992).

Pain Disability Index

The Pain Disability Index (PDI; Pollard, 1984) was developed as a brief self-report measure of pain related disability. The inventory consists of seven questions designed to measure the degree to which patients believe that their pain interferes with functioning in the areas of family/home responsibilities, recreation, social activities, occupation, sexual behavior, self-care, and life support activity. Patients respond to each item on 0–10 scales anchored with the descriptors "no disability" to "total disability."

In an extensive examination of the measure's psychometric properties, Tait, Chibnall, and Krause (1990) examined a sample of 444 patients with chronic pain who completed the PDI and several other pain-relevant measures as part of a comprehensive evaluation prior to participation in a rehabilitation program. Factor analysis of the PDI revealed a single factor that accounted for 56% of the variance in the data. Internal consistency for this single factor as measured by Cronbach's alpha was .86. Since previous research had discovered a two-factor solution, these same data were forced into a two-factor solution. Two reliable factors were again discovered, one described as assessing voluntary or discretionary activities, while the second was thought to assess disability in obligatory activities (self-care and life support). Patients were then grouped into high versus low levels of disability on the PDI and compared on the other standardized measures. Results generally supported the concurrent validity of the PDI. More recent work on a larger sample (n = 1,059) of patients with chronic pain supports the one-factor solution (Chibnall & Tait, 1994).

A subset of the original sample also completed the PDI a second time prior to their participation in treatment. Test–retest reliability was statistically significant, but lower than would be expected or desired (r = .44). Using this subsample, investigators found significant differences in observed pain behaviors among high versus low scorers on the PDI—findings that further support the validity of the measure. Studies have also demonstrated that the PDI discriminates between patients immediately after surgery (high disability) and those several months removed from surgery (low disability) (Pollard, 1984); outpatients (low disability) and inpatients (high disability) with pain (Tait, Pollard, Margolis, Duckro, & Krause, 1987); employed and unemployed patients with pain (Chibnall & Tait, 1994; Tait, Chibnall, & Richardson, 1990); patients injured at work (high disability) and those with pain of other origins (Chibnall & Tait, 1994); and patients involved in litigation and those who are not (Chibnall & Tait, 1994; Tait, Chibnall, & Richardson, 1990). Jerome and Gross (1991) found that the factor consisting of discretionary activities was more likely to discriminate between working and nonworking people with pain, and also between depressed and nondepressed patients, than the obligatory factor was.

The PDI has shown a discriminative ability in a study of Holocaust survivors compared to a control group with chronic pain (Yaari, Eisenberg, Adler, & Birkhan, 1999). While the Holocaust survivors reported higher levels of pain, more pain sites, and more depression that chronic pain controls, they reported less disability on the PDI. Similarly, the PDI was found to be useful in discriminating patients with cancer and pain from patients with chronic pain but without cancer (Turk et al., 1998). The PDI has also been translated into at least one other language: Finnish (Gronblad, Hurri, & Kouri, 1997).

The measure has strengths related to its brevity and its theoretical and practical importance. Evaluations of its psychometric properties largely support its reliability and utility, but questions about its face-apparent nature (i.e., patients are clearly aware of its intended use) and possible systematic biases in reporting (e.g., desire of some patients to distort their reports toward an appearance of increased disability) should be examined before it is accepted as a valid measure of disability.

Reports by Others

The operant conditioning model of chronic pain emphasizes the important role that social contingencies for demonstrations of pain and disability may play in the perpetuation of the chronic pain experience. Although the model emphasizes the importance of direct observation of behavior as the ideal method for exploring hypotheses informed by the model, the expense, awkwardness, and marginal reliability of most direct observation methods generally preclude their practical use in clinical and clinical–research settings. The development of reliable self-report measures holds potential promise as an alternative to direct observation in many clinical and research settings.

Significant-Other WHYMPI

As noted above, the WHYMPI includes a section designed to assess pain-relevant social interactions from the patient's perspective. More recently, Kerns and Rosenberg (1995) reported on a version of the same measure, but from the perspective of a significant other of the person experiencing pain.

The items included in the initial stage of development of the significant-other version of the WHYMPI pain-relevant response scales were the same 21 items used in the initial phases of development of the patient version of the measure. Instructions call for partners of individuals experiencing chronic pain to record the frequency with which they respond to expressions of pain by the patient with a specific behavior. Each item is followed by a 7-point scale anchored by 0 = "never" and 6 = "very often."

Items were administered to a sample of 123 partners of individuals who had been referred to a pain rehabilitation program. An additional 31 individuals who were approached to participate in the study either refused or provided incomplete data. These individuals were also administered a measure of marital satisfaction and communication in order to assess criterion-related validity of the significant-other WHYMPI. The patients with chronic pain also participated and completed the patient version of the WHYMPI and these same measures of marital functioning.

Of the 21 items administered to partners, 3 items were skewed as a result of low item endorsement and were subsequently dropped from further consideration. The remaining 18 items were grouped into the three hypothesized subscales in a manner consistent with the content of the three subscales from the patient version. One item in the Negative subscale was found to have a particularly low item-to-total correlation and was also eliminated.

The final version of the significant-other form of the WHYMPI consists of 17 items, including 10 items constituting the Solicitous response subscale, 3 items composing the Distracting subscale, and four items composing the Negative response subscale. Indices of internal consistency for the three subscales range from .75 to .80. Correlations between the patient and significant-other versions of the three subscales range from .42 to .49. As expected, Solicitous responding has been found to be significantly and positively related to measures of both marital/couple satisfaction and positive communication, whereas Negative responding has

been demonstrated to have significant inverse relationships with these same variables.

Additional support for the validity of the measure comes from a study previously reported by Romano, Turner, Friedman, and colleagues (1992) involving direct observation of pain-relevant communication between individuals reporting chronic pain and their spouses. In that study, the investigators demonstrated that observed solicitous behavior was significantly correlated with spouse reports, but not patient reports, of solicitous behavior.

It should be noted that several investigators have modified the WHYMPI, either in its entirety or in part, in order to administer it to significant others. See, for example, the work of Lousberg, Schmidt, and Groenman (1992). Unfortunately, basic psychometric work to evaluate the internal consistency, stability, or validity of these versions of the measure, other than that described above for Section II, has not been reported. Therefore, significant-other versions of this measure should be used with caution, in the absence of demonstrations of their psychometric properties.

Diaries

In the psychosocial assessment of the experience of pain, interviews and inventories provide an overview, a historical perspective, and composite measures of critical variables. The interview also provides an opportunity to interact extensively with a patient, and to gather impressions concerning his or her psychological readiness for rehabilitation. Additional valuable information can be acquired with the use of pain, mood, activity and sleep diaries, because they allow an investigation into the actual temporal relationship between psychosocial variables and pain, rather than self reports of such. Affleck, Tennen, Urrows, and Higgins (1991), for example, report on the use of a daily events diary to examine relationships between negative events and pain in patients with rheumatoid arthritis.

Support for the reliability and validity of diary methodology is available from a number of investigators. Follick, Ahern, and Laser-Wolston (1984) investigated the psychometric properties of an activity diary for patients with low back pain by comparing the patients' diary reports with those of spouses (n = 20) and with data from an automated, electromechanical "uptime/downtime" device (n = 8). The diary asked for ratings to be made three times a day for each preceding half hour, in the following categories: position (lying, sitting, standing walking, asleep); time spent alone, with family, with others; time at home; medication use; use of pain relief activities or devices; and average daily ratings of pain, tension, and mood. Pearson product–moment correlations were used to determine the relationships between patient ratings and spouse and mechanical data. The correlations were all positive and statistically significant. The strongest correlations were in areas that were most clearly behaviorally defined, like medication use; the weakest were in the most subjective areas, like mood and pain intensity ratings. The authors note that one way in which these findings are useful is to validate diary reports as pretreatment and outcome measures of functional impairment.

Haythornthwaite, Hegel, and Kerns (1991) have reported on the use of daily diaries to monitor sleep of patients with pain. In that study, 46 patients admitted for inpatient treatment for chronic pain kept diaries every morning after waking. Items were derived from clinical experience and from the literature, and included both specific incidents (such as the number of times one awoke) and subjective reports (e.g., sleep quality). Patients also reported on sleep in the last week; completed measures of pain severity, depression, and anxiety; and reported average level of activity, as well as wore a pedometer during the admission. Haythornthwaite and colleagues report that for patients with pain, poor sleep is only partly a function of pain; it is more reliably related to mood. They also report results suggesting acceptable levels of reliability and stability, and present some helpful comments on the special issue of assessing stability in diary studies.

Wilson, Watson, and Currie (1998) have also reported on the use of diary assessment of sleep. They had 40 patients use sleep diaries in combination with ambulatory activity monitoring with an actigraph. Similar results were found between the diaries and the actigraphs for total sleep time, time awake after sleep onset, and sleep efficiency, but not for sleep onset latency and nocturnal awakenings. They found that the two methods of assessment gathered different but complementary information, and they argue for multimethod assessment practices.

Combined Measures

McGill Comprehensive Pain Questionnaire

We have noted in our earlier discussion that a comprehensive evaluation generally makes use of both interviews and self-report measures. An instrument that combines a questionnaire packet with a semistructured interview is the McGill Comprehensive Pain Questionnaire (MCPQ), offered by Monks and Taenzer (1983). The MCPQ is a self-report inventory complemented by an interview. The inventory is meant to inquire into the pain, its history, and its treatments; other physical symptoms; psychosocial concomitants; and personal variables, for the purposes of treatment planning, program evaluation, and research. The interview is used to clarify responses on the inventory, and to investigate personal and subjective variables (e.g., the patient's expectations, changes in sexual activity due to pain). The interviewer guide also contains the MPQ (Melzack, 1975; see Melzack & Katz, Chapter 3, this volume), an inventory easily completed by patients alone. Monks and Taenzer report that the MCPQ was derived from clinical experience and from previously published instruments.

The MCPQ appears to be easy to use, and the authors report success in having patients complete the inventory part prior to their first appointments. It is probably most helpful in eliciting the patient's report of the pain history and its effect on work, finances, leisure, sleep, and weight. It is less clear how the sections on parents and family are to be used, particularly by workers who are not mental health professionals. The interview itself explores a number of pertinent areas, but offers no guidance in recording data that would allow pre–post comparisons or tests of research hypotheses, if properly quantified. Davis (1989) does report a study in which she used the MCPQ with patients with rheumatic disease and patients with acute surgical pain. She reports that it was time-consuming to use and difficult to score, but that it was helpful in understanding the experience of the individual. Davis (1988) has also reported on a short form of the MCPQ, in which the patient inventory and the interview are combined. Also of concern is the emphasis in both the inventory and the interview on the effects of pain on other variables, rather than vice versa or both.

In summary, the MCPQ is a combined inventory and follow-up interview meant to be comprehensive in nature. It is rather long and difficult to score reliably or at all (depending on the question). It may be very useful to the neophyte pain management clinician trying to get a feel for the population, but less useful in a busy clinic, where routine evaluation should point fairly reliably at appropriate and measurable targets for intervention.

Multiperspective Multidimensional Pain Assessment Protocol

An example of a multidisciplinary and multi-instrument perspective can be found in the Multiperspective Multidimensional Pain Assessment Protocol (MMPAP; Rucker, Metzler, & Kregel, 1996). The MMPAP was designed to be a comprehensive assessment tool for use in the disability determination process and was developed under contract to the Social Security Administration. It was developed following a literature review and with the help of two expert panels. Completion of the MMPAP requires information from the patient, the medical record, direct physical examination, and physician assessment of patient behavior. As such, it is an instrument that includes psychosocial information in addition to other important variables. The seven domains covered are Demographic Information, Pain Dimensions, Medical Information, Mental Health, Social Support Networks, Functional Limitations, and Employment or Rehabilitation. Questions are all forced-choice. The patient completes part of the instrument, and physicians complete the remainder. The MMPAP was standardized on a sample of 651 patients with chronic pain of at least 6 months' duration. Ninety-nine patients were assessed twice and completed two full MMPAPs, at least 31 days apart. Some patients were assessed by the same medical team (to evaluate test–retest reliability) and some were not (to test interrater reliability). Concurrent validity was assessed using a variety of well-accepted instruments such as the MPQ (Melzack, 1975) and the WHYMPI (Kerns et al., 1985). Overall, the reliability was acceptable to good, and concurrent validity was demonstrated.

The final version of the MMPAP is 23 pages long; it may require 2–4 hours to complete, and is expected to be completed on a single day. The authors note that many pain centers use a variety of instruments and approaches that take as long. They suggest that using a comprehensive and standardized assessment such as the MMPAP allows for early identification of problem areas, permits standardization across treatment centers, and facilitates working with insurance companies and workers compensation claims.

CONCLUSIONS

Consideration of psychosocial factors has become a routine component of the assessment of chronic pain conditions. Most would agree that to ignore the possible deleterious effects of chronic pain on an individual's life, or to fail to take into account possible psychological, interpersonal, and sociological contributors to the development and maintenance of the pain complaint, leaves the clinician vulnerable to erroneous assumptions about the extent of the problem, its etiology, and possible solutions. Similarly, systematic investigation of psychosocial factors will continue to have an enormous impact on understanding chronic pain conditions and their possible treatment.

This chapter has provided a brief introduction into the broad domain of relevant psychosocial factors, an overview of the psychosocial assessment process, and descriptions of some of the widely used or promising clinical and research measures of psychosocial functioning available. The review of the measures is intended to provide the interested reader with enough information to make preliminary decisions about the choice of instruments. More critical discussion of the measures is beyond the scope of this chapter.

Selection of individual measures should be based on the specific needs of the clinician or clinical setting or on the goals of the investigator, but should balance the desire to be thorough with the needs and abilities of patients. Use of measures that have been validated on the specific population being served is always desirable. In the end, clinicians and researchers alike will do well to avoid relying on information from only one source, regardless of the presumed reliability or validity of the measure. Clinicians are reminded to incorporate selected psychosocial measures into a more comprehensive (and, optimally, interdisciplinary) evaluation. Investigators should consider a multivariate approach that incorporates multiple measures of single constructs in order to minimize measurement error and bias. This is particularly important, given the self-report nature of most of these measures. Continued examination of the psychometric properties and utility of the measures offered in this chapter, as well as the development of alternative methods and measures, is strongly encouraged.

REFERENCES

Anonymous. (1978). *The Sickness Impact Profile: A brief summary of its purpose, uses, and administration.* Unpublished manuscript.

Affleck, G., Tennen, H., Urrows, S., & Higgins, P. (1991). Individual differences in the day-to-day experience of chronic pain: A prospective daily study of rheumatoid arthritis patients. *Health Psychology, 10*(6), 419–426.

Banks, S. M., & Kerns, R. D. (1996). Explaining high rates of depression in chronic pain: A diathesis–stress framework. *Psychological Bulletin, 119*(1), 95–110.

Beck, A. T., & Beamesderfer, A. (1974). Assessment of depression: The depression inventory. In P. Pichot (Ed.), *Psychological measurements in psychopharmacology* (pp. 151–169). Basel: S. Karger.

Beck, A. T., Ward, C. H., Mendelson, M., Mock, J., & Erbaugh, J. (1961). An inventory for measuring depression. *Archives of General Psychiatry, 4*, 561–571.

Bergner, M., Bobbitt, R. A., Carter, W. B., & Gilson, B. S. (1981). The Sickness Impact Profile: Development and final revision of a health status measure. *Medical Care, 19*, 787–805.

Bergner, M., Bobbitt, R. A., Kressel, S., Pollard, W. E., Gilson, B. S., & Morris, J. R. (1976). The Sickness Impact Profile: Conceptual formulation and methodology for the development of a health status measure. *International Journal of Health Services, 6*, 393–415.

Bergner, M., Bobbitt, R. A., Pollard, W. E., Martin, D. P., & Gilson, B. S. (1976). The Sickness Impact Profile: Validation of a health status measure. *Medical Care, 14*, 57–67.

Black, R. G. (1975). The chronic pain syndrome. *Surgical Clinics of North America, 55*, 999–1011.

Blumer, D., & Heilbronn, M. (1982). Chronic pain and a variant of depressive disease: The pain-prone disorder. *Journal of Nervous and Mental Disease, 170*, 381–394.

Bruehl, S., Lofland, K. R., Sherman, J. J., & Carlson, C. R. (1999). The Variable Responding Scale for detection of random responding on the Multidimensional Pain Inventory. *Psychological Assessment, 10*(1), 3–9.

Byrne, D. (1982). Illness behaviour and psychosocial outcome after a heart attack. *British Journal of Clinical Psychology, 21*, 145–146.

Chibnall, J. T., & Tait, R. C. (1994). The Pain Disability Index: Factor structure and normative data. *Archives of Physical Medicine and Rehabilitation, 75*(10), 1082–1086.

Chwalow, A. J., Lurie, A., Bean, K., Parent du Chatelet, I., Venot, A., Dusser, D., Douot, Y., & Strauch, G. (1992). A French version of the Sickness Impact Profile (SIP): Stages in the cross cultural validation of a generic quality of life scale. *Fundamental and Clinical Pharmacology, 6*(7), 319–326.

Davis, G. C. (1988). McGill Comprehensive Pain Questionnaire—"modified version." In C. F. Waltz & O. L. Strickland (Eds.), *Measurement of nursing outcomes* (Vol. 1, pp. 160–184). New York: Springer.

Davis, G. C. (1989). The clinical assessment of chronic pain in rheumatic disease: Evaluating the use of two instruments. *Journal of Advanced Nursing, 14*, 397–402.

De Gagne, T. A., Mikail, S. F., & D'Eon, J. L. (1995). Confirmatory factor analysis of a four-factor model of chronic pain evaluation. *Pain, 60*(2), 195–202.

Deyo, R. A. (1986). Comparative validity of the Sickness Impact Profile and shorter scales for functional assessment in low-back pain. *Spine, 11*, 951–954.

Deyo, R. A., & Centor, R. M. (1986). Assessing the responsiveness of functional scales to clinical change: An analogy to diagnostic test performance. *Journal of Chronic Diseases, 39*, 897–906.

Ehde, D. M., Holm, J. E., & Metzger, D. L. (1991). The role of family structure, functioning, and pain modeling in headache. *Headache, 31*(1), 35–40.

Engel, G. L. (1959). "Psychogenic" pain and the pain-prone patient. *American Journal of Medicine, 26*, 899–918.

Faucett, J. A., & Levine, J. D. (1991). The contributions of interpersonal conflict to chronic pain in the presence or absence of organic pathology. *Pain, 44*, 35–43.

Flor, H., Kerns, R. D., & Turk, D. C. (1987). The role of spouse reinforcement, perceived pain, and activity levels of chronic pain patients. *Journal of Psychosomatic Research, 31*, 251–259.

Flor, H., Turk, D. C., & Rudy, T. E. (1987). Pain and families: I. Etiology, maintenance and psychosocial impact. *Pain, 30*, 3–27.

Flor, H., Turk, D. C., & Rudy, T. E. (1989). Relationship of pain impact and significant other reinforcement of pain behaviors: The mediating role of gender, marital status and marital satisfaction. *Pain, 38*, 45–50.

Follick, M. J., Ahern, D. K., & Laser-Wolston, N. (1984). Evaluation of a daily activity diary for chronic pain patients. *Pain, 19*, 373–382.

Fordyce, W. E. (1974). Pain viewed as a learned behavior. In J. J. Bonica (Ed.), *Advances in neurology* (Vol. 4, pp. 415–422). New York: Raven Press.

Fordyce, W. E. (1976). *Behavioral methods for chronic pain and illness.* St. Louis, MO: Mosby.

Getto, C. J., & Heaton, R. K. (1985). Assessment of patients with chronic pain. In D. P. Swiercinsky (Ed.), *Testing adults: A reference guide for special psychodiagnostic assessments* (pp. 113–122). Kansas City, MO: Test Corporation of America.

Getto, C. J., Heaton, R. K., & Lehman, R. A. W. (1983). PSPI: A standardized approach to the evaluation of psychosocial factors in chronic pain. In J. J. Bonica, U. Lindblom, & A. Iggo (Eds.), *Advances in pain research and therapy* (Vol. 5, pp. 885–890). New York: Raven Press.

Gilson, B. S., Gilson, J. S., Bergner, M., Bobbitt, R. A., Kressel, S., Pollard, W. E., & Vesselago, M. (1975). Sickness Impact Profile: Development of an outcome measure of health care. *American Journal of Public Health, 65*, 1304–1310.

Gordon, R. L. (1975). *Interviewing: Strategy, techniques, and tactics.* Homewood, IL: Dorsey Press.

Gronblad, M., Hurri, H., & Kouri, J. (1997). Relationships between spinal mobility, physical performance tests, pain intensity and disability assessments in chronic low back pain patients. *Scandinavian Journal of Rehabilitation Medicine, 29*, 17–24.

Hadler, N. M., Curtis, P., Gillings, D. B., & Stinnett, S. (1987). A benefit of spinal manipulation as adjunctive therapy for acute low-back pain: A stratified controlled trial. *Spine, 12*, 703–706.

Haynes, S. N. (1978). *Principles of behavioral assessment.* New York: Gardner Press.

Haythornthwaite, J. A., Hegel, M. T., & Kerns, R. D. (1991). Development of a sleep diary for chronic pain patients. *Journal of Pain and Symptom Management, 6*(2), 65–72.

Heaton, R. K., Getto, C. J., Lehman, R. A. W., Fordyce, W. E., Brauer, E., & Groban, S. E. (1981). A standardized evaluation of psychosocial factors in chronic pain. *Pain*, Suppl. 1, S154.

Heaton, R. K., Getto, C. J., Lehman, R. A. W., Fordyce, W. E., Brauer, E., & Groban, S. E. (1982). A standardized evaluation of psychosocial factors in chronic pain. *Pain*, *12*, 165–174.

Heaton, R. K., Lehman, R. A. W., & Getto, C. J. (1985). *A manual for the psychosocial pain inventory.* Odessa, FL: Psychological Assessment Resources.

Holmes, J. A., & Stevenson, C. A. Z. (1990). Differential effects of avoidant and attentional coping strategies on adaptation to chronic and recent-onset pain. *Health Psychology*, *9*, 577–584.

Holzman, A. D., Kerns, R. D., & Turk, D. C. (1981). *Pain assessment report.* Unpublished manuscript.

Jensen, M. P., Strom, S. E., Turner, J. A., & Romano, J. M. (1992). Validity of the Sickness Impact Profile Roland scale as a measure of dysfunction in chronic pain patients. *Pain*, *50*(2), 157–162.

Jerome, A., & Gross, R. T. (1991). Pain Disability Index: Construct and discriminant validity. *Archives of Physical Medicine and Rehabilitation*, *72*(11), 920–922.

Joyce, P. R., Bushnell, J. A., Walshe, J. W. B., & Morton, J. B. (1986). Abnormal illness behaviour and anxiety in acute non-organic pain. *British Journal of Psychiatry*, *149*, 57–62.

Kames, L. D., Naliboff, B. D., Heinrich, R. L., & Schag, C. C. (1984). The Chronic Illness Problem Inventory: Problem-oriented psychosocial assessment of patients with chronic illness. *International Journal of Psychiatry in Medicine*, *14*(1), 65–75.

Kames, L. D., Rapkin, A. J., Naliboff, B. D., Afifi, S., & Ferrer-Brechner, T. (1990). Effectiveness of an interdisciplinary pain management program for the treatment of chronic pelvic pain. *Pain*, *41*, 41–46.

Karoly, P. (1985). The assessment of pain: Concepts and procedures. In P. Karoly (Ed.), *Measurement strategies in health psychology* (pp. 461–515). New York: Wiley.

Karoly, P., & Jensen, M. P. (1987). *Multimethod assessment of chronic pain.* New York: Pergamon Press.

Keefe, F. J., Crisson, J. E., Maltbie, A., Bradley, L., & Gil, K. M. (1986). Illness behavior as a predictor of pain and overt behavior patterns in chronic low back pain patients. *Journal of Psychosomatic Research*, *30*(5), 543–551.

Kerns, R. D. (1995). Family assessment and intervention in chronic illness. In P. M. Nicassio & T. W. Smith (Eds.), *Managing chronic illness: A biopsychosocial perspective* (pp. 207–244). Washington, DC: American Psychological Association.

Kerns, R. D. (1999). Family therapy for adults with chronic pain. In R. J. Gatchel & D. C. Turk (Eds.), *Psychosocial factors in pain: Critical perspectives* (pp. 445–456). New York: Guilford Press.

Kerns, R. D., & Haythornthwaite, J. A. (1988). Depression among chronic pain patients: Cognitive-behavioral analysis and effect on rehabilitation outcome. *Journal of Consulting and Clinical Psychology*, *56*(6), 870–876.

Kerns, R. D., Haythornthwaite, J., Southwick, S., & Giller, E. L., Jr. (1990). The role of marital interaction in chronic pain and depressive symptom severity. *Journal of Psychosomatic Research*, *34*(4), 401–408.

Kerns, R. D., & Jacob, M. C. (1992). Assessment of the psychosocial context of the experience of chronic pain.

In D. C. Turk & R. Melzack (Eds.), *Handbook of pain assessment* (pp. 235–253). New York: Guilford Press.

Kerns, R. D., & Payne, A. (1996). Treating families of chronic pain patients. In R. J. Gatchel & D. C. Turk (Eds.), *Psychological approaches to pain management: A practitioner's handbook* (pp. 283–304). New York: Guilford Press.

Kerns, R. D., & Rosenberg, R. (1995). Pain relevant responses from significant others: Development of a significant-other version of the WHYMPI scales. *Pain*, *61*(2), 245–249.

Kerns, R. D., Southwick, S., Giller, E. L., Haythornthwaite, J. A., Jacob, M. C., & Rosenberg, R. (1991). The relationship between reports of pain-related social interactions and expressions of pain and affective distress. *Behavior Therapy*, *22*, 101–111.

Kerns, R. D., Turk, D. C., Holzman, A. D., & Rudy, T. E. (1986). Comparison of cognitive-behavioral and behavioral approaches to the outpatient treatment of chronic pain. *Clinical Journal of Pain*, *1*, 195–203.

Kerns, R. D., Turk, D. C., & Rudy, T. E. (1985). The West Haven–Yale Multidimensional Pain Inventory (WHYMPI). *Pain*, *23*, 345–356.

Kerns, R. D., & Weiss, L. H. (1994). Family influences on the course of chronic illness: A cognitive-behavioral transactional model. *Annals of Behavioral Medicine*, *16*(2), 116–121.

Klein, R. G., & Eek, B. C. (1990). Low-energy laser treatment and exercise for chronic low back pain: Double-blind controlled trial. *Archives of Physical Medicine and Rehabilitation*, *71*, 34–37.

Linton, S. J., Jensen, I. B., Bodin, L., Nygren, A. L., & Carlsson, S. G. (1998). Reliability and factor structure of the Multidimensional Pain Inventory—Swedish Language Version (MPI-S). *Pain*, *75*(1), 101–110.

Lousberg, R., Schmidt, A. J., & Groenman, N. H. (1992). The relationship between spouse solicitousness and pain behavior: Searching for more experimental evidence. *Pain*, *51*(1), 75–79.

Lousberg, R., Schmidt, A. J. N., Groenman, N. H., Vendrig, L., & Dijkman-Caes, C. I. (1997). Validating the MPI-DLV using experience sampling data. *Journal of Behavioral Medicine*, *20*(2), 195–206.

Lousberg, R., van Breukelen, G. J., Groenman, N. H., Schmidt, A. J., Arntz, A., & Winter, F. A. (1999). Psychometric properties of the Multidimensional Pain Inventory, Dutch language version (MPI-DLV). *Behaviour Research and Therapy*, *37*(2), 167–182.

Mechanic, D., & Volkart, E. H. (1960). Illness behavior and medical diagnosis. *Journal of Health and Human Behavior*, *1*, 86–96.

Melzack, R. (1975). The McGill Pain Questionnaire: Major properties and scoring methods. *Pain*, *1*, 277–299.

Melzack, R., & Wall, P. D. (1965). Pain mechanisms: A new theory. *Science*, *150*, 971–979.

Miller, R. J., & Hafner, R. J. (1991). Medical visits and psychological disturbance in chronic low back pain: A study of a back education class. *Psychosomatics*, *32*(3), 309–316.

Monks, R., & Taenzer, P. (1983). A comprehensive pain questionnaire. In R. Melzack (Ed.), *Pain measurement and assessment* (pp. 233–237, 1A–14A). New York: Raven Press.

Moos, R., & Moos, B. (1986). *Family Environment Scale: Manual* (2nd ed.). Palo Alto, CA: Consulting Psychologists Press.

Okifuji, A., Turk, D. C., & Eveleigh, D. J. (1999). Improving the rate of classification of patients with the Multidimensional Pain Inventory (MPI): Clarifying the meaning of "significant other." *Clinical Journal of Pain*, 15, 290–296.

Parsons, T. (1951). *The social system*. New York: Free Press.

Patterson, J. M. (1988). Families experiencing stress: The family adjustment and adaptation response model. *Family Systems in Medicine*, 5, 202–237.

Patterson, J. M., & Garwick, A. W. (1994). The impact of chronic illness on families: A family systems perspective. *Annals of Behavioral Medicine*, 16, 131–142.

Payne, B., & Norfleet, M. A. (1986). Chronic pain and the family: A review. *Pain*, 26, 1–22.

Pilowsky, I. (1967). Dimensions of hypochondriasis. *British Journal of Psychiatry*, 113, 89–93.

Pilowsky, I. (1970). Primary and secondary hypochondriasis. *Acta Psychiatrica Scandinavica*, 46, 273–285.

Pilowsky, I., & Barrow, C. G. (1990). A controlled study of psychotherapy and amitriptyline used individually and in combination in the treatment of chronic intractable, 'psychogenic' pain. *Pain*, 40, 3–19.

Pilowsky, I., & Spence, N. D. (1975). Patterns of illness behaviour in patients with intractable pain. *Journal of Psychosomatic Research*, 19, 279–287.

Pilowsky, I., & Spence, N. D. (1983). *Manual for the Illness Behavior Questionnaire (IBQ)* (2nd ed.). Adelaide, Australia: University of Adelaide, Department of Psychiatry.

Pollard, C. A. (1984). Preliminary validity study of the Pain Disability Index. *Perceptual and Motor Skills*, 59(3), 974.

Pollard, W. E., Bobbitt, R. A., Bergner, M., Martin, D. P., & Gilson, B. S. (1976). The Sickness Impact Profile: Reliability of a health status measure. *Medical Care*, 14, 146–155.

Riley, J. L., III, Zawacki, T. M., Robinson, M. E., & Geisser, M. E. (1999). Empirical test of the factor structure of the West Haven–Yale Multidimensional Pain Inventory. *Pain*, 15(1), 24–30.

Robinson, M. E., Myers, C. D., Sadler, I. J., Riley J. L., III, Kvaal, S. A., & Geisser, M. E. (1997). Bias effects in three common self-report pain assessment measures. *Clinical Journal of Pain*, 13(1), 74–81.

Roland, M., & Morris, R. (1983a). A study of the natural history of back pain: Part I. Development of a reliable and sensitive measure of disability in low-back pain. *Spine*, 8(2), 141–144.

Roland, M., & Morris, R. (1983b). A study of the natural history of low-back pain: Part II. Development of guidelines for trials of treatment in primary care. *Spine*, 8(2), 145–150.

Romano, J. M., & Turner, J. A. (1985). Chronic pain and depression: Does the evidence support a relationship? *Psychological Bulletin*, 97(1), 18–34.

Romano, J. M., Turner, J. A., Friedman, L. S., Bulcroft, R. A., Jensen, M. P., Hops, H., & Wright, S. F. (1992). Sequential analysis of chronic pain behaviors and spouse responses. *Journal of Consulting and Clinical Psychology*, 60(5), 777–782.

Romano, J. M., Turner, J. A., & Jensen, M. P. (1992). The Chronic Illness Problem Inventory as a measure of dysfunction in chronic pain patients. *Pain*, 49(1), 71–75.

Rucker, K. S., Metzler, H. M., & Kregel, J. (1996). Standardization of chronic pain assessment: A multi-

perspective approach. *Clinical Journal of Pain*, 12(2), 94–110.

Rudy, T. E. (1989). *Multiaxial assessment of pain: Multidimensional Pain Inventory. Computer program users' manual. Version 2.1*. Pittsburgh, PA: Pain Evaluation and Treatment Institute.

Rudy, T. E., Turk, D. C., Zaki, H. S., & Curtin, H. D. (1989). An empirical taxometric alternative to traditional classification of temporomandibular disorders. *Pain*, 36(3), 311–320.

Sanders, S. H., & Brena, S. F. (1993). Empirically derived chronic pain patient subgroups: The utility of multidimensional clustering to identify differential treatment effects. *Pain*, 54(1), 51–56.

Sanders, S. H., Brena, S. F., Spier, C. J., Beltrutti, D., McConnell, H., & Quintero, O. (1992). Chronic low back pain patients around the world: Cross-cultural similarities and differences. *Clinical Journal of Pain*, 8(4), 317–323.

Schanberg, L. E., Keefe, F. J., Lefebvre, J. C., Kredick, D. W., & Gil, K. M. (1998). Social context of pain in children with juvenile primary fibromyalgia syndrome: Parental pain history and family environment. *Clinical Journal of Pain*, 14(2), 107–115.

Schnurr, R. F., Brooke, R. I., & Rollman, G. B. (1990). Psychosocial correlates of temporomandibular joint pain and dysfunction. *Pain*, 42, 153–165.

Sternbach, R. A. (1974). *Pain patients: Traits and treatment*. New York: Academic Press.

Tait, R. C., Chibnall, J. T., & Krause, S. (1990). The Pain Disability Index: Psychometric properties. *Pain*, 40, 171–182.

Tait, R. C., Chibnall, J. T., & Richardson, W. D. (1990). Litigation and employment status: Effects on patients with chronic pain. *Pain*, 43, 37–46.

Tait, R. C., Pollard, C. A., Margolis, R. B., Duckro, P. N., & Krause, S. J. (1987). The Pain Disability Index: Psychometric properties and validity data. *Archives of Physical Medicine and Rehabilitation*, 68, 438–441.

Turk, D. C., Flor, H., & Rudy, T. E. (1987). Pain and families: II. Assessment and treatment. *Pain*, 30, 29–46.

Turk, D. C., & Kerns, R. D. (1985). Assessment in health psychology: A cognitive-behavioral perspective. In P. Karoly (Ed.), *Measurement strategies in health psychology* (pp. 335–372). New York: Wiley.

Turk, D. C., Meichenbaum, D., & Genest, M. (1983). *Pain and behavioral medicine: A cognitive-behavioral perspective*. New York: Guilford Press.

Turk, D. C., & Rudy, T. E. (1988). Toward an empirically derived taxonomy of chronic pain patients: Integration of psychological assessment data. *Journal of Consulting and Clinical Psychology*, 56(2), 233–238.

Turk, D. C., & Rudy, T. E. (1990). The robustness of an empirically derived taxonomy of chronic pain patients. *Pain*, 43, 27–36.

Turk, D. C., & Rudy, T. E. (1992). Classification logic and strategies in chronic pain. In D. C. Turk & R. Melzack (Eds.), *Handbook of pain assessment* (pp. 409–428). New York: Guilford Press.

Turk, D. C., Sist, T. C., Okifuji, A., Miner, M. F., Florio, G., Harrison, P., Massey, J., Lema, M. L., & Zevon, M. A. (1998). Adaptation to metastatic cancer pain, regional/local cancer pain and non-cancer pain: Role of psychological and behavioral factors. *Pain*, 74(2–3), 247–256.

Turk, D. C., Sobel, H. J., Follick, M. J., & Youkilis, H. D. (1980). A sequential criterion analysis for assessing coping with chronic illness. *Journal of Human Stress, 6*, 35-40.

Turkat, I. D., & Pettegrew, L. S. (1983). Development and validation of the Illness Behavior Inventory. *Journal of Behavioral Assessment, 5*(1), 35-47.

Turner, J. A. (1982). Comparison of group progressive-relaxation training and cognitive-behavioral group therapy for chronic low back pain. *Journal of Consulting and Clinical Psychology, 50*, 757-765.

Turner, J. A., & Clancy, S. (1988). Comparison of operant behavioral and cognitive-behavioral group treatment of chronic low back pain. *Journal of Consulting and Clinical Psychology, 56*, 261-266.

Waddell, G., Pilowsky, I., & Bond, M. R. (1989). Clinical assessment and interpretation of abnormal illness behaviour in low back pain. *Pain, 39*(1), 41-53.

Wade, J. B., Dougherty, L. M., Hart, R. P., Rafii, A., & Price, D. D. (1992). A canonical correlation analysis of the influence of neuroticism and extraversion on chronic pain, suffering, and pain behavior. *Pain, 51*, 67-73.

Weinstein, J., Spratt, K. F., Lehmann, T., McNeill, T., & Hejna, W. (1986). Lumbar disc herniation: A comparison of the results of chemonucleolysis and open discectomy after ten years. *Journal of Bone and Joint Surgery, 68*, 43-54.

Williams, R. C. (1988). Toward a set of reliable and valid measures for chronic pain assessment and outcome research. *Pain, 35*, 239-251.

Wilson, K. G., Watson, S. T., & Currie, S. R. (1998). Daily diary and ambulatory activity monitoring of sleep in patients with insomnia associated with chronic musculoskeletal pain. *Pain, 75*(1), 75-84.

Wolinsky, F. D., & Wolinsky, S. R. (1981). Expecting sick-role legitimation and getting it. *Journal of Health and Social Behavior, 22*, 229-242.

Yaari, A., Eisenberg, E., Adler, R., & Birkhan, J. (1999). Chronic pain in Holocaust survivors. *Journal of Pain and Symptom Management, 17*(3), 181-187.

APPENDIX 19.A. WEST HAVEN–YALE MULTIDIMENSIONAL PAIN INVENTORY (WHYMPI)

BEFORE YOU BEGIN, PLEASE ANSWER TWO PRE-EVALUATION QUESTIONS BELOW:

1. Some of the questions in this questionnaire refer to your "significant other." A significant other is *the person with whom you feel closest*. This includes anyone that you relate to on a regular or frequent basis. It is very important that you identify someone as your "significant other." Please indicate below who your significant other is (check one):

☐ Spouse   ☐ Partner/Companion   ☐ Housemate/Roommate
☐ Friend   ☐ Neighbor   ☐ Parent/Child/Other Relative
☐ Other (please describe):

2. Do you currently live with this person?   YES ☐   NO ☐

When you answer questions in the following pages about "your significant other," always respond in reference to the specific person you just indicated above.

Section 1

In the following 20 questions, you will be asked to describe your pain and how it affects your life. Under each question is a scale to record your answer. Read each question carefully and then *circle* a number on the scale under that question to indicate how that specific question applies to you.

1. Rate the level of your pain at the present moment.

0	1	2	3	4	5	6
No pain						Very intense pain

2. In general, how much does your pain problem interfere with your day-to-day activities?

0	1	2	3	4	5	6
No interference						Extreme interference

3. Since the time you developed a pain problem, how much has your pain changed your ability to work?

0	1	2	3	4	5	6
No change						Extreme change

_ Check here, if you have retired for reasons other than your pain problem.

4. How much has your pain changed the amount of satisfaction or enjoyment you get from participating in social and recreational activities?

0	1	2	3	4	5	6
No change						Extreme change

5. How supportive or helpful is your spouse (significant other) to you in relation to your pain?

0	1	2	3	4	5	6
Not at all supportive						Extremely supportive

6. Rate your overall mood during the *past week*.

0	1	2	3	4	5	6
Extremely low mood						Extremely high mood

7. On the average, how severe has your pain been during the *last week*?

0	1	2	3	4	5	6
Not at all severe						Extremely severe

8. How much has your pain changed your ability to participate in recreational and other social activities?

0	1	2	3	4	5	6
No change						Extreme change

9. How much has your pain changed the amount of satisfaction you get from family-related activities?

0	1	2	3	4	5	6
No change						Extreme change

10. How worried is your spouse (significant other) about you in relation to your pain problem?

0	1	2	3	4	5	6
Not at all worried						Extremely worried

11. During the *past week*, how much control do you feel that you have had over your life?

0	1	2	3	4	5	6
Not at all in control						Extremely in control

12. How much *suffering* do you experience because of your pain?

0	1	2	3	4	5	6
No suffering						Extreme suffering

13. How much has your pain changed your marriage and other family relationships?

0	1	2	3	4	5	6
No change						Extreme change

14. How much has your pain changed the amount of satisfaction or enjoyment you get from work?

0	1	2	3	4	5	6
No change						Extreme change

— Check here, if you are not presently working.

15. How attentive is your spouse (significant other) to your pain problem?

0	1	2	3	4	5	6
Not at all attentive						Extremely attentive

16. During the *past week*, how much do you feel that you've been able to deal with your problems?

0	1	2	3	4	5	6
Not at all						Extremely well

17. How much has your pain changed your ability to do household chores?

0	1	2	3	4	5	6
No change						Extreme change

18. During the *past week*, how irritable have you been?

0	1	2	3	4	5	6
Not at all irritable						Extremely irritable

19. How much has your pain changed your friendships with people other than your family?

0	1	2	3	4	5	6
No change						Extreme change

20. During the *past week*, how tense or anxious have you been?

0	1	2	3	4	5	6
Not at all tense or anxious						Extremely tense or anxious

Section 2

In this section, we are interested in knowing how your significant other (this refers to the person you indicated above) responds to you when he or she knows that you are in pain. On the scale listed below each question, *circle a number* to indicate *how often* your significant other generally responds to you in that particular way *when you are in pain.*

1. Ignores me.

0	1	2	3	4	5	6
Never						Very often

2. Asks me what he/she can do to help.

0	1	2	3	4	5	6
Never						Very often

3. Reads to me.

0	1	2	3	4	5	6
Never						Very often

(cont.)

4. Expresses irritation at me.

0	1	2	3	4	5	6
Never						Very often

5. Takes over my jobs or duties.

0	1	2	3	4	5	6
Never						Very often

6. Talks to me about something else to take my mind off the pain.

0	1	2	3	4	5	6
Never						Very often

7. Expresses frustration at me.

0	1	2	3	4	5	6
Never						Very often

8. Tries to get me to rest.

0	1	2	3	4	5	6
Never						Very often

9. Tries to involve me in some activity.

0	1	2	3	4	5	6
Never						Very often

10. Expresses anger at me.

0	1	2	3	4	5	6
Never						Very often

11. Gets me some pain medications.

0	1	2	3	4	5	6
Never						Very often

12. Encourages me to work on a hobby.

0	1	2	3	4	5	6
Never						Very often

13. Gets me something to eat or drink.

0	1	2	3	4	5	6
Never						Very often

14. Turns on the T.V. to take my mind off my pain.

0	1	2	3	4	5	6
Never						Very often

Section 3

Listed below are 18 common daily activities. Please indicate *how often* you do each of these activities by *circling* a number on the scale listed below each activity. Please complete *all* 18 questions.

1. Wash dishes.

0	1	2	3	4	5	6
Never						Very often

2. Mow the lawn.

0	1	2	3	4	5	6
Never						Very often

3. Go out to eat.

0	1	2	3	4	5	6
Never						Very often

4. Play cards or other games.

  0   1   2   3   4   5   6
  Never   Very often

5. Go grocery shopping.

  0   1   2   3   4   5   6
  Never   Very often

6. Work in the garden.

  0   1   2   3   4   5   6
  Never   Very often

7. Go to a movie.

  0   1   2   3   4   5   6
  Never   Very often

8. Visit friends.

  0   1   2   3   4   5   6
  Never   Very often

9. Help with the house cleaning.

  0   1   2   3   4   5   6
  Never   Very often

10. Work on the car.

  0   1   2   3   4   5   6
  Never   Very often

11. Take a ride in a car.

  0   1   2   3   4   5   6
  Never   Very often

12. Visit relatives.

  0   1   2   3   4   5   6
  Never   Very often

13. Prepare a meal.

  0   1   2   3   4   5   6
  Never   Very often

14. Wash the car.

  0   1   2   3   4   5   6
  Never   Very often

15. Take a trip.

  0   1   2   3   4   5   6
  Never   Very often

16. Go to a park or beach.

  0   1   2   3   4   5   6
  Never   Very often

17. Do a load of laundry.

  0   1   2   3   4   5   6
  Never   Very often

18. Work on a needed house repair.

  0   1   2   3   4   5   6
  Never   Very often

(cont.)

WHYMPI Scoring

Section 1:

Interference:	(Question 2 + 3 + 4 + 8 + 9 + 13 + 14 + 17 + 19)/9
Support:	(Question 5 + 10 + 15)/3
Pain Severity:	(Question 1 + 7 + 12)/3
Life-Control:	(Question 11 + 16)/2
Affective Distress:	((6- Question 6) + 18 + 20)/3

Section 2:

Negative Responses:	(Question 1 + 4 + 7 + 10)/4
Solicitous Responses:	(Question 2 + 5 + 8 + 11 + 13 + 14)/6
Distracting Responses:	(Question 3 + 6 + 9 + 12)/4

Section 3:

Household Chores:	(Question 1 + 5 + 9 + 13 + 17)/5
Outdoor Work:	(Question 2 + 6 + 10 + 14 + 18)/5
Activities Away from Home:	(Question 3 + 7 + 11 + 15)/4
Social Activities:	(Question 4 + 8 + 12 + 16)/4
General Activity:	(Sum of all questions in Section 3)/18

Note. Copyright 1985/2000 by Robert D. Kerns, Dennis C. Turk, and Thomas E. Rudy. Reprinted by permission.

Chapter 20

Presurgical Psychological Screening

MICHAEL E. ROBINSON
JOSEPH L. RILEY III

Surgery is one of the treatment options for a variety of chronic pain conditions, including (but not limited to) various spine disorders, wrist and hand injuries, pelvic pain conditions, and temporomandibular disorders. In most cases, the patients' goal is to obtain relief from the pain, though that is clearly not the only indication for surgery, nor is it the only desirable outcome. In addition to relief from pain, stabilizing a joint to avoid additional injury or damage or to reduce progression of a disease process, returning to work, and/or increasing functional ability are also objectives of surgical treatment.

Regardless of the desired outcome, surgical interventions for chronic pain conditions are frequent occurrences. Surgeries for back pain conditions alone account for upwards of 300,000 procedures annually (Taylor, Deyo, Cherkin, & Kreuter, 1994; Taylor et al., 1995). Other pain-related surgeries account for hundreds of thousands of additional surgeries for pelvic pain, temporomandibular disorders, complex regional pain syndromes, and carpal tunnel syndrome or other hand/wrist injuries (AbuRahma, Robinson, Powell, Bastug, & Boland, 1994; Dolwick & Dimitroulis, 1994; Feuerstein, Huang, & Pransky, 1999; Reiter, 1998; Wilcox et al., 1994). In addition to the sheer number of these procedures, the costs of performing surgery and of subsequent recovery and rehabilitation are substantial. Estimates for back surgery costs suggest an average cost in the area of $18,000 to $50,000, depending on

the procedure (Block, 1999). Hand surgeries (primarily carpal tunnel), though less expensive, are estimated to cost a total of $2 billion annually (Palmer & Hanrahan, 1995). Additional costs for the rehabilitation of these individuals are those for incurred physical and occupational therapy, and for a variety of assistive devices (e.g., braces, canes, bone stimulators). The potential financial costs for failed or less than optimal outcomes of these types of surgeries can therefore be substantial. More difficult to quantify are the personal and social costs of repeated failed surgical attempts at relieving patients' pain and suffering.

A number of surgical outcome studies exist for the treatment of a variety of spine surgeries; these are explored in more detail in a later section. Reviews of the literature on certain spine surgeries (fusion) indicate only modest success rates, ranging from 15% to 95% with an average of 68% (Turner, Ersek, Herron, & Deyo, 1992). Spinal fusion tends to be one of the more expensive spine surgeries, suggesting that failed surgeries incur considerable cost. Multiple surgeries for pelvic pain and temporomandibular disorders are also common (Reiter, 1998; Widmark, 1997).

Recent reviews suggest that patients with chronic pain conditions also have a significant co-occurrence of psychological symptoms (e.g., Robinson & Riley, 1999). Although it is beyond the scope of this chapter to discuss the etiological precedence of pain and negative affect in people with chronic pain, this affective disturbance is very likely to be existent in individuals facing the possibility of surgery for a pain condition. Negative affect is a considerable influence on patients' adjustment, coping, and decision-making ability, and should be assessed with respect to potential candidacy for surgery. In addition to affective disturbance, personality features and disorders, environmental influences, social learning effects, and compensation and litigation factors are all likely contributors to the status of patients being considered for pain-related surgery.

In the following sections, we review the empirical basis for employing psychological assessments for people who are being considered as candidates for surgical amelioration of their chronic pain conditions. First, we review the outcome studies available for several types of high-frequency pain-related surgeries, with an emphasis on surgery for the spine. Then we review common assessment approaches used in evaluation of people being considered for surgery. Finally, we suggest additional research that could clarify the validity and efficacy of presurgical screening for pain-related surgery.

TYPES OF SURGERIES

Surgery for the Spine

The experience of back pain is a common occurrence, with approximately 40%–50% of people suffering some form of back pain each year (Von Korff, Dworkin, Le Resche, & Kruger, 1988). Although most people recover within the first several days of pain onset, patients with chronic back pain are often frustrated about the lack of effective treatment, seek care from multiple health caregivers, and receive multiple treatments. In a study of industrial injuries (Spengler et al., 1986), back injury constituted 19% of all workers' compensation claims but accounted for 41% of the total costs. Furthermore, 10% of the back injury claims were associated with 79% of the total back injury costs. The data suggest that a small proportion of those who experience back pain do not recover, but become chronic sufferers from back pain and subsequently are very costly to society.

The etiology of chronic back pain is varied, with common causes including degenerative processes of the spine or disc herniation (see Waddell & Turk, Chapter 23, this volume). However, many patients do not demonstrate identifiable organic pathophysiology, and the source of their pain remains undetermined. Moreover, radiographic results frequently show that many asymptomatic individuals display abnormal findings (Boos et al., 1995; Deyo, 1996). Diagnosis can be difficult because of the lack of pathognomonic signs. For patients seeking relief from chronic back pain, there are many treatment modalities available. Current conservative treatments include drug therapy (Deyo, 1996), electrical stimulation (Meyler, de Jongste, & Rolf, 1994), exercise (Rodriquez, Bilkey, & Agre, 1992), acupuncture (Lewith & Vincent, 1996), biofeedback and relaxation training (DeGood, 1993), and cognitive-behavioral interventions (Bradley, 1996). Of the population of patients suffering from chronic back pain, approximately 1% ultimately receive spine surgery.

Although we use the single term *surgery*, there are several common surgical procedures available, with technology constantly evolving. One of the most common procedures is discectomy, which involves removal of the portion of the disc that is impinging on the nerve root. This procedure typically also involves removing part or all of the lamina. A good example of the evolution of spine surgical procedures is arthroscopic discectomy, which reduces the invasiveness of the procedure by allowing the surgeon to perform the procedure with the aid of fiber optics. A spinal fusion is a procedure in which bone fragments are placed into unstable segments of the spine in such a way that the bones fuse together, stabilizing the spine. Devices such as plates, rods, or screws may be inserted to provide additional stability, and this procedure is also used to treat scoliosis (curvature of the spine). Rhizotomy is a procedure to sever the neural pathway believed to be transmitting pain signals from irritated or damaged facet joints. The surgical implantation of spinal cord stimulators to block nerve transmissions and implantation of morphine pumps are other surgical procedures for the treatment of back pain.

Overall, how effective are these surgical procedures? Determining outcome is a complex process (Deyo, 1996). Assessment of success can be defined by technical aspects of the procedure, improvement in function, increased quality of life, improved mental health, reduced medication use, patient satisfaction, return to work, reduced health care expenditures, or reduction in perceived pain. Additional variability in outcome comes from procedural or patient selection differences and variability in follow-up duration. Generally, the results of outcome studies indicate that surgery is effective but not always so, with unsatisfactory outcome estimated to be in the range of 30% for spinal fusion (Turner, Ersek, Herron, Haselkorn, et al., 1992) or laminectomy/discectomy (Hoffman, Wheeler, & Deyo, 1993).

Another way to assess effectiveness is to compare surgery with other treatment modalities. One study (Malter, Larson, Urban, & Deyo, 1996) suggests that surgery can be a cost-effective alternative for patients with herniated lumbar discs that are unresponsive to conservative management. However, conservative treatment is typically preferred for those with only moderate pathology, particularly with male patients (Herno, Airaksinen, Saari, & Luukkonen, 1996). In all probability, the most appropriate question is not whether or not a particular procedure is successful, but for which patients is it successful.

Poor outcome from surgical procedures has an impact on the health care system through increased use of medication and possibly the need for a second surgical procedure (Hoffman et al., 1993). It has been suggested that surgery for disc herniation may be performed two to four times more often than necessary in the United States (Nachemson, 1993). Given that the outcomes from surgical procedures are inconsistent, and that the requisite resources to permit surgery are substantial, prediction of outcome is of considerable interest. Hoffman and colleagues (1993) have stated that the primary reason for poor outcome is inappropriate patient selection. Successfully identifying patients with a high likelihood of poor surgical outcome could save resources while avoiding the trauma and risk of surgery. There is strong evidence that psychosocial variables significantly influence the development and chronicity of back pain (Burton, Tillotson, Main, & Hollis, 1995) and are among the strongest predictors of spinal surgery outcome (Block, 1996; Schade, Semmer, Main, Hora, & Boos, 1999).

Psychological Distress/Personality Factors

Given that pain is a subjective experience, it is not surprising that an individual's personality traits could influence outcome from surgical treatment for chronic back pain. The first study of surgical outcome using psychosocial variables (Wiltse & Rocchio, 1975) evaluated the efficacy of Minnesota Multiphasic Personality Inventory (MMPI) scale scores as predictors of surgical success. High scores on the MMPI Hysteria (Hs) and Hypochondriasis (Hy) scales were predictive of the result of chemonucleolysis. Patient demographic variables (e.g., age, sex) were not related to postoperative outcome. Further evidence of the utility of psychological

variables was demonstrated in a study showing that patients with elevated MMPI scores were more likely to report pain on the injection of a non-disrupted disc than were patients without high scores (Block, Vanharanta, Ohnmeiss, & Guyer, 1996). This suggests that discographic pain reports are not only related to anatomical abnormalities, but are influenced by a patient's personality. The authors concluded that patients with elevated scores on the Hy, Hs, and Depression (D) scales of the MMPI may tend to overreport pain during discographic injection.

Regardless of the assessment methodology used (Cashion & Lynch, 1979; Riley, Robinson, Geisser, Wittmer, & Smith, 1995), studies have generally found the MMPI scales Hs, Hy, and frequently D to be the most predictive of surgical outcome. The Hs and Hy scales consist of items reflecting somatic preoccupation, with the Hy scale also containing items indicative of social discomfort and the underreporting of emotion (Graham, 1990). The composition of the D scale reflects the syndrome of depression: subjective depression, psychomotor retardation, mental dullness, and brooding. Differences in premorbid psychological factors have been shown to be meaningful contributors to the variations in the patients' eventual outcome (Spengler, Ouellette, Battie, & Zeh, 1990). It has been hypothesized that the Hs and Hy scales are associated with an excessive focus on physical symptoms and pain (Graham, 1990) and may be associated with a focus on a medical cure and denial of psychological distress related to pain (Riley & Robinson, 1998).

Other MMPI scales have also been predictive of the outcome of spinal surgery. The Psychopathic Deviate (Pd) scale, which assesses hostility and rebelliousness (Graham, 1990), has predicted outcome in several studies (Long, Brown, & Engelberg, 1980; Riley et al., 1995; Spengler et al., 1990). Others have suggested that patients with excessive anger tend to blame others for their problems and are less likely to comply with treatment regimens (Fernandez & Turk, 1995). Elevations on the Psychasthenia (Pt) scale are also associated with poor outcome (Doxey, Dzioba, Mitson, & Lacroix, 1988). This scale is considered a measure of worry and obsessive thoughts, and may relate to poor outcome because these people are rigid and unable to adapt to lifestyle changes. However, as none of these studies administered the MMPI before the onset of back pain, it is likely that the MMPI scores reflect both the individuals' responses to back pain and dimensions of personality.

Although most studies have relied on the MMPI in prediction of spine surgery outcome, other measures of psychological distress are also used in the assessment of patients with chronic pain. Depression has been consistently associated with poor outcome for back pain (Gatchel, Polatin, & Mayer, 1995). Studies using a prediction equation that included Beck Depression Inventory scores have been able to discriminate between good and bad surgical outcomes (Hasenbring, Marienfeld, Kuhlendahl, & Soyka, 1994). Another study linked depression to surgical outcome as measured by postoperative pain relief and return to work, but not subjective disability, following discectomy (Schade et al., 1999).

Clinical studies have shown that chronic pain and psychopathology are frequently associated; however, few studies have used designs that allow inferences about the temporal relationship between pain and negative emotion. Negative emotion can result from the experience of chronic pain, and negative emotion also causes some pain (Robinson & Riley, 1999). Consequently, if the latter is true and negative emotion contributes to pain, the probability of positive outcome from treatment should decrease, given a premorbid history of psychopathology. One study used a composite score that included a measure of psychological history, and found that a significant psychological history predicted poor outcome from surgery (Manniche et al., 1994). Unfortunately, few studies differentiate between co-occurring emotional distress and a formal psychiatric diagnosis prior to pain onset.

Cognitive Factors

Many studies have documented an association between pain coping and chronic pain (Jensen, Turner, Romano, & Karoly, 1991); however, few studies have examined the association between pain coping and spine surgical outcome. Gross (1986) assessed the preferred pain coping strategies of patients with back pain prior to a laminectomy procedure. She found that self-reliance (believing that one could decrease pain) and engaging in catastrophic thinking prior to undergoing surgery were predictive of reduced pain ratings and poorer postsurgical adjustment, respectively. Patients with postoperative complaints differed in their modes of coping with back pain, and had substantially less satisfactory occupational, family, and social lives than complaint-free patients (Dvorak, Valach, Fuhrimann, & Heim, 1988). Using a psychodynamic model of coping (e.g., defense mecha-

nisms), one group found that patients with poor and good lumbar discectomy outcome differed significantly in their use of rationalization and regression (Fulde, Junge, & Ahrens, 1995).

Historical/Behavioral Issues

1. *Physical/sexual abuse.* There is some evidence that a history of physical and sexual abuse may predispose individuals toward the development of chronic back pain. One study found that the probability of developing chronic back pain was four to five times greater for women with a history of physical or sexual abuse (Linton, 1997). A second study tested for an association between childhood traumas in general and outcome following lumbar spine surgery (Schofferman, Anderson, Hines, Smith, & White, 1992). Patients who had three or more of a possible five serious childhood traumas, which included abuse, had an 85% likelihood of an unsuccessful surgical outcome compared to a 5% failure rate for those without a trauma history. This study demonstrates that a history of childhood traumas may be a risk factor for unsuccessful outcome from lumbar spine surgery.

2. *Substance abuse.* Although the excessive use of alcohol or opioid pain medication would seem to exert a negative influence over the recovery and rehabilitation of patients following surgery, there is little research to document this relationship. One such study (Spengler, Freeman, Westbrook, & Miller, 1980) reported that more than 75% of patients with spine surgery failures were involved in medication and alcohol abuse. Another study (Uomoto, Turner, & Herron, 1988) also reported that alcohol abuse was associated with poor surgical outcome. Unfortunately, it is not possible to determine whether the substance abuse reported in these two studies was directly related to surgical failure or the effect of continued pain.

3. *Number of past surgeries.* When a surgery has failed to accomplish the intended outcome, additional surgeries are often undertaken. It has been reported that 23% of patients receiving a spinal fusion underwent an additional procedure within 2 years (Franklin, Haug, Heyer, McKeefrey, & Picciano, 1994). Studies consistently indicate that the probability of a satisfactory outcome decreases with multiple surgical procedures (Turner, Ersek, Herron, & Deyo, 1992).

4. *Pain duration.* Chronicity of the back pain complaint is thought to be associated with poor outcome of treatment, including surgery (Franklin et al., 1994; Junge, Dvorak, & Ahrens, 1995).

Longer duration is associated with poorer outcome. Decreased strength and reduced physical ability from lack of conditioning because of increased fear and avoidance of painful movements have been suggested as the mechanisms for this relationship.

5. *Smoking.* Several studies of spine surgery outcome suggest that use of nicotine is predictive of poor outcome. The relationship of patients' smoking with the rate of failure in fusion or laminectomy has been demonstrated (Brown, Orme, & Richardson, 1986). Examination 1–2 years following surgery revealed that 40% of the patients who smoked had developed a pseudarthrosis, whereas in those who did not smoke the rate was 8%. Another study (Manniche et al., 1994) also reported that smoking was associated with poor outcome. Suggested mechanisms include that tobacco use is detrimental to delayed healing through decreased bone density and reduced vascularization (Daftari et al., 1994).

Environmental Factors

1. *Social environment.* Fordyce (1976) has speculated that family responses to the behavior of patients with back pain (or other chronic pain) may contribute to the maintenance of pain behavior and disability. This relationship has been documented in numerous studies (Flor, Turk, & Rudy, 1987; Romano et al., 1995; Williamson, Robinson, & Melamed, 1997). The family is also an important source of emotional support, and studies have demonstrated that the spouse of a patient with chronic pain is at risk for emotional and marital maladjustment (Romano, Turner, & Clancy, 1989). Marital conflict and stress may be associated with an increased display of pain behaviors, which in turn is associated with greater negative affective responses and more punitive behaviors by the spouse (Schwartz, Slater, & Birchler, 1996). Reduced social support and increased depression have been associated with less improvement following hip replacement surgery (Mutran, Reitzes, Mossey, & Fernandez, 1995). Possible mechanisms through which social support could affect outcome include poor compliance (O'Brien, 1980) and the attribution of pain to psychological causes (Block & Boyer, 1984). One recent study has linked social support from the spouse to surgical outcome as measured by reduced pain following discectomy (Schade et al., 1999).

2. *Work environment.* Vocational factors such as job satisfaction (Bigos et al., 1992) and job demands (Davis, 1994; Junge et al., 1995) have

been shown to be associated with back injury and/or spine surgery outcome. Greenough and Fraser (1989) examined the influence of compensation on recovery from low back pain. Compensation has been shown to be related to poor outcome as measured by increased pain and disability, psychological disturbance, and length of time off work (Greenough & Fraser, 1989). The duration of sick leave prior to surgery was reported in one study to be significantly longer in the group with unsatisfactory outcome (Nygaard, Romner, & Trumpy, 1994). Individuals with a history of compensation-related lawsuits and disability pension claims also have poorer surgical outcomes (Finneson & Cooper, 1979; Junge et al., 1995; Manniche et al., 1994). Compensation has been associated with poor outcomes in lumbar surgery but not cervical disc surgery (Kaptain et al., 1999).

Spine Surgery Conclusions

As stated earlier, it is difficult to draw conclusions about the relative value of the psychosocial variables reviewed as predictors of spine surgery outcome, because of the lack of standardized methodology. This lack of standardization is particularly problematic with regard to the inclusion of a restricted range of predictors in particular models (i.e., limited psychosocial variables) and with regard to the dimensions of outcome assessed. A common, problematic practice in these studies has been the development of a composite predictor of weighted variables (Junge et al., 1995; Spengler et al., 1990), with no rationale stated for the weights chosen.

In closing, we discuss a recent study that has addressed some of these criticisms. Schade and colleagues (1999) examined the predictive utility of three categories of variables assessed presurgically—medical signs, including magnetic resonance imaging (MRI) abnormalities; psychological factors; and psychosocial aspects of work—in a well-controlled prospective study involving 46 patients undergoing discectomy. Evaluators who were unaware of the patients' surgical status assessed the patients postoperatively. Outcome was measured 2 years following surgery in four ways: reported pain relief, disability in daily activities, return to work, and a composite measure of surgical outcome commonly reported in other studies (Stauffer & Coventry, 1972). Using stepwise regression methodology, Schade and colleagues found that pain reduction was predicted by reduced neural compromise as viewed on MRI and less social support by the spouse. Reduction in disability was predicted by neural compromise and work-related satisfaction, and return to work was predicted by low levels of presurgical depression and occupational stress. The composite outcome was predicted by depression and the extent of initial disc herniation. This study demonstrates the interplay between medical signs and psychosocial factors as predictors of outcome. It further demonstrates that predictors were differentially valuable, depending on the outcome being considered. Additional complex studies incorporating predictors from multiple domains need to be tested simultaneously in multivariate models before the true predictive mechanisms of spine surgery outcome can be determined.

Surgery for Upper-Extremity Pain (Especially Hand/Wrist Disorders)

Recent estimates suggest that upper-extremity injuries (especially carpal tunnel and other hand/wrist disorders) are a significant public health problem (Feuerstein, Burrell, et al., 1999; Feuerstein, Huang, & Pransky, 1999). In their review of the literature on work-related upper-extremity injuries, Feuerstein, Huang, and Pransky (1999) note that carpal tunnel syndrome diagnoses resulted in 29,000 cases sufficient to warrant lost days from work in 1996 alone. Over 400,000 vocationally related upper-extremity injury cases were reported for the same time period. With respect to psychological distress, disability status, and work days lost, patients with upper-extremity injuries appear quite similar to patients with other chronic pain conditions (Feuerstein, Huang, & Pransky, 1999). Despite the high frequency of these diagnoses, our review of the literature found very little information regarding the prediction of surgical outcome for these disorders.

One study (Bessette et al., 1997) found that the use of a hand diagram specifying the areas of pain and workers' compensation status predicted carpal tunnel surgery outcome. Their results indicated that involvement with workers' compensation was associated with more poor treatment outcome following surgery. Their analyses controlled for presurgical pain, symptom severity, and other predictors, making conclusions about the interaction of these variables with the hand diagram and compensation status difficult to interpret. It also precluded the analysis of these controlled variables themselves as predictors. Similar results are available suggesting that psychosocial variables and

workers' compensation status also prolong disability and return to work in patients with carpal tunnel syndromes (Bonzani, Millender, Keelan, & Mangieri, 1997). Patient satisfaction with carpal tunnel surgery has been shown to be associated with age, level of functional ability, motor latency, and environmental exposure to vibration (Atroshi, Johnsson, & Ornstein, 1998). Despite the large number of cases and the high cost to patients, employers, and society, little work has been done to determine the predictors of surgical outcome in the highly prevalent upper-extremity pain conditions.

Orofacial Surgery

Surgery related to the orofacial region typically involves the jaw or temporomandibular joint. Patients experiencing orofacial pain have been shown to differ significantly across a number of psychosocial factors, even though they may not differ on the basis of physical signs and symptoms (Rudy, Turk, Kubinski, & Zaki, 1995). Psychosocial variables such as emotional response to pain, beliefs about pain, and coping are typically related to outcome of conservative treatment for orofacial pain (Dworkin et al., 1994; Turner, Whitney, Dworkin, Massoth, & Wilson, 1995). Although many of the psychosocial predictors of surgical outcome for operative procedures at other musculoskeletal sites should predict success from orofacial surgery, few studies have tested these hypotheses.

We found two studies that tested for psychosocial variables associated with outcome to orthognathic surgery. One study (Holman, Brumer, Ware, & Pasta, 1995) found that the availability of support and satisfaction with social support were associated with ratings of patient satisfaction. Another study reported that presurgical expectations of problems were significant predictors of postsurgical reports of dissatisfaction and mood disturbances (Kiyak, Vitaliano, & Crinean, 1988). Patients who anticipated few problems with surgery (avoidant copers) reported better psychological outcomes than patients who expected numerous problems (vigilant copers) before undergoing surgery. Consistent with these studies, another study has shown that poor postoperative recovery from removal of all four third molars was significantly predicted by anxiety, expectations about recovery, coping behaviors, and health locus of control (George, Scott, Turner, & Gregg, 1980). Furthermore, the effects of these psychosocial variables were largely independent of the surgeon's rating of trauma.

TYPES OF ASSESSMENT TYPICALLY EMPLOYED IN PRESURGICAL SCREENING

Clinical Interview

A clinical interview conducted by a psychologist familiar with the area of chronic pain and the specific surgical procedure being considered can yield considerable useful information. The number of previous surgeries for the same condition is an obvious and reasonably well-validated predictor of success, with increasing previous surgeries a negative prognostic sign. Less obvious, perhaps, are other pain-related surgeries (especially those that have failed), which may suggest that the patient has a relatively passive approach to managing his or her pain condition. Previous failed surgeries may also be an indication that the patient has unrealistic expectations for pain relief, functional restoration, or other global outcome from the surgery.

It is important to remember that patients' perspective for treatment outcome is often heavily weighted toward pain relief or pain elimination. They are less interested in the quality of the surgical technique, or status of the anatomy being surgically addressed. In the clinical interview, success is defined by the patient, and a significant mismatch between the patient's historical expectations of success and the obtained results from surgery is a potential poor prognostic sign.

The interview is also one arena for the diagnosis of psychopathology. Negative affect, particularly depression, has been shown to be a negative prognostic indicator for surgery (Herron, Turner, Clancy, & Weiner, 1986). Excessive anxiety or worry and excessive anger may also be poor prognostic signs, though less research has been conducted on these emotional states than on depression (Robinson & Riley, 1999). All of these negative affective states have the potential of clouding the judgment of patients who are being asked to understand and consent to what are often complex but elective surgeries. The identification of clinically significant negative affect should be a sign to the astute clinician that extra care should be taken in explaining the rationale and expectations of surgery to optimize surgical outcome; it may even be an indication that surgery should be delayed for psychological or psychiatric treatment. Severe indications of psychopathology (suicidal depression, psychotic disorders) would appear to be a strong contraindication for surgery, at least until effective treatment of these conditions can be attempted. (See Sullivan, Chapter 15, this volume).

Assessing a surgical candidate's previous satisfaction with employment is critical if return to work is a key surgical outcome variable being considered (Bigos et al., 1992; Gatchel, Polatin, & Mayer, 1995). Although not typically a standardized assessment of job satisfaction, the interview is one source of such information, and clear indications that the patient has a history of low job satisfaction suggests that he or she will not respond well to surgical treatment (especially when outcome is measured by return to work).

Litigation and compensation status are typically obtained during interview and supplemented by other sources (e.g., attorneys, court documents, insurance adjusters). There is increasing evidence that litigation and compensation status are significant predictors of treatment outcome for a variety of pain conditions and treatments for chronic pain (Glassman et al., 1998; Hadjistavropoulos, 1999). The nature of the relationship between litigation status and outcome is complex (Hadjistavropoulos, 1999), but the general direction of findings is that involvement in litigation is a sign that outcome will be poorer, or at least prolonged, compared to that of patients who are not involved in litigation.

As noted previously, a number of investigators have shown that a history of physical or sexual abuse is associated with greater negative affect, more somatic symptoms, and higher pain report (Fillingim, Maixner, Sigurdsson, & Kincaid, 1997; Linton, 1997; Riley, Robinson, Kvaal, & Gremillion, 1998). This history has not been investigated with respect to surgery prediction, but given the relationship to adjustment to chronic pain, and the potential influence on treatment in general, a few questions during the clinical interview are warranted. There is a large literature on the assessment of abuse, and it is not without controversy with respect to assessment or definition of what constitutes abuse (Riley, Robinson, Kvaal, & Gremillion, 1998). Careful, compassionate inquiry need not cause undue distress to the patient. In our practice we have interviewed hundreds of patients with abuse histories without incident, and find that most people are more than willing to talk about the history and show interest in how it might influence their current pain condition.

A structured interview approach such as that conducted by Gatchel, Polatin, and Kinney (1995) suggests that the presence of a personality disorder may indicate the potential for poor outcome from surgery. In their study, Gatchel and his colleagues demonstrated that the presence of a personality disorder as defined by *Diagnostic and Statistical Manual of Mental Disorders*, third edition (DSM-III) criteria was indicator of increased probability of developing chronic low back pain from an acute back injury. Although not specifically addressing surgical outcome, these data are consistent with data from self-report assessment of personality (Riley et al., 1995) that will be reviewed later. Although often time-consuming, the structured interview approach yields more reliable and standardized information than less structured approaches do. Whether the information is obtained via a structured or unstructured interview, the presence of personality disorders should be considered an indication to proceed with caution with respect to any invasive procedures. The motivations to undergo surgery, the expectations for surgery to "cure" more problems than what the surgeon intends, and the reliability of a patient's self-report of symptoms and previous outcomes all come into question in the presence of a personality disorder.

Clinical lore and a few studies also support the assessment of health behaviors, particularly smoking, as a predictor of surgical outcome (Lavernia, Sierra, & Gomez-Marin, 1999; Silcox et al., 1995; Weis, Betz, Clements, & Balsara, 1997). Poor outcomes from joint replacement surgery and spinal fusion have both been associated with smoking status. The clinical interview of the patient is one of the most efficient means of obtaining this information, though it is less likely to yield standardized, metric data on smoking level.

Personality Assessment by Means of Questionnaire or Inventory

Without doubt, the most investigated test used in the prediction of surgery outcome has to be the MMPI. (See Bradley & McKendree-Smith, Chapter 16). Two types of approaches to the interpretation of the MMPI have been employed in the prediction of surgical outcome for pain, particularly spine pain (Riley et al., 1995; Riley, Robinson, Geisser, & Wittmer, 1993). These approaches involve either interpreting scores from single scales and comparing these scales with continuous measures of outcome, or comparing success or failure categories on the MMPI scales. Multiple studies have shown that three scales from the MMPI are significant predictors of surgical outcome (Block & Callewart, 1999; Herron et al., 1986; Riley et al., 1995; Spengler et al., 1990). The best predictors

appear to be clinical elevations on the *Hy* and *Hs* scales, with these scales being better predictors of success than medical imaging diagnostics or neurological signs (Spengler et al., 1990). Consistent with other literatures on surgical outcome, the *D* scale has also been found to be a poor sign for surgical outcome (Herron et al., 1986; Turner, Ersek, Herron, & Deyo, 1992; Turner, Ersek, Herron, Haselkorn, et al., 1992).

More statistically sophisticated approaches have interpreted profiles of MMPI scales to compare profile type to surgical outcome (Riley et al., 1995). In particular, we (Riley et al., 1995) showed that elevations on the *Hy* and *Hs* scales were not necessarily a poor prognostic sign. Patients who had elevations on these scales, but not on the *D* scale, tended to be dissatisfied with lumbar fusion outcome. However, those patients who had moderate elevations on the *Hy*, *Hs*, and *D* scales had outcomes similar to those patients with no clinical elevations. A fourth group that showed significant psychopathology also had poor outcome from surgery. The results were interpreted to indicate that patients with no significant clinical elevations had the best outcome odds. Those with elevations suggestive of and adjustment reaction to their pain condition had similar favorable odds of good surgical outcome. Patients with elevations on the *Hy* and *Hs* scales alone (the conversion V-type profile) had poor odds for positive outcome. The fourth group, with significant elevations on most clinical scales, had similar poor odds. The significance of this research is the additional refinement of prognostic predictions for patients with elevations on the *Hy* and *Hs* scales of the MMPI: An additional positive outcome group was identified in the Riley and colleagues (1995) study—one that with other analytical approaches would have been considered to have poor odds of successful outcome. Although receiving far less investigation, the Millon Behavioral Health Inventory and Symptom Checklist-90 Revised are other instruments that have similar multidimensional approaches to assessing personality and distress and may have promise for surgical prediction (Herron, Turner, Ersek, & Weiner, 1992).

Assessment of Distress and Negative Affect

As mentioned previously, negative affect has frequently been shown to be associated with chronic pain conditions (Robinson & Riley, 1999). In addition to the assessment of negative mood via interview, the MMPI, Beck Depression Inventory, and Hamilton Rating Scale are probably the most frequent means of assessing depression in patients with chronic pain. The diagnosis or assessment of depression in patients with pain is controversial because of potential problems in symptom overlap, though more recent research has allayed these concerns somewhat (Geisser, Roth, & Robinson, 1997). There are consistent findings between studies employing the Beck Depression Inventory and the MMPI D scale (Block, 1999), suggesting that the presence of significant depressive symptomatology is a negative prognostic sign for pain-related surgery. There is some evidence that a chronic dysthymia or depression that predates the onset of pain will also predict poor outcome from surgery (Riley et al., 1995). The assessment of depression by means of questionnaire should always be conducted in conjunction with a careful clinical interview to confirm the precedence of depression or pain symptoms and to evaluate the influence of symptom overlap in the diagnosis.

Anger and anxiety are often assessed by means of questionnaire, but fewer data are available to adequately assess the impact each has on surgical outcome. Clinical lore suggests that an excessive level of either anger or anxiety is an indicator of poor outcome. One relatively new measure of pain-specific anxiety is the Pain Anxiety Symptoms Scale (PASS), which has much promise for the assessment of anxiety in patients with pain conditions (McCracken, Faber, & Janeck, 1998; McCracken, Zayfert, & Gross, 1992). This instrument is multidimensional (it includes dimensions reflecting pain avoidance, cognitive anxiety, physiological anxiety, and fearful appraisal), with good psychometrics. An examination of the content of the PASS suggests that it may have significant overlap with one construct that has been shown to be repeatedly associated with poor outcome from variety of treatments for pain—namely, catastrophic thoughts about pain.

There is some evidence that the Pd and Ps scales of the MMPI predict poor outcome from spine surgery (Block, 1999). However, the interpretation of either of these scales as primarily measures of anger or anxiety is controversial. Other evidence (Brown, Robinson, Riley, & Gremillion, 1996) does suggest that the three major negative affect constructs (depression, anger, anxiety) form a higher-order construct, best labeled *negative affect* or *negative mood*. These results provide some indirect evidence that the predictive value of depression is likely to hold for anger and anxiety as well. As noted previously, the profile approaches derived from MMPI scales may also represent a form of this higher-order construct.

Assessment of Coping Responses to Pain

A large literature has accumulated over the last several years that demonstrates the relationship between coping and chronic pain conditions (see DeGood & Tait, Chapter 17). *Coping* has been defined in a variety of ways, but generally refers to thoughts or behaviors that people use in attempts to alter their pain or the emotional effects associated with pain. The most widely used coping strategies assessment is the Coping Strategies Questionnaire (CSQ; Rosenstiel & Keefe, 1983) and a recent revision of it, the Coping Strategies Questionnaire—Revised (CSQ-R; Riley & Robinson, 1997). The CSQ scale most frequently associated with negative affect, pain, or outcome in a variety of treatment studies is the Catastrophizing scale. It is also the scale that is most robust in the factor-analytic studies of the CSQ and CSQ-R (Riley & Robinson, 1997; Robinson et al., 1997). Catastrophic self-statements tend to be face-valid descriptions of negative outcome, low expectations for pain control, expectation of "the worst," and so forth. There is continuing controversy regarding the definition of catastrophizing as a coping strategy versus an attribute of pain (Geisser, Robinson, & Riley, 1999). Although the Catastrophizing scale is associated with depression, at least one study has shown that it accounts for unique variance in pain report after depression is controlled for (Geisser, Robinson, Keefe, & Weiner, 1994).

Very little work has been done on assessing the predictive ability of the CSQ with surgical outcomes. A search of the literature revealed only a few studies directly testing the relationship between coping and pain surgery outcome prediction. Gross (1986) found that the Control scale from the CSQ appeared to predict better outcome from spine surgery, suggesting that individuals who had higher feelings of control and self-efficacy responded better to surgery. Though there is little current evidence that coping style is predictive of pain surgery outcome, it may simply be the result of a lack of studies addressing this issue. Coping style has been associated with MMPI profiles and with outcome in conservative treatment approaches (Swimmer, Robinson, & Geisser, 1992; Turner &

Clancy, 1986). Given the robust, repeated findings associated with catastrophizing in particular (Geisser et al., 1999), this construct needs assessment and further study.

Pain as a Predictor

Extensive coverage of the assessment of pain is available in other chapters of this book. However, a brief review of the predictive ability of pain assessment with respect to surgical outcome is warranted. Most studies investigating pain surgery outcomes do not use preoperative pain as a predictor variable and understandably use pain as an outcome variable alone. There is some reason to investigate preoperative pain level as a potential marker for outcome. Preoperative pain has been shown to be a significant negative predictor of outcome for sympathectomy (Walker & Johnston, 1980). As is often the case, however, it is not clear whether higher levels of preoperative pain are a marker for greater pathology (tissue damage) or represent an idiosyncratic response pattern of the patient. From a prediction standpoint, there is limited evidence to assume that higher preoperative pain levels will be associated with higher postoperative pain scores.

Disability Assessment

Like pain assessment, when disability status is used as both predictor and outcome variable, some association is expected from presurgery to postsurgery (Gatchel, Mayer, Dersh, Robinson, & Polatin, 1999; Gatchel, Polatin, & Kinney, 1995). Gatchel and colleagues have demonstrated such relationships with conservative treatment outcomes, with the direction of the relationship as expected: The higher the pretreatment disability, the higher the posttreatment disability and the less successful the treatment outcome. A number of scales exist for the assessment of disability or functional status that may have some as yet unknown predictive validity for surgery. A representative but not exhaustive list of scales commonly used for this purpose includes the Roland and Morris Disability Scale, the Oswestry Low-Back Pain Disability Questionnaire (Leclaire, Blier, Fortin, & Proulx, 1997), the Medical Outcome Study 36-Item Short-Form Health Survey (Ware & Sherbourne, 1992), and the Pain Disability Index (Tait, Pollard, Margolis, Duckro, & Krause, 1987).

Battery or Profile Approaches to Surgical Screening

As should be evident from the preceding sections, the presurgical assessment needs to be multidimensional to capture the complex nature of the constellation of predictive variables. Those presurgical assessment approaches that are multidimensional are likely to show the most promise and to obtain some empirical support as providing higher predictive validity. Block (1999) has proposed probably the most comprehensive approach to this multidimensional assessment, which he has named the Presurgical Psychological Screening (PPS) approach. The name is a slight misnomer, since the PPS includes medical, health behavior, and social factors as well as psychological variables. The approach appears to be a sound one and includes all of the factors that have been empirically supported in prediction studies. At present it is designed for spine surgery, but could be adapted for other types of surgery as well.

The general approach of the PPS is to use a "scorecard" to tally risk factors obtained from the medical domain (chronicity, previous surgeries, destructiveness of proposed surgery, nonorganic signs, non-spine-related treatments, smoking status, and obesity), the clinical interview (litigation and compensation status, job dissatisfaction, heavy-lifting job, substance abuse, family reinforcement of pain behavior, marital dissatisfaction, physical and sexual abuse, preinjury psychopathology) and testing results (MMPI, CSQ). Not all of the items in the PPS have the same level of empirical support, but all of the factors have been discussed and at least suggested in the literature as potential predictors of spine surgery outcome.

A recent study conducted by Block, Ohnmeiss, Guyer, Rashbaum, and Hochschuler (2001) has tested the predictive validity of the PPS system, with promising results. In their study, the researchers employed the PPS with 204 patients who were being evaluated for spine surgery (laminectomy, discectomy, or fusion). All of the patients underwent spine surgery. Surgical effectiveness was assessed by means of the Oswestry Low-Back Pain Disability Questionnaire, medication use, and pain ratings at least 6 months after surgery. Overall, the results indicated significant improvements in pain, functional ability, and medication use. Psychological and medical risk factors associated with the PPS were significantly predictive of surgery outcome. To compare the PPS classification with categories of surgery outcome, classification of outcome was derived from a combination of Oswestry scores, pain report, and medication use. The overall accuracy of the PPS was 82% correct classification, with only 9 of 53 patients predicted to have poor outcome actually having a fair or good outcome. Thus it would appear that the sensitivity of the PPS to poor outcome is relatively good as is the overall correct classification rate. Additional analyses of these data (A. R. Block, personal communication, November 4, 1999) indicate significant contributions to outcome from each of the major domains of the PPS (interview, testing, and medical).

Another profile approach worth mentioning is represented by the cluster-analytic approach employed with the West Haven–Yale Multidimensional Pain Inventory (WHYMPI; Turk & Rudy, 1990; see also Jacob & Kerns, Chapter 19). One study has shown that the profile types derived from the WHYMPI are associated with differential outcomes of both conservative and surgical treatments for temporomandibular disorders (Dahlstrom, Widmark, & Carlsson, 1997). In their study, Dahlstrom et al. showed that Dysfunctional profiles obtained from the WHYMPI were associated with a higher frequency of surgery failures, whereas patients with Adaptive Coper profiles were shown to have a greater frequency of successful temporomandibular surgery. The WHYMPI has many of the characteristics of other multidimensional batteries and shows promise as an initial screening instrument for surgical candidates.

SUMMARY

Despite a considerable amount of time since the initial studies on presurgical screening, the state of the empirical support for its practice remains scarce for most surgical procedures. The strongest evidence by far comes from the literature on spine surgeries. For fusions especially, the data seem quite consistent, with robust and repeatable results; in these surgeries, psychosocial factors predominate as the best predictors of outcome. Similar though less extensive support is available for discectomy. For other high-frequency surgeries (carpal tunnel release, temporomandibular surgery), there is very little currently available empirical support specifically for these types of surgeries. The available studies have significant limitations that prohibit firm conclusions about the efficacy of treatments or the prognostic values of many measures (Feuerstein, Burrell, et al., 1999) for carpal tunnel syndrome and related hand surgeries.

The best available evidence suggests, however, that most if not all of the data from the literature on spine surgery outcome should be relevant to other forms of pain-related surgery. The majority of studies that have assessed the psychological factors associated with chronic pain of nearly any type show remarkable consistency with respect to psychological distress, the relationship of psychosocial factors to conservative and multidisciplinary treatment, and typical descriptions of sufferers from chronic pain. These similarities suggest that the same predictors of outcome for spine surgery have considerable promise as predictors of other pain-related surgery outcome. The prudent clinician should, of course, proceed with caution when applying these criteria with candidates for nonspinal surgery until more direct evidence of the predictive validity is obtained and reported.

Given the major gaps in our knowledge of prediction specific to surgery outcome and specific to surgeries other than spine surgeries, recommendations about what methods and measures the average clinician should employ in assessment is difficult. The present state of the art suggests that an approach similar to that proposed by Block (1999) shows the greatest promise. At a bare minimum, it is suggested that a careful clinical interview be conducted to obtain the information described earlier. Of paper-and-pencil assessments, the MMPI clearly has several advantages and a large body of literature to support its use for surgical prediction. The MMPI is time-consuming, however, and should clinicians opt not to administer it, more brief questionnaires to assess negative affect are a limited substitute.

FUTURE DIRECTIONS

There is a great need of additional prospective studies aimed at evaluating the predictive validity of presurgical screening for all industrial injuries, but particularly hand injuries, repetitive strain injuries, and temporomandibular disorders. More studies that combine psychosocial, medical and environmental variables as predictors are likely to yield a more complete picture of accurate prediction. The profile approaches that have begun to be employed (Block, 1996, 1999; Block & Callewart, 1999) are good examples of such an approach.

Given the recent research on sex differences in pain perception and epidemiology of pain (Riley, Robinson, Wise, Myers, & Fillingim, 1998), additional work on potential sex differences in surgical outcome is warranted.

Finally, there is little information available on what should be done for the patient who appears to be a poor candidate for surgery. Most practitioners associated with chronic pain treatment find that they have many patients who have "failed" multiple conservative treatments, may also have failed previous surgeries, and have exhausted the repertoires of their treating professionals. Additional studies to determine which if any of the poor prognostic signs can be ameliorated through targeted treatments (cognitive-behavioral, psychotherapy, physical therapy) or alteration of a patient's environment (home, work, litigation status, financial status, etc.) are needed to best treat the entire population of sufferers from chronic pain. To date, we are not aware of any studies that have first attempted to identify those individuals at risk for surgery failure and then employed specific interventions to attempt to make these patients better candidates who subsequently receive successful surgical interventions. The high financial and time costs of conducting such studies are likely to be the major reasons for the paucity of these studies.

Some of the research suggests that at least some of the factors associated with poor treatment outcome (e.g., personality disorder, history of previous surgeries) are not particularly amenable to current forms of treatment. Other treatment options need to be considered for these patients, including multidisciplinary functional restoration programs and perhaps long-term opioid treatments.

Despite our criticisms of the literature and reservations about the state of the art in surgery outcome prediction, much good work has been done that represents a strong foundation for additional work to build upon and refine. Given the attention to managed care and related cost concerns, greater attention may be paid to this problem in the near future, and with luck future publications reviewing this topic will have resolutions to many of the gaps in our present knowledge.

REFERENCES

AbuRahma, A. F., Robinson, P. A., Powell, M., Bastug, D., & Boland, J. P. (1994). Sympathectomy for reflex sympathetic dystrophy: Factors affecting outcome. *Annals of Vascular Surgery, 8,* 372-379.

Atroshi, I., Johnsson, R., & Ornstein, E. (1998). Patient satisfaction and return to work after endoscopic carpal tunnel surgery. *Journal of Hand Surgery (American), 23,* 58-65.

Bessette, L., Keller, R. B., Lew, R. A., Simmons, B. P., Fossel, A. H., Mooney, N., & Katz, J. N. (1997). Prognostic value of a hand symptom diagram in surgery for carpal tunnel syndrome. *Journal of Rheumatology, 24,* 726-734.

Bigos, S. J., Battie, M. C., Spengler, D. M., Fisher, L. D., Fordyce, W. E., Hansson, T., Nachemson, A. L., & Zeh, J. (1992). A longitudinal, prospective study of industrial back injury reporting. *Clinical Orthopaedics and Related Research, 279,* 21-34.

Block, A. R. (1996). *Presurgical psychological screening in chronic pain syndromes.* Hillsdale, NJ: Erlbaum.

Block, A. R. (1999). Presurgical psychological screening in chronic pain syndromes: Psychosocial risk factors. In R. J. Gatchel & D. C. Turk (Eds.), *Psychosocial factors in pain: Critical perspectives* (pp. 390-400). New York: Guilford Press.

Block, A. R., & Boyer, S. L. (1984). The spouse's adjustment to chronic pain: Cognitive and emotional factors. *Social Science and Medicine, 19,* 1313-1317.

Block, A. R., & Callewart, C. (1999). Surgery for chronic spine pain: Procedures for patient selection and outcome enhancement. In A. R. Block, E.F. Kremer, & E. Fernandez (Eds.), *Handbook of pain syndromes* (pp. 191-212). Mahwah, NJ: Erlbaum.

Block, A. R., Ohnmeiss, D. D., Guyer, R. D., Rashbaum, R., & Hochschuler, S. N. (2001). *The use of presurgical psychological screening to predict the outcome of spine surgery.* Manuscript in review.

Block, A. R., Vanharanta, H., Ohnmeiss, D. D., & Guyer, R. D. (1996). Discographic pain report: Influence of psychological factors. *Spine, 21,* 334-338.

Bonzani, P. J., Millender, L., Keelan, B., & Mangieri, M. G. (1997). Factors prolonging disability in work-related cumulative trauma disorders. *Journal of Hand Surgery (American), 22,* 30-34.

Boos, N., Rieder, R., Schade, V., Spratt, K. F., Semmer, N., & Aebi, M. (1995). The diagnostic accuracy of magnetic resonance imaging, work perception, and psychosocial factors in identifying symptomatic disc herniations. *Spine, 20,* 2613-2625.

Bradley, L. A. (1996). Cognitive-behavioral therapy for chronic pain. In R. J. Gatchel & D. C. Turk (Eds.), *Psychological approaches to pain management: A practitioner's handbook* (pp. 131-147). New York: Guilford Press.

Brown, C. W., Orme, T. J., & Richardson, H. D. (1986). The rate of pseudarthrosis (surgical nonunion) in patients who are smokers and patients who are nonsmokers: A comparison study. *Spine, 11,* 942-943.

Brown, F. F., Robinson, M. E., Riley, J. L., & Gremillion, H. A. (1996). Pain severity, negative affect, and microstressers as predictors of life interference in TMD patients. *Journal of Craniomandibular Practice, 14,* 63-70.

Burton, A. K., Tillotson, K. M., Main, C. J., & Hollis, S. (1995). Psychosocial predictors of outcome in acute and subchronic low back trouble. *Spine, 20,* 722-728.

Cashion, E. L., & Lynch, W. J. (1979). Personality factors and results of lumbar disc surgery. *Neurosurgery, 4,* 141-145.

Daftari, T. K., Whitesides, T. E., Jr., Heller, J. G., Goodrich, A. C., McCarey, B. E., & Hutton, W. C. (1994).

Nicotine on the revascularization of bone graft: An experimental study in rabbits. *Spine, 19*, 904–911.

Dahlstrom, L., Widmark, G., & Carlsson, S. G. (1997). Cognitive-behavioral profiles among different categories of orofacial pain patients: Diagnostic and treatment implications. *European Journal of Oral Science, 105*(5, Pt. 1), 377–383.

Davis, R. A. (1994). A long-term outcome analysis of 984 surgically treated herniated lumbar discs. *Journal of Neurosurgery, 80*, 415–421.

DeGood, D. E. (1993). What is the role of biofeedback in the treatment of chronic pain patients? *American Pain Society Bulletin, 3*, 1–5.

Deyo, R. A. (1996). Drug therapy for back pain: Which drugs help which patients? *Spine, 21*, 2840–2849; discussion, 2849–2850.

Dolwick, M. F., & Dimitroulis, G. (1994). Is there a role for temporomandibular joint surgery? *British Journal of Oral and Maxillofacial Surgery, 32*, 307–313.

Doxey, N. C., Dzioba, R. B., Mitson, G. L., & Lacroix, J. M. (1988). Predictors of outcome in back surgery candidates. *Journal of Clinical Psychology, 44*, 611–622.

Dvorak, J., Valach, L., Fuhrimann, P., & Heim, E. (1988). The outcome of surgery for lumbar disc herniation: II. A 4–17 years' follow-up with emphasis on psychosocial aspects. *Spine, 13*, 1423–1427.

Dworkin, S. F., Turner, J. A., Wilson, L., Massoth, D., Whitney, C., Huggins, K. H., Burgess, J., Sommers, E., & Truelove, E. (1994). Brief group cognitive-behavioral intervention for temporomandibular disorders. *Pain, 59*, 175–187.

Fernandez, E., & Turk, D. C. (1995). The scope and significance of anger in the experience of chronic pain. *Pain, 61*, 165–175.

Feuerstein, M., Burrell, L. M., Miller, V. I., Lincoln, A., Huang, G. D., & Berger, R. (1999). Clinical management of carpal tunnel syndrome: A 12-year review of outcomes. *American Journal of Industrial Medicine, 35*, 232–245.

Feuerstein, M., Huang, G. D., & Pransky, G. (1999). Workstyle and work related upper extremity disorders. In R. J. Gatchel & D. C. Turk (Eds.), *Psychosocial factors in pain: Critical perspectives* (pp. 175–192). New York: Guilford Press.

Fillingim, R. B., Maixner, W., Sigurdsson, A., & Kincaid, S. (1997). Sexual and physical abuse history in subjects with temporomandibular disorders: Relationship to clinical variables, pain sensitivity, and psychologic factors. *Journal of Orofacial Pain, 11*, 48–57.

Finneson, B. E., & Cooper, V. R. (1979). A lumbar disc surgery predictive score card: A retrospective evaluation. *Spine, 4*, 141–144.

Flor, H., Turk, D. C., & Rudy, T. E. (1987). Pain and families: II. Assessment and treatment. *Pain, 30*, 29–45.

Fordyce, W. E. (1976). *Behavioral methods for chronic pain and illness.* St. Louis, MO: Mosby.

Franklin, G. M., Haug, J., Heyer, N. J., McKeefrey, S. P., & Picciano, J. F. (1994). Outcome of lumbar fusion in Washington State workers' compensation. *Spine, 19*, 1897–1903; discussion, 1904.

Fulde, E., Junge, A., & Ahrens, S. (1995). Coping strategies and defense mechanisms and their relevance for the recovery after discectomy. *Journal of Psychosomatic Research, 39*, 819–826.

Gatchel, R. J., Mayer, T., Dersh, J., Robinson, R., & Polatin, P. (1999). The association of the SF-36 health status survey with 1-year socioeconomic outcomes in a chronically disabled spinal disorder population. *Spine, 24*, 2162–2170.

Gatchel, R. J., Polatin, P. B., & Kinney, R. K. (1995). Predicting outcome of chronic back pain using clinical predictors of psychopathology: A prospective analysis. *Health Psychology, 14*, 415–420.

Gatchel, R. J., Polatin, P. B., & Mayer, T. G. (1995). The dominant role of psychosocial risk factors in the development of chronic low back pain disability. *Spine, 20*, 2702–2709.

Geisser, M. E., Robinson, M. E., Keefe, F. J., & Weiner, M. L. (1994). Catastrophizing, depression and the sensory, affective and evaluative aspects of chronic pain. *Pain, 59*, 79–83.

Geisser, M. E., Robinson, M. E., & Riley, J. L. (1999). Pain beliefs, coping, and adjustment to chronic pain: Let's focus more on the negative. *Pain Forum, 8*, 161–168.

Geisser, M. E., Roth, R. S., & Robinson, M. E. (1997). Assessing depression among persons with chronic pain using the Center for Epidemiological Studies—Depression Scale and the Beck Depression Inventory: A comparative analysis. *Clinical Journal of Pain, 13*, 163–170.

George, J. M., Scott, D. S., Turner, S. P., & Gregg, J. M. (1980). The effects of psychological factors and physical trauma on recovery from oral surgery. *Journal of Behavioral Medicine, 3*, 291–310.

Glassman, S. D., Minkow, R. E., Dimar, J. R., Puno, R. M., Raque, G. H., & Johnson, J. R. (1998). Effect of prior lumbar discectomy on outcome of lumbar fusion: A prospective analysis using the SF-36 measure. *Journal of Spinal Disorders, 11*, 383–388.

Graham, J. R. (1990). *MMPI-2: Assessing personality and psychopathology.* New York: Oxford University Press.

Greenough, C. G., & Fraser, R. D. (1989). The effects of compensation on recovery from low-back injury. *Spine, 14*, 947–955.

Gross, A. R. (1986). The effect of coping strategies on the relief of pain following surgical intervention for lower back pain. *Psychosomatic Medicine, 48*, 229–238.

Hadjistavropoulos, T. (1999). Chronic pain on trial: The influence of litigation and compensation on chronic pain syndromes. In A. R. Block, E. F. Kremer, & E. Fernandez (Eds.), *Handbook of pain syndromes* (pp. 59–76). Mahwah, NJ: Erlbaum.

Hasenbring, M., Marienfeld, G., Kuhlendahl, D., & Soyka, D. (1994). Risk factors of chronicity in lumbar disc patients: A prospective investigation of biologic, psychologic, and social predictors of therapy outcome. *Spine, 19*, 2759–2765.

Herno, A., Airaksinen, O., Saari, T., & Luukkonen, M. (1996). Lumbar spinal stenosis: A matched-pair study of operated and non-operated patients. *British Journal of Neurosurgery, 10*, 461–465.

Herron, L. D., Turner, J. A., Clancy, S., & Weiner, P. (1986). The differential utility of the Minnesota Multiphasic Personality Inventory: A predictor of outcome in lumbar laminectomy for disc herniation versus spinal stenosis. *Spine, 11*, 847–850.

Herron, L. D., Turner, J. A., Ersek, M., & Weiner, P. (1992). Does the Millon Behavioral Health Inventory (MBHI) predict lumbar laminectomy outcome?: A comparison with the Minnesota Multiphasic Personality Inventory (MMPI). *Journal of Spinal Disorders, 5*, 188–192.

Hoffman, R. M., Wheeler, K. J., & Deyo, R. A. (1993). Surgery for herniated lumbar discs: A literature synthesis. *Journal of General Internal Medicine, 8,* 487–496.

Holman, A. R., Brumer, S., Ware, W. H., & Pasta, D. J. (1995). The impact of interpersonal support on patient satisfaction with orthognathic surgery. *Journal of Oral and Maxillofacial Surgery, 53,* 1289–1297; discussion, 1297–1299.

Jensen, M. P., Turner, J. A., Romano, J. M., & Karoly, P. (1991). Coping with chronic pain: A critical review of the literature. *Pain, 47,* 249–283.

Junge, A., Dvorak, J., & Ahrens, S. (1995). Predictors of bad and good outcomes of lumbar disc surgery: A prospective clinical study with recommendations for screening to avoid bad outcomes. *Spine, 20,* 460–468.

Kaptain, G. J., Shaffrey, C. I., Alden, T. D., Young, J. N., Laws, E. R., Jr., & Whitehill, R. (1999). Secondary gain influences the outcome of lumbar but not cervical disc surgery. *Surgical Neurology, 52,* 217–223; discussion, 223–225.

Kiyak, H. A., Vitaliano, P. P., & Crinean, J. (1988). Patients' expectations as predictors of orthognathic surgery outcomes. *Health Psychology, 7,* 251–268.

Lavernia, C. J., Sierra, R. J., & Gomez-Marin, O. (1999). Smoking and joint replacement: Resource consumption and short-term outcome. *Clinical Orthopaedics and Related Research, 367,* 172–180.

Leclaire, R., Blier, F., Fortin, L., & Proulx, R. (1997). A cross-sectional study comparing the Oswestry and Roland–Morris Functional Disability scales in two populations of patients with low back pain of different levels of severity. *Spine, 22,* 68–71.

Lewith, G. T., & Vincent, C. (1996). On the evaluation of the clinical effects of acupuncture: A problem reassessed and a framework for future research. *Journal of Alternative and Complementary Medicine, 2,* 79–90; discussion, 91–100.

Linton, S. J. (1997). A population-based study of the relationship between sexual abuse and back pain: Establishing a link. *Pain, 73,* 47–53.

Long, C. J., Brown, D. A., & Engelberg, J. (1980). Intervertebral disc surgery: Strategies for patient selection to improve surgical outcome. *Journal of Neurosurgery, 52,* 818–824.

Malter, A. D., Larson, E. B., Urban, N., & Deyo, R. A. (1996). Cost-effectiveness of lumbar discectomy for the treatment of herniated intervertebral disc. *Spine, 21,* 1048–1054; discussion, 1055.

Manniche, C., Asmussen, K. H., Vinterberg, H., Rose-Hansen, E. B., Kramhoft, J., & Jordan, A. (1994). Analysis of preoperative prognostic factors in first-time surgery for lumbar disc herniation, including Finneson's and modified Spengler's score systems. *Danish Medical Bulletin, 41,* 110–115.

McCracken, L. M., Faber, S. D., & Janeck, A. S. (1998). Pain-related anxiety predicts non-specific physical complaints in persons with chronic pain. *Behaviour Research and Therapy, 36,* 621–630.

McCracken, L. M., Zayfert, C., & Gross, R. T. (1992). The Pain Anxiety Symptoms Scale: Development and validation of a scale to measure fear of pain. *Pain, 50,* 67–73.

Meyler, W. J., de Jongste, M. J., & Rolf, C. A. (1994). Clinical evaluation of pain treatment with electrostimulation: A study on TENS in patients with different pain syndromes. *Clinical Journal of Pain, 10,* 22–27.

Mutran, E. J., Reitzes, D. C., Mossey, J., & Fernandez, M. E. (1995). Social support, depression, and recovery of walking ability following hip fracture surgery. *Journals of Gerontology: Series B. Psychological Sciences and Social Sciences, 50,* S354–S361.

Nachemson, A. L. (1993). Evaluation of results in lumbar spine surgery. *Acta Orthopedica Scandinavica,* Suppl. 251, 130–133.

Nygaard, O. P., Romner, B., & Trumpy, J. H. (1994). Duration of symptoms as a predictor of outcome after lumbar disc surgery. *Acta Neurochirurgica, 128*(1–4), 53–56.

O'Brien, M. E. (1980). Effective social environment and hemodialysis adaptation: A panel analysis. *Journal of Health and Social Behavior, 21,* 360–370.

Palmer, D. H., & Hanrahan, L. P. (1995). Social and economic costs of carpal tunnel surgery. *Instructional Course Lectures, 44,* 167–172.

Reiter, R. C. (1998). Evidence-based management of chronic pelvic pain. *Clinical Obstetrics and Gynecology, 41,* 422–435.

Riley, J. L., III, & Robinson, M. E. (1997). CSQ: Five factors or fiction? *Clinical Journal of Pain, 13,* 156–162.

Riley, J. L., III, & Robinson, M. E. (1998). Validity of MMPI-2 profiles in chronic back pain patients: Differences in path models of coping and somatization. *Clinical Journal of Pain, 14,* 324–335.

Riley, J. L., III, Robinson, M. E., Geisser, M. E., & Wittmer, V. T. (1993). Multivariate cluster analysis of the MMPI-2 in chronic low-back pain patients. *Clinical Journal of Pain, 9,* 248–252.

Riley, J. L., III, Robinson, M. E., Geisser, M. E., Wittmer, V. T., & Smith, A. G. (1995). Relationship between MMPI-2 cluster profiles and surgical outcome in low-back pain patients. *Journal of Spinal Disorders, 8,* 213–219.

Riley, J. L., III, Robinson, M. E., Kvaal, S. A., & Gremillion, H. A. (1998). Effects of physical and sexual abuse in facial pain: Direct or mediated? *Journal of Craniomandibular Practice, 16,* 259–266.

Riley, J. L., III, Robinson, M. E., Wise, E. A., Myers, C. D., & Fillingim, R. B. (1998). Sex differences in the perception of noxious experimental stimuli: A meta-analysis. *Pain, 74,* 181–187.

Robinson, M. E., & Riley, J. L., III. (1999). The role of emotion in pain. In R. J. Gatchel & D. C. Turk (Eds.), *Psychosocial factors in pain: Critical perspectives* (pp. 74–88). New York: Guilford Press.

Robinson, M. E., Riley, J. L., III, Myers, C. D., Sadler, I. J., Kvaal, S. A., Geisser, M. E., & Keefe, F. J. (1997). The Coping Strategies Questionnaire: A large sample, item level factor analysis. *Clinical Journal of Pain, 13,* 43–49.

Rodriquez, A. A., Bilkey, W. J., & Agre, J. C. (1992). Therapeutic exercise in chronic neck and back pain. *Archives of Physical Medicine and Rehabilitation, 73,* 870–875.

Romano, J. M., Turner, J. A., & Clancy, S. L. (1989). Sex differences in the relationship of pain patient dysfunction to spouse adjustment. *Pain, 39,* 289–295.

Romano, J. M., Turner, J. A., Jensen, M. P., Friedman, L. S., Bulcroft, R. A., Hops, H., & Wright, S. F. (1995). Chronic pain patient–spouse behavioral interactions predict patient disability. *Pain, 63,* 353–360.

Rosenstiel, A. K., & Keefe, F. J. (1983). The use of coping strategies in chronic low back pain patients: Relationship to patient characteristics and current adjustment. *Pain, 17,* 33–44.

Rudy, T. E., Turk, D. C., Kubinski, J. A., & Zaki, H. S. (1995). Differential treatment responses of TMD patients as a function of psychological characteristics. *Pain, 61,* 103–112.

Schade, V., Semmer, N., Main, C. J., Hora, J., & Boos, N. (1999). The impact of clinical, morphological, psychosocial and work-related factors on the outcome of lumbar discectomy. *Pain, 80,* 239–349.

Schofferman, J., Anderson, D., Hines, R., Smith, G., & White, A. (1992). Childhood psychological trauma correlates with unsuccessful lumbar spine surgery. *Spine, 17*(6, Suppl.), S138–S144.

Schwartz, L., Slater, M. A., & Birchler, G. R. (1996). The role of pain behaviors in the modulation of marital conflict in chronic pain couples. *Pain, 65,* 227–233.

Silcox, D. H., III, Daftari, T., Boden, S. D., Schimandle, J. H., Hutton, W. C., & Whitesides, T. E., Jr. (1995). The effect of nicotine on spinal fusion. *Spine, 20,* 1549–1553.

Spengler, D. M., Bigos, S. J., Martin, N. A., Zeh, J., Fisher, L., & Nachemson, A. (1986). Back injuries in industry: A retrospective study. I. Overview and cost analysis. *Spine, 11,* 241–245.

Spengler, D. M., Freeman, C., Westbrook, R., & Miller, J. W. (1980). Low-back pain following multiple lumbar spine procedures: Failure of initial selection? *Spine, 5,* 356–360.

Spengler, D. M., Ouellette, E. A., Battie, M., & Zeh, J. (1990). Elective discectomy for herniation of a lumbar disc: Additional experience with an objective method. *Journal of Bone and Joint Surgery* (American), *72,* 230–237.

Stauffer, R. N., & Coventry, M. B. (1972). Anterior interbody lumbar spine fusion. Analysis of Mayo Clinic series. *Journal of Bone and Joint Surgery* (American), *54,* 756–768.

Swimmer, G. I., Robinson, M. E., & Geisser, M. E. (1992). Relationship of MMPI cluster type, pain coping strategy, and treatment outcome. *Clinical Journal of Pain, 8,* 131–137.

Tait, R. C., Pollard, C. A., Margolis, R. B., Duckro, P. N., & Krause, S. J. (1987). The Pain Disability Index: Psychometric and validity data. *Archives of Physical Medicine and Rehabilitation, 68,* 438–441.

Taylor, V. M., Deyo, R. A., Cherkin, D. C., & Kreuter, W. (1994). Low back pain hospitalization: Recent United States trends and regional variations. *Spine, 19,* 1207–1212.

Taylor, V. M., Deyo, R. A., Goldberg, H., Ciol, M., Kreuter, W., & Spunt, B. (1995). Low back pain hospitalization in Washington State: Recent trends

and geographic variations. *Journal of Spinal Disorders, 8,* 1–7.

Turk, D. C., & Rudy, T. E. (1990). The robustness of an empirically derived taxonomy of chronic pain patients. *Pain, 43,* 27–35.

Turner, J. A., & Clancy, S. (1986). Strategies for coping with chronic low back pain: Relationship to pain and disability. *Pain, 24,* 355–364.

Turner, J. A., Ersek, M., Herron, L., & Deyo, R. (1992). Surgery for lumbar spinal stenosis: Attempted meta-analysis of the literature. *Spine, 17,* 1–8.

Turner, J. A., Ersek, M., Herron, L., Haselkorn, J., Kent, D., Ciol, M. A., & Deyo, R. (1992). Patient outcomes after lumbar spinal fusions. *Journal of the American Medical Association, 268,* 907–911.

Turner, J. A., Whitney, C., Dworkin, S. F., Massoth, D., & Wilson, L. (1995). Do changes in patient beliefs and coping strategies predict temporomandibular disorder treatment outcomes? *Clinical Journal of Pain, 11,* 177–188.

Uomoto, J. M., Turner, J. A., & Herron, L. D. (1988). Use of the MMPI and MCMI in predicting outcome of lumbar laminectomy. *Journal of Clinical Psychology, 44,* 191–197.

Von Korff, M., Dworkin, S. F., Le Resche, L., & Kruger, A. (1988). An epidemiologic comparison of pain complaints. *Pain, 32,* 173–183.

Walker, P. M., & Johnston, K. W. (1980). Predicting the success of a sympathectomy: A prospective study using discriminant function and multiple regression analysis. *Surgery, 87*(2), 216–221.

Ware, J. E., Jr., & Sherbourne, C. D. (1992). The MOS 36-Item Short-Form Health Survey (SF-36): I. Conceptual framework and item selection. *Medical Care, 30,* 473–483.

Weis, J. C., Betz, R. R., Clements, D. H., III, & Balsara, R. K. (1997). Prevalence of perioperative complications after anterior spinal fusion for patients with idiopathic scoliosis. *Journal of Spinal Disorders, 10,* 371–375.

Widmark, G. (1997). On surgical intervention in the temporomandibular joint. *Swedish Dental Journal,* Suppl. 123, 1–87.

Wilcox, L. S., Koonin, L. M., Pokras, R., Strauss, L. T., Xia, Z., & Peterson, H. B. (1994). Hysterectomy in the United States, 1988–1990. *Obstetrics and Gynecology. 83,* 549–555.

Williamson, D., Robinson, M. E., & Melamed, B. (1997). Pain behavior, spouse responsiveness, and marital satisfaction in patients with rheumatoid arthritis. *Behavior Modification, 21,* 97–118.

Wiltse, L. L., & Rocchio, P. D. (1975). Preoperative psychological tests as predictors of success of chemonucleolysis in the treatment of the low-back syndrome. *Journal of Bone and Joint Surgery* (American), *57,* 478–483.

Chapter 21

Matching Treatment to Assessment of Patients with Chronic Pain

DENNIS C. TURK
AKIKO OKIFUJI

Chronic pain syndromes are extremely prevalent. Some of the most common of these syndromes are back pain, fibromyalgia syndrome (FMS), temporo-mandibular disorder (TMD), complex regional pain syndrome (CRPS), tension-type headaches, chronic pelvic pain, and irritable bowel syndrome. Although differing in location and other features, these diverse pain syndromes have something important in common. All are characterized by a lack of information regarding the etiological mechanisms. Thus the diagnostic criteria rely on historical and current signs and symptoms. The specificity of these criteria across different pain disorders is poorly understood. It is quite possible that these diagnoses are general rubrics into which patients with diverse features may be assigned, primarily on the basis of some similarities in location and symptoms rather than of known etiology. In short, a heterogeneous group of patients may be treated as if they are homogeneous.

Lack of understanding of the underlying mechanisms of these syndromes has not inhibited attempts to treat patients with diverse modalities. Although treatments have spanned the entire spectrum of surgical, pharmacological, rehabilitation, and psychological approaches, these syndromes remain recalcitrant. In fact, the lack of understanding of the etiology and maintaining factors may have facilitated an empirical approach in which diverse treatments without clear rationales result in conflicting outcomes. Perhaps what is most peculiar is that despite the very different targets of treatment (muscular

deconditioning, immunological defects, emotional distress), positive outcomes for at least some of these patients are reported with each treatment modality. We can ask the question "How is this possible?"

In the traditional clinical model, the intervention is matched to a diagnosis that is derived from specific pathological findings. This is logical when there is a known etiology, but it has no basis when the cause is unknown, as is so commonly the case with the prevalent chronic pain syndromes.

Consider FMS as an illustration. FMS is a prevalent musculoskeletal pain disorder with no known etiology, estimated to affect 3–6 million Americans (Goldenberg, 1987) and to make up approximately 20% of the practice of rheumatologists (White, Speechley, Harth, & Ostbye, 1995). It is characterized by widespread pain; pain upon palpation of at least 11 of the 18 specific locations ("tender points"); and a range of associated symptoms, including nonrestorative sleep, fatigue, stiffness, and mood disturbance (Wolfe et al., 1990). Patients with FMS have been treated with steroidal and nonsteroidal anti-inflammatory agents, antidepressants, muscle relaxants, infusions of local anesthetics, aerobic exercises, chiropractic manipulations, bright-light therapy, biofeedback, relaxation, hypnosis, cognitive-behavioral therapy, and various combinations of these treatments (Okifuji & Turk, 1999), not to mention many home remedies and nonprescription dietary supplements. The results appear fairly consistent. That is, a significant minority of patients appear to achieve favorable results regardless of the treatment, although none of the treatments works for all or even the majority of patients.

In the absence of known pathology, one of the determinants for the selection of treatment modalities seems to be the therapist's training and preferred intervention rather than on specific characteristics of the patients or the syndrome. For example, patients with TMD have been treated with a variety of intraoral appliances, biofeedback, oral surgery, psychoanalysis, and so forth, depending upon the conceptualization of the cause of the symptoms and the practitioner's training and experience (Turk, Penzien, & Rains, 1995).

At least two explanations, which are not mutually exclusive, may account for the perplexing observation that treatments that may seem contradictory are reported to be equally effective. One explanation is the faith in the treatment provided. This is not just the familiar placebo effect based on patients' beliefs and expectations; it is also the result of the confidence of the health care professional who promotes the treatment (Volinn, 1999). A second possibility is that the patients diagnosed with one of the common chronic pain disorders are a disparate group, sharing only some characteristics. When diverse treatments are provided, a subset of patients receiving a treatment that addresses the underlying etiology for the symptoms, whereas others (although having similar symptoms and thus the same diagnosis) do not share the same etiology. That is, although the symptoms making up the syndrome are common to all of the patients, there may be more than one cause for these symptoms. Combining heterogeneous groups of patients into broad diagnostic groups may inappropriately take the place of making a differential diagnosis with treatments matched to specific etiological factors. We focus on the heterogeneity explanation in the remainder of this chapter. Patient heterogeneity, however, is not necessarily independent of patient and provider faith in a treatment, but is likely to be synergistic with it.

CURRENT PROBLEMS: THE PATIENT UNIFORMITY MYTH AND THE SHOTGUN VERSUS RIFLE APPROACH

Classifications of many chronic pain syndromes are "expert-based," where pain complaints with common parameters (e.g., body systems, anatomical

ranges) are lumped together as forming a syndrome. Consequently, we can observe rather peculiar phenomena. On the one hand, patients with chronic pain who have the same diagnosis (e.g., low back pain) are often treated as a homogeneous group (Gallagher et al., 1989), as though the same treatment is appropriate for all patients who fit loosely within the diagnostic category. On the other hand, multidisciplinary pain clinics (MPCs) that treat a diverse sample of patients with chronic pain may prescribe a generic, multimodal therapy to all patients. This issue is further complicated by the fact that there is no consensus as to what should be included in the "multidisciplinary treatment" program. That is, the conceptual basis for the MPC treatment packages range from those based predominantly on the principles of operant conditioning (Anderson, Cole, Gullickson, Hudgens, & Roberts, 1977) to those with a heavy emphasis on physical conditioning–functional restoration (Mayer et al., 1987). All types have been prescribed to patients with various pain conditions. This might be referred to as an MPC *treatment uniformity myth.*

In the absence of clear information regarding the underlying pathology of the condition, and in the absence of empirical evidence to support the effectiveness of a particular treatment, the health care provider is left with the difficult decision of selecting an intervention among the array of treatments options available. If the rationale for using nonsteroidal anti-inflammatory agents is that an inflammatory process plays an underlying role in the symptoms, then these drugs should only be prescribed in the presence of inflammation. If the rationale for treating tension-type headaches with biofeedback is related to the presence of maladaptive muscular activity, then biofeedback should only be offered to patients who demonstrate some degree of maladaptive muscular activity. If the use of operant conditioning treatment is predicated on alteration of maladaptive environmental contingencies reinforcing pain behaviors, then some effort should be made to offer this form of treatment only to those patients in whom such reinforcement contingencies have been demonstrated, as originally proposed by Fordyce (1976). Few attempts, however, have been made to customize treatments for common, generic chronic pain syndromes to unique patient characteristics. In short, we have adopted a *patient uniformity myth,* as well as a treatment uniformity myth. All patients with the same diagnosis, no matter how vague, are treated in a similar fashion. Clinical trials based upon this "one size fits all" approach, however carefully designed, tend to yield only a modest level of efficacy, and hence minimize advances in our clinical knowledge.

Another implicit assumption of the rehabilitation-oriented programs offered at many MPCs is that when multicomponent treatments are provided to all patients with chronic pain, some component(s) will prove effective for each patient, and perhaps different ones will be effective for patients with different characteristics—a *shotgun* as opposed to a *rifle* approach. Thus the rehabilitation offered at an MPC may include physical exercise (which can vary in aggressiveness as well as in nature), education in body mechanics, assertion training, systematic medication reduction, stress management, biofeedback, family counseling, transcutaneous nerve stimulation, nerve blocks, and so forth. This is akin to treating patients with a range of different vitamin deficiencies with multivitamins—in the hope that each patient will derive benefits from the appropriate vitamin contained in the collection of vitamins making up the multivitamin regimen—rather than prescribing specific vitamin therapy based on individual patients' needs. The rationale behind this shotgun approach seems to be that chronic pain is a multifactorial problem requiring treatment strategies that address various aspects of pain. However, rarely do we understand either how each component of the treatment influences specific aspects of the disorder or how each component of the treatment interacts with the other components. Without understanding the relationship between treatment strategies and treatment target, we have no choice but to resort to the shotgun approach, hoping that *something* in the treatment program works on *something* in a patient with chronic pain.

IDENTIFICATION OF SUBGROUPS OF PATIENTS

For chronic pain syndromes, physical and anatomical factors are often the decisive ones used for assigning a patient a diagnosis. However, prescribing somatic treatments, intended to address those factors, do not typically provide amelioration of symptoms for a significant number of patients with diverse chronic pain syndromes (Osterweis, Kleinman, & Mechanic, 1987). Those with the same medical diagnosis and ostensibly the same level of physical findings often respond quite differently to the same treatment. For example, approximately

59% of patients with back pain in one study who were carefully selected to receive a spinal cord stimulator reported at least a 50% reduction in pain, 58% reported improvements in the ability to perform activities, and 13% returned to work (Turner, Loeser, & Bell, 1995). Such disparity in responses has led to calls for research to identify predictors of outcomes. Many physical, demographic, and personal variables have been examined to determine the characteristics of those who benefit from a specific form of treatment. The usual strategy has been to examine retrospectively criteria differentiating those patients who have been successfully treated via a particular method of treatment from those who have not (King & Snow, 1989; Maruta, Swanson, & McHardy, 1990).

Interestingly, the evidence does not support the importance of physical factors in predicting response to treatment for many chronic pain syndromes. Numerous studies have reported that initial medical diagnosis had little predictive or prognostic value (e.g., Cairns, Mooney, & Crane, 1984). In the past two decades, there have been growing awareness of and empirical support for the importance of psychological factors in reports of pain, suffering, and disability (Gallagher et al., 1989; Waddell, Main, Morris, Di Paola, & Gray, 1984). For example, Flor and Turk (1988) found that physical factors in patients with low back pain and rheumatoid arthritis did not predict pain severity, life interference, or physician visits, whereas cognitive appraisals of helplessness and hopelessness were predictive of both self-report of pain impact and behavior in response to pain. However, despite the importance of nonphysical factors in chronic pain experience, specific demographic information, disease status, pain history, prior treatment, litigation and compensation, and psychological features that consistently predict successful treatment outcome have yet to be determined (Turk & Rudy, 1990b).

There is no doubt a need to identify the characteristics of patients who improve and those who fail to improve with different treatments, and not just to look at the overall treatment effects. The goal should be to prescribe a specific treatment only for those patients who are likely to derive a significant benefit from that treatment. Furthermore, identifying the characteristics of patients who do not benefit from a specific treatment will facilitate the development of innovative treatment approaches targeting the needs of those patients who do not benefit from any existing treatment programs. The ability to predict outcome should therefore lead to a reduction in costs and an improvement in the overall cost-effectiveness of the treatments programs. Thus, rather than asking whether a particular treatment is effective for patients with a generic pain diagnosis such as back pain, FMS, or CRPS, we should ask, "What treatments are most effective for patients with this particular subset of characteristics?" (Turk, 1990).

In order to counteract the patient uniformity myth, a number of investigators have suggested the need to identify subgroups of patients based on specific characteristics. One way may be to incorporate subgroups into the diagnostic system. For example, based on expert judgments, Dworkin and LeResche (1992) classified patients with TMD into eight different subtypes. Others have attempted to identify subgroups of patients with chronic pain on the basis of single factors such as physical mobility (Moffroid, Haugh, Henry, & Short, 1994), litigation (Rohling, Binder, & Langhinrichsen-Rohling, 1995), race (Jordan, 1999), attitudinal patterns (Tait & Chibnall, 1998), and behavioral expression (Keefe, Bradley, & Crisson, 1990). Rehabilitative outcomes, however, are likely to be determined by the interactive effects of multiple factors, as single factors will not account for a statistically significant or clinically meaningful proportion of the variance in outcome. Several studies that included measures of both physical and psychological functioning have reported interactive effects of biopsychosocial factors on the outcome of patients with low back pain (Frymoyer, Rosen, Clements, & Pope, 1985; Reesor & Craig, 1988).

A number of authors (Dworkin & LeResche, 1992; Turk & Rudy, 1988) have suggested that multidimensional rather than unidimensional classifications should be attempted for a problem as complex as chronic pain. That is, patients with chronic pain can vary in both physical factors and psychosocial/behavioral factors that may characterize how they adapt and respond to their chronic pain state. This approach might be viewed as a dual-diagnostic one, in which each patient with chronic pain is assigned to two diagnoses: one based on physical pathology, and a second based on psychosocial/behavioral characteristics. We focus on the classification of patient on only one of the dimensions, psychosocial/behavioral; however, the logic and methodology we describe can be readily applied to the physical dimension as well.

CLASSIFICATION OF PATIENTS WITH CHRONIC PAIN ON THE BASIS OF PSYCHOLOGICAL VARIABLES

A number of studies have focused on empirically identifying patient subgroups based on psychological characteristics and psychopathology. Investigators have assumed that the most important and discriminating factor in the clinical outcome of patients with chronic pain will be psychological distress and personality features. Consequently, the attempts to identify subgroups have relied primarily on the use of traditional psychological measures such as the Minnesota Multiphasic Personality Inventory (MMPI) (Bradley, Prokop, Margolis, & Gentry, 1978; Watkins, O'Brien, Draugelis, & Jones, 1986) and the Symptom Checklist-90 Revised (Butterworth & Deardorff, 1987; Jamison, Rock, & Parris, 1988), as well as on the basis of different sets of pain behaviors (Keefe et al., 1990).

The "So What" Question

Calling for studies concerning the responses of different subgroups to various pharmacological, medical, and behavioral treatments is nothing new (e.g., Bradley & Van der Heide, 1984). However, few attempts have been made to address the "so what" question. That is, there are many ways to classify groups, but the real issue is whether or not there is any benefit to such a classification. One way to establish the clinical utility of a classification system is to demonstrate the differential efficacy of treatments customized to patient characteristics once the subgroups of patients are identified. The vast majority of the studies that have been conducted to date have used retrospective methods, rather than looking prospectively at differential response to the same treatment. Using the MMPI clustering, these retrospective studies (Guck, Meilman, Skultety, & Poloni, 1988; McGill, Lawlis, Selby, Mooney, & McCoy, 1983; Moore, Armentrout, Parker, & Kivlahan, 1986) have failed to delineate the differential treatment responses based upon the MMPI subgroups. This body of research has not gone on to address the "so what" question.

McGill and colleagues (1983) and Moore and colleagues (1986) have speculated that different patients may benefit from different components of a comprehensive multidisciplinary program—the shotgun explanation discussed previously. That is, since the usual MPC treatment is not individualized, differential effects may be washed out as each patient finds some aspect of the program to be helpful. For example, McGill and colleagues have suggested that patients with elevated scores on the MMPI neurotic triad scales might respond best to a treatment program of respondent conditioning and antidepressant medication, whereas patients with elevated scores on the more pathological scales might benefit most from an individualized reinforcement program and antipsychotic medication. Furthermore, they have speculated that those patients who produce MMPI scale scores within one standard deviation of the mean "would be most likely to respond to 'traditional' management or to an operant program designed to identify and reinforce positive coping styles" (p. 91). Although this speculation may be accurate, no attempt to evaluate the effects of matching treatments to the groups identified has been published.

In considering the lack of evidence supporting the predictive nature of subgroups for treatment success, Guck and colleagues (1988) have offered an alternative proposal—that despite clear initial differences in MMPI scores, all patients may have received comparable benefits from the same components of the program. That is, the treatment has nonspecific effects (e.g., patient and provider faith; Volinn, 1999). Perhaps an equally plausible interpretation of the results, however, is that subgroups, based on general personality characteristics are not useful for identifying a specific response to treatment. At this point, each of these explanations must be viewed as only suggestive, because only a handful of studies have directly examined these speculations.

Another potential reason why the MMPI-based subgroups do not provide any guidance for differential treatments for patients with pain is the applicability of the measure itself. The fundamental assumption in using those measures that were developed with the intention of identifying psychiatric problems or severe psychological distress in populations with pain is that there may be distinct types of psychosocial and behavioral pathology that are differentially related to patients' pain disorders. Studies that classify patients based on responses to the MMPI yield several subgroups, although the nature of groups across these studies is variable. The most critical issue, however, is the absence of data supporting the predictive validity of the classifications (Moore et al., 1986). Thus there seems to be a need to develop an instrument that addresses multiple areas of psychosocial domains specifically related to chronic pain.

EMPIRICALLY DERIVED CLASSIFICATION OF PATIENTS WITH PAIN

The psychological assessment of pain requires incorporation of cognitive, affective, and behavioral information (Turk & Rudy, 1988). Using the West Haven–Yale Multidimensional Pain Inventory (WHYMPI; Kerns, Turk, & Rudy, 1985), Turk and Rudy (1988) classified patients with chronic pain into three relatively homogeneous sets. The version of the WHYMPI used in this research consists of 60 questions, in which each item is pain-relevant and is rated on a 7-point scale. Based upon the item response, separate scores on 12 scales can be obtained. The scales are designed to assess the following characteristics of patients with chronic pain: (1) pain severity and suffering, (2) perceptions of how pain interferes with their lives, including interference with family and marital/couple functioning, work, and social and recreational activities; (3) dissatisfaction with present levels of functioning in family relationships, marital/couple relationship, work, and social life; (4) appraisals of support received from significant others; (5) perceived life control, incorporating perceived ability to solve problems and feelings of personal mastery and competence; (6) affective distress, including depressed mood, irritability, and tension; and (7) activity levels.

The WHYMPI has been shown to have good psychometric properties (Kerns et al., 1985; Mikail, DuBreuil, & D'Eon, 1993) and has been used in numerous studies with diverse medical syndromes (Turk, Okifuji, Sinclair, & Starz, 1996; Turk & Rudy, 1988; Turk, Sist, et al., 1998; Widar & Ahlstrom, 1999). The factor structure has been replicated in several studies in the United States (Bernstein, Jaremko, & Hinkley, 1995) and in other countries, such as Germany (Flor, Rudy, Birbaumer, & Schugers, 1990), the Netherlands (Lousberg, Schmidt, Groenman, Vendrig, & Dijkman-Caes, 1997; Lousberg et al., 1999), and Sweden (Bergstrom et al., 1998). For more details, see Jacob and Kerns (Chapter 19, this volume).

Using cluster-analytic and multivariate classification methods, and a statistical procedure designed to identify commonalities across groups of subjects, Turk and Rudy (1988) identified three distinct and homogeneous subgroups of patients with chronic pain based on their responses on the WHYMPI. The three groups were as follows: (1) Dysfunctional (DYS), patients who perceived the severity of their pain to be high, reported that pain interfered with much of their lives, reported a higher degree of psychological distress due to pain, and reported low levels of activity; (2) Interpersonally Distressed (ID), patients with a common perception that significant others were not very supportive of their pain problems; and (3) Adaptive Copers (AC), patients who reported high levels of social support, relatively low levels of pain and perceived interference, and relatively high levels of activity. Reliable external scales supported the uniqueness of each of the three subgroups of patients.

To establish the external validity of the WHYMPI patient subgroups, multivariate and univariate analyses of variance for reliable, conceptually related measures not used in the original clustering solutions—for instance, the McGill Pain Questionnaire (Melzack, 1975), the Pain Behavior Checklist (Turk, Wack, & Kerns, 1985), and the Beck Depression Inventory, (Beck, Ward, Mendelson, Mock, & Erbaugh, 1961)—were used to test for significant differences among the three subgroups. Patient demographic characteristics and medical findings were included in these analyses. The patient subgroups were found to be independent of age, gender, and duration of pain. There remained significant subgroup differences even when the effects of physical pathology were statistically controlled for.

As hypothesized, significant subgroup differences were found in (1) the frequency of using prescription analgesic medication, (2) the amount of time spent in bed, (3) employment status, and (4) scores on the Pain Behavior Checklist (Turk et al., 1985). The patients in the DYS subgroup used pain medications more frequently, spent more time in bed due to pain, were more likely to be unemployed, and displayed more pain behaviors than those in the other two subgroups (i.e., ID and AC). The ID subgroup differed significantly from the other two groups in terms of marital satisfaction.

A caution should be noted about the use of cluster analysis. This statistical procedure is designed to "find" subgroups. Thus it is possible that entering almost any set of data can lead to the identification of subgroups (see the chapter by Turk & Rudy, 1992, in the first edition of this text for a detailed discussion). It is therefore important to replicate the generation of subgroups with a different sample. If the initial sample is large enough, it can be split into two groups, and the second sample can be used to confirm that the same subgroups would be identified in both sets of patients.

Alternatively, Bayesian posterior probabilities can be used to determine whether or not a significant proportion of patients in a second sample can be classified into one of the subgroups identified in the original sample. That is, would the same results have been obtained (replicated) if the study was conducted in a different setting?

Several studies have indeed replicated the three subgroups of patients identified in the Turk and Rudy (1988) study. These replication studies were conducted in a large study in multiple MPCs across the United States (Jamison, Rudy, Penzien, & Mosley, 1994), as well as in the Netherlands (Lousberg, Groenman, & Schmidt, 1996). Talo, Rytokoski, and Puukka (1992) attempted to replicate the three subgroups based on WHYMPI responses in a rehabilitation sample in Finland. The interesting point of the Talo and colleagues study was that the authors used a different set of measures, which were, however, matched to the same dimensions contained in the WHYMPI. The authors found virtually the same three subgroups of patients, even though the scales used were different from those in the original study. These results provide strong support for the presence of three subgroups of patients with chronic pain, which can be labeled as DYS, ID, and AC.

In the studies described above, all of the samples consisted of patients with chronic back pain being evaluated at pain rehabilitation programs. This raises the question of whether or not similar subgroups are common in chronic pain syndromes other than back pain.

Generalizability of Subgroups across Chronic Pain Diagnoses: TMD, Low Back Pain, Headache, and FMS

In order to evaluate the generalizability of the subgroups of patients with chronic pain previously identified (Turk & Rudy, 1988), we and our colleagues have conducted a set of studies that have evaluated the presence of these subgroups across a range of chronic pain syndromes. As noted below, the majority (70%–92%) of the patients with diverse chronic pain syndromes can be classified into one of the primary WHYMPI profiles. However, the proportions of each profile vary across pain disorders.

Turk and Rudy (1988) examined the WHYMPI scale patterns of the WHYMPI profile groups in several different chronic pain syndromes—

specifically, chronic low back pain (CLBP), headache (HA), and TMD. As would be expected, the mean scores on each of the MPI scales were significantly different for each of the three patient samples. When group mean scores were controlled for, a higher percentage of patients with CLBP were classified as DYS than in the other two patient samples; a greater percentage of patients with TMD and HA than patients with CLBP were classified as AC; and no between-group differences were observed for the ID profile. In contrast to the samples with TMD, CLBP, and HA, we (Turk et al., 1996) found that the percentage of patients with FMS in the DYS group was substantially lower (26%) and the percentage in the ID group (39%) was substantially higher. Thus, although all of these four syndromes were represented in each of the subgroups, the percentages varied substantially.

These results provide support for the dual-diagnostic approach proposed earlier. Thus it is possible that patients with TMD, HA, CLBP, and FMS who are classified within the same subgroup may be psychologically more similar to each other than patients with the same diagnosis but who are classified in different subgroups. It follows that patients within a specific medical diagnosis may vary substantially in their psychosocial and behavioral responses to the presence of their symptoms. Thus the psychosocial subgroups appear to be relatively independent of the physically based diagnoses.

Up to this point, the pain syndromes that we have discussed might be viewed as having a significant psychological component. That is, these are vague syndromes for which the physical basis is not well understood and often no objective physical factors can be identified. Consequently, perhaps what have been identified are psychosocial subgroups that are unique to these syndromes. Would there be similar subgroups for patients with pain syndromes with a definitive physical basis?

Generalization beyond "Nonmalignant" Pain: Cancer Pain versus Noncancer Pain

We have replicated the WHYMPI-based subgroup results with patients who have cancer pain. Figure 21.1 shows the mean WHYMPI scale scores for three groups of patients: patients with cancer, patients with FMS, and patients with non-FMS, noncancer chronic pain (CP). A multivariate analysis of variance (MANOVA) with the WHYMPI scale scores as the dependent variables and pain diagnosis as the independent variable was computed. The MANOVA produced significant results. Furthermore, the results indicate that the three groups of patients reported different mean scores on the scales of the WHYMPI. However, the covariance structures among the WHYMPI scales (subgroup patterns) were remarkably consistent among the three WHYMPI subgroups, despite the differences in physical diagnoses and mean scale scores (see Figure 21.1).

We interpret these results as indicating that although there may be variability in the mean scale scores of the WHYMPI, all three subgroups are present in each biomedical diagnostic group. From Figure 21.1, we hypothesize that patients with FMS, cancer, and CP who are classified within the same WHYMPI subgroup may be more similar to each other in subjective experience and response to symptoms than patients who have the same pain diagnosis but are classified as belonging to a different WHYMPI subgroup. These results suggest that although different physical diagnostic groups may require common biomedical treatment targeting the pathophysiological mechanisms underlying each disorder, they may also benefit from specific psychosocial interventions tailored to their psychosocial and behavioral characteristics that are specifically relevant to chronic pain.

We are still left with the "so what" question posed earlier. The results reported up to this point appear to provide strong support for the existence of at least three subgroups of patients with chronic pain across a diverse group of chronic pain syndromes. The important question remains as to whether assessment and classification of patients can lead to differential treatment planning and improved outcomes.

Treatment Responses by the WHYMPI Subgroups: TMD

Based upon the previous findings of three subgroups of patients with TMD who exhibited dis-

TABLE 21.1. Distributions of the WHYMPI Profiles in Various Pain Disorders

| WHYMPI subgroups | Pain syndromes | | | |
	FMS (n = 91)	CLBP (n = 200)	HA (n = 245)	TMD (n = 200)
DYS	26%	62%	44%	46%
ID	39%	18%	26%	22%
AC	35%	20%	30%	32%

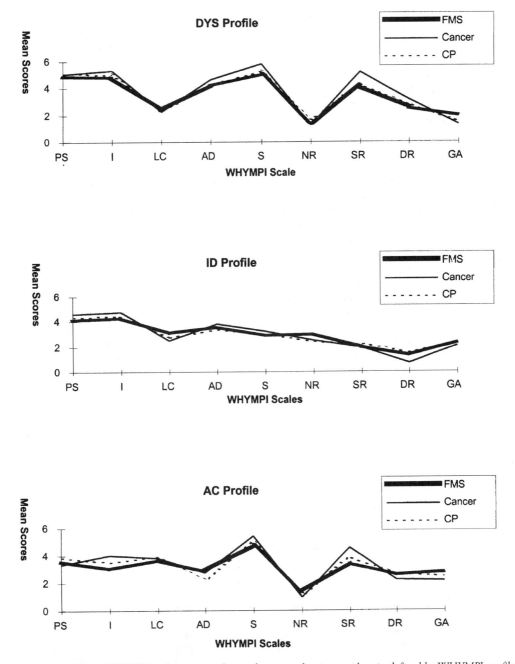

FIGURE 21.1. Mean WHYMPI scale scores in three subgroups of patients with pain defined by WHYMPI profile.

tinctive psychological profiles, Turk and colleagues (Turk, Rudy, Kubinski, Zaki, & Greco, 1996; Turk, Zaki, & Rudy, 1993) developed a treatment program specifically tailored to the clinical needs of the DYS patients. Fifty patients with TMD classified as belonging to the DYS group were randomly assigned to one of two treatment conditions: (1) interocclusal appliance (IA), biofeedback-assisted relaxation (BF), and supportive counseling (IA + BF + SC), and (2) IA + BF treatment plus cognitive therapy (CT) for depression (IA + BF + CT). Both groups received six once-weekly treatment sessions, followed by posttreatment and 6-month follow-up evaluations.

MANOVAs of nine indices measuring physical, psychosocial, and behavioral changes indicated that groups receiving both treatment protocols (IA + B + SC and IA + BF + CT) displayed significant improvements at the follow-up. Compared with the patients in the IA + BF + SC group, patients in the IA + BF + CT group displayed significantly greater changes, particularly in pain and depression. It appears then that DYS patients with TMD generally demonstrate and maintain significant improvement in physical, psychosocial, and behavioral measures following treatment that targets specific problems of the DYS subgroup. Thus including a component tailored to the DYS patients, especially in the areas of depression and pain, added incrementally to the outcome.

The differential responses of the three WHYMPI subgroups of patients with TMD when given a conservative treatment consisting of IA, BF, and stress management were evaluated (Rudy, Turk, Kubinski, & Zaki, 1995). The results demonstrated that, as a group, patients significantly improved and maintained the improvements in physical, psychosocial, and behavioral measures.

The DYS patients showed significantly greater improvements in measures of pain intensity, perceived impact of TMD on their lives, and depression ($p < .01$), compared with the ID and AC patients. ID patients also displayed treatment effects that were different from those for the AC patients (see Figure 21.2). Overall, then, the treatment may have been effective, but *only* for a subset of patients. These findings support the clinical utility of the psychosocial/behavioral classification system, and

suggest that individualizing treatments based upon patients' adaptation to pain may improve treatment efficacy. In addition, these findings have important methodological implications for TMD treatment outcome studies. That is, combining heterogeneous samples without statistically controlling for subgroup differences may result in nonsignificant findings.

Treatment Responses by the WHYMPI Subgroups: FMS

Given the multiple symptoms of FMS, many have advocated the importance of employing a multicomponent rehabilitation approach (Masi & Yunus, 1991). In a preliminary study, Turk, Rudy, and colleagues (1996) examined the efficacy of an interdisciplinary treatment program for 67 patients with FMS, including 6-month follow-up. The treatment program consisted of six half-day sessions, spaced over 4 weeks. Each session included medical (education, medication management), physical (aerobic and stretching exercise), occupational (pacing, body mechanics), and psychological (pain and stress management) components.

The comparisons between the pretreatment and posttreatment scores revealed significant improvement in the targeted areas of pain severity, sense of control, depression, and fatigue, but remained at the pretreatment levels for nontargeted variables such as support from significant others. The results at the follow-up revealed that the majority of treatment gains were sustained for 6 months following the completion of the treatment, although there was a statistically significant relapse in reported fatigue.

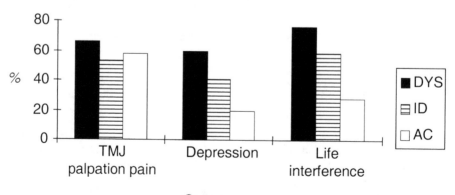

Outcomes

FIGURE 21.2. Percentages of patients in WHYMPI-based subgroups showing clinically significant improvement.

The psychosocial distinctiveness of the WHYMPI subgroups was tested (Turk, Okifuji, Starz, & Sinclair, 1998). The areas of interest included observed physical functioning, pain, depressive moods, perceived functional limitation, and quality of interpersonal relationships. These variables were measured via the standardized self-report instruments or protocols (physical functioning). As expected, the three groups did not differ in the observed physical functioning such as lumbar flexion, "fingertips to floor," straight-leg raise, and cervical range of motion. However, the analyses revealed that (1) the DYS patients reported significantly higher levels of pain than the AC patients; (2) the DYS and ID groups reported significantly higher levels of depressed mood and perceived disability; and (3) the ID patients rated their interpersonal relationships with significant others to be significantly lower in quality than the DYS and AC patients rated their relationships. Post hoc analyses of the co-occurring symptoms demonstrated that the three groups did not differ in the prevalence of various symptoms. Once again, the results reinforce the suggestion that the psychosocial dimension of chronic pain syndromes may be independent of the biomedical/physical dimension.

From the significant differences in adaptation to the chronic pain condition across psychosocial subgroups of patients with FMS (Turk, Okifuji, Starz, & Sinclair, 1998), it was hypothesized that the WHYMPI subgroups would respond differently to a standard rehabilitation treatment protocol. Patients who completed the FMS program were classified into one of the three WHYMPI profiles on the basis of their pretreatment WHYMPI scores. Planned comparisons were conducted to evaluate whether the differences between pretreatment and posttreatment evaluation were significant. Overall, the patients in the DYS group improved in most areas, whereas the ID patients, who reported levels of pain and disability comparable to those of the DYS group, failed to respond to the treatment. There were minor changes in the AC patients, possibly due to a a relative lack of room for improvement. The results further support the need for different treatments targeting specific characteristics of subgroups, and suggest that psychosocial characteristics of patients with FMS are important predictors of treatment responses and may be used to customize treatment. For example, whereas the ID patients may require additional treatment components addressing clinical needs specific to this group (e.g., inter-

personal skills), some components of the standard interdisciplinary treatment may not be essential for the AC patients.

POTENTIAL FOR CUSTOMIZING TREATMENT

The results of the studies reviewed above support our contention that there are different subgroups of patients with pain and that treating them all the same may dilute the ability to demonstrate treatment efficacy. That is, specific interventions may have their greatest utility with particular subgroups of patients. Combining heterogeneous patients into a single treatment condition without addressing the key clinical individual differences may result in nonsignificant or only modest therapeutic gains.

Failure to customize the treatments may lead to erroneous conclusions regarding treatment efficacy. For example, Moore and Chaney (1985) reported that the addition of patients' spouses to behavioral treatment groups did not add to the efficacy of a cognitive-behavioral intervention. However, no effort was made to address individual differences in the quality of the marital relationship. Turk's previous work (Turk & Rudy, 1988) demonstrated that approximately 25% of patients with chronic pain could be characterized by the perceived lack of support from significant others in their environment. Moreover, the extent to which behavioral principles are relevant to marital/couple relationship seems to depend upon the quality of the relationship. Flor, Turk, and Rudy (1989) reported that operant reinforcement factors were only related to reports of pain and activity levels in those married couples for whom the marital relationship was rated as satisfactory or better. These data raise the question of whether Moore and Chaney (1985) would have observed different outcomes had they matched the inclusion of spouses with marital satisfaction or whether different types of spouse involvement, tailored to the patients' marital characteristics, would have led to differential outcome.

One of the critical issues related to subgrouping is knowing the clinically relevant component by which we group patients. The number of potential variables is infinite—height, income, Social Security number, primary pain locations, psychopathology, and so forth. It is important to ensure that the key criterion of subgrouping is clinically valid. Thus it makes the most sense to use the WHYMPI to subgroup patients with pain when different strategies to address psychosocial adaptation are to be used. The delineation of homogeneous subgroups among patients with pain provides a framework for the development of optimal treatment regimens for specific patient subgroups (1) when treatment can be matched to assessment of relevant variables that are reasonably distinct and not consistently correlated, (2) when valid measures of these response classes are available, and (3) when treatments that affect these response classes are available.

DUAL-DIAGNOSTIC APPROACH

Some have suggested that physical assessment and treatment should be directed toward the disease classification (Merskey, 1986), and that other treatments should focus on a psychosocial/behavioral taxonomy that is complementary to a physical taxonomy. However, several groups of investigators (Dworkin & LeResche, 1992; Scharff, Turk, & Marcus, 1995; Turk, 1990) have proposed the use of a dual-diagnostic approach, whereby two separate and distinct diagnoses are assigned concurrently—physical and psychosocial/behavioral. Treatment could then be directed toward both simultaneously.

A patient with chronic pain might have diagnoses on two different but complementary taxonomies—for example, an International Association

for the Study of Pain (IASP) classification and a WHYMPI-based classification. Thus a patient might be classified as having CRPS, Type 2 (203.91, Axis 1 Region = Upper Shoulder and Upper Limbs, Axis II System = Nervous, Axis III Temporal Characteristics of Pain: Pattern of Occurrence = none of the codes listed, Axis IV Intensity and Time of Onset = Severe, More Than 6 months, Axis V Aetiology = Genetic or Congenital) according to the IASP taxonomy, and might be classified as belonging to the DYS subgroup in the WHYMPI-based taxonomy. Note that not all patients with CRPS would be classified as DYS, and not all DYS patients would have CRPS. A second patient might have the same IASP diagnosis, CRPS, but might be profiled as ID in the WHYMPI-based classification. Conversely, patients might have quite different classifications on the IASP but have the identical WHYMPI-based classification. The most appropriate treatment for these different groups might vary, with different complementary components of treatments addressing the physical diagnosis (IASP) and the psychosocial diagnosis (WHYMPI-based). In Figure 21.3, we present a heuristic view of the dual-diagnosis or dual-axis approach.

Adopting a dual-diagnostic approach provides a promising clinical algorithm that serves the valuable function of encouraging clinicians as well as researchers to think concurrently in terms of two

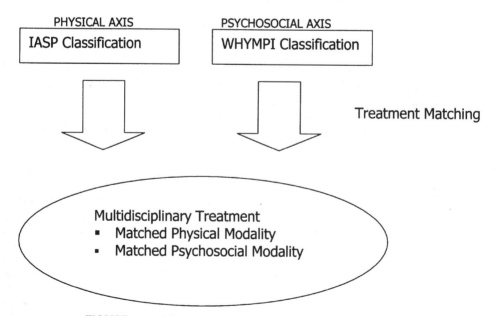

FIGURE 21.3. Schematic view of dual-axis approach to chronic pain.

different (biomedical and psychosocial/behavioral), but complementary, diagnostic systems. Empirical studies are needed to evaluate the efficacy of individualized treatments based on the dual-diagnostic approach.

CONCLUSION

The strategy of combining very different groups of patients with chronic pain into generic chronic pain diagnostic groups may have impeded progress in the understanding and treatment of these perplexing conditions. Delineation of homogeneous subgroups among patients with chronic pain may provide an important basis for the development of specific, optimal treatment regimens for the different subgroups of patients—the rifle versus the shotgun approach. Of course, the notion of matching treatment to diagnosis is not new; it is the foundation of clinical medicine and psychological therapy. However, given the complexity of chronic pain and its impact on patients' lives, establishing a better link between the dual-diagnostic approach we have proposed and treatment planning remains a significant challenge.

In this chapter we have focused on using an empirical approach—namely, cluster analysis—to identify subgroups of patients with chronic pain based on psychosocial and behavioral responses. We have suggested that these psychosocial/behavioral subgroups are largely independent of physical diagnosis. Although we have discussed the psychosocial/behavioral subgroups, the logic and methodology used with psychosocial and behavioral data can be adapted for use with physical data as well. For example, a number of symptoms commonly co-occur in patients diagnosed with FMS, in addition to the criteria used for the formal diagnosis. Many studies have attempted to identify neurohormonal, immunological, and endocrinological factors that underlie this syndrome. It is possible that physically based subgroups of patients with FMS could be identified in the same way that we have identified psychosocial/behavioral subgroups. Empirical approaches such as cluster analysis could be used to determine whether there are indeed subgroups of such patients based on patterns of signs and symptoms. In the same way that treatment can be targeted at subgroups based on psychosocial and behavioral characteristics, they might be aimed at underlying physical perturbations that characterize subgroups. If, as we believe, the physical and psychological characteristics are

relatively independent, then in the future treatments matched to both relevant dimensions should lead to improved outcomes.

Many studies, using a range of different assessment instruments, have identified subgroups of patients with chronic pain. To date, however, there have been only few attempts to customize treatment to patients' characteristics. The studies described above support the potential value of treatment matching. It no longer seems sufficient simply to provide all patients with a common medical diagnosis the same treatment or to identify differences among patients in response to treatment; rather, there is a critical need to make use of these results in designing treatments and evaluating their differential efficacy.

Clinical investigations should be conducted to determine the relative utility of different treatment modalities based on the match of treatment to patient characteristics and classification, and to predict which patients are most likely to benefit from what combination of therapeutic modalities. Thus, rather than accepting the patient homogeneity myth, researchers and clinicians might advance the field by asking a set of questions first proposed for psychotherapy treatment—namely, "What treatment, by whom, is most effective for this person, with that specific problem, under this set of circumstances?"

Treatments might be provided in a modular fashion, where separate components are woven into an overall treatment regimen fabric of individual patient characteristics. For example, all patients with back pain may require physical therapy and psychological support and encouragement; however, some may need additional modules such as treatment for depression (Bradley et al., 1978; Bradley & Van der Heide, 1984). The combination of physical therapy and specific psychological interventions may provide unique and complementary advantages in addressing different symptoms.

It is important to acknowledge that the identification of subgroups, regardless of the methods used, does not mean that the resulting classification will incorporate all features of the patients. Subgroups should be viewed as prototypes, with significant room for individual variability with the subgroup. Thus treatments designed to match subgroup characteristics will also need to consider and address the unique characteristics of individual patients. The subgroup customization fits somewhere between the exclusively idiographic approach evaluated by single-case treatment designs and the generic patient homogeneity approach that has characterized many of the pain treatment outcome studies.

At this point, whether treatment tailoring will produce greater effects than providing completely idiographic or generic treatments can only be viewed as a plausible hypothesis. Until a greater number of prospective studies matching treatment to patient characteristics is conducted, all that can be said is that the matching hypothesis is reasonable, albeit intriguing. The fact that a significant proportion of patients with chronic pain are not successfully treated by current general approaches (Flor, Fydrich, & Turk, 1992; Holroyd & Penzien, 1990; Turk & Rudy, 1990a), together with the identification of various subgroups of patients, makes investigation of treatment matching of particular importance.

ACKNOWLEDGMENTS

Preparation of this chapter was supported in part by grants from the National Institute of Arthritis and Musculoskeletal and Skin Diseases (No. AR/AI44724) and the National Institute of Child Health and Human Development (No. HD33989) to Dennis C. Turk, and by Grant No. AR44230 from the National Institute of Arthritis and Musculoskeletal and Skin Diseases to Akiko Okifuji. We wish to thank Emily Anderson for her careful reading and helpful comments of an earlier version of this chapter.

REFERENCES

Anderson, T., Cole, T., Gullickson, G., Hudgens, A., & Roberts, A. (1977). Behavior modification of chronic pain: A treatment program by a multidisciplinary team. *Journal of Clinical Orthopedics, 129,* 96–100.

Beck, A., Ward, C., Mendelson, M., Mock, J., & Erbaugh, J. (1961). An inventory for measuring depression. *Archives of General Psychiatry, 4,* 561–571.

Bergstrom, G., Jensen, I. B., Bodin, L., Linton, S. J., Nygren, A. L., & Carlsson, S. G. (1998). Reliability and factor structure of the Multidimensional Pain Inventory–Swedish Language Version (MPI-S). *Pain, 75,* 101–110.

Bernstein, I. H., Jaremko, M. E., & Hinkley, B. S. (1995). On the utility of the West Haven–Yale Multidimensional Pain Inventory. *Spine, 20,* 956–963.

Bradley, L., Prokop, C., Margolis, R., & Gentry, W. (1978). Multivariate analyses of the MMPI profiles of low back pain patients. *Journal of Behavioral Medicine, 1,* 253–272.

Bradley, L., & Van der Heide, L. (1984). Pain-related correlates of MMPI profile subgroups among back pain patients. *Health Psychology, 3,* 57–74.

Butterworth, J. C., & Deardorff, W. W. (1987). Psychometric profiles of craniomandibular pain patients: Identifying specific subgroups. *Cranio, 5,* 225–232.

Cairns, D., Mooney, V., & Crane, P. (1984). Spinal pain rehabilitation: Inpatient and outpatient treatment results and development of predictors for outcome. *Spine, 9,* 91–95.

Dworkin, S., & LeResche, L. (1992). Research diagnostic criteria for temporomandibular disorders: Review, criteria, examinations and specifications, critique. *Journal of Craniomandibular Disorders, 6,* 301–355.

Flor, H., Fydrich, T., & Turk, D. C. (1992). Efficacy of multidisciplinary pain treatment centers: A meta-analytic review. *Pain, 49,* 221–230.

Flor, H., Rudy, T., Birbaumer, N., & Schugers, M. (1990). Zur anwend bar keit des West Haven–Yale Multidimensional Pain Inventory in Deutschen sprachraum. *Der Schmerz, 4,* 82–87.

Flor, H., & Turk, D. C. (1988). Chronic back pain and rheumatoid arthritis: Predicting pain and disability from cognitive variables. *Journal of Behavioral Medicine, 11,* 251–265.

Flor, H., Turk, D. C., & Rudy, T. E. (1989). Relationship of pain impact and significant other reinforcement of pain behaviors: The mediating role of gender, marital status and marital satisfaction. *Pain, 38,* 45–50.

Fordyce, W. (1976). *Behavioral methods for chronic pain and illness.* St. Louis, MO: Mosby.

Frymoyer, J. W., Rosen, J. C., Clements, J., & Pope, M. H. (1985). Psychologic factors in low-back-pain disability. *Clinical Orthopaedics and Related Research, 195,* 178–184.

Gallagher, R., Rauh, V., Haugh, L., Milhous, R., Callas, P., Langelier, R., McClallen, J., & Frymoyer, J. (1989). Determinants of return-to-work among low back pain patients. *Pain, 39,* 55–67.

Goldenberg, D. L. (1987). Fibromyalgia syndrome: An emerging but controversial condition. *Journal of the American Medical Association, 257,* 2782–2787.

Guck, T., Meilman, P., Skultety, F., & Poloni, L. (1988). Pain-patient Minnesota Multiphasic Personality Inventory (MMPI) subgroups: Evaluation of long-term treatment outcome. *Journal of Behavioral Medicine, 11,* 159–169.

Holroyd, K., & Penzien, D. (1990). Pharmacological versus non-pharmacological prophylaxis of recurrent migraine headache: A meta-analytic review of clinical trials. *Pain, 42,* 1–13.

Jamison, R. N., Rock, D. L., & Parris, W. C. (1988). Empirically derived Symptom Checklist 90 subgroups of chronic pain patients: A cluster analysis. *Journal of Behavioral Medicine, 11,* 147–158.

Jamison, R. N., Rudy, T. E., Penzien, D. B., & Mosley, T. H., Jr. (1994). Cognitive-behavioral classifications of chronic pain: Replication and extension of empirically derived patient profiles. *Pain, 57,* 277–292.

Jordan, J. (1999). Effect of race and ethnicity on outcomes in arthritis and rheumatic conditions. *Current Opinion in Rheumatology, 11,* 98–103.

Keefe, F. J., Bradley, L. A., & Crisson, J. E. (1990). Behavioral assessment of low back pain: Identification of pain behavior subgroups. *Pain, 40,* 153–160.

Kerns, R. D., Turk, D. C., & Rudy, T. E. (1985). The West Haven–Yale Multidimensional Pain Inventory (WHYMPI). *Pain, 23,* 345–356.

King, S., & Snow, B. (1989). Factors for predicting premature termination from a multidisciplinary inpatient chronic pain program. *Pain, 39,* 281–287.

Lousberg, R., Groenman, N., & Schmidt, A. (1996). Profile characteristics of the MPI-DLV clusters of pain patients. *Journal of Clinical Psychology, 52,* 161–167.

Lousberg, R., Schmidt, A. J., Groenman, N. H., Vendrig, L., & Dijkman-Caes, C. I. (1997). Validating the MPI-DLV using experience sampling data. *Journal of Behavioral Medicine, 20,* 195–206.

Lousberg, R., Van Breukelen, G. J., Groenman, N. H., Schmidt, A. J., Arntz, A., & Winter, F. A. (1999). Psychometric properties of the Multidimensional Pain Inventory, Dutch Language Version (MPI-DLV). *Behaviour Research and Therapy, 37,* 167–182.

Maruta, T., Swanson, D., & McHardy, M. (1990). Three year follow-up of patients with chronic pain who were treated in a multidisciplinary pain management center. *Pain, 41,* 47–53.

Masi, A. T., & Yunus, M. B. (1991). Fibromyalgia—which is the best treatment?: A personalized, comprehensive, ambulatory, patient-involved management programme. *Baillière's Clinical Rheumatology, 4,* 333–370.

Mayer, T. G., Gatchel, R. J., Mayer, H., Kishino, N. D., Keeley, J., & Mooney, V. (1987). A prospective two-year study of functional restoration in industrial low back injury: An objective assessment procedure. *Journal of the American Medical Association, 25,* 1763–1767.

McGill, J., Lawlis, G., Selby, D., Mooney, V., & McCoy, C. (1983). The relationship of Minnesota Multiphasic Personality Inventory (MMPI) profile clusters to pain behaviors. *Journal of Behavioral Medicine, 6,* 77–92.

Melzack, R. (1975). The McGill Pain Questionnaire: Major properties and scoring methods. *Pain, 1,* 277–299.

Merskey, H. (1986). Classification of chronic pain: Descriptions of chronic pain syndromes and definitions. *Pain,* Suppl. 3, S1–S225.

Mikail, S., DuBreuil, S., & D'Eon, J. (1993). A comparative analysis of measures used in the assessment of chronic pain patients. *Psychological Assessment, 5,* 117–120.

Moffroid, M., Haugh, L., Henry, S., & Short, B. (1994). Distinguishable groups of musculoskeletal low back pain patients and asymptomatic control subjects based on physical measures of the NIOSH Low Back Atlas. *Spine, 19,* 1350–1358.

Moore, J., & Chaney, E. (1985). Outpatient group treatment of chronic pain: Effects of spouse involvement. *Journal of Consulting and Clinical Psychology, 53,* 326–334.

Moore, J. E., Armentrout, D. P., Parker, J. C., & Kivlahan, D. R. (1986). Empirically derived pain-patient MMPI subgroups: Prediction of treatment outcome. *Journal of Behavioral Medicine, 9,* 51–63.

Okifuji, A., & Turk, D. C. (1999). Fibromyalgia: Search for mechanisms and effective treatments. In R. Gatchel & D. C. Turk (Eds.), *Psychosocial factors in pain: Critical perspectives* (pp. 227–246). New York: Guilford Press.

Osterweis, M., Kleinman, A., & Mechanic, D. (1987). *Pain and disability: Clinical, behavioral, and public policy perspectives.* Washington, DC: National Academy Press.

Reesor, K. A., & Craig, K. D. (1988). Medically incongruent chronic back pain: Physical limitations, suffering, and ineffective coping. *Pain, 32,* 35–45.

Rohling, M., Binder, L., & Langhinrichsen-Rohling, J. (1995). Money matters: A meta-analytic review of the association between financial compensation and the experience and treatment of chronic pain. *Health Psychology, 14,* 537–547.

Rudy, T. E., Turk, D. C., Kubinski, J. A., & Zaki, H. S. (1995). Differential treatment responses of TMD patients as a function of psychological characteristics. *Pain, 61,* 103–112.

Scharff, L., Turk, D. C., & Marcus, D. A. (1995). Psychosocial and behavioral characteristics in chronic headache patients: Support for a continuum and dual-diagnostic approach. *Cephalalgia, 15,* 216–223.

Tait, R., & Chibnall, J. (1998). Attitude profiles and clinical status in patients with chronic pain. *Pain, 78,* 49–57.

Talo, S., Rytokoski, U., & Puukka, P. (1992). Patient classification, a key to evaluate pain treatment: A psychological study in chronic low back pain patients. *Spine, 17,* 998–1011.

Turk, D. C. (1990). Customizing treatment for chronic pain patients: Who, what, and why. *Clinical Journal of Pain, 6,* 255–270.

Turk, D. C., Okifuji, A., Sinclair, J. D., & Starz, T. W. (1996). Pain, disability, and physical functioning in subgroups of patients with fibromyalgia. *Journal of Rheumatology, 23,* 1255–1262.

Turk, D. C., Okifuji, A., Starz, T., & Sinclair, J. (1998). Differential responses by psychosocial subgroups of fibromyalgia syndrome patients to an interdisciplinary treatment. *Arthritis Care and Research, 11,* 397–404.

Turk, D. C., Penzien, D. B., & Rains, J. C. (1995). Temporomandibular disorders. In A. J. Goereczny (Ed.), *Handbook of recent advances in behavioral medicine* (pp. 55–77). New York: Plenum Press.

Turk, D. C., & Rudy, T. E. (1988). Toward an empirically derived taxonomy of chronic pain patients: Integration of psychological assessment data. *Journal of Consulting and Clinical Psychology, 56,* 233–238.

Turk, D. C., & Rudy, T. E. (1990a). Neglected factors in chronic pain treatment outcome studies: Referral patterns, failure to enter treatment, and attrition. *Pain, 43,* 7–25.

Turk, D. C., & Rudy, T. E. (1990b). The robustness of an empirically derived taxonomy of chronic pain patients. *Pain, 43,* 27–35.

Turk, D. C., & Rudy, T. E. (1992). Classification logic and strategies in chronic pain. In D. C. Turk & R. Melzack (Eds.), *Handbook of pain assessment* (pp. 409–428). New York: Guilford Press.

Turk, D. C., Rudy, T. E., Kubinski, J. A., Zaki, H. S., & Greco, C. M. (1996). Dysfunctional patients with temporomandibular disorders: Evaluating the efficacy of a tailored treatment protocol. *Journal of Consulting and Clinical Psychology, 64,* 139–146.

Turk, D. C., Sist, T. C., Okifuji, A., Miner, M. F., Florio, G., Harrison, P., Massey, J., Lema, M. L., & Zevon, M. A. (1998). Adaptation to metastatic cancer pain, regional/local cancer pain and non-cancer pain: Role of psychological and behavioral factors. *Pain, 74,* 247–256.

Turk, D. C., Wack, J., & Kerns, R. (1985). An empirical examination of the "pain-behavior" construct. *Journal of Behavioral Medicine, 8,* 119–130.

Turk, D. C., Zaki, H. S., & Rudy, T. E. (1993). Effects of intraoral appliance and biofeedback/stress management alone and in combination in treating pain and depression in patients with temporomandibular disorders. *Journal of Prosthetic Dentistry, 70*, 158–164.

Turner, J., Loeser, J., & Bell, K. (1995). Spinal cord stimulation for chronic low back pain: A systematic literature synthesis. *Neurosurgery, 37*, 1088–1095.

Volinn, E. (1999). Do workplace interventions prevent low-back disorders? If so, why?: A methodologic commentary. *Ergonomics, 42*, 258–272.

Waddell, G., Main, C., Morris, E., Di Paola, M., & Gray, I. (1984). Chronic low-back pain, psychologic distress, and illness behavior. *Spine, 9*, 209–213.

Watkins, R., O'Brien, J., Draugelis, R., & Jones, D. (1986). Comparisons of preoperative and postoperative MMPI data in chronic back patients. *Spine, 11*, 385–390.

White, K. P., Speechley, M., Harth, M., & Ostbye, T. (1995). Fibromyalgia in rheumatology practice: A survey of Canadian rheumatologists. *Journal of Rheumatology, 22*, 722–726.

Widar, M., & Ahlstrom, G. (1999). Pain in persons with post-polio: The Swedish version of the Multidimensional Pain Inventory (MPI). *Scandinavian Journal of Caring Sciences, 13*, 33–40.

Wolfe, F., Smythe, H. A., Yunus, M. B., Bennett, R. M., Bombardier, C., Goldenberg, D. L., Tugwell, P., Campbell, S. M., Abeles, M., Clark, P., Fam, A. G., Farber, S. J., Fiechtner, J. J., Franklin, C. M., Gatter, R. A., Hamaty, D., Lessard, J., Lichtbroun, A. S., Masi, A. T., McCain, G. A., Reynolds, W. J., Romano, T. J., Russell, I. J., & Sheon, R. P. (1990). The American College of Rheumatology 1990 Criteria for the Classification of Fibromyalgia: Report of the Multicenter Criteria Committee [see comments]. *Arthritis and Rheumatism, 33*, 160–172.

Part V

SPECIFIC PAIN STATES
AND SYNDROMES

Chapter 22

Assessment of Acute Pain, Pain Relief, and Patient Satisfaction

JENNIFER A. HAYTHORNTHWAITE
JAMES A. FAUERBACH

Since the first edition of this volume was published in 1992, a number of groups and organizations have developed guidelines and policies pertaining to the assessment of acute pain. In February 1992, the Agency for Health Care Policy and Research (AHCPR) issued the clinical practice guideline *Acute Pain Management: Operative or Medical Procedures and Trauma*, which was also summarized in the pain literature (Pain Management Guideline Panel, 1992). In the executive summary, the AHCPR cited the "widespread inadequacy of pain management" (p. 1) as the primary catalyst for developing these clinical guidelines. Incorporated into the AHCPR guidelines was earlier work conducted by the American Pain Society (APS) Committee on Quality Assurance Standards for Acute Pain and Cancer Pain, which developed and published its own set of standards (Max, 1991). These standards include the following: (1) assessing pain, pain relief, and patient satisfaction; (2) making information about analgesics easily available; (3) promising patients attentive analgesic care; (4) defining policies for using advanced analgesic technologies; and (5) monitoring adherence to standards.

Specific strategies for implementing these guidelines have also been published (Miaskowski & Donovan, 1992). Data obtained from systematically implementing the guidelines revealed some interesting, and puzzling, findings. Patient satisfaction with pain management was generally high, even when patients reported high levels of pain (Miaskowski, Nichols, Brody, & Synold, 1994; Ward & Gordon, 1994). A large-scale implementation of the guidelines increased patient satisfaction ratings, despite no substantial change in ratings of the worst pain experienced during the past 24 hours during the early phase of the program (Bookbinder et al., 1996).

The APS Quality of Care Committee (1995) later published an updated set of guidelines focusing on quality improvement. The assessment of patient outcomes expanded to include the impact of pain on function, direct questions as to whether the patient would like stronger pain medication, an assessment of patient-related barriers to using pain medications, and ratings of the clarity of information provided for outpatient pain management. A year later, the president of the APS, James Campbell, promoted "Pain as the Fifth Vital Sign" in his presidential address in order to increase awareness of pain assessment and treatment among health care professionals (Campbell, 1995). In a large multicenter study of postoperative intensive care units, Carroll and colleagues (1999) observed that only 54% of patients had a numerical rating of pain documented in their medical record during the first 24 hours following surgery, although

91% of the records included a description of pain. Documentation of pain increases when pain assessment is included in the vital sign sheet (Bookbinder et al., 1996; Carroll et al., 1999).

The integration of pain as a vital sign has become the theme for the U.S. Veterans Health Administration's (VHA's) implementation of a nationwide program addressing the inconsistent and often inaccessible pain management services throughout the VHA system. The VHA is currently finalizing a tool kit titled *Pain Assessment: The Fifth Vital Sign*, which guides implementation of systematic pain assessment and its documentation, education for health care providers, and education for patients and families. In late March 1999, the Joint Commission on the Accreditation of Healthcare Organizations (JCAHO) expanded existing standards to apply across the continuum of care. The JCAHO standards, which were implemented in 2001, require accredited health care organizations to monitor and manage pain and to educate staff and patients about the importance of effective pain management.

In any assessment of acute pain, either for a clinical trial or in routine clinical care, measurement considerations include feasibility, convenience, and speed of completion; sensitivity to treatment effects; and clinical utility (Max & Laska, 1991). As discussed by Jensen and Karoly in Chapter 2 of this volume, no single measure of pain intensity can be considered universally valid across clinical settings. Strengths and weaknesses of each measure have been identified and must be weighed during decision making, since errors in using pain scales occur with almost every scale (Jensen, Karoly, O'Riordan, Bland, & Burns, 1989; Jensen, Miller, & Fisher, 1998). Clinical factors to consider include the patient's age, educational level, and level of consciousness; the availability of the patient's writing hand; the frequency of assessment; and the burden of the assessment process relative to the amount of information obtained. (For a discussion of special populations, the reader is referred to McGrath & Gillespie, Chapter 6; Gagliese, Chapter 7; and Hadjistavropoulos, von Baeyer, & Craig, Chapter 8. For a discussion of the assessment of pain quality and location, the reader is referred to Chapter 2 by Jensen & Karoly.)

Since the limitations of most clinical settings demand use of self-report rather than behavioral observation, the clinician must also consider environmental factors that influence self-report (Jensen, 1997). Environmental and social factors shown to influence pain ratings (Jensen, 1997) include the

sex of the experimenter (Levine & DeSimone, 1991), the presence of a solicitous spouse (Block, Kremer, & Gaylor, 1980), and whether the clinician selectively attends to well behavior or pain behavior (White & Sanders, 1986). In addition, cognitive factors such as expectancies can also influence reported pain intensity and are particularly relevant in a clinical setting that includes the use of placebos (Montgomery & Kirsch, 1997). Of note, expectancies, but not desire for relief, appear to mediate between conditioning and the placebo analgesia response (Price et al., 1999).

PAIN INTENSITY

Three types of pain intensity scales are most commonly used in clinical settings: Visual Analogue Scales (VASs), Numerical Rating Scales (NRSs), and Verbal Rating Scales (VRSs). The psychometric properties and relative strengths of these scales are discussed in more detail by Jensen and Karoly in Chapter 2. Pain intensity scales are used for varying periods of time, including pain right now, lowest pain during a period of time (e.g., since last medication dose), highest pain, and typical pain. Acute pain assessment needs to target both resting pain, or *tonic pain*, and activity-related pain, or *phasic pain*.

VASs provide a line, usually 100 mm long, that includes anchors from "no pain" to " the most intense pain sensation imaginable." The patient places a mark on the line that indicates the intensity of pain experienced during a period of time. The patient's rating is the distance (in millimeters) from 0. These scales are sensitive to treatment effects (Littman, Walker, & Schneider, 1985; Seymour, 1982; Wallenstein, Heidrich, Kaiko, & Houde, 1980). However, a VAS, because it requires a clear visuospatial estimation and a precise motoric response by the patient, may be of only limited use in some clinical settings where the patient's writing hand is not free or easily accessible (Jensen et al., 1998; see also Hadjistavropoulos et al., Chapter 8). The need to measure the distance adds an additional step that may limit the feasibility of this scale in some clinical settings. Mechanical measures, such as Price's slide algometer, produce similar responses to written measures and eliminate the extra step of measuring the patient's mark (Price, Bush, Long, & Harkins, 1994), but still require manipulation by the patient.

NRSs ask patients to rate their pain using numbers ranging from 0 ("no pain") to 10 or 100 ("the worst pain imaginable") and typically require written or oral ratings. Patients' use of numbers between whole numbers on 11-point scales (e.g., 7.5; Jensen, Turner, & Romano, 1994) led Jensen and colleagues (1998) to recommend a 21-point scale over the 11-point scale in their study of acute pain assessment scales. The 21-point scale was as sensitive as a VAS in detecting changes in pain. Information is not lost when 101-point scales are recoded to be 21-point scales, and most patients use the 101-point scale as a 21-point scale, reporting responses that are multiples of 5 (Jensen et al., 1994). Unlike VASs, NRSs do not show ratio properties (i.e., equal intervals between response categories). Although NRSs are widely used in clinical settings, their interpretation is limited to relative changes in pain (e.g., increase or decrease) rather than percentage of increase or decrease (Price et al., 1994).

VRSs include a list of adjectives that reflect the extremes of pain (e.g., "none" to "severe"). These scales have demonstrated validity relative to other pain scales and are generally sensitive to treatment effects. However, patients may have difficulty selecting an appropriate adjective to describe their pain, and these scales generally do not show ratio properties. For example, in an early study comparing different pain scales, Downie and colleagues (1978) demonstrated that the modal numerical rating for a rating of "none" was 0, for "mild" was 3 (ranging from 1 to 5), for "moderate" was 5 (ranging from 3 to 7), and for "severe" was 10 (ranging from 7 to 10). Other investigators demonstrated in more detail that the relationship between VRS and VAS pain severity ratings is best described using power functions rather than linear models (Wallenstein et al., 1980).

The three commonly used types of pain intensity rating scales described above place different demands on the patient and show different scaling properties. No one method will be superior across all clinical settings with all types of patients, and other types of scales may be more appropriate with special populations. Although VAS methods show the strongest scaling characteristics and the greatest sensitivity to treatment, not all patients understand how to use this type of scale, and its utility may be severely limited with special populations (e.g., patients with hand injuries, patients with visual or cognitive impairments, or children; see Hadjistavropoulos et al., Chapter 8). The NRSs are probably the most widely used pain intensity assessment measures in clinical settings, and scales using 11 or 21

points are sensitive to treatment effects (Jensen et al., 1994). Of the three types of scales, VRSs show the poorest scale properties and should be avoided when possible.

PAIN RELIEF

The most common strategies for assessing pain relief include VASs, typically anchored with descriptors of "no relief" and "complete relief," and VRSs that provide categories (e.g., "none," "slight," "moderate," "lots," "complete"). Some VRSs include "worse" as an additional anchor. The scaling characteristics of VRS ratings of pain relief are similar to those of VAS ratings of pain relief. These two measures show linear associations, such that increments in VAS ratings of pain relief are proportional to increments in verbal ratings (Wallenstein, 1984).

The correspondence between pain relief ratings and changes in pain intensity ratings can be inconsistent. Studies note instances of patients reporting increases in pain ratings while simultaneously indicating some degree of pain relief. For example, in a study examining a large database from a series of analgesic trials, a significant minority of patients (12%) reported at least moderate relief when there was no change over 1 hour in their verbal description of moderate pain (Littman et al., 1985). Among another group of patients whose pain actually increased from moderate to severe, more than one-third of these people (38%) rated "none" (rather than "worse") or "moderate" pain relief (Littman et al., 1985). Todd, Funk, Funk, and Bonacci (1996) used a bipolar relief scale ("much less," "a little less," "about the same," "a little more," "much more") to establish the typical VAS rating change that corresponded with "a little less" or "a little more." Some patients presenting in an emergency department reported pain relief when sequential VAS pain ratings actually increased. In the context of a clinical trial, despite an increase in present pain early in the trial (28%), some patients with chronic dental pain (90%) also reported some degree of relief on a VAS (Feine, Lavigne, Dao, Morin, & Lund, 1998). Thus these inconsistencies occur in a significant minority of patients in a variety of clinical settings.

Unlike pain intensity measures, different types of pain relief measures—VRSs and VASs—show similar scaling characteristics. However, the discordance at times between ratings of pain relief and actual changes in pain intensity raises questions about which of these outcome measures is more accurate and which should be used in determining the outcome of a pain treatment intervention. Research on these scales identifies factors that will influence the accuracy of pain reports, including both pain intensity and pain relief, following a therapeutic intervention.

FACTORS THAT INFLUENCE THE RECALL OF PAIN

Clinical assessment of pain often requires a patient to describe pain experienced during past episodes and relief obtained from past treatments. The accurate recall of painful episodes is of significant clinical import, since the decision to undergo potentially painful diagnostic, dental, or surgical procedures may depend on recall of pain experienced during prior episodes of the same or similar events. Furthermore, the treatment prescribed to a patient in pain often depends on the accurate retrospective ratings of previous acute pain episodes. Finally, if patients cannot accurately describe their previous acute pain episodes, then clinical trials that investigate the effectiveness of anesthetic agents need real-time measures of pain intensity and pain relief.

Pain Intensity Ratings

Data on the accuracy of pain recall are inconsistent, but studies identify circumstances associated with increased accuracy. Some evidence suggests that ratings of pain intensity and many pain behaviors can be accurately recalled over periods as long as 30 days (Salovey, Smith, Turk, Jobe, & Willis, 1993). The accurate recall of peak pain and average pain up to 1 week later has been observed in children as young as 5, although accuracy increased as age approached 16 years (Zonnefeld, McGrath, Reid, & Sorbi, 1997). Other studies suggest that patients with chronic pain overestimate average pain over 1 week compared to hourly ratings of pain intensity (Jamison, Sbrocco, & Parris, 1989) and overestimate pretreatment levels of pain intensity at the end of treatment (Linton & Melin, 1982). Inconsistencies in these studies may be due to the use of small sample sizes, heterogeneous groups of participants, and measurements taken in the clinic versus the laboratory (Salovey et al., 1993). In addition, measurement strategies differ across these studies, although two discrepant studies used hourly ratings on validated NRSs.

The method of assessment—VAS or VRS— may also influence the accuracy of pain recall. VASs of pain intensity overestimate baseline pain, whereas VRSs yield both overestimates and underestimates of baseline pain (Linton & Gotestam, 1983). Inaccuracies in retrospective ratings of pain intensity are influenced by present pain intensity (Eich, Reeves, Jaeger, & Graff-Radford, 1985; Feine et al., 1998), elapsed time since recording baseline pain, and baseline pain intensity (Feine et al., 1998). Overestimation of pain also correlates with emotional distress, female sex, less education, and disability status (Jamison et al., 1989).

Phenomena studied in the memory literature, including recency, salience, and state-dependent effects, provide information on factors that can influence constructions of pain memories. When patients are asked to describe pain during a medical procedure or a period of time, it is clear that they do not simply compute an arithmetic average of their pain experienced during the relevant period. In other words, all pain experiences are not equally weighted in the computational formula used.

Recency Effects

Evidence for these patterns in memory comes from studies that obtained serial pain ratings during painful medical procedures and compared these to summary ratings made after completion of the procedures. Participants' recollections of their total pain during a procedure was highly related to the pain experienced during the last few moments of the painful episode (i.e., a recency effect). For example, retrospective ratings of total pain intensity made by patients who had undergone colonoscopy and lithotripsy were strongly related to the pain intensity recorded in real time during the last 3 minutes of these procedures (called end pain; Redelmeier & Kahneman, 1996). Patients made these retrospective ratings of total pain on an 11-point scale (0 = "no discomfort" to 10 = "awful discomfort"). The same high correlation between end pain and recall of total pain was obtained within 1 hour of the procedure and again at 1 month (after colonoscopy) and 1 year (after lithotripsy). Physicians' recall of the patients' total pain during the procedure also followed this same pattern, suggesting that the effect was not attributable to anesthesia, to gradual forgetting, or to recording in real-time; rather, it was a function of the way in which the judgments were first constructed.

Salience Effects

These same studies provide support for the phenomenon of a *salience effect*, which is the tendency to recall most accurately that part of a stimulus with the strongest positive or negative valence. Retrospective ratings of pain intensity made by patients after colonoscopy and lithotripsy had been completed were also strongly related to the peak pain intensity recorded during the procedure (Redelmeier & Kahneman, 1996). As with end pain, the same pattern of high correlation between peak pain intensity and recall of total pain was obtained within 1 hour of each procedure and again at 1 month and 1 year.

State and Assimilation Effects

The accuracy and completeness of memory have been shown to be functions of *state effects* (e.g., pain or mood) present during memory acquisition across some studies. Two days after delivering, new mothers retrospectively rated the pain of delivery as lower than had been actually recorded during labor (Norvell, Gastron-Johansson, & Fridh, 1987). This has been attributed to the effects of negative mood during labor, which would increase pain ratings at the time of labor, and the effects of positive mood after completion of labor, which would decrease pain ratings after labor (Salovey et al., 1993). State-dependent effects of mood on recalled pain were not observed during laboratory manipulations of mood in community volunteers who were asked to recall average or maximum pain from their most recent pain episode over the previous year (Salovey et al., 1993). The artificial moods induced in the Salovey and colleagues (1993) study were probably less intense and less salient than the moods experienced by women in the two clinical studies, suggesting state-dependent mood effects on pain memories.

Some investigators have demonstrated that a participant's current pain level affects the accuracy of recall for prior painful episodes. This effect has been termed an *assimilation effect*, in that recollections of pain are assimilated to current experiences of pain (Salovey et al., 1993). For example, high levels of present pain intensity were associated with retrospective *over*estimation of usual, maximum, and minimum pain, whereas low levels of present pain intensity were associated with retrospective *under*estimation of real-time pain ratings (Eich et al., 1985). As another example, patients with chronic pain completing a physical therapy session that reduced pain underestimated their pain re-

corded during the previous week, whereas patients assessed prior to this therapy accurately recalled the levels of pain they had previously recorded (Smith & Safer, 1993). Among patients with cancer exposed to a similar procedure, present pain intensity positively correlated with recalled pain intensity (Smith, Gracely, & Safer, 1998). This was seen as evidence of the assimilation effect, in that memories were reconstrued to be more consistent with (i.e., assimilated to) current status of pain and affect (Smith et al., 1998, p. 127).

A study of women after surgery for breast cancer provides further evidence for the assimilation effects of present pain and the state-dependent effects of current mood on memories for pain. Women who reported chronic pain following surgery recalled higher levels of baseline pain than women who did not experience chronic pain following surgery (Tasmuth, Estlanderb, & Kalso, 1996). Depression was higher in the group with chronic pain, and correlated with retrospective overestimates of postsurgical pain.

Duration Effects

In constructing summary ratings of pain, it is perhaps intuitively appealing to suggest that the duration of acute pain contributes to one's remembered pain intensity. That is, longer duration may contribute to higher ratings, and shorter duration may contribute to lower ratings of intensity. The data are not consistent on this issue. *Duration neglect* has been described, whereby subsequent recollections of acute pain are not related to the duration of the painful episode.

Laboratory manipulations of mood documented duration neglect in global retrospective ratings of affective response to negative and positive movie segments (Fredrickson & Kahneman, 1993). When peak and end ratings of mood were controlled for, no effects of duration of exposure on global ratings were observed. The authors concluded that retrospective evaluations appeared to be determined by a weighted average of "snapshots" of the actual emotional experience, as if duration did not matter (Fredrickson & Kahneman, 1993). The study of pain ratings during and after colonoscopy and lithotripsy found that retrospective ratings of pain were only weakly related to the duration of the procedure (Redelmeier & Kahneman, 1996). Although a weak correlation between recalled peak pain intensity and duration was found, the authors attributed this effect to the increased opportunity for a high peak pain intensity, given more time.

That is, more time never results in a lower peak pain rating, but may occasionally result in a higher rating. Thus duration itself did not account for the correlation between memory for total pain and duration (Redelmeier & Kahneman, 1996). Alternatively, the patients who underwent breast cancer surgery showed a *duration effect*, such that retrospective ratings of postoperative pain worsened as duration of chronic pain continued in the year following surgery (Tasmuth et al., 1996). This effect can be interpreted in the context of laboratory data, which show that positive mood decreases with continued exposure to a positive stimulus and that negative mood increases with continued exposure to a negative stimulus (Fredrickson & Kahneman, 1993).

Summary

There are circumstances under which the recall of pain can be relatively accurate. These conditions include the use of validated instruments and short periods of recall (e.g., less than 30 days) and when specific episodes of acute pain are to be recalled (Salovey et al., 1993). In addition, under certain circumstances it does not appear that small changes in mood affect the accuracy of memory for either pain or pain behavior (Salovey et al., 1993). On the other hand, there are conditions that are known to erode the accuracy of reports of recalled pain, including high levels of present pain intensity (Redelmeier & Kahneman, 1996), a successful pain-focused intervention (Linton & Melin, 1982), marked shifts in mood (Norvell et al., 1987), and differences between current pain and pain at the point in time being recalled (Feine et al., 1998). Retrospective pain reports are subject to many of the same effects that are observed in all learning-based studies. These include recency (i.e., end pain), salience (i.e., peak pain), and assimilation (i.e., past experience reconstructed to be consistent with present pain intensity). That is, pain remembered will be influenced by pain experienced near the end of an episode, by the peak pain during the episode, and by the individual's present pain intensity.

Pain Relief Ratings

The rating of pain relief entails remembering an earlier pain state, evaluating the current pain state, subtracting the current state from that remembered earlier state, and selecting a rating from the scale

provided (Mackie, 1989). Studies suggest that the process of rating relief involves different parameters or cognitive factors from those involved in rating present pain intensity. The memory effects outlined above may explain the complicated relationship between changes in pain intensity and ratings of pain relief.

Factors that influence pain relief ratings include baseline pain, present pain, remembered pain, and time since baseline. When patients in an emergency department initially reported a high level of pain on an NRS, ratings of significant or complete relief were associated with an average of 84% reduction in VAS pain scores. When patients started at lower levels of pain, similar ratings of relief were associated with an average of 29% reduction in VAS pain intensity ratings (Stahmer, Shofer, Marino, Shepherd, & Abbuhl, 1998). Feine and colleagues (1998) used a series of VAS pain relief scales to assess the responses of patients with oral pain to a 10-week trial of oral appliances. Patients first used a VAS with a bipolar scale to rate relief ("the worst it could become," "no relief," "complete relief"). When a rating was above "no relief," then patients rated relief on a unipolar scale ("no relief" to "complete relief"). Multivariate analyses indicated that actual change in pain intensity did not significantly predict ratings of relief. Other factors, including the type of treatment received, present pain, remembered pain (10 weeks earlier), and the length of time patients had been in the treatment, were significant predictors of ratings of relief. The higher the present pain, the lower the rating of relief; the higher the remembered pain, the higher the rating of relief. Interestingly, the effect of time amounted to an average increase in rating of relief of 2 mm each week. Thus, regardless of treatment received, patients rated greater relief each week they were involved in the treatment (Feine et al., 1998).

The relationship between ratings of pain intensity and pain relief appears also to change as a function of analgesia. Angst, Brose, and Dyck (1999) described the impact of methadone and hydromorphone infusions on VAS ratings of resting pain and pain relief. The relationship between pain intensity ratings and pain relief ratings changed after maximum analgesia was achieved and became stronger, such that time plots of the two scales were almost mirror images—when pain intensity decreased, pain relief increased. Before maximum analgesia was achieved, however, larger increases in pain relief were reported relative to the magnitude of the decrease in pain intensity ratings (Angst et al., 1999). As discussed below, expectancies of a continued downward trend in present pain intensity during the period prior to maximum analgesia may contribute to an estimation of greater relief. Present pain intensity ratings may depend more on ongoing nociceptive input.

Measurement Sensitivity

Retrospective ratings of clinical improvement, such as pain relief, are often used in clinical research to ascertain outcome and these ratings have tremendous relevance to clinical settings. As global measures, ratings of change are meaningful, efficient, cost-effective, and broadly applicable to most patients and most clinical settings (Gotzsche, 1990). Regardless of scaling technique (e.g., VAS or categorical), global evaluations of improvement show greater sensitivity than measures of pain across numerous trials and scaling techniques in clinical trials with patients who have arthritis (Gotzsche, 1990). Ratings of pain relief have been shown to be more sensitive to treatment effects than changes in ratings of pain intensity.

Littman and colleagues (1985) combined data from a large number of analgesic clinical trials and examined the consistency and sensitivity of a VRS of pain relief ("worse," "none," "a little," "moderate," "a lot," and "complete") to relative changes in VAS and VRS ratings of pain intensity. During the first hour after medication administration, the pain relief VRS showed the largest treatment effects across a number of clinical trials, suggesting slightly greater sensitivity than changes in the pain intensity VAS (Littman et al., 1985). Others have also argued that pain relief scales may be more sensitive to treatment outcome than pain intensity ratings (Stahmer et al., 1998). Similarly, among a large group of patients with chronic arthritis who were treated with a range of interventions for pain and disability, retrospective ratings of improvement were consistently higher than difference scores calculated from serial measures (e.g., posttreatment rating minus pretreatment rating; Fischer et al., 1999). Further analyses revealed that retrospective ratings scaled from "very much worse" to "very much better" showed greater efficiency in detecting change due to treatment (i.e., sensitivity) than did changes in serial measures (Fischer et al., 1999). Although categorical ratings are proportional to VAS ratings of pain relief, the pain relief VAS is more sensitive to drug and dose effects in analyses combining multiple clinical trials (Wallenstein, 1991).

Summary

Multiple factors influence summary ratings of pain relief, including present pain intensity, remembered pain intensity, baseline pain intensity, and duration of treatment. These complex ratings are similar to other global judgments of improvement and appear to be more sensitive to treatment effects than simple (arithmetic) pain intensity change scores. Some data indicate greater sensitivity of VAS pain relief ratings over categorical ratings of relief.

Theoretical Mechanisms

Certain metaphenomena may account for the inaccuracies in ratings of pain relief and memory for pain that have been observed and reported as the effects of present state, salience, recency and duration neglect. Although there are no data to suggest the involvement of these mechanisms in the construction of pain memories, they provide possible explanations for the effects observed.

Response Shift Bias

Retrospective ratings are based on the twin assumptions that (1) respondents have an internal metric for evaluating the construct, and (2) the metric is stable over time. The discordance between real-time pain ratings and retrospective pain ratings, including pain relief, may be due to an instability in the metric used to rate pain. Recalibration or reconceptualization of the personal metric used to rate pain intensity or total pain will cause significant shifts in ratings. Such changes in calibration or conceptualization are not the same as actual changes in pain as experienced. Errors attributable to this sort of change in the metric have been termed *response shift bias* (Howard et al., 1979). Norman and Parker (1996) have adapted a typology of change from organizational psychology (Golembiewski, Billingsley, & Yeager, 1976). Applied to the assessment of acute pain, this model identifies three levels of change that may occur. A change in the actual pain state is the *alpha level*, a change in the metric or scaling of pain is the *beta level*, and a change in the meaning or conceptualization of the pain is the *gamma level*.

Psychological interventions, such as cognitive-behavioral interventions (Caudill, 1995; Turk, Meichenbaum, & Genest, 1983) or hypnosis (Patterson, Everett, Burns, & Marvin, 1992), often operate on the scaling (beta) or conceptualization (gamma) levels. For example, reductions in the frequency of catastrophizing, a negative thought pattern in response to pain, often enable the patient to attend to the actual fluctuations in the level of present pain intensity rather than always perceiving it to be "as bad as it could be." This is an example of changing the scaling or metric used by the patient. Alternatively, reconceptualizing the pain as due to temporary, specific, and malleable causes (e.g., poor pacing during activity) rather than permanent, global and fixed causes (e.g., cancer metastases) is an example of changing the meaning of the pain.

Changing the scaling or the conceptualization of pain is seen both as an important goal in and of itself and as a means of affecting the actual pain state (alpha level). In cases where changes in calibration or conceptualization occur, it is quite possible that retrospective ratings of pain will be made with a different metric than was employed for rating the pain intensity or pain affect during the real-time event as experienced (Sprangers, 1996). This change in metric, or response shift bias, not only may account for inconsistencies in previous research but may lead to erroneous conclusions as well. For example, response shift bias may account for the anomalous finding that pain relief is experienced when present pain intensity ratings actually increase (Feine et al., 1998; Littman et al., 1985). Patients undergoing treatment for pain may alter their conceptualization of the pain and its meaning, thereby shifting the metric or scale they use for evaluating pain. Hence, although pain intensity is rated higher, the meaning may have become more benign—therefore leading to higher perceived relief. If these interpretations of these studies are viable, then the discrepancy between ratings of pain intensity and pain relief may be attributable to systematic, post hoc reconstructions leading to shifts in the scaling of pain.

Attentional Limitations

Present pain intensity degrades the accuracy of memory for pain. The effect of present pain intensity may be to serve as a distractor that interferes with cognitive processes such as recall. A study investigating cold pressor pain found that pain intensity affected recall and recognition memory in general, but did not differentially affect recall or recognition memory for positive or negative words (Kuhajda, Thorn, & Klinger, 1998). These authors concluded that pain interferes with attentional resources, limiting the ability to engage in other cog-

nitive activities simultaneously, but that this effect is not specific to positively or negatively valenced memories.

Both theory (Melzack & Wall, 1965) and research (McCaul & Malott, 1984) suggest that attentional limitations are important determinants of acute pain perception. The limits of attention serve as the rationale for using distraction to influence pain perception, since certain stimuli can distract attention away from the perception of pain (McCaul & Malott, 1984). The use of distraction is a common clinical intervention in some acute pain settings. One recent study suggests that the timing of pain assessment can alter the efficacy of a distraction intervention. Undergraduates exposed to a cold pressor task for 90 seconds were randomly assigned to low-distraction and high-distraction conditions and to immediate recall versus 10-minute delayed recall (Christenfeld, 1997). The group exposed to a high level of distraction and asked to rate pain after a delay reported significantly less pain than the other groups. These findings point to the potential impact of pain assessment on the efficacy of a treatment intervention.

Expectancy Effects

What one expects to happen (i.e., *expectancies*) can have either a direct or an indirect effect on memory for painful episodes. Expectancies guide perception such that people focus on, and hence remember, stimuli consistent with their expectations (Anderson & Pitchert, 1978). Similarly, studies have shown that people remember experiences consistent with their expectations while forgetting inconsistent information (Lord, Ross, & Lepper, 1979). Furthermore, ratings of past events have been shown to be sensitive to the effects of the present. For example, judges recalled midterm grades to be higher when final exam grades were high and lower when final exam grades were low (Hirt, 1990, study 1). When participants expected that grades would improve, they recalled lower midterm grades relative to final grades, and when a decline was expected in grades, then higher midterm grades were recalled relative to final exam grades (Hirt, 1990). If this is the case, in general as well as in the recall of pain, then it may be that expectancies are an integral part of the mechanism by which memory of pain is systematically reconstructed (i.e., a change at the gamma level, or change in meaning). Supporting this, retrospective placebo responses (i.e., retrospective ratings of pain in the presence of a placebo cream) were three to four times greater than the placebo responses observed immediately after conditioning trials, and correlated with expectancies but not with desire for relief (Price et al., 1999).

This expectancy effect closely resembles the assimilation effect, whereby present pain intensity degrades the accuracy of memory for pain (Salovey et al., 1993; Smith et al., 1998). A model of reconstructive memory has been proposed that suggests that at recall, information is integrated and weighted from three sources: (1) the present (e.g., present pain intensity); (2) the expectancy of the relationship between the present and the past; and (3) the original memory trace of the pain (Hirt, 1990). Factors such as salience and recency can determine the strength of the effect of expectancies on memory (Hirt, Reickson, & McDonald, 1993). Support for this model comes from studies demonstrating that end pain, salience, and the original memory correlate with inaccuracies in retrospective ratings of baseline pain intensity (Feine et al., 1998; Redelmeier & Kahneman, 1996).

Summary

Response shift bias, distraction, and expectancies may explain some of the inaccuracies observed in retrospective reports of pain. Response shifts can alter the metric with which pain and its meaning are evaluated, thus providing retrospective ratings that are unrelated to real-time recordings (Sprangers, 1996). Distraction can interfere with the accurate encoding or recall of phenomena such as pain (Kuhajda et al., 1998). And finally, expectancies can influence people to ignore information that is inconsistent (Lord et al., 1979) and to attend selectively to confirmatory information (Anderson & Pitchert, 1978), thus distorting the completeness of the data available for encoding.

PATIENT SATISFACTION

Patient satisfaction is another general index of outcome that is gaining increased attention in clinical settings as health care systems attempt to address the undertreatment of pain and establish pain management quality assurance programs. As noted above, the APS encourages assessment of patient satisfaction as part of quality assurance efforts (see Okifuji & Turk, Chapter 33). In general, specific questions yield more reliable and valid information than general questions do (Herrmann, 1995). Unfortunately, the assessment of patient satisfac-

tion typically uses broad, general questions rather than specific questions about the dimensions relevant to satisfaction (McCracken, Klock, Mingay, Asbury, & Sinclair, 1997). Some studies of patient satisfaction generally indicate high levels of satisfaction despite concurrent high levels of pain (Bookbinder et al., 1996; Miaskowski et al., 1994; Ward & Gordon, 1994, 1996). Other studies find an inverse correlation between satisfaction ratings and level of pain (Carroll et al., 1999; Jamison et al., 1997; McNeill, Sherwood, Starck, & Thompson, 1998).

Early measures of patient satisfaction focused on global ratings of satisfaction with physician and nursing care, and reported delays in getting pain medications. Using a questionnaire modeled after the standards recommended by the APS, Ward and Gordon (1994) examined patient satisfaction with how pain was treated during an inpatient admission. High levels of satisfaction with both nurses and physicians were observed, ranging from 90% to 95% among adults, despite periods of relatively high levels of pain. Most patients reported quick responsiveness on the part of the treatment team when they reported inadequate pain management, with 75% of the sample reporting a change in treatment plan within 2 hours of reporting inadequate pain control. The satisfaction ratings suggested high-quality pain management; however, the actual pain ratings indicated relatively high levels of "worst" pain during the previous 24 hours. Similar levels of satisfaction in the context of high levels of pain were observed by Miaskowski and colleagues (1994) in another clinical setting. If used in isolation, positive ratings could mislead clinicians about the quality of pain reduction and management achieved (Ward & Gordon, 1994). In a later study using a revised patient satisfaction questionnaire, Ward and Gordon (1996) reported similar levels of pain and satisfaction in two new samples, one inpatient and one outpatient.

Despite institutional efforts to improve the quality of pain management, no reduction in experienced pain was observed in Ward and Gordon's (1994, 1996) sequential studies, or in a large-scale study of acute and cancer pain management (Bookbinder et al., 1996). Building upon this work, Jamison and colleagues (1997) developed a similar 13-item questionnaire to measure satisfaction with postoperative pain management. Questions about expectations for pain, usefulness of preoperative preparation, and treatment helpfulness were added. Test–retest stability of preoperative pain, worst postoperative pain, expectations, treatment helpfulness, and delay in getting medication were acceptable over a 1- to 5-hour period (coefficients ranged from .76 to .92). Similar to earlier studies, they found high levels of patient satisfaction. Factor analysis of this scale revealed five factors (Pain Intensity, Satisfaction with Care, Helpfulness of Treatment, a tendency toward Dissatisfaction, and Expected Postoperative Pain).

The APS Quality of Care Committee (1995) published a revised patient outcome survey that included an assessment of the impact of pain on function, patient beliefs about pain management and perceived barriers to pain management, and clarity of guidelines for using medications for outpatients. Many of the new items were taken from existing scales. Using this updated measure with inpatients, McNeill and colleagues (1998) demonstrated acceptable levels of internal consistency for the subscales—Pain Intensity, Impact of Pain, Satisfaction with Pain Management, and Barriers to Pain Management (coefficient alphas ranging from .68 to .82). A factor analysis of the slightly modified satisfaction items (Calvin, Becker, Biering, & Grobe, 1999) revealed a single factor (although one item showed a worrisomely low intercorrelation, $r = 0.24$) that showed somewhat higher internal consistency than the McNeill and colleagues study. This slightly modified scale showed convergent validity with other measures of patient satisfaction (Calvin et al., 1999).

McCracken and his colleagues (1997) took a broader perspective on patient satisfaction, operationalizing this construct as having behavioral, emotional, and verbal dimensions that should show convergence. After pilot testing demonstrated that a 7-point NRS format produced a positively skewed distribution of summary scores, a multiple-choice format that included 20 items was developed. Patients seen in an outpatient chronic pain service completed the scale, which demonstrated high internal consistency. Validity coefficients indicated convergence with physician ratings of patient satisfaction and another measure of global treatment satisfaction.

Correlates of Patient Satisfaction

As noted above, inconsistent relationships between pain intensity and patient satisfaction have been observed. Early studies showed no relationship between pain intensity and patient satisfaction (Bookbinder et al., 1996; Miaskowski et al., 1994; Ward & Gordon, 1994, 1996), but more recent studies have found that patient satisfaction de-

creases as pain intensity increases (Carroll et al., 1999; Jamison et al., 1997; McNeill et al., 1998). In addition to pain intensity, the reported frequency of moderate to severe pain predicts level of patient satisfaction (Carroll et al., 1999).

Other aspects of treatment outcome also predict level of satisfaction. In the McCracken and colleagues (1997) study, satisfaction scores were unrelated to present pain intensity, but highly correlated with ratings of pain reduction and improvements in daily living resulting from treatment. Among hospitalized patients who wanted more pain medication, dissatisfied patients reported higher levels of present pain, worst pain, and general level of pain and higher levels of interference with daily activities and sleep, compared to patients who were satisfied with pain management (McNeill et al., 1998). The only demographic correlate of this group—dissatisfied and wanting more pain medication—was age: Younger patients generally wanted more pain medication (McNeill et al., 1998). Other studies have also demonstrated that age and gender influence ratings of satisfaction, with younger patients and females reporting lower levels of satisfaction (Thomas, Robinson, Champion, McKell, & Pell, 1998).

Not surprisingly, aspects of the clinical care received also influence ratings of patient satisfaction. Whether staff members communicate the importance of pain management (Ward & Gordon, 1996) and whether they show their concern to patients (Jamison et al., 1997) predict levels of patient satisfaction. Having to wait longer for medications (Bookbinder et al., 1996; Carroll et al., 1999), appointments (McCracken et al., 1997), or telephone calls (McCracken et al., 1997) predicts lower levels of satisfaction. Although having a dedicated area for documenting pain raises documentation rates, this aspect of care does not appear to influence patient satisfaction ratings (Carroll et al., 1999).

Ward and Gordon (1996) have raised the provocative idea that the use of "as-needed" dosing of pain medications results in a cyclical pattern in which the patient experiences pain, requests medication, experiences some reduction in pain, and then waits for the level to rise before again requesting pain medication. The authors speculate that this cyclical pattern of pain is consistent with patients' expectations; thus they are satisfied. Although this conceptualization has not been empirically tested, studies of patient expectations have found that, among other factors, having more pain than expected (Carroll et al., 1999) or having expectations that pain will be low (Thomas et al., 1998) predicts low ratings of satisfaction. Perceptions of control over pain may also mediate patient satisfaction. Pellino and Ward (1998) used sophisticated data-analytic techniques to examine psychological factors associated with pain experience and patient satisfaction. In a group of patients followed after orthopedic surgery, perceptions of control over pain were more strongly related to patient satisfaction than were ratings of pain severity.

Barriers to Reporting Pain

Patients vary widely in their openness to reporting pain and their subsequent willingness to use pain medications. A growing literature has examined specific attitudes about pain, the use of pain medications, correlates of negative attitudes, and the impact these attitudes have on compliance. The Barriers Questionnaire (Ward et al., 1993) was developed to assess patients' concerns about reporting pain and using pain medications. This 27-item instrument includes items assessing fear of addiction, fear of tolerance, concerns about the side effects of pain medications, the belief that pain is an inevitable consequence of cancer, the belief that good patients do not complain of pain, fear that discussions of pain will distract the physician from addressing cancer, the belief that pain signifies disease progression, and fear of injections. The internal consistency of the scales has been shown to be acceptable, ranging from .54 to .91. Except for the scale assessing concern about injections, a group of patients who were undermedicated for their pain scored consistently higher on each of the scales than to a group of patients who were adequately medicated for pain (Ward et al., 1993). Whether this reflected the patients' willingness to report pain, their physicians' prescriptions, or the patients' willingness to fill and use the prescriptions was not identified. Of note, the scale assessing concerns about addiction received the highest score of all the scales, suggesting that these beliefs are strong and common.

A later study of Puerto Rican patients with cancer found similar results (Ward & Hernandez, 1994). A slightly modified version of the Barriers Questionnaire was adapted for patients with AIDS, and the relationship between higher total scores and undertreatment of pain was replicated (Breitbart et al., 1998). In this study, total scores correlated with global distress and depression. Using multivariate analyses that controlled for gender, education, and injection drug use, Breitbart and colleagues (1998) found that each increment of 1 point on the Barriers Questionnaire was associated with a twofold increase in the likelihood of undermedication.

Summary

The measurement of patient satisfaction with pain management is a relatively new area, and existing scales have evolved with experience. Multiple modifications have been made to the APS-recommended scales, and the extent to which these modifications alter the psychometric properties of the scales has been only partially examined. Patient satisfaction is best regarded as a multidimensional construct that includes behavioral, emotional, and verbal dimensions (McCracken et al., 1997). Unfortunately, most existing measures have focused primarily on the emotional dimension (i.e., satisfaction) and ignored the behavioral (i.e., patients would return to the same pain management service or clinic) and verbal (i.e., patients would recommend the service or clinic to a family member or friend). Moreover, since most existing measures are global measures of outcome, it is not surprising that the correlations with pain intensity are inconsistent. The importance of measuring and improving patient satisfaction is indicated by McCracken and colleagues' (1997) finding that greater patient satisfaction correlated with reduced use of the health care system, including physician consultations and visits for pain.

CONCLUSIONS AND RECOMMENDATIONS

The assessment of acute pain requires consideration of such factors as feasibility, convenience, and clinical utility. No one type of pain intensity scale will be appropriate for all settings, and each type has strengths and weaknesses. When appropriate, VASs are recommended, since they show the strongest scaling properties and generally are more sensitive to treatment effects than the alternatives. However, in many clinical settings NRSs with 11 or 21 points will be adequate and easily implemented. The inclusion of pain relief scales (either categorical or VAS) may improve clinical decision making, since these scales often detect changes not detected by serial measures of pain intensity.

Ratings of pain relief and many ratings of pain intensity require the patient to remember pain. Retrospective ratings of pain intensity, even over as short a period as an hour, are strongly weighted by peak pain experience and end pain experience.

As broader measures of outcome, pain relief ratings may have greater immediate relevance to the clinical environment than do retrospective pain intensity ratings. Furthermore, disparities between changes in pain intensity and ratings of pain relief are likely due to a complex interplay of such factors as response shift bias, attentional limitations, and patient expectations.

Patient satisfaction is a growing area of outcome assessment, but high levels of patient satisfaction do not always indicate adequate pain management. Greater understanding of the factors that influence patient satisfaction, including patient attitudes about pain and adequate pain management, may elucidate the seeming paradox of high satisfaction in the context of high pain. The psychometric properties of currently available measures of patient satisfaction have not been widely explored, particularly since these measures continue to evolve. Existing measures have generally incorporated a limited multidimensional perspective, and further development of these scales is warranted before they are widely adopted in clinical outcome assessment.

The clinician conducting painful procedures will be challenged by two conflicting goals—the accurate measurement of pain versus the optimal treatment of pain. The combined effects on memory of peak pain intensity, end-of-episode pain intensity, and duration neglect have clinical relevance. Clinicians wanting to optimally lower patients' subsequent memories for pain should focus on reducing the peak intensity experienced during the episode (Redelmeier & Kahneman, 1996). If the peak anesthetic effect coincides with the end of the procedure, memory for pain will also be minimized. However, these suggestions may counter the clinician's natural tendency to try to minimize the duration of exposure to pain, sometimes at the "price" of heightening peak pain. Similarly, interventions based on diverting attention away from pain (i.e., distraction) are less likely to be effective if the patient is required to attend to the pain in order to rate its intensity for the purposes of assessment. Therefore, clinicians need to consider the potentially deleterious impact of pain assessment itself when certain types of pain management interventions are used.

ACKNOWLEDGMENTS

The writing of this chapter was supported in part by grants from the National Institutes of Health (No. P01 HD33990) and the U.S. Department of Education (No. H133A700025).

REFERENCES

Agency for Health Care Policy and Research (AHCPR). (1992). *Acute pain management: Operative or medical procedures and trauma* (DHHS Publication No. AHCPR 92-0032). Rockville, MD: U.S. Department of Health and Human Services,.

American Pain Society (APS) Quality of Care Committee. (1995). Quality improvement guidelines for the treatment of acute pain and cancer pain. *Journal of the American Medical Association, 274,* 1874–1880.

Anderson, R. C., & Pitchert, J. W. (1978). Recall of previously unrecallable information following a shift in perspective. *Journal of Verbal Learning and Verbal Behavior, 17,* 1–12.

Angst, M. S., Brose, W. G., & Dyck, J. B. (1999). The relationship between the visual analog pain intensity and pain relief scale changes during analgesic drug studies in chronic pain patients. *Anesthesiology, 91,* 34–41.

Block, A. R., Kremer, E. F., & Gaylor, M. (1980). Behavioral treatment of chronic pain: The spouse as a discriminative cue for pain behavior. *Pain, 9,* 243–252.

Bookbinder, M., Coyle, N., Kiss, M., Goldstein, M. L., Holritz, K., Thaler, H., Gianella, A., Derby, S., Brown, M., Racolin, A., Ho, M. N., & Portenoy, R. K. (1996). Implementing national standards for cancer pain management: Program model and evaluation. *Journal of Pain and Symptom Managment, 12,* 334–347.

Breitbart, W., Passik, S., McDonald, M. V., Rosenfeld, B., Smith, M., Kaim, M., & Funesti-Esch, J. (1998). Patient-related barriers to pain management in ambulatory AIDS patients. *Pain, 76,* 9–16.

Calvin, A., Becker, H., Biering, P., & Grobe, S. (1999). Measuring patient opinion of pain management. *Journal of Pain and Symptom Management, 18,* 17–26.

Campbell, J. (1995). *Pain as the fifth vital sign.* Presidential address to the meeting of the American Pain Society, Los Angeles, CA.

Carroll, K. C., Atkins, P. J., Herold, G. R., Mlcek, C. A., Shively, M., Clopton, P., & Glaser, D. N. (1999). Pain assessment and management in critically ill postoperative and trauma patients: A multisite study. *Americal Journal of Critical Care, 8,* 105–117.

Caudill, M. A. (1995). *Managing pain before it manages you.* New York: Guilford Press.

Christenfeld, N. (1997). Memory for pain and the delayed effects of distraction. *Health Psychology, 16,* 327–330.

Downie, W. W., Leatham, P. A., Rhind, V. M., Wright, V., Branco, J. A., & Anderson, J. A. (1978). Studies with pain rating scales. *Annals of Rheumatic Diseases, 37,* 378–381.

Eich, E., Reeves, J. L., Jaeger, B., & Graff-Radford, S. B. (1985). Memory for pain: Relation between past and present pain intensity. *Pain, 23,* 375–379.

Feine, J. S., Lavigne, G. J., Dao, T. T., Morin, C., & Lund, J. P. (1998). Memories of chronic pain and perceptions of relief. *Pain, 77,* 137–141.

Fischer, D., Stewart, A. L., Bloch, D. A., Lorig, K., Laurent, D., & Holman, H. (1999). Capturing the patient's view of change as a clinical outcome measure. *Journal of the American Medical Association, 282,* 1157-1162.

Fredrickson, B. L., & Kahneman, D. (1993). Duration neglect in retrospective evaluations of affective episodes. *Journal of Personality and Social Psychology, 65,* 45-55.

Gotzsche, P. C. (1990). Sensitivity of effect variables in rheumatoid arthritis: A meta- analysis of 130 placebo controlled NSAID trials. *Journal of Clinical Epidemiology, 43,* 1313-1318.

Golembiewski, R. T., Billingsley, K., & Yeager, S. (1976). Measuring change and persistence in human affairs: Types of change generated by OD designs. *Journal of Applied Behavioral Science, 12,* 133-157.

Herrmann, D. (1995). Reporting current, past, and changed health status: What we know about distortion. *Medical Care, 33*(4, Suppl.), AS89-AS94.

Hirt, E. R. (1990). Do I see only what I expect?: Evidence for an expectancy-guided retrieval model. *Journal of Personality and Social Psychology, 58,* 937-951.

Hirt, E. R., Reickson, G. A., & McDonald, H. E. (1993). The role of expectancy timing and outcome consistency in expectancy-guided retrieval. *Journal of Personality and Social Psychology, 65,* 640-656.

Howard, G. S., Ralph, K. M., Gulanick, N. A., Maxwell, S. E., Nance, S. W., & Gerber, S. K. (1979). Internal validity in pretest–posttest self-report evaluations and a re-evaluation of retrospective pretests. *Applied Psychological Measurements, 3,* 1-23.

Jamison, R. N., Ross, M. J., Hoopman, P., Griffin, F., Levy, J., Daly, M., & Schaffer, J. L. (1997). Assessment of postoperative pain management: Patient satisfaction and perceived helpfulness. *Clinical Journal of Pain, 13,* 229-236.

Jamison, R. N., Sbrocco, T., & Parris, W. C. V. (1989). The influence of physical and psychosocial factors on accuracy of memory for pain in chronic pain patients. *Pain, 37,* 289-294.

Jensen, M. (1997). Validity of self-report. In T. S. Jensen, J. A. Turner, & Z. Wiesenfeld-Hallin (Eds.), *Proceedings of the VIII World Congress on Pain* (pp. 637-661). Amsterdam: Elsevier.

Jensen, M. P., Karoly, P., O'Riordan, E. F., Bland, F., Jr., & Burns, R. S. (1989). The subjective experience of acute pain: An assessment of the utility of 10 indices. *Clinical Journal of Pain, 5,* 153-159.

Jensen, M. P., Miller, L., & Fisher, L. D. (1998). Assessment of pain during medical procedures: A comparison of three scales. *Clinical Journal of Pain, 14,* 343-349.

Jensen, M. P., Turner, J. A., & Romano, J. M. (1994). What is the maximum number of levels needed in pain intensity measurement? *Pain, 58,* 387-392.

Joint Commission on Accreditation of Healthcare Organizations. (1999). New standards to assess and manage pain. *Joint Commission Perspectives, 19*(5), 5.

Kuhajda, M. C., Thorn, B. E., & Klinger, M. R. (1998). The effect of pain on memory for affective words. *Annals of Behavioral Medicine, 20,* 31-35.

Levine, F. M., & DeSimone, L. L. (1991). The effects of experimenter gender on pain report in male and female subjects. *Pain, 44,* 69-72.

Linton, S. J., & Gotestam, K. G. (1983). A clinical comparison of two pain scales: Correlation, remembering chronic pain, and a measure of compliance. *Pain, 17,* 57-65.

Linton, S. J., & Melin, L. (1982). The accuracy of remembering chronic pain. *Pain, 13,* 281-285.

Littman, G. S., Walker, B. R., & Schneider, B. E. (1985). Reassessment of verbal and visual analog ratings in analgesic studies. *Clinical Pharmacolology and Therapeutics, 38,* 16-23.

Lord, C. G., Ross, L., & Lepper, M. (1979). Biased assimilation and attitude polarization: The effects of prior theories on subsequently considered evidence. *Journal of Personality and Social Psychology, 37,* 2098-2109.

Mackie, A. (1989). Further thoughts on analgesia and pain relief. In C. R. Chapman & J. D. Loeser (Eds.), *Issues in pain measurement* (pp. 183-185). New York: Raven Press.

Max, M. (1991). American Pain Society quality assurance standards for relief of acute pain and cancer pain. In M. R. Bond, J. E. Charlton, & C. J. Woolf (Eds.), *Proceedings of the VI World Congress on Pain* (pp. 186-189). Amsterdam: Elsevier.

Max, M., & Laska, E. M. (1991). Single-dose analgesic comparisons. In M. Max, R. Portenoy, & E. Laska (Eds.), *Advances in pain research and therapy* (Vol. 18, pp. 55-95). New York: Raven Press.

McCaul, K. D., & Malott, J. M. (1984). Distraction and coping with pain. *Psychological Bulletin, 95,* 516-533.

McCracken, L. M., Klock, A., Mingay, D. J., Asbury, J. K., & Sinclair, D. M. (1997). Assessment of satisfaction with treatment for chronic pain. *Journal of Pain and Symptom Management, 14,* 292-299.

McNeill, J. A., Sherwood, G. D., Starck, P. L., & Thompson, C. J. (1998). Assessing clinical outcomes: Patient satisfaction with pain management. *Journal of Pain and Symptom Management, 16,* 29-40.

Melzack, R., & Wall, P. D. (1965). Pain mechanisms: A new theory. *Science, 150,* 971-979.

Miaskowski, C., & Donovan, M. (1992). Implementation of the American Pain Society quality assurance standards for relief of acute pain and cancer pain in oncology nursing practice. *Oncology Nursing Forum, 19,* 411-415.

Miaskowski, C., Nichols, R., Brody, R., & Synold, T. (1994). Assessment of patient satisfaction utilizing the American Pain Society's quality assurance standards on acute and cancer-related pain. *Journal of Pain and Symptom Management, 9,* 5-11.

Montgomery, G. H., & Kirsch, I. (1997). Conditioned placebo effects: Stimulus substitution or expectancy change. *Pain, 72,* 107-113.

Norman, P., & Parker, S. (1996). The interpretation of change in verbal reports: Implications for health psychology. *Psychology and Health, 11,* 301-314.

Norvell, K. T., Gaston-Johansson, F., & Fridh, G. (1987). Remembrance of labor pain: How valid are retrospective pain measurements? *Pain, 31,* 77-86.

Pain Management Guideline Panel. (1992). Clinicians' quick reference guide to postoperative pain management in adults: Agency for Health Care Policy and Research, US Department of Health and Human Services. *Journal of Pain and Symptom Management, 7,* 214-228.

Patterson, D. R., Everett, J. J., Burns, G. L., & Marvin, J. A. (1992). Hypnosis for the treatment of burns. *Journal of Consulting and Clinical Psychology, 60,* 1-5.

Pellino, T. A., & Ward, S. E. (1998). Perceived control mediates the relationship between pain severity and patient satisfaction. *Journal of Pain and Symptom Management, 15,* 110–116.

Price, D. D., Bush, F. M., Long, S., & Harkins, S. W. (1994). A comparison of pain measurement characteristics of mechanical visual analogue and simple numerical rating scales. *Pain, 56,* 217–226.

Price, D. D., Milling, L. S., Kirsch, I., Duff, A., Montgomery, G. H., & Nicholls, S. S. (1999). An analysis of factors that contribute to the magnitude of placebo analgesia in an experimental paradigm. *Pain, 83,* 147–156.

Redelmeier, D. A., & Kahneman, D. (1996). Patients memories of painful medical treatments: Real-time and retrospective evaluations of two minimally invasive procedures. *Pain, 66,* 3–8.

Salovey, P., Smith, A. F., Turk, D. C., Jobe, S., & Willis, G. B. (1993). The accuracy of memory for pain: Not so bad most of the time. *American Pain Society Journal, 2,* 184–191.

Seymour, R. A. (1982). The use of pain scales in assessing the efficacy of analgesics in post-operative dental pain. *Euopean Journal of Clinical Pharmacology, 23,* 441–444.

Smith, W. B., Gracely, R. H., & Safer, M. A. (1998). The meaning of pain: Cancer patients' rating and recall of pain intensity and affect. *Pain, 78,* 123–129.

Smith, W. B., & Safer, M. A. (1993). Effects of present pain level on recall of chronic pain and medication use. *Pain, 55,* 355–361.

Sprangers, M. A. G. (1996). Response-shift bias: A challenge to the assessment of patients' quality of life in cancer clinical trials. *Cancer Treatment Reviews, 22*(Suppl.), 55–62.

Stahmer, S. A., Shofer, F. S., Marino, A., Shepherd, S., & Abbuhl, S. (1998). Do quantitative changes in pain intensity correlate with pain relief and satisfaction? *Academy of Emergency Medicine, 5,* 851–857.

Tasmuth, T., Estlanderb, A. M., & Kalso, E. (1996). Effect of present pain and mood on the memory of past postoperative pain in women treated surgically for breast cancer. *Pain, 69,* 343–347.

Thomas, T., Robinson, C., Champion, D., McKell, M., & Pell, M. (1998). Prediction and assessment of the severity of post-operative pain and of satisfaction with management. *Pain, 75,* 177–185.

Todd, K. H., Funk, K. G., Funk, J. P., & Bonacci, R. (1996). Clinical significance of reported changes in pain severity. *Annals of Emergency Medicine, 27,* 485–489.

Turk, D. C., Meichenbaum, D., & Genest, M. (1983). *Pain and behavioral medicine: A cognitive-behavioral perspective.* New York: Guilford Press.

Wallenstein, S. L. (1984). Scaling clinical pain and pain relief. In B. Bromm (Ed.), *Pain measurement in man: Neurophysiological correlates of pain* (pp. 389–396). Amsterdam: Elsevier.

Wallenstein, S. L. (1991). The VAS relief scale and other analgesic measures. In M. Max, R. Portenoy, & E. Laska (Eds.), *Advances in pain research and therapy* (Vol. 18, pp. 97–103). New York: Raven Press.

Wallenstein, S. L., Heidrich, G., III, Kaiko, R., & Houde, R. W. (1980). Clinical evaluation of mild analgesics: The measurement of clinical pain. *British Journal of Clinical Pharmacology, 10*(Suppl. 2), 319S–327S.

Ward, S. E., Goldberg, N., Miller-McCauley, V., Mueller, C., Nolan, A., Pawlik-Plank, D., Robbins, A., Stormoen, D., & Weissman, D. E. (1993). Pain-related barriers to management of cancer pain. *Pain, 52,* 319–324.

Ward, S. E., & Gordon, D. B. (1994). Application of the American Pain Society quality assurance standards. *Pain, 56,* 299–306.

Ward, S. E., & Gordon, D. B. (1996). Patient satisfaction and pain severity as outcomes in pain management: A longitudinal view of one setting's experience. *Journal of Pain and Symptom Management, 11,* 242–251.

Ward, S. E., & Hernandez, L. (1994). Pain-related barriers to management of cancer pain in Puerto Rico. *Pain, 58,* 233–238.

White, B., & Sanders, S. H. (1986). The influence on patients' pain intensity ratings of antecedent reinforcement of pain talk or well talk. *Journal of Behavior Therapy and Experimental Psychiatry, 17,* 155–159.

Zonnefeld, L. N. L., McGrath, P. J., Reid, G. J., & Sorbi, M. J. (1997). Accuracy of children's pain memories. *Pain, 71,* 297–302.

Chapter 23

Clinical Assessment of Low Back Pain

GORDON WADDELL
DENNIS C. TURK

Back pain is one of the most common symptoms presenting for health care. A number of epidemiological surveys have reported that from 50% to 70% of people have back pain at some time in their adult lives (Andersson, Pope, & Frymoyer, 1984; Frymoyer, Pope, Rosen, & Goggin, 1980; Nagi, Riley, & Newby, 1973; Waddell, 1998). Based on the U.S. National Health and Nutrition Survey, Deyo and Tsui-Wu (1987) found that almost 14% reported that they had experienced back pain lasting more than 2 weeks. Fortunately, for the large majority the pain is relatively mild and transient. When asked to rate the intensity of pain, only 18%–22% of those reporting back pain reported that it was severe to excruciating (Frymoyer et al., 1990; Nagi et al., 1973).

Perhaps more important than the prevalence of symptoms is the impact of back pain on the ability to function. Holbrook, Grazier, Kelsey, and Staufer (1984) estimated that 11.7 million Americans are significantly impaired by back pain, with 2.6 million permanently disabled and another 2.6 million temporarily disabled at any one time (National Center for Health Statistics, 1981).

The costs of back pain are staggering. For example, Waddell (1998) estimated the health care costs of spinal disorders in the United States at approximately $33 billion each year, while the annual cost of surgery alone may exceed $8 billion. There are no good estimates of the societal costs of back pain in the United States, but European data suggest that sickness absence, social security and compensation, and other social costs

may far outweigh the health care costs and account for 80%–90% of the total costs of back pain.

A serious problem exists when the statistics cited above are considered in light of current methods available to assess back pain. It is widely accepted that in 70%–90% of cases of back pain, it is not possible to identify or localize any pathological lesion, and in many cases there may be minimal objective evidence of any significant abnormality. Contributing to the failure to identify the etiology of back pain may be the dubious reliability, sensitivity, specificity, and utility of many common examination and laboratory tests used in back pain (Bernard & Kirkaldy-Willis, 1987). Conversely, sensitive imaging procedures may reveal abnormalities that we might assume would be associated with pain; yet these are equally common in asymptomatic people. So, even when such abnormalities are identified in symptomatic patients, they may not necessarily be the source of patients' pain. Thus we must be cautious not to overinterpret either the presence or absence of clinical and radiological findings.

ASSESSING THE PHYSICAL CONTRIBUTION TO THE REPORT OF PAIN

Difficulties in assessing the physical contributions to chronic pain are well recognized, and there are no universal criteria for scoring the presence, absence, or importance of a particular sign (e.g., positive radiographs, distorted gait, limitation of spinal mobility); quantifying the degree of disability; or establishing the association of these findings to treatment outcome (Rudy, Turk, & Brena, 1988; Rudy, Turk, & Brody, 1992; however, see Polatin & Mayer, Chapter 11, this volume). This should hardly be surprising when we consider, for example, that functional assessment of a patient with back pain may include such physical examination procedures as active forward flexion and straight-leg raising (SLR) without specific instructions regarding how these procedures should be conducted, how motivation should be maximized, or how the patient's performance should be scored.

The inherent subjectivity of physical examination is most evident when we note that agreement between physicians may be better for items of patient history than for some items included in the physical examination (Wood, Diehr, Wolcott, Slay, & Tompkins, 1979). The reproducibility of clinical findings even among experienced physicians is low (e.g., Nelson, Allen, Clamp, & deDombal, 1979). Medical attempts to judge whether pain is "organic" or "nonorganic" are particularly unreliable, which is perhaps not surprising, given the lack of conceptual basis for such a distinction (see, e.g., Agre, Magness, Hull, Wright, & Baxter, 1987; Waddell et al., 1982). Yet interobserver agreement in such fundamental clinical measures as spine motion and muscle strength, even when inclinometers or dynamometers are used, may be surprisingly poor (Agre et al., 1987). The discriminative power of many clinical and radiological signs has also been called into question. For example, Rowe (1969) reported that the prevalence of leg length differences, increased lumbosacral angles, spondylolisthesis, transitional lumbosacral vertebrae, and spina bifida occulta were not significantly different in patients with back pain and an asymptomatic control group.

Some of the variability in the results of physical examination is related to patients' behavior during assessment. Measures of flexibility, strength, or timed activities (e.g., time to transverse an obstacle course or cover a specified distance) often reflect nonphysical, highly subjective states as much as physical capabilities. Thus, although physical measurements are more "objective" than patient self-reports, in many instances they are still likely to be influenced by patients' motivation, effort, and psychological state (Pope, Rosen, Wilder, & Frymoyer, 1980; see Polatin & Mayer, Chapter 11).

Frustration with the unavoidable, inherent subjectivity in clinical examination has often led to overreliance on radiological investigations and laboratory tests, but this is unjustified. Substantial interobserver variability has also been documented for more "objective" imaging and laboratory tests, including lumbar spine radiographs (Deyo, McNiesh, & Cone, 1985; Koran, 1975). The sensitivity, specificity, and predictive value of X-rays (Rockey, Tompkins, Wood, & Wolcott, 1978; Torgerson & Dotter, 1976), myelography (Hitselberger & Witten, 1968; Hudgens, 1970), and magnetic resonance imaging (MRI) (Boden, Davis, Dina, Patronas, & Wiesel, 1990; Jensen, Brant-Zawadzki, & Obuchowski, 1994) in the evaluation of patients with back pain—all common strategies for assessing pathology—have been questioned. A significant practical problem with imaging procedures is the high rate of false positives, particularly in older patients.

In short, routine clinical assessment of a patient with low back pain is frequently subjective and unreliable (AHCPR, 1994; McCombe, Fairbank, Cockersole, & Pynsent, 1989). It is usually not possible to make any precise pathological diagnosis or even to identify the anatomical source of the pain. Yet, despite these limitations, a careful clinical history and physical examination remain the best defenses against overinterpreting results from imaging procedures.

In this chapter we consider three aspects of clinical assessment of patients with low back pain, with a specific emphasis on strategies for improving the physical examination. First, we outline an algorithm for making a differential diagnosis of nonspecific low back pain, nerve root pain, and possible serious spinal pathology. The remainder of the chapter concentrates on the clinical assessment of the patient with nonspecific low back pain. In the second section we consider assessment of severity in terms of pain, disability, and physical impairment. Finally, we consider a broader biopsychosocial assessment of cognitive factors, affective disturbance, and illness behavior. Throughout this chapter, the emphasis is on methods suitable for routine clinical assessment rather than research techniques.

DIFFERENTIAL DIAGNOSIS

Most medical textbooks provide a long list of differential diagnoses for low back pain, but many of these conditions are rare. Moreover, attempting to match the presentation of a particular patient to a vaguely recalled series of such "thumbnail" clinical sketches is an illogical and inefficient clinical strategy.

Analysis of a series of 900 patients referred to an orthopedic outpatient clinic (Waddell, 1982) suggests that an alternative approach based on clinical history and examination can be used to separate patients into three broad diagnostic groups: (1) those with nonspecific, mechanical low back pain, (2) those with nerve root pain, and (3) those with possible serious spinal pathology. The term *mechanical* is used simply to indicate that the pain is related to physical activity. The term *serious pathology* includes tumor, infection or inflammatory conditions. Major structural deformities such as scoliosis or kyphosis, and widespread neurological disorders involving more than one nerve root, should be obvious in even the most cursory clinical assessment and examination. Such deformities or major neurological disorders introduce completely different differential diagnoses and are not considered further here. The differential diagnosis among low back pain, nerve root pain, and possible serious pathology, however, is fundamental to the management and prognosis of low back disorders.

Most patients with low back disorders present to the physician with symptoms of pain located in the lower back, with or without radiation of pain to the leg(s), and less commonly with neurological symptoms or spinal deformity. Neurological symptoms or findings are commonly confined to a single dermatome or myotome. Similarly, the common deformity associated with low back pain is a simple sciatic list due to muscle spasm. Differentiation of these presenting symptoms depends on two fundamental decisions that are based largely on careful assessment of the symptoms supplemented by the clinical examination. The first question to consider is whether any leg pain is an indication of nerve root involvement or is simply referred pain. The second question is whether there is any suspicion of possible serious spinal pathology. We address these two questions below.

The Interpretation of Leg Pain and Identification of Nerve Root Involvement

It is wrong to assume that all leg pain is "sciatica," and that it is due to pressure on a nerve root or

that it must be due to a disc prolapse. Percutaneous needle stimulation of most of the structures of the back (either electrically or by injection of hypertonic saline solution) can generate referred pain spreading to the buttocks and thighs, usually posterior and only occasionally spreading much below the knees (Kellgren, 1938, 1939). This dull, aching, and poorly localized referred pain arising from the ligaments, muscles, facet joints, peridural structures, or disc itself (but not due to pressure on the nerve root) may be regarded simply as a spread of low back pain.

Clinically, this radiating pain is usually quite different from the root pain produced when a needle hits a nerve, which is described as sharper and shooting. Moreover, it at least approximates a dermatomal pattern, often contains an element of paresthesia, and at the common L5 and S1 levels usually radiates to the ankle or foot. The first clinical decision, then, is to decide whether leg pain is root pain or simply referred pain. Referred pain can be classified, investigated, and treated together with low back pain. Note that this is based on the anatomical distribution of pain, and that the severity of pain is of little diagnostic value. Referred pain can be every bit as painful as nerve root pain.

Examination findings of root irritation and root compression signs provide additional evidence of nerve root involvement. The earliest signs are those of nerve root irritation, which can be demonstrated by maneuvers that stretch or press upon an irritable nerve to reproduce radiating root pain and paresthesia.

Despite its widespread use, the SLR test is still commonly misinterpreted. Limitation of SLR due to low back pain is simply an index of severity of low back pain and is not in itself a sign of nerve involvement. The specific sign of nerve irritation on SLR is limitation due to reproduction of radiating leg pain. Root irritation may also be demonstrated through reproduction of symptomatic leg pain by direct pressure on the irritable nerve in the bowstring test or by crossover pain from SLR of the asymptomatic leg.

Actual compression of the nerve interferes with electrical function to give muscle wasting, motor weakness, sensory disturbance, or depressed tendon reflexes that approximate the myotome and dermatome supplied by a single nerve root. Nerve function is usually only depressed rather than absent, and classical anesthesia or total paralysis is rare, so that examination for minor neurological changes should be based on comparison with the normal leg.

Final confirmation of nerve root involvement depends on integration of clinical and radiological criteria:

1. Pattern of root pain
2. Root irritation signs
3. Root compression signs
4. Matching radiology by MRI or computed tomography (CT)

In a prospective surgical series of 175 patients, Morris, DiPaola, Vallance, and Waddell (1986) demonstrated that diagnosis based on logical interpretation of these four key criteria provides more accurate prediction of surgical findings than either a "total clinical picture" or overreliance on radiology alone.

Screening for Possible Spinal Pathology

The second essential for differential diagnosis is to have a simple, rapid, yet reliable method of identifying patients who require further investigation for possible spinal pathology—or, alternatively, a method of providing confident reassurance that there is no sign of any serious disease. Both the U.S. (Agency for Health Care Policy and Research, 1994) and U.K. (Clinical Standards Advisory Group, 1994; Royal College of General Practitioners, 1999) clinical guidelines suggest that this should be based on the identification of clinical "red flags":

- Presentation age < 20 years or onset > 55 years
- Violent trauma (e.g., fall from a height, motor vehicle accident)
- Constant, progressive, nonmechanical pain
- Thoracic pain
- Previous history of carcinoma, use of systemic steroids, drug abuse, or HIV
- Systematically unwell (weight loss)
- Persisting severe restriction of lumbar flexion
- Widespread neurology
- Structural deformity
- Investigations when required:
  - Sedimentation rate (ESR) > 25
  - Plain X-ray—vertebral collapse or bone destruction

Summary of Clinical Approach

These basic clinical observations and decisions described above allow differential diagnosis of the three main categories of simple mechanical low back pain, nerve root problems, and possible spinal pathology—each with quite different significance for prognosis, investigation, and management. Several studies have confirmed the reliability, validity, and clinical utility of both the methods of clinical history and examination and the diagnostic classification (Waddell et al., 1982).

We suggest that the approach to low back pain described above and outlined in Figure 23.1 provides a logical basis for clinical assessment that is simple, reliable, and safe. From the most basic medical student level to a specialized back pain clinic, it forms a fundamental framework for clinical decision making and helps to remove some of the confusion and doubt that too often obscure the approach to low back pain.

ASSESSMENT OF SEVERITY

Assessment of the severity of low back disorders is fundamental to making decisions about treatment, assessing clinical progress, and providing social support. Severity can be assessed in terms of pain, disability, and physical impairment. Unfortunately, although these are related, the relationship is weak, and correlations are generally only about .30–.40 (Waddell, Somerville, Henderson, & Newton, 1992). Pain is a symptom; disability is restricted function. Physicians are often requested to undertake disability evaluation, but that is really only an assessment of physical impairment, and the ultimate determination of disability is an administrative rather than a medical responsibility (American Medical Association, 1993; see also Robinson, Chapter 14). It is therefore important to make a very clear conceptual and clinical distinction between pain and disability, and between disability and physical impairment (Waddell, 1998).

Definitions

Pain is "an unpleasant sensory and emotional experience associated with actual or potential tissue damage, or described in terms of such damage" (Merskey, 1979). Impairment and disability are

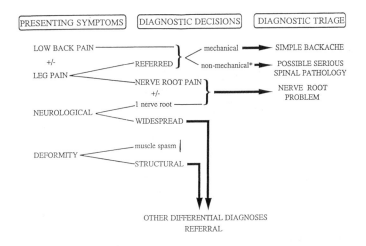

FIGURE 23.1. Differential diagnosis of low back pain. From Waddell (1998, p. 13). Copyright 1998 by Churchill Livingstone. Reprinted by permission.

fundamentally different concepts. *Physical impairment* is "pathological, anatomical or physiological abnormality of structure or function leading to loss of normal bodily ability," while *disability* is the resulting "diminished capacity for everyday activities and gainful employment" or the "limitation of a patient's performance compared to a fit person's of the same age and sex" (Waddell, Allan, & Newton, 1991; Waddell & Main, 1984). Thus the concept of impairment is traditionally based on tissue damage, whereas the concept of disability is task-oriented.

Assessment Techniques

Pain

We have found it useful to consider the following set of aspects of pain in the routine assessment of patients with low back pain. It is important to assess the anatomical distribution, the pattern over time, the intensity of pain, and the quality of the pain.

As suggested by the Quebec Task Force on Spinal Disorders (1987), the simplest and most reliable strategy for assessing back pain is based on its anatomical distribution. This corresponds to the diagnostic classification above into low back pain alone, low back pain with referred pain into the thigh but not below the knee, nerve root pain, and nerve root pain with neurological deficit.

The pattern of pain over time is also a useful distinction. Traditionally, low back pain is classified clinically as acute, recurrent, or chronic. Acute and chronic pain are fundamentally different in kind (Turk & Okifuji, 2001). Acute pain bears a relatively straightforward relationship to peripheral stimulus and tissue damage. There may be some anxiety about the meaning and consequences of the pain, but acute pain, acute disability, and acute illness behavior are usually highly associated with physical findings. Appropriate treatment directed at the underlying physical problem usually relieves acute pain. Chronic pain, chronic disability, and chronic illness behavior, in contrast, may become dissociated from the physical problem, and there may be very little evidence of any remaining tissue damage. Instead, chronic pain and disability become increasingly associated with psychological distress, depression, disease conviction, and illness behavior. The patient seems to adapt to chronic invalidism.

Chronic pain may become a self-sustaining condition that does not respond to traditional medical management (Fordyce, 1976). Physical treatment directed to hypothetical but unidentified tissue damage is not only unsuccessful but may cause further damage. Failed treatment may then reinforce and aggravate pain, psychological distress, illness behavior, and disability.

The distinction between acute and chronic pain is less clear, however, than it was previously thought to be. Earlier views relied primarily on a linear dimension of time; however, there is a growing body of evidence that rather than there being a simple cutoff of time, back pain may be more episodic, with recurrence and exacerbation being the norm. For example, Bergquist-Ullman and Larsson (1977) reported a 1-year recurrence rate for back pain of 62%, and in a prospective study of industrial back injuries reported by Troup, Martin, and Lloyd (1981), there was a recurrence of back trouble requiring further treatment in almost 50% of injured workers during the first year. First return to work is often taken as a measure of successful outcome, but this measure may not reflect recurrent problems. Baldwin, Johnson, and Butler (1996) noted that using first return to work after back injury as a proxy for recovery would lead to the conclusion that 85% of workers in their study recovered from their injuries, when in fact 61% had subsequent episodes of work disability. Thus it cannot be assumed that resolution of symptoms is an indication that a person does not have a persistent problem.

Perhaps the simplest and most useful clinical method for measuring the intensity of pain is some form of Visual Analogue Scale (VAS). We have found that a diagram of a thermometer may be more readily understood by some patients (Figure 23.2). It is simple to administer and to score. The major difficulty lies in interpreting exactly what the pain scale measures.

Verbal Rating Scales (VRSs) are also frequently used to describe the intensity of pain. It is, however, difficult to define the exact meaning of each adjective used, and the "steps" on the scale may not be equal. The fundamental limitation of both VASs and VRSs is that no unidimensional scale can adequately reflect the complexity of the pain experience (see Jensen & Karoly, Chapter 2).

The quality of pain can be assessed to some extent by the use of descriptive adjectives. The most widely used method is the McGill Pain Questionnaire (MPQ; Melzack, 1975). This was originally administered as an interview, but is now generally used as a self-report questionnaire. The adjectives used to describe the pain can be separated into Sensory, Affective, and Evaluative dimensions that provide some assessment of different qualities of the pain. The Affective and Evaluative dimensions bear similarities to other clinical measures of psychological distress. The short-form MPQ (Melzack, 1987) is much simpler and more practical for routine clinical use. (See Melzack & Katz, Chapter 3, for a full discussion of both forms of the MPQ.)

Ratings on any self-report pain scale are in no sense absolute or objective measures of pain, and the patient's report of pain may bear very little

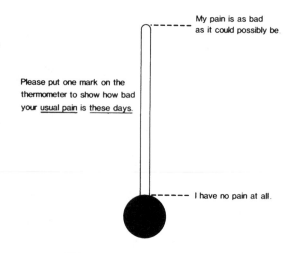

FIGURE 23.2. Pain thermometer.

relationship to any physiological or pathological change. The patient's self-report of pain may include physical sensation, distress, pain behavior, and communication. With these qualifications, it is obviously important not to overinterpret patients' ratings of their pain, but to accept them simply as indicators of how patients choose to communicate their pain experience. Pain communication is important because it serves as a cue for responses from significant others and health professionals. We return to the importance of patient communication when we discuss pain behaviors and illness behaviors below.

Disability

Disability is a complex phenomenon that incorporates physical pathology, the individual's response to that physical insult, and environmental factors that can serve to maintain the disability and associated pain even after the initial physical cause has been resolved. It is important to keep in mind Cailliet's (1969) assertion that "Evaluation is not of disability; it is evaluation of a patient who is disabled" (p. 1380). Clinical assessment of disability must concentrate on loss of function rather than pain. The question is not "Is that activity painful?", but rather "Are you actually restricted in that activity?"

Although disability is predicated on objective determination of what patients can or cannot do, this usually depends on what patients report, and their reports are determined as much by their attitudes, beliefs, and motivations as by objectively determined physical pathology. Consequently, disability determination will always be highly subjective—based on both physicians' attitudes and beliefs concerning the associations between physical pathology and ability to engage in specific physical functions, and the credibility they give to patients' subjective reports (Turk, 1991; see also Robinson, Chapter 14).

To illustrate the subjectivity of physicians making disability determinations, the results of a study reported by Carey, Hadler, Gillings, Stinnett, and Wallsten (1988) can be examined. These investigators asked physicians to rate disability of simulated case vignettes of U.S. Social Security Administration disability claimants. The vignettes were constructed so that the simulated claimant did not even *approximate* the statutory prerequisites for a disability award under the then-current Social Security guidelines. The mean certainty of disability for the individual vignettes ranged from .08 to .43. In addition, the mean certainty estimates across physicians ranged from 0 to .61, indicating substantial variability in how the physicians determined disability. This was likely to have been related to the physicians' interpretation and their conceptualizations of impairment and consequent disability. For example, Carey and colleagues reported that approximately one-half of the physicians surveyed indicated that disability applicants tended to exaggerate their symptoms, and that they could work if they "tried hard enough."

The common or usual level of functioning should be assessed, discounting occasional limitations or special efforts. Waddell and Main (1984) have shown that disability in activities of daily living can be assessed reliably from information obtained in a routine clinical history, and that the following limits are most applicable in low back disorders:

• *Lifting:* Help is required with, or the patient avoids, heavy lifting (30 to 40 pounds—e.g., a heavy suitcase or a 3- to 4-year-old child).

• *Sitting:* Sitting in an ordinary chair is generally limited to less than 30 minutes at a time before the patient needs to get up and move around.

• *Standing:* Standing in one place is generally limited to less than 30 minutes at a time before the patient needs to move around.

• *Walking:* Walking is generally limited to less than 30 minutes or 1–2 miles at a time before the patient needs to rest.

• *Traveling:* Traveling in a car or bus is generally limited to less than 30 minutes at a time before the patient needs to stop and have a break.

• *Social life:* The patient regularly misses or curtails social activities and normal social mobility (not sports, which involve a very different level of disability).

• *Sleep:* Sleep is regularly disturbed by pain (i.e., two or three times per week).

• *Sex life:* Frequency of sexual activity is reduced because of pain.

• *Dressing:* Help is regularly required with footwear (tights, socks, or shoelaces).

Alternatively, disability in activities of daily living can be assessed by self-report questionnaires. The two most widely used measures of low back disability are the Oswestry Low-Back Pain Disability Questionnaire (Fairbank, Couper, Davies, & O'Brien, 1980) and the Roland and Morris Disability Questionnaire (Roland & Morris, 1983). The latter questionnaire (see Appendix 23.A) was developed from the Sickness Impact Profile (SIP; Bergner, Bobbitt, Carter, & Gilson, 1981), which is a widely used general disability questionnaire. Several independent studies have confirmed the value of the Roland and Morris Disability Questionnaire. Deyo (1986) and Jensen, Strom, Turner, and Romano (1992) compared this questionnaire with the original SIP. They found that it was simpler, quicker, and easier to use than the SIP, but gave very similar results in both acute and chronic low back pain. It gave a sensitive measure of change both during recovery from the acute attack and following treatment of chronic pain.

Roberts (1991) directly compared the Roland and Morris instrument with the Oswestry questionnaire. He found that the former was simpler, faster and more acceptable to patients. He agreed with Deyo (1986) that it provides a more sensitive measure of early and acute disability. It gives the best measure of recovery or the early development of chronic pain and disability. Its main disadvantage is that it is less able to measure very severe levels of chronic disability.

Physical Impairment

The aim of physical assessment is to provide objective medical evidence of impairment that is reliable, is distinguishable from nonorganic and behavioral features, distinguishes patients with low back pain from normal asymptomatic subjects, and is related to functional disability. Waddell and Main (1984) identified the following structural factors that were associated with permanent impairment: structural deformity of the spine, structural damage such as fracture or spondylolisthesis, surgical damage and scarring, and long-standing neurological deficit. However, none of these is applicable to the patient with nonspecific low back pain with no nerve root involvement and no previous surgery.

More recently Waddell and colleagues (1992) have developed a comprehensive clinical evaluation of current physical impairment applicable to the patient with simple low back pain. It is essential to standardize the examination technique carefully to obtain reliable results. It should be stressed that this is a measure of current rather than permanent impairment (Cox, Keeley, Barnes, Gatchel, & Mayer, 1988). Moreover, although it is based on objective clinical findings, it assesses restriction of function due to pain rather than any anatomical or structural impairment. In terms of the World Health Organization's (1980) definition, it may be best regarded as a measure of physiological impairment.

Examination Technique for Physical Impairment

The first step is for you, the examiner, to identify the anatomical landmarks (Ohlen, 1989; E. V. Spangfort, personal communication, 1989; J.D.G. Troup, personal communication, 1989). They can be palpated most easily with the patient lying prone with relaxed muscles. Horizontal marks are made on the skin in the midline at S2 and T12/L1. For S2, palpate the inferior border of the posterior superior iliac spines, which lie at the bottom of the posterior part of the iliac crest just below and lateral to the dimples of Venus. Then count up to the spinous processes of T12/L1, checking that the iliac crests approximate to the L4/L5 level. Make vertical marks in the midline over the spinous processes of T12 and T9.

The next step is to have the patient perform warm-up exercises (Keeley et al., 1986): flexion–extension twice, left–right rotation twice, left–right lateral flexion twice, and one more full flexion–extension.

It is then necessary to standardize the examination positions (Ohlen, 1989; Spangfort, personal communication, 1989; Troup, personal communication, 1989). Waddell and his colleagues found particular difficulty in having patients achieve a consistent erect position, but this is essential, as reliable measurement of movement depends on a standard starting point. After personal discussion

with Spangfort and Troup, the most satisfactory position was finally determined to be the following: bare feet, heels together, knees straight with the weight borne evenly on the two legs, looking straight ahead, arms hanging at the sides, relaxed. If there is severe muscle spasm, then ask the patient to get as close to that position as he or she can hold comfortably for several minutes. The supine position is lying relaxed flat on the back, head lying on the couch without a pillow, arms at the sides, and hips and knees extended as fully as possible without tension. The prone position is lying with no pillow, head and shoulders relaxed on the table, and arms by the side.

The only pieces of equipment required are a ballpoint pen, a small spring-loaded centimeter tape from any haberdashery store, and an inclinometer. Although it is not essential, an electronic inclinometer (manufactured by Cybex Division of Lumex, Inc., 100 Spence Street, Bay Shore, NY 11706) may be more convenient.

The following tests can be carried out in any order, but we generally arrange them in sequence in the erect, prone, and supine positions.

1. *Lumbar flexion* is measured with the inclinometer (Mayer, Tencer, Kristoferson, & Mooney, 1984). With the patient in the erect position, make recordings at S2 and then at T12/L1. Next, instruct the patient to bend forward and reach down with the fingertips of both hands as far as possible toward the toes. Make sure the patient keeps his or her knees straight. Keep the patient fully flexed, and obtain the third recording at T12/L1 and the fourth recording at S2. These four readings permit simple calculation of true lumbar flexion, pelvic flexion, and total combined flexion.

2. *Lumbar extension* is measured at T12/L1 (Mayer et al., 1984). Obtain the first reading with the patient in the erect position. Then instruct the patient to arch backward as far as possible, looking up to the ceiling. Support the patient with your free hand on one shoulder to maintain his or her balance and give some feeling of security. Hold this position and obtain the second reading. Simple subtraction gives the measure of total extension.

3. *Lateral lumbar flexion* is also measured at T12/L1. A longer bar is needed on the inclinometer. Obtain the first inclinometer reading with the inclinometer bar lined up tangentially with the spine processes at T9 and T12. Then instruct the patient to lean straight over to one side as far as possible, with fingertips reaching straight down the side of the thigh. The patient should avoid flexing forward

or twisting round. Support the patient's shoulder with a hand and make sure that both feet stay flat on the ground. Repeat on the other side.

4. Reliable examination of *tenderness* can only be achieved by particularly careful standardization. This is carried out with the patient prone, and it is important to make sure the muscles are relaxed. Palpation should be done slowly, without sudden pressure and without hurting the patient unduly. Begin by making sure that there is no superficial tenderness to light skin pinch; this is behavioral in nature and invalidates palpation for deep tenderness (Waddell, McCulloch, Kummel, & Venner, 1980). Local tenderness is then sought to firm pressure, with the ball of the thumb over the spinous process or interspinous ligaments within 1 cm of the midline from T12 to S2. It is important to use specific wording: "Is that painful?" Any response apart from a specific "No" is taken as positive. Any qualified response such as "Only a little bit" is counted positive. If the patient is doubtful or does not answer, then repeat the question "Is it painful when I do that?" Widespread non-anatomical tenderness is again discounted as behavioral (Waddell et al., 1980).

5. *SLR* is carried out with the patient supine, making sure that the head remains relaxed and that the patient does not look up to watch what is happening (modified from Breig & Troup, 1979; Mayer et al., 1984). Hold the foot with one hand, and make sure that the hip is in neutral rotation. Position the inclinometer on the tibial crest just below the tibial tubercle with the other hand and set it at 0. Passively raise the leg, and at the same time hold the inclinometer in position with the other hand, which also holds the knee fully extended. Raise the leg slowly to the maximum tolerated SLR (not the onset of pain) and record the maximum reading obtained. If SLR is less than 75 degrees, then note whether it is limited by back pain, hamstring discomfort, or radiating leg pain (Edgar & Park, 1974). Limited SLR on formal examination should always be checked with distraction at a later stage of the examination (Waddell et al., 1980).

6. *Bilateral active SLR* is tested in the supine position (modified from Biering-Sorensen, 1984). Ask the patient to lift both legs together 6 inches off the couch and to hold that position for 5 seconds. Only count as positive if both calves and heels are clear of the couch. Do not count aloud or use verbal encouragement. Do not allow the patient to use his or her hands to lift the legs. Record whether the patient fails to lift his or her legs clear of the couch at all, can lift them clear but for less than 5 seconds, or manages to hold the position for a full 5 seconds.

7. *Active sit-up* is again tested in the supine position (modified from Biering-Sorensen, 1984; Lloyd & Troup, 1983; National Institute for Occupational Safety and Health, 1988). Have the patient flex the knees to 90 degrees and place the soles of the feet flat on the couch. Hold down both feet with one hand. Instruct the patient to reach up with the fingertips of both hands to touch (not hold) both knees and to hold that position for 5 secs. Only count as successful if the fingertips of both hands reach the patellae. Again record whether the patient fails to reach their knees, is able to reach the knees but for less than 5 seconds, or is able to hold the position for the full 5 seconds.

These seven items are each scored 0 or 1, for a total score of 0–7 (see Table 23.1).

Summary of Assessment of Severity

When pain, physical impairment, and disability are all proportionate, then together they provide an unequivocal measure of the clinical severity of a low back disorder. However, when there is significant disproportion among the patient's report of pain, disability and work loss, and the physician's assessment of the underlying pathology and objective physical impairment, then a more comprehensive assessment is required of the cognitive, affective, and behavioral dimensions of the disorder.

TABLE 23.1. Objective Clinical Evaluation of Physical Impairment

Total flexion	<87°
Total extension	<18°
Average lateral flexion (left and right)	<24°
Average SLR	
Female	<71°
Male	<66°
Spinal tenderness	Positive
Bilateral active SLR	<5 seconds
Sit-up	<5 seconds

Note. Each item is scored 0 or 1, to give a total score of 0–7. Reprinted from Waddell, G., Somerville, D., Henderson, I., and Newton, M. (1992). Objective clinical evaluation of physical impairment in chronic low back pain. *Spine, 17,* 617–628. Copyright 1992 by Harper & Row. Reprinted by permission of Lippincott Williams & Wilkins.

BIOPSYCHOSOCIAL ASSESSMENT

It is important to acknowledge that by its very nature, chronic pain extends over time. Biomedical factors, in the majority of cases, appear to be most important in the acute phase. If the condition becomes more chronic, psychosocial factors may serve to exacerbate and maintain levels of pain and disability. Moreover, secondary physical factors may come to play an important role, with physical deconditioning contributing to weakened muscles, loss of muscle flexibility, and reduced physical endurance. The longer the pain persists, the greater the disability. Thus, pain that persists over time should not be viewed as solely physical or as solely psychologically caused; rather, a set of biomedical and psychosocial factors all contribute to the experience of pain.

Clinical assessment of the patient with low back pain should provide not only a physical assessment and diagnosis but also a comprehensive evaluation of the patient's pain, his or her attitudes and beliefs about the pain, the affective dimension of the pain, the pattern of illness behavior that has developed, and the resulting disability. The most systematic approach is to consider each component of a biopsychosocial model of illness: cognitive, affective, and behavioral (see Figure 23.3).

In clinical practice, however, these generally present and are assessed in the reverse order. Behavioral symptoms and signs present at clinical interview and examination, and often provide the first clinical clue that further psychological assessment is required. Affective disturbance may be detected

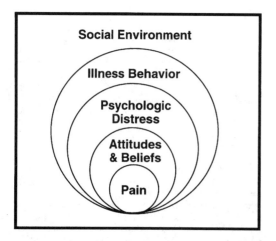

FIGURE 23.3. A biopsychosocial model of chronic pain and disability.

on closer clinical assessment and may be measured by standard psychological assessment or instruments. The underlying cognitive factors are buried most deeply and have been hardest to elucidate.

Illness Behavior

All good clinicians use the clinical interview and examination not only to diagnose physical disease, but also to learn about the patient and his or her response to illness. First, we must recognize that the patient is ill—not only by what he or she tells us, but also by changes in the whole pattern of behavior that we recognize as "sick" or "illness behavior." Unfortunately, traditional clinical training concentrates on disease, whereas assessment of the patient is learned by experience and is largely based on subconscious impressions that are unreliable, difficult to validate, and impossible to teach. What we need to do now is to distinguish the symptoms and signs of illness behavior from those of physical disease.

The Pain Drawing

Clinical observation of illness behavior is most simply illustrated by the pain drawing (Figure 23.4). Patients willingly record their pain on an outline of the body, but the *way* they draw their pain is strongly influenced by emotional distress (Ransford, Cairns, & Mooney, 1976). Poorly localized, widespread, and nonanatomical drawings; expansion or magnification of pain to other areas of the body or outside the body outline; and additional emphasis or comment on the severity of the pain all reflect a patient's distress rather than the physical characteristics of the pain. So the patient's description of pain communicates both physical information about the pain and psychological information about his or her response to the pain. (Contrast drawings A and B in Figure 23.4.) It is not a question of deciding whether the pain is physical or psychogenic and has nothing to do with the origin of the pain, but rather of recognizing which parts of the clinical description of pain are physical and which other parts are emotional in nature, and interpreting them appropriately.

Behavioral Symptoms

Interpretation of a medical history is based on the occurrence of common and hence recognizable patterns of symptoms. The way most patients de-

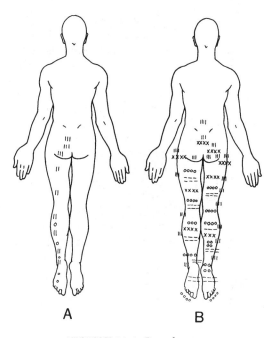

A   **B**

FIGURE 23.4. Pain drawing.

scribe their symptoms approximates anatomical and pathological patterns of disease. Occasionally, however, patients offer descriptions that clearly do not fit clinical experience. These "behavioral" symptoms and signs are vague and ill localized, and fit what Walters (1961) has described as *regional* or *body image* patterns rather than neuroanatomical patterns. They lack the normal relationship to time and physical activity, and are difficult to fit to any reasonable anatomical or pathological mechanism.

Of course, our knowledge is limited, and the fact that we can not understand a physical problem does not in itself mean that it is psychological. Nevertheless, there are some symptoms that do not fit any anatomical, pathological, or neurophysiological explanation, and that have been demonstrated to be more closely related to psychological distress (Waddell, Main, Morris, DiPaola, & Gray, 1984):

1. *Pain at the tip of the tailbone.* Coccydynia can be caused by local direct injury. Coccydynia in a patient with low back pain, however, is often associated with other behavioral symptoms.

2. *Whole-leg pain.* The whole leg is reported to be painful in a stocking distribution, usually from the groin down or below the knee. Such regional patterns of pain do not fit any neuroanatomy or neurophysiology.

3. *Whole-leg numbness.* The whole leg goes numb or dead in a stocking distribution. It usually comes and goes. The distribution again do not fit any normal neuroanatomy or neurophysiology.

4. *Whole leg giving way.* The whole leg gives way or collapses, although very few patients actually fall to the ground. Again, the essential feature is the regional nature of the symptoms, which is clearly different from a localized muscle weakness.

5. *Complete absence of any spells without pain.* The patient's pain has persisted for many years and become progressively worse, without the normal variation and remissions with time.

6. *Intolerance of and reactions to treatments.* Our treatment for low back pain is not very effective, so we should not blame the patient if the pain does not improve. Side effects of treatment are also quite common, but are usually minor or short-lived. One should look more closely, however, at the patient in whom every treatment has to be stopped because it aggravates the pain or causes severe side effects or complications.

7. *Emergency admissions to a hospital.* Non-specific low back pain is so severe that the patient has to be rushed into a hospital as an emergency case. This may be inappropriate behavior on the part of the physician who refers the patient to the hospital or the one who admits him or her, rather than by the patient him- or herself. Nevertheless, it is a measure of the patient's distress and emotional reaction to the pain.

These behavioral symptoms are clearly separate from the common symptoms of physical disease and are closely related to psychological distress (Waddell et al., 1984). They are simple and reliable to assess as part of the routine clinical history. Indeed, most of them are elicited by the standard medical interview, and it is simply a matter of recognizing that these are behavioral rather than physical symptoms. They form a closely interrelated, homogeneous group of symptoms that must be considered as a whole. Assessment should be based on the whole clinical picture, and isolated symptoms should be ignored. No doctor would diagnose a disc prolapse solely on the basis of an absent ankle reflex, and it is equally important not to make a psychological diagnosis on isolated clinical observations. In rare cases these behavioral symptoms can occur in relation to serious spinal pathology, such as tumor, infection, or paraparesis. This particular group of symptoms is therefore only inappropriate to simple low back pain or sciatica and may not be inappropriate in other situations. The symptoms should not be regarded as behavioral until spinal pathology has been excluded.

Nonorganic Signs or Behavioral Responses to Examination

In the same way, Waddell and colleagues (1980) have identified and standardized a group of nonorganic signs—or, more precisely, behavioral responses to examination. Physical findings on medical examination are frequently regarded as objective. But when one human being examines another human being who is in pain, and in the process may deliberately elicit pain—for example, when looking for tenderness or testing SLR—then the examination should not only detect objective physical abnormality, but also provide information about the patient's response to pain. Behavioral responses to examination include the following:

1. *Tenderness.* Tenderness related to physical disease is usually localized to a particular skeletal or neuromuscular structure. Nonorganic tenderness may be superficial or nonanatomical (Figure 23.5).

a. *Superficial tenderness.* The skin is tender to light pinch over a wide area of lumbar skin. A localized band in a posterior primary ramus distribution may be caused by nerve irritation and should be accepted as physical.

b. *Nonanatomical tenderness.* Deep tenderness over a wide area is not localized to any musculoskeletal anatomy, but extends to the thoracic spine, sacrum, or pelvis.

2. *Simulation tests.* These give the impression that a particular maneuver is being carried out when in fact it is not. Usually this is based on movement producing pain. On formal examination, a particular movement causes the patient to report pain. That movement is then simulated without actually being performed. If pain is reported, it is physically inappropriate. It is essential to minimize suggestion.

a. *Axial loading.* Low back pain may be reported on vertical loading over the patient's skull by the examiner's hands (Figure 23.6). Neck pain is common and should be accepted as physical, but organic lumbar pain is surprisingly rare even in the presence of serious spinal pathology such as tumor or infection.

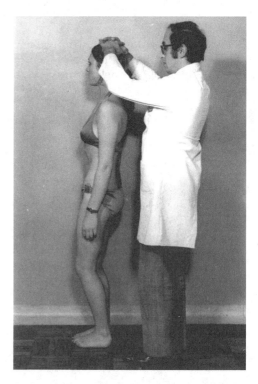

FIGURE 23.6. Axial loading: Back pain on vertical loading on the standing patient's head. From Waddell, G., McCulloch, J. A., Kummel, E., and Venner, R. M. (1980). Nonorganic physical signs in low back pain. *Spine*, 5, 117–125. Copyright 1980 by Harper & Row. Reprinted by permission of Lippincott Williams & Wilkins.

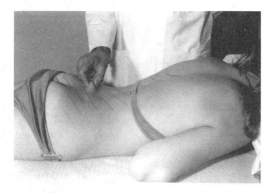

FIGURE 23.5. Nonorganic tenderness showing technique of testing superficial skin tenderness and the area (shaded) frequently involved in widespread nonorganic tenderness. From Waddell, G., McCulloch, J. A., Kummel, E., and Venner, R. M. (1980). Nonorganic physical signs in low back pain. *Spine*, 5, 117–125. Copyright 1980 by Harper & Row. Reprinted by permission of Lippincott Williams & Wilkins.

b. *Simulated rotation*. Back pain is reported when the shoulders and pelvis are passively rotated together in the same plane as the patient stands relaxed with the feet together (Figure 23.7). In the presence of nerve irritation, leg pain may be produced and should be accepted as physical.

3. *Distraction tests*. A positive physical finding is demonstrated in the routine manner, and this finding is then checked while the patient's attention is distracted. Distraction must be nonpainful, nonemotional, and nonsurprising. In its simplest and most effective form, this consists of indirect observation—simply observing the patient throughout the period that he or she is in the examiner's presence, while the patient is unaware of being examined. During examination, parts of the body other than the particular part being formally tested should also be observed. Any finding that is consistently present is likely to be physically based. Findings that are present only on formal examination and disappear at other times are behavioral.

a. *SLR*. SLR is the most useful distraction test (Figure 23.8). A patient with distress or limited pain tolerance may show marked improvement in SLR on distraction compared with formal testing. There are several varia-

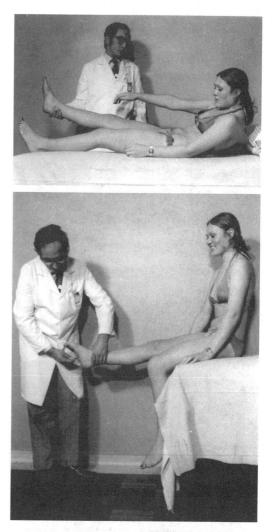

FIGURE 23.8. *Top*: Overreaction to examination: Disproportionate verbalization, facial expression, muscle tension and tremor, collapsing or sweating. *Bottom*: Straight-leg raising improving with distraction. From Waddell, G., McCulloch, J. A., Kummel, E., and Venner, R. M. (1980). Nonorganic physical signs in low back pain. *Spine*, *5*, 117–125. Copyright 1980 by Harper & Row. Reprinted by permission of Lippincott Williams & Wilkins.

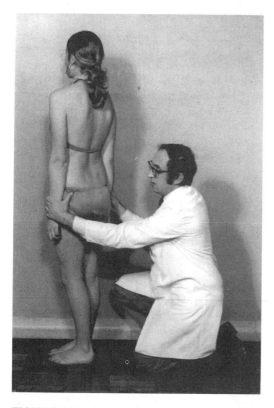

FIGURE 23.7. Simulated rotation: Back pain when shoulders and pelvis are passively rotated in the same plane. From Waddell, G., McCulloch, J. A., Kummel, E., and Venner, R. M. (1980). Nonorganic physical signs in low back pain. *Spine*, *5*, 117–125. Copyright 1980 by Harper & Row. Reprinted by permission of Lippincott Williams & Wilkins.

tions based on sitting. This is commonly known in North America as the "flip test."

4. *Regional disturbances.* Regional disturbances involve a widespread region of neighboring parts such as the leg below the knee. The essential feature is divergence from accepted neuroanatomy.

a. *Weakness.* Weakness is demonstrated on formal testing by jerky "giving way" of many muscle groups that cannot be explained on a localized neurological basis.

b. *Sensory disturbances.* Sensory disturbances include altered sensation to light touch, pinprick, and sometimes other modalities, fitting a "stocking" rather than a dermatomal pattern (Figure 23.9).

Giving way and sensory changes commonly affect the same area, and there may be associated

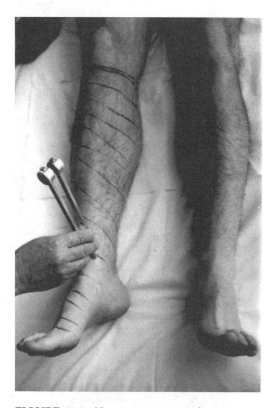

FIGURE 23.9. Nonorganic sensory alteration in a "stocking" distribution affecting light touch, pinprick, and sometimes other modalities. From Waddell, G., McCulloch, J. A., Kummel, E., and Venner, R. M. (1980). Nonorganic physical signs in low back pain. *Spine, 5,* 117–125. Copyright 1980 by Harper & Row. Reprinted by permission of Lippincott Williams & Wilkins.

nonanatomical regional tenderness. Care must be taken, particularly in patients with spinal stenosis or patients who have had repeated spinal surgery, not to mistake multiple nerve root involvement for a regional disturbance.

These nonorganic or behavioral signs are again clearly separable from the standard signs of physical disease and are closely related to emotional distress. Although they can occur in a medicolegal context, they are also commonly seen in the Problem Back Clinic in patients with no legal proceedings or compensation claims. They form part of complex emotional and behavioral patterns. They must not be overinterpreted simplistically as faking, and it is essential to assess the whole clinical picture before drawing conclusions. Rather, they should be regarded as the clinical presentation of psychological distress—as a form of patient–doctor communication or the patient's cry for help.

Overt Pain Behavior

The operant model of chronic pain proposes that when a person is exposed to a nociceptive stimulus that creates tissue damage, the immediate responses are withdrawal and attempts to escape from the pain. These may be accomplished by avoidance of activity believed to cause or exacerbate pain (e.g., work, exercise, movement) or help seeking (e.g., complaining) to reduce the symptoms. The operant model does not concern itself with the subjective experience of pain, but with pain behaviors. *Pain behaviors* are observable communications of pain, distress, and suffering (e.g., moaning, grimacing, limping). Over time, avoidance of activity, distorted ambulation and posture, or both may lead to even greater disability. Moreover, attention to these behavioral reactions by environmental reinforcers (e.g., attention from significant others, monetary compensation) may lead to maintenance of the pain behaviors even when the initial cause of the pain is no longer present (Fordyce, 1976).

Waddell and colleagues (1980) originally included clinical judgment of overreaction to examination as one of the nonorganic signs, but found that this was open to considerable observer bias. The most systematic approach to the assessment of overt pain behaviors is reflected in the work of Keefe and his colleagues (Keefe & Block, 1982; Keefe, Wilkins, & Cook, 1984; see also Keefe, Williams, & Smith, Chapter 10). Keefe and Block (1982) have developed a coding system for the observation of five overt pain behaviors commonly displayed by patients with low back pain in static and dynamic situations. Waddell and Richardson (1992) have confirmed that after careful training these can be assessed by physicians during routine clinical examination. Briefly, these consist of the following:

- *Guarding.* Abnormally stiff, interrupted, or rigid movement while moving from one position to another.
- *Bracing.* A stationary position in which a fully extended limb supports and maintains an abnormal distribution of weight.
- *Rubbing.* Any contact between hand and back (e.g., touching, rubbing, or holding the affected area of pain).
- *Grimacing.* Obvious facial expression of pain, which may include furrowed brow, narrowed eyes, tightened lips, corners of mouth pulled back, and clenched teeth.
- *Sighing.* Obvious exaggerated exhalation of air, usually accompanied by shoulders first rising and then falling; cheeks may be expanded.

These are all methods of assessing illness behavior, or, more specifically, illness presentation in the context of a medical interview and examination. Illness behavior in low back pain can now be assessed in a variety of ways, which can be combined in factor analysis (Waddell & Richardson, 1992):

- Pain drawing (Ransford et al., 1976)
- Behavioral symptoms (Waddell et al., 1984)
- Nonorganic or behavioral signs (Waddell et al., 1980)
- Overt pain behavior (Keefe & Block, 1982; see also Keefe et al., Chapter 10)
- Use of walking aids
- Downtime—the average number of hours spent lying down between 7 A.M. and 11 P.M. (Rosenstiel & Keefe, 1983)

Interpretation of Illness Behavior

In both clinical practice and medicolegal assessment, these methods of observing illness behavior must not be overinterpreted or misinterpreted. Waddell (1998) and Waddell and Main (1984) have listed a number of important caveats:

1. Always carry out diagnostic triage first. Exclude serious spinal pathology or a widespread neurological disorder before considering any question of illness behavior.

2. Clinical observation of illness behavior depends on careful technique. It is particularly important to avoid observer bias and provocation of illness behavior.

3. Isolated behavioral symptoms and signs are of no significance. Many normal patients show a few such symptoms and signs. Only a complete pattern of various types of illness behavior is significant.

4. Behavioral symptoms and signs do not provide any information about the initial cause of the pain and do not mean that a patient does not have "real" physical pain or that the pain is "psychogenic." Most back pain starts with a physical problem in the back, and illness behavior is only one dimension of the patient's current clinical presentation.

5. There is no differential diagnosis between physical disease on the one hand and illness behavior on the other. Most patients have both a physical problem in their backs *and* varying degrees of illness behavior.

6. Illness behavior is not a diagnosis. Clinical observations of illness behavior do not provide a complete psychological assessment and do not provide a psychological or psychiatric diagnosis. They are only screening tests that demonstrate the need for more thorough clinical and psychological assessment of the patient.

7. Behavioral symptoms and signs are not medicolegal tests, but observations of normal human behavior in illness. They do not necessarily mean that a patient is acting or faking or malingering. Most illness behavior occurs in patients with pain who are not in a compensation or adversarial legal situation.

Psychological Distress

Fordyce (1988) has emphasized the distinction between *pain* and *suffering*. The best definition and measure of suffering may be psychological distress. From an extensive review of previous work (Engel, 1959; Merskey & Spear, 1967; Szasz, 1968) and his own detailed clinical studies (Sternbach, 1974, 1977; Sternbach & Timmermans, 1975; Sternbach, Wolf, Murphy, & Akeson, 1973a, 1973b), Sternbach concluded that the most important psychological disturbances associated with pain were anxiety in acute pain and depression in chronic pain.

In their own analysis of chronic low back pain and disability (Main & Waddell, 1982; Waddell et al., 1984), Waddell and his colleagues also found that the most important psychological features were increased bodily awareness (as assessed by the Modified Somatic Perception Questionnaire, or MSPQ; Main, 1983), which appears to be related to anxiety and depressive symptoms (as assessed by the Zung Self-Rating Depression Scale; Zung, 1965). These completely overshadowed other psychological measures of personality traits or fears and beliefs about illness. In particular, increased awareness and reporting of bodily functioning appeared to be a much more powerful clinical concept than theories of hypochondriasis, whereas depressive symptoms appeared to be part of a normal affective dimension of pain rather than a primary psychiatric illness (Sternbach & Timmermans, 1975; Waddell, Morris, DiPaola, Bircher, & Finlayson, 1986). Anxiety, increased bodily awareness, and depression are best regarded clinically as forms of distress—a simple emotional reaction to pain and disability (see Sullivan, Chapter 15, and Bradley & McKendree-Smith, Chapter 16).

Psychological distress cannot be assessed reliably by the general clinician's "clinical impression." One of us (GW) is a spinal surgeon who has a quarter of a century clinical and research experience of back pain, with a particular interest in psychological issues and illness behavior. Recently he studied a series of 120 patients and attempted to rate depression from his routine clinical interview. This rating was then compared with each patient's score on a psychological questionnaire measuring depressive symptoms. His experienced clinical judgment was *hopelessly inaccurate*. Psychological distress can, however, be measured easily and reliably by simple questionnaires such as the MSPQ (Main, 1983; see Appendix 23.B) and either the Beck Depression Inventory (Beck, Ward, Mendelson, Mock, & Erbaugh, 1961) or the Zung Self-Rating Depression Scale (Zung, 1965).

Cognition

Patients' beliefs, appraisals, and expectations about their pain, their ability to cope, their social supports, their disorder, the medicolegal system, the health care system, and their employers are all important, as they may either facilitate or disrupt the patients' sense of control and ability to manage pain. These factors also influence patients' investment in treatment, acceptance of responsi-

bility, perceptions of disability, adherence to treatment recommendations, support from significant others, expectancies for treatment, and acceptance of treatment rationale (Turk & Rudy, 1991).

Cognitive interpretations also will affect how patients present symptoms to significant others, including health care providers and employers. Overt communication of pain, suffering, and distress (i.e., pain behaviors) will enlist responses that may reinforce the pain behaviors and impressions about the seriousness, severity, and uncontrollability of the pain. That is, complaints of pain may lead physicians to prescribe more potent medications (Turk & Okifuji, 1997), order additional diagnostic tests, and initiate treatments (e.g., surgery, increases in analgesic prescription, nerve blocks). Family members may express sympathy, excuse a patient from usual responsibilities, and encourage passivity, thereby fostering further physical deconditioning.

A number of specific attitudes and beliefs have been identified that relate to symptom presentation and adaptation. A patient's beliefs about the effectiveness of his or her coping skills and about whether he or she can execute such skills (*self-efficacy beliefs*) are essential in adaptive coping with pain. It has been suggested that individuals' choice of action and the amount of effort they expend on the action are largely determined by the self-efficacy beliefs. In chronic pain, a belief that pain is uncontrollable is commonly observed (Turk & Rudy, 1992). Such beliefs appear to have a direct impact on functioning and mood, as well as influence patients' willingness to engage in coping efforts.

Cognitive errors or *maladaptive cognitions* are beliefs about oneself and situations that are distorted in a way that they emphasize negative aspects and imply pessimistic sequels (e.g., "My case is hopeless," "I'll never get any better," "I can't do anything I used to do"). Maladaptive cognitions are commonly observed among patients with chronic pain who exhibit "medically incongruent" signs (Reesor & Craig, 1988), suggesting that maladaptive thoughts may adversely affect pain experience. Cognitive errors and distortions have been shown to be associated with depression (Gil, Williams, Keefe, & Beckham, 1990), pain severity (Gil et al., 1990), and disability (Smith, Follick, Ahern, & Adams, 1986).

Psychological factors may also act indirectly on pain and disability by reducing physical activity, and consequently reducing muscle flexibility, strength, tone, and endurance. Fear of reinjury, fear of loss of disability compensation, and job dissatisfaction can also influence the extent of patients' disability (Crombez, Vlaeyen, Heuts, & Lysens, 1999; Vlaeyen, Kole-Snijders, Boeren, & Van Eek, 1995). Clinically, the most important cognitive factor identified from self-report measures of cognitive factors and coping strategies questionnaires (see, e.g., Flor & Turk, 1988; Main, Wood, Spanswick, Roberts, & Robson, 1991; see also DeGood & Tait, Chapter 17) appears to be *catastrophizing* (Rosenstiel & Keefe, 1983), which is closely linked to depressive symptoms (Rudy, Kerns, & Turk, 1988) and low back disability (Main & Waddell, 1991).

It has, however, been argued that these cognitive measures are still too general; thus Waddell, Newton, Henderson, Somerville, and Main (1993) have developed a Fear–Avoidance Beliefs Questionnaire (FABQ). The FABQ is based on fear theory and avoidance behavior (Lenthem, Slade, Troup, & Bentley, 1983) and focuses specifically on the patient's beliefs about how physical activity and work would or might affect his or her low back pain. Fear–avoidance beliefs about work appeared in this study to be the most specific and powerful cognitive factor yet identified to explain work loss due to low back pain. Fear–avoidance beliefs may be detected by a few simple questions in routine clinical interview, or measured more accurately by a self-report questionnaire such as the FABQ (Waddell et al., 1993; see Appendix 23.C).

Psychosocial Risk Factors for Chronicity: "Yellow Flags"

To put the concepts described in this chapter into routine clinical practice, Kendall and colleagues (1997) have described psychosocial "yellow flags" that may help to identify a patient at risk of developing chronic pain and disability at an early stage. A patient may be considered at risk if his or her clinical presentation includes one or more very strong indicators of risk, or several less important factors that combine cumulatively. Kendall and colleagues suggest that the following features consistently predict poor outcomes:

- Presence of a belief that back pain is harmful or potentially severely disabling
- Fear–avoidance behavior (avoiding a movement or activity due to misplaced anticipation of pain) and reduced activity levels
- Tendency toward low mood and withdrawal from social interaction

- An expectation that passive treatments rather than active participation will help

They also suggest the following exploratory questions, which can be phrased in the interviewer's own words:

- "Have you had time off work in the past with back pain?"
- "What do you understand is the cause of your back pain?"
- "What are you expecting will help you?"
- "How is your employer responding to your back pain? Your coworkers? Your family?"
- "What are you doing to cope with back pain?"
- "Do you think that you will return to work? If so, when?"

CONCLUSION

Assessment of back pain requires care and systematic physical examination to arrive at a diagnosis and treatment plan. It is essential that reliable and valid procedures be employed. In order to accomplish this, a great deal of attention has to be given to the manner in which the physical examination is performed. In this chapter we have described a detailed strategy for physical examination.

It is important to acknowledge that for *chronic* back pain, physical examination by itself is not sufficient. A number of psychological and behavioral factors also need to be considered, as there is no simple one-to-one association among physical pathology, pain, and disability. Various psychological assessment instruments are available and many of these are discussed throughout this volume. For both medical and psychological assessment of patients with back pain, clinicians should be careful to select instruments and procedures that have demonstrated good reliability, validity, and utility.

REFERENCES

Agency for Health Care Policy and Research. (1994). *AHCPR 1994 management guidelines for acute low back pain.* Rockville, MD: U.S. Department of Health and Human Services.

Agre, J. C., Magness, J. L., Hull, M., Wright, K. C., & Baxter, T. L. (1987). Strength testing with portable dynamometer: Reliability for upper and low extremities. *Archives of Physical Medicine and Rehabilitation,* 69, 454–458.

American Medical Association. (1993). *Guides to the evaluation of permanent impairment* (4th ed.). Chicago: Author.

Andersson, G. B. J., Pope, M. H., & Frymoyer, J. W. (1984). Epidemiology. In M. H. Pope & J. W. Frymoyer (Eds.), *Occupational low back pain* (pp. 115–124). New York: Praeger.

Baldwin, M. L., Johnson, W. G., & Butler, R. J. (1996). The error of using return-to-work to measure the outcome of health care. *American Journal of Industrial Medicine, 29*, 632–641.

Beck, A. T., Ward, C. H., Mendelson, M. M., Mock, J., & Erbaugh, J. (1961). An inventory for measuring depression. *Archives of General Psychiatry, 4*, 561–571.

Bernard, T. N., Jr., & Kirkaldy-Willis, W. H. (1987). Recognizing specific characteristics of nonspecific low back pain. *Clinical Orthopaedics and Related Research, 217*, 266–280.

Bergner, M., Bobbitt, R. A., Carter, W. B., & Gilson, B. S. (1981). The Sickness Impact Profile: Validation of a health status measure. *Medical Care, 19*, 561–571.

Bergquist-Ullmann, M., & Larsson, U. (1977). Acute low back pain in industry. *Acta Orthopedica Scandinavica, 170*(Suppl.), 1–117.

Biering-Sorensen, F. (1984). Physical measurements at risk indicators for low back trouble over a one year period. *Spine, 9*, 106–119.

Boden, S. D., Davis, D. O., Dina, T. S., Patronas, N. J., & Wiesel, S. W. (1990). Abnormal magnetic-resonance scans of the lumbar spine in asymptomatic subjects. *Journal of Bone and Joint Surgery (American), 72*, 403–408.

Breig, A., & Troup, J. D. G. (1979). Biomechanical considerations in the straight-leg-raising test. *Spine, 3*, 242–250.

Cailliet, R. (1969). Disability evaluation. *Southern Medical Journal, 62*, 1380–1382.

Carey, T. S., Hadler, N. M., Gillings, D., Stinnett, S., & Wallsten, T. (1988). Medical disability assessment of the back pain patient for the Social Security Administration: The weighting of presenting clinical features. *Journal of Epidemiology, 41*, 691–697.

Clinical Standards Advisory Group. (1994). *CSAG 1994 report on back pain*. London: Her Majesty's Stationery Office.

Cox, R., Keeley, J., Barnes, D., Gatchel, R., & Mayer, T. (1988). *Effects of functional restoration treatment upon Waddell impairment/disability ratings in chronic low back pain patients*. Paper presented at the meeting of the International Society for the Study of the Lumbar Spine, Miami, FL.

Crombez, G., Vlaeyen, J. W. S., Heuts, P. H. T. G., & Lysens, R. (1999). Pain related fear is more disabling than pain itself: Evidence on the role of pain-related fear in chronic back pain disability. *Pain, 80*, 329–340.

Deyo, R. A. (1986). Comparative validity of the Sickness Impact Profile and shorter scales for functional assessment in low-back pain. *Spine, 11*, 951–954.

Deyo, R. A., McNiesh, L. M., & Cone, R. O., III. (1985). Observer variability in interpretation of lumbar spine radiographs. *Arthritis and Rheumatism, 28*, 1066–1070.

Deyo, R. A., & Tsui-Wu, Y. J. (1987). Descriptive epidemiology of low back pain and its related medical care in the United States. *Spine, 12*, 264–271.

Edgar, M. A., & Park, W. M. (1974). Induced pain patterns on passive straight-leg raising in low lumbar disc protrusion. *Journal of Bone and Joint Surgery (British), 56*, 658–667.

Engel, G. L. (1959). "Psychogenic" pain and the pain-prone patient. *American Journal of Medicine, 26*, 899–918.

Fairbank, J. C. T., Couper, J., Davies, J. B., & O'Brien, J. P. (1980). The Oswestry Low-Back Pain Disability Questionnaire. *Physiotherapy, 66*, 271–273.

Flor, H., & Turk, D. C. (1988). Chronic back pain and rheumatoid arthritis: Predicting pain and disability from cognitive variables. *Journal of Behavioral Medicine, 11*, 251–265.

Fordyce, W. E. (1976). *Behavioral methods for chronic pain and illness*. St. Louis, MO: Mosby.

Fordyce, W. E. (1988). Pain and suffering: A reappraisal. *American Psychologist, 43*, 267–282.

Frymoyer, J. W., Pope, M. H., Rosen, J., & Goggin, J. (1980). Epidemiologic studies of low back pain. *Spine, 5*, 419–428.

Gil, K. M., Williams, D. A., Keefe, F. J., & Beckham, J. C. (1990). The relationship of negative thoughts to pain and psychological distress. *Behavior Therapy, 21*, 349–352.

Hitselberger, W. E., & Witten, R. M. (1969). Abnormal myelograms in asymptomatic patients. *Journal of Neurosurgery, 28*, 204–208.

Holbrook, T. L., Grazier, K., Kelsey, J. L., & Stauffer, R. N. (1984). *The frequency of occurrence, impact and cost of selected musculoskeletal conditions in the United States*. Park Ridge, IL: American Academy of Orthopedic Surgeons.

Hudgens, R. W. (1970). The predictive value of myelography in the diagnosis of uptured lumbar disc. *Journal of Neurosurgery, 32*, 151–161.

Jensen, M. C., Brant-Zawadzki, M. N., & Obuchowski, N. (1994). Magnetic resonance imaging of the lumbar spine in people without back pain. *New England Journal of Medicine, 331*, 69–73.

Jensen, M. P., Strom, S. E., Turner, J. A., & Romano, J. M. (1992). Validity of the Sickness Impact Profile Roland Scale as a measure of dysfunction in chronic pain patients. *Pain, 50*, 157–162.

Jensen, M. P., Turner, J. A., Romano, J. M., & Karoly, P. (1991). Coping with chronic pain: A critical review of the literature. *Pain, 47*, 249–284.

Keefe, F. J., & Block, A. R. (1982). Development of an observation method for assessing pain behavior in chronic low back pain patients. *Behavior Therapy, 13*, 363–375.

Keefe, F. J., Wilkins, R. H., & Cook, W. A. (1984). Direct observation of pain behavior in low back pain patients during physical examination. *Pain, 20*, 59–68.

Keeley, J., Mayer, T. G., Cox, R., Gatchel, R. J., Smith, J., & Mooney, V. (1986). Quantification of lumbar function: Part 5. Reliability of range of motion measures in the sagittal plane and *in vivo* torso rotation measurement technique. *Spine, 11*, 31–35.

Kellgren, J. H. (1938). Observations on referred pain arising from muscle. *Clinical Science, 3*, 173–190.

Kellgren, J. H. (1939). On the distribution of pain arising from deep somatic structures with charts of segmental pain areas. *Clinical Science, 4*, 35–46.

Kendall, N. A. S., Linton, S. J., & Main, C. J. (1997). *Guide to assessing psychosocial yellow flags in acute low* back pain: Risk factors for long-term disability and work loss. Wellington, New Zealand: Accident Rehabilitation and Compensation Insurance Corporation of New Zealand and the National Health Committee.

Koran, L. M. (1975). Reliability of clinical methods, data, and judgements. *New England Journal of Medicine, 293*, 642-646, 695-701.

Lethem, J., Slade, P. D., Troup, J. D. G., & Bentley, G. (1983). Outline of a fear avoidance model of exaggerated pain perception. *Behaviour Research and Therapy, 21*, 401-408.

Lloyd, D. C., & Troup, J. D. G. (1983). Recurrent back pain and its prediction. *Journal of Social and Occupational Medicine, 33*, 66-74.

Main, C. J. (1983). The Modified Somatic Perception Questionnaire. *Journal of Psychosomatic Research, 27*, 503-514.

Main, C. J., & Waddell, G. (1982). Chronic pain, distress and illness behavior. In C. J. Main (Ed.), *Clinical psychology and medicine* (pp. 1-52). New York: Plenum Press.

Main, C. J., & Waddell, G. (1991). A comparison of cognitive measures in low back pain: Statistical structure and clinical validity at initial assessment. *Pain, 46*, 287-298.

Main, C. J., Wood, P. L. R., Spanswick, C. C., Roberts, A. P., & Robson, J. (1991). *The Pain Locus of Control Questionnaire.* Unpublished manuscript.

Mayer, T. G., Tencer, A. F., Kristoferson, S., & Mooney, V. (1984). Use of noninvasive techniques for quantification of spinal range-of-motion in normal subjects and chronic low-back dysfunction patients. *Spine, 9*, 588-595.

McCombe, P. F., Fairbank, J. C. T., Cockersole, B. C., & Pynsent, P. B. (1989). Reproducibility of physical signs of low-back pain. *Spine, 14*, 908-918.

Melzack, R. (1975). The McGill Pain Questionnaire: Major properties and scoring methods. *Pain, 1*, 277-299.

Melzack, R. (1987). The short-form McGill Pain Questionnaire. *Pain, 30*, 191-197.

Merskey, H. (1979). Pain terms: A list with definitions and notes on usage. *Pain, 6*, 249-252.

Merskey, H., & Spear, F. G. (1967). *Pain: Psychological and psychiatric aspects.* London: Ballière, Tindall, & Cassell.

Morris, E. W., DiPaola, M., Vallance, R., & Waddell, G. (1986). Diagnosis and decision making in lumbar disc prolapse and bony entrapment. *Spine, 11*, 436-439.

Nagi, S. Z., Riley, L. E., & Newby, L. G. (1973). A social epidemiology of back pain in a general population. *Journal of Chronic Disease, 26*, 769-773.

National Center for Health Statistics. (1981). *Prevalence of selected impairments, United States–1977* (Series 10, No. 134; DHHS Publication No. PHS 81-1562). Washington, DC: U.S. Government Printing Office.

National Institute for Occupational Safety and Health. (1988). *National Institute for Occupational Safety and Health low back atlas.* Morgantown, WV: U.S. Department of Health and Human Services.

Nelson, M. A., Allen, P., Clamp, S. E., & deDombal, F. T. (1979). Reliability and reproducibility of clinical findings in low-back pain. *Spine, 4*, 97-101.

Ohlen, G. (1989). *Spinal sagittal configuration and mobility: A kyphometer study.* Unpublished doctoral dissertation, Karolinska Institute, Stockholm, Sweden.

Pope, M. H., Rosen, J. C., Wilder, D. G., & Frymoyer, J. W. (1980). Relation between biomechanical and psychological factors in patients with low back pain. *Spine, 5*, 173-178.

Quebec Task Force on Spinal Disorders. (1987). Scientific approach to the assessment and management of activity-related spinal disorders. *Spine, 12*(Suppl. 1), S1-S59.

Ransford, A. O., Cairns, D., & Mooney, V. (1976). The pain drawing as an aid to the psychological evaluation of patients with low back pain. *Spine, 1*, 127-134.

Reesor, K. A., & Craig, K. (1988). Medically incongruent chronic back pain: Physical limitations, suffering and ineffective coping. *Pain, 32*, 35-45.

Roberts, A. (1991). *The conservative treatment of low back pain.* Unpublished doctoral dissertation, University of Nottingham.

Rockey, J. S., Tompkins, R. W., Wood, R. W., & Wolcott, B. W. (1978). The usefulness of X-ray examinations in the evaluation of patients with back pain. *Journal of Family Practice, 7*, 455-465.

Roland, M., & Morris, R. (1983). A study of the natural history of back pain: Part I. Development of a reliable and sensitive measure of disability in low back pain. *Spine, 8*, 141-144.

Rosenstiel, A. K., & Keefe, F. J. (1983). The use of coping strategies in chronic low back pain: Relationships to patient characteristics and current adjustment. *Pain, 17*, 33-44.

Rowe, M. L. (1969). Low back pain in industry: A position paper. *Journal of Occupational Medicine, 11*, 161-169.

Royal College of General Practitioners. (1999). *RCGP 1999 clinical guidelines for the management of acute low back pain* (2nd ed.). London: Author.

Rudy, T. E., Kerns, R. D., & Turk, D. C. (1988). Chronic pain and depression: Toward a cognitive-behavioral mediational model. *Pain, 35*, 129-140.

Rudy, T. E., Turk, D. C., & Brena, S. F. (1988). Differential utility of medical procedures in the assessment of chronic pain patients. *Pain, 34*, 53-60.

Rudy, T. E., Turk, D. C., & Brady, M. C. (1992). Quantification of biomedical findings in chronic pain: Problems and solutions. In D. C. Turk & R. Melzack (Eds.), *Handbook of pain assessment* (pp. 447-469). New York: Guilford Press.

Smith, T. W., Follick, M. J., Ahern, D. L., & Adams, A. (1986). Cognitive distortion and disability in chronic low back pain. *Cognitive Therapy and Research, 10*, 201-210.

Sternbach, R. A. (1974). *Pain patients: Traits and treatment.* New York: Academic Press.

Sternbach, R. A. (1977). Psychological aspects of chronic pain. *Clinical Orthopaedics and Related Research, 129*, 150-155.

Sternbach, R. A., & Timmermans, G. (1975). Personality changes associated with reduction of pain. *Pain, 1*, 177-182.

Sternbach, R. A., Wolf, S. R., Murphy, R. W., & Akeson, W. H. (1973a). Aspects of chronic low back pain. *Psychosomatics, 14*, 226-229.

Sternbach, R. A., Wolf, S. R., Murphy, R. W., & Akeson, W. H. (1973b). Traits of pain patients: The low-back "loser." *Psychosomatics, 14*, 226-229.

Szasz, T. S. (1968). The psychology of persistent pain: A portrait of l'homme douloureux. In A. Souairac,

J. Cahm, & J. Charpentier (Eds.), *Pain* (pp. 93–113). New York: Academic Press.

Torgerson, W. R., & Dotter, W. E. (1976). Comparative roentgenographic study of the asymptomatic and symptomatic lumbar spine. *Journal of Bone and Joint Surgery (American), 58,* 850.

Troup, J. D. G., Martin, J. D., & Lloyd, D. C. (1981). Back injury in industry: a prospective study. *Spine, 6,* 61–69.

Turk, D. C. (1991). Evaluation of pain and dysfunction. *Journal of Disability, 2,* 1–20.

Turk, D. C., & Okifuji, A. (1997). What factors affect physicians' decisions to prescribe opioids for chronic non-cancer pain patients? *Clinical Journal of Pain, 13,* 330–336.

Turk, D. C., & Okifuji, A. (2001). Pain terms and taxonomies. In J. D. Loeser, C. R. Chapman, S. D. Butler, & D. C. Turk (Eds.), *Bonica's management of pain* (3rd ed., pp. 17–25). Philadelphia: Lippincott Williams & Wilkins.

Turk, D. C., & Rudy, T. E. (1991). Chronic pain and the injured worker: Integrating physical, psychosocial, and behavioral factors. *Journal of Occupational Rehabilitation, 1,* 159–179.

Turk, D. C., & Rudy, T. E. (1992). Cognitive factors and persistent pain: A glimpse into Pandora's box. *Cognitive Therapy and Research, 16,* 99–122.

Vlaeyen, J. W. S., Kole-Snijders, A. M. J., Boeren, R. G. B., & Van Eek, H. (1995). Fear of movement/(re)injury in chronic low back pain and its relation to behavioral performance. *Pain, 62,* 363–372.

Waddell, G. (1982). An approach to backache. *British Journal of Hospital Medicine, 28,* 187–219.

Waddell, G. (1998). *The back pain revolution.* Edinburgh: Churchill Livingstone.

Waddell, G., Allan, D. B., & Newton, M. (1991). Clinical evaluation of disability in low back pain. In J. W. Frymoyer (Ed.), *The adult spine* (pp. 155–166). New York: Raven Press.

Waddell, G., & Main, C. J. (1984). Assessment of severity in low back pain disorders. *Spine, 9,* 204–298.

Waddell, G., Main, C. J., Morris, E. W., DiPaola, M., & Gray, I. C. (1984). Chronic low-back pain, psychologic distress, and illness behavior. *Spine, 9,* 209–213.

Waddell, G., Main, C. J., Morris, E. W., Venner, R. M., Rae, P. S., Sharmy, S. H., & Galloway, H. (1982). Normality and reliability in the clinical assessment of backache. *British Medical Journal, 284,* 1519–1523.

Waddell, G., McCulloch, J. A., Kummel, E., & Venner, R. M. (1980). Nonorganic physical signs in low back pain. *Spine, 5,* 117–125.

Waddell, G., Morris, E. W., DiPaola, M. P., Bircher, M., & Finlayson, D. (1986). A concept of illness tested as an improved basis for surgical decisions in low back disorders. *Spine, 11,* 712–719.

Waddell, G., Newton, M., Henderson, I., Somerville, D., & Main, C. (1993). A Fear-Avoidance Beliefs Questionnaire (FABQ) and the role of fear-avoidance beliefs in chronic low back pain and disability. *Pain, 52,* 157–168.

Waddell, G., & Richardson, J. (1992). Observation of overt pain behavior by physicians during routine clinical examination of patients with low back pain. *Journal of Psychosomatic Research, 36,* 77–87.

Waddell, G., Somerville, D., Henderson, I., & Newton, M. (1992). Objective clinical evaluation of physical impairment in chronic low back pain. *Spine, 17,* 617–628.

Walters, A. (1961). Psychogenic regional pain alias hysterical pain. *Brain, 84,* 1–18.

Wood, R. W., Diehr, P., Wolcott, B. W., Slay, L., & Tompkins, R. K. (1979). Reproducibility of clinical data and decisions in management of upper respiratory illness: Comparison of physician and nonphysician providers. *Medical Care, 17,* 767–779.

World Health Organization. (1980). *International classification of impairment, disability and handicaps.* Geneva: Author.

Zung, W. W. K. (1965). A Self-Rating Depression Scale. *Archives of General Psychiatry, 12,* 63–70.

APPENDIX 23.A. THE ROLAND AND MORRIS DISABILITY QUESTIONNAIRE

When your back hurts, you may find it difficult to do some of the things you normally do. This list contains some sentences that people have used to describe themselves when they have back pain. When you read them, you may find that some stand out because they describe you *today*. As you read the list, think of yourself *today*. When you read a sentence that describes you today, put a tick against it. If the sentence does not describe you, then leave the space blank and go to the next one. Remember, only tick the sentence if you are sure it describes you today.

1. I stay at home most of the time because of my back.
2. I change position frequently to try and get my back comfortable.
3. I walk more slowly than usual because of my back.
4. Because of my back I am not doing any of the jobs that I usually do around the house.
5. Because of my back, I use a handrail to get upstairs.
6. Because of my back, I lie down to rest more often.
7. Because of my back, I have to hold on to something to get out of an easy chair.
8. Because of my back, I try to get other people to do things for me.
9. I get dressed more slowly than usual because of my back.
10. I only stand for short periods of time because of my back.
11. Because of my back, I try not to bend or kneel down.
12. I find it difficult to get out of a chair because of my back.
13. My back is painful almost all the time.
14. I find it difficult to turn over in bed because of my back.
15. My appetite is not very good because of my back pain.
16. I have trouble putting on my socks (or stockings) because of the pain in my back.
17. I only walk short distances because of my back pain.
18. I sleep less well because of my back.
19. Because of my back pain, I get dressed with help from someone else.
20. I sit down for most of the day because of my back.
21. I avoid heavy jobs around the house because of my back.
22. Because of my back pain, I am more irritable and bad-tempered with people than usual.
23. Because of my back, I go upstairs more slowly than usual.
24. I stay in bed most of the time because of my back.

Note. From Roland, M., and Morris, R. (1983). A study of the natural history of back pain: Part I. Development of a reliable and sensitive measure of disability in low back pain. *Spine, 8,* 141–144. Copyright 1983 by Harper & Row. Adapted by permission of Lippincott Williams & Wilkins.

APPENDIX 23.B. MODIFIED SOMATIC PERCEPTION
QUESTIONNAIRE (MSPQ)

Please describe how you have felt during the PAST WEEK by making a check mark (✔) in the appropriate box. Please answer all questions. Do not think too long before answering.

	Not at all	A little / slightly	A great deal / Quite a lot	Extremely / Could not have been worse
Heart rate increasing				
Feeling hot all over*	0	1	2	3
Sweating all over*	0	1	2	3
Sweating in a particular part of the body				
Pulse in neck				
Pounding in head				
Dizziness*	0	1	2	3
Blurring of vision*	0	1	2	3
Feeling faint*	0	1	2	3
Everything appearing unreal				
Nausea*	0	1	2	3
Butterflies in stomach				
Pain or ache in stomach*	0	1	2	3
Stomach churning*	0	1	2	3
Desire to pass water				
Mouth becoming dry*	0	1	2	3
Difficulty swallowing				
Muscles in neck aching*	0	1	2	3
Legs feeling weak*	0	1	2	3
Muscles twitching or jumping*	0	1	2	3
Tense feeling across forehead*	0	1	2	3
Tense feeling in jaw muscles				

Note. The questionnaire as given to patients does not include the scoring. From Main (1983, p. 114). Copyright 1983 by Pergamon Press. Reprinted by permission.

*Only these items are scored and added to give a total score.

APPENDIX 23.C. THE FEAR-AVOIDANCE BELIEFS QUESTIONNAIRE (FABQ)

Here are some of the things which other patients have told us about their pain. For each statement please circle any number from 0 to 6 to say how much physical activities such as bending, lifting, walking or driving affect or would affect *your* back pain.

	COMPLETELY DISAGREE			UNSURE			COMPLETELY AGREE
1 My pain was caused by physical activity	0	1	2	3	4	5	6
2 Physical activity makes my pain worse	0	1	2	3	4	5	6
3 Physical activity might harm my back	0	1	2	3	4	5	6
4 I should not do physical activities which (might) make my pain worse	0	1	2	3	4	5	6
5 I cannot do physical activities which (might) make my pain worse	0	1	2	3	4	5	6

The following statements are about how your normal work affects or would affect your back pain.

	COMPLETELY DISAGREE			UNSURE			COMPLETELY AGREE
6 My pain was caused by my work or by an accident at work	0	1	2	3	4	5	6
7 My work aggravated my pain	0	1	2	3	4	5	6
8 I have a claim for compensation for my pain	0	1	2	3	4	5	6
9 My work is too heavy for me	0	1	2	3	4	5	6
10 My work makes or would make my pain worse	0	1	2	3	4	5	6
11 My work might harm my back	0	1	2	3	4	5	6
12 I should not do my normal work with my present pain	0	1	2	3	4	5	6
13 I cannot do my normal work with my present pain	0	1	2	3	4	5	6
14 I cannot do my normal work till my pain is treated	0	1	2	3	4	5	6
15 I do not think that I will be back to my normal work within 3 months	0	1	2	3	4	5	6
16 I do not think that I will ever be able to go back to that work	0	1	2	3	4	5	6

Scoring:
Scale 1: Fear-avoidance beliefs about work—items 6, 7, 9, 10, 11, 12, 15.
Scale 2: Fear-avoidance beliefs about physical activity—items 2, 3, 4, 5.

Note. Reprinted from *Pain, 52,* G. Waddell, M. Newton, I. Henderson, D. Somerville, and C. Main, A Fear-Avoidance Beliefs Questionnaire (FABQ) and the role of fear-avoidance beliefs in chronic low back pain and disability, 157–168. Copyright 1993, with permission from Elsevier Science.

Chapter 24

Assessment of Patients with Headache

FRANK ANDRASIK

Headache, like other pain disorders covered in this volume, is subjective, without reliable objective markers; is multidetermined; and calls for a comprehensive, multifactorial assessment approach. I begin by addressing the following aspects of assessment: psychological needs of the patient with headache, the importance of a physical/neurological evaluation, various classification and diagnostic considerations, and the biopsychological model of headache as a guiding framework for assessment. I then review the varied approaches used to measure head pain.

PSYCHOLOGICAL NEEDS OF PATIENTS WITH HEADACHE: HEADACHE THROUGH THE EYES OF PATIENTS

By the time a patient is motivated to seek treatment, headache complaints may be embedded within strong emotional reactions. Chief among these are frustration; anger at the headache, oneself, or others; tension and nervousness; depression; helplessness; and fear (Barnat & Lake, 1983). It is important for the practitioner to be cognizant of these concerns and the questions that patients bring with them to the first interview, and to realize that these may be at variance with the clinician's own thinking. Results from Packard's (1979; see also Packard, 1987) survey of the expectations of patients and physicians at the initial interview are instructive. When patients were asked to list what they sought

most from the initial visit, an explanation for what was causing the headache was mentioned foremost (by about one-half). Physicians, on the other hand, stated that they believed patients most wanted pain relief (mentioned by two-thirds). Thus patients and physicians held markedly opposed views about chief needs to be addressed in the initial evaluation. Only a minority of patients felt it might be helpful to have additional medical consultations (eye examinations, laboratory test, etc.). Neither patients nor physicians described psychological evaluation as important, indicating the need for tact when this type of referral is being considered. Packard (1979) aptly summarized the significance of these findings:

> If we believe patients are mainly seeking pain relief, that will be our goal. However, if the patient is mainly concerned about knowing what is wrong, or about his eyes, or simply wants a doctor who is willing to follow him for his headaches, our pill may well be doomed to failure and we may miss our greatest opportunity of providing relief: a simple explanation and reassurance. (p. 373)

Thus patience, reflective listening, support, and education merit high priorities at the initial visit.

MEDICAL EVALUATION

It is imperative that patients be evaluated for the presence of underlying permanent structural defects or diagnosable physical conditions other than a primary headache disorder. Neurological examination and select laboratory evaluations are seen as essential components of the initial workup of the patient with headache, and these should be arranged at the outset. Nonphysician practitioners are urged to refer all potential patients to a physician who is experienced with headache prior to accepting such patients into treatment. In many cases, a close collaboration needs to be maintained with a physician throughout treatment. Even after arranging a medical evaluation, the nonphysician therapist must be continually alert for evidence of a developing underlying physical problem. Table 24.1 contains a list of some "danger signs" that may suggest a need for immediate referral to a physician.

HEADACHE CLASSIFICATION AND DIAGNOSIS

Prior to the 1980s, there was little consensus about headache classification and diagnosis. In 1985 the International Headache Society (IHS) assembled headache experts from around the world to enumerate the various types and subtypes of headache, and to develop explicit inclusion and exclusion diagnostic criteria. Their recommendations were published in 1988 (see IHS Headache Classification Committee, 1988), and have since been endorsed by all national headache societies within IHS, by the World Federation of Neurology, and by the World Health Organization for inclusion in the 10th revision of the *International Classification of Diseases* (see Olesen, 2000, for further discussion). Thirteen different categories resulted (see Table 24.2 on page 456), with categories 1, 2, and 3 (termed *primary headache disorders*) and 5 and 8 (termed *secondary headaches*) being the most likely to be presented for treatment at pain specialty facilities. Diagnostic criteria for categories 1–3 and 5 are listed in Table 24.3 on page 457 (IHS Headache Classification Committee, 1988). It is not uncommon for migraine headache and tension-type headache to "coexist" within the same individual and to warrant separate diagnoses (which in the past had been termed variously *mixed headache, tension–vascular headache,* or *combination headache*).

The IHS classification system and criteria departed markedly from those available previously (e.g., Ad Hoc Committee on the Classification of Headache, 1962). This new system came about from efforts to incorporate previously unacknowledged headache types (headaches associated with

TABLE 24.1. "Danger Signs" in Patients with Headache Pain That May Suggest the Need for Immediate Referral to a Physician

1. Headache is a new symptom for the individual in the past 3 months, or the nature of the headache has changed markedly in the past 3 months.
2. Presence of any sensory or motor deficits preceding or accompanying headache other than the typical visual prodromata of migraine with aura. Examples include weakness or numbness in an extremity, twitching of the hands or feet, aphasia, or slurred speech.
3. Headache is one-sided and has always been on the same side of the head.
4. Headache is due to trauma, especially if it follows a period of unconsciousness (even if only momentary).
5. Headache is constant and unremitting.
6. For a patient reporting tension-type headache-like symptoms:
   a. Pain intensity has been steadily increasing over a period of weeks to months with little or no relief.
   b. Headache is worse in the morning and becomes less severe during the day.
   c. Headache is accompanied by vomiting.
7. Patient has been treated for any kind of cancer and now has a complaint of headache.
8. Patient or significant other reports a noticeable change in personality or behavior or a notable decrease in memory or other intellectual functioning.
9. The patient is over 60 years of age, and the headache is a relatively new complaint.
10. Pain onset is sudden and occurs during conditions of exertion (such as lifting heavy objects), sexual intercourse, or "heated" interpersonal situation.
11. Patient's family has a history of cerebral aneurysm, other vascular anomalies, or polycystic kidneys.

Note. List developed in consultation with Lawrence D. Rodichok, MD. Diagnoses have been modified to be compatible with the classification system developed by the International Headache Society (IHS Headache Classification Committee, 1988). From Andrasik and Baskin (1987, p. 327). Copyright 1987 by Plenum Publishing Corporation. Reprinted by permission.

substances or their withdrawal and those resulting from trauma), to apply advances in etiological understanding, to reclassify certain subtypes (with cluster headache now being recognized as a separate diagnostic entity), and to sharpen overall inclusion and exclusion criteria in the hopes of improving diagnostic accuracy. Accumulated evidence suggests that diagnostic precision has been improved considerably (Weeks, 1992), although problems re-

TABLE 24.2. Classification of Headache

1. Migraine
    1.1 Migraine without aura
    1.2 Migraine with aura
    1.5 Childhood periodic syndromes that may be precursors to or associated with migraine

2. Tension-type headache
    2.1 Episodic tension-type headache
        2.1.1 Episodic tension-type headache associated with disorder of pericranial muscles
        2.1.2 Episodic tension-type headache unassociated with disorder of pericranial muscles
    2.2 Chronic tension-type headache
        2.2.1 Chronic tension-type headache associated with disorder of pericranial muscles
        2.2.2 Chronic tension-type headache unassociated with disorder of pericranial muscles

3. Cluster headache and chronic paroxysmal hemicrania
    3.1 Cluster headache
        3.1.1 Cluster headache periodicity undetermined
        3.1.2 Episodic cluster headache
        3.1.3 Chronic cluster headache

4. Miscellaneous headaches unassociated with structural lesion

5. Headache associated with head trauma
    5.1 Acute posttraumatic headache
        5.1.1 With significant head trauma and/or confirmatory signs
        5.1.2 With minor head trauma and no confirmatory signs
    5.2 Chronic posttraumatic headache
        5.2.1 With significant head trauma and/or confirmatory signs
        5.2.2 With minor head trauma and/or confirmatory signs

6. Headache associated with vascular disorders

7. Headache associated with nonvascular intracranial disorder

8. Headache associated with substances or their withdrawal
    8.1 Headache induced by acute substance use or exposure
        8.1.1 Nitrate/nitrite-induced headache
        8.1.2 Monosodium glutamate-induced headache
        8.1.3 Carbon monoxide-induced headache
        8.1.4 Alcohol-induced headache
        8.1.5 Other substances
    8.2 Headache induced by chronic substance use or exposure
        8.2.1 Ergotamine induced headache
        8.2.2 Analgesics abuse headache
        8.2.3 Other substances
    8.3 Headache from substance withdrawal (acute use)
        8.3.1 Alcohol withdrawal headache (hangover)
        8.3.2 Other substances
    8.4 Headache from substance withdrawal (chronic use)
        8.4.1 Ergotamine withdrawal headache
        8.4.2 Caffeine withdrawal headache
        8.4.3 Narcotics abstinence headache
        8.4.4 Other substances
    8.5 Headache associated with substances but with uncertain mechanism
        8.5.1 Birth control pills or estrogens
        8.5.2 Other substances

9. Headache associated with noncephalic infection

10. Headache associated with metabolic disorder

11. Headache or facial pain associated with disorder of cranium, neck, eyes, ears, nose, sinuses, teeth, mouth, or other facial or cranial structures

12. Cranial neuralgias, nerve trunk pain, and deafferentation pain

13. Headache nonclassifiable

Note. From International Headache Society Headache Classification Committee (1988). Reprinted from *Cephalalgia,* 8(Suppl. 7), 1988, pp. 1–96, by permission of Scandinavian University Press. Copyright is held by Scandinavian University Press.

main in need of attention (Marcus, Nash, & Turk, 1994).

The revised classification system upholds traditional etiological distinctions between migraine headache and tension-type headache, although some argue that the two are simply manifestations of similar underlying physiological processes and differ only with respect to severity of involvement (see, e.g., Raskin, 1988; Saper, 1986). As research unfolds, migraine is being found to be much more complex and multidetermined than was previously thought. In addition to the peripheral vascular abnormalities once thought to be the key causal factors, research has shown that biochemical imbalances, neurotransmitter/receptor dysfunction, and neuronal suppression play pivotal roles as well (Olesen & Goadsby, 2000).

TABLE 24.3. Headache Diagnostic Criteria

1.0   Migraine

1.1   Migraine without aura

   A.   At least 5 attacks fulfilling B–D

   B.   Headache attacks lasting 4–72 hours (2–48 hours for children below age 15), untreated or unsuccessfully treated

   C.   Headache has at least two of the following characteristics:
     1.   Unilateral location
     2.   Pulsating quality
     3.   Moderate or severe intensity (inhibits or prohibits daily activities)
     4.   Aggravation by walking stairs or similar routine physical activity

   D.   During headache at least one of the following:
     1.   nausea and/or vomiting
     2.   photophobia and phonophobia

   E.   At least one of the following:
     1.   History, physical, and neurological examinations do not suggest 1 of the disorders listed in groups 5–11 (see Table 24.2)
     2.   History and/or physical, and/or neurological examinations do suggest such disorder, but is ruled out by appropriate investigations
     3.   Such disorder is present, but migraine attacks do not occur for the first time in close temporal relation to the disorder

1.2   Migraine with aura

   A.   At least 2 attacks fulfilling B

   B.   At least 3 of the following 4 characteristics:
     1.   One or more fully reversible aura symptoms indicating focal cerebral cortical and/or brain stem dysfunction
     2.   At least 1 aura symptom develops gradually over more than 4 minutes or 2 or more symptoms occur in succession
     3.   No aura symptom lasts more than 60 minutes. If more than 1 aura symptom is present, accepted duration is proportionally increased
     4.   Headache follows with a free interval of less than 60 minutes. It may also begin before or simultaneously with the aura

   C.   Same as migraine without aura, criteria E

2.0   Tension-type

2.1   Episodic tension-type headache

   A.   At least 10 previous headache episodes fulfilling criteria B–D. Number of days with such headache < 180/year (< 15/month)

   B.   Headache lasting from 30 minutes to 7 days

   C.   At least 2 of the following pain characteristics:
     1.   Pressing/tightening (nonpulsating) quality
     2.   Mild or moderate intensity (may inhibit, but does not prohibit activities)
     3.   Bilateral location
     4.   No aggravation by walking stairs or similar routine physical activity

   D.   Both of the following:
     1.   No nausea or vomiting (anorexia may occur)
     2.   Photophobia and phonophobia are absent, or one but not the other is present

   E.   Same as migraine without aura, criteria E

2.1.1   Episodic tension-type headache associated with disorder of pericranial muscles

   A.   Fulfills criteria for 2.1

   B.   At least one of the following:
     1.   Increased tenderness of pericranial muscles demonstrated by manual palpation or pressure algometer
     2.   Increased EMG level of pericranial muscles at rest or during physiological tests

2.1.2   Episodic tension-type headache unassociated with disorder of pericranial muscles

   A.   Fulfills criteria for 2.1

   B.   No increased tenderness of pericranial muscles. If studied, EMG of pericranial muscles shows normal levels of activity

2.2   Chronic tension-type headache

   A.   Average headache frequency ≥ 15 days/month (180 days/year) for ≥6 months fulfilling criteria B–D listed below

   B.   Same as criteria B, episodic tension-type headache

   C.   Both of the following:
     1.   No vomiting
     2.   No more than 1 of the following: nausea, photophobia, or phonophobia

   D.   Same as migraine without aura, criteria E

2.2.1   Chronic tension-type headache associated with disorder of pericranial muscles

   A.   Fulfills criteria for 2.2

   B.   Same as criteria B for 2.1.1

(cont.)

TABLE 24.3. (*cont.*)

2.2.2 Chronic tension-type headache unassociated with disorder of pericranial muscles

    A. Fulfills criteria for 2.2

    B. Same as criteria B for 2.1.2

3.1 Cluster headache

    A. At least 5 attacks fulfilling B–D

    B. Severe unilateral orbital, supraorbital, and/or temporal pain lasting 15–180 minutes untreated

    C. Headache is associated with at least 1 of the following signs, which have to be present on the pain side:
      1. Conjunctival injection
      2. Lacrimation
      3. Nasal congestion
      4. Rhinorrhea
      5. Forehead and facial sweating
      6. Miosis
      7. Ptosis
      8. Eyelid edema

    D. Frequency of attacks from 1 every other day to 8 per day

    E. Same as criteria E for 1.1

5.2 Chronic posttraumatic headache

5.2.1 With significant head trauma and/or confirmatory signs

    A. Significance of head trauma documented by at least 1 of the following:
      1. Loss of consciousness
      2. Posttraumatic amnesia lasting more than 10 minutes
      3. At least 2 of the following exhibit relevant abnormality: clinical neurological examination, X-ray of skull, neuroimaging, evoked potentials, spinal fluid examination, vestibular function test, neuropsychological testing

    B. Headache occurs less than 14 days after regaining consciousness (or after trauma, if there has been no loss of consciousness). Headache continues more than 8 weeks after regaining consciousness (or after trauma, if there has been no loss of consciousness).

5.2.2 With minor head trauma and no confirmatory signs

    A. Head trauma that does not satisfy 5.2.1.A

    B. Headache occurs less than 14 days after injury

    C. Headache continues more than 8 weeks after injury

Note. From International Headache Society Headache Classification Committee (1988). Reprinted from *Cephalalgia, 8*(Suppl. 7), 1988, pp. 1–96, by permission of Scandinavian University Press. Copyright is held by Scandinavian University Press.

Tension-type headache has received a number of labels over the years (*muscle contraction headache, psychogenic headache, depression headache, stress headache, conversion headache, psychomyogenic headache,* and the like), which reflect the varied views and confusion about its etiology. Also, it was increasingly noted by clinicians that symptom presentation had a bearing on treatment response (the more chronic the condition, the poorer the response) and that muscular involvement was often not readily detectable. The IHS classification committee proposed a creative four-group scheme to help investigators and clinicians sort out the roles of various causative factors. Patients with tension-type headache are now sorted on the basis of chronicity (episodic vs. chronic) and the presence of identifiable muscle involvement (evidence of pericranial muscle tenderness upon palpation or elevated electromyographic readings vs. the absence of this evidence), resulting in a 2 × 2 classification table. This expanded coding format asks diagnosticians to identify the most likely causative factors by specifying whether one or more of the following factors are present: oromandibular dysfunction, psychosocial stress, anxiety, depression, delusion, muscular stress, drug overuse, or other headache condition.

Unfortunately, researchers have rarely used the level of precision described above when conducting investigations of the pathophysiology of tension-type headache. Thus progress in partialing out the role of the numerous suspected causes has been slow. Researchers continue to pursue actively the role of stress, appraisal, and psychophysiological involvement in the genesis and maintenance of tension-type headache (Andrasik & Passchier, 2000; Jensen, 1999). Use of a bilateral frontal-posterior neck electrode placement, muscle scanning protocols, dynamic recordings (taken during movement and postural changes as well as during rest; e.g., Ahles et al., 1988; Hudzinski & Lawrence, 1988, 1990), and musculoskeletal assessment approaches (Marcus, Scharff, Mercer, & Turk, 1999; Okifuji, Turk, & Marcus, 1999) show promise. (More detailed discussion of psychophysiological assessment approaches that may be helpful with headache patients is provided by Flor in Chapter 5 of this volume.)

A new diagnostic entity that had not been formally recognized previously is *headache associated with substances or their withdrawal.* Research that began to appear in the 1980s suggested that two types of medication commonly prescribed for patients with headache—namely, analgesics (Kudrow, 1982; Rapoport, 1988; Worz, 1983) and ergotamine preparations (Saper, 1987; Saper & Jones, 1986; Worz, 1983)—could lead to rebound headaches if overused. The term *rebound* refers both to the worsening of the headache as the medication wears off and to the fact that the patient goes through a marked exacerbation after abrupt discontinuation of the medication (a withdrawal-like phenomenon). It is this sequence of symptoms that "seduces" patients into taking ever-increasing amounts of medication, establishing a vicious cycle. Saper (1987) describes the typical course of ergotamine dependency syndrome, which is summarized in Table 24.4.

Kudrow (1982) described a similar course in patients with tension-type headache: A patient takes increasing amounts of analgesics, which subsequently increase pain symptomatology and then render the headache refractory to treatments that formerly would have been of benefit. Kudrow conducted one of the few empirical tests of this concept by randomly assigning patients who abused analgesics to one of four conditions (see Table 24.5). Patients were either withdrawn from or allowed to continue analgesics, and simultaneously were assigned to either placebo or amitriptyline (the most commonly prescribed prophylactic drug for

TABLE 24.5. Treatment Outcome

	Amitriptyline	Placebo
Analgesics withdrawn	72%	43%
Analgesics continued	30%	18%

Note. Data from Kudrow (1982).

this form of headache at that time). He found that mere withdrawal from analgesics led to measurable improvement (approximately 40%); that withdrawal combined with a proven medication led to the greatest improvement (nearly 75%); and, perhaps most importantly, that allowing patients to continue analgesics at an abusively high level markedly interfered with the effectiveness of the medication (effectiveness was reduced by approximately two-thirds, or from 72% to 30%). Subsequent research has confirmed these findings regarding medication overuse and its interference potential (Blanchard, Taylor, & Dentinger, 1992; Mathew, Kurman, & Perez, 1990; Michultka, Blanchard, Appelbaum, Jaccard, & Dentinger, 1989).

Clinicians assessing patients with headache need to be familiar with criteria for medication abuse; to inquire carefully about current and past medication consumption; and to arrange, in close collaboration with a physician, a medication reduction/detoxification plan for patients suspected of experiencing medication rebound headache. Ergotamine withdrawal can be difficult to accomplish on an outpatient basis and may require a brief hospital stay. Saper (1987) reports that within 72 hours of ergotamine withdrawal patients may experience their most intense headache, which may last up to 72 hours (often necessitating a 6- or 7-day hospital stay). Saper suggests that dosage days per week are the more critical variable in determining whether ergotamine is being abused. He suggests any patient consuming ergotamine on more than 2 days per week is a candidate for medication withdrawal (when ergotamine is taken 3 or more days per week, significant enough amounts remain in the body to perpetuate the problem). Kudrow (1982) had patients who abused analgesics withdraw on their own (in the absence of therapist contact) and encountered high rates of dropout in the process. Regular therapist contact and support, concurrent provision of appropriate prophylactic medication as necessary, and beginning instruction in behavioral coping skills may help patients to be more successful in completing a needed medication washout period (Worz, 1983).

TABLE 24.4. Clinical Features and Evolution of Ergotamine Dependency Syndrome

History:	Intermittent migraine or mixed migraine tension headache
Ergotamine:	Insidious increase to greater than 2 dosage days per week
Headache:	Parallel increase in migraine frequency
Ergotamine:	Use becomes irresistible and predictable
Headache:	Becomes refractory to other appropriate treatment
Ergotamine:	Patient demands increasing amounts of medicine
Ergotamine:	Withdrawal following continuation
Other:	Concurrent symptoms of depression, sleep disturbance, and loss of well-being

The criteria initially developed by the IHS for drug-induced headache, as well as a revised set developed at the Second International Workshop on Drug-Induced Headache (Diener & Wilkinson, 1988), are listed in Table 24.6. The latter criteria (Wilkinson, 1988) give primary emphasis to days of consumption (consistent with Saper's [1987] theorizing for ergotamine abuse), whereas the former primarily emphasize amount or quantity of consumption. Additional discussion of abuse and abuse-proneness may be found in Saper and Sheftell (2000).

For the typical patient with migraine or tension-type headache (uncomplicated by medication overuse and episodic in presentation), both pharmacological and nonpharmacological approaches appear to be of similar effectiveness (see Bogaard & ter Kuile, 1994; Haddock et al., 1997; Holroyd, 1993; Holroyd & Penzien, 1990; and Holroyd,

Penzien, & Cordingley, 1991, for examples of descriptions and discussions of relaxation, biofeedback, and cognitive-behavioral/stress coping treatment procedures, as well as results from meta-analyses of outcomes including those for certain medications). Behavioral treatments have been found to be especially effective for pediatric patients with headache (Attanasio et al., 1985; Hermann, Kim, & Blanchard, 1995; Holden, Deichmann, & Levy, 1999). For elderly patients with headache, outcomes from behavioral treatments can be quite favorable as well, provided that protocols are adjusted to compensate for any age-related declines in information-processing capabilities (see, e.g., Arena, Hannah, Bruno, & Meador, 1991; Nicholson & Blanchard, 1993).

Attempts to treat patients diagnosed as having cluster headache (see Table 24.3) chiefly via nonpharmacological methods have proven to

TABLE 24.6. Competing Diagnostic Criteria for Drug-Induced Headache

IHS initial criteria[a]	Second International Workshop criteria[b]
8.2 Headache induced by chronic substance use or exposure	
A. Occurs after daily doses of a substance for ≥3 months	1. More than 20 headache days per month
B. A certain required minimum dose should be indicated	2. Daily headache duration exceeding 10 hours
C. Headache is chronic (15 days or more a month)	3. Increase in the severity and frequency of headaches after discontinuation of drug intake (rebound headache)
D. Headache disappears within 1 month after withdrawal of the substance	4. The nature of the underlying headache (e.g., migraine, tension-type headache, cluster headache, posttraumatic headache, or cervicogenic headache) is not related to the syndrome
8.2.1 Ergotamine-induced headache	
A. Is preceded by daily ergotamine intake (oral ≥ 2 mg, rectal ≥ 1 mg)	1. Intake of migraine drugs on more than 20 days per month
B. Is diffuse, pulsating, or distinguished from migraine by absent attack pattern and/or absent associated symptoms	2. Regular intake of ergotamine preparations in combination with barbiturates, codeine, caffeine, antihistamines, or tranquilizers
8.2.2 Analgesics abuse headache	
A. One or more of the following: 1. ≥50 g aspirin a month or equivalent of other mild analgesics 2. ≥100 tablets a month of analgesics combined with barbiturates or other nonnarcotic compounds 3. One or more narcotic analgesics	1. Intake of analgesic drugs on more than 20 days per month 2. Regular intake of analgesics in combination with barbiturates, codeine, caffeine, antihistamines, or tranquilizers

[a]From International Headache Society Headache Classification Committee (1988). Reprinted from *Cephalalgia*, 8(Suppl. 7), 1988, pp. 1–96, by permission of Scandinavian University Press. Copyright is held by Scandinavian University Press.
[b]Based on Wilkinson (1988).

be minimally successful (Blanchard, Andrasik, Jurish, & Teders, 1982). Nonpharmacological approaches may still be of value to some patients with cluster headaches, however, in helping them cope more effectively with the sometimes overwhelming distress that results from having to endure repeated, intense attacks of this type of headache. Patients whose headaches occur following trauma typically experience a multitude of problems that make treatment particularly difficult (Andrasik & Wincze, 1994; Ramadan & Keidel, 2000). A coordinated, interdisciplinary approach, similar to that found in place at most comprehensive pain centers, is typically required (Duckro, Tait, Margolis, & Silvermintz, 1985; Medina, 1992). Inpatient headache specialty units have sprouted across the country to handle complicated cases, such as patients whose headaches are related to both medication abuse and trauma headache (see Table 24.7 for a listing of typical inpatient admission criteria).

Despite the best efforts of the IHS to identify, characterize, and define all basic types of headache, some headache types have still not been addressed adequately. The first of these is daily or near-daily headache, which is widespread, particularly in pain specialty clinics. Studies have shown that a sizeable number of people presenting with chronic daily headache cannot be classified according to the IHS criteria (see Silberstein, Lipton, Solomon, & Mathew, 1994). The diagnostic challenge is distinguishing a migraineous headache that has been "transformed" into a continuous presentation (first discussed by Mathew, Reuveni, & Perez, 1987) from a chronic form of tension-type headache that is due in part to medication rebound, as well as from other rare forms of short-duration daily pain (chronic cluster headache, chronic paroxysmal hemicrania, SUNCT syndrome (an acronym for Short-Lasting, Unilateral, Neuralgia form headaches with Conjunctivitis and Tearing), hypnic headache, idiopathic stabbing headache, or cranial neuralgia; Guitera, Muñoz, Castillo, & Pascual, 1999). Several sets of criteria have been proposed, with the latest being reproduced in Table 24.8. This distinction (migraine vs. other) is especially important when pharmacological treatment is being pursued (see Mathew & Bendtsen, 2000, and Tfelt-Hansen & Welch, 2000a, 2000b, for guidelines for pharmacological management). It has similarly been found that individuals with daily or near-daily high-intensity headache do not respond well to behavioral treatment alone (Blan-

TABLE 24.7. Criteria for Admission to Headache Inpatient Unit

1. Prolonged, unrelenting headache with associated symptoms, such as nausea and vomiting that, if allowed to continue, would pose a further threat to the patient's welfare.
2. Status migraine.
3. Dependence on analgesics, caffeine, narcotics, barbiturates, and/or tranquilizers.
4. Habituation to ergots; if taken on a daily basis, ergots cause a rebound headache when stopped.
5. Pain that is accompanied by serious adverse reactions or complications from therapy; continued use of such therapy aggravates or induces further illness.
6. Pain that occurs in the presence of significant medical disease; appropriate treatment of headache symptoms aggravates or induces further illness.
7. Chronic cluster that is unresponsive to treatment.
8. Treatment requiring co-pharmacy with drugs that may cause a drug interaction and necessitating careful observation within a hospital environment (monoamine oxidase inhibitors and ß-blockers).
9. Patients with probable organic cause of their headache requiring appropriate consultations and perhaps neurosurgical interventions.
10. Severe intractable pain in the presence of dehydration, electrolyte loss, or prostration.
11. Severe pain in association with severe psychiatric disease.
12. Pain necessitating frequent parenteral medication.

Note. From Freitag, F. G. (1999), Headache clinics and inpatient treatment units for headache. In M. L. Diamond and G. D. Solomon (Eds.), *Diamond and Dalessio's the practicing physician's approach to headache* (6th ed., pp. 243–256). Philadelphia: Saunders. Copyright 1992 by Williams & Wilkins. Reprinted by permission of Lippincott Williams & Wilkins.

chard, Appelbaum, Radnitz, Jaccard, & Dentinger, 1989).

Although a sizeable number of females experience all or a portion of their migraine symptoms during a menstrual cycle, little attention has been given to study of such headaches (MacGregor, 1997; Massiou & Bousser, 2000). Indeed, the IHS has not listed menstrual migraine as a diagnostic entity, leaving those who have investigated this topic to develop their own criteria. Early investigations suggested that headaches linked to the menstrual cycle were not as responsive to behavioral treatment as were those migraines occurring at other times. More recent research questions whether this is so (Holroyd & Lipchik, 1997). Clearly, further study of this headache type is warranted.

TABLE 24.8. Proposed Diagnostic Criteria for Transformed Migraine

A. Daily or almost daily (more than 15 days per month) head pain for more than 1 month.
B. Average duration of more than 4 hours per day.
C. History of episodic migraine meeting any IHS criteria 1.1 to 1.6.
D. At some time current headache meets IHS criteria for migraine 1.1 to 1.6 other than duration.
E. At least one of the following:
    1. There is no suggestion of one of the disorders listed in groups 5 to 11.
    2. Such a disorder is suggested, but is ruled out by appropriate investigations.
    3. Such a disorder is present, but first migraine attacks do not occur in close temporal relation to the disorder.

Note. From Guitera, V., Muñoz, P., Castillo, J., and Pascual, J. (1999). Transformed migraine: A proposal for the modification of its diagnostic criteria based on recent epidemiological data. *Cephalalgia, 19,* 847–850. Copyright 1999 by Blackwell Science Ltd. Reprinted by permission.

A BIOPSYCHOLOGICAL FRAMEWORK FOR HEADACHE ASSESSMENT

The biopsychological model of headache states that the likelihood of any individual experiencing headache depends upon the specific pathophysiological mechanisms that are "triggered" by the interplay of the individual's physiological status (e.g., level of autonomic arousal); environmental factors (e.g., stressful circumstances, certain foods, alcohol, toxins, hormonal fluctuations); the individual's ability to cope with these factors (both cognitively and behaviorally); and consequential factors that may serve to reinforce, and thus increase, the person's chances of reporting head pain (Martin, 1993; Waggoner & Andrasik, 1990). The main determinant for the resulting headache is the pathophysiological biological response system that is activated. Psychological factors do not play a causal role per se. Rather, psychological factors contribute to headache as (1) triggering factors; (2) maintaining or exacerbating factors (to illustrate, ask a patient which is worse—onset of a headache when the patient is refreshed and rested, or when work and family frustrations are at a peak); and (3) sequelae to continued head pain and subsequent life disruption.

The prolonged presence of headache begins to exert a psychological toll on the patient over time, such that the patient becomes "sick and tired of

feeling sick and tired." The negative thoughts and emotions arising from the repeated experience of headache can thus become further stressors or trigger factors in and of themselves (referred to as *headache-related distress*), serving at that point both to help maintain the disorder and to increase the severity and likelihood of future attacks. Pointing out the direct and indirect psychological influences on headache may make it easier for the patient to understand and accept the role of psychological factors, and can often facilitate referral for adjunctive psychological/psychiatric care when needed. This model points out the various areas to address in interviewing patients with headache.

A number of behavioral, lifestyle, hormonal, environmental, and dietary factors may precipitate headaches (see the following sources for more extended discussion: Gallagher, 1990; Holroyd, Lipchik, & Penzien, 1998; Paiva & Hering-Hanit, 2000). Systematic record keeping can be helpful in identifying such triggers. Relationships, however, are not always obvious. A given stimulus does not always serve as a precipitant, and multiple stimuli may have to operate in concert in order to trigger a headache. When it is possible to identify precipitants, avoiding or limiting exposure to them can be quite helpful in staving off headaches. A more involved form of monitoring—typically, that utilized in cognitive-behavioral or stress coping training—may be necessary for identifying behavioral and lifestyle factors to target for treatment. Intensive self-monitoring skills are used to enable participants to identify the covert and overt events that precede, accompany, and follow stressful or headache-eliciting transactions. Patients seek to identify the sensations, feelings, thoughts, and behaviors associated with stressful events and headache attacks. As a patient becomes adept at self-monitoring, the therapist assists the patient in identifying relationships among situational variables (e.g., criticism from significant other); thoughts (e.g., "I can't do anything right"); and emotional, behavioral, and symptomatic responses (e.g., depression, withdrawal, and headache).

Figure 24.1 summarizes a day of recording by a patient being treated with cognitive-behavioral therapy (Holroyd & Andrasik, 1982). This patient's diary provides fertile ground for hypotheses for intervention. Headache onset, it is noted, is preceded by resentment and anxiety over work demands and by the apparent sexual overtures of a fellow employee, as well as by nausea and sensations of tingling and lightheadedness. The patient does not appear to be able to resolve these con-

Time	Situation	Physical sensations	Thoughts	Feeling (0–100)	Behavior
8:00 AM	Breakfast, husband says I look "scattered"	—	Worry about getting to work on time (e.g., If I'm late Mr. _____ will notice)	Anxiety (25) Hurt (20)	Rush through breakfast, leave dishes in sink
10:00 AM	Given too many technical letters to type	Upset stomach from coffee, tense muscles	Everybody assumes I'm superwoman. No one takes account of other demands on my time	Anxiety (30) Annoyance (20)	Rushed typing, curt on telephone, take extra long break to calm down
12:00 noon	Jerry (fellow employee and supervisor) asks me to lunch. Talks suggestively about recent divorce	Lightheaded, tingling sensations in head and face, nausea	Jerry in on the make. I don't like fending him off—so why am I here? Am I seductive?	Anxiety (50) Awkwardness (40) Is that a feeling?	Try and offer sympathy but resent ulterior motive. Probably curt
2:00 PM	Spencer gives me long report with 5 tables to be done by 5:00	Headache—back of neck	F--- him—he didn't even ask what else I had to do. Fantasize Spencer stuck in elevator. No time to relax	Anger (60) Anxiety (60)	Typing report— distractedly
4:00 PM	Report completed	Headache worsening, nausea	If I could quit ruminating and was more organized I would get more work done	Anger (40) Anxiety (50)	Give report for correction. Complain to Susan. Type letters

FIGURE 24.1. Sample from self-monitoring record of events associated with onset of headache. From Holroyd and Andrasik (1982, p. 303). Copyright 1982 by Academic Press, Inc. Reprinted by permission.

flicts and the accompanying emotional distress in an effective manner, in part due to her persistent negative self-talk and rumination. Poor nutrition and problems with time management may be serving as further contributing factors that need attention. Not all self-monitoring yields such rich assessment data, and most patients with headache experience at least some of their headaches as appearing without warning or identifiable precipitants. These headaches are dealt with by attempting to modify the psychological correlates of headache and altering factors in the patients' lives that may increase vulnerability to headache, even when they do not occur in close proximity to the headache attacks themselves.

The psychological status of a patient deserves special attention, in order to identify conditions (e.g., formal thought disorder, certain personality disorders) that may interfere with treatment and need to be handled prior to treatment of the headache per se, or that may otherwise compromise

treatment (see Merikangas & Stevens, 1997, and Radat et al., 1999; see also Sullivan, Chapter 15, and Bradley & McKendree-Smith, Chapter 16, this volume). For example, studies have consistently shown that patients displaying only minor elevations on a scale commonly used to assess depression (the Beck Depression Inventory) have a diminished response to self-regulatory treatments (Blanchard et al., 1985; Jacob, Turner, Szekely, & Eidelman, 1983) and even abortive courses of medication (Holroyd et al., 1988). Other variables (anxiety; scales 1, 2, and 3 of the Minnesota Multiphasic Personality Inventory) have been suggested as predictive of response to behavioral treatments as well (Blanchard et al., 1985; Werder, Sargent, & Coyne, 1981).

The relationship between stress and headache has long been noted in the literature (Henryk-Gutt & Rees, 1973; Howarth, 1965). Stress-induced migraine may occur not at the peak of stress, but during a period of relaxation immediately following stress (e.g., April 16 for tax accountants, the end of the term for teachers). Stress probably interacts with other precipitants to increase vulnerability to migraine, without necessarily precipitating any particular migraine episode. It is important to realize that a patient's stress experience is idiosyncratic; stress rests within the individual's cognitive interpretive framework. That is, what determines whether any given event is stressful is more a function of how the patient appraises the event.

Lazarus and Folkman (1984) distinguish two types of appraisal: *primary* (whether a given event is judged to be significant to the patient's well-being) and *secondary* (whether the patient possesses the available resources or options to respond successfully to the event). What is appraised as significant by one individual may not be appraised as such by another. For any given patient with headache, stress is likely to be operating in one or more ways and in concert with other various biological influences. Take as an example, the headache sufferer who is able to drink a glass or two of red wine and escape headache when feeling "on top of the world," but is not able to do so when overworked, eating on the run, and so on. Therapists need to recognize that major stressful life events are not always the main culprit. Rather, more recent evidence indicates that everyday "ups and downs" or "hassles" are sufficient to engage biological headache mechanisms (De Benedittis & Lorenzetti, 1992; Holm, Holroyd, Hursey, & Penzien, 1986; Levor, Cohen, Naliboff, McArchur, & Heuser, 1986). (For more discussion of psychological and cognitive aspects, see Sullivan, Chapter 15; Bradley & McKendree-Smith, Chapter 16; and DeGood & Tait, Chapter 17.)

Fordyce (1976) has pointed out how pain complaints can be maintained by environmental consequences. Fowler (1975) has applied this perspective to patients with headache. A patient is most likely to "learn" pain behavior when (1) pain behavior is positively reinforced or rewarded, or (2) "well" behavior is insufficiently reinforced, punished, or aversive (see Keefe, Williams, & Smith, Chapter 10). Therapists can unwittingly become a part of the learned pain behavior process in several different ways. Attention from others is a near-universal reinforcer; the sympathetic ear of a therapist can be especially powerful. Medication-prescribing practices can foster untoward learning effects as well. Palliative medications are often prescribed on an "as-needed" basis, accompanied by the caution "Take this only when you really need it; it is powerful and may be addicting." When instructed in this

manner, many patients will delay taking the medication until their pain becomes barely tolerable or approaches maximum level. If the medication effectively relieves the headache, medication-taking behavior has become strongly reinforced and is likely to become more frequent in the future (according to principles of learning theory).

A final trap can occur when treating patients whose headache severity has markedly compromised their day-to-day functioning (a common occurrence with posttraumatic headache). Such patients are typically instructed, "Do only what you can," or "Continue your activities until the pain becomes unbearable." The patient begins an activity, experiences increased pain, and then stops. Stopping the activity reduces discomfort and makes the patient less likely to engage in activity in the future. Consequently, a therapist needs to probe for environmental conditions, including familial factors (see Romano & Schmaling, Chapter 18, and Jacob & Kerns, Chapter 19), that may be serving to maintain headache pain behavior, and to be aware of how he or she may subtly begin to contribute to the headache problem itself.

Some ways out of these traps are to lessen (gradually) the attention given to pain symptoms; to encourage and reinforce efforts to cope with head pain (e.g., asking "How are you trying to manage your headaches?" rather than "How is your headache today?"); to encourage an inactive patient to set daily goals and stick to them despite the pain level; and to arrange for needed analgesic medications to be taken on a time-contingent, as opposed to a pain-contingent, basis. Fordyce (1976) presents a detailed format for questions to ask of patients and family members being treated for chronic pain. Such questions are also appropriate to consider in evaluating with headache patients (see, as well, Romano & Schmaling, Chapter 18, and Jacob & Kerns, Chapter 19).

When significant cognitive deficits or diminished cognitive capacities are observed or suspected (as in the case of posttraumatic headache), it may be helpful to conduct a structured neuropsychological screening to determine whether referral to a clinical neuropsychologist is warranted. Penzien, Rains, and Holroyd (1993) recommend use of the Cognitive Capacities Screening Examination (Jacobs, Bernhard, Delgado, & Strain, 1977) or the Mini-Mental State (Folstein, Folstein, & McHugh, 1975) for this purpose. However, these measures seem to have little utility on a routine basis in a headache practice. When tested in such a setting, only

2 of 88 patients scored in the range suggesting significant organic involvement (Lawson et al., 1988).

MEASUREMENT OF HEADACHE PAIN

The Headache Diary/Log

Pain is a private event, and no method yet exists that can reliably objectify any headache parameters. By default, subjective ratings of head pain, sampled daily, have come to be regarded as the "gold standard." In early research on headache (Budzynski, Stoyva, Adler, & Mullaney, 1973), patients completed very detailed self-monitoring records like the one depicted in Figure 24.2 on a daily basis. The recording grid was typically reproduced on a 3 × 5-inch index card; and participants were asked to make hourly determinations of their head pain on a graded intensity scale, and also to record any medications consumed. Because change in headache can occur along varied dimensions (change in frequency, duration, or severity), data from the records were summarized in various ways: (1) frequency—number of discrete headaches over a specified interval; (2) duration—length of time between headache onset and offset; (3) intensity/severity—rated on a preset scale, and summarized as either the mean or the peak (or highest) intensity value for a given period, which allowed the therapist to determine whether the "edge" was being taken off headaches; and (4) headache index/activity—a composite measure that incorporated all dimensions, calculated by summing all intensity values (which would yield a value of 53 for the sample record in Figure 24.2). This was felt to reflect the total burden or suffering of patients.

In behavioral treatment studies, the composite diary measure has been utilized most consistently. However, committees recently tasked by the IHS to develop guidelines for conducting and evaluating pharmacological agents have recommended that composite measures no longer be used (IHS Committee on Clinical Trials in Migraine, 1999; IHS Committee on Clinical Trials in Tension-Type Headache, 1999). This index is seen as weighting severity and duration in an arbitrary manner, which renders it of little value when comparisons are being made across subjects. Furthermore, the clinical meaning of changes is noted to be unclear. Rather, these committees recommend that the following serve as the primary diary measures of headache pain:

1. *Number of days with headache in a 4-week period.* (The specification of measurement intervals that last at least 4 weeks departs from the recommendations of Blanchard, Hillhouse, Appelbaum, & Jaccard, 1987, who, in comparing baseline periods of varied intervals, concluded that 2 weeks were adequate for research investigations and 1 week was adequate for clinical purposes for tension-type headache, and that 3 weeks were adequate for research investigations and 2 weeks were adequate for clinical purposes for migraine headache or the two types combined. They concluded further that a single week of monitoring was adequate for gauging improvement at follow-up assessment.)

2. *Severity of attacks.* This is rated on either a 4-point scale—where 0 = no headache; 1 = mild headache (allowing normal activity); 2 = moderate headache (disturbing but not prohibiting normal activity, bed rest is not necessary); and 3 = severe headache (normal activity has to be discontinued, bed rest may be necessary)—or a Visual Analogue Scale (VAS), with one end anchored as "none" and the other as "very severe."

3. *Headache duration in hours.*

4. *Responder rate.* This rate is defined as the number or percentage of patients achieving a reduction in headache days or headache duration per day that is equal to or greater than 50%. This definition is in accord with the recommendations of Blanchard and Schwarz (1988).

Several modifications to the intensive, hourly recording format have been proposed in order to improve adherence and accuracy. Epstein and Abel (1977), when directly observing patients, noted that most did not record continuously; rather, they would periodically fill in omitted recordings later by recall. Their modified procedure asked patients to make ratings only four times per day: wakeup/breakfast, lunch, evening meal, and bedtime. These events tend to occur at fairly regular times during a patient's day and are times that are easily discriminated. Collins and Martin (1980) compared this reduced-demand format to a bihourly monitoring schedule and found that they yielded fairly equivalent results. Epstein and Abel additionally asked patients to record situational variables and methods used to manage pain. They also attempted to evaluate possible extralaboratory indications of headache by conducting clinical interviews or engaging in telephone conversations with persons in the patient's natural environment (spouse, personal physician, etc.), hoping to find information that

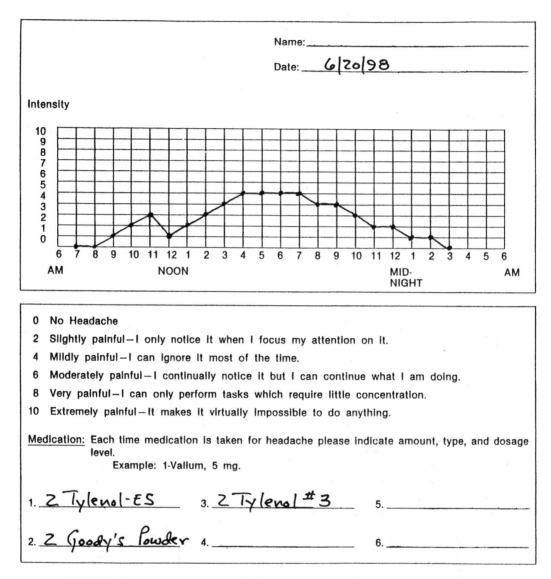

Name: _____

Date: _6/20/98_____

Intensity

0   No Headache

2   Slightly painful—I only notice it when I focus my attention on it.

4   Mildly painful—I can ignore it most of the time.

6   Moderately painful—I continually notice it but I can continue what I am doing.

8   Very painful—I can only perform tasks which require little concentration.

10 Extremely painful—It makes it virtually impossible to do anything.

<u>Medication:</u> Each time medication is taken for headache please indicate amount, type, and dosage level.
    Example: 1-Valium, 5 mg.

1. _2 Tylenol-ES_   3. _2 Tylenol #3_   5. _____

2. _2 Goody's Powder_   4. _____   6. _____

FIGURE 24.2. Front (top panel) and back side (bottom panel) of a sample headache diary.

would provide additional insights for treatment planning and progress assessment.

Although a time-sampling format (such as four times per day) is less demanding for patients and is likely to yield more reliable and valid data, it does have some shortcomings. With this type of approach, it is not possible to obtain true measures for frequency and duration of headache. If either of these are of prime interest to the therapist or researcher, then the format will have to be altered. Chronic or unwavering pain lends itself quite nicely to either format, but a clinician may want to make alterations for people with infrequent, but discrete

and prolonged, migraine attacks. In the latter case, a patient can make ratings repeatedly throughout an attack or, alternatively, can note the time of onset and offset and then perform a single rating of peak headache intensity. This will allow the therapist to keep track of all key parameters. We have used this procedure successfully in an investigation of self-regulatory treatment for pediatric migraines (Andrasik, Burke, Attanasio, & Rosenblum, 1985). If patients resist recording on multiple occasions throughout the day, then a single recording at the end of the day is most advisable. Occasionally a patient's symptoms will display "reactivity" when being recorded systematically and will worsen because of this increased symptom focus. These reactions are typically short-lived, but if they persist, many alternatives can be substituted.

A critical concern with any type of daily monitoring record is the level of patient adherence. In an analogue sample of college students, approximately 40% of subjects evidenced some degree of nonadherence. The most common form of noncompliance involved subjects' recalling and completing ratings at a later time (Collins & Thompson, 1979). Reviewing pain records regularly, socially praising efforts to comply (yet refraining from punishing noncompliance), and having the patient mail records to the office when gaps between appointments are large may help emphasize the importance of and facilitate accurate record keeping.

It is common for clinicians to have their patients monitor headache on a systematic basis during treatment, but to conduct follow-up evaluations by interview or questionnaire completion. Several studies have examined correspondence between these two approaches: prospective, daily monitoring versus retrospective, global determinations (Andrasik et al., 1985; Andrasik & Holroyd, 1980; Cahn & Cram, 1980). Very different results emerge, with the latter believed to yield biased overestimates of improvement. The clinician needs to be aware of bias when it is necessary to alter measures midstream, and should not be lulled into uncritical acceptance of biased global reports of benefit.

Alternative or Supplementary Approaches

A number of supplementary and alternative approaches have been developed to assess headaches. Four may be easily adopted by practitioners and researchers: (1) measurement of multiple aspects of pain, (2) social validation of patient improvement, (3) measurement of pain behavior or behavior motivated by pain, and (4) assessment of impact on other aspects of functioning.

Multiple Dimensions of Head Pain

The experience of pain is complex and includes several dimensions or aspects, such as sensory, affective, and evaluative (see Jensen & Karoly, Chapter 2; Price, Riley, & Wade, Chapter 4; and Dworkin & Sherman, Chapter 32). The sensory component, for example, includes stimulus attributes such as intensity, location, and quality of the

pain; the affective (or reactive) component involves a patient's emotional reaction to the pain, fears about what the pain may signal, and concerns about ability to cope in a socially acceptable manner. Research suggests that the headache diary as typically used is sensitive primarily to the sensory (or intensity) dimension and is not all that effective for tapping into the affective dimension (Andrasik, Blanchard, Ahles, Pallmeyer, & Barron, 1981). We adapted Tursky's (1976) idiographic multidimensional measurement technique for separating the two dimensions of pain (sensory and affective) in the aforementioned study (Andrasik et al., 1981). Although effective, Tursky's procedure requires considerable patient time for administration and therapist time for scoring, which restricts its utility for everyday clinical application. Items contained in the McGill Pain Questionnaire (Melzack, 1975; see also Melzack & Katz, Chapter 3) are similarly designed to access varied components of pain, and these items may be more practical for use by therapists.

Price, McGrath, Rafii, and Buckingham (1983) successfully piloted a procedure for assessing the sensory and affective aspects of chronic pain by use of VASs (see Jensen & Karoly, Chapter 2). Their approach could be adapted for use by patients with headache and repeated at various times during the day. In their procedure, the VASs were anchored as follows: "no sensation" and "the most intense sensation imaginable" for the sensory dimension, and "not bad at all" and "the most intense bad feeling possible for me" for the affective dimension.

The clinical utility of considering multiple aspects of the pain experience is illustrated by the following. When standard headache diary measures are used alone, it is common for a patient to complete treatment with no appreciable change being reflected in pain ratings. Upon interview, such patients often describe marked improvement, most notably in the level of distress now experienced. Although it is possible that such comments result from efforts or perceived demands to please the therapist, it seems more likely that even though the sensory aspects of pain have not changed, significant change has occurred in the affective realm. In support of this notion, patients may report "Even though my head hurts just as much, I don't let it bother me so," or "It still hurts a lot, but I can cope with it better now." Failure to incorporate aspects other than the sensory dimension may lead to a loss of much clinically important information.

Social Validation of Improvement

Another approach we have found useful is based on the notions of social validity (Kazdin, 1977; Wolf, 1978). In a supporting investigation, we administered a brief questionnaire to a significant other identified by each patient (parent, spouse, child, roommate) upon completion of treatment, and asked the significant other to complete these forms and return them to us without conferring with the patient (Blanchard, Andrasik, Neff, Jurish, & O'Keefe, 1981). One part of the questionnaire asked the significant other to rate the degree of change in the patient's headache activity since the patient entered treatment.

Ratings were made on a 100-mm VAS, which was anchored at the left end by "unchanged or worse" and at the right by "extremely improved or completely cured." Measuring the distance between the left end of the scale and the point indicated by the significant other yielded a percentage improvement score (ranging from 0% to 100%). Ratings provided by significant others correlated modestly (r = .44) with actual diary ratings completed by the patients, suggesting some usefulness to this approach. When the line of best fit was plotted for data collected from 62 patients, it was noted to

intercept the Y axis above the 0 point; at the point at which patient diaries reflected 0% improvement, ratings by significant others reflected about 30% improvement (see Figure 24.3). Based on this, it is possible that the data provided by significant others are positively biased, or that the significant others may be reacting to another aspect of pain (such as the affective component). Yet another possible explanation is that measurement biases could be operating because the two measures that were compared had different endpoints (ratings by significant others could not reflect deterioration, whereas the diary measures could). If clinicians decide to use this type of approach, it is recommended that the description for the left end of the VAS be modified to read something like "markedly worse," and that "no change/no improvement" be centered midway between the two endpoints (Andrasik, 2001).

Behavior Motivated by Head Pain

Philips (1983a, 1983b) has pointed out the limitations of measurement approaches that rely solely on subjective reports of patients with headache. The fundamental problem is that the physiological, subjective, and behavioral aspects are not perfectly

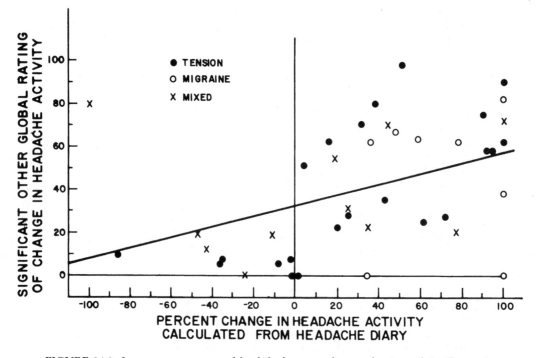

FIGURE 24.3. Improvement as assessed by daily diary recordings and ratings of significant others.

correlated. Attention to all dimensions is needed to provide the most helpful assessment. Philips and Hunter (1981) reported on the preliminary development of a behavioral checklist for use with headache patients, which was subsequently refined by Philips and Jahanshahi (1986). The revised checklist is composed of 49 items, with items designed to yield three different subscores (Avoidance Behavior, Verbal and Nonverbal Complaints, and Help-Seeking Behavior) and a total score. In the 1986 study, several psychometric properties were investigated (test–retest reliability, factor structure, and construct validity). One-week test–retest coefficients were acceptable for all scores except Help-Seeking Behavior ($r = .53$). Thirteen rather than the hypothesized three factors emerged, and they, along with item loadings, are presented in Table 24.9. Although numerous factors emerged, the majority were subcomponents of three general cate-

TABLE 24.9. PA2 Varimax-Rotated Factor Matrix Including Only Items with Loadings > 0.30

Factor 1. Social Avoidance (21.9%)[a]

Item 44	Avoid discos/dances	0.76
Item 32	Avoid party-going	0.71
Item 36	Avoid cinema	0.68
Item 26	Avoid pub-going	0.53
Item 31	Avoid travel in cars	0.51
Item 48	Avoid having visitors	0.50
Item 29	Avoid visiting	0.49
Item 27	Avoid sex	0.41

Factor 2. Housework Activities (27.2%)

Item 11	Avoid heavy housework	0.69
Item 42	Avoid light housework	0.61
Item 24	Avoid shopping	0.54
Item 38	Avoid odd jobs in house	0.50
Item 45	Slow down in physical movements	0.48
Item 5	Avoid cooking	0.47
Item 25	Limp, drag yourself	0.38

Factor 3. Daily Mobility Avoidance (31.6%)

Item 2	Avoid lifting objects	0.70
Item 3	Avoid public transportation	0.56
Item 8	Avoid walking stairs	0.54
Item 7	Avoid restaurants	0.53
Item 49	Avoid carrying	0.48
Item 16	Avoid bending	0.41
Item 46	Avoid stretching	0.34

Factor 4. Activities Avoidance (35.6%)

Item 18	Avoid gardening	0.64
Item 23	Avoid cleaning car	0.54
Item 22	Avoid time on hobbies	0.44

Factor 5. Daily Exercise Avoidance (39.2%)

Item 20	Avoid standing	0.53
Item 19	Avoid walking	0.46
Item 39	Avoid spending time with cohabiters	0.40
Item 9	Avoid gentle exercise	0.38

Factor 6. Stimulation Avoidance (42.6%)

Item 34	Avoid loud noise	0.63
Item 33	Lie down/rest/sleep	0.50
Item 12	Avoid bright lights	0.30
Item 15	Avoid going to work	0.27

Factor 7. Nonverbal Complaint (45.7%)

Item 47	Grimace, frown, pull face	0.60
Item 30	Sigh, moan, cry out	0.54
Item 37	Change posture	0.46
Item 10	Grip, rub, stroke site of pain	0.36

Factor 8. Verbal Complaint (48.5%)

Item 21	Tell a friend	0.67
Item 43	Tell acquaintance	0.62
Item 6	Tell someone in family	0.54

Factor 9. Self-Help Strategies A (51.2%)

Item 40	Have alcohol	0.51
Item 35	Go swimming	0.49
Item 13	Sit on hard chair	0.30

Factor 10. Self-Help Strategies B (53.8%)

Item 41	Have back massaged	0.50
Item 4	Apply heat	0.37

Factor 11. Medication (56.1%)

Item 1	Take prescribed pill	0.57
Item 28	Take unprescribed pill	0.51

Factor 12. Cry (58.4%)

Item 14	Cry	0.44

Factor 13. Distract (60.5%)

Item 17	Distract yourself by reading, etc.	0.57

Note. Reprinted from *Behaviour Research and Therapy*, 24, H. C. Philips and M. Jahanshahi, The components of pain behaviour report, 117–125. Copyright 1986, with permission from Elsevier Science.

[a]The cumulative percentage of variance is given in parentheses.

gories. Avoidance behaviors predominated the first six factors, complaint behaviors characterized the next two factors, while self-help behaviors comprised the next two factors. Thus only six unique domains emerged (Avoidance, Complaints, Self-Help, Medication, Crying, and Distraction). Caution is suggested in interpreting the latter two factors, as each of these factors contain only one item. Overall, construct validity was supported.

Philips and Jahanshahi (1986) point out that the practical use of this revised checklist calculation of the factor scores permits more precise specification of the type of pain behavior emitted by patients, which then can be used for planning treatment. For example, patients receiving high Verbal and Nonverbal Complaint factor scores may be especially prone to secondary gain and may require certain environmental modifications. Those scoring high on the Medication factor may be more prone to problems from medication rebound. It is important to remember that the scale as used by Philips and Jahanshahi is completed by patients themselves, and thus constitutes *self-report* of behavior (not actual behavior). Several of the factors could be adapted to permit actual behavior observations, with information provided by treatment staff, significant others, and so on. Appelbaum, Radnitz, Blanchard, and Prins (1988) conducted an investigation very similar to that of Philips and Jahanshahi, and readers may find their more abbreviated scale of interest.

Medication consumption has frequently been monitored, as another way to assess behavior motivated by pain. The most direct way to assess this aspect is to ask patients to record or count the number of pills consumed. Simple pill counts become problematic when patients take more than one medication, when they switch medications during treatment, or when comparison across patients is desired. Coyne, Sargent, Segerson, and Obourn (1976) had medical experts rate the potency for various analgesic preparations used to control migraine. We (Blanchard & Andrasik, 1985) subsequently added to this list and grouped the medications by potency values that ranged from 1 to 7. A medication index could then be obtained by multiplying and then summating the number of pills taken by their respective potency value. More recently, due chiefly to the proliferation of medications with varied modes of action, researchers have shied away from attempts to weight and then combine medications. The IHS guidelines committees recommend that patients record the number of attacks for which symptomatic medications were taken (or the number of tablets taken, if feasible), and that this measure be considered as a secondary effect parameter.

Even when it is viewed as only a secondary parameter, it is important to monitor medication consumption for several reasons. The first is to be on guard for excessive use that may be triggering rebound headache. Second, many patients specifically request nonpharmacological treatment because of a desire to reduce or eliminate their need for medication; systematic measures are necessary to evaluate progress toward this goal. Finally, concurrent tracking of pain parameters and medication allows the therapist to determine whether observed improvements in pain level are due in part to increased use of medications or enhanced compliance with a prescribed prophylactic regimen.

Functional Consequences of Headache

It is only within the last decade that researchers have begun to assess the impact of chronic headache on a patient's functioning and well-being—aspects that go beyond the previously described work of Philips and colleagues. Osterhaus and Townsend (1991) administered an updated version of a quality-of-life scale used in the Medical Outcomes Study (Stewart et al., 1989) to over 500 patients with migraines. When the obtained data were compared to data previously collected from patients with various other medical disorders (hypertension, diabetes, arthritis myocardial infarction, and gastrointestinal disorders), it was found that the personal impact of migraines was more serious for several of the indices. Overall, results showed that although the patients with migraines functioned better physically, their behavioral functioning was at a level well below their physical capabilities. A number of scales are currently available for assessing functional impairment, but until recently most of them targeted chronic, stable conditions and were of questionable value for recurrent, episodic disorders such as headache.

Most recently, researchers have begun to focus on scales specific to migraine or to headache in general (e.g., Davies, Santanello, Gerth, Lerner, & Block, 1999; Martin et al., 2000; Stewart, Lipton, Kolodner, Liberman, & Sawyer, 1999; Stewart, Lipton, Simon, Von Korff, & Liberman, 1998). These scales seek to quantify the functional consequences of headache in terms of three dimensions: (1) impairment (pain, limitations to range of motion, etc.); (2) functional limitations (ability to ambulate, etc.); and (3) disability (work and function in other roles) (Stewart et al., 1999). Such scales have the potential to be of considerable value in screening patients and research participants, developing treatment approaches, and assessing outcome.

SUMMARY

Headache is multidetermined, requiring a comprehensive, multifactorial assessment approach. The assessor of a patient with headache needs to be mindful of the patient's need for information, understanding, and reassurance. Thus patient education and information exchange become an important part of the assessment process early. Assessment begins with a thorough physical and neurological evaluation to rule out permanent structural defects or diagnosable physical conditions other than a primary headache disorder. Clinicians need to remain alert for a developing physical problem, and to maintain close medical collaboration throughout treatment to monitor such problems and to obtain assistance with medication management and modification as needed. Determination of specific headache type is necessary to determine the proper medication approach; to identify patients whose headaches may be occurring in part because of medication abuse; to identify headache types that have been found to be resilient to nonpharmacological approaches alone (cluster and chronic daily headache); and to decide when a comprehensive, multidisciplinary approach (posttraumatic headache) or even hospitalization is needed.

A biopsychological model points out the need to search for trigger, environmental, coping, and reinforcement factors that may be linked to headache. Assessment of the psychological status of the patient deserves special attention in order to identify conditions that might preclude direct treatment of headache at the moment (a significant Axis I psychiatric problem or a personality disorder) or complicate current treatment and compromise progress (e.g., depression). Identification of stress factors, both major and minor, are often helpful in suggesting targets for intervention. A minority of patients may require specialized neuropsychological assessment.

Finally, various approaches to measurement are recommended. The main approach ("gold standard") at present involves use of daily headache pain diaries, from which multiple parameters may be obtained (headache frequency, duration, intensity, and medication consumption). More recent approaches concern measurement of separate aspects of the pain experience (reactive as well as sensory component), validation by contact with significant others, assessment of pain behaviors or behaviors assumed to be motivated by pain, and determination of the impact upon nonheadache variables (such as quality of life and functional impairment).

REFERENCES

Ad Hoc Committee on Classification of Headache. (1962). Classification of headache. *Journal of the American Medical Association, 179,* 717–718.

Ahles, T. A., Martin, J. B., Gaulier, B., Cassens, H. L., Andres, M. L., & Shariff, M. (1988). Electromyographic and vasomotor activity in tension, migraine, and combined headache patients: The influence of postural variation. *Behaviour Research and Therapy, 26,* 519–525.

Andrasik, F. (2001). *Another look at social validation of the headache diary.* Manuscript in preparation.

Andrasik, F., & Baskin, S. (1987). Headache. In R. L. Morrison & A. S. Bellack (Eds.), *Medical factors and psychological disorders: A handbook for psychologists* (pp. 325–349). New York: Plenum Press.

Andrasik, F., Blanchard, E. B., Ahles, T. A., Pallmeyer, T., & Barron, K. D. (1981). Assessing the reactive as well as the sensory component of headache pain. *Headache, 21,* 218–221.

Andrasik, F., Burke, E. J., Attanasio, V., & Rosenblum, E. L. (1985). Child, parent, and physician reports of a child's headache pain: Relationships prior to and following treatment. *Headache, 25,* 421–425.

Andrasik, F., & Holroyd, K. A. (1980). Reliability and concurrent validity of headache questionnaire data. *Headache, 20,* 44–46.

Andrasik, F., & Passchier, J. (2000). Psychological mechanisms of tension-type headache. In J. Olesen, P. Tfelt-Hansen, & K. M. A. Welch (Eds.), *The headaches* (2nd ed., pp. 599–603). Philadelphia: Lippincott Williams & Wilkins.

Andrasik, F., & Wincze, J. P. (1994). Emotional and psychological aspects of mild head injury. *Seminars in Neurology, 14,* 60–66.

Appelbaum, K. A., Radnitz, C. L., Blanchard, E. B., & Prins, A. (1988). The Pain Behavior Questionnaire (PBQ): A global report of pain behavior in chronic headache. *Headache, 28,* 53–58.

Arena, J. G., Hannah, S. L., Bruno, G. M., & Meador, K. J. (1991). Electromyographic biofeedback training for tension headache in the elderly: A prospective study. *Biofeedback and Self-Regulation, 16,* 379–390.

Attanasio, V., Andrasik, F., Burke, E. J., Blake, D. D., Kabela, E., & McCarran, M. S. (1985). Clinical issues in utilizing biofeedback with children. *Clinical Biofeedback and Health, 8,* 134–141.

Barnat, M. R., & Lake, A. E., III. (1983). Patient attitudes about headache. *Headache, 23,* 229–237.

Blanchard, E. B., & Andrasik, F. (1985). *Management of chronic headaches: A psychological approach.* New York: Pergamon Press.

Blanchard, E. B., Andrasik, F., Evans, D. D., Neff, D. F., Appelbaum, K. A., & Rodichok, L. D. (1985). Behavioral treatment of 250 chronic headache patients: A clinical replication series. *Behavior Therapy, 16,* 308–327.

Blanchard, E. B., Andrasik, F., Jurish, S. E., & Teders, S. J. (1982). The treatment of cluster headache with relaxation and thermal biofeedback. *Biofeedback and Self-Regulation, 7,* 185–191.

Blanchard, E. B., Andrasik, F., Neff, D. F., Jurish, S. E., & O'Keefe, D. M. (1981). Social validation of the headache diary. *Behavioral Therapy, 12,* 711–715.

Blanchard, E. B., Appelbaum, K. A., Radnitz, C. L., Jaccard, J., & Dentinger, M. P. (1989). The refractory headache patient: I. Chronic daily, high intensity headache. *Behaviour Research and Therapy, 27,* 403–410.

Blanchard, E. B., Hillhouse, J., Appelbaum, K. A., & Jaccard, J. (1987). What is an adequate length of baseline in research and clinical practice with chronic headache? *Biofeedback and Self-Regulation, 12,* 323–329.

Blanchard, E. B., & Schwarz, S. P. (1988). Clinically significant changes in behavioral medicine. *Behavioral Assessment, 10,* 171–188.

Blanchard, E. B., Taylor, A. E., & Dentinger, M. P. (1992). Preliminary results from the self-regulatory treatment of high medication consumption headache. *Biofeedback and Self-Regulation, 17,* 179–202.

Bogaard, M. C., & ter Kuile, M. M. (1994). Treatment of recurrent tension headache: A meta-analytic review. *Clinical Journal of Pain, 10,* 174–190.

Budzynski, T. H., Stoyva, J. M., Adler, C. S., & Mullaney, D. J. (1973). EMG biofeedback and tension headache: A controlled outcome study. *Psychosomatic Medicine, 35,* 484–496.

Cahn, T., & Cram, J. R. (1980). Changing measurement instrument at follow-up: A potential source of error. *Biofeedback and Self-Regulation, 5,* 265–273.

Collins, F. L., & Martin, J. E. (1980). Assessing self-report of pain: A comparison of two recording procedures. *Journal of Behavioral Assessment, 2,* 55–63.

Collins, F. L., & Thompson, J. K. (1979). Reliability and standardization in the assessment of self-reported headache pain. *Journal of Behavioral Assessment, 1,* 73–86.

Coyne, L., Sargent, J., Segerson, J., & Obourn, R. (1976). Relative potency scale for analgesic drugs: Use of psychophysical procedures with clinical judgments. *Headache, 16,* 70–71.

Davies, G. M., Santanello, N., Gerth, W., Lerner, D., & Block, G. A. (1999). Validation of a migraine work and productivity loss questionnaire for use in migraine studies. *Cephalalgia, 19,* 497–502.

De Beneditttis, G., & Lorenzetti, A. (1992). Minor stressful life events (daily hassles) in chronic primary headache: Relationship with MMPI personality patterns. *Headache, 32,* 330–332.

Diener, H.-C., & Wilkinson, M. (Eds.). (1988). *Drug-induced headache.* Berlin: Springer-Verlag.

Duckro, P. N., Tait, R., Margolis, R. B., & Silvermintz, S. (1985). Behavioral treatment of headache following occupational trauma. *Headache, 25,* 328–331.

Epstein, L. H., & Abel, G. G. (1977). An analysis of biofeedback training effects for tension headache patients. *Behavior Therapy, 8,* 37–47.

Folstein, M. F., Folstein, S. E., & McHugh, P. R (1975). "Mini-Mental State": A practical method for grading the cognitive state of patients for the clinician. *Journal of Psychiatric Research, 12,* 189–198.

Fordyce, W. E. (1976). *Behavioral methods for chronic pain and illness.* St. Louis, MO: Mosby.

Fowler, R. S. (1975). Operant therapy for headaches. *Headache, 15,* 1–6.

Freitag, F. G. (1992). Headache clinics and inpatient units for treatment of headache. In S. Diamond & D. J. Dalessio (Eds.), *The practicing physician's approach to headache* (5th ed., pp. 270–280). Baltimore: Williams & Wilkins.

Gallagher, R. M. (1990). Precipitating cause of migraine. In S. Diamond (Ed.), *Migraine headache prevention and management* (pp. 31–44). New York: Marcel Dekker.

Guitera, V., Muñoz, P., Castillo, J., & Pascual, J. (1999). Transformed migraine: A proposal for the modification of its diagnostic criteria based on recent epidemiological data. *Cephalalgia, 19,* 847–850.

Haddock, C. K., Rowan, A. B., Andrasik, F., Wilson, P. G., Talcott, G. W., & Stein, R. J. (1997). Home-based behavioral treatments for chronic benign headache: A meta-analysis of controlled trials. *Cephalalgia, 17,* 113–118.

Henryk-Gutt, R., & Rees, W. C. (1973). Psychological aspects of migraine. *Journal of Psychosomatic Research, 17,* 141–153.

Hermann, C., Kim, M., & Blanchard, E. B. (1995). Behavioral and prophylactic pharmacological intervention studies of pediatric migraine: An exploratory meta-analysis. *Pain, 20,* 239–256.

Holden, E. W., Deichmann, M. M., & Levy, J. D. (1999). Empirically supported treatments in pediatric psychology: Recurrent pediatric headache. *Journal of Pediatric Psychology, 24,* 91–109.

Holm, J. E., Holroyd, K. A., Hursey, K. G., & Penzien, D. (1986). The role of stress in recurrent tension headaches. *Headache, 26,* 160–167.

Holroyd, K. A. (1993). Integrating pharmacologic and non-pharmacologic treatments. In C. D. Tollison & R. S. Kunkel (Eds.), *Headache: Diagnosis and treatment* (pp. 309–320). Baltimore: Williams & Wilkins.

Holroyd, K. A., & Andrasik, F. (1982). A cognitive-behavioral approach to recurrent tension and migraine headache. In P. C. Kendall (Ed.), *Advances in cognitive-behavioral research and therapy* (Vol. 1, pp. 275–320). New York: Academic Press.

Holroyd, K. A., Holm, J. E., Hursey, K. G., Penzien, D. B., Cordingley, G. E., Theofanous, A. G., Richardson, S. C., & Tobin, D. L. (1988). Recurrent vascular headache: Home-based behavioral treatment vs. abortive pharmacological treatment. *Journal of Consulting and Clinical Psychology, 56,* 218–223.

Holroyd, K. A., & Lipchik, G. L. (1997). Recurrent headache disorders. In S. J. Gallant, G. P. Keita, & R. Royak-Shaler (Eds.), *Health care for women: Psychological, social, and behavioral influences* (pp. 365–384). Washington, DC: American Psychological Association.

Holroyd, K. A., Lipchik, G. L., & Penzien, D. B. (1998). Psychological management of recurrent headache disorders: Empirical basis for clinical practice. In K. S. Dobson & K. D. Craig (Eds.), *Empirically supported therapies* (pp. 187–236). Thousand Oaks, CA: Sage.

Holroyd, K. A., & Penzien, D. (1990). Pharmacological versus non-pharmacological prophylaxis of recurrent migraine headache: A meta-analytic review of clinical trials. *Pain, 42,* 1–13.

Holroyd, K. A., Penzien, D. B., & Cordingley, G. A. (1991). Propranolol in the prevention of recurrent migraine: A meta-analytic review. *Headache, 31,* 333–340.

Howarth, E. (1965). Headache, personality, and stress. *British Journal of Psychiatry, 111,* 1193–1197.

Hudzinski, L. G., & Lawrence, G. S. (1988). Significance of EMG surface electrode placement models and headache findings. *Headache, 28,* 30–35.

Hudzinski, L. G., & Lawrence, G. S. (1990). EMG surface electrode normative data for muscle contraction headache and biofeedback therapy. *Headache Quarterly, 1,* 224–229.

International Headache Society (IHS) Committee on Clinical Trials in Migraine. (1999). Guidelines for controlled trials of drugs in migraine. In IHS (Ed.), *Members' handbook 2000* (pp. 111–133). Oslo: Scandinavian University Press.

International Headache Society (IHS) Committee on Clinical Trials in Tension-Type Headache. (1999). Guidelines for trials of drug treatments in tension-type headache. In IHS (Ed.), *Members' handbook 2000* (pp. 134–160). Oslo: Scandinavian University Press.

International Headache Society (IHS) Headache Classification Committee. (1988). Classification and diagnostic criteria for headache disorders, cranial neuralgias, and facial pain. *Cephalalgia, 8* (Suppl. 7), 1–96.

Jacob, R. G., Turner, S. M., Szekely, B. C., & Eidelman, B. H. (1983). Predicting outcome of relaxation therapy in headaches: The role of "depression." *Behavior Therapy, 14,* 457–465.

Jacobs, J. W., Bernhard, M. R., Delgado, A., & Strain, J. J. (1977). Screening for organic mental syndromes in the medically ill. *Annals of Internal Medicine, 86,* 40–46.

Jensen, R. (1999). Pathophysiological mechanisms of tension-type headache: A review of epidemiological and experimental studies. *Cephalalgia, 19,* 602–621.

Kazdin, A. E. (1977). Assessing the clinical or applied importance of behavior change through social validation. *Behavior Modification, 1,* 427–452.

Kudrow, L. (1982). Paradoxical effects of frequent analgesic use. *Advances in Neurology, 33,* 335–341. New York: Raven Press.

Lawson, P., Kerr, K., Penzien, D. B., Hursey, K. G., Ray, S. E., Arora, R, Marcus-Mendoza, S., & Holm, J. E. (1988, November). *Caveats in using mental status examinations: Factors that influence performance.* Paper presented at the annual meeting of the Association for Advancement of Behavior Therapy, New York.

Lazarus, R. S., & Folkman, S. (1984). Coping and adaption. In W. D. Gentry (Ed.), *Handbook of behavioral medicine* (pp. 282–325). New York: Guilford Press.

Levor, R. M., Cohen, M. J., Naliboff, B. D., McArchur, D., & Heuser, G. (1986). Psychosocial precursors and correlates of migraine headache. *Journal of Consulting and Clinical Psychology, 54,* 347–353.

MacGregor, E. A. (1997). Menstruation, sex hormones, and migraine. *Neurologic Clinics, 15,* 125–141.

Marcus, D. A., Nash, J. M., & Turk, D. C. (1994). Diagnosing recurring headaches: IHS criteria and beyond. *Headache, 34,* 329–336.

Marcus, D. A., Scharff, L, Mercer, S., & Turk, D. C. (1999). Musculoskeletal abnormalities in chronic headache: A controlled comparison of headache diagnostic groups. *Headache, 39,* 21–27.

Martin, B. C., Pathak, D. S., Sharfman, M. I., Adelman, J. U., Taylor, F., Kwong, W. J., & Jhingran, P. (2000). Validity and reliability of the Migraine-Specific Quality of Life Questionnaire (MSQ Version 2.1). *Headache, 40,* 204–215.

Martin, P. R. (1993). *Psychological management of chronic headaches.* New York: Guilford Press.

Massiou, H., & Bousser, M.-G. (2000). Influence of female hormones on migraine. In J. Olesen, P. Tfelt-

Hansen, & K. M. A. Welch (Eds.), *The headaches* (2nd ed., pp. 261–267). Philadelphia: Lippincott Williams & Wilkins.

Mathew, N. T., & Bendtsen, L. (2000). Prophylactic pharmacotherapy of tension-type headache. In J. Olesen, P. Tfelt-Hansen, & K. M. A. Welch (Eds.), *The headaches* (2nd ed., pp. 667–673). Philadelphia: Lippincott Williams & Wilkins.

Mathew, N. T., Kurman, R., & Perez, F. (1990). Drug induced refractory headache: Clinical features and management. *Headache, 30,* 634–638.

Mathew, N. T., Reuveni, U., & Perez, F. (1987). Transformed or evolutive migraine. *Headache, 27,* 102–106.

Medina, J. L. (1992). Efficacy of an individualized outpatient program in treatment of chronic post-traumatic headache. *Headache, 32,* 180–183.

Melzack, R. (1975). The McGill Pain Questionnaire: Major properties and scoring methods. *Pain, 7,* 277–299.

Merikangas, K. R., & Stevens, D. E. (1997). Comorbidity of migraine and psychiatric disorders. *Neurologic Clinics, 15,* 115–123.

Michultka, D. M., Blanchard, E. B., Appelbaum, K. A., Jaccard, J., & Dentinger, M. P. (1989). The refractory headache patient: II. High medication consumption (analgesic rebound) headache. *Behaviour Research and Therapy, 27,* 411–420.

Nicholson, N. L., & Blanchard, E. B. (1993). A controlled evaluation of behavioral treatment of chronic headache in the elderly. *Behavior Therapy, 24,* 395–408.

Okifuji, A., Turk, D. C., & Marcus, D. A. (1999).Comparison of generalized and localized hyperalgesia in recurrent headache and fibromyalgia patients. *Psychosomatic Medicine, 61,* 212–219.

Olesen, J. (2000). Classification of headache. In J. Olesen, P. Tfelt-Hansen, & K. M. A. Welch (Eds.), *The headaches* (2nd ed., pp. 9–15). Philadelphia: Lippincott Williams & Wilkins.

Olesen, J., & Goadsby, P. J. (2000). Synthesis of migraine mechanisms. In J. Olesen, P. Tfelt-Hansen, & K. M. A. Welch (Eds.)., *The headaches* (2nd ed., pp. 331–336). Philadelphia: Lippincott Williams & Wilkins.

Osterhaus, J. T., & Townsend, R. J. (1991, June–July). *The quality of life of migraineurs: A cross sectional profile.* Paper presented at the 5th International Headache Congress, Washington, DC.

Packard, R. C. (1979). What does the headache patient want? *Headache, 19,* 370–374.

Packard, R. C. (1987). Differing expectations of headache patients and their physicians. In C. S. Adler, S. M. Adler & R. C. Packard (Eds.), *Psychiatric aspects of headache* (pp. 29–33). Baltimore: Williams & Wilkins.

Penzien, D. B., Rains, J. C., & Holroyd, K. A. (1993). Psychological assessment of the recurrent headache sufferer. In C. D. Tollison & R. S. Kunkel (Eds.), *Headache: Diagnosis and interdisciplinary treatment* (pp. 39–49). Baltimore: Williams & Wilkins.

Paiva, T., & Hering-Hanit, R. (2000). Headache and sleep. In J. Olesen, P. Tfelt-Hansen, & K. M. A. Welch (Eds.), *The headaches* (2nd ed., pp. 967–973). Philadelphia: Lippincott Williams & Wilkins.

Philips, C. (1983a). Assessment of chronic headache behavior. In R. Melzack (Ed.), *Pain measurement and assessment* (pp. 155–163). New York: Raven Press.

Philips, C. (1983b). Chronic headache experience. In R. Melzack (Ed.), *Pain measurement and assessment* (pp. 97–103). New York: Raven Press.

Philips, C., & Hunter, M. (1981). Pain behaviour in headache sufferers. *Behaviour Analysis and Modification, 4,* 257–266.

Philips, H. C., & Jahanshahi, M. (1986). The components of pain behaviour report. *Behaviour Research and Therapy, 24,* 117–125.

Price, D. D., McGrath, P. A., Rafii, A., & Buckingham, B. (1983). The validation of visual analog scale as ratio scale measures for chronic and experimental pain. *Pain, 17,* 45–56.

Radat, F., Sakh, D., Lutz, G., El Amrani, M., Ferreri, M., & Bousser, M.-G. (1999). Psychiatric comorbidity is related to headache induced by chronic substance use in migraineurs. *Headache, 39,* 477–480.

Ramadan, N. M., & Keidel, M. (2000). Chronic posttraumatic headache. In J. Olesen, P. Tfelt-Hansen, & K. M. A. Welch (Eds.), *The headaches* (2nd ed., pp. 771–780). Philadelphia: Lippincott Williams & Wilkins.

Rapoport, A. M. (1988). Analgesic rebound headache. *Headache, 28,* 662–665.

Raskin, N. H. (1988). *Headache* (2nd ed.). New York: Churchill Livingstone.

Saper, J. R. (1986). Changing perspectives on chronic headache. *Clinical Journal of Pain, 2,* 19–28.

Saper, J. R. (1987). Ergotamine dependency: A review. *Headache, 27,* 435–438.

Saper, J. R., & Jones, I. M. (1986). Ergotamine dependency. *Clinical Neuropharmacology, 9,* 244–256.

Saper, J. R., & Sheftell, F. D. (2000). Headache in the abuse-prone individual. In J. Olesen, P. Tfelt-Hansen, & K. M. A. Welch (Eds.), *The headaches* (2nd ed., pp. 953–958). Philadelphia: Lippincott Williams & Wilkins.

Silberstein, S. D., Lipton, R. B., Solomon, S., & Mathew, N. T. (1994). Classification of daily and near-daily headaches: Proposed revisions to the IHS criteria. *Headache, 34,* 1–7.

Stewart, A. L., Greenfield, S., Hays, R. D., Wells, K., Rogers, W. H., Berry, S. D., Mcglynn, E. A., & Ware, J. E. (1989). Functional status and well-being of patients with chronic conditions. *Journal of the American Medical Association, 262,* 907–913.

Stewart, W. F., Lipton, R. B., Kolodner, K., Liberman, J., & Sawyer, J. (1999). Reliability of the migraine disability assessment score in a population-based sample of headache sufferers. *Cephalalgia, 19,* 107–114.

Stewart, W. F., Lipton, R. B., Simon, D., Von Korff, M., & Liberman, J. (1998). Reliability of an illness severity measure for headache in a population sample of migraine sufferers. *Cephalalgia, 18,* 44–51.

Tfelt-Hansen, P., & Welch, K. M. A. (2000a). General principles of pharmacological treatment of migraine. In J. Olesen, P. Tfelt-Hansen, & K. M. A. Welch (Eds.), *The headaches* (2nd ed., pp. 385–389). Philadelphia: Lippincott Williams & Wilkins.

Tfelt-Hansen, P., & Welch, K. M. A. (2000b). Prioritizing prophylactic treatment of migraine. In J. Olesen, P. Tfelt-Hansen, & K. M. A. Welch (Eds.), *The headaches* (2nd ed., pp. 499–500). Philadelphia: Lippincott Williams & Wilkins.

Tursky, B. (1976). The development of a pain perception profile: A psychophysical approach. In M. Weisenberg & B. Tursky (Eds.), *Pain: New perspectives in therapy and research* (pp. 171–194). New York: Plenum Press.

Waggoner, C. D., & Andrasik, F. (1990). Behavioral assessment and treatment of recurrent headache. In T. W. Miller (Ed.), *Chronic pain* (Vol. 1, pp. 319–361). Madison, CT: International Universities Press.

Weeks, R. E. (1992, March). *Controversies in the diagnostic classification of headache: Toward a clinically meaningful, reliable system.* Paper presented at the annual meeting of the Association for Applied Psychophysiology and Biofeedback, Colorado Springs, CO.

Werder, D. S., Sargent, J. D., & Coyne, L. (1981). MMPI profiles of headache patients using self-regulation to control headache activity. *Headache, 21,* 164–169.

Wilkinson, M. (1988). Introduction. In H.-C. Diener & M. Wilkinson (Eds.), *Drug-induced headache* (pp. 1–2). Berlin: Springer-Verlag.

Wolf, M. M. (1978). Social validity: The case for subjective measurement or how applied behavior analysis is finding its heart. *Journal of Applied Behavior Analysis, 11,* 203–214.

Worz, R. (1983). Analgesic withdrawal in chronic pain treatment. In K. A. Holroyd, B. Schlote, & H. Zenz (Eds.), *Perspectives in research on headache* (pp. 137–144). Toronto: Hogrefe.

Chapter 25

Assessment of Orofacial Pain

SAMUEL F. DWORKIN
RICHARD OHRBACH

OROFACIAL PAIN: AN OVERVIEW

Orofacial pain is generally considered to encompass pain located in and around the mouth, the facial regions, and the preauricular regions. Orofacial pain arises primarily from, and is often categorized in terms of, the following (Okeson, 1995):

1. Dentoalveolar structures—teeth and periodontium, in association with inflammation secondary to infection or trauma.
2. Neuropathological conditions, in decreasing order of frequency of occurrence, of the trigeminal (Vth) cranial nerve, of the glossopharyngeal (IXth) cranial nerve, and of the facial (VIIth) cranial nerve.
3. Hard and soft tissue pathology associated with intra- or perioral tumor (e.g., carcinoma of the tongue or salivary glands), mucosal lesions (e.g., oral mucositis), and secondary oral manifestations of systemic disease (e.g., AIDS, metastatic bone cancer).
4. Musculoskeletal pain associated with the muscles of mastication and/or the temporomandibular joints (TMJs), collectively referred to as *temporomandibular disorder* (TMD) pain.

Table 25.1 summarizes the International Association for the Study of Pain (IASP) classification of conditions (excluding those associated with the teeth) that can give rise to acute or chronic orofacial pain, including a number of syndromes that are not addressed in this chapter but that demonstrate the breadth of conditions associated with orofacial pain.

Orofacial pain assessment can require consideration of a large number of etiological and contributing factors, such that the use of two basic dichotomies helps organize the collection of orofacial pain assessment data. The first dichotomy is between acute and chronic orofacial pain conditions; the second is between orofacial pain associated with iatrogenic (i.e., treatment) factors and endogenously arising pain associated with pathobiological processes such as infection, inflammation, or tumor. After addressing these two dichotomies, thorough orofacial pain assessment—like assessment of all pain conditions—entails evaluation of behavioral, psychological, and psychosocial levels of functioning, in order to differentiate etiological and contributing factors associated with onset of the orofacial pain problem from factors that serve to exacerbate or maintain pain.

For present purposes, *acute* orofacial pain can be defined as pain of an emergent, suddenly arising nature for which a suitable remedy has not been initiated—toothache is a classic example. *Chronic* pain can be defined as orofacial pain that persists beyond the time a biologically plausible remedy can be expected to be effective or beyond the time when healing processes are expected to have occurred. Chronic orofacial pain persists, by definition, either because accurate assessment and hence accurate diagnosis cannot be made (e.g., due to unreliability

475

TABLE 25.1. International Association for the Study of Pain (IASP) Diagnostic Classification of Chronic Pain: Orofacial Pain

	Code
II. Neuralgias of the Head and Face	
1. Trigeminal Neuralgia (Tic Douloureux)	006.X8a
2. Secondary Neuralgia (Trigeminal) from Central Nervous System Lesions	006.X4 (tumor)
	006.X0 (aneurysm)
3. Secondary Trigeminal Neuralgia from Facial Trauma	006.X1
4. Acute Herpes Zoster (Trigeminal)	002.X2a
5. Post-Herpetic Neuralgia (Trigeminal)	003.X2b
6. Geniculate Neuralgia (VIIth Cranial Nerve): Ramsay Hunt Syndrome	006.X2
7. Glossopharyngeal Neuralgia (IXth Cranial Nerve)	006.X8b
8. Neuralgia of the Superior Laryngeal Nerve (Vagus Nerve Neuralgia)	006.X8c
9. Occipital Neuralgia	004.X8 or 004.X1 if subsequent to trauma
III. Craniofacial Pain of Musculoskeletal Origin	
1. Acute Tension Headache	034.X7a
2. Tension Headache: Chronic Form (Scalp Muscle Contraction Headache)	033.X7b
3. Temporomandibular Pain and Dysfunction Syndrome	034.X8a
4. Osteoarthritis of the Temporomandibular Joint	033.X6
5. Rheumatoid Arthritis of the Temporomandibular Joint	032.X3b
VI. Pain of Psychological Origin in the Head and Face (code only)	
1. Delusional or Hallucinatory Pain (code only)	01X.X9a
2. Hysterical or Hypochondriacal (code only)	01X.X9b

Note. Reprinted from *Pain* (Suppl. 3), International Association for the Study of Pain (IASP) Subcommittee on Taxonomy and H. Merskey (Eds.), Classification of chronic pain syndromes and definitions of pain terms, S1–S226. Copyright 1986, with permission from Elsevier Science.

of clinical measures), or because diagnostic assessment does not point to available treatments that are enduringly effective. Table 25.2 briefly summarizes these well-known considerations in the differential diagnosis of acute versus chronic orofacial pain.

Although there exists (as Tables 25.1 and 25.2 attest) an extensive array of conditions potentially associated with pain in the orofacial region, the purpose of this chapter is to present current information with regard to assessment of the most prevalent orofacial conditions associated with pain, and to include some attention to those orofacial pain problems whose assessment remains problematic for clinicians. The vast preponderance of orofacial pain complaints for which people seek treatment stem from acutely arising pain conditions associated with dentoalveolar infectious and inflammatory processes—specifically, acute toothache, acute periodontal pain, and pain from alveolar and periodontal infectious abscesses. Identifiable infectious processes as the initiating etiological factors, and resultant inflammatory processes in response to infection, are the proximate etiology for these acute orofacial pains. Assessment and management

of such highly prevalent orofacial pain conditions fall within the purview of clinical dentistry, especially because of the difficulties in differential diagnosis, and it is neither appropriate nor possible to present a full discussion of the differential diagnosis of acute orofacial pain in general or acute dentoalveolar pain more specifically. Table 25.3, discussed below, presents an overview of the most important features of such pains, as well as of the orofacial pains that are dealt with at greater length below. The interested reader is referred to clinical texts (American Academy of Orofacial Pain [AAOP] & Okeson, 1996; Ohrbach & Burgess, 1999) for a fuller elaboration of the orofacial pains addressed here, and to standard clinical dental texts for more information regarding acute dental pains. The latter conditions were historically a scourge of humankind. They are now, however, readily controllable by operative and pharmacological methods that dentistry has pioneered and made widely available.

The major orofacial pain conditions that remain challenging to assess and to diagnose differentially constitute a cluster of neuropathic and musculoskeletal chronic pain conditions, to which

TABLE 25.2. Acute and Chronic Orofacial Pain States: Sources of Pain and Related Psychological and Psychosocial Factors

Type of orofacial pain	Source of orofacial pain		Psychological and psychosocial factors		
	Pathological endogenous	Exogenous/ iatrogenic	Emotional states	Cognitive processes	Pain behaviors
Acute					
• Recent onset, brief	Inflammation (dental caries, dentoalveolar-alveolar abscess)	Traumatic	Anxiety	Anticipation and apprehension over threat or harm	Agitation
• Typically of known etiology		Intra- and post-operative states	Panic		Autonomic nervous system arousal
• Clinical course consistent with known biological mechanisms of action	Malignancy		Phobia		Sleep problems
• Extent, duration, and quality of pain typically consistent with physical findings	Neuropathy				
• Resolved with dental/surgical intervention and/or medication					
• Psychological and behavioral pain-related sequelae usually resolved with resolution of etiological factors					
Chronic					
• Persistent, recurrent	Neuropathic (including atypical odontalgia)	Postsurgery	Depression	Negativity	Isolation
• Typically of indeterminate etiology		After medical treatment	Anxiety	Hopelessness	Avoidance
• Clinical course generally not consistent with confirmed biological mechanisms of action	Malignancy		Anger	Worry	Sleep problems
• Extent, duration, and quality of pain often inconsistent with physical findings	Musculoskeletal				Extensive use of health care
• Frequently unresolved with dental/surgical intervention and/or medication					
• Psychological and behavioral pain-related sequelae persisting in apparently poor relation to course of etiological factors (if known)					

this chapter is devoted. Chronic orofacial neuropathic pain conditions (including atypical odontalgia) are much less prevalent than chronic musculoskeletal pains of the orofacial region. As is the case for all chronic pain conditions, each of these persistent orofacial pain conditions can be a source of minor inconvenience for some patients, whereas for others they can become a decades-long major disorganizing force associated with significant depression and disruption of their everyday lives. Typically, these conditions have no detectable, let alone diagnosable (i.e., objectively confirmable), physical changes to distinguish either those with recent TMD onset or those suffering from TMD for a long time. Because musculoskeletal orofacial pain conditions, primarily TMD, are so much more widespread and have the capacity for becoming associated with appreciable psychological and psychosocial disability, the largest part of this chapter is devoted to the multidimensional assessment of these conditions.

Before we turn to assessment of chronic musculoskeletal orofacial pain, however, it is necessary to point out that all orofacial pain complaints present unique assessment and diagnostic challenges. The orofacial region contains structures of diverse embryonic origin that develop into highly specialized organs subserving the senses of taste and smell, while immediately adjacent are the specialized organs for vision and hearing. The region contains an intricate network of cranial and cervical innervation. It also contains a comparably rich vascular network supplying not only the specialized sense organ systems, but a complex musculoskeletal system (referred to in dentistry as the *stomatognathic system*), which supports the critical life functions of respiration and mastication (food intake, chewing, and initiation of digestion). Moreover, the orofacial region carries profound psychological and emotional intra- and interpersonal significance for people because of its critical role in establishing verbal and nonverbal communication, facial appearance, and sexual attractiveness, as well as the initiation of other complex interpersonal behaviors, including those that constitute sexuality.

At least in part because the anatomical, physiological, and psychological characteristics of the orofacial region are so complexly intertwined with many functions vital to physical and emotional well-being, it is probably not surprising that assessing signs and symptoms of orofacial pain can be especially complex, and that differential diagnosis of orofacial pain—the ultimate goal of pain assessment—can be elusive. Assessment difficulties are encountered because comorbid pathological conditions may exist in closely adjoining structures (e.g., in both joints and muscles, or in both teeth and supporting soft and hard tissues). These structures are all innervated by the same few major cranial nerves that carry both sensory and motor information and that lie in close proximity to a rich vascular supply.

In addition, genetically determined patterns underlying referred pain (i.e., neural convergence) and developmentally acquired neural plasticity changes in innervation (i.e., underlying sensitization) make possible a confusing array of overlapping patterns of pain signs and symptoms. Under some circumstances, it is hard even to distinguish whether an acute pain condition has been superimposed upon a more enduring chronic one.

Finally, the complexity of the area is compounded by the impact on the person of his or her orofacial pain condition, which depends so heavily for its clinical assessment on subjective self-report of pain perception and pain behavior. Because chronic orofacial pain conditions are not commonly associated with readily identifiable pathology, the validity of the individual's self-reported symptomatology is often not regarded seriously by health care providers; this can lead to further escalation of distress and to comorbidity with other conditions, such as depression, loss of hopefulness, and illness behavior in the form of further treatment seeking.

It is generally agreed that careful history taking is the most important factor in the assessment of both acute and chronic pain, followed by physical examination and use of imaging methods for visualizing hard and soft structures, the latter most commonly including routine intraoral radiographic assessment for acute dental pains but also including extraoral radiography and nonradiographic imaging methods, principally magnetic resonance imaging (MRI). An overview of the major findings from history and physical examination for orofacial pain conditions is presented in Table 25.3. As a further guide to assessing the most commonly encountered forms of orofacial pain, Table 25.3 also summarizes the most common orofacial pain symptom presentations and identifies distinguishing characteristics to be assessed in the service of arriving at a differential diagnosis and rational basis for selecting treatment for the orofacial pain disorder.

Despite the biological and psychological complexity of the orofacial region, it is generally possible to establish an accurate assessment and differential diagnosis in the majority of cases presenting with an orofacial pain problem, especially for the vast majority of cases that present with an acute pain problem. Careful history, physical examination, and appropriate use of other physical diagnostic methods (imaging, diagnostic nerve blocks, drug trials, etc.) can lead to a clinically useful assessment. This assessment should lead to a rational choice of treatment for the pain problem. The result should yield a satisfactory resolution of many acute and chronic orofacial pain conditions. From current clinical perspectives, it appears that a relatively small number of chronic pain conditions continue to present assessment and management challenges that are frustrating for clinicians. These conditions are associated with appreciable suffering. The resistant orofacial pain problems fall within the following three categories: (1) orofacial neuralgias; (2) neuropathic pains, either associated with the teeth and commonly labeled *atypical odontalgia*, or associated with the tongue and labeled *burning tongue* or *burning mouth syndrome* (BMS); and (3) musculoskeletal pain, primarily TMD.

OROFACIAL PAIN CONDITIONS

For the purposes of this chapter, clinical characteristics of the primary orofacial pain conditions are presented in order to highlight the complexity of diagnosis, coupled with the interlinking of behavior (and other variables of psychological interest) with the physical pathology—or, in some cases, with the lack of observable or measurable physical pathology.

Orofacial Neuralgias

Primary Trigeminal Neuralgia (Tic Douloureux)

The assessment of primary trigeminal neuralgia is fairly straightforward. Although its etiology is ascribed to pathology in the distribution of the trigeminal nerve, the basic etiological mechanism still remains somewhat controversial. Adequate epidemiological data are lacking. The assessment of trigeminal neuralgia takes into consideration that onset before the age of 20 is rare, with the modal age of onset generally thought to be in the fifth decade of life, and with females at higher risk. Pain is most frequently unilateral and right-sided, unrelated to handedness. The first (ophthalmic) division of the trigeminal nerve is almost never involved, and pain follows the distribution of the second (maxillary) or third (mandibular) divisions with about equal frequency; simultaneous involvement of both the second and third divisions is also possible.

The assessment and diagnosis of trigeminal neuralgia is primarily by history and secondarily by examination. The classic pathognomonic physical indicator is the presence of one or more trigger areas on the face, which, when tested by examination with even the mildest non-noxious levels of physical stimulation, gives rise to paroxysms of excruciatingly intense pain. The pain is described as "searing," "shooting," and "like an electric shock." The pain is typically localized unilaterally and follows the anatomical distribution of the maxillary and mandibular divisions of the trigeminal nerve without sensory loss as evaluated by neurological examination. Diagnostic trials of medications that aid in assessment include carbamazepine (probably the most common medication used for primary trigeminal neuralgia), phenytoin, and mephenesin.

Secondary Trigeminal Neuralgia

Secondary trigeminal neuralgia is orofacial neuralgia arising from conditions other than primary pathology in the trigeminal nerve itself. It is often difficult to assess accurately.

Other pathological conditions give rise to neuralgia pain that follows the distribution of the trigeminal system. These conditions include multiple sclerosis, posttraumatic neuralgia, postherpetic neuralgia, tumors or other lesions of the nasal and paranasal sinuses, dental pathology, and disorders of the TMJ. Although pain following the distribution of the trigeminal nerve can result from these conditions, careful clinical assessment will differentially attribute pain etiology to pathophysiology outside the trigeminal nerve.

Atypical Facial Neuralgia

Atypical facial neuralgia has also been labeled *lower-half headache*, and tends to be described as arising from deeper structures of the midface and orofacial region, including the teeth. Clinical assessment distinguishes atypical facial neuralgia from primary and secondary trigeminal neuralgia because the classic hallmarks of trigeminal neuralgia (i.e., exquisitely sensitive trigger areas and brief paroxysms of shooting pains that follow the anatomical distribution of the two lower divisions of the trigeminal nerve) are absent or only ambiguously present. Instead, pain is described as diffuse or ache-like in character, poorly localized, and not following the distribution of trigeminal nerve innervations. The more diffuse pain is fairly constant, can be longstanding (often hours to days in duration), and is

TABLE 25.3. Assessment of Orofacial Pain: Distinguishing Characteristics Contributing to Differential Diagnosis

	Oral				TMD	Vascular	Neuropathy	
	Dental	Periodontal	Mucosal/tongue	Salivary glands			Neuralgias	Atypical odontalgia
Location	Mouth, ear, jaws, cheek	Defined to affected tooth	Oral mucosa/deep in tongue	Area of gland	Temple, ear, jaws, teeth	Orbit or upper face	Nerve distribution	Diffuse, deep, sometimes across midline
Localization	Poor, diffuse, radiating, does not cross midline	Good	Usually good/diffuse	Usually good	Poor, but usually unilateral	Usually good	Fair to good	Poor
Duration	Seconds to days	Hours to days	Hours to days/months/years	Hours to days	Weeks to years	Minutes to hours	Seconds	Weeks to years
Character of pain	Intermittent, sharp, paroxysmal	Same level, boring	Burning, sharp/burning, ache	Drawing, pulling	Dull, continuous	Throbbing, deep	Lancinating, paroxysmal	Dull, boring, continuous
Precipitating factors	Hot and cold foods	Chewing	Sour and sharp foods/chewing, thermal, sharp foods	Eating	Yawning, chewing	Alcohol	Touch, wind, vibration	Stress, fatigue

Associated signs	Caries, exposed dentine	Periodontal abscess	Erosive or ulcerative lesion/ typically no visible signs	Salivary gland swelling	Limited mouth opening, click in TMJ	Lacrimation, injected eye, nasal discharge	Facial tic	None
Etiological factors	Caries, abrasion, gingival recession	Acute periodontal inflammation	Bacterial, viral, fungal, autoimmune/ unknown etiology	Saliva retention, ascending infection	Stress, para-function	Vasomotor, allergic	Idiopathic, multiple sclerosis	Depression, peripheral nerve injury
Imaging	Intraoral radiographs for interproximal caries, periapical infection	Intraoral radiographs for alveolar supporting bone loss	Typically NA	Sialography, MRI / CT, ultrasound	MRI, panoramic radiograph		MRI, panoramic radiograph	Intraoral and/or panoramic radiographs, CT, MRI
Treatment	Tooth restoration, endodontics	Endodontics of tooth extraction	Medical/surgical/ palliative, anti-depressants	Blockage removal, antibiotics	Physiotherapy, CBT, NSAIDs, antidepressants	Methysergide, lithium carbonate	Tegretol, nerve block, neuro-surgery	Tricyclic antidepressants, CBT

Note. NA, not applicable; MRI, magnetic resonance imaging; CT, computed tomography; CBT, cognitive-behavioral therapy; NSAIDs, nonsteroidal anti-inflammatory drugs. From Sharav, Y. (1989). Orofacial pain. In P. D. Wall & R. Melzack (Eds.), *Textbook of pain* (2nd ed., pp. 441–454). Edinburgh: Churchill Livingstone. Copyright 1989 by Churchill Livingstone. Adapted by permission.

not influenced by external stimulation of the face. The condition may be confused with pain resulting from pathology in the teeth or periodontal tissues and other forms of headache, as well as with primary and secondary trigeminal neuralgia.

The etiological mechanism is unknown, but some workers view atypical facial neuralgia as a reflex sympathetic dystrophy because it is often accompanied by lacrimal tearing, rhinorrhea, and facial flushing, and frequently it is not relieved by sensory nerve blocks. Depression has been implicated as an etiological factor, but without much empirical support other than the fact that antidepressant medication in noncontrolled trials has been reported as beneficial.

Glossopharyngeal and Facial Neuralgia

Glossopharyngeal neuralgia is viewed as a true or primary neuralgia of the glossopharyngeal nerve, with virtually all of the same distinguishing characteristics as primary trigeminal neuralgia except for the location of the pain, which is described as deep in the tongue and throat. For facial neuralgia, the same similarity holds, except that the pain is located in the relatively superficial muscles of facial expression. Glossopharyngeal neuralgia seems to affect males more frequently, unlike primary trigeminal neuralgia and facial neuralgia.

Neuropathic Pain Conditions

Atypical Odontalgia

Accurate assessment of atypical odontalgia is most critical, because the presenting symptom is intense, long-lasting toothache in the absence of any clinical signs of tooth pulp pathology, and inappropriate assessment may lead to unnecessary and irreversible loss of healthy tooth pulp tissue and loss of normal healthy teeth. Atypical odontalgia represents one of the most perplexing intraoral pain conditions; agreement is lacking concerning which clinical parameters are critical to assess, and the significance attached to clinical findings seems extremely varied. Pain is most typically located in the premolar and molar area, and is about twice as common in the maxillary arch as in the mandibular arch. Often pain continues to be identified as arising from specific teeth even after endodontic (tooth pulp removal) therapy of the putative offending teeth.

Numerous case reports document this type of pain persisting after endodontic therapy as well as after removal of the offending teeth themselves. The

surgical procedures often continue not only with removal of adjacent teeth, but also sometimes with removal of all teeth in the arch. When the pain condition is associated with teeth that no longer have pulpal innervation, or is located in dentoalveolar sites that have become edentulous, the condition has in the past been labeled *phantom tooth pain*; currently, however, this type of pain is more often termed simply neuropathic since it is not related to peripheral somatic pathology (e.g., tooth).

Indications that a patient may be assigned the diagnosis of atypical odontalgia (*typical odontalgia* is defined as classic toothache) or neuropathic pain include the following: (1) presence of dentoalveolar pain with no obvious local or other known systemic pathology; (2) continuous pain of greater than 4 months' duration; (3) hyperesthesia; and (4) equivocal somatosensory block. Atypical odontalgia arises predominantly in females in the fourth and fifth decades of life. Etiological theories, all unsubstantiated, include deafferentation pain (probably the favored theory); however, vascular and psychogenic etiological theories have also been offered, at least in part because of reports from uncontrolled trials that sympathetic blocks are sometimes effective, as are serotonergic antidepressive medications. Again, accurate assessment is critical, because of the risk that unwarranted (or at least unfounded) invasive therapies will result in loss of healthy biological tissues and structures.

The differential diagnosis for such conditions should also include the possibility of referred pain due to convergence of spinal-level neurons (Fields, 1987) from adjacent structures that allow a common projection pathway to higher centers in the pain transmission system. Thus pain that appears to be musculoskeletal, for example, may be due to pain arising from neuropathy but referred to adjacent musculoskeletal structures. It is critical that assessment of orofacial pain (following guidelines presented below) include evaluation of the known possibilities for referred pain, based on increased understanding of the complex pain transmission system.

Burning Mouth Syndrome

BMS (Bogetto, Maina, Ferro, Carbone, & Gandolfo, 1998; Miyamoto & Ziccardi, 1998; Mott, Grushka, & Sessle, 1993; Ship et al., 1995), also known as *glossodynia*, is characterized by spontaneous onset of burning, stinging pain—in the tip of the tongue most commonly, and (in equal prevalence) in the lips, the lateral border of the tongue, the dorsum of the tongue, and the palate. More than one site is common. The pain does not follow anatomical boundaries, and there are no visible mucosal lesions. Pain patterns have been characterized as follows:

Type I (none in morning, gradual worsening as day progresses).
Type II (continuous pain).
Type III (days of remission and recurrence with no identified pattern).

Pain intensity appears to be reported as mild, moderate, and severe at equal prevalences. Putative causes of BMS are multiple, with little evidence confirming most of them, but they have been organized as *local, systemic,* and *psychogenic* (a term we do not favor). Associated local symptoms include persistent taste alteration (bitter, metallic), thirst, xerostomia (not associated with altered salivary flow rate), dysgeusia, and dysphagia. Other symptoms reported in association with this condition include poor sleep, mood changes, and social isolation. There is a much higher prevalence in females in the menopausal and postmenopausal periods. Patients are typically described in the literature as seeking consultation from a wide variety of practitioners, with 50%-67% of patients eventually terminating care seeking and adapting to the problem within 6-7 years after onset, especially when the care provider is supportive.

Putative local causes of BMS include poorly fitting dental appliances, allergic reactions to dental appliances, and candidiasis. Evidence is negligible for these; furthermore, correction of the identified problem does not resolve BMS symptoms. Another local cause cited is carcinoma, but in this case, local tissue destruction can be identified. Putative systemic causes include menopause, iron deficiency anemia, B-complex vitamin deficiency, and diabetes mellitus. Findings such as treatment response with the appropriate agent fail to provide strong support for the putative cause.

There is a high comorbidity of BMS with primary mental disorders (over 70%, with the primary diagnoses in the mood disorders and anxiety disorders groups) and, to some degree, with life stress. The role of primary mental disorders has been recognized across multiple studies, and the best evidence suggests that the BMS onset occurs prior to either the current mental disorder or even the lifetime disorder. The latter possibility is often suggested but only recently has garnered any evidence (Bogetto et al., 1998).

Mechanisms to explain the pain associated with BMS have been few. Because of the nature of the pain complaint, peripheral mechanisms would seem reasonable in the form of tonic peripheral nociceptive afferent input, such as from inflammation or nerve injury; however, clinical signs are negative for inflammatory processes, and trauma history is generally negative. The other mechanism, central changes, would also appear sensible, with an unmasking of nociceptive afferent input accompanied by changes in somatosensory function; however, the latter are largely absent in BMS. Reliable findings do indicate that patients with BMS have slightly lowered pain tolerance and modest changes in taste. This could suggest, then, that there is an interaction between the gustatory and the nociceptive neurons, leading to the pain complaints.

Most of the literature describing treatment for BMS contains only anecdotal reports of treatment efficacy. The remaining treatment literature demonstrates that any treatment that works in one study is not replicated in subsequent studies. The only treatment that appears to be reported as reliably effective is antidepressant medication. Antidepressants appear to be as effective at low as at high dosages, and equally so whether or not the patient meets *Diagnostic and Statistical Manual of Mental Disorders* (DSM) criteria for a mood disorder (Ship et al., 1995; see also Sullivan, Chapter 15, this volume). Part of the problem in evaluating treatment effects relates to poor diagnostic criteria. Their improvement, along with improvements in systemic assessment, would be likely to improve this unfortunate situation.

Assessment for BMS, then, lies in performing a standard clinical soft tissue intraoral examination (in order to rule out obvious disease)—coupled with the appropriate laboratory tests deemed generally important, despite their frequent noncontributory nature, in order to provide reassurance. But the assessment procedures likely to be useful will include current and lifetime history of psychological functioning, life events at time of onset, and current coping and illness behavior as it relates to the pain condition, setting the stage for a positive helping relationship between health care provider and patient.

Musculoskeletal Pain

Overview

Musculoskeletal pain—that is, pain of muscle and articular origin—is by far the most common pain problem encountered in the orofacial region. Pain is presumed to derive from pathophysiological processes active in the hard and soft tissue components of the stomatognathic system. These components include the following:

1. The temporal bones of the skull.
2. The mandible.
3. Bilateral major bony articulations, the TMJs, containing the fixed glenoid fossa of the temporal bone and the movable condylar process of the mandible.
4. Articular discs that separate the condylar processes from the temporal bones.
5. Articular capsules enclosing the bony components and the articular discs of the TMJs.
6. The muscles of mastication, which allow the mandible to open and close; the major masticatory muscles act to close the mandible. These have their origins on the temporal bone and their insertions on the mobile mandible, forming a sling suspending the mandible from the skull and allowing great pressure to be exerted during mandibular function (e.g., biting, chewing).
7. The teeth and their supporting periodontal structures.

Each of the components of the stomatognathic system can generate pain during mandibular function, or pain originating from presumed pathology in one of the components can be referred to adjacent regions, as discussed above. Furthermore, sensitization known to arise from peripheral inflammatory processes as well as from noninflammatory means (e.g., myofascial trigger point phenomena) can yield the perception of pain arising in a widely dispersed area that may not reflect the actual extent of local physical pathological change. Thus many different musculoskeletal pain conditions are possible in the region, and indeed many have been identified and systematically labeled.

Although Table 25.1 lists the major pain conditions associated with the hard and soft tissue components of the orofacial region, a more recent classificatory and diagnostic scheme for musculoskeletal pain in the orofacial region has been offered by the American Academy of Orofacial Pain (AAOP) and is summarized in Table 25.4 (see also Andrasik, Chapter 24). The AAOP diagnostic scheme (AAOP & Okeson, 1996), which uses guidelines consistent with those recommended for the classification of headache by the International Headache Society (IHS), is highly regarded and has received widespread acceptance by clinicians (primarily dentists) in the field because of its clinical utility. However, neither the IHS nor the AAOP diagnostic scheme for musculoskeletal orofacial pain includes enough operational criteria to allow scientific assessment of (1) the reliability of clinical examiners; (2) the reliability, and hence validity, of clinical findings or of the diagnosis; or (3) the proposed diagnostic subtypes as a taxonomic group. Although the AAOP guidelines clearly advocate the inclusion of the assessment of biobehavioral factors, they do not provide a sufficiently clear specification of how a reliable assessment can be performed for pain-related behavioral and emotional factors, as implicated and recommended by current biopsychosocial models of pain.

Temporomandibular Disorders

As noted earlier, the most commonly occurring musculoskeletal pain disorders in the orofacial region are collectively referred to as TMD. TMD constitutes a cluster of related TMJ and masticatory muscle pain disorders characterized by the following major clinical signs and symptoms, which may occur singly or in combination:

1. Persistent pain in the region of the masticatory muscles or TMJs.
2. Physical limitations in mandibular function.
3. TMJ sounds possibly denoting pathology or denoting a pathological TMD risk factor.

Additional signs and symptoms co-occur with some regularity, including tooth wear as evidence of jaw clenching or grinding (bruxism), and referred or radiating pain to adjacent muscles in the head and neck.

Although a large number of pathological states and diseases that include pain as a prominent feature affect the tissues of the face and jaws (see Table 25.1), the term TMD is generally restricted to painful and dysfunctional conditions affecting the muscles of mastication and the TMJs. Multiple labels have been applied to the condition, including myofascial pain dysfunction, temporomandibular joint syndrome or simply TMJ, and craniomandibular disorder. We prefer the relatively neutral (with regard to etiology and presumed site of pathology) and all-inclusive term TMD, as recommended by the American Dental Association (1983).

Epidemiological data confirm that TMD occurs in countries on every continent, and the occurrence of TMD has been well documented throughout the developed world. However, it has

TABLE 25.4. International Headache Society (IHS) and American Academy of Orofacial Pain (AAOP) Recommended Diagnostic Classification

11. Headache or facial pain associated with disorder of cranium, neck, eyes, ears, nose, sinuses, teeth, mouth, or other facial or cranial structures

11.1 Cranial bones including the mandible	11.5 Nose and sinuses
11.2 Neck	11.6 Teeth and related oral structures
11.3 Eyes	11.7 Temporomandibular joint
11.4 Ears	11.8 Masticatory muscle

11.1 Cranial bones including the mandible

11.1.1 Congenital and developmental disorders	11.1.2 Acquired disorders
11.1.1.1 Aplasia	11.1.2.1 Neoplasia
11.1.1.2 Hypoplasia	11.1.2.2 Fracture
11.1.1.3 Hyperplasia	
11.1.1.4 Dysplasia	

11.7 Temporomandibular joint articular disorders

11.7.1 Congenital or developmental disorders	11.7.4 Inflammatory disorders
11.7.1.1 Aplasia	11.7.4.1 Capsulitis/synovitis
11.7.1.2 Hypoplasia	11.7.4.2 Polyarthritides
11.7.1.3 Hyperplasia	11.7.5 Osteoarthritis (noninflammatory disorders)
11.7.1.4 Neoplasia	11.7.5.1 Osteoarthritis: primary
11.7.2 Disc derangement disorders	11.7.5.2 Osteoarthritis: secondary
11.7.2.1 Disc displacement with reduction	11.7.6 Ankylosis
11.7.2.2 Disc displacement without reduction	11.7.7 Fracture (condylar process)
11.7.3 Temporomandibular joint dislocation	

11.8 Masticatory muscle disorders

11.8.1 Myofascial pain	11.8.4 Local myalgia—unclassified
11.8.2 Myositis	11.8.5 Myofibrotic contracture
11.8.3 Myospasm	11.8.6 Neoplasia

Note. From American Academy of Orofacial Pain (AAOP) and Okeson, J. P. (Eds.). (1996). *Orofacial pain: Guidelines for assessment, diagnosis, and management.* Chicago: Quintessence. Copyright 1996 by Quintessence. Reprinted by permission.

been repeatedly observed that lack of a consistent methodology for conducting either population-based studies or assessment of clinical samples has significantly limited research, and hence progress toward prevention and amelioration of this important chronic orofacial pain condition (Carlsson & LeResche, 1995). As a result, early reports implied wildly divergent distributions of pain and related signs and symptoms, both in the general population and in clinics. Recent careful reviews (LeResche, 1997) of epidemiological studies indicate a much narrower range of variability in distribution of relevant signs and symptoms when studies using similar measurement methods are compared. For instance, TMD-related pain was reported with a prevalence of 12.1% in a well-designed population-based study of adults conducted in the United States (Von Korff, Dworkin, LeResche, & Kruger, 1988).

A significant gender factor has emerged, demonstrating that the most dependable risk factors for TMD are being female and being in the reproductive years of the life span. The gender ratio for prevalence of TMD-related pain in the population hovers around 2:1, favoring females. The gender discrepancy is much greater in clinic patient populations around the world, where the ratio of women to men ranges from 3:1 to 6:1; however, nearly all the population-based data are from Europe or North America.

It is fair to say that TMD is by far the most commonly occurring chronic orofacial pain condition around the world. This is true from the perspective of numbers of people reporting the condition, extent of treatment provided (largely by dentists), and numbers of reports in the scientific and clinical literature. The impact on health care delivery systems, especially dentistry, of TMD as a clinical problem dwarfs that of all other chronic orofacial pain-related conditions taken together, including neuropathic pain conditions (e.g., trigeminal neuralgia and traumatic neuropathies) and oral malignancy.

Data comparing TMD with other common chronic pain conditions in the United States indicate that TMD is perceived as comparable in intensity and persistence to back pain, abdominal pain, and headache. As with all commonly occurring chronic pain conditions, available data indicate that TMD is associated not only with appreciable pain that can extend over years or even decades, but for many patients with significant personal suffering in the form of behavioral disturbance, psychological distress, and psychosocial disability (Dworkin, 1990). *Psychosocial disability* or disability in psychosocial functioning, as it is commonly termed in the biobehavioral literature, refers to disability at the level of societal or interpersonal interactions, relating to what the World Health Organization originally termed *handicap* and has more recently labeled *participation*.

Few data have been reported from other locations around the world that shed comparable light on the relative distribution of psychological disturbance and psychosocial disability associated with TMD. Moreover, the relationship between extent of physical pathology and pain patterns or severity is not well understood, and much controversy exists over the short-term and long-term significance of physical signs as etiological agents for pain and enduring pathology.

Even more controversial is the relation between physical parameters of TMD and behavioral, psychological, and psychosocial factors. Although it is generally acknowledged, at least in much of the developed world, that TMD is associated with appreciable personal distress, heated controversies remain concerning whether psychosocial factors (singly or in combination) are causes or consequences of TMD-related chronic pain and physical limitations in mandibular function (Dworkin, 1995).

All TMD nosology systems are in agreement that the predominant clinical subtypes of TMD be classified as (1) masticatory muscle disorders; (2) internal derangements (i.e., displacements) of the articular discs of the TMJs; and (3) degenerative joint changes typically classified as arthralgia, arthritis, and arthrosis of the joint. Muscle dis-

orders constitute by far the most common form of TMD, whereas internal derangements rarely occur as solitary diagnoses of clinical importance. Within the degenerative joint changes, arthritis and arthrosis are also quite rare, but arthralgia (representing a painful or inflamed TMJ) is common among those diagnosed with TMD. Although many patients with TMD carry more than one of these physical diagnoses, the most common multiple diagnosis is that of a muscle disorder together with TMJ arthralgia—therefore, a clinical disorder characterized primarily by pain.

Since behavioral, psychological, and psychosocial factors often play an important role in shaping the behavior, thinking, and emotions of all patients with chronic pain, these personal and interpersonal factors require attention in formulating a diagnosis or treatment plan for patients with TMD. Characteristics of TMD found in common with other chronic pain conditions include the following:

1. Poor correspondence between the nature or extent of pathophysiological change and global severity of pain and suffering.
2. Dysfunctional behaviors that directly affect the pain condition, such as oral parafunctional habits.
3. Transient psychological distress.
4. The potential for clinically meaningful depression, anxiety, and presence of nonspecific physical symptoms.
5. Interference with ability to perform usual activities at home, work, or school.
6. Frequent use of the health care system, with potential for excessive treatment seeking and abuse of medications, and iatrogenic complications from inappropriate or excessive treatment.

ASSESSMENT OF TMD

Observational Methods

Reliable and valid observational methods have been developed for assessing pain-related behaviors—primarily behaviors relevant to back pain rather than behaviors associated with orofacial pain, however. These observational measures have gained widespread acceptance and are discussed in several chapters throughout this book (see Craig, Prkachin, & Grunau, Chapter 9, and Keefe, Williams, & Smith, Chapter 10). At this point, however, observational methods applied to TMD have been limited to recording facial expressions of TMD-related pain (Craig, 1989; LeResche & Dworkin,

1988; Prkachin & Mercer, 1990; see also Craig et al., Chapter 9). LeResche, Dworkin, Wilson, and Ehrlich (1992) have shown that people with recent-onset TMD emit few facial expressions of pain overall, but that facial expressions increase in frequency as a function of chronicity of the disorder. These results imply that facial expressions become increasingly important to patients with more chronic TMD as a means for communicating pain and suffering. However, at present, the coding and analysis of facial expression data for pain and other emotions remain a relatively specialized and labor-intensive undertaking, limiting its clinical utility.

Critical Dimensions and Related Assessment

Typically, self-report methods for assessment of orofacial pain are similar in principle and often in substance to those used to assess all other pain conditions. These include use of interview schedules, symptom checklists, psychological and biobehavioral rating scales, and psychological tests assessing mental and emotional status, psychosocial adaptation, coping behaviors, and health care utilization (see Bradley & McKendree-Smith, Chapter 16; DeGood & Tait, Chapter 17; Romano & Schmaling, Chapter 18; and Jacob & Kerns, Chapters 19). It is beyond our present scope to review the many published measures that have received at least some attention from biobehaviorally oriented TMD clinical researchers. The most common self-report measures used for biobehavioral assessment of chronic orofacial pain conditions are discussed below.

Minnesota Multiphasic Personality Inventory

Perhaps the best known and most widely used instrument for assessing psychological status, the Minnesota Multiphasic Personality Inventory (MMPI; Hathaway & McKinley, 1983), is not intended as a diagnostic instrument; rather, it provides a profile of psychological function. The test requires 1–2 hours by patients, and highly specialized training is needed by clinicians to interpret it. Hence it is not deemed suitable for use by many dental clinicians.

The clinical value of the MMPI to many biomedical and other non-mental-health clinicians remains somewhat problematic. Standardization samples used for MMPI scale construction are reported in several independent studies as not

appropriate for patients with chronic pain. However, using clustering methods to identify MMPI scale profiles that characterize patients with pain, including those with TMD, has proven somewhat more useful.

Generally, whether on the MMPI or the more recently revised and restandardized MMPI-2, elevations on scales 1, 2, and 3 (Hypochondriasis, Depression, and Hysteria) are associated with perceptions of severe pain and excessive concern about bodily functioning, affective disturbance, and maladaptive patterns of psychosocial functioning. When elevations on Psychopathic Deviate and Schizophrenia scales are found accompanying elevations on scales 1, 2, and 3, not surprisingly, higher levels of psychopathology and resistance to modification of pain behavior are observed (see Bradley & McKendree-Smith, Chapter 16).

Although it was originally anticipated that distinct MMPI profiles would be confirmed for patients with chronic pain, these have not clearly emerged. Nevertheless, the MMPI has been used in many studies of patients with TMD, and these studies support the conclusion that clinical psychopathology is present in an appreciable number of patients with TMD presenting for treatment (Deardorff, 1995).

Using the MMPI in a study predicting response to treatment for TMD, McCreary, Clark, Oakley, and Flack (1992) found that the presence of multiple somatic symptoms, measured in the MMPI as somatization, was related to jaw function problems at long-term follow-up, but not at early follow-up. They reported that "somatization was a significant predictor of outcome" for patients with chronic TMD, and they concluded that "if treatment does not address this somatization process, there is an increased risk there will be no improvement" (McCreary et al., 1992, p. 168).

Symptom Checklist-90 Revised

The Symptom Checklist-90 Revised (SCL-90R; Derogatis, 1983) is a 90-item checklist that yields 10 major scales, of which the most relevant for use in chronic pain assessment are the scales assessing Depression, Anxiety, and Somatization. The SCL-90R is much briefer than the MMPI, but, like the MMPI, its overall usefulness with patients with chronic pain has also not been unequivocally established. Furthermore, some problems have emerged with its use in populations with chronic pain. For example, there has been difficulty in replicating the original 10-factor structure of the full SCL-90R (see

Bradley & McKendree-Smith, Chapter 16). Nevertheless, the SCL-90R has been used extensively to study populations with all types of chronic pain, including TMD.

In research comparing responses of patients with chronic pain to those of psychiatric populations, the patients with chronic pain were distinguished by reports of psychological distress limited to somatic, as opposed to emotional or cognitive, symptoms of anxiety and depression (Buckelew, DeGood, Schwartz, & Kerler, 1986; Dworkin, Von Korff, & LeResche, 1990, 1992; Wilson, Dworkin, Whitney, & LeResche, 1994). Taken together, the studies cited find both appreciable psychological distress in samples of patients at TMD clinics, and a poor relationship between physical signs or extent of physical jaw impairment and extent of psychological distress in patients with TMD.

Nonspecific Physical Symptoms

Increased relevance has been attached to assessing in patients with chronic pain the presence of co-existing physical symptoms of a nonspecific nature (e.g., night sweats, tremors, heart palpitation), commonly referred to as *somatization*. Assessment is aided by the use of symptom checklists or somatization scales (e.g., the Somatization scale of the SCL-90R). Furthermore, it is recommended that assessment of somatization be extended to include quantity of health care use—specifically, numbers of health care visits (Raustia & Pyhtinen, 1990), and numbers and types of medications prescribed for pain. A spectrum of severity has been described for somatization (Fordyce, Brockway, Bergman, & Spengler, 1986), with one end of the spectrum occupied by somatoform psychiatric disorders that are recognized in the *Diagnostic and Statistical Manual of Mental Disorders*, fourth edition (DSM-IV; American Psychiatric Association, 1994), and that require the presence of at least eight physical symptoms, distributed over multiple organ systems and not explained by a diagnosable medical condition. More relevant to clinicians working with chronic pain problems is that part of the somatization spectrum represented by four or five similarly nonspecific physical symptoms that are perceived as distressful, such as trembling, night sweats, and heart palpitations (American Academy of Pediatric Dentistry & University of Texas Health Science Center at San Antonio Medical School, 1990; Helmy, Timmis, Sharawy, Abdelatif, & Bays, 1990).

Of related interest, it is very difficult to qualify for a formal (DSM-IV) diagnosis of mood or anxiety disorder without identifying a number of nonspecific physical symptoms as frequently present and distressing. In other words, anxious and depressed persons experience many dysphoric symptoms, including aches and pains as well as other nonspecific physical symptoms. It is also noteworthy that somatization consistently emerges as a major predictor or correlate of such pain behaviors as treatment seeking and prevalence of physical symptoms (Dao, Knight, Tenenbaum, Lue, & Ton-That, 1996). Thus there is some question regarding the nature of the distress that patients with chronic pain experience. It may be that considerable overlap exists in physical symptoms and psychosocial responses exhibited by persons experiencing significant emotional disturbance and those experiencing common chronic pain conditions. These commonalities include self-reported pains, as well as limitations in behavior, social withdrawal, and avoidance of responsibilities; again, the latter psychosocial factors are observed in persons experiencing both mood and anxiety disorders and persistent chronic pain conditions such as headache, back pain, and TMD.

It is interesting to speculate that assessment of somatization is important because it may represent a common factor shared by these apparently diverse responses to life's physical, environmental, and social stressors. These theoretical distinctions could be extended clinically with respect to how the distress should be primarily managed—specifically, whether the management of chronic pain should include the management of mood or anxiety disorders when the latter are detected. Clearly, this is an important area for further research.

Graded Chronic Pain Scale

The Graded Chronic Pain Scale (GCPS), developed on populations with chronic headache, back pain, and TMD, assesses chronic pain severity from grade 0 to grade IV (Von Korff, Dworkin, & LeResche, 1990; Von Korff, Ormel, Keefe, & Dworkin, 1992; see also Von Korff, Chapter 31). The GCPS was created not only to provide a meaningful quantitative index of the extent to which pain is perceived as mild or severe in intensity, but to capture, in a single quantitative index, the extent to which pain is psychosocially disabling. Since the GCPS was derived from population-based studies of chronic pain in the community and not from a pain clinic population, it can be used for data collection under a variety of research designs (ranging from random sample surveys to clinical intervention studies), and it has proven to be a very useful clinical measure to assess the impact of chronic TMD on our patients.

The development of the GCPS and its psychometric properties have been described in detail elsewhere (Von Korff et al., 1992; see also Von Korff, Chapter 31). In summary, however, it measures psychosocial disability by assessing both pain intensity *and* extent of pain-related interference with daily activities and number of lost activity days (e.g., days unable to go to work or school, attend to household responsibilities, etc.) attributed to TMD (or other chronic) pain. Grade I is defined as pain of low intensity, averaging less than 5.0 on a 10-point scale, and associated with little pain-related interference in daily living. Grade II is defined as high-intensity pain, above 5.0 on a 10-point scale, also associated with little pain-related interference in daily living. Grades III and IV are associated with increasing levels of pain-related psychosocial disability regardless of pain level, indicating appreciable impact on activities, including days lost to work or school due to pain interference. For clinical purposes, therefore, functional patients (individuals not significantly disabled by their TMD or other chronic pain condition) are defined as having grade I or II pain. By contrast, we define dysfunctional patients as having grade III or IV chronic pain on the GCPS.

These demarcations of functional and dysfunctional grades of chronic pain have received empirical support (Foreman, Harold, & Hay, 1994; Turner, Whitney, Dworkin, Massoth, & Wilson, 1995), including cross-validation of their clinical utility through studies involving randomized clinical trials of TMD treatments based on level of psychosocial functioning as determined by the GCPS (Dworkin, Sherman, et al., 1999; Dworkin, Turner, et al., 1999; Huggins et al., 1999; Ohrbach, Dworkin, & Truelove, 1999). Similarly, it is important to note that despite widespread agreement regarding its public health, research, and treatment implications, the concept of dysfunctional chronic pain (i.e., behavioral participation in relation to an impairment or disease) has been extended only minimally to TMD research and clinical application.

West Haven–Yale Multidimensional Pain Inventory

Turk and colleagues (Rudy, Turk, Zaki, & Curtin, 1989; Turk & Rudy, 1988) have developed the West Haven–Yale Mulidimensional Pain Inventory (WHYMPI), perhaps the most widely used self-report measure for the assessment of psychosocial and cognitive responses of patients with chronic pain (see Jacob & Kerns, Chapter 19). It has been extensively investigated for its psychometric properties, demonstrating acceptable levels of reliability, validity, and predictability of pain response pattern. Like the other scales reviewed to this point, and unlike the IMPATH and TMJ Scales (see below), its use is not limited to patients with TMD. The measure was developed with pain clinic populations and has been found to yield three distinct patient clusters that appear consistently across diverse chronic pain conditions, including back pain, headache, cancer pain, and TMD.

These three clusters of chronic pain groups distinguished by the multiaxial WHYMPI are labeled Adaptive Copers, Interpersonally Distressed, and Dysfunctional, and reflect a continuum of increasing disability and pain-related psychosocial dysfunction. For example, Rudy and colleagues (1989) have demonstrated that patients with TMD characterized as Dysfunctional by the WHYMPI show significantly elevated depression, report receiving less effective support, and report significantly more physical symptoms, compared to those patients with TMD categorized as Adaptive Copers. However, Dysfunctional patients with TMD did not differ from adaptive copers in physical parameters (proportion of positive computed tomography scan findings, objective findings from a TMD clinical exam, etc.). More recently, Rudy, Turk, Kubinski, and Zaki (1994) have used the WHYMPI to assess the relative efficacy of a cognitive-behavioral treatment intervention compared to a physical treatment that involved use of an intraoral occlusal splint. Specifically, they found biofeedback to be more effective than intraoral appliances, in the long run, for maintaining lower levels of pain and better adaptation to the TMD condition. They presented evidence indicating that Dysfunctional patients versus Adaptive Copers and Interpersonally Stressed patients responded differentially to these treatments, supporting their conclusion that clinical treatment decisions for TMD should include not only assessment of biobehavioral status but assignment of patients to treatment interventions specifically designed according to the assessed level of psychosocial function. It seems fair to say that the WHYMPI is one of the most carefully designed and well-studied self-report measures for assessing biobehavioral and psychosocial functioning in patients with chronic pain. (See Jacob & Kerns, Chapter 19, and Turk & Okifuji, Chapter 21, for more extensive discussion of this topic.)

TMJ Scale

The TMJ Scale (Levitt, 1990, 1991; Levitt, Lundeen, & McKinney, 1988, 1994), developed as a self-report measure for use in the home or office, assesses three domains: Physical, Psychosocial, and Global. The Physical domain includes assessment of pain, while the Psychosocial domain assesses psychological factors and stress. The scale, which the developers report has been used quite extensively, requires scoring and interpretation by its developers. It yields information that may be useful to guide clinicians treating TMD, although some questions of its validity as a psychological assessment tool have been noted by Rugh, Woods, and Dahlstrom (1993), Deardorff (1995), and others (e.g., Glaros & Glass, 1993).

Findings from research on the TMJ Scale indicate that women with TMD report a higher level of severity of all physical and psychological symptoms than do men, and that a relationship between severity of psychological problems and chronicity of TMD is noted. It is important to note, as the authors readily acknowledge, that the TMJ Scale has not been the subject of longitudinal studies. That is, cohorts of patients have not been repeatedly assessed with the TMJ Scale over time, but substantial data are available as cross-sectional data collected over a number of years.

IMPATH Scale

The IMPATH Scale for TMD (Fricton & Schiffman, 1987) is an interactive, computer-based assessment instrument developed for use as a screening and personal history instrument. In contrast to the TMJ Scale, the IMPATH Scale does include a carefully constructed component allowing it to be used to derive physical diagnoses of TMD subtypes. It has the advantage of instantaneous feedback, but, unfortunately, the psychometric characteristics of its illness behavior components have not yet been well established. It is mentioned here because, like the TMJ Scale, it may serve as a useful guide to clinicians wishing to obtain a clinical impression of how their patients are doing psychologically and assist them in making treatment decisions.

Multiaxial Evaluation and Classification

Until relatively recently, a critical obstacle to a broader and deeper understanding of TMD was the lack of a standardized method for conducting a reliable physical assessment of TMD signs and symptoms that could yield evidence-based diagnostic criteria for defining clinical subtypes of TMD, as well as a theoretically driven set of assessment parameters for describing a person with the pain. The rationale for assessment criteria and for integrating these two obvious dimensions—the physical diagnosis and the person—is clearly established by the success of the DSM approach for mental diseases (i.e., identifying unambiguous diagnostic criteria for each disorder, coupled with a systematic multiaxial approach for organizing comorbid factors deemed theoretically important and relevant to the specific individual).

Within the domain of pain, a number of systems have attempted an integrated multiaxial approach. These systems include the five-axis IASP pain classification system; the WHYMPI, mentioned above; and a two-dimensional system for organizing pain-related physical pathology and pain behavior (Brena & Chapman, 1983; Sanders & Brena, 1993). Although the use of each of these systems was organized centrally around pain, none has achieved widespread acceptance and usage except the WHYMPI, which has been very well received by the pain research and clinical communities and is in extensive use around the world (see Jacob & Kerns, Chapter 19, and Turk & Okifuji, Chapter 21). Nevertheless, none of these systems, including the WHYMPI, addresses a paramount concern—namely, the ability, within a single diagnostic and classification system, to integrate parameters of physical disease status *and* parameters reflecting levels of personal functioning within the context of chronic pain.

Research Diagnostic Criteria for TMD

The two of us were involved in the development of a pain diagnostic and classification system that is described in detail in the remainder of this chapter, not only because of its relevance to TMD, but also because it represents an approach that is applicable to other chronic pain disorders. It is, at present, the only comprehensive approach to assessment and diagnosis of both disease and person parameters for any of the orofacial pain disorders.

The Research Diagnostic Criteria for TMD (RDC/TMD; Dworkin & LeResche, 1992) system, resulting from an international collaboration of leading clinical researchers, allows standardization and replication of clinical TMD assessment, both for research purposes and to aid in determining diagnostic subtypes of TMD. The RDC/TMD system has been very well received and has been accepted as a standard research instrument by many sectors of the clinical research community around the world. The *American Pain Society Bulletin* reproduced the RDC/TMD examination forms and specifications in their entirety, and in the accompanying article, the RDC/TMD was held out as a model system applicable to the assessment of all chronic pain conditions (Garofalo & Wesley, 1997).

The critical features incorporated into the RDC/TMD that have been deemed valuable and innovative include the following:

1. *An interdisciplinary effort.* The RDC/TMD represents the working agreement of an international team of recognized researchers in the field whose areas of interest and expertise range from basic biological sciences to clinical dental and biobehavioral sciences.

2. *Use of a biopsychosocial theoretical model.* Because psychological and psychosocial disability have been assessed in significant numbers of patients experiencing all forms of chronic pain, it was deemed essential to describe the current behavioral, psychological, and psychosocial status of such a patient in quantifiable terms, so that the immediate and longer-term relationship between physical findings and extent of psychosocial dysfunction could be better understood.

3. *Operational definition of terms.* The RDC/TMD system's criteria are stated in operational, or measurable, terms to maximize reproducibility among investigators, hence facilitating their adoption for research and allowing comparison of results among researchers.

4. *Use of epidemiological data.* The researchers developing the RDC/TMD utilized epidemiological data to guide the selection and operationalization of these criteria.

5. *Specification of examination methods.* Detailed examination specifications are provided to allow clinical data associated with each RDC/TMD criterion to be gathered through standardized clinical examination and interview methods.

6. *Reliability of measurement.* The reliability of clinical methods and measures was established and served as the basis for selecting specific clinical measurement methods.

7. *Dual-axis system.* A two-axis approach has been used that allows physical diagnosis, placed on Axis I, to be coordinated with operationalized

assessment of psychological distress and psychosocial dysfunction associated with chronic TMD pain and orofacial disability, placed on Axis II.

A synopsis of the RDC/TMD's domains of assessment, methods for its use, and selected supporting data are provided below. A full description of the rationale and relevant empirical support for the creation of the RDC/TMD, as well as a detailed description of the complete assessment methods underlying its use, is available (Dworkin & LeResche, 1992).

Axis I: Physical Domain

The physical domain is concerned with the clinical examination and diagnostic classification for common subtypes of TMD. The results of the RDC/TMD clinical assessment examination yield Axis I diagnoses that differentiate the many physical characteristics of the disorders. Detailed specifications are provided for conducting a reliable clinical examination to yield RDC/TMD diagnoses of the most common types of TMD (Dworkin & LeResche, 1992).

TMD Signs and Symptoms. The RDC/TMD clinical examination involves clinical assessment of the following TMD signs and symptoms:

1. *Pain site.* Presenting pain is assessed as ipsi- or contralateral to pain provoked by clinical examination of masticatory muscles and by tests of jaw function;

2. *Mandibular range of motion* (*in millimeters*) *and associated presence and location of pain.* Three modes of assessment are used:

> *Jaw opening patterns* to assess for corrected/uncorrected deviations in jaw excursions during vertical jaw opening.
> *Vertical range of motion* of the mandible to assess extent of unassisted opening without pain, maximum unassisted opening, and maximum assisted opening.
> *Extent of mandibular excursive movements* to assess extent of lateral and protrusive jaw excursions.

3. *TMJ sounds.* Palpation is used to assess clicking, grating, and/or crepitus joint sounds during vertical, lateral, and protrusive jaw excursions.

4. *Muscle and joint palpation for pain or tenderness.* This includes bilateral palpation of extra-

oral and intraoral masticatory and related muscles (18 muscle sites) and bilateral palpation of TMJs (4 joint sites).

5. *TMJ imaging.* The RDC/TMD relies on clinical findings for arriving at a diagnosis, due to the high reliability of the clinical procedures (Schiffman, Anderson, Fricton, Burton, & Schellhas, 1989). However, for certain diagnostic categories related to arthroses and internal derangements of the articular disc, imaging is also recommended to confirm RDC/TMD diagnoses.

The tomographic specifications for a positive diagnosis of osteoarthrosis are that tomograms show one or more of the following: (a) erosion of normal cortical delineation, (b) sclerosis of parts or all of the condyle and articular eminence, (c) flattening of joint surfaces, or (d) osteophyte formation. The MRI specifications recommended by the RDC/TMD for disc displacement without reduction are as follows: (a) In the intercuspal occlusal position, the posterior band of the disc is clearly located at or anterior to the 11:30 position; and (b) on full opening, the posterior band remains clearly anterior to the 12:00 position.

Axis I Diagnostic Groups. The RDC/TMD groups the most common forms of TMD into three Axis I diagnostic categories and allows multiple diagnoses to be made for a given patient. The RDC/TMD Axis I diagnostic groups are as follows:

Group I. Muscle Disorders (one diagnosis permitted)
a. Myofascial Pain
b. Myofascial Pain with limited opening
Group II. Disc Displacements (one diagnosis per joint permitted)
a. Disc Displacement with reduction
b. Disc Displacement without reduction, with limited opening
c. Disc Displacement without reduction, without limited opening
Group III. Arthralgia, Arthritis, Arthrosis (one diagnosis per joint permitted)
a. Arthralgia
b. Osteoarthritis of the TMJ
c. Osteoarthrosis of the TMJ

Several independent studies (Dworkin, Sherman, et al., 1999; Ohrbach, Dworkin, & Truelove, 1999; Sherman, Dworkin, LeResche, Huggins, & Truelove, 1999) confirm the reliability of the RDC/TMD examination and the clinical validity or utility.

Axis II: Psychosocial Assessment (Self-Report Questionnaire)

The RDC/TMD Axis II assessment involves evaluation of patients' TMD-pain-related behavioral functioning, psychological status, and psychosocial level of adaptation to their TMD condition. A profile derived from self-reported ratings and endorsement of symptoms or limitations reflects perceived pain intensity, pain-related disability, orofacial limitations, depression, and nonspecific physical symptoms.

The incorporation of Axis II was guided by a multidimensional biopsychosocial model of chronic pain, which advocates classifying patients with chronic pain, including patients with TMD, according to their level of psychosocial function (Rudy et al., 1989; Turk, 1990). Although pain conditions differ in terms of the location, severity, and etiology of the pain itself, all chronic pain conditions—regardless of body site or peripheral nociceptive mechanisms—tend to be associated with similar cognitive, affective, and behavioral characteristics. For example, many patients with chronic pain have negative expectations regarding the abatement of their pain and exhibit many symptoms of depression (Dworkin & Massoth, 1994; Gatchel, Garofalo, Ellis, & Holt, 1996). The Axis II profile of the RDC/TMD taps into these characteristics, making further exploration possible.

Specifically, the RDC/TMD Axis II questionnaire includes 31 questions covering the following information devoted to demographics and Axis II psychosocial assessment.

Demographics. Demographic information includes age, gender, ethnicity, education level, marital status, and income level.

Pain Characteristics. Pain intensity is assessed with Visual Analogue Scales or Numerical Rating Scales, and temporal patterns of TMD-related pain are determined.

Parafunctional Behaviors and Jaw Disability. The domain of parafunctional behaviors and jaw disability associated with the pain disorder has been the least well-developed area, but it was important enough to capture that it was subsumed into a single dimension in the original RDC/TMD. Current thinking, however, clearly supports the separation of parafunctional behaviors (as factors that contribute to the pain problem) from disability (which is related to the behavioral or functional consequences of the problem). Note, however, that these two constructs may be confounded in their assessment. Here we provide our latest thinking on these two areas, along with preliminary data supportive of some new approaches.

1. *Parafunctional behaviors.* The major theories of TMD etiology include the possibility that parafunctional oral behaviors may represent opportunities for masticatory muscle physical abuse and physiological impairment to occur—the latter primarily manifested as prolonged and painful nociceptive reactions in response to muscle overuse (American Academy of Orofacial Pain & Okeson, 1996; Fricton, Kroening, & Hathaway, 1987; Ohrbach & Gale, 1989). Although there is little evidence for peripheral inflammation in the masticatory muscle as causal to chronic muscle pain, a precise understanding of how such pain (and presumably nociception) arises remains elusive (Lund, Dong, Widmer, & Stohler, 1991; Mense, 1991). Nevertheless, it is widely accepted on epidemiological, experimental, and theoretical grounds that parafunctional oral behaviors are significantly associated with chronic TMD pain (Flor & Turk, 1989; Glaros, Tabacchi, & Glass, 1998; Goulet, Lavigne, & Lund, 1995; Ohrbach, Blascovich, Gale, McCall, & Dworkin, 1998; Velly, Philippe, & Gornitsky, 1999), with the mechanism linking parafunction to pain being unclear (Ohrbach & McCall, 1996). Thus tooth grinding and jaw clenching are factors contributing to TMD-related pain for many patients, and the presence of persistent daytime and nocturnal jaw clenching or bruxism is a critical obstacle to improvement, especially for those patients with TMD diagnosed with a primary muscle disorder and/or joint pain (e.g., RDC/TMD Axis I, Group I Muscle Disorders and Group IIIa Arthralgia Disorders).

The assessment of maladaptive behaviors affecting the use of the jaw represents one of the two least quantified aspects of the RDC/TMD, and it is an assessment dimension that requires substantial additional development. The traditional approach is to use a behavioral checklist (inquiring whether the patient is aware of such behaviors during the daytime, whether symptoms indicative of nocturnal bruxism are present, whether a sleeping partner has observed the behavior during sleep) and self-monitoring.

Self-monitoring includes the use of a diary for the patient to record target behaviors, and it is particularly appropriate for behaviors such as oral parafunction that are often outside conscious awareness but can be brought into awareness via intentional monitoring. Although self-monitoring is a well-established method in the behavioral literature (Hedges, Krantz, Contrada, & Rozanski, 1990; Kerns, Finn, & Haythornthwaite, 1988), we believe that it is underutilized in the assessment of parameters intrinsic or related to chronic pain. Furthermore, we believe that self-monitoring of behaviors such as oral parafunction constitutes an opportunity for research into conscious processes.

The fact that oral parafunction often occurs outside conscious awareness not only makes its reliable detection problematic, but also leads to serious problems in estimating its causal role. For example, how much parafunctional behavior is required for it to be dysfunctional? How much of such behavior needs to be brought under conscious control in order for pain to change? Finally, is the behavior autonomous, stress-related, or a concomitant of certain emotional states, and do these various predictors lead to differential ability to reliably assess the presence and extent of the behavior? These are all issues that need to be addressed in the RDC approach to TMD.

2. *Jaw disability.* The assessment of disability during use of the jaw in the presence of orofacial pain has, curiously, not been well developed to date. Part of the problem may be a confounding of assessing limitations in jaw use as a consequence of TMD-related pain, with alterations in jaw use reflected as parafunctional jaw behaviors as a causal factor for the disorder, although parafunctional jaw behaviors are frequently observed in the absence of any orofacial pain condition.

There is only one published instrument for assessing jaw disability in terms of reported limited ability to use the jaws: the Mandibular Function Impairment Questionnaire (MFIQ; Stegenga, de Bont, de Leeuw, & Boering, 1993). The MFIQ has excellent face validity, inquiring about difficulties in eating hard food, smiling, and kissing; a strength is the presence of six items assessing difficulties in eating specific items (e.g., an apple or a raw carrot). Its validity with respect to clean and simple factors, however, is problematic: There are two reasonably strong factors and a weak third factor; the authors combine without explanation the third largely independent factor into the second, with the resultant factor labels of "Masticatory" and "Nonmasticatory." The Nonmasticatory factor is a combination of jaw behaviors such as yawning and of social and work activities. Validity was further assessed through the use of self-administration versus interview administration over a 2-hour period; the Pearson coefficient was greater than .90. No test–retest reliability and no assessment of construct validity were provided by the authors.

We have recently used an alternative approach to the assessment of jaw disability (Horrell, Ohrbach, Markello, & Granger, 1999; Ohrbach, Dworkin, & Granger, 1999), and although it is still in development, it may be useful to describe it briefly. The approach is based on a Rasch measurement model, allowing development of a successful measure of functional limitations for use in inpatient rehabilitation medicine settings, the Functional Independence Measure.

Applying Rasch measurement methodology to self-reported jaw disability, our analyses of the highly face-valid terms for assessing such disability, such as eating hard food, yawning, smiling, or talking, have resulted in a hierarchy of these items that makes sense physiologically. That is, with jaw pain, difficulty in eating hard food would be an item associated with minimal disability. In contrast, difficulty in drinking or swallowing would be associated with appreciable disability, because normally those behaviors are easily performed. Thus the Rasch modeling approach produces a scale in which items, across diverse samples of patients, will be graded from least difficult (minimally disabling) to most difficult (appreciably disabling). Compared to classical test theory (where it does not matter which items were endorsed to create a particular score, and where the same score can be obtained by endorsing different combinations of the same number of items), in Rasch modeling the particular items endorsed matter very much, because they are arranged in an empirically validated hierarchy from least to most difficult. We believe that this measurement model has much merit for exploring the complex domain of TMD-related disability.

Psychological Status. Depression, Anxiety, and nonspecific physical symptoms (Somatization) scores are measured with subscales of the SCL-90R (Derogatis, 1983), although the RDC/TMD does not require use of these measures only to screen for psychological status; indeed, any well-validated measure for which relevant population norms are available (e.g., the Beck Depression Inventory or the Spielberger State–Trait Anxiety Inventory) may be used to accomplish the intended purpose of identifying whether the patient may be at risk for an important mood or anxiety disorder. The scales incorporated into the RDC/TMD for assessing psychological status have been normed on relevant populations through large-scale population-based studies of individuals with chronic pain, including TMD.

Psychosocial Functioning. The domain of psychosocial functioning is assessed in the RDC/TMD through use of a version of the GCPS (discussed above). This yields a 0–IV score reflecting the severity and psychosocial impact of TMD in terms of interference with usual functioning at home, work, or school and incorporating disability days (loss of work days) due to TMD-related pain.

CONCLUSIONS

The conceptual approach and methods employed by the RDC/TMD allow assessment of pathophysiological and psychosocial factors demonstrated to be relevant to management of TMD. Because much more attention has typically been directed at the pathophysiological processes that might account for TMD, attention is directed in this concluding section to the four biobehavioral domains assessed by the RDC/TMD, with a view to guiding more rational decisions concerning management of TMD. From a practical treatment perspective, it should be noted that the assessment of these biobehavioral domains is accomplished largely through routine history and examination methods incorporated into the RDC/TMD—methods that are generally familiar and typically used by the clinician following the standard biomedical assessment model—and requires no special measuring instruments or questionnaires. Where specialized measures may be useful, they have been indicated.

Patient's Self-Assessment

Included in the patient's self-assessment is recording of *pain complaint* (with special attention to consistency of subjective report with relevant anatomy and physiology); *treatment history* (with attention to record of prior successful and unsuccessful treatments and experiences with health care professionals); and the patient's *explanatory model* for his or her condition (with attention to physical vs. behavioral factors, such as stress, in perceived etiology, maintenance, and exacerbation of the condition). Patients with a rigidly held physical or biomedical model of their condition will be more resistant to consideration of behavioral change strategies that may help them cope more adequately with their chronic pain problem (Massoth et al., 1994).

Oral Parafunction and Jaw Disability

Assessment of the second biobehavioral domain includes assessment of parafunctional oral behaviors such as nocturnal and diurnal bruxism (tooth grinding) and jaw clenching. Because the principal treatment for these maladaptive jaw behaviors is, in effect, to change the behavior, it is reasonable to include assessment of parafunctional behaviors as part of the full psychosocial assessment of the patient with TMD. Again, more attention seems to have been directed by dentists and psychologists and other mental health workers at modifying maladaptive parafunctional oral behaviors than at any other clinical aspect of the TMD condition. At the same time, as mentioned earlier, this domain has received very little systematic attention with regard to development of reliable and valid measures for determining whether and when parafunctional jaw behaviors are associated with orofacial pain conditions, and whether and when jaw disability arises in association with or is independent of abusive patterns of jaw use.

Psychological Status

Assessment of the third biobehavioral domain includes depression, anxiety, and the presence of multiple nonspecific physical symptoms (somatization). Formal assessment of psychological status requires specialized measurement instruments and diagnostic interview schedules (see Sullivan, Chapter 15, and Bradley & McKendree-Smith, Chapter 16). However, the inclusion of relatively straightforward measures such as the SCL-90R in a clinical database used routinely with all patients minimizes resistance to the perception that undue attention is being given to psychological factors while the patient feels that a physical pain problem is being presented. Such measures are more appropriate as screening aids, allowing clinical impressions to be formed concerning the need for more specialized psychological assessment, which is generally achieved through referral to a psychiatrist or clinical psychologist. Depression commonly co-occurs with chronic pain conditions and has been documented as present in patients attending TMD clinics. Similarly, somatization is present in

a significant minority of patients with TMD, and there is ample evidence that even moderately elevated levels of long-standing somatization represent an important obstacle to successful treatment outcome.

Psychosocial Status

The fourth biobehavioral domain, current level of psychosocial function, is generally reflected for patients with chronic pain in extent of interference with activities of daily living attributed to TMD, as well as extent of health care utilization (see also Jacob & Kerns, Chapter 19). Prognosis is more guarded when self-reported activity limitations due to TMD are high, and when pain interferes appreciably with ability to discharge responsibilities at home, school, or work and/or limits socializing activities. The assessment of both psychological status and level of psychosocial function is viewed as essential to allowing rational clinical decisions to be made in the management of TMD. The most useful measures for assessing level of psychosocial functioning are the WHYMPI, and the version of the GCPS contained within the RDC/TMD.

The most compelling rationale for conducting a thorough, multidimensional assessment of patients with pain is to gather a rational evidence base for making treatment and long-term management decisions. Management of all chronic pain conditions, including TMD, emphasizes a rehabilitation approach to treatment rather than a cure model (Melzack & Wall, 1982). Consistent with such an approach, reliance is placed on a patient's acquiring a useful set of self-management strategies that facilitate more adaptive pain coping behaviors, emotional responses, and thought patterns.

REFERENCES

American Academy of Orofacial Pain (AAOP) & Okeson, J. P. (Eds.). (1996). *Orofacial pain: Guidelines for assessment, diagnosis, and management.* Chicago: Quintessence.

American Academy of Pediatric Dentistry & University of Texas Health Science Center at San Antonio Dental School. (1990). Treatment of temporomandibular disorders in children: Summary statements and recommendations. *Journal of the American Dental Association, 120,* 265–269.

American Dental Association. (1983). *The President's Conference on the Dentist–Patient Relationship and the Management of Fear, Anxiety and Pain.* Chicago: Author.

American Psychiatric Association. (1994). *Diagnostic and statistical manual of mental disorders* (4th ed.). Washington, DC: Author.

Bogetto, F., Maina, G., Ferro, G., Carbone, M., & Gandolfo, S. (1998). Psychiatric comorbidity in patients with burning mouth syndrome. *Psychosomatic Medicine, 60,* 378–385.

Brena, S. F., & Chapman, S. L. (1983). An algorithm for decision-making in patients with pain. In S. F. Brena & S. L. Chapman (Eds.), *Management of patients with chronic pain* (pp. 111–120). New York: SP Medical & Scientific Books.

Buckelew, S. P., DeGood, D. E., Schwartz, D. P., & Kerler, R. M. (1986). Cognitive and somatic item response pattern of pain patients, psychiatric patients, and hospital employees. *Journal of Clinical Psychology, 42,* 852–860.

Carlsson, G. E., & LeResche, L. (1995). Epidemiology of temporomandibular disorders. In B. J. Sessle, P. S. Bryant, & R. A. Dionne (Eds.), *Progress in pain research and management* (pp. 211–226). Seattle, WA: International Association for the Study of Pain Press.

Craig, K. D. (1989). Emotional aspects of pain. In P. D. Wall & R. Melzack (Eds.), *Textbook of pain* (2nd ed., pp. 220–230). Edinburgh: Churchill Livingstone.

Dao, T. T. T., Knight, K., Tenenbaum, H. C., Lue, F., & Ton-That, V. (1996). Influence of oral contraceptives on the fluctuations of myofascial pain over three consecutive menstrual cycles: A preliminary report. *Abstracts of the 8th World Congress on Pain,* 278.

Deardorff, W. H. (1995). TMJ scale. In J. C. Conoley & J. C. Impara (Eds.), *The twelfth mental measurements yearbook* (pp. 1070–1071). Lincoln: Buros Institute of Mental Measurements, University of Nebraska.

Derogatis, L. R. (1983). *SCL-90-R: Administration, scoring and procedures manual–II for the Revised Version.* Towson, MD: Clinical Psychometric Research.

Dworkin, S. F. (1990). Illness behavior and dysfunction: Review of concepts and application to chronic pain. *Canadian Journal of Physiology and Pharmacology, 69,* 662–671.

Dworkin, S. F. (1995). Personal and societal impact of orofacial pain. In J. R. Fricton & R. B. Dubner (Eds.), *Orofacial pain and temporomandibular disorders* (pp. 15–32). New York: Raven Press.

Dworkin, S. F., & LeResche, L. (Eds.). (1992). Research Diagnostic Criteria for Temporomandibular Disorders: Review, criteria, examinations and specifications, critique. *Journal of Craniomandibular Disorders: Facial and Oral Pain, 6,* 301–355.

Dworkin, S. F., & Massoth, D. L. (1994). Temporomandibular disorders and chronic pain: Disease or illness? *Journal of Prosthetic Dentistry, 72,* 29–38.

Dworkin, S. F., Sherman, J., Ohrbach, R., Truelove, E., Huggins, K. H., & LeResche, L. (1999, March). *Validity for research and clinical utility of RDC/TMD Axis II* [Abstract]. Paper presented at the annual meeting of the International Association for Dental Research, Vancouver, British Columbia, Canada.

Dworkin, S. F., Turner, J., Huggins, K. H., Massoth, D., Wilson, L., Mancl, L., & Truelove, E. (1999, August). *Tailoring TMD treatment: Cognitive-behavioral therapy (CBT) with usual treatment for dysfunctional cases* [Abstract]. Paper presented at the International Association for the Study of Pain 9th World Congress on Pain, Vienna.

Dworkin, S. F., Von Korff, M. R., & LeResche, L. (1990). Multiple pains and psychiatric disturbance: An epidemiologic investigation. *Archives of General Psychiatry, 47,* 239–244.

Dworkin, S. F., Von Korff, M., & LeResche, L. (1992). Epidemiologic studies of chronic pain: A dynamic-ecologic perspective. *Annals of Behavioral Medicine, 14,* 3–11.

Fields, H. (1987). *Pain.* New York: McGraw-Hill.

Flor, H., & Turk, D. C. (1989). Psychophysiology of chronic pain: Do chronic pain patients exhibit symptom-specific psychophysiologic responses? *Psychological Bulletin, 105,* 215–259.

Fordyce, W. E., Brockway, J. A., Bergman, J. A., & Spengler, D. (1986). Acute back pain: A control-group comparison of behavioral vs. traditional management methods. *Journal of Behavioral Medicine, 9,* 127–140.

Foreman, P. A., Harold, P. L., & Hay, K. D. (1994). An evaluation of the diagnosis, treatment, and outcome of patients with chronic orofacial pain. *New Zealand Dental Journal, 90,* 44–48.

Fricton, J. R., Kroening, R. J., & Hathaway, K. M. (1987). *TMJ and craniofacial pain: Diagnosis and management.* St. Louis, MO: Ishiyaku EuroAmerica.

Fricton, J. R., & Schiffman, E. L. (1987). The craniomandibular index: Validity. *Journal of Prosthetic Dentistry, 58,* 222–228.

Garofalo, J. P., & Wesley, A. L. (1997, May–June). Research Diagnostic Criteria for Temporomandibular Disorders: Reflection of the physical–psychological interface. *American Pain Society Bulletin,* pp. 4–16.

Gatchel, R. J., Garofalo, J. P., Ellis, E., & Holt, C. (1996). Major psychological disorders in acute and chronic TMD: An initial examination. *Journal of the American Dental Association, 127,* 1365–1374.

Glaros, A. G., & Glass, E. G. (1993). Temporomandibular disorders. In R. J. Gatchel & E. B. Blanchard (Eds.), *Psychophysiological disorders* (pp. 299–356). Washington, DC: American Psychological Association.

Glaros, A. G., Tabacchi, K. N., & Glass, E. G. (1998). Effect of parafunctional clenching on TMD pain. *Journal of Orofacial Pain, 12,* 145–152.

Goulet, J.-P., Lavigne, G. J., & Lund, J. P. (1995). Jaw pain prevalence among French-speaking Canadians in Quebec and related symptoms of temporomandibular disorders. *Journal of Dental Research, 74,* 1738–1744.

Hathaway, S. R., & McKinley, J. C. (1983). *Manual for administration and scoring of the MMPI.* Minneapolis, MN: National Computer Systems.

Hedges, S., Krantz, D. S., Contrada, R. J., & Rozanski, A. R. (1990). Development of a diary for use with ambulatory monitoring of mood, activities, and physiological function. *Journal of Psychopathology and Behavioral Assessment, 12,* 203–217.

Helmy, E. S., Timmis, D. P., Sharawy, M. H., Abdelatif, O., & Bays, R. A. (1990). Fatty change in the human temporomandibular joint disc: Light and electron microscopy study. *International Journal of Oral and Maxillofacial Surgery, 19,* 38–43.

Horrell, B. M., Ohrbach, R., Markello, S., & Granger, C. (1999). Validity of a self-report scale for TMD-related disability [Abstract]. *Journal of Dental Research, 78,* 292.

Huggins, K. H., Dworkin, S. F., Turner, J., Wilson, L., Massoth, D., Lane, M., Mancl, L., & Truelove, E. (1999, August). *Tailoring TMD treatment: Self-*

management vs. usual treatment for psychosocially functional patients [Abstract]. Presented at the International Association for the Study of Pain 9th World Congress on Pain, Vienna.

International Association for the Study of Pain (IASP) Subcommittee on Taxonomy & Merskey, H. (Eds.). (1986). Classification of chronic pain syndromes and definitions of pain terms. *Pain*, Suppl. 3, S1–S226.

Kerns, R. D., Finn, P., & Haythornthwaite, J. (1988). Self-monitored pain intensity: Psychometric properties and clinical utility. *Journal of Behavioral Medicine*, 11, 71–82.

LeResche, L. (1997). Epidemiology of temporomandibular disorders: Implications for the investigation of etiologic factors. *Critical Reviews in Oral Biology and Medicine*, 8, 291–305.

LeResche, L., & Dworkin, S. F. (1988). Facial expressions of pain and emotions in chronic TMD patients. *Pain*, 35, 71–78.

LeResche, L., Dworkin, S. F., Wilson, L., & Ehrlich, K. J. (1992). Effect of temporomandibular disorder pain duration on facial expressions and verbal report of pain. *Pain*, 51, 289–295.

Levitt, S. R. (1990). Predictive value of the TMJ Scale in detecting clinically significant symptoms of temporomandibular disorders. *Journal of Craniomandibular Disorders: Facial and Oral Pain*, 4, 177–185.

Levitt, S. R. (1991). Predictive value: A model for dentists to evaluate the accuracy of diagnostic tests for temporomandibular disorders as applied to the TMJ Scale. *Journal of Prosthetic Dentistry*, 66, 385–390.

Levitt, S. R., Lundeen, T. F., & McKinney, M. W. (1988). Initial studies of a new assessment method for temporomandibular joint disorders. *Journal of Prosthetic Dentistry*, 59(4), 490–495.

Levitt, S. R., Lundeen, T. F., & McKinney, M. W. (1994). *The TMJ Scale manual*. Durham, NC: Pain Resource Center.

Lund, J. P., Dong, R., Widmer, C. G., & Stohler, C. S. (1991). The pain-adaptation model: A discussion of the relationship between chronic pain and musculoskeletal pain and motor activity. *Canadian Journal of Physiology and Pharmacology*, 69, 683–693.

Massoth, D. L., Dworkin, S. F., Whitney, C. W., Harrison, R. G., Wilson, L., & Turner, J. (1994). Patient explanatory models for temporomandibular disorders. In G. F. Gebhart, D. L. Hammond, & T. S. Jensen (Eds.), *Proceedings of the 7th World Congress on Pain* (pp. 187–200). Seattle, WA: International Association for the Study of Pain Press.

McCreary, C. P., Clark, G. T., Oakley, M. E., & Flack, V. (1992). Predicting response to treatment for temporomandibular disorders. *Journal of Craniomandibular Disorders: Facial and Oral Pain*, 6, 161–169.

Melzack, R., & Wall, P. D. (1982). *The challenge of pain*. New York: Basic Books.

Mense, S. (1991). Considerations concerning the neurobiological basis of muscle pain. *Canadian Journal of Physiology and Pharmacology*, 69, 610–616.

Miyamoto, S. A., & Ziccardi, V. B. (1998). Burning mouth syndrome. *Mount Sinai Journal of Medicine*, 65, 343–347.

Mott, A. E., Grushka, M., & Sessle, B. J. (1993). Diagnosis and management of taste disorders and burning mouth syndrome. *Dental Clinics of North America*, 37, 33–71.

Ohrbach, R., Blascovich, J., Gale, E. N., McCall, W. D., Jr., & Dworkin, S. F. (1998). Psychophysiological assessment of stress in chronic pain: Comparisons of stressful stimuli and of response systems. *Journal of Dental Research*, 77(10), 1840–1850.

Ohrbach, R., & Burgess, J. (1999). Temporomandibular disorders and orofacial pain. In R. E. Rakel (Ed.), *Conn's current therapy* (pp. 97–104). Philadelphia: Saunders.

Ohrbach, R., Dworkin, S. F., & Granger, C. V. (1999, August). *Cross-validation of a disability scale for chronic temporomandibular disorder pain* [Abstract]. Paper presented at the International Association for the Study of Pain 9th World Congress on Pain, Vienna.

Ohrbach, R., Dworkin, S. F., & Truelove, E. (1999, March). *Domains of measurement in chronic TMD pain: Psychometric properties* [Abstract]. Paper presented at the annual meeting of the International Association for Dental Research, Vancouver, British Columbia, Canada.

Ohrbach, R., & Gale, E. N. (1989). Pressure pain thresholds in normal muscles: Reliability, measurement and topographic differences. *Pain*, 37, 257–263.

Ohrbach, R., & McCall, W. D., Jr. (1996). The stress-hyperactivity-pain theory of myogenic pain: Proposal for a revised theory. *Pain Forum*, 5, 51–66.

Okeson, J. P. (1995). *Bell's orofacial pains* (5th ed.). Chicago: Quintessence.

Prkachin, K., & Mercer, S. R. (1990). Pain expression in patients with shoulder pathology: Validity, properties and relationship to sickness impact. *Pain*, 39, 257–265.

Raustia, A. M., & Pyhtinen, J. (1990). Computed tomography of the temporomandibular joint. In A. M. DelBalso (Ed.), *Maxillofacial imaging* (pp. 653–673). Philadelphia: Saunders.

Rudy, T., Turk, D., Kubinski, J., & Zaki, H. (1994). Efficacy of tailoring treatment for dysfunctional TMD patients [Abstract]. *Journal of Dental Research*, 73, 439.

Rudy, T. E., Turk, D. C., Zaki, H. S., & Curtin, H. D. (1989). An empirical taxometric alternative to traditional classification of temporomandibular disorders. *Pain*, 36, 311–320.

Rugh, J. D., Woods, B. J., & Dahlstrom, L. (1993). Temporomandibular disorders: Assessment of psychosocial factors. *Advances in Dental Research*, 7, 127–136.

Sanders, S. H., & Brena, S. F. (1993). Empirically derived chronic pain patient subgroups: The utility of multidimensional clustering to identify differential treatment effects. *Pain*, 54, 51–56.

Schiffman, E., Anderson, G., Fricton, J., Burton, K., & Schellhas, K. (1989). Diagnostic criteria for intraarticular T.M. disorders. *Community Dentistry and Oral Epidemiology*, 17(5), 252–257.

Sharav, Y. (1989). Orofacial pain. In P. D. Wall & R. Melzack (Eds.), *Textbook of pain* (2nd ed., pp. 441–454). Edinburgh: Churchill Livingstone.

Sherman, J. J., Dworkin, S. F., LeResche, L., Huggins, K. H., & Truelove, E. (1999, August). *The validity and clinical utility of the RDC/TMD Axis II* [Abstract]. Paper presented at the International Association for the Study of Pain 9th World Congress on Pain, Vienna.

Ship, J. A., Grushka, M., Lipton, J. A., Mott, A. E., Sessle, B. J., & Dionne, R. A. (1995). Burning mouth syndrome: An update. *Journal of the American Dental Association*, 126, 842–853.

Stegenga, B., de Bont, L. G. M., de Leeuw, R., & Boering, G. (1993). Assessment of mandibular function impairment associated with temporomandibular joint osteoarthrosis and internal derangement. *Journal of Orofacial Pain, 7,* 183–195.

Turk, D. C. (1990). Strategies for classifying chronic orofacial pain patients. *Anesthesia Progress, 37,* 155–160.

Turk, D. C., & Rudy, T. E. (1988). Toward an empirically derived taxonomy of chronic pain patients: Integration of psychological assessment data. *Journal of Consulting and Clinical Psychology, 56,* 233–238.

Turner, J. A., Whitney, C., Dworkin, S. F., Massoth, D. L., & Wilson, L. (1995). Do changes in patient beliefs and coping strategies predict temporomandibular disorder treatment outcomes? *Clinical Journal of Pain, 11,* 177–188.

Velly, A. M., Philippe, P., & Gornitsky, M. (1999). Case-control study of risk factors for temporomandibular disorders [Abstract]. *Journal of Dental Research, 78,* 491.

Von Korff, M., Dworkin, S. F., & LeResche, L. (1990). Graded chronic pain status: An epidemiologic evaluation. *Pain, 40,* 279–291.

Von Korff, M., Dworkin, S. F., LeResche, L., & Kruger, A. (1988). An epidemiologic comparison of pain complaints. *Pain, 32,* 173–183.

Von Korff, M., Ormel, J., Keefe, F. J., & Dworkin, S. F. (1992). Grading the severity of chronic pain. *Pain, 50,* 133–149.

Wilson, L., Dworkin, S. F., Whitney, C., & LeResche, L. (1994). Somatization and pain dispersion in chronic temporomandibular pain. *Pain, 57,* 55–61.

Chapter 26

The Diagnosis of Myofascial Pain Syndromes

ROBERT D. GERWIN

Physicians are frequently asked to see persons with a primary complaint of pain. The nature of the pain must be determined so that it may be treated specifically, if possible. At times this can be a difficult task, especially when the cause is obscure or the pain is poorly defined. When pain occurs in a region of the body but no structural or pathological cause is found, the physician and the patient are both frustrated. Symptomatic treatment may be given reluctantly without a firm diagnosis. Psychological causes for the pain are often diagnosed or implied to exist. The problem can be irksome when the patient has undergone surgery—for example, for a herniated disc with radiculopathy—but still complains of pain in the previously affected arm or leg despite normal postoperative magnetic resonance scanning and no new neurological impairment. The patient may be labeled a malingerer or thought to be drug-seeking. Muscle pain or myofascial pain should be considered in such cases.

Patients do not often identify muscle as the source of the pain. Rather, they are likely to identify an area or region of the body (e.g., the shoulder, the hip, or the low back) as the site of pain. The ability of the clinician to diagnose the condition causing such pain is often dependent on the skill with which muscle is examined and the familiarity of the examiner with the pain patterns caused by myofascial or muscle trigger points.

TWO CASE EXAMPLES

Pain syndromes caused by tender zones in muscle can be simple in an acute injury if only a single muscle is involved. On the other hand, chronic syndromes can be complex when there are multiple muscles involved and when there are underlying or comorbid conditions that impede the recovery process. Two case histories illustrate these different presentations.

Case 1

History

R. W. was a 20-year-old college student who developed acute left chest pain while playing varsity football. He was sent home for an evaluation for a suspected heart attack or other cardiac problem. Cardiac evaluation, including a 24-hour Holter monitor, echocardiogram, and treadmill stress test, was normal. He was referred for evaluation of noncardiac chest pain. The history was of an acute injury on the playing field. He had not had any previous similar chest pain, and was otherwise healthy. He was doing well in school.

Examination

Tight, tender bands were found in the left pectoralis major muscle, as well as restricted extension and abduction of the left arm because of pain. Palpation of the tender bands of muscle in the pectoralis major muscle reproduced R. W.'s chest pain. Strumming palpation of the bands caused them to contract sharply or to twitch. No other abnormality was found.

Treatment

Trigger point injections using local anesthetic were given in the tender areas on the taut bands. His pain was relieved immediately. The muscle was stretched, and he was taught a self-stretching routine.

Follow-Up

R. W. had no further chest pain, and returned to school 2 weeks later. He was reinstated on the football team and played the remainder of the season with no recurrence. He remained well throughout the school year.

Comment

R. W. illustrates a single muscle syndrome, with pain that is local (rather than referred to a distance), acute in nature, and referable to a specific incident, without confounding perpetuating factors to impede recovery. Diagnosis and treatment were straightforward and successful.

Case 2

History

A. P. was a 45-year-old woman who complained of bilateral shoulder and neck pain, as well as severe fatigue. She worked for an international corporation and traveled widely. She had been stationed in Africa on and off for 15 years. She had traveled extensively in rural Africa 12 years previously; she had contracted amoebiasis at that time, but had been treated and considered parasite-free. She had recently been assigned to open a new branch office, but found the job daunting because of pain and fatigue. She had no history of injury. She was a highly effective career woman, with a strong sense of duty and a strong drive to succeed. She often worked 12- to 14-hour days. Her job required hours at the computer, long stretches of reading and editing, and long periods of time on the telephone, in addition to dealing with personnel issues and establishing new contacts and procedures. She complained of vague abdominal pains, which were ascribed to stress by her primary phy-

sician. She was also constipated, and felt cold when others felt comfortable. She wore sweaters in the summer. She was easily tired, felt exhausted after working 4–6 hours, often read in bed because she was too tired to stay at the office, and never felt rested even after a night's sleep.

Examination

There was widespread muscle tenderness in the muscles of the neck and shoulder, including both the right and left splenius capitis muscles, the trapezius muscles, the levator scapulae, the infraspinatus muscles, the sternocleidomastoid muscles, the pectoral muscles, the teres major and minor muscles, the latissimus dorsi muscles, and the subscapularis muscles. These muscles contained multiple taut bands that were tender to palpation. Palpation of these muscles reproduced the pain that she usually experienced. Muscle twitch responses were readily elicited when the taut bands were manually strummed. Range of motion of the neck was restricted in rotation and extension. Range of motion of the arms was restricted in internal rotation on the hand-to-scapula test, where the person is asked to reach behind the back and touch the opposite scapula. The general physical examination was normal except for a nodular thyroid gland that was twice the normal size. The neurological examination was normal except for reduction of upper-extremity strength because of pain.

Treatment

A. P. was treated in physical therapy and given trigger point injections with local anesthetic. There was transient relief of some muscle pain, but she never reached an optimal level of comfort or felt free of pain in her neck, shoulders, or arms. She continued to feel fatigued, and also became deeply depressed over her condition. She felt that she was letting the company down by not being able to perform at her best and was stressed by the certainty that she would lose her job, despite assurances by her superiors that they were willing to give her whatever time she needed to recover her health. Attention was turned to investigating the causes of her persistent pain, in an effort to understand why she did not respond as expected. Laboratory studies were performed to evaluate tissue iron stores, thyroid function, and vitamin B_{12} and folic acid levels; a complete blood count and serum chemistries were also done. She was found to have depleted tissue iron stores, with a ferritin level of

21 ng/ml. Despite a normal thyroid-stimulating hormone (TSH) level the previous year, her TSH was now elevated to 20 MIU/L. The hematocrit and hemoglobin, and the erythrocyte size and hemoglobin, were normal. She was diagnosed as having iron deficiency and hypothyroidism. Iron supplementation and thyroxin were prescribed. She was evaluated by an endocrinologist for the cause of her hypothyroidism, subsequently diagnosed as Hashimoto's thyroiditis. Her ferritin level rose to 41 ng/ml, and the TSH dropped to 7.0, then 4.9, and finally 2.6 ISU. She improved somewhat, and her fatigue lessened but was still a limiting factor in her work. She could work longer hours, but she had to go home to bed after work and was unable to attend social functions in the evening. She no longer felt as cold. The treatment of her muscle pain and the elimination of the painful trigger points was more effective, and she improved functionally, becoming better able to carry out her work activities. Nevertheless, she did not feel well and continued to be affected by recurrent and disabling upper body pain. The history of amoebiasis was reviewed, and the possibility that she still harbored an amoebic infestation was evaluated by examining her stools for ova and parasites, and obtaining serological studies for amoeba. These studies showed active infection with *Dientamoeba fragilis* and *Entamoeba histolytica*. She underwent treatment for amoebiasis. Her abdominal pains ceased after treatment; she was also no longer as fatigued, and she responded quite well to physical therapy and to muscle trigger point injection therapy. However, she found the ordeal of her long illness draining and took a leave of absence from her job. She felt less stress, slept better, and felt rested upon awakening. Her pain was now minimal and did not interfere with her daily activities.

Follow-up

A. P. was able to begin a physical conditioning program. She continued with this regimen, (including a regular exercise program) and remained relatively pain-free throughout the next year, with only minor relapses that were easily treated. She was successful at free-lance consulting during that year.

Comment

This was an unusually complex situation. A. P. complained of pain that on examination was readily found to be caused by widespread muscle trigger points. She had no obvious injury or biomechani-

cal stresses to account for the degree of pain and widespread nature of the myofascial syndrome. There was a tendency for her primary physicians to blame the pain on the psychological stress of her new position. However, she was found to have two common perpetuating factors associated with persistent, chronic myofascial pain syndromes—hypothyroidism and iron deficiency, both capable of producing a state of easy fatigue associated with a sense of inner coldness. She also had an uncommon cause of persistent myofascial pain syndrome—amoebiasis. Treatment of all of these conditions allowed her muscles to respond to treatment. The leave of absence from her job further reduced her psychological stress, and undoubtedly contributed to her recovery as well.

These two case histories illustrate the diagnostic principles of myofascial pain management. The identification of the pain problem as being caused by muscle is the necessary first step. Localization of the muscles involved in the pain syndrome is the second step. Reevaluation of the problem to identify causes for persistent pain is the third step, which leads in turn to a comprehensive treatment program. Each step is a complex process requiring the solution of particular problems.

DIAGNOSTIC EVALUATION

Identification of the problem as being caused by muscle requires the usual history and physical examination that all clinicians use daily. The peculiar adaptations of history taking required by investigating pain problems are discussed below. The physical examination starts with a general assessment, as in any examination. A basic neurological examination is also necessary to assess motor and sensory function. The musculoskeletal examination starts with the assessment of the skeletal structure, and proceeds to a muscle-by-muscle examination of relevant regions for myofascial trigger points. Finally, laboratory examinations are made to evaluate associated comorbid conditions that either initiate or perpetuate the myofascial pain syndrome. Reexamination is always in order when the response is not as expected, and the patient is not recovering.

History

The history of the pain problem (see Table 26.1 on page 505) begins with a description of the present complaint, to help focus the physician on the problem at hand. A pain diagram (Figure 26.1A) is very helpful in understanding the patient's complaint. When used on subsequent follow-up visits, it dramatically illustrates improvement or lack of improvement. For example, a young woman came to the clinic with a 2-week history of pain "where I sit" in the right buttock. She was not comfortable sitting down at all, and preferred to stand while telling her story. She was well until she sat on a stony beach during her vacation. The stones made walking uncomfortable, causing her to scoot across the stones on her buttocks to the water in order to swim, and to reverse the process when she came out of the water to sunbathe. She did this for several days. The flight back home from her holiday was quite uncomfortable, and she walked up and down the aisle of the plane as much as possible, in contrast to the com-

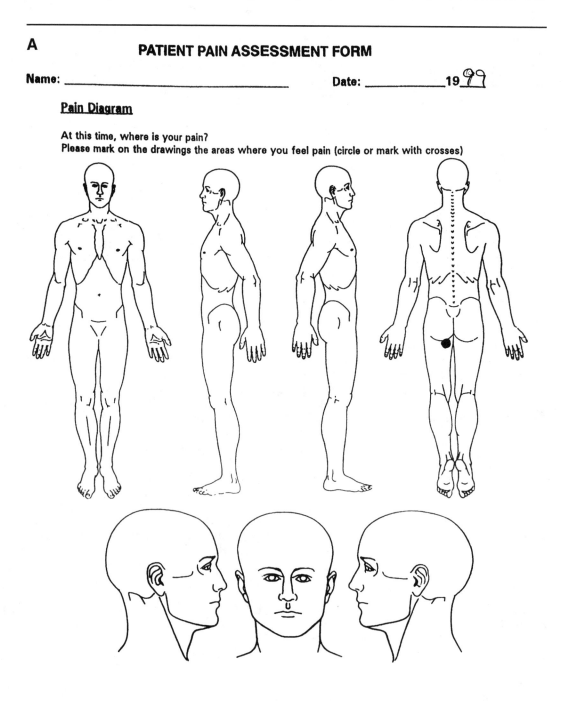

A   **PATIENT PAIN ASSESSMENT FORM**

Name: _____   **Date:** _____ 19__

Pain Diagram

At this time, where is your pain?
Please mark on the drawings the areas where you feel pain (circle or mark with crosses)

B

PATIENT PAIN ASSESSMENT FORM

Name: _____   **Date:** __6–15__ 19__98__

Pain Diagram

At this time, where is your pain?
Please mark on the drawings the areas where you feel pain (circle or mark with crosses)

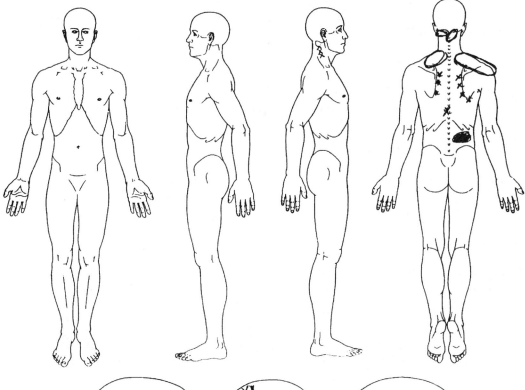

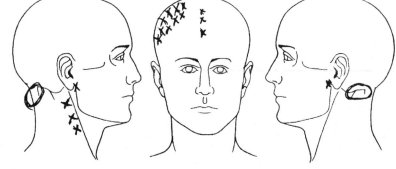

C

PATIENT PAIN ASSESSMENT FORM

Name: _____   Date: _____19____

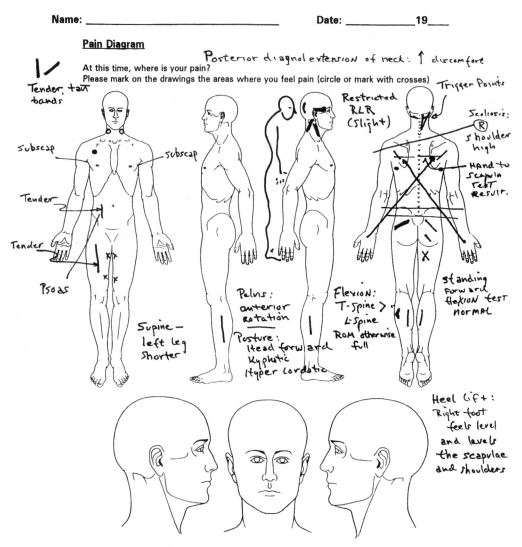

FIGURE 26.1. Patient pain diagrams. A shows the pain drawing of a woman with an acute, relatively simple muscle pain syndrome involving trigger points in the left semitendinosus and semimembranosus muscles, which referred the pain proximally to just distal to the ischial tuborosity. B shows a more complex pain drawing in a woman complaining of shoulder pain, middle and low back pain, and headache. C is the doctor's worksheet, showing the findings at examination of scoliosis (left shoulder low); a hyperlordotic, kyphotic standing posture; notations for the standing forward flexion test; spinal rotation; the results of a right heel lift; and the finding of pelvic rotation and leg length inequality. The doctor's worksheet is completed on each visit. The patient's pain drawing is repeated whenever there is a change in symptoms, and at intervals during the treatment to document progress or regression.

TABLE 26.1. History of the Pain Complaint

1. Description of the present complaint, including duration and limitation of activities by pain.
2. Details of the initiating events, if known.
3. Factors that worsen or lessen the pain.
4. Previous treatment, including surgery, physical therapy, and pharmaceutical therapy.
5. Description of work or other activities that may create ergonomic stresses contributing to the pain.
6. Family and social history, to identify both the support available to the patient and the stresses felt by the patient.
7. Psychological history of possible emotional stresses, including history of abuse.

fortable flight she had going to the coastal resort. Once home, she was comfortable lying down, standing, or walking, but sitting increased the pain in her right buttock region. She had no back pain. Coughing and sneezing did not aggravate the pain. She had no difficulty going up or down stairs, no weakness of which she was aware, and no numbness or tingling. She saw no swelling or discoloration in the leg or foot. The pain was new for her. She had no other illnesses, and was otherwise in good health. She took no medications for the pain. Her pain drawing showed only the one area of pain, in contrast to the more complex pain drawing of Figure 26.1B on page 503.

This history was one of an acute illness, with a possible source for the pain in a specific stressful activity. Peripheral nerve compression and radiculopathy were not suggested by this history. This problem was clearly acute, not likely to be related to any systemic illness, and very localized. Vascular or joint disease was unlikely. The relationship of pain to sitting was consistent with a compression-induced pain. The only structures likely to be compressed in this situation were the posterior thigh muscles and the sciatic nerve. The absence of weakness and parasthesias turned attention away from the sciatic nerve (although the possibility was not completely eliminated) and to the muscle. The localization of pain to the "sitting region" of the buttock, and the aggravation of the pain by sitting, implicated either the hamstring muscles or the gluteus maximus muscle. Of the medial and lateral hamstring muscles, the two medial hamstring muscles (semitendinosus and semimembranosus) refer pain to the ischial region. The subsequent examination identified trigger points only in these muscles. The remainder of the examination was normal. Elimination of the medial

hamstring trigger points completely resolved her problem.

The description of the major pain complaint is enhanced by asking the patient to draw his or her pain on a diagram of the body (see A and B in Figure 26.1). The description of the present pain problem is followed by a review of the onset of the symptoms, and then a description of those factors that worsen or improve the pain. The effects of particular exercises or activities, such as walking, sitting, or standing, are important. Onset of pain immediately on standing or only after walking a distance, or improvement or worsening with walking, help to differentiate hip joint pain, claudication, radiculopathy, and myofascial pain.

The impact of pain on daily activities, both within the family or social structure and at work, is ascertained. Possible secondary gains or distortions of the usual family relationships caused by loss of earning capacity or change in caregiver or care receiver status are explored. Activities such as exercise, and postures or medication that improve or worsen pain, are also identified. The history of drug usage must be ascertained carefully, as patients sometimes hide or forget about drug usage. More than once a patient has denied past or current narcotic drug use, only to ask for a prescription for paregoric, used 2–4 ounces daily "to control diarrhea" or to stop abdominal pain. The use of acetaminophen may be admitted, but the fact that it is in combination with codeine, hydrocodone, or oxycodone may be omitted. Direct questions about specific medication usage and about the use of alcohol or recreational drugs are necessary.

Sleep disturbance is important, as pain can disturb sleep, and lack of sleep can worsen pain during the day. Unrestful sleep is a characteristic often seen in persons with fibromyalgia (Moldofsky & Walsh, 1978), but usually not in persons with myofascial pain. Persons with myofascial pain report that they usually sleep well once pain is controlled. The chronic use of sedatives or hypnotics can result in middle-of-the-night insomnia or rebound insomnia.

Cold intolerance, or a sense of being "cold to the core," is frequently reported by persons with chronic myofascial pain (Gerwin & Gevirtz, 1995). The importance of this symptom is that it is indicative of conditions that perpetuate symptomatic myofascial trigger points by impairing the ability of muscle to recover. It is commonly seen in hypothyroidism, where it can be associated with increased discomfort in rainy weather. The incidence of cold intolerance in persons with iron deficiency or depleted tissue iron stores as determined by low serum ferritin levels is high (Gerwin & Gevirtz, 1995). The association of depleted tissue iron stores to coldness as a symptom or to cold intolerance may be related to the role of iron in temperature regulation or its role in the conversion of inactive T_4 (tetraiodothyronine) to active T_3 (triiodothyronine). The role of iron in perpetuating myofascial trigger points is possibly through its obligate requirement in energy-producing cytochrome oxidase reactions that generate adenosine triphosphate (ATP). A limitation in the production of ATP could produce a metabolic stress resulting in the development or persistence of abnormal muscle bands and tenderness (trigger points) (Hong & Simons, 1998; Simons, Travell, & Simons, 1999).

A history of headaches is very common in a person with chronic myofascial pain syndrome of shoulder, head, and neck muscles. The pain description varies from a unilateral headache to a bilateral or a band-like headache, or a pain that runs from the back of the head to the front, above or behind the eye. Location, frequency, and intensity do not distinguish these headaches from myofascial trigger points from the more commonly diagnosed migraine headache without aura. Migraine with aura is not typically seen as a result of myofascial trigger points. The two headache types may coexist in the same individual, however. Headaches tend to be chronic, frequently daily or nearly daily, and often marked by a paroxysmal increase in headache described by the patient as "migraine"; this can be accompanied by nausea or vomiting, photophobia, and phonophobia, requiring the person to seek a quiet, dark room in which to rest.

An often-heard complaint is of weekly migraine headaches with in-between daily headaches. Side-of-the-head pain occurs in persons with myofascial trigger points in the muscles of the jaw—the masseter, temporalis, and pterygoid muscles. Trigger points in these muscles cause pain to be felt in the teeth, as well as in the jaw, in the temple, and above the ipsilateral eye. A history of dental treatment or tooth extraction in an attempt to relieve local jaw pain may be a tipoff that these muscles harbor trigger points that aggravate a myofascial headache syndrome. Persons with neck and shoulder trigger points that refer pain to the parietal region of the scalp complain that the scalp or hair is tender, and they do not want to brush their hair or rest that side of the head against the pillow or bed.

Headache that is better on Monday morning and worse toward the end of the week may be the result of work-related mechanical stresses on the neck and shoulder muscles. Headaches that occur on the weekend and improve during the work week suggest psychological stresses within the family. The distinction may be made by computerized surface electromyography that documents increased tension in the trapezius muscles either progressively into the work week in the first instance, or increased muscle tension Monday morning and progressive relaxation as the work week progresses in the second instance. A history of a change in hearing or tinnitus, or a complaint of imbalance and even of true vertigo, is characteristic of persons who have symptomatic sternocleidomastoid trigger points.

A history of recurrent vaginal yeast infections, often the result of repeated antibiotic administration for the sore throat or ear pain associated with sternocleidomastoid and masseter muscle trigger points, is seen in some women with widespread myofascial trigger point pain syndromes. The number of women presenting with this history has been too small to develop a statistical correlation. Diagnostic evaluation to verify recurrent vaginal infection is often difficult, and the suspicion of yeast infection may be based on circumstantial evidence. Of course, all that itches is not *Candida albicans*; nevertheless, treatment with antifungal drugs has resulted in marked improvement in many of these women.

A travel history is important in identifying those persons who may have parasitic infections that act as perpetuating factors for trigger points. Amoebiasis is the most frequent of these infections seen in the United States, but giardia and trematodes have been identified as well. A reliable laboratory is needed to examine stool, including fresh samples for amoebic antigen.

Previous surgery is important to note. Postlaminectomy pain can be caused by scar tissue, by recurrent disc herniation with nerve root compression, or by untreated myofascial trigger point pain syndromes that mimic radiculopathy. In some cases, there may never have been a period of postoperative pain relief, suggesting that the original pain for which the surgery was performed was myofascial and not discal herniation at all. Patients whose pain returned as soon as they began to ambulate postoperatively, and whose pain is sciatic in distribution, may have a piriformis muscle syndrome with compression of the sciatic nerve by a contracted piriformis muscle. The suspected diagnosis can be confirmed by a diagnostic piriformis muscle trigger point injection with local anesthetic. Fusion of L5 to S1 can result in the loss of the normal reciprocal rotational movement of L5 on S1 when walking; this loss shifts the movement to the sacroiliac joints, causing sacroiliac joint pain and pain from myofascial trigger points in the related gluteal muscles.

A careful work history can identify work-related mechanical stresses. Computer stations have been notorious for poor ergonomic design, though that situation is rapidly changing. Jobs can require awkward postures such as repeated reaching overhead or twisting and lifting motions, prolonged bending, or repeated activities that have led to the controversial, but undoubtedly real, repetitive strain syndrome (Armstrong & Martin, 1997). Certain activities, such as cradling the telephone between the ear and the shoulder, are becoming less common as hands-free telephones are more frequently used. Stressful postures may be adopted by workers and passed on from one "generation" of workers to another as "the way it is done" without regard to the physical consequences of the activity, even though workers may complain of back or shoulder pain. This has been seen in hospital technicians performing echocardiograms who work with the equipment behind them and the patient in front of them, requiring them to constantly twist to look at the monitor, instead of working with the monitor across the bed in direct frontal view (J. Dommerholt, personal communication, 1998). Photographs taken of the patient at work can be of great help in identifying work-related mechanical stresses.

Psychological stresses that result in increased muscle tension, particularly in the shoulder, neck, and jaw muscles, are often difficult to elicit and require sensitive questioning and empathetic listening. Occasionally the psychological stresses will result in somatization disorders that are not really conversion reactions, but may prevent use of a part because of pain caused by myofascial trigger points. For instance, a young college student transferred from an elite music conservatory, unable to play the instrument that previously was played well enough to win competitions. Not only was the person unable to play or even to practice, but writing and use of the computer for schoolwork were impossible. Complaint of forearm pain was associated with a variable degree of myofascial trigger point involvement of the forearm muscles, including the pronator, the finger flexor, the supinator, and the extensor muscles alike. The patient's parents accompanied the student to each clinic and therapy session, expressing concern that their child would not be able to pursue a desired concert ca-

reer. Only when the patient came to a physical therapy session alone did the desire to pursue an entirely different career become known. The therapist added counseling to physical therapy, and validated the patient's wish to give up musical performance for other pursuits. The somatic complaints subsided within 2 weeks, and myofascial trigger points ceased to be found. Full use of the forearms in all activities was achieved within 1 month, including writing and the use of the computer. In other cases, conflicts with the spouse/ partner or with coworkers or superiors at work lead to myofascial trigger-point-related headaches or back pain that will not improve until the conflicts are resolved.

Physical Examination

The physical examination of patients with myofascial pain syndrome is predicated on the identification of the unique features of the myofascial trigger point, as discussed later in this chapter. It is nevertheless necessary to perform a general physical examination and an examination of the skeletal structures as well, as discussed here. Dental and neurological examinations may also be done. (See Table 26.2.)

General Physical Examination

The general physical examination is performed specifically to identify comorbid conditions that may be the primary cause of myofascial trigger point development or activation, or that may perpetuate trigger points' existence when present, impeding recovery when a patient has been appropriately treated. All conditions cannot be given as examples, as the list is extensive. Common conditions associated with

---

TABLE 26.2. Physical Examination Protocol

1. General physical examination, including vital signs; skin; head and neck (including tongue and thyroid gland); heart, lungs, and abdomen; and extremities (including joints, pretibial edema, and length of second metatarsal bone).
2. Dental examination, if relevant.
3. Neurological examination, including trigeminal and facial nerve function, motor tone, bulk, strength and coordination, sensation, deep tendon reflexes, gait, stance, and Romberg test.
4. Skeletal examination (see Table 26.3).
5. Muscle examination for trigger points (see Table 26.4).

myofascial pain syndromes are presented here (see Gerwin, 1995, for a fuller discussion).

Hypothyroidism is among the four most common medical conditions associated with chronic myofascial pain syndromes (Gerwin, 1995; Simons, Travell, & Simons, 1999). It is associated with widespread myofascial trigger points. Physical examination features suggestive of hypothyroidism include dry skin and hair, hair loss, thyroid gland nodularity, a doughy feel to muscle, pretibial edema, and slowing of the second or recovery phase of the tendon reflex. Vitamin B_{12} deficiency was the most common disorder in the study cited above (Gerwin, 1995). Optic nerve atrophy and a beefy, depapillated tongue are late signs of vitamin B_{12} deficiency, whereas peripheral sensory loss, especially when vibration and position sense are decreased out of proportion to the loss of pain and temperature sense, is common in the earlier stages of the condition. An increase in tendon reflex activity at the ankles and knees despite peripheral sensory loss is strongly suggestive of vitamin B_{12} deficiency, because of the involvement of the lateral corticospinal tracts of the spinal cord. Diffuse muscle tenderness in the upper and in the lower halves of the body, without the presence of myofascial trigger points sufficient to explain the pain, and of 3 or more months' duration, is indicative of fibromyalgia, a syndrome of chronic muscle pain that often has myofascial trigger points as a complication. Joint enlargement or tenderness indicates one of the arthritides, which can be a initiating or perpetuating factor. Lyme disease may also be associated with joint pain or arthritis. The malar rash of systemic lupus erythematosus may also be associated with signs of arthritis, peripheral neuropathy, and myofascial trigger points. Gouty tophi are other signs associated with a metabolic abnormality (in this case, in uric acid and purine metabolism) that can aggravate muscle trigger points. (Uric acid elevation with normal purine metabolism is seen in the use of thiazide diuretics, and can be a factor in the perpetuation of trigger point pain.) The point of this listing is that the general physical examination, like the medical history, gives clues to the identification of conditions that predispose patients to the development of myofascial trigger point pain syndromes or to their perpetuation.

Dental Examination

Dental examination is highly useful for headache and for facial and jaw pain complaints, if the dentist is familiar with the concepts of myofascial trig-

ger points and their referred pain patterns. Lack of adequate dental support for the jaw, clenching, posterior retrusion of the jaw, and forward head posture can lead to the development and persistence of myofascial trigger points in the masseter and temporalis muscles. Trigger points in the superior portion of the lateral pterygoid muscle can displace the articular disc of the temporomandibular joint anteriorly, causing a palpable and audible click, or limiting the opening of the mouth. Jaw movement during chewing and talking is always accompanied by changes in head position, and in that sense the jaw and its associated muscles form a postural unit with the neck and the muscles that control neck and head position. Changes in the movement of the jaw resulting from trigger points that alter the contraction, relaxation, and length of the masseter, temporalis, and pterygoid muscles alter tension in the muscles of the neck, such as the sternocleidomastoid, the scalene, and the splenius cervicis and splenius capitis muscles. Hence, when symptomatic trigger points are found in the muscles that move the jaw, or in muscles that control neck movement and neck and head posture, trigger points are usually found in the other components of these functionally related muscles.

Neurological Examination

The neurological examination shows no abnormality of cognitive function, in contrast to the memory loss and inability to concentrate claimed by individuals with fibromyalgia. Cranial nerve function is normal, except in those instances of severe vestibular dysfunction associated with sternocleidomastoid or upper posterior cervical muscle trigger points, where nystagmus can be seen. Motor function may be impaired, there being weakness without atrophy as a result of the shortening of muscle by the contracted, taut bands of the trigger points. A flaccid paralysis with atrophy is characteristic of late poliomyelitis. A study of 54 patients who had survived polio showed that 50% of them had symptomatic myofascial pain syndrome (Gerwin, 1993). Coordination can likewise be impaired, as reciprocal inhibition is abnormal in the functional muscle units affected by symptomatic trigger points. *Functional muscle units* are muscles related to each other as agonists or antagonists, or as synergists exerting force in certain vectors or stabilizing body parts such as the scapula. Repetitive and rapidly alternating movements are poorly performed when reciprocal inhibition is impaired. Loss of sensory function is seen in nerve entrapment syndromes caused by myofascial trigger points, such as sciatic nerve entrapment in the piriformis muscle syndrome, or the impairment of brachial plexus function in anterior and medial scalene muscle trigger point syndrome. However, trigger point pain syndromes associated with nerve root (radicular) irritation can produce segmental, dermatomal patterns of hypersensitivity (Fischer, 1997). Parasthesias associated with trigger point referred pain occur without sensory loss. Muscle tone is normal. There is no limb ataxia. The Romberg test and tandem walking may be abnormal when trigger points in the sternocleidomastoid create cervical vertigo and cause truncal imbalance.

Skeletal Examination

Examination of the skeletal system (see Table 26.3) is performed to identify abnormalities of skeletal function that lead to muscle imbalance and mechanical stress, and the development or perpetuation of trigger points. These conditions need to be corrected or alleviated if possible, for optimum resolution of the myofascial pain syndrome. Skeletal dysfunction can also occur as a result of muscle shortening that occurs as a consequence of trigger points, and both the muscle and the skeletal dysfunction must be corrected.

Segmental spinal hypomobility can result from local increase in muscle tension associated with trigger points in the deep paraspinal muscles. Segmental hypomobility also loads the segments above and below the level of dysfunction, as greater movement occurs in these segments in order to compensate for the loss of mobility at affected segments. Trigger points can occur in these areas, as muscles can be mechanically overloaded at the levels of compensation. Release of the trigger points in the deep paraspinal muscles may facilitate the restoration of normal mobility at the hypomobile segments.

Pelvic torsion and sacroiliac joint dysfunction are seen in persons with low back and pelvic region myofascial pain syndromes. These conditions can result in functional leg length inequalities and scoliosis. The tilted or rotated pelvis will directly or indirectly tilt the spine, resulting in a compensatory curve of the spine to the midline, in order to level the eyes. Muscles are in a state of chronic contraction to effect the correction of spinal tilt. Chronically shortened muscles develop trigger points and create regional myofascial pain syndrome.

Pelvic torsion occurs when one iliac bone is rotated to a relatively anterior or posterior position with respect to the opposite side. Anterior iliac rotation results in lowering the acetabulum, which is located eccentrically in the ilium. The effect is to functionally lengthen the leg, producing a leg length discrepancy and a pseudoscoliosis that is corrected by rotating the ilium posteriorly. The standing and sitting forward flexion tests, measurement of the relative heights of the posterior and anterior iliac spines, and the relative changes in leg length on the supine-to-sitting test identify this condition. The standing forward flexion test is performed by asking the patient to bend forward at the waist while standing. The examiner's thumbs are placed under the posterior superior iliac spines (PSISs). The PSISs should move symmetrically on forward bending. If not, one side will rise more than the other, indicating torsion of the pelvis. This can occur as a result of iliac rotation or because of true leg length inequality. The movement of the PSISs is also assessed while the patient is sitting—the so-called sitting or sacral forward flexion test. The iliac bone is fixed in position when sitting, and will not rotate asymmetrically in forward flexion. If asymmetry persists during forward flexion while the patient is sitting, the problem is fixation or hypomobility at the sacroiliac joint. If the PSISs are not level when standing, the pelvis is either tilted or rotated. The anterior superior iliac spines (ASISs) are then compared by placing the thumbs under them. When both the PSIS and the ASIS on one side are either higher or lower than those on the other side, there is a pelvic tilt signifying true leg length inequality. If one PSIS is low and the ipsilateral ASIS is high, then there is pelvic

TABLE 26.3. Skeletal Examination

1. Stance, for posture and scoliosis: kyphosis or round-shouldered, head-forward posture, loss of cervical or lumbar lordosis, paraspinal muscle spasm.
2. Gait, for scoliosis, external or internal rotation of legs, pronation or supination of feet, pelvic stability.
3. Range of motion of waist and neck.
4. Standing and sitting forward flexion tests, for pelvic torsion.
5. Trendelenberg test, for gluteus medius strength and pelvic stability.
6. Spinal movement, for segmental hypomobility.
7. Range of motion of the joints in the extremities, including the glenohumeral joint and the hip joint.
8. Evaluation of joints for arthritic changes (e.g., rheumatoid arthritis or osteoarthritis).

rotation, and a pseudoscoliosis is likely to be present. True leg length inequality is corrected by a heel lift. When apparent inequality is associated with a shortened hemipelvis causing scoliosis sitting, it may be corrected by an ischial or "butt" lift. Correction of these conditions often relieves chronic muscle overload with associated trigger points in the muscles that return the tilted spine to the midline, and reduces low back pain.

Leg length inequality will tilt the pelvis when standing, producing a pseudoscoliosis. This should be corrected with a heel lift. Shortening of the psoas muscle or of the quadratus lumborum muscle by myofascial trigger points will also tilt the pelvis, bringing the rib cage down and hiking the ipsilateral pelvis. These muscles should be examined for trigger points, and if found they should be released and the muscles returned to their full length by stretching, before any attempt is made to correct a pseudoscoliosis with a heel lift. True scoliosis caused by structural asymmetries in the spine will not be corrected with a heel lift, and may actually worsen when a heel lift is placed under one foot.

Muscle Examination

There is no consensus on the features required to diagnosis myofascial pain syndrome (Russell, 1999b). The trigger point or trigger zone must be identified in order to diagnosis the condition by definition. We infer that the trigger point is responsible for the pain when the trigger point is stimulated and reproduces the patient's pain, and then is inactivated by treatment and the pain is eliminated. This has yet to be documented in a properly controlled study. There is lack of agreement about the critical features that uniquely define the trigger point and allow diagnosis to be made. This issue has been addressed by a consensus conference held at the Fourth World Congress on Myofascial Pain and Fibromyalgia in Italy in 1998. The consensus committee was charged with the task of developing a study protocol and conducting a study that would determine which features associated with the trigger point were essential, specific, and sensitive in diagnosing myofascial pain syndrome (Russell, 1999b). The examination for myofascial trigger points that is used in the clinic is a manual (hands-on) examination. Other techniques have been used to aid in the identification of the trigger point, or to confirm its presence or location. These include electromyography (Hubbard & Berkoff, 1993), algometry (Fischer, 1994), and diagnostic ultrasound (Gerwin & Duranleau, 1997). Identification of the trigger point by electromyographic demonstration of the characteristic spontaneous activity of the trigger zone has been used to direct the injection of trigger-point-inactivating substances experimentally, but the technique is time-consuming and not practical for general clinical evaluation or for following the progress of a patient. Algometry measures the pressure required to produce pain, and therefore is a measure of tenderness. Diagnostic ultrasound combined with electromyography correlates the contraction of a mechanically stimulated muscle fascicle as seen on ultrasound, with the polyphasic burst of the local twitch response, and as such records these trigger point phenomena for later review.

Trigger points can be identified by palpation of the muscle. The features of the trigger point, listed in Table 26.4, are readily found by examiners trained in trigger point palpation. As in any aspect of physical diagnosis, practice and training enhance the skills needed to detect the changes in the muscle that signify a myofascial trigger zone. When the nature of the physical features are well understood, and examiners have been adequately trained, interrater reliability of trigger point physical feature identification is high (Gerwin, Shannon, Hong, Hubbard, & Gevirtz, 1997).

Taut Band

One must become familiar with the consistency of muscle between or under the fingers in order to appreciate the subtilties of the myofascial trigger point and trigger zone. The taut band (Simons et al., 1999) is the most constant feature of the trigger zone. It is the primary motor dysfunction

---

TABLE 26.4. Features of the Myofascial Trigger Point to Be Identified by Physical Examination

1. Taut bands in muscle.
2. Tenderness associated with taut bands.
3. Referred pain.
4. Reproduction of the usual pain problem by mechanical stimulation of the tender, taut band.
5. Local twitch response or contraction of the taut band in response to mechanical stimulation.
6. Restricted range of motion.
7. Weakness without atrophy or other neurological impairment.
8. Autonomic dysfunction (changes in skin temperature or sweating, piloerection, lacrimation).
9. Trophic skin changes (skin edema, decreased sweating) indicating segmental neural dysfunction.

of the trigger point. The mechanism underlying the development of the taut band is not definitely known at this time, but current evidence points to the excessive release of acetylcholine at the motor end plate, causing intense sarcomere contraction in the end plate region. Since a muscle fiber extends from one tendinous insertion of a muscle to the other, contraction of the midfiber at the end plate zone will result in increasing the distance between the sarcomere I-bands on either side, thus putting a stretch on these segments of the muscle fiber. A grouping of muscle fibers with myofascial trigger zones can give rise to a long, taut band running the length of the muscle. The taut band distinguishes myofascial pain syndrome from other causes of muscle pain, such a fibromyalgia or myalgia induced by cholesterol-lowering "-statin" drugs.

Taut bands are not confined to symptomatic, painful muscles, but are found in asymptomatic muscles as well. There has to be an activation of the taut band to release noxious substances by or in the region of the trigger zone to convert an asymptomatic band into a tender, symptomatic taut band that produces pain when stimulated.

Taut bands are readily identified in superficial muscles as tight strings or cords of muscle, or sometimes as broad bands that are a centimeter or more across, standing out against the background of normal muscle. The bands roll beneath or between the fingers. Some muscles, like the biceps brachii and the sternocleidomastoid, can have many taut bands that are generally very accessible to palpation. The bands will be tender and painful to palpation when they are associated with active trigger points that cause pain spontaneously (at rest) or with activity, or with inactive trigger points that are painful when stimulated mechanically. The bands are more difficult to palpate in muscular or obese individuals, or in deeper muscles like the piriformis muscle. The band feels more like a linear region of increased muscle resistance or hardness in these situations. It is as if one is palpating a pencil beneath several inches of polyurethane foam. Confirmation that this is indeed a relevant trigger point comes when palpation of such a firm muscle band reproduces the person's pain. The taut band contracts sharply when needled—a certain sign that the taut band or trigger zone has been entered, as no other structure will produce a local twitch response.

Tenderness

Whereas the taut band is the motor manifestation of the trigger point, tenderness is the sensory com-

ponent of the trigger point related to pain. The trigger zone is very tender to mildly noxious stimulation and is exquisitely tender to noxious palpation (hypersensitivity), and is often tender to usually nonpainful palpation (allodynia). These are manifestations both of spinal cord sensitization and of peripheral nociceptive receptor sensitization that occurs in response to a peripheral noxious stimulus (Mense, 1997; Simons et al., 1999). The taut band is not always tender; or, put another way, all taut bands are not tender all of the time. Peripheral sensitization of central pain-related structures and functions must occur. There must be a local release of endogenous substances that are noxious and that sensitize peripheral nociceptors and central dorsal horn neurons (e.g., bradykinin and prostaglandins) to lead to activation of the central dorsal horn nociceptive neuron—for example, by decreasing spinal release of nitric oxide.

Muscles are palpated carefully to identify tender spots and to exam the relationship of tender spots to taut bands. When tenderness is greater on a taut band, there should be adjacent areas of nontender or less tender spots. Fibromyalgia, in contrast, has tender spots that are not found primarily in taut bands, but are diffusely represented in muscle. An overwhelming association of tenderness with taut bands distinguishes myofascial pain syndrome from fibromyalgia. The force required to identify tender, taut bands varies with the build of the patient and the state of the muscle. There is no predetermined pressure that must be applied, as has been recommended for fibromyalgia (4 kg pressure) (McCain, 1994). Superficial muscles like the sternocleidomastoid require very little pressure in order to identify tender, taut bands. Deep muscles, like the piriformis muscle, require greater pressure to elicit tenderness. Muscular people and individuals with edematous skin that is difficult to roll between the fingers require more force to palpate muscle. It is necessary only to elicit tenderness and to determine whether a taut band is present; it is not necessary to be so forceful as to create great discomfort or pain.

Referred Pain

Referred pain (Simons et al., 1999; see Figure 26.2) occurs spontaneously, and can also be induced by palpation and other mechanical stimulation, such as needling or injecting the trigger point. Stimulation of the muscle trigger zone elicits pain and sometimes parasthesias locally, but can also do so at a distance. When distant pain or discom-

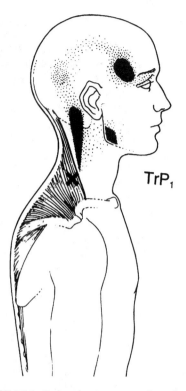

TrP₁

FIGURE 26.2. Referred pain patterns from the trapezius muscle. The ✕ in the upper trapezius muscle represents a common site for trigger points to appear. The solid areas in the neck, jaw, and temple represent the more common sites for referred pain to be felt from the trigger point in the upper trapezius. The stippled areas are less common sites of pain referral, although they can be just as intense as the more common sites of referral.

fort, or parasthesias, are felt, the sensation is termed *referred pain*. It is often a confusing aspect of myofascial pain syndromes, because it does not conform to dermatomal, myotomal, or vascular patterns. The receptive field for a particular nociceptor dorsal horn neuron or related cortical region is potentially much larger than is seen under usual circumstances (Mense & Hoheisel, 1999). The expanded receptive fields may include remote body sites (Schultz & Melzack, 1999). A likely spinal cord mechanism is convergence of sensory inputs from different sites to one dorsal horn neuron, sometimes by splitting of a peripheral nerve fiber into two axons going to two sites, or the activation of normally nonfunctioning axons by central or spinal cord excitation. Each dorsal horn neuron "sees" a unique receptive field from which it receives sensory input. A specific neuron

has the potential of responding to sensory input from other fields that usually activate a second dorsal horn neuron. The afferent nerve from the second receptive field that goes to the second neuron also has connecting axons to the first neuron, but these are usually nonfunctional, so that the first neuron does not "see" the second receptive field. When there is central sensitization as a result of peripheral painful input, the nonfunctioning connections become activated. The first neuron now receives input from two or more receptive fields. This has been called *unmasking*. Input from one field may be interpreted as coming from all of the potentially active receptive fields. Unmasking is also hypothesized for thalamo-cortical and cortico-cortical connections (Doetsch, 1997). The basis of referred pain is therefore most likely central or spinal cord activation (Devor & Wall, 1981) and sensitization.

Referred pain is an extremely important component of the trigger point, as it explains many of the clinical presentations that mimic other conditions. Thoracic outlet presentations of pain in the shoulder radiating down the arm to the fingers can occur with trigger points in the infraspinatus, scalene, and latissimus dorsi muscles. Sciatic or lumbar radiculopathy pain patterns can occur with trigger points in the gluteus minimus muscle, and from trigger points in other low back and pelvic region pain. Pain in the region of the ischial tuberosity can arise from trigger points in the medial hamstring muscles, the semimembranosus and semitendinosus muscles. Pain in the anterior chest wall can be referred pain from trigger points in the paraspinal muscles in the posterior thorax. Pain in the head is frequently referred pain from posterior neck muscle trigger points, or from trigger points in the trapezius or sternocleidomastoid muscles.

Referred pain from trigger points is identified clinically by palpation of muscle. Referred pain must be suspected as a cause of pain in a given region. The suspected muscle or muscles are palpated for trigger points. When a tender, taut band is identified, pressure is applied to the tender spot and held for 5–10 seconds. Time is required for referred pain to develop, perhaps because central activation is required. Referred pain can be missed if pressure is held on the trigger point for only a few seconds. The patient is questioned about the occurrence of pain away from the area being palpated. Care is taken not to lead the patient with questions asking whether pain is felt in particular areas, until the patient has had an opportunity to respond spontaneously. Even then, the questions should be as open-ended as possible; the examiner should ask whether pain is felt in the chest, back, or arm, for example, rather than asking whether pain is felt "here" while pointing to a specific location. Patients may point only to one of several referral sites if not questioned closely. Activation of the trigger point by needling or by injection commonly elicits a patient's typical referred pain pattern, which can be diagnostic, relating the trigger point to the patient's pain. Inactivation of the trigger point either by manual treatment or by injection or dry needling eliminates the referred pain symptoms.

Reproduction of Pain

The reproduction of the patient's pain complaint by activation of the trigger point through palpation or through needling or injecting the trigger zone is convincing to both the patient and the examiner that the trigger point is related to the presenting complaint. Reproduction of the presenting pain by manual stimulation of the tender site of the taut band is the most important feature relating the patient's pain to the trigger point (Gerwin & Dommerholt, 1998). Manual stimulation of muscle away from the tender, taut band does not reproduce usual pain. The role of the trigger point in producing the person's pain is established when inactivation of the trigger point abolishes the pain.

A tender spot is palpated, and the patient is asked whether the usual pain is elicited either directly by pressing on the tender spot or indirectly by induced referred pain. The patient is asked whether pressing on the muscle causes the usual pain to appear, or whether it produces a familiar pain, either in the region being examined or elsewhere in the body. Compression of the upper trapezius, for example, may lead patients to say that it recreates their usual headache pain in the temple or their constant pain in the back of the neck.

Local Twitch or Contraction Response

The taut band will contract sharply when stimulated manually or by a needle. The taut band is most likely maintained by local leakage of excessive acetylcholine release at the motor end plate, but is not the result of alpha motor neuron activity. In this regard, the trigger point is electrically silent. However, the sharp contraction of the trigger point taut band when stimulated is mediated primarily by a spinal cord reflex that involves anterior horn cell discharge (Hong, Torigoe, & Yu,

1995). The local twitch response is electrically manifested by a high-amplitude (2–6 mV), polyphasic discharge that can last up to 200 milliseconds. The discharge is best elicited from the trigger zone on the taut band. It is attenuated by moving the stimulating needle off the taut band even a few millimeters, or by stimulating the taut band several centimeters away from the trigger zone. Severing or blocking the peripheral nerve to the muscle eliminates most of the response, there being only a small component of local muscle activity contributing to the reflex (Hong & Torigoe, 1994). The reflex is not dependent on descending spinal cord influences. The twitch is not a tendon reflex. The local twitch response is a confirmatory sign that a taut band is identified. It does not occur from stimulation of non-taut-band muscle. It is seen in asymptomatic individuals as well as symptomatic persons, so that it is not confined to active trigger points.

The local twitch response is elicited by manual palpation or by inserting a needle into the taut band at or near the trigger zone. The taut band will contract sharply when it is strummed, much as a violin or guitar string does when it is plucked. The contracting band may be felt, and it may be seen as a distinct contraction within the larger muscle. When elicited either by dry needling or by injecting the trigger zone, or when an electromyogram is being performed, the twitch response is obtained by a firm insertion of the needle. The insertion movement need not be quick, but neither should it be tentative. The characteristic electromyographic activity of the trigger zone described earlier in this chapter is obtained by a very slow, twisting motion of the needle, which avoids triggering the twitch response. The patient is often very much aware of the twitch, as it has a distinct feel. The contraction extends the entire length of the muscle fiber. It is possible to stimulate the longissimus thoracis in the upper thoracic spinal region and see it contract in the lumbar region. The contraction is commonly accompanied by referred pain and re-creation of the patient's usual pain. The taut band relaxes along with inactivation of the trigger point when it is entered with an examining or treating needle, and the twitch response is obtained. This does not happen when the band is stimulated manually.

Restricted Range of Motion

The taut band of the trigger point restricts the full extension of its muscle. This is a cause for mechanical dysfunction of the muscle and of its functional motor unit. For example, the arm cannot be fully abducted at the shoulder if the subscapularis and latissimus dorsi muscles do not lengthen fully. A substitute movement involving elevation of the shoulder by the trapezius and levator scapulae muscles attempts to compensate for the limitation imposed by shortening of the two adductor muscles. The restriction of range of motion is not captured by the often used orthopedic maneuvers (American Academy of Orthopedic Surgeons, 1965; Macnab & McCulloch, 1994; Patla & Paris, 1993). A useful assessment of range of motion as it applies to myofascial restrictions caused by the taut band is performed by taking the movement to its end range, which should be painless. An end range that is painful is either joint-related or related to a myofascial trigger point restriction. The individual can often point to or identify the region of pain, which frequently harbors a trigger point with a palpable taut band. This concept of assessing end range has been proposed by David Simons (personal communication, 1999) and remains to be tested for reliability and validity.

Restriction of movement caused by shortening of muscles is nevertheless a useful means of identifying muscles that have trigger points. It is usually less to the point to note how many degrees of movement remain (although that information is frequently required for recording impairment and documenting subsequent function) than it is to know which muscles produce the restriction. For example, restriction in rotation of the head to the right occurs with trigger points in the right sternocleidomastoid muscle, the left splenius capitis, the left oblique capitis inferior, and the right upper trapezius. The restrictions, once found, direct the examiner to the muscles that need to be carefully examined and treated. Autonomic changes such as piloerection or changes in skin temperature can be seen in referral zones of trigger points. Lacrimation and coryza can be seen with sternocleidomastoid trigger points. Trophic skin changes such as skin edemas and local changes in sweating are manifestions of Neural impairment seen in segmental spinal dysfunction.

Adjunctive Examination Techniques

Adjunctive testing methods are listed in Table 26.5. Algometry has been used to identify tender areas and to quantitate the pressure required to produce pain (Fischer, 1994; Jaeger & Reeves, 1986). It is useful to record the pain pressure threshold before, during, and after treatment, to document the severity of the trigger point pain (how tender it is)

TABLE 26.5. Adjunctive Testing Methods for Documentation of Myofascial Trigger Point Features

1. Algometry to measure pain pressure thresholds at the trigger point and normal control sites.
2. Electromyography for the characteristic spontaneous electrical activity at the trigger point.
3. Tissue compliance or hardness over the taut band.
4. Ultrasound (?) to document the taut band and twitch response.

and the success of the treatment in reducing myofascial pain. Algometry of myofascial trigger points requires identification of the taut band initially. Algometry permits the determination of taut band tenderness, once the taut band is identified. Algometry does not identify a trigger point by itself.

Electromyographic determination of the characteristic, spontaneous activity described by Hubbard and Berkoff (1993) and further studied by Simons, Hong, and Simons (Hong & Simons, 1998; Simons, 1996; Simons, Hong, & Simons, 1995; Simons et al., 1999) can definitively identify the trigger zone. It is being explored as a tool to direct injection of drugs into the trigger zone. However, it has not achieved sufficient ease of use generally to permit its employment clinically, and it is time-consuming when applied to widespread myofascial pain syndromes. Furthermore, it is invasive and therefore uncomfortable to the patient. The trigger point is intensely painful when entered by the examining or treating needle, and this limits the extent of the examination. The use of diagnostic ultrasound, combined with the identification of the local twitch response to locate and document the trigger zone, has been proposed and is being further explored (Gerwin & Duranleau, 1997).

Laboratory Tests

The general laboratory tests listed in Table 26.6 (imaging by magnetic resonance, computerized tomography, or X-ray; blood chemistries and hemogram) are of no positive benefit in making the diagnosis of myofascial pain syndrome. They are most useful in looking for coexisting or complicating conditions such as disc herniation or Lyme disease, tumors, bone fractures, osteoporosis, hypothyroidism, or other metabolic, hormonal, infectious, or degenerative disorders. The diagnosis of myofascial pain syndrome still requires the identification of the tender, taut band that reproduces the patient's pain by manual palpation.

TABLE 26.6. Laboratory Tests Useful
for Identifying Causes of Persistent
Myofascial Trigger Point Pain Syndromes

1. Imaging by magnetic resonance, computerized
   tomography, or X-ray.
2. Complete blood count.
3. Serum ferritin level.
4. Serum vitamin B_{12} level.
5. TSH level, free tetraiodothyronine (T_4).
6. Serum and erythrocyte folate.
7. Uric acid and serum calcium levels.
8. Stools for ova and parasites, amoebic antigen.

PERPETUATING FACTORS

When myofascial pain becomes chronic (chronicity is variously defined as 3 or 6 months' duration), the cause of the persistent pain must be sought. In early chronic myofascial pain, the problem may simply be that the patient was not effectively treated. In long-standing chronic myofascial pain, which have lasted for years, specific causes should be considered. The challenge lies in identifying the problems that have interfered with expected recovery. These issues have already been alluded to in the case of A. P. at the beginning of this chapter. Travell and Simons have called these problems *perpetuating factors*. They are discussed in detail in Chapter 4 of the second edition of their text (Simons et al., 1999). Perpetuating factors can conveniently be divided into two main categories: *structural* and *medical*. The structural factors initially described by Travell and Simons emphasize those conditions that place muscles under chronic or recurrent stress or physical tension. Thus leg length inequality contributes to chronic trigger point pain by causing chronic contraction of unilateral gluteal, quadratus lumborum, paraspinal, levator scapula, trapezius, and scalene muscles, in an alternating, zig-zag fashion up the body axis, in order to correct the spinal column tilt and level the eyes. Leg length pseudoinequality does the same thing: A shortened quadratus lumborum muscle will raise the hip and lower the rib cage on the ipsilateral side, producing a functional (not a fixed structural) scoliosis. In both cases, the demands on axial musculature exceed the ability of the muscle to meet them without trouble, the trouble being the development of trigger points. This may reflect the inability of the muscle to supply the energy demands required by chronic contraction. Muscle that can handle this kind of demand may fail if it is otherwise injured.

Structural Perpetuating Factors

Pelvic rotation and segmental spinal hypomobility are being recognized more frequently as the causes of persistent myofascial pain. The acetabulum is located eccentrically in the ilium, so that anterior rotation of the ilium will drop the acetabulum, and the ipsilateral leg will appear to be longer. Once recognized, the condition is treated by rotating the pelvis back to its normal position. Conditions in which shortened muscles cause restriction of joint movements and thereby disrupt normal muscle function should be identified and corrected early in the course of treatment. Tightened or shortened muscles need to be identified and corrected in order to improve articular dysfunction and unload the muscles that harbor active or latent trigger points. One protocol that does this in the low back combines manual medicine or osteopathic techniques with muscle-lengthening or stretching techniques that are intended to restore more normal body mechanics. The protocol is as follows:

1. The rotation of the pelvis is examined on forward bending, with the physician behind the patient.
2. Iliac crest heights are compared. If they are asymmetrical, the examiner should note which shoulder is high, which PSIS is higher posteriorly, and which ASIS is higher anteriorly. If one PSIS is high and the ipsilateral ASIS is low, then the ilium is anteriorly rotated. If both the PSIS and the ipsilateral ASIS are high, then either a true inequality or a pseudoinequality of leg length is associated with pelvic obliquity. Rotation of the ilium is corrected with muscle energy techniques. True leg length inequality is corrected with a heel lift. Leg length pseudoinequality is corrected by identifying the muscles that produce pelvic tilting, inactivating their trigger points, and restoring them to their normal length.
3. The hamstring muscles are examined in the supine position for limited straight-leg raising, which indicates that there is downward pull on the ischial tuberosity.
4. The iliopsoas muscle is likewise examined for shortening that can cause an anterior rotation of the ilium.
5. The iliopsoas and hamstring muscles are then stretched if they were found to be shortened, in order to reduce muscle imbalances that influence pelvic movement and symmetry, and that secondarily affect low back and pelvic region muscle function.

6. Sacral base movement and the sacral axis are evaluated for an abnormal or fixed sacral base. The PSIS movement in the standing forward flexion test (flexion at the waist while standing) is compared with PSIS movement in the sitting forward flexion test (bending forward while sitting). If the movement of the right and left PSISs is asymmetrical, the side that moves cephalad is the freely moving side, and the opposite side is fixed. The sacral axis is named for the fixed side. Thus, if the right PSIS moves upward when the patient bends forward at the waist, the sacrum has a left axis. This means that rotation of the sacrum will occur around the left axis, which runs from the left upper sacral angle to the right inferior sacral angle, the axis being on the diagonal. It is now possible to determine whether the freely moving sacral base is rotated anteriorly or posteriorly by sliding the palpating thumb from the PSIS into the sacral sulcus, and appreciating which side is deeper (anterior).

7. The pubic symphysis is evaluated for tenderness and for asymmetry in height of the two pubic rami. The pelvis is a ring of bone with three joints. If asymmetrical forces are applied to the pelvis by the muscles attached to the pelvic bones, as a result of myofascial taut bands that shorten those muscles, there will be torsion of the pelvic ring and shear forces across pubic symphysis and sacroiliac joints. Restoring the normal length to the muscles by inactivating the trigger points and stretching them to their full length reduces the mechanical stress to the pelvis and allows correction of the pelvic torsion. Muscle energy techniques are applied through forceful abduction and adduction of the knees to alter pubic symphysis and sacroiliac joint relationships and reduce pain.

Mechanical stresses that perpetuate trigger points and impede recovery are not confined to long-standing myofascial trigger points. They can occur or reoccur during the course of the treatment. Therefore, it is prudent to examine for scoliosis, pelvic tilt and rotation, leg length inequalities, and weakness of the gluteus minimus and gluteus medius muscles by the Trendelenberg test prior to initiating any further treatment at each visit.

The cervical facet joint syndrome that occurs after a whiplash injury likewise perpetuates muscle trigger points in the neck and shoulders (Bogduk & Simons, 1993; Lord, Barnsley, Wallis, & Bogduk, 1996). The pain referral patterns of the muscles are similar to the pain referral patterns of the facet joints, and the two may be confused. However, they should be considered complementary, since they may coexist, and an individual with chronic whiplash pain may have a combined pain referral syndrome. Persistent neck or shoulder pain, or recurrent headache, should initiate an evaluation of the facet joints through diagnostic evaluation of the cervical zygapophyseal (facet) joints. Relief of pain for the duration of action of a local anesthetic applied to the medial branch of the posterior rami supplying the joint is evidence for the facet joint syndrome.

Medical Perpetuating Factors

Fibromyalgia is a commonly diagnosed condition of widespread muscle pain (Bennett, 1995). It is too often diagnosed as the cause of chronic, widespread muscle pain when the condition is in fact myofascial pain syndrome (Gerwin, 1999). The difference is of importance, since fibromyalgia is characterized as a condition that requires lifelong treatment, but is not curable. Myofascial pain, on the other hand, either is curable or can be greatly ameliorated, depending on the presence of correctable or incorrectable associated perpetuating factors (e.g., scoliosis or degenerative arthritis). Fibromyalgia syndrome is a disorder of chronic (greater than 3 months) widespread pain, usually associated with a sleep disturbance (nonrestorative sleep), morning stiffness, and severe chronic fatigue. Other associated complaints include headache, dyspareunia, irritable bowel syndrome, Raynaud's phenomenon, orthostatic hypotension, interstitial cystitis, arthritis, and a cognitive impairment called "fibrofog" by the patients. These multiple symptoms have led to a concept that there is a more widespread dysregulation of body function in fibromyalgia, including hormonal and autonomic dysfunction.

Widespread tenderness is a manifestation of a hypersensitivity syndrome or hypervigilance syndrome, in which there is a lowered threshold for the perception of pain from a variety of stimulation, not just pressure. The finding of increased levels of substance P in spinal fluid (Russell, 1999a) is consistent with a more generalized central hypersensitization at the spinal cord level, caused by a hyperexcitability of dorsal horn sensory neurons, that results in the diffuse muscle tenderness seen in fibromyalgia (Hoheisel, Mense, & Ratkai, 1996; Mense & Hoheisel, 1999).

The necessary diagnostic feature of fibromyalgia syndrome is widespread muscle tenderness of at least 3 months' duration. Tenderness must be present in muscles in the upper and lower halves of the body, as well as on the right and left sides. One widely adopted criterion recommended for clinical research studies but adopted for general clinical use is that 11 of 18 specified points must be tender (Wolfe et al., 1990). The criteria have been recommended as inclusive rather than exclusionary (Bennett, 1995). That is, if there is widespread tenderness of 3 months' duration, then the condition is fibromyalgia syndrome. There is no need to exclude other conditions, therefore. However, other medical conditions can produce widespread muscle tenderness that is chronic. Most notable is myofascial pain that is widespread (three or four body quadrants) in 45% of patients with myofascial pain syndrome (Gerwin, 1995). Other causes include the myalgia associated with the "-statin" type of cholesterol-lowering drugs; hypothyroidism, which can produce a widespread myalgia; and myoadenylate deaminase deficiency (Marin & Connick, 1997). Sporadic cases of other conditions that can cause widespread myalgia are discussed below.

Suffice it to say that fibromyalgia is not a diagnosis to be made by inclusion alone; at least the above-mentioned conditions must be excluded. A competent examination of muscle by palpation to exclude taut bands and referred tenderness must be part of the evaluation before the diagnosis of fibromyalgia can be made with confidence. Other medical perpetuating factors include nutritional deficiency states, metabolic and endocrine dysfunction, chronic infections and infestations, allergic disorders, and nerve impingement or compression. These problems are also discussed in detail in Chapter 4 of the Simons and colleagues (1999) text on myofascial pain.

Ferritin levels of 20 ng/ml or less were found in 50% of 70 individuals with chronic muscle pain, 90% of whom had myofascial pain syndrome (Gerwin & Gevirtz, 1995). Muscle, bone marrow, and liver are depleted of freely mobilizable, non-essential iron stores at 15–20 ng/ml, thus potentially limiting the energy-producing iron-requiring cytochrome oxidase enzymatic reactions in muscle. Vitamin B_{12} deficiency was found in 16% of subjects with chronic myofascial pain syndrome, and folic acid and hypothyroidism were each found in 10% of persons with myofascial pain syndrome (Gerwin, 1995). Sporadic cases of recurrent candidias are associated with widespread myofascial pain. The numbers are too small to develop a statistical analysis, but treatment of candidiasis as primary therapy of chronic myofascial pain syndrome has been associated with resolution of the widespread myalgia and myofascial trigger points. Gouty

diathesis, amoebiasis, and allergic rhinitis have all been associated with persistent myofascial pain syndrome that clears or improves significantly when the underlying condition is treated. Psychological stress should not be overlooked, as trigger points can develop in association with anxiety, stress, and adjustment disorders, and clear when the stress is resolved (Banks, Jacobs, Gevirtz, & Hubbard, 1998; McNulty, Gevirtz, Berkoff, & Hubbard, 1994). An appropriate first step in evaluating a person with chronic myofascial pain for medical perpetuating factors is to obtain a complete blood count, a serum ferritin level, serum vitamin B_{12} and folic acid levels, erythrocyte folic acid levels, and serum TSH and free T_4 levels.

CONCLUSION

The diagnosis of myofascial pain syndrome can be made reliably by trained clinicians using manual palpation to identify the tender, taut muscle bands that reproduce the patient's pain, either directly or by producing referred pain patterns that reproduce the patient's usual pain. Myofascial pain syndrome should be considered in situations where pain persists and the cause is not readily apparent. These situations include chronic, recurrent headaches and postlaminectomy syndromes, among other conditions. Mechanical and structural perpetuating factors must be sought when initial treatment fails to eliminate the painful trigger points and maintain the patient in a pain-free state.

REFERENCES

American Academy of Orthopedic Surgeons. (1965). *Joint motion: Method of measuring and recording.* Chicago: Author.

Armstrong, T. J., & Martin, B. J. (1997). Adverse effects of repetitive loading and sequential relaxation. In M. Nordin, G. B. J. Andersson, & M. H. Pope (Eds.), *Musculoskeletal disorders in the workplace: Principles and practice* (pp. 134–151). St. Louis, MO: Mosby.

Banks, S. L., Jacobs, D. W., Gevirtz, R., & Hubbard, D. R. (1998). Effects of autogenic relaxation training in active myofascial trigger points. *Journal of Musculoskeletal Pain, 6,* 23–32.

Bennett, R. M. (1995). Fibromyalgia: The commonest cause of widespread pain. *Comprehensive Therapy, 21,* 269–275.

Bogduk, N., & Simons, D. G. (1993). Neck pain: Joint pain or trigger points. In H. Vaeroy & H. Merskey (Eds.), *Progress in fibromyalgia and myofascial pain* (pp. 267–273). Amsterdam: Elsevier.

Devor, M., & Wall, P. (1981). Plasticity in the spinal cord sensory map following peripheral nerve injury in rats. *Journal of Neuroscience, 1*, 679–684.

Doetsch, G. (1997). Progressive changes in cutaneous trigger zones for sensation referred to a phantom hand: A case report with implications for cortical reorganization. *Somatosensory and Motor Research, 14*, 6– 16.

Fischer, A. A. (1994). Pressure algometry (dolorimetry) in the differential diagnosis of muscle pain. In E. S. Rachlin (Ed.), *Myofascial pain and fibromyalgia* (pp. 121–141). St. Louis, MO: Mosby.

Fischer, A. A. (1997). New developments in diagnosis of myofascial pain and fibromyalgia. In A. A. Fischer (Ed.), *Myofascial pain: Update in diagnosis and treatment* (Vol. 8, pp. 1–21). Philadelphia: Saunders.

Gerwin, R. D. (1993). [Myofascial pain syndrome in polio survivors]. Unpublished raw data.

Gerwin, R. D. (1995). A study of 96 subjects examined for both fibromyalgia and myofascial pain. *Journal of Musculoskeletal Pain, 3*(Suppl. 1), 121.

Gerwin, R. D. (1999). Differential diagnosis of myofascial pain syndrome and fibromyalgia. *Journal of Musculoskeletal Pain, 7*(1–2), 209–215.

Gerwin, R. D., & Dommerholt, J. (1998). [Trigger point indentification]. Unpublished raw data.

Gerwin, R. D., & Duranleau, D. (1997). Ultrasound identification of the myofascial trigger point. *Muscle and Nerve, 20*, 767–768.

Gerwin, R. D., & Gevirtz, R. (1995). Chronic myofascial pain: Iron insufficiency and coldness as risk factors. *Journal of Musculoskeletal Pain, 3*(Suppl. 1), 120.

Gerwin, R. D., Shannon, S., Hong, C.-Z., Hubbard, D., & Gevirtz, R. (1997). Interrater reliability in myofascial trigger point examination. *Pain, 69*, 65–73.

Hoheisel, H., Mense, S., & Ratkai, M. (1996). Effects of spinal cord superfusion with substance P on the excitability of rat dorsal horn neurons processing input from deep tissues. *Journal of Musculoskeletal Pain, 3*(3), 23–45.

Hong, C.-Z., & Simons, D. G. (1998). Pathophysiologic and electrodiagnostic mechanisms of myofascial trigger points. *Archives of Physical Medicine and Rehabilitation, 79*, 863–872.

Hong, C.-Z., & Torigoe, Y. (1994). Electrophysiologic characteristics of localized twitch responses in responsive taut bands of rabbit skeletal muscle. *Journal of Musculoskeletal Pain, 2*(2), 17–43.

Hong, C.-Z., Torigoe, Y., & Yu, J. (1995). The localized twitch responses in responsive taut bands of rabbit skeletal muscle are related to the reflexes at spinal cord level. *Journal of Musculoskeletal Pain, 3*(1), 15–33.

Hubbard, D. H., & Berkoff, G. M. (1993). Myofascial trigger points show spontaneous needle EMG activity. *Spine, 18*, 1803–1807.

Jaeger, B., & Reeves, J. L. (1986). Quantification of changes in myofascial trigger point sensitivity with the pressure algometer following passive stretch. *Pain, 27*, 203–210.

Lord, S. M., Barnsley, L., Wallis, B. J., & Bogduk, N. (1996). Chronic cervical zygapophysial joint pain after whiplash: A placebo controlled prevalence study. *Spine, 21*, 1737–1744.

Macnab, I., & McCulloch, J. (1994). *Anatomy and biomechanics of the shoulder joint, neck ache and shoulder pain.* Baltimore: Williams & Wilkins.

Marin, R., & Connick, E. (1997). Tension myalgia versus myoadenylate deaminase deficiency: A case report. *Archives of Physical Medicine and Rehabilitation, 78*, 95–97.

McCain, G. (1994). A clinical overview of the fibromyalgia syndrome. *Journal of Musculoskeletal Pain, 4*(1–2), 9–34.

McNulty, W., Gevirtz, R., Berkoff, G., & Hubbard, D. G. (1994). Needle electromyographic evaluation of trigger point response to a psychological stressor. *Psychophysiology, 31*, 313–316.

Mense, S. (1997). Pathophysiologic basis of muscle pain syndromes. In A. A. Fischer (Ed.), *Myofascial pain: Update in diagnosis and treatment* (Vol. 8, pp. 23–55). Philadelphia: Saunders.

Mense, S., & Hoheisel, U. (1999). New developments in the understanding of the pathophysiology of muscle pain. *Journal of Musculoskeletal Pain, 7*(1–2), 13–24.

Moldofsky, H., & Walsh, J. J. (1978). Plasma tryptophane and musculoskeletal pain in nonarticular rheumatism ("fibrositis syndrome"). *Pain, 5*, 65–71.

Patla, C. E., & Paris, S. V. (1993). Reliability of interpretation of the Paris classification of normal end feel for elbow flexion and extension. *Journal of Manual and Manipulative Therapy, 1*, 60–66.

Russell, I. J. (1999a). Neurochemical pathogenesis of fibromyalgia syndrome. *Journal of Musculoskeletal Pain, 7*(1–2), 183–191.

Russell, I. J. (1999b). Reliability of clinical assessment measures for the classification of myofascial pain syndrome. *Journal of Musculoskeletal Pain, 7*(1–2), 309–324.

Schultz, G., & Melzack, R. (1999). Referred pain evoked by remote light touch after partial nerve injury. *Pain, 81*, 199–202.

Simons, D. G. (1996). Clinical and etiological update of myofascial pain from trigger points. *Journal of Musculoskeletal Pain, 4*(1–2), 93–121.

Simons, D. G., Hong, C.-Z., & Simons, L. S. (1995). Prevalence of spontaneous electrical activity at trigger spots and control sites in rabbit muscle. *Journal of Musculoskeletal Pain, 3*(1), 35–48.

Simons, D. G., Travell, J. G., & Simons, L. S. (1999). *Myofascial pain and dysfunction: The trigger point manual* (Vol. 1, 2nd ed.). Baltimore: Williams & Wilkins.

Wolfe, F., Smythe, H. A., Yunus, M. B., Bennett, R. M., Bombadier, C. L., Goldenberg, D. L., Tudwell, P., Campbell, S. M., Abeles, M., Clark, P., Fam, A. G., Fiechter, J. J., Franklin, C. M., Gatter, R. A., Hamaty, D., Lessard, J., Lichtbroun, A. S., Masi, A. T., McCain, G. A., Reynolds, W. J., Romano, T. J., Russell, I. J. & Sheon, R. P. (1990). The American College of Rheumatology criteria for the classification of fibromyalgia. *Arthritis and Rheumatism, 33*, 160–172.

Chapter 27

Assessment of Neuropathic Pain

ROBERT H. DWORKIN
ELNA M. NAGASAKO
BRADLEY S. GALER

Neuropathic pain has been defined by the International Association for the Study of Pain (IASP) as pain "initiated or caused by a primary lesion or dysfunction in the nervous system" (Merskey & Bogduk, 1994, p. 212). Depending on where the lesion or dysfunction is located within the nervous system, neuropathic pain is subdivided into *peripheral* and *central* neuropathic pain. As with other types of pain, a distinction is also made between *acute* and *chronic* neuropathic pain. Following the convention established by the IASP, neuropathic pain can be considered chronic when it has persisted beyond the normal time of healing; with nonmalignant pain, "three months is the most convenient point of division between acute and chronic pain," whereas for cancer pain, "three months is sometimes too long to wait before regarding a pain as chronic" (Merskey & Bogduk, 1994, p. xi). Unfortunately, many patients suffering from neuropathic pain have chronic pain.

In this chapter, we emphasize assessment methods developed specifically for neuropathic pain. Methods more commonly used for other types of pain are also discussed, with an emphasis on their role in the assessment of neuropathic pain. Although the research we discuss has been conducted primarily in patients with peripheral neuropathic pain, many of the techniques and results are also relevant to patients with central neuro-

pathic pain and neuropathic pain associated with cancer (e.g., Allen, 1998; Berić, 1998). We devote more attention to the assessment of chronic, rather than acute, neuropathic pain, which reflects the greater emphasis on chronic pain in the literature as well as in the clinic. We do not review research on complex regional pain syndrome (CRPS) or the unique issues associated with it, because Chapter 28 by Bruehl, Steger, and Harden is devoted to this condition. Table 27.1 lists the more common neuropathic pain syndromes, distinguishing nonmalignant peripheral and central neuropathic pain from neuropathic pain found in patients with cancer. Bennett (1997) has provided estimates of the incidence of many of these neuropathic pain syndromes, and concludes that almost 1.7 million individuals suffer from neuropathic pain in the United States (if neuropathic back pain is included, the total becomes 3.8 million).

We begin by discussing general issues in the assessment of neuropathic pain, including the different models, contexts, and goals of assessment. Next, we review the aspects of neuropathic pain that should be included in a comprehensive assessment. We then discuss the methods most commonly used in assessing neuropathic pain—specifically, the history and neurological examination, patient self-report questionnaires, and various procedures (with an emphasis on quantitative sensory testing, or QST).

TABLE 27.1. Common Types of Neuropathic Pain

Peripheral neuropathic pain	Central neuropathic pain	Cancer-associated neuropathic pain
Carpal tunnel syndrome	Central poststroke pain	Chemotherapy-induced polyneuropathy
Complex regional pain syndrome (CRPS)	HIV myelopathy	Neuropathy secondary to tumor infiltration or nerve compression
HIV sensory neuropathy	Multiple sclerosis pain	Phantom breast pain
Meralgia paresthetica	Parkinson's disease pain	Postmastectomy pain
Painful diabetic neuropathy	Spinal cord injury pain	Postradiation plexopathy and myelopathy
Phantom limb pain	Syringomyelia	
Postherpetic neuralgia (PHN)		
Postthoracotomy pain		
Trigeminal neuralgia		

GENERAL ISSUES

Disease versus Mechanism Models of Neuropathic Pain

Until recently, the primary goal of pain assessment has been diagnosis—that is, determining what disease or condition is responsible for the patient's pain complaint. During the past several years, however, an alternative perspective for how best to conceptualize a patient's pain has emerged from the basic science literature and from the relatively limited clinical advances that have been made with the traditional disease-based approach. This alternative to classifying patients based on disease is a classification based on pain mechanisms. In this approach, the major goal of assessment is to attempt to identify the specific pathophysiological mechanisms of the patient's pain and to use these mechanisms to identify appropriate treatments (Arnér, 1998; Max, 1990, 1991; Meyerson, 1997; Woolf et al., 1998; Woolf & Decosterd, 1999; Woolf & Mannion, 1999).

The impetus for this novel approach comes from the identification of a large number of pain mechanisms in research on animals and humans (see, e.g., Bennett, 1994; Fields & Rowbotham, 1994; Fields, Rowbotham, & Baron, 1998; Wiesenfeld-Hallin, Hao, & Xu, 1997). In addition, there is a growing recognition that pain syndromes identified by disease—for example, postherpetic neuralgia (PHN) or painful diabetic neuropathy— most likely have mutiple distinct underlying pain mechanisms. There are several implications of this perspective. One is that patients with the same disease typically have differing pathophysiologies that result in different patterns of symptoms and physical findings. In other words, neuropathic pain syndromes include heterogeneous groups of patients who differ in their symptoms, treatment response, and prognosis. This heterogeneity may be conceptualized in terms of different subtypes of patients (see, e.g., Rowbotham, Petersen, & Fields, 1998) or as the co-existence of different mechanisms within patients that vary between patients in the extent to which they account for pain. It follows that patients with different diseases may be more similar to each other with respect to the mechanisms of their pain than they are to other patients with the same disease. For example, a patient with PHN may share underlying pain mechanisms with a patient with painful diabetic neuropathy, but not with another patient with PHN.

At present, it is not possible to directly identify the specific pathophysiological mechanisms that account for a report of pain or a patient's findings on physical examination. Therefore, although it is based on a considerable body of research, there is limited evidence that the mechanism-based approach to pain assessment has greater value than the disease-based approach. No large prospective clinical studies have been reported that assess whether mechanism-based assessment and treatment lead to improved patient outcomes. Clinical researchers are currently examining the extent to which pain mechanisms can be identified from patterns of symptoms, pain quality, physical findings, sensory testing, and response to pharmacological challenges (Galer & Jensen, 1997; Rowbotham, Petersen, & Fields, 1998; Woolf & Decosterd, 1999).

Because this mechanism-based perspective is becoming increasingly important in research on neuropathic pain and on its treatment, we discuss assessment from both the traditional disease-based perspective and the perspective of this new alternative conceptualization. It will be apparent that these different models of pain have important implications not only for understanding pathophysiology, but also for assessing pain, predicting treatment response, and examining the natural history of a patient's pain.

The Context and Goals of Neuropathic Pain Assessment

The assessment of neuropathic pain occurs within two broad contexts. One is the clinical context, in which patients are evaluated and treated. The second is the context of clinical research, in which typical studies seek to evaluate the efficacy of treatments or to describe the characteristics of patients and the natural histories of their pain syndromes. These different contexts are accompanied by different but partially overlapping sets of goals for the assessment of patients. In the clinic, the predominant goals are diagnosis and treatment. Thus a physician's goals in this context are to provide a thorough and precise assessment that will (1) improve the chances of making the correct diagnosis of a patient's pain condition (e.g., is this patient's chest pain PHN or Tietze's syndrome?), (2) guide the tailoring of treatment to a specific pain condition (e.g., will a tricyclic antidepressant or a series of nerve block injections provide the most pain relief?), (3) provide information regarding prognosis, and (4) provide a means of evaluating treatment outcome.

In clinical research, the goals of patient assessment often differ from the goals of assessment in the clinic. In clinical trials of treatment, for example, a major goal of assessment is to determine whether a patient meets criteria for inclusion in a particular study. Depending on whether the study has a disease-based or a mechanism-based perspective, criteria for inclusion in a study would include either the patient's diagnosis or the mechanism of the patient's pain. The mechanism-based approach to determining eligibility for a study can involve mechanisms at different levels of specificity—for example, neuropathic versus non-neuropathic pain, peripheral versus central neuropathic pain, central hyperactivity versus central reorganization, large-fiber versus small-fiber loss.

A second major goal of clinical research overlaps with an important goal in the clinical setting: that is, to reliably assess symptoms and physical findings as a means of establishing treatment efficacy or the natural history of a disease. In the traditional disease-based model of pain, the assessment of treatment outcome evaluates various aspects of the patient's pain syndrome—for example, pain intensity, pain quality, the staged severity of the disorder, and the impact of the pain syndrome on quality of life. In a mechanism-based approach, on the other hand, treatment outcome is assessed by evaluating the specific mechanisms of the patient's pain. For example, once pain mechanisms have been identified at a baseline visit, subsequent assessments will evaluate these mechanisms and determine whether they have been affected by treatment.

Although in the following review we emphasize the assessment of neuropathic pain in clinical research, much of what we discuss also has applicability within the clinic. One major reason for this is the steadily increasing attention to the necessity of documenting patient outcomes as a routine part of the daily evaluation and treatment of patients with pain.

WHAT SHOULD BE ASSESSED?

Continuous Pain and Abnormal Sensation

Before we describe specific measures and methods, it is important to review the types of pain (and other abnormal sensations) that should be included in a comprehensive assessment of neuropathic pain. In evaluating neuropathic pain, an initial distinction must be made between *stimulus-evoked* pain and *spontaneous* pain that is stimulus-independent (Bennett, 1994). Spontaneous pain and sensations are present in the absence of any stimulation, and can be further subdivided into *continuous* and *intermittent* types. Continuous pain is present all or almost all of the time, although patients usually report that it varies in intensity. Moreover, most patients describe more than one type of spontaneous pain; that is, their pain has several different qualities (e.g., burning, throbbing, cold-like; Galer & Jensen, 1997). The predominant qualities of continuous pain, which are discussed below, not only vary within patients but also between patients. The second type of spontaneous pain is intermittent pain, which is episodic and typically has a relatively short duration when it occurs. Intermittent neuropathic pain is often paroxysmal and described as shooting, stabbing, or electric-like in quality.

In addition to these two broad types of spontaneous pain, patients with neuropathic pain frequently report other spontaneous abnormal sensations. The term *dysesthesia* refers to an abnormal sensation that is unpleasant, whereas *paresthesia* refers to an abnormal sensation that is not unpleasant; each of these types of abnormal sensation can be either spontaneous or evoked (Merskey & Bogduk, 1994). Examples of dysesthesias and paresthesias commonly reported by patients with neuropathic pain are itching, numbness, tingling, and pins-and-needles sensations. It is unfortunate that so little research has been devoted to these abnormal sensations in patients with neuropathic pain. The distinction between the sensations labeled as "painful" and the sensations that the same individual labels "unpleasant" or just "abnormal" is of particular interest in clinical trials. It is not uncommon that patients being screened for a neuropathic pain trial will describe disabling spontaneous and evoked sensations, but will refuse to call these symptoms "pain." Interestingly, this seems to occur most frequently in patients with polyneuropathy, as compared to, for example, patients with PHN. Identifying the physiological and psychological reasons why one patient refers to sensations as "pain" and another does not is an important area for future research—one that will have direct effects on patient care. It is possible that the sensory phenomena of paresthesias, dysesthesias, and pain lie on a continuum, and that individuals have different thresholds for what they consider painful along this continuum of abnormal sensation and perception. If this is true, then the most informative approach to the assessment of neuropathic pain would include a comprehensive assessment of all the abnormal sensations experienced by the patient, regardless of whether the patient calls them "painful," "unpleasant," or "abnormal."

Spontaneous continuous and intermittent pain (and abnormal sensations) vary not only in their intensity and quality, but also in their location and area, frequency, and duration. A comprehensive assessment of neuropathic pain must attend to each of these characteristics, which vary within patients as a function of time and treatment, as well as between patients. Although methods for assessing the intensity, quality, and location of spontaneous continuous pain have been the focus of a substantial number of studies, considerably less attention has been paid to the systematic assessment and interpretation of the frequency and duration of spontaneous intermittent neuropathic pain. In addition, relatively few studies have systematically examined the different qualities of neuropathic pain that patients describe. Many older textbooks differentiate *constant persistent pains* from *lancinating pains* and use this distinction for determining treatment (i.e., tricyclic antidepressants to treat the former and anticonvulsants to treat the latter); however, as we discuss below, the few prospective controlled clinical trials that have systematically assessed these pain qualities find little evidence of a differential treatment response.

Stimulus-Evoked Pain and Abnormal Sensation

The second broad type of neuropathic pain and abnormal sensation is *stimulus-evoked* pain (also termed *stimulus-dependent* pain). There is a consensus that the multiple types of stimulus-evoked pain present in patients with neuropathic pain provide important information about pathophysiology. Unfortunately, however, there is still a great deal of inconsistency in the terminology used to refer to the different types of stimulus-evoked pain. It is beyond the scope of this chapter to review these variations in terminology, and we adhere to the IASP definitions in discussing stimulus-evoked pain and abnormal sensation (Merskey & Bogduk, 1994).

As can be seen from Table 27.2, the different types of stimulus-evoked pain and abnormal sensation vary with respect to whether the provoking stimulus is normally nonpainful (i.e., *innocuous*) or normally painful (i.e., *noxious*). They also vary with respect to whether the patient's response is a report of pain or another sensation. These various types of stimulus-evoked pain and abnormal sensation can be conceptualized in terms of the stimulus–response curves relating stimulus intensity to the subject's response. These evoked sensations involve abnormal changes in the intercept and/or the slope

TABLE 27.2. International Association for the Study of Pain (IASP) Definitions of Pain Terms

Pain term	Definition[a]
Allodynia	Pain due to a stimulus which does not normally provoke pain.
Analgesia	Absence of pain in response to stimulation which would normally be painful.
Hyperalgesia	An increased response to a stimulus which is normally painful.
Hyperesthesia	Increased sensitivity to stimulation, excluding the special senses.
Hyperpathia	A painful syndrome characterized by an abnormally painful reaction to a stimulus, especially a repetitive stimulus, as well as an increased threshold.
Hypoalgesia	Diminished pain in response to a normally painful stimulus.
Hypoesthesia	Decreased sensitivity to stimulation, excluding the special senses.

[a]The definitions are from Merskey and Bogduk (1994).

of these stimulus–response curves, as depicted in Figure 27.1.

The response portion of these stimulus–response curves involves the patient's report of normal sensation or pain, and relatively similar assessments of these responses can be used for different evoking stimuli. The stimuli that have been used in assessing stimulus-evoked pain are of many types, including thermal (cold or heat), vibration, static (punctate or blunt), dynamic (moving brush-evoked), and chemical (e.g., capsaicin, mustard oil). Importantly, it has become clear from research on the neurophysiology of pain that distinct mechanisms are involved in the response to these different types of stimuli. One broad and oversimplified distinction is between stimuli that normally activate Aβ-fiber mechanoreceptors and stimuli that normally activate Aδ- and C-fiber nociceptors. The characteristics of the major sensory fibers that are relevant to neuropathic pain and its assessment are presented in Table 27.3. The typical stimuli that

normally activate each of these fiber types, and the different sensations that are normally experienced as a result of this activity, are also presented in the table. In patients with neuropathic pain, these relationships among evoking stimuli, activity in primary afferents, and sensory experience are often abnormal and can provide important information about the mechanisms of their pain (Bennett, 1994; Fields et al., 1998; Koltzenburg, 1995, 1996).

A comprehensive assessment of the different types of stimulus-evoked neuropathic pain and abnormal sensations must attend to their intensity, quality, location and area, frequency, and duration—all of which vary within patients as a function of time and treatment, as well as between patients. However, a comprehensive assessment of stimulus-evoked pain is not typically performed in clinical practice, and unfortunately has not often been conducted in clinical research. Separate analyses of intensity, duration, and area have rarely been reported in either the experimental or clinical literature;

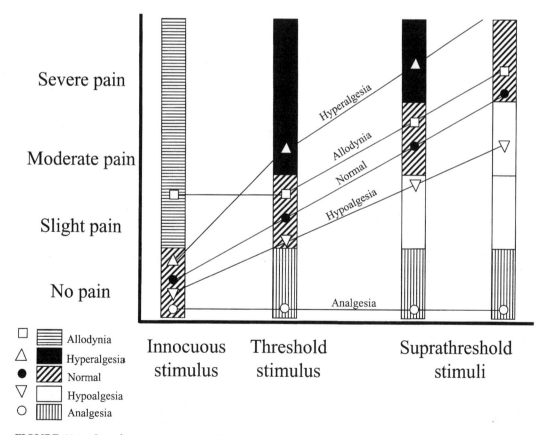

FIGURE 27.1. Stimulus–response curves for sensory abnormalities associated with neuropathic pain. Shaded regions indicate ranges of abnormal response to different stimulus intensities.

TABLE 27.3. Characteristics of Primary Sensory Neurons

Fiber class	Receptor type	Adequate stimulus	Perceived sensation	Myelination
Aβ	Low-threshold mechanoreceptor (e.g., Ruffini, Merkel receptors)	Maintained displacement	Sustained pressure	Myelinated
	Low-threshold mechanoreceptor (e.g., Meissner corpuscle)	Velocity of displacement	Flutter	Myelinated
	Low-threshold mechanoreceptor (e.g., Pacinian corpuscle)	Vibration	Vibration	Myelinated
Aδ	Low-threshold mechanoreceptor	Velocity of displacement		Myelinated
	Cooling thermoreceptor	Innocuous cooling	Cooling	Myelinated
	Mechanical nociceptor	Noxious mechanical stimuli	Sharp pain	Myelinated
	Thermal nociceptor	Noxious thermal stimuli	Sharp pain	Myelinated
C	Warming thermoreceptor	Innocuous warming	Warmth	Unmyelinated
	Cooling thermoreceptor	Innocuous cooling	Cooling	Unmyelinated
	Polymodal nociceptor	Noxious mechanical stimuli	Burning pain	Unmyelinated
		Noxious thermal stimuli		
		Noxious chemical stimuli		
	Mechanical nociceptor	Noxious mechanical stimuli		Unmyelinated
	Thermal nociceptor	Noxious thermal stimuli	Burning pain	Unmyelinated

Note. The information presented in this table has been drawn from Light and Perl (1993) and from Martin and Jessell (1991).

Bennett (1994) notes that this is unfortunate, because there is evidence that abnormalities in the intensity of stimulus-evoked neuropathic pain can be distinguished from abnormalities in its duration.

CLINICAL EVALUATION OF NEUROPATHIC PAIN

A careful history and physical examination play an essential role in the comprehensive assessment of neuropathic pain, and are as important in clinical research as in the clinic. There is a great deal of information relevant to the assessment of a patient's neuropathic pain that cannot be obtained from questionnaires or procedures such as quantitative sensory testing. Although clinical practice has evolved and refined the history-taking procedures and physical examinations conducted in patients with neuropathic pain, a systematic description of the information that should be obtained is not available. Because no standardized approach to assessment exists, there is undoubtedly a great deal of variability among individuals who conduct assessments of neuropathic pain. This variability makes it very likely that the reliability of these clinical assessments is modest at best.

In psychiatry, inadequate interrater reliability among diagnosticians has been improved by the use of standardized diagnostic criteria (American Psychiatric Association, 1994) and structured clinical interviews to assess these criteria (e.g., First, Gibbon, Spitzer, & Williams, 1997). The IASP *Classification of Chronic Pain* (Merskey & Bogduk, 1994), based on the consensus of the expert members of a task force, is the first step in the direction of standardized diagnostic criteria for pain syndromes. This taxonomy includes many neuropathic pain syndromes, but few of the diagnostic criteria have stimulated research intended to refine them (for important exceptions, see Bruehl et al., 1999; Galer, Bruehl, & Harden, 1998; Harden et al., 1999). Much less effort has been devoted to systematically describing how to obtain the information in the history and physical examination that is needed to make these diagnostic evaluations. An interview guide for the assessment of chronic pain was published a number of years ago (Melzack, 1983), but it does not include information that is now known to be important in assessing neuropathic pain. Fortunately, several recent publications provide guidance on the clinical assessment of neuropathic pain from both disease- and mechanism-based perspectives (Backonja & Galer, 1998; Galer, 1998; Koltzenburg, 1998; Woolf & Decosterd, 1999), and efforts to specify the symptoms and signs that characterize different types of neuropathic pain can be expected to continue.

In recent research on diabetic neuropathy, considerable attention has been paid to the standardization of diagnostic criteria and the neurological history and physical examination (e.g., Diabetes Control and Complications Trial Research Group, 1995; Dyck, Melton, O'Brien, & Service, 1997). Pain is only one of the symptoms of diabetic neuropathy, and it is not present in all patients. Unfortunately, neither spontaneous nor stimulus-evoked pain has received a great deal of attention in these efforts to standardize diagnostic criteria and assessments in diabetic neuropathy. Typically, a detailed assessment of pain is not required, nor is the effect of pain on the patient's quality of life evaluated. Nevertheless, this research provides valuable examples of how the assessment of symptoms and signs that occur

in patients with neuropathic pain could be standardized. We hope that future revisions of these instruments will include more comprehensive pain assessments.

The Total Symptom Score (TSS; Ziegler et al., 1995) is the briefest of these measures and the least comprehensive, but it nevertheless provides a clear example of how neuropathic symptoms may be assessed in a standardized manner when taking a patient's history. Four symptoms—pain, burning, paresthesias, and numbness—are each rated with respect to their intensity ("absent," "slight," "moderate," "severe") and their frequency ("occasional," "frequent," "[almost] continuous"). Each of the 12 combinations of the four levels of intensity with the three levels of frequency has been assigned a score ranging from 0 to 3.66, and each of the four symptoms receives one of these scores based on its intensity and frequency ratings. Scores on the TSS therefore range from 0 (no symptoms are present) to a maximum of 14.64 (all four symptoms are severe in intensity and [almost] continuously present). Although this measure assesses several important symptoms of diabetic neuropathy in a structured and efficient manner, the basis for the scores given to the various combinations of intensity and frequency is unclear (e.g., a severe symptom that is ocasionally present is assigned a score of 3.00, whereas a moderately intense symptom that is [almost] continuously present is assigned a score of 2.66). The TSS has not been used in clinical trials in which the primary endpoint is pain, but its separate assessment of symptom intensity and frequency is noteworthy and may provide important information that is not obtained with other measures.

The Neuropathy Symptoms and Change (NSC) questionnaire (Dyck, Peroutka, et al., 1997) provides a more comprehensive assessment of neuropathy symptoms than the TSS. The NSC instrument contains a series of 38 symptoms that are assessed as present or absent, and, if present, are rated as "slight," "moderate," or "severe." For each of these symptoms, a rating can also be made of whether the symptom is "the same," "better," or "worse" than was found in a previous assessment; for ratings of better or worse, the degree of change is rated as "slight," "moderate," or "much." The ratings are made for symptoms of weakness (e.g., "weakness of fingers when clasping or grasping objects"), sensory symptoms (e.g., "decrease or inability to feel pain, cuts, bruises, or injuries"), and autonomic symptoms (e.g., "dryness of the eyes which is not due to use of medication or known eye disease"). For each of the sensory symptoms rated as present, a further rating is made of the part of the body that is affected. The NSC questionnaire provides relatively detailed instructions for the neurologist who is making these ratings, and it is an example of how the symptom assessments that are made during a history can be standardized with respect to both content and methods. However, because the NSC instrument is a measure of a variety of neuropathy symptoms, its assessment of neuropathic pain is not as comprehensive as would be desirable in a measure designed specifically for this purpose.

The Neuropathy Impairment Score (NIS; Dyck et al., 1995) contains a series of items in which muscle weakness, reflexes, and sensory function are rated on the right and left sides on the basis of a neurological examination. Each of the ratings of muscle weakness (e.g., wrist flexion, shoulder abduction) is made on a scale ranging from "normal" through varying degrees of weakness and movement to paralysis. The ratings of reflexes (e.g., biceps brachii, quadriceps femoris) and finger and toe sensation (e.g., pinprick, vibration) are made on a scale of "normal," "decreased," or "absent." Instructions are provided to the examiner indicating that anatomical site, age, gender, height, weight, and physical fitness should be considered when making the ratings. Although these ratings are based on the examiner's judgment of what is normal, the methods used in assessing touch pressure, pinprick, vibration sensation, and joint position are standardized. This approach to the neurological examination undoubtedly provides increased consistency in the content and methods of the assessments that are conducted. The NIS, however, does not include ratings of neuropathic pain signs such as allodynia and hyperalgesia, and it will need to be supplemented if a comprehensive assessment of neuropathic pain is required.

We have described the NSC and NIS measures in detail because we believe that these comprehensive and systematic measures of the symptoms and signs of neuropathy could serve as a guide in developing a similar approach to assessing neuropathic pain. To date, no structured history or physical examination has been developed for the comprehensive assessment of the symptoms and signs of neuropathic pain, although these would certainly be of great value. Fortunately, Backonja and Galer (1998) have provided a detailed review of the major components of an evaluation of patients with neuropathic pain. They emphasize that

the assessment of pain is based on a traditional history, including a review of the chief complaint and a review of systems. In addition, they underscore the importance of paying particular attention to the specific elements of neuropathic pain, such as intensity, location, and quality of spontaneous and stimulus-evoked pain, as well as findings on physical examination of mechanical allodynia, thermal allodynia, and hyperalgesia. They also stress the importance of noting the temporal course of these symptoms.

In taking the history of a patient with neuropathic pain, there is much important clinical information that should be gathered, in addition to that which is specific to pain. This information is essential in conducting a comprehensive evaluation, and is needed to evaluate prognosis and develop a treatment plan. As with all other types of chronic pain conditions, the following should be assessed: psychiatric comorbidity (e.g., depression, anxiety disorder, posttraumatic stress disorder), sleep, work-related issues, illness conviction, rehabilitative needs, and the availability of a support system. Each of these factors can have a direct effect on symptoms, quality of life, and response to various therapies. For example, a patient with a work-related painful nerve injury who is also experiencing posttraumatic stress disorder, insomnia, depression, and the stresses of being unemployed in the workers' compensation system needs a very different therapeutic approach from that required by a retired person with PHN and no significant comorbid conditions.

The physical examination of the patient with neuropathic pain should include detailed sensory testing as well as a general neurological evaluation (Backonja & Galer, 1998). Positive and negative sensory signs, such as mechanical allodynia, thermal allodynia, and hyperalgesia, should be assessed. As Backonja and Galer (1998) stress, it is important for examiners to ask patients unambiguous questions and to observe and record patients' behavioral responses when stimuli are administered. *Mechanical allodynia*, which refers to the abnormal perception of pain evoked by a normally nonnoxious stimulus, can be subdivided into *dynamic* allodynia, which is pain evoked by a moving stimulus across the skin, and *static* allodynia, which is pain evoked by pressure applied to a single focus with a blunt object. Although the presence of mechanical allodynia can be elicited from a patient during the history, it is important to evaluate the patient's response to actual stimuli. In both clinical and research settings, dynamic allodynia can be elicited by lightly rubbing the painful skin with a finger, cotton swab, or foam paintbrush. Static allodynia can be elicited by blunt pressure with a finger or von Frey filaments. *Thermal allodynia* is evoked by normally non-noxious thermal stimuli, either cold or hot, and it can be assessed in the clinic simply by heating or cooling a tuning fork or by applying ice briefly to the involved region. A more detailed and quantitative assessment of thermal sensation and perception can be performed via QST, which is discussed later in this chapter.

Hyperalgesia, by definition, is an exaggerated pain response evoked by a normally noxious stimulus. Unlike mechanical allodynia, the presence of hyperalgesia cannot be elicited during the history. *Summation* is an abnormally increasing painful sensation in response to a repeated stimulus while the actual stimulus remains constant; for example, as one continues to administer pinpricks to the involved skin, the perception of pain increases and becomes more painful than what would normally be experienced. *Aftersensation* is the abnormal persistence of a sensory perception provoked by a stimulus even though the stimulus has ceased, which may last for several seconds or even several minutes. In addition, patients who experience aftersensations may describe an enlarged region of pain (e.g., "The pain area got bigger and spread like a starburst").

Patients with neuropathic pain also frequently experience motor symptoms and signs, and these should be routinely assessed. Backonja and Galer (1998) point out that such patients may suffer disability from weakness, hypotonia, tremor, dystonia, incoordination, ataxia, apraxia, and motor neglect. Although motor dysfunction is less common in certain neuropathic pain conditions, such as PHN (although it may occur when PHN involves a limb), motor abnormalities are not uncommon in polyneuropathies and CRPS. In fact, several recent studies of CRPS have shown that motor dysfunction is one of the most common symptoms in this disorder (Bruehl et al., 1999; Galer, Hendersen, Perander, & Jensen, in press; Galer & Jensen, 1999; Harden et al., 1999; Veldman, Reynen, Arntz, & Goris, 1993).

In their discussion of both the history and the physical examination, Backonja and Galer (1998) highlight the critical importance of a careful musculoskeletal and myofascial evaluation in all patients with chronic pain. *Myofascial pain syndrome* is defined as chronic pain that is maintained by chronic tightness and spasm of soft

muscles and tissues. Patients who have this pain syndrome

> may describe their pain similarly as those with neuropathic pain, using terms such as burning, shooting, and aching. Myofascial pain may develop as a secondary phenomenon, evolving from disuse or overuse of musculature being caused by the primary neuropathic pain syndrome, although in some patients it is the primary origin of the chronic pain. Thus, even in patients with definite neuropathic pain syndromes, myofascial examination is critical to assess whether a secondary myofascial component is present, because myofascial pain requires a distinct treatment strategy. (Backonja & Galer, 1998, pp. 783–784)

If the clinician or clinical researcher fails to identify the presence of a myofascial component, then the evaluation of treatment outcome of a therapy for neuropathic pain would be misleading. (For a fuller discussion of myofascial pain syndrome, see Gerwin, Chapter 26.)

Backonja and Galer (1998) conclude their discussion of the assessment of patients with neuropathic pain by noting that the diagnosis is usually straightforward and is often based on a history of nerve injury, the patient's description of symptoms, and the presence of one or more neuropathic pain sensory signs on physical examination. Nevertheless, the diagnosis of neuropathic pain may also be given without a definite history of nerve injury in patients with symptoms and physical findings that are consistent with this diagnosis. For example, Backonja and Galer note that specific symptoms and signs are associated with a diagnosis of CRPS, and that these should be assessed whether or not there is a history of nerve injury, especially if a limb is involved. We have not reviewed these symptoms and their assessment, because they are discussed in detail by Bruehl and colleagues in Chapter 28. Patients with a painful polyneuropathy do not have a definite history of nerve injury and may also present with only paresthesia, dysesthesia, or pain in the toes or feet. If such a patient has a known exposure to a neurotoxin, such as the chemotherapeutic agent paclitaxel (Forsyth et al., 1997), or has a known medical condition where polyneuropathy is a complication, such as diabetes mellitus or HIV, then diagnosis is facilitated. However, making a diagnosis of polyneuropathy in a patient with painful feet without known risk factors for polyneuropathy can be more difficult. Yet, in patients with a history and examination findings consistent with this diagnosis, it is recommended that a diagnosis of polyneuropathy should be made.

SELF-REPORT METHODS FOR ASSESSING NEUROPATHIC PAIN

Pain Intensity

What comes to mind most often when pain specialists think of pain assessment are the diverse measures available for rating the intensity of pain and describing its quality. It is as important to assess the intensity of neuropathic pain as it is to assess the intensity of other kinds of pain, and this is no less true in the clinic than it is in research. There are a large number of measures of pain intensity available; these are comprehensively reviewed by Jensen and Karoly in Chapter 2, as well as in other chapters of this volume. These measures may be grouped into three broad types: Verbal Rating Scales (VRSs; e.g., "none," "mild," "moderate," "severe"), Numerical Rating Scales (NRSs; e.g., an 11-point scale anchored by "no pain" and "worst pain imaginable"), and Visual Analogue Scales (VASs; e.g., a 10-cm line anchored by "no pain" and "pain as bad as it could be"). Some measures of pain intensity do not fit readily into one of these categories (e.g., facial scales, pain thermometers), and others (e.g., the Descriptor Differential Scale; Gracely & Kwilosz, 1988) combine aspects of more than one of these types of measures. Nevertheless, most assessment of pain intensity is conducted with either VRSs, NRSs, or VASs.

The choice of one of these measures is most often based on the experience of the investigator. Although there are a number of studies in the literature that compare two or more of these different methods (e.g., Duncan, Bushnell, & Lavigne, 1989; Jensen, Karoly, & Braver, 1986; Price, Bush, Long, & Harkins, 1994), to our knowledge no study of this design has been conducted specifically with patients who have neuropathic pain. After reviewing this literature and comparing the advantages and disadvantages of different methods of measuring pain intensity in diverse samples of patients with chronic pain, Jensen and Karoly (1992) concluded in the first edition of this volume that "unless a particular clinician or researcher has a very strong rationale for using a VAS over other scales, we recommend against using the VAS as a *primary* (or sole) measure of pain intensity in adult clinical populations" (p. 140, original emphasis). They reach a similar conclusion in Chapter 2 of this volume.

This recommendation is based primarily on the difficulty that some patients have in understanding and using VAS measures of pain intensity. This problem may be particularly prevalent in elderly individuals (see, e.g., Carlsson, 1983; Kremer, Atkinson, & Ignelzi, 1981; Max, 1991), perhaps as a result of increased difficulty with abstraction (Walsh, 1984), which is consistent with our experience in using a VAS with older individuals. Because many common neuropathic pain syndromes are more prevalent in the elderly (e.g., PHN, painful diabetic neuropathy, central poststroke pain), use of a VAS may be limited in the assessment of neuropathic pain. Another obvious problem with using the VAS is that it cannot be administered in a telephone interview or to subjects who cannot indicate their pain with a written response (either because of limited motor function or because of the specific assessment situation—for example, during functional magnetic resonance imaging [MRI]).

Jensen and colleagues have conducted a series of studies comparing different measures of pain intensity (e.g., Jensen et al., 1986; Jensen, Miller, & Fisher, 1998; Jensen, Turner, & Romano, 1994). The results of these studies suggest that NRS methods of assessing pain intensity are somewhat superior to other approaches in the extent to which they are used accurately by subjects. In addition, it appears that a 21-point scale with numbers ranging from 0 to 100 in multiples of 5 may be the optimal measure. This is certainly consistent with our clinical and research experience, in which patients often respond with two adjacent numbers when administered a 0–10 scale orally, or indicate a point midway between two adjacent numbers when administered an 11-point scale in a written format. We therefore recommend the use of NRS methods (in preference to VAS and VRS methods) to assess pain intensity in research on neuropathic pain (see, e.g., Anderson, Syrjala, & Cleeland, Chapter 30, this volume; Jensen et al., 1998; but see also Price et al., 1994).

An important question regarding the assessment of pain intensity involves whether the pain rated by the patient is current, usual (average), worst, or least pain. In addition, when usual, worst, and least pain are assessed, a time frame for the ratings must be selected (e.g., past week, past 24 hours, today, since previous rating). Often these decisions will be determined by the specific clinical or research question. However, there are many situations in which the investigator must decide among these options, and there is unfortunately not a great deal of guidance in the literature in making these choices.

Pain Location, Frequency, and Duration

As noted above, less attention has been devoted to the systematic assessment of pain location and area, pain frequency, and pain duration. In assessing pain location and area, a common approach is to ask patients to indicate the area of their pain on drawings of the front and back of the human body. Such drawings may be analyzed in various ways, including total area of pain, number of body regions affected, and anatomical appropriateness or abnormality (for a review, see Jensen & Karoly, Chapter 2). With respect to neuropathic pain, it is possible to examine the total affected area not only of spontaneous pain but also of stimulus-evoked pain (e.g., the area of allodynia). There are various methods for doing this, including ratings by the investigator of the percentage of the dermatome(s) affected, and assessments of change in area using body maps, tracings of the affected area, and/or a polar planimeter. The most accurate assessment of variables such as total affected area and percentage of dermatome affected would be obtained by analyzing digital photographs, and the use of this approach is certain to increase in the coming years. Unfortunately, no published clinical trial has prospectively evaluated change in the size of the painful area with treatment. Yet, based on the evidence that prolonged neuropathic pain can be accompanied by an enlargement in receptive fields (e.g., Coderre, Katz, Vaccarino, & Melzack, 1993), it may be expected that a positive response to treatment could be manifested as the shrinkage of a painful area.

The systematic assessment of neuropathic pain frequency and duration has received little attention, although their importance has been emphasized by Bennett (1994). When measured, these aspects of pain have typically been assessed on an ad hoc basis. Several examples of questions for assessing pain frequency and duration are provided by Von Korff (Chapter 31). These could be readily adapted for use with both spontaneous and stimulus-evoked neuropathic pain.

Pain Quality

The assessment of different pain qualities has been an integral component of the assessment of neuropathic pain for many years, and has been emphasized in descriptive surveys (e.g., Bhala, Ramamoorthy, Bowsher, & Yelnoorker, 1988; Chan et al., 1990), clinical trials (e.g., Max et al., 1992;

Watson & Babul, 1998), and research on pathophysiology (Baron & Saguer, 1993; Rowbotham, Petersen, & Fields, 1998). Often the quality of spontaneous and stimulus-evoked neuropathic pain has been assessed with simple questions and procedures (e.g., pinprick, cotton swab) developed specifically for a particular study. During the past several years, there has been an increased interest in improving the accuracy of assessments of pain quality. The reasons for this include the need for measures of treatment response that may be more sensitive than overall ratings of pain intensity, and the expectation that different pain qualities may reflect distinct pathophysiological mechanisms.

For the past 25 years, the preeminent method for systematically assessing the quality of a patient's spontaneous pain has been the McGill Pain Questionnaire (MPQ), which includes sensory, affective, and evaluative descriptors of pain (Melzack, 1975; see Melzack & Katz, Chapter 3). The MPQ has been as frequently used in the assessment of neuropathic pain as in the assessment of all other types of acute and chronic pain. Indeed, one of the earliest efforts to demonstrate the ability of the MPQ to discriminate among different types of pain included two examples of neuropathic pain, PHN and phantom limb pain (Dubuisson & Melzack, 1976).

Later studies using the MPQ included demonstrations that it could discriminate trigeminal neuralgia from atypical facial pain (Melzack, Terrence, Fromm, & Amsel, 1986), symptomatic diabetic neuropathy from non-neuropathic leg and/or foot pain (Masson, Hunt, Gem, & Boulton, 1989), diverse types of peripheral neuropathic pain from chronic benign pain (Boureau, Doubrère, & Luu, 1990), and chronic pain following complete spinal cord injury from chronic pain following partial injury (Defrin, Ohry, Blumen, & Urca, 1999). In the study conducted by Boureau and colleagues (1990), six MPQ Sensory adjectives were significantly more frequently chosen by patients with neuropathic pain ("electric shock," "burning," "cold," "pricking," "tingling," "itching"); of these, electric shock, burning, and tingling were the most common in the patients with neuropathic pain (53%, 54%, and 48%, respectively). These results provide important support for clinical observations that these adjectives are particularly valuable in identifying patients with neuropathic pain. However, several other adjectives typically considered characteristic of neuropathic pain did not discriminate the two groups (e.g., "lancinating," "shooting"). One very interesting finding in this study was that all of the MPQ Affective adjectives were less frequently chosen by the patients with neuropathic pain, and in some cases the differences were large (e.g., "fearful" was endorsed by 48% of the patients with non-neuropathic pain, but only 3% of the patients with neuropathic pain).

The MPQ has also been used to characterize changes in the quality of pain in specific neuropathic pain syndromes. For example, the quality of acute neuropathic pain in herpes zoster has been compared with the quality of chronic pain in PHN (Bhala et al., 1988; Bowsher, 1993). Sharp, stabbing pain was found to be more common in patients with acute herpes zoster than in patients with PHN, whereas burning pain was found to be more common in patients with PHN and was much less likely to be reported by patients with acute herpes zoster. Unfortunately, these results were based on cross-sectional studies of different groups of patients and not a prospective study of the same individuals. Interestingly, other data suggest that throbbing and burning pain should be examined separately in PHN. Patients with PHN who had received the antiviral agent acyclovir for treatment of their acute herpes zoster infection were found to be much less likely to report burning pain than patients with PHN who had not received acyclovir; reports of throbbing pain in these two groups, however, did not differ (Bowsher, 1992, 1993). Given the strong association between the adjective "burning" and neuropathic pain found in the study conducted by Boureau and colleagues (1990), one interpretation of these data is that antiviral treatment attenuates the development of one of the mechanisms of neuropathic pain in PHN.

Because the MPQ can be relatively time-consuming for some patients, Melzack (1987) has developed a short form of the MPQ (SF-MPQ). The initial studies of the reliability and validity of the SF-MPQ examined postsurgical, labor, and musculoskeletal pain, but did not include patients with neuropathic pain (Melzack, 1987). In subsequent research, however, this measure has been used in what are the two largest placebo-controlled clinical trials ever conducted for neuropathic pain. These studies reported beneficial effects of gabapentin treatment on SF-MPQ Total, Sensory, and Affective scores in patients with PHN (Rowbotham, Harden, Stacey, Bernstein, & Magnus-Miller, 1998) and painful diabetic neuropathy (Backonja et al., 1998). In additional analyses of the data from the PHN trial in which the individual SF-MPQ items were examined, treatment with gabapentin was

associated with significantly greater pain relief for 10 of the 11 Sensory items and all four of the Affective items (Stacey, Rowbotham, Harden, Magnus-Miller, & Bernstein, 1999). In the results of a parallel series of analyses in which the SF-MPQ data from the diabetic neuropathy trial were examined, gabapentin treatment was associated with significantly greater pain relief for 9 of the 11 Sensory items, and nonsignificant improvement in all four of the SF-MPQ Affective items (Dworkin, 1999).

The results of these studies demonstrate the value of the MPQ and SF-MPQ in the assessment of patients with neuropathic pain. For assessing neuropathic pain, the greatest value of these measures may lie less in the Total, Sensory, and Affective scores and more in the ratings of the 11 Sensory descriptors. A similar conclusion was reached by the investigators of a multicenter study of the MPQ in 1,700 patients with chronic pain, who concluded that combining the MPQ descriptors into subscales may seriously limit the information obtained, because "information concerning the specific pain qualities endorsed by the patient is lost" (Holroyd et al., 1992, p. 309).

One possible interpretation of the results of the SF-MPQ analyses in the PHN and painful diabetic neuropathy gabapentin clinical trials, in which little discrimination among pain qualities in treatment response was found, is that the MPQ must be supplemented by more specific and sensitive measures when neuropathic pain is being assessed. Of course, the MPQ and the SF-MPQ were not developed specifically for the assessment of neuropathic pain. Galer and Jensen (1997) recently developed the Neuropathic Pain Scale (NPS; see Appendix 27.A), which was specifically designed to assess the different qualities of neuropathic pain in a questionnaire format. In initial studies of the validity of the NPS (Galer & Jensen, 1997), the measure discriminated patients with PHN from patients with three other types of neuropathic pain (i.e., complex regional pain syndrome, diabetic neuropathy, and peripheral nerve injury). The NPS also successfully assessed the treatment response to intravenous lidocaine and phentolamine infusions in a group of patients with central and peripheral neuropathic pain.

In a more recent study, the NPS was used to assess the prevalence of pain in patients with Charcot–Marie–Tooth (CMT) disease and to compare pain quality in CMT disease and several peripheral neuropathic pain syndromes (Carter et al., 1998). The results of this study demonstrated that pain intensity and pain quality in CMT disease and in PHN, CRPS, diabetic neuropathy, and peripheral nerve injury were generally comparable, and they provided additional support for the value of the NPS in the assessment of neuropathic pain. Although the NPS is being widely used as a treatment outcome measure in neuropathic pain clinical trials, it remains to be seen whether the NPS is a more sensitive measure of treatment outcome than the MPQ or even a single overall pain intensity measure. In addition, future research will need to determine whether the different pain qualities assessed by self-report questionnaires such as the MPQ or the NPS actually reflect distinct pain mechanisms in patients with neuropathic pain.

It is important to emphasize that no measure of pain quality, whether the MPQ or NPS, was designed as a diagnostic tool for neuropathic pain. Studies using both of these measures have provided data suggesting that patients with different neuropathic pain syndromes may have significantly different profiles of pain qualities. For neither measure, however, are there data that support its use as a diagnostic tool to differentiate neuropathic pain from other types of pain, such as myofascial pain or arthritis. Such studies are currently being conducted for the NPS.

QUANTITATIVE SENSORY TESTING

The assessment of sensory thresholds provides a method of examining the function of peripheral nerve fibers and their central connections (Yarnitsky, 1997). Because different fiber groups participate in the perception of different stimulus modalities, the assessment of several modalities allows the characterization of function across a variety of fiber populations. Small fibers, whose function is not readily assessed by nerve conduction studies, are one of the fiber groups that can be readily examined (Triplett & Ochoa, 1990). The information that can be obtained from an assessment of sensory function can be used to document symptoms—for example, thermal testing in a region of reported heat allodynia. In addition, as understanding of different pain mechanisms has increased, sensory testing has become increasingly useful in identifying these mechanisms and differentiating between them (see, e.g., Dyck, Peroutka, et al., 1997; Fields et al., 1998). Sensory testing can also play a role in the diagnosis and staging of painful conditions (see, e.g., Dyck, 1988; Dyck et al., 1992); in research on the natural history of neuropathic pain syndromes (see, e.g., Cheng et al., 1999; Dyck,

Davies, Litchy, & O'Brien, 1997); and in evaluating treatment response in patients with neuropathic pain (see, e.g., Attal, Brasseur, Parker, Chauvin, & Bouhassira, 1998; Eisenberg, Alon, Ishay, Daoud, & Yarnitsky, 1998; Zaslansky & Yarnitsky, 1998). In small-fiber neuropathies, thermal detection threshold may be the only means by which to document a neuropathy.

QST is a variant of conventional sensory testing wherein the goal is the quantification of the level of stimulation needed to produce a particular sensation. Measures for which there are normative data (based on age, sex, and body location) include warm and cold threshold, vibration threshold, and heat and cold pain threshold. In many cases, computer-controlled devices, which allow precise control of stimulus parameters, have made quantification possible. An example of this is the use of Peltier junctions in computer-controlled thermodes for the delivery of stimuli with known temperature and duration (Fruhstorfer, Lindblom, & Schmidt, 1976). However, the testing apparatus need not be complicated for stimulus quantification; von Frey filaments allow the estimation of tactile thresholds without the need for complicated instrumentation (Bell-Krotoski & Tomancik, 1987).

An important aspect of QST findings that must be considered in their interpretation is that the obtained thresholds reflect the functioning of the entire sensory system, including not only the peripheral sensory nerve but also central sensory and motor pathways. Although it has often been assumed that abnormal thresholds reflect abnormalities in specific peripheral afferent fibers, in order to obtain a threshold the stimulus energy must be transduced into energy in the peripheral nerve, which must then be perceived by the sensory cortex, which must then activate the motor system so that the subject can respond (typically by pressing a button). Although the major application of QST has been the identification of abnormal sensory thresholds, QST can also provide information regarding abnormal sensory perceptions, such as when cold stimulation causes an abnormal perception of burning and shooting pain that lasts for several minutes (aftersensations). Unfortunately, a standard method for assessing the abnormal sensory perceptions that can be evoked by different QST stimuli has not been developed.

In addition to the choice of stimulus modality and stimulus delivery method, another important element of QST is the choice of testing protocol (Gruener & Dyck, 1994; Yarnitsky, 1997). One example is the method of limits, which is commonly used with vibration and thermal modalities. In this method, the stimulus intensity is increased from a baseline value until the subject indicates that the stimulus is perceived. Although this method generally takes less time than other approaches and is straightforward with respect to patient instruction, it also includes a reaction time artifact (Dyck et al., 1993; Yarnitsky & Ochoa, 1990). There are many other testing protocols, each varying in complexity, repeatability, and test length. For a quantitative sensory test to be completely characterized, the modality, stimulus delivery method, and the testing protocol must be specified.

Types of Stimuli and Peripheral Nerve Fibers

QST typically encompasses use of the following stimulus modalities: warmth, cooling, heat pain, cold pain, vibration, static pressure, and brush-like stimuli. These modalities can be subdivided into the two broad categories of thermal and mechanical stimulation. Each stimulus modality can be tested either to locate the detection threshold or to determine the suprathreshold stimulus–response curve. Different receptor and fiber subpopulations are activated by the different stimulus modalities (Light & Perl, 1993; Triplett & Ochoa, 1990). In QST, the choice of the stimulus modality to be examined depends on the specific fiber subpopulation or symptom quality of interest. Although the focus of this section is on the relationship between stimulus modality and nerve fiber function in the periphery, it is important to recognize that the choice of stimulus modality also influences which central nervous system (CNS) pathway is preferentially activated. The measurement of patient response across various stimulus types is one method of investigating the function of different somatosensory pathways. Thermal and pain sensation thresholds are associated with the integrity of the spino-thalamic tract; vibration and tactile thresholds reflect the function of the dorsal column–medial lemniscal pathway. QST has been used in this context for the investigation of central pain (see, e.g., Berić, Dimitrijević, & Lindblom, 1988; Boivie, 1994).

Sensory fibers can be divided on the basis of the type of stimuli to which they preferentially respond (Light & Perl, 1993). Fibers are commonly classified as *low-threshold mechanoreceptors*, which respond preferentially to non-noxious skin displacement, velocity of displacement, or vibration; *thermo-*

receptors, which respond preferentially to skin temperature changes; and *nociceptors*, which respond to noxious levels of skin deformation, heating, or cooling. Nociceptors may also respond preferentially to noxious chemical stimuli. Within these classes, fibers can be further divided according to the related properties of conduction velocity and fiber diameter. In order of decreasing fiber diameter and decreasing conduction velocity, the sensory fiber classes are Aα, Aβ, Aδ, and C. The A fibers are myelinated, and the C fibers are unmyelinated. As can be seen from Table 27.3, the primary thermoreceptors include C-fiber warm receptors and Aδ and C cool receptors. Noxious heat and noxious cold stimulate C and Aδ nociceptors. In specifications of these relationships between fiber types and the stimuli to which they respond, the integrity and function of the CNS is assumed to be normal.

After a fiber has been classified by modality and diameter, further divisions are possible based on the specific type of receptor with which it is associated. For example, low-threshold mechanoreceptors are predominantly Aβ fibers. Among the Aβ low-threshold mechanoreceptors are Pacinian corpuscles, Ruffini endings, and Meissner corpuscles. These fibers are respectively associated with preferential responses to high-frequency skin displacement (i.e., vibration), maintained skin displacement (i.e., static mechanical stimuli), and velocity of displacement (i.e., dynamic mechanical stimuli). Although each subgroup of fibers has an optimal mode of stimulation, other modes of stimulation can still cause excitation (e.g., fibers with Ruffini endings will also respond to cooling). This excitation may contribute to the perception of stimulus presence, but may not contribute to the perception of stimulus quality (e.g., warmth, cold). It is important to recognize that fiber populations grouped by stimulus modality or diameter are not homogeneous, and that even when a single modality is used, a variety of fiber subtypes can be activated.

Methods of Stimulus Delivery

Thermal Testing

Thermal testing is typically performed with a computer-controlled thermode. Thermodes can vary in size, temperature range, and rates of cooling and heating (Fruhstorfer et al., 1976; Gruener & Dyck, 1994). Although the thermode size and temperature range are typically fixed for a given thermode, the rates of heating and cooling can usually be set by the user. A common thermode size is 3 cm × 3 cm; smaller stimulus areas are available, and these may be advantageous when one is testing restricted areas such as a single dermatome. It is important to recognize that the size of the thermode is critical when data from studies using different instruments are being compared; larger thermodes may activate greater numbers of fibers, and in so doing may lower the threshold that is obtained.

To prevent injury to the patient, the thermode's temperature is restricted, with a typical range being from 5° to 50°C. Rates of heating and cooling can usually be set by the user and range from 0.1°C/ second to 4°C/second. When a testing protocol is used that is influenced by the subject's reaction time (e.g., the method of limits), a fast rate of stimulus change may lead to an overestimate of the threshold (Dyck et al., 1993; Yarnitsky & Ochoa, 1990). Although a slower rate is advantageous from this standpoint, a slow rate of stimulus change lengthens the testing protocol. Rates on the order of 4°C/second have been used in protocols in which reaction time artifact is not present (Dyck et al., 1993). As with thermode size, it is critical that the rates of temperature change be considered when the results of studies using different protocols are being compared.

Mechanical Testing

Mechanical stimuli may be divided into three categories—*static mechanical*, *dynamic mechanical*, and *vibration*. Static mechanical stimuli are those in which the deformation of the skin is maintained over time. With dynamic mechanical stimuli, the skin displacement changes with time (e.g., moving stimuli). Vibration stimuli also have a skin displacement that changes with time, but with a rapidly changing velocity. Low-threshold mechanoreceptors are predominantly Aβ fibers and less commonly Aδ fibers. As discussed above, each type of mechanical stimulus is optimally transduced by a different cutaneous receptor type. Although all of these mechanical stimuli involve excitation of Aβ low-threshold mechanoreceptors, a particular stimulus may be more suitable in a given situation, based on the symptoms described by the patient or the specifics of the testing environment.

Static Mechanical Stimuli. Various static mechanical stimuli have been used in QST, including von Frey filaments and pressure algometers.

Stimuli vary in applied force and may also vary in surface area. The von Frey filaments consist of flexible filaments (initially horsehairs of different strength, but now plastic) of increasing diameters attached to a rigid rod (Bell-Krotoski & Tomancik, 1987). The free end of the filament is applied to the skin, and a force is applied to the rod until the filament begins to bend. This bending force increases with increasing filament diameter, allowing the application of a range of forces. Although the pressure applied is typically calculated by dividing the bending force by the contact area, the actual contact area may not be equal to the surface area of the fiber tip because of the bending of the fiber. Pressure algometers are another type of static mechanical stimulus used in QST.

A distinction is often made between sharp, punctate, or pinprick stimuli and pressure stimuli. However, the quality of a stimulus is not a fixed characteristic and depends on the amount of force used (Greenspan & McGillis, 1991). A given probe can produce sensations of dull pressure, sharp pressure, or sharp pain, depending on the force that is applied. The force needed for a perception of sharp pressure from a given probe falls between those needed for the perceptions of dull pressure and of sharp pain. When one is measuring mechanical allodynia in evaluating treatment outcome, it is critical that exactly the same body location is tested with the subject in the same position; for example, assessing allodynia on the dorsum of the foot may yield different results, depending on whether the person is standing or recumbent.

Vibration. Vibration thresholds are another measure of Aβ-fiber function (Goldberg & Lindblom, 1979). Vibration stimulators vary in surface area, applied frequency, range of displacement, and load weight. They usually consist of a small probe connected to a control unit, which is itself computer-controlled. A typical probe size is 1 cm². The applied frequency may be fixed (a typical value is 125 Hz) or controlled by the user. The frequency used may be chosen empirically as the frequency that gives the best test–retest reliability in the patient group of interest, or may be varied as one of the test parameters (Koltzenburg, Torebjork, & Wahren, 1994). The range of possible displacements is usually determined by the choice of stimulator. The load weight, which is determined by the stimulator configuration, is the amount of static force applied by the stimulator to the skin surface independent of the vibratory stimulation (Dyck et al., 1990; Goldberg & Lindblom, 1979). With stimulators in which the probe is suspended over the area tested, the load weight can be reliably set to the same value over multiple tests. The load weight cannot be reliably determined with hand-held stimulators, although a constant load weight can be approximated by allowing the stimulator to rest on the skin without additional applied pressure. A fixed load weight is desirable so that the static mechanical component of the stimulus is the same over repeated testing sessions. However, because it may not be feasible to suspend the stimulator over certain areas of the body, such as the back, a fixed load weight is not always possible.

Dynamic Mechanical (Brush-Evoked) Stimuli. The parameters involved in dynamic mechanical stimulation are the rate at which the source of stimulation is moved across the skin, the surface area that is applied to the skin, and the pressure applied to the skin. Although not specified in current testing protocols, another parameter that may be important in assessing dynamic allodynia is the direction in which the stimulus is moved. As in the visual system, it is possible that different movement directions are encoded differently in the brain. One method that is widely used in clinical trials for generating a dynamic stimulus makes use of a small paintbrush with a firm handle and a foam tip; camel's hair brushes have also been used. The surface area is determined by the dimensions of the tip, and the pressure is held approximately constant by pressing on the brush until the foam tip just begins to bend. The rate is determined by the administrator, who attempts to move the brush at the specified rate across the skin. Similarly, a cotton swab attached to a flexible metal strip has also been used to produce a dynamic mechanical stimulus (LaMotte, Shain, Simone, & Tsai, 1991), as has an electric toothbrush (see, e.g., Eide & Rabben, 1998; Nurmikko & Bowsher, 1990). All of these methods of producing dynamic mechanical stimuli can be applied to a predetermined area, or can be used to map out the borders of an area of abnormal sensation. Dynamic mechanical stimuli are preferentially transduced by Aβ low-threshold mechanoreceptors.

Stimulus Delivery and Response Collection Protocols

Although QST is defined with respect to the quantification of sensory stimuli, the protocols used for sensory testing are equally important. Many differ-

ent aspects of the testing protocol influence the results obtained with QST, including subject and stimulus factors. For example, the subject's attentiveness and understanding of the protocol can play an important role; these may be monitored by the introduction of null stimuli. In addition, the magnitude and repeatability of the thresholds obtained may depend on the order in which the stimuli are presented (i.e., ascending, descending, random). In choosing a protocol, many other factors must also be considered, including the required accuracy of the results and pragmatic concerns such as the time available for testing and patient fatigue (for reviews of QST protocols, see Gruener & Dyck, 1994; Yarnitsky, 1997).

QST protocols also define the responses from which a subject can choose. In the case of threshold determination, the responses are usually limited (e.g., "yes" or "no"). For suprathreshold protocols, the subject is given a range of response choices. For example, an 11-point NRS or a VRS (e.g., "nothing," "slightly warm," "warm," "hot," "very hot") may be used.

The selection of a specific protocol for QST depends on the goals of the assessment. Protocols may be divided into *threshold determination* protocols and *suprathreshold* protocols. Threshold determination protocols are designed to quantify the stimulus intensity needed for detection of the stimulus, whereas suprathreshold protocols are designed to determine the magnitude of the subject's responses to a set of stimulus intensities above the perception threshold. The sensation of interest may either be a pain sensation or an innocuous sensation.

Threshold Determination Protocols

Method of Limits. In the method of limits (Fruhstorfer et al., 1976), the stimulus intensity is increased or decreased until the subject indicates that the stimulus is perceived. Typically, the average of 3–10 trials is taken as the threshold value. This method has the advantage of relatively straightforward subject instructions and a short testing time. Its primary disadvantage is the influence of the subject's reaction time on the threshold value, which can cause spuriously elevated thresholds at fast rates of stimulus increase (Dyck et al., 1993; Yarnitsky & Ochoa, 1990).

Method of Constant Stimuli. In methods in which constant stimuli are used, the stimuli are increased or decreased to fixed target values (Yarnitsky & Ochoa, 1990). At the termination of each stimulus, the subject indicates whether the stimulus was perceived or not. Subsequent stimulus values depend on the subject's response—values ascend until perception is indicated, then descend until perception is lost—and the step sizes used vary with the specific protocol (Dyck et al., 1993; Yarnitsky & Ochoa, 1990). The threshold can be defined as the mean of the intensities where ascending or descending perception occurred, the mean of the "turnaround" points (where perception is achieved and lost), or the value where perception occurs with a specified probability (e.g., greater than 50% of the time). Null stimuli may also be presented; repeated indications that a null stimulus has been perceived suggest subject inattention or lack of comprehension of the instructions. Subject response time is not a factor in this method. Although the testing time using the method of constant stimuli will vary, depending on the criterion for threshold, in general this method takes longer than the method of limits (but less time than the forced-choice method).

Forced-Choice Method. The forced-choice method is one of the most robust protocols used in QST (Dyck et al., 1990). In this protocol, the stimulus is presented in one of two intervals. After both intervals conclude, the subject is asked to select the interval in which the stimulus occurred. There is a 50% chance of guessing correctly without any stimulus perception. The threshold value is defined as the stimulus intensity at which the subject's "hit" rate reaches a predefined level above 50%. Reaction time is not a factor in this protocol, and random presentation of stimuli can reduce the subject's anticipation of stimuli. The primary disadvantages of the protocol are the length of time it can take to achieve the desired accuracy level and the complexity of the task. The length of the test session depends on the accuracy level selected and on the subject's sensitivity.

Suprathreshold Protocols

In suprathreshold protocols, the focus is on the determination of the subject's stimulus–response curve for the specific stimulus modality examined. For this reason, the subject's responses must be derived from a rating scale. Suprathreshold testing protocols differ in the order of stimulus presentation and in the scales used for the subject's responses.

Stimuli may be presented in ascending order or in random order. In principle, although a de-

scending order may be used, this is not usually done because of the possibility of sensitization from the initial presentation of high-intensity stimuli. In the nonrepeating ascending stimulus protocol (Dyck et al., 1996), the stimulus intensity is increased in discrete steps, and the subject response is collected at each step. When a predetermined level of response is reached, the test is terminated. This test is useful for heat pain stimuli when multiple presentations of moderately painful stimuli are not required. With randomly presented stimuli, the test is not terminated at a particular response level, although a maximum response level is often set and no stimuli are administered that would produce responses greater than that level (Attal, Brasseur, Parker, et al., 1998). In suprathreshold protocols, subject responses are collected for each stimulus presentation, and any one of the different methods of rating pain intensity can be used.

Signal Detection Theory Protocols

One of the major ways in which signal detection theory (SDT) protocols differ from the other QST methods is that the subject's ability to discriminate stimuli is assessed in addition to the subject's criterion for response (Green & Swets, 1966). In these protocols, stimuli of fixed intensity are presented randomly, and the subject is asked to choose a response from a preselected rating scale. This approach distinguishes the sensory-discriminative aspects of subjects' responses from the extent to which subjects report their sensory experience as painful. SDT methods yield two measures: an index of sensory discrimination (d' or $P(A)$), which is interpreted as reflecting the functioning of the neurosensory system, and a measure of response criterion (Lx or B), which is interpreted as reflecting the subject's affective response to the sensory experience—that is, how readily he or she reports pain (Clark, 1974). Clark and Yang (1983) propose that the major advantage of these methods is that "at a descriptive, or qualitative, level, the sensory and emotional components of pain have long been recognized. SDT now permits the quantification of these two components into indices of discriminability and pain report criterion" (p. 23).

Interpretation of Findings

QST may be conducted for a variety of reasons. These include clarifying the nature of the sensory abnormalities present (Bouhassira, Attal, Willer, &

Brasseur, 1999); documenting the extent of the abnormalities for comparisons over time (Apfel et al., 1998; Attal, Brasseur, Parker, et al., 1998; Eisenberg et al., 1998); suggesting pain mechanisms that may be present in the patient (Rowbotham, Petersen, & Fields, 1998); and indicating possible diagnoses (Borg & Lindblom, 1986; Dyck et al., 1987). The role of QST will continue to evolve as more is discovered about the mechanisms of neuropathic pain and as more is learned about selectively treating pain symptoms, whether from a disease- or mechanism-based perspective. If the traditional disease-based treatment of pain continues to predominate in the future, the goals of symptom documentation and disease diagnosis will remain primary. If a mechanism-based model of pain treatment becomes more widespread, however, the goal of identifying the mechanisms of the patient's pain will become paramount.

Quantifying Symptoms

Neuropathic pain may be associated with a variety of sensory abnormalities (e.g., for PHN, see Nurmikko & Bowsher, 1990; Rowbotham, Petersen, & Fields, 1998). Some deficits may only become apparent on sensory testing, although other abnormalities may form a large part of the patient's complaint. Alterations of sensory function that are distressing to the patient can be quantified with respect to both their area and their severity, and these measures can be used to monitor treatment efficacy (see, e.g., Apfel et al., 1998; Attal, Brasseur, Parker, et al., 1998; Eisenberg et al., 1998; Lang et al., 1995). Less prominent alterations of sensory function can assist in diagnosis (Borg & Lindblom, 1986) or may predict disease course (Baron, Haendler, & Schulte, 1997).

The patient's responses to a given set of stimuli may be characterized using a stimulus–response curve (see Figure 27.1). The stimulus intensity axis will have the units of the relevant stimulus parameter (e.g., force or pressure, temperature, displacement). The response axis may have a numerical scale (e.g., VAS length in millimeters, NRS numerical ratings) or may be anchored by categorical descriptors. Multiple points on the curve may be determined via suprathreshold testing; alternatively, only a single feature, such as the detection threshold, may be assessed. Although the details of the stimulus–response curve will differ by testing method, modality, and subject, some broad characteristics of these curves may be defined.

The slope of the stimulus–response curve determines how much the patient's response increases for a given increase in stimulus intensity. *Hyperesthesia*, an increased responsiveness to stimuli, would be reflected in a curve with a steeper slope. If the stimuli under consideration are normally noxious, the steeper slope indicates an increased pain response to normally noxious stimuli, and the more specific term *hyperalgesia* can be used. A reported or observed increase in stimulus-evoked pain response can be investigated by performing a suprathreshold measurement of response to painful stimuli. Thermal hyperalgesia is often documented in such a manner, with protocols such as the heat pain nonrepeating ascending stimulus algorithm (Dyck et al., 1996). The use of von Frey filaments allows mechanical hyperalgesia to be documented in a similar manner (Attal, Brasseur, Parker, et al., 1998). Because calibrated dynamic mechanical stimuli have been less available, most QST approaches to the assessment of dynamic mechanical allodynia have used a single stimulus intensity to map out the affected area (e.g., a foam brush with fixed bending force and approximately constant rate of movement). Rather than a suprathreshold mapping of the stimulus–response curve, such an approach maps out the size of the area of the body where allodynia in response to a single stimulus is present or absent.

Sensory thresholds correspond to the minimum level of sensation that can be detected by the subject. In practice, sensory thresholds are specified in terms of the minimum stimulus level needed to produce a particular sensation. Typical thresholds used are the sensation detection threshold and the pain detection threshold, but thresholds can also be defined in terms of the stimulus needed to reach a particular pain rating. Threshold changes may be referred to directly or may be described with the same terms used for changes in the slope of the stimulus–response curve. Raised thresholds may be referred to as *hypoesthesia* and lowered thresholds may be referred to as *allodynia* or *hyperesthesia*, depending on whether the threshold in question is a pain threshold or a detection threshold. Thresholds for dynamic mechanical stimulation are less easily determined than thresholds for thermal, static mechanical, and vibration stimuli, because of the lack of calibrated methods for administering dynamic stimuli.

The quantitative documentation of sensory abnormalities allows a comparison between subgroups of patients with a given syndrome, which may help illuminate pathophysiology (e.g., Bouhassira et al., 1999; Eide & Rabben, 1998). In one recent example, QST has been used to compare patients with painful and painless HIV sensory neuropathy (Bouhassira et al., 1999). Mechanical allodynia and hyperalgesia were found in the patients with painful neuropathy but not in the patients without pain, and these abnormalities correlated with the intensity of spontaneous pain. Such findings can provide a basis for evaluating the contribution of peripheral and central mechanisms to the altered processing of mechanical stimuli in this peripheral neuropathic pain syndrome.

Using QST to compare painful and painless subtypes within a particular syndrome has also been done in the context of central pain (Andersen, Vestergaard, Ingeman-Nielsen, & Jensen, 1995; Vestergaard et al., 1995). A consecutive series of patients with acute stroke was examined in the first week after admission, with follow-up testing at 1 and 6 months and 1 year after stroke. Patients with sensory deficits but without pain were compared to patients with both sensory deficits and pain. It was found that although some sensory deficits, such as decreased tactile sensation, were present in both the pain and nonpain groups, thermal abnormalities were significantly more frequent in the pain group. This result suggests that central poststroke pain is associated with injury to the spino-thalamic tract.

Identification of Mechanisms

As attention to the mechanism-based approach to pain assessment and treatment continues to increase, the use of QST for the identification of pain mechanisms can be expected to increase as well. At the present time, however, there is limited evidence to support the use of QST in everyday practice to identify pain mechanisms in individual patients and then select treatments based on these mechanisms. Although patterns of QST findings in patients with the same diagnosis have been used to identify different pain mechanisms and thereby to define different subgroups of patients (e.g., Rowbotham, Petersen, & Fields, 1998), few prospective studies have been reported in which treatments are matched to pain mechanisms. Furthermore, although numerous mechanisms of neuropathic pain have been identified in studies of animal models and human clinical syndromes (see, e.g., Bennett, 1994; Fields & Rowbotham, 1994; Woolf & Mannion, 1999), the role of QST in identifying many of these pain mechanisms requires further clarification.

There is considerable evidence that in many patients stimulus-independent neuropathic pain reflects abnormal activity in primary afferent nociceptors (e.g., for reviews, see Bennett, 1994; Koltzenburg, 1996). QST is commonly used to examine fiber function in the periphery, and can provide information about mechanisms of both stimulus-independent and stimulus-dependent neuropathic pain. As discussed above, however, QST findings do not simply reflect abnormalities in the peripheral nervous system, but also reflect sensory and perhaps motor function at peripheral, spinal, and cortical levels in the nervous system. Moreoever, the results of a QST assessment are very likely to be affected by more than one of the pain mechanisms occurring at a given level. For this reason, it is possible to have the same pattern of QST findings arising from very different neuropathic pain mechanisms. For example, dynamic mechanical allodynia occurring together with thermal sensory deficits may indicate deafferentation-induced sprouting of non-nociceptive Aβ fibers within the dorsal horn. Alternatively, it is possible that nociceptors disconnected from the skin are spontaneously active, and maintain a state of central sensitization while being unresponsive to cutaneous pain stimuli (Fields et al., 1998). In addition, the well-documented alterations that occur throughout the neuraxis following peripheral nerve injury suggest that a single pathophysiological event in the periphery results in a cascade of CNS alterations that can also become mechanisms of pain. Because multiple mechanisms can generate similar patterns of QST findings, it is essential that other sources of information be used in the interpretation of the results of a QST assessment.

Additional important complications in the interpretation of QST findings are that several different pain mechanisms may be involved in a single disease, and that the same pain mechanism may arise from more than one disease. It is for precisely these reasons that mechanism-based models of pain treatment are currently attracting a great deal of attention (Woolf et al., 1998). However, these multiple and overlapping relationships among diseases, symptoms, signs, and pain mechanisms make the identification of mechanisms with QST difficult to implement in practice. A particular patient may have several mechanisms active at a given time. Each of these mechanisms can contribute to the QST results, leading to an amalgam that may be difficult to interpret. In addition, the mechanisms present in a particular patient may change over time as the disease progresses or is modified by treatment.

At the most general level, QST evaluates whether there are any abnormalities in the patient's stimulus–response curve for a relatively standard selection of stimulus modalities. In the interpretation of the results of a QST assessment (see Table 27.4), several more specific questions should be addressed, including these:

• *Are any nonpainful detection thresholds elevated?* The presence of sensory deficits in these thresholds provides information about losses in various fiber populations.

• *Is dynamic mechanical allodynia present?* Dynamic mechanical sensation normally activates non-nociceptive Aβ low-threshold mechanoreceptors. The presence of pain in response to normally non-noxious dynamic mechanical stimuli suggests that central changes may be present that make second-order pain transmission neurons responsive to stimulation of Aβ low-threshold mechanoreceptors (Koltzenberg et al., 1994).

• *Is cold allodynia present?* Cold allodynia accompanied by an increase in the cold detection threshold may indicate disinhibition due to a selective loss of cool-specific Aδ fibers (LaMotte & Thalhammer, 1982).

• *Is static mechanical hyperalgesia or heat hyperalgesia present?* These symptoms are generally thought to reflect peripheral sensitization of nociceptors (Koltzenburg, Lundberg, & Torebjork, 1992; LaMotte, Lundberg, & Torebjork, 1992).

• *Are there abnormal perceptions associated with the stimuli?* For example, a cold stimulus that evokes the perception of sharp, shooting pains that last for several minutes may reflect different pathophysiological mechanisms in the nervous system from those associated with abnormalities in sensory thresholds.

The results of QST provide information regarding both central and peripheral mechanisms of neuropathic pain. These mechanisms may be further distinguished according to whether existing connections are maintained, but with altered function of pre- and postsynaptic neurons, or whether new structural connections have developed. In Table 27.5, we present several important mechanisms of neuropathic pain and representative patterns of QST findings that are thought to reflect them. Peripheral sensitization occurs when primary sensory fibers increase their firing rate or their responsiveness to stimuli changes due to injury or environmental factors (LaMotte et al., 1992). Nociceptor sensitization is believed to contribute to static mechanical hyperalgesia (Koltzenburg et al., 1992) and to heat hyperalgesia (LaMotte et al., 1992). If there is decreased input from peripheral neurons to the dorsal horn instead of increased input, and if the involved neurons play a regulatory role in the perception of another sensory modality, disinhibition can occur. For example, cold allodynia in the presence of an elevated

TABLE 27.4. Putative Peripheral and Central Mechanisms of Sensory Abnormalities

Stimulus type	Response to innocuous stimuli		Response to painful stimuli	
	Hypoesthesia	Hyperesthesia/allodynia	Hypoalgesia	Hyperalgesia
Mechanical				
Static mechanical	Aβ loss	Peripheral sensitization		Peripheral sensitization
Dynamic mechanical		Central sensitization Central reorganization Disinhibition Phenotypic switching		
Punctate		Central sensitization	Aδ loss	Central sensitization
Vibration	Aβ loss			
Thermal				
Heating	C loss	Peripheral sensitization		Peripheral sensitization
Cooling	Aδ loss	Aδ cool-specific loss Central sensitization		Aδ cool-specific loss Central sensitization

TABLE 27.5. **Examples of Patterns of Sensory Abnormalities Associated with Proposed Peripheral and Central Mechanisms of Neuropathic Pain**

Mechanism	Thermal sensory abnormalities	Mechanical sensory abnormalities	Anesthetic infiltration
1. Central sensitization (maintained by sustained nociceptor input)	Minimal deficit or heat hyperalgesia	Dynamic mechanical allodynia	Decreased pain
2. Deafferentation-induced central reorganization	Thermal sensory deficits	Dynamic mechanical allodynia	Decreased allodynia (short duration)
3. Differential loss of cool-specific fibers	Cooling detection deficit Cold allodynia		
4. Deafferentation-induced central hyperactivity	Thermal sensory deficits	No dynamic mechanical allodynia	No change
5. Spino-thalamic tract injury	Thermal sensory deficits	None or less marked than thermal deficits	

Note. Some of the information presented in this table has been drawn from Rowbotham, Petersen, and Fields (1998).

cool detection threshold may be explained by disinhibition (LaMotte & Thalhammer, 1982). Because cooling-sensitive Aδ fibers determine the cool detection threshold and also inhibit the response to cold-responsive nociceptors, a disproportionate loss of Aδ fibers relative to C nociceptors will raise the cool detection threshold while decreasing the cold pain threshold.

Central sensitization of neurons in the spinal cord can be caused by sustained nociceptive input from the periphery. When this nociceptive activity is a result of neurons that have remained connected to the skin, the resulting symptoms will be associated with preserved thresholds in the relevant stimulus modality (Fields et al., 1998). The nociceptive input may also arise from activity in injured neurons that are no longer connected to the skin surface, which would be associated with sensory deficits in the relevant modality. The central sensitization that is maintained by these types of abnormal peripheral input causes central pain transmission neurons to become responsive to afferent neurons that normally transduce non-noxious stimuli, and this is believed to be an important mechanism of dynamic mechanical allodynia (Kolzenburg et al., 1994; Simone et al., 1991).

Central reorganization is another putative mechanism of dynamic mechanical allodynia (Devor & Wall, 1981). A loss of peripheral nociceptive input caused by damage or destruction of primary nociceptors can cause Aβ fibers to sprout

into areas of the dorsal horn associated with pain transmission (Woolf, Shortland, & Coggeshall, 1992). The pattern of QST findings that would be expected from this mechanism is dynamic mechanical allodynia accompanied by decreased sensitivity to thermal stimuli (Fields et al., 1998).

The use of QST to investigate pain mechanisms is not restricted to peripheral neuropathic pain syndromes. Sensory thresholds have been used in conjunction with laser-evoked potentials to investigate the mechanisms responsible for central pain following cerebral or brainstem infarction. One hypothesis attributes central pain to a lesion-induced increase in the excitability of spino-thalamic tract neurons. In one study, thermal and static mechanical thresholds and laser-evoked potentials were assessed in patients with unilateral pain (Casey et al., 1996). Comparison of the results from both sides showed that many patients with thermal and pain sensation deficits also had a reduction in laser-evoked potential amplitude on the affected side. The authors suggested that these results reflect a reduction in spino-thalamic tract function rather than increased CNS responsivity.

The Role of QST in the Comprehensive Assessment of Neuropathic Pain

The results of a QST assessment, no matter how extensive, do not alone provide a basis for diagnosing or evaluating neuropathic pain (Dyck et al., 1998). When included with other methods for evaluting a patient's symptoms and signs, however, QST provides valuable information that can be used in a variety of research and clinical situations. Zaslansky and Yarnitsky (1998) have reviewed the clinical applications of QST across a range of disorders, including endocrine, metabolic, compression, toxic, infection-associated, immune-related, and hereditary neuropathies, as well as CNS diseases and trauma.

Of these diverse disorders, diabetes is the one in which the role of QST has been most frequently studied and most clearly elaborated. This research has examined the prevalence and natural history of sensory deficits in patients with diabetes, the relationships between QST and other methods of assessing diabetic neuropathy, and the role of QST in predicting prognosis and evaluating therapeutic reponse (see, e.g., Dyck et al., 1992; Zaslansky & Yarnitsky, 1998). Importantly, in a number of studies various methodological aspects of QST have been examined, including the determination of normal values and differences in sensitivity and test–retest reliability between testing protocols (e.g., Dyck, 1993; Dyck et al., 1991, 1995; Zaslansky & Yarnitsky, 1998). We believe that this research on diabetic neuropathy and QST serves as an excellent example of how QST can be incorporated in research on other types of neuropathic pain.

The results of recent open-label studies of the effectiveness of anticonvulsant medications provide an additional example of how QST can augment the information obtained in an assessment of neuropathic pain. In these studies, spontaneous continuous pain, spontaneous intermittent pain, stimulus-evoked pain, and QST were examined. Attal and colleagues reported that 6 weeks of open-label gabapentin treatment reduced continuous pain, intermittent pain, and dynamic allodynia, and increased cold pain thresholds in patients with peripheral and central neuropathic pain (Attal, Brasseur, Parker, et al., 1998). There were, however, no changes in heat and tactile detection thresholds or in heat and punctate pain thresholds. A somewhat similar pattern of findings was reported by Eisenberg and colleagues (1998) in an open-label study of lamotrigine in painful diabetic neuropathy. As in the research reported by Attal and colleagues (1998), continuous pain decreased (as did cold allodynia), cold pain thresholds increased (although this was not statistically significant), and there were no changes in heat and tactile detection thresholds and heat and punctate pain

thresholds (intermittent pain was not assessed in this study). However, because mechanical allodynia was minimal, the effect of lamotrigine on dynamic allodynia could not be assessed, in contrast to the reduction in dynamic allodynia reported in two gabapentin studies (Attal, Brasseur, Parker, et al., 1998; Caracenti, Zecca, Martini, & De Conno, 1999). Although the results of these studies must be interpreted with caution because they were not placebo-controlled, such patterns of findings can provide valuable information about mechanisms and treatment response of neuropathic pain.

In concluding this section, it is important to emphasize that although QST allows clinicians and researchers to obtain important information regarding the functional status of different parts of the nervous system, its ability to identify distinct pain mechanisms in individual patients has not been established. Indeed, it is possible that the mechanisms involved in the development and maintenance of human neuropathic pain are so complex that additional approaches to the assessment of such pain will need to be developed before pain mechanisms can be reliably determined in individual patients. Certainly, more research is needed before QST can be recommended for routine use in the daily clinical care of patients with neuropathic pain.

OTHER PROCEDURES

Various other procedures can provide valuable information in the assessment of neuropathic pain. These include skin punch biopsies (Holland et al., 1997; Oaklander et al., 1998; Rowbotham et al., 1996); electromyography and nerve conduction studies (see, e.g., Benedetti et al., 1998; Dyck, 1988; Wolfe et al., 1999); nerve blocks and infusions (see, e.g., Dellemijn, Fields, Allen, McKay, & Rowbotham, 1994; Galer & Jensen, 1997; Galer, Miller, & Rowbotham, 1993); laser Doppler flowmetry (Baron & Saguer, 1993, 1994; Kurvers et al., 1996); and positron emission tomography and MRI (see, e.g., Attal, Brasseur, Chauvin, & Bouhassira, 1998; Baron, Baron, Disbrow, & Roberts, 1999; Iadarola et al., 1995).

All of these procedures can provide important information regarding mechanisms of neuropathic pain. However, all require specialized training for administration and interpretation. In addition, these procedures are generally more invasive and considerably more expensive than the other approaches to the assessment of neuropathic pain discussed in this chapter. For these reasons, these approaches should not currently be used on a routine basis in the assessment of neuropathic pain, either in the clinic or in research. Nevertheless, it can be expected that as research using these procedures in patients with neuropathic pain continues, their use will contribute to our understanding of neuropathic pain and have greater application in its assessment. Although detailed discussion of these procedures is beyond the scope of this chapter, many of them are discussed elsewhere in this volume.

CONCLUSIONS

The assessment of neuropathic pain requires that the person conducting the assessment evaluate his or her specific needs. What is the setting of the assessment—patient care or research? What should be assessed? What is the level of detail required for this particular assessment? Such questions must be answered prior to the actual assessment. It has only been over the last decade, and especially in the past several years, that specific tools to evaluate neuropathic pain have been developed and systematically studied. The continued development of neuropathic pain measures—such as sensory symptom questionnaires (e.g., the NPS; Galer & Jensen, 1997), sensory examination procedures (e.g., for assessing dynamic mechanical allodynia), and QST—will increase our understanding of the mechanisms of neuropathic pain. Furthermore, the identification of subgroups of patients who share the same symptoms, physical examination findings, or QST profiles has the potential to dramatically alter the way neuropathic pain is treated.

The point we would most like to emphasize in concluding this chapter is that a comprehensive assessment of neuropathic pain must examine a variety of symptoms and signs, and that the use of a single measure or method is inadequate. Although this is undoubtedly obvious to many readers, we believe that it must be emphasized, because it can be tempting to assess neuropathic pain in a less comprehensive manner. One recent example of an inadequate assessment of neuropathic pain is provided by a randomized, double-blind, placebo-controlled clinical trial of the analgesic effect of lamotrigine (McCleane, 1999). In this otherwise generally well-designed study, patients were diagnosed as having neuropathic pain and were enrolled in the trial if they had three of the following five "cardinal symptoms" of neuropathic pain: shooting/lancinating, burning, numbness, allodynia, and paresthesia/dysesthesia. No informa-

tion was provided regarding the methods used for assessing these five symptoms. Although the results of studies reviewed above suggest that many (perhaps all) of these symptoms may be more common in patients with neuropathic pain, we have also emphasized that all of these symptoms can be found in patients with non-neuropathic pain. The validity of the diagnoses of neuropathic pain made in this study are therefore questionable, and the results must be considered uninformative with respect to the efficacy of lamotrigine in neuropathic pain.

In this chapter, we have discussed the assessment of neuropathic pain and not the assessment of patients with neuropathic pain. The assessment of such patients involves much more than the assessment of their neuropathic pain. As with the comprehensive evaluation of any patient with chronic pain, the assessment of a patient with neuropathic pain should include an evaluation of the impact of the pain on psychological function (e.g., depression, coping) and quality of life (e.g., sleep, occupational disability, activities of daily living, social relationships), and may also include an examination of health care utilization and costs, depending on the assessment context and goals (see, e.g., Dworkin, 1997a, 1997b; Dworkin et al., 1997). We have not discussed these aspects of the assessment of the patient with neuropathic pain, because they are comprehensively reviewed elsewhere in this volume.

A fitting conclusion to this chapter is to underscore the complex nature of neuropathic pain and its impact on the patient. As Backonja and Galer (1998) emphasize,

It is the rule rather than [the] exception that patients who have chronic neuropathic pain have more than one type of pain. For example, a man who has PHN at high and midthorax may have constant ongoing pain that keeps him awake all night; mechanical allodynia and hyperalgesia that prevent him from wearing any clothing so he cannot be active and socialize; secondary myofascial pain in the shoulder so that use of that arm is limited; and after a few short weeks of his pain, the patient is by now sleep deprived, depressed, anxious, and very irritable. (p. 785)

ACKNOWLEDGMENT

Preparation of this chapter was supported in part by the U.S. Army Medical Research and Materiel Command under Grant No. DAMD17-98-1-8238.

REFERENCES

Allen, R. R. (1998). Neuropathic pain in the cancer patient. *Neurologic Clinics, 16,* 869–887.

American Psychiatric Association. (1994). *Diagnostic and statistical manual of mental disorders* (4th ed.). Washington, DC: Author.

Andersen, G., Vestergaard, K., Ingeman-Nielsen, M., & Jensen, T. S. (1995). Incidence of central post-stroke pain. *Pain, 61,* 187–193.

Apfel, S. C., Kessler, J. A., Adornato, B. T., Litchy, W. J., Sanders, C., Rask, C. A., & the NGF Study Group. (1998). Recombinant human nerve growth factor in the treatment of diabetic neuropathy. *Neurology, 51,* 695–702.

Arnér, S. (1998). Pain analysis in prediction of treatment outcome. *Acta Anaesthesiologica Scandinavica, 42*(Suppl. 113), 24–28.

Attal, N., Brasseur, L., Chauvin, M., & Bouhassira, D. (1998). A case of 'pure' dynamic mechano-allodynia due to a lesion of the spinal cord: Pathophysiological considerations. *Pain, 75,* 399–404.

Attal, N., Brasseur, L., Parker, F., Chauvin, M., & Bouhassira, D. (1998). Effects of gabapentin on the different components of peripheral and central neuropathic pain syndromes: A pilot study. *European Neurology, 40,* 191–200.

Backonja, M., Beydoun, A., Edwards, K. R., Schwartz, S. L., Fonseca, V., Hes, M., LaMoreaux, L., & Garofalo, E. (1998). Gabapentin for the symptomatic treatment of painful neuropathy in patients with diabetes mellitus. *Journal of the American Medical Association, 280,* 1831–1836.

Backonja, M.-M., & Galer, B. S. (1998). Pain assessment and evaluation of patients who have neuropathic pain. *Neurologic Clinics, 16,* 775–789.

Baron, R., Baron, Y., Disbrow, E., & Roberts, T. P. (1999). Brain processing of capsaicin-induced secondary hyperalgesia: A functional MRI study. *Neurology, 53,* 548–557.

Baron, R., Haendler, G., & Schulte, H. (1997). Afferent large fiber polyneuropathy predicts the development of postherpetic neuralgia. *Pain, 73,* 231–238.

Baron, R., & Saguer, M. (1993). Postherpetic neuralgia: Are C-nociceptors involved in signalling and maintenance of tactile allodynia? *Brain, 116,* 1477–1496.

Baron, R., & Saguer, M. (1994). Axon-reflex reactions in affected and homologous contralateral skin after unilateral peripheral injury of thoracic segmental nerves in humans. *Neuroscience Letters, 165,* 97–100.

Bell-Krotoski, J., & Tomancik, E. (1987). The repeatability of testing with Semmes-Weinstein monofilaments. *Journal of Hand Surgery (American), 12,* 155–161.

Benedetti, F., Vighetti, S., Ricco, C., Amanzio, M., Bergamasco, L., Casadio, C., Cianci, R., Giobbe, R., Oliaro, A., Bergamasco, B., & Maggi, G. (1998). Neurophysiologic assessment of nerve impairment in posterolateral and muscle-sparing thoracotomy. *Journal of Thoracic and Cardiovascular Surgery, 115,* 841–847.

Bennett, G. J. (1994). Neuropathic pain. In P. D. Wall & R. Melzack (Eds.), *Textbook of pain* (3rd ed., pp. 201–224). Edinburgh: Churchill Livingstone.

Bennett, G. J. (1997). Neuropathic pain: An overview. In D. Borsook (Ed.), *Progress in pain research and man-*

agement: Vol. 9. Molecular neurobiology of pain (pp. 109–113). Seattle, WA: International Association for the Study of Pain Press.

Berić, A. (1998). Central pain and dysesthesia syndrome. *Neurologic Clinics, 16,* 899–918.

Berić, A., Dimitrijević, M. R., & Lindblom, U. (1988). Central dysesthesia syndrome in spinal cord injury patients. *Pain, 34,* 109–116.

Bhala, B. B., Ramamoorthy, C., Bowsher, D., & Yelnoorker, K. N. (1988). Shingles and postherpetic neuralgia. *Clinical Journal of Pain, 4,* 169–174.

Boivie, J. (1994). Sensory abnormalities in patients with central nervous system lesions as shown by quantitative sensory tests. In J. Boivie, P. Hansson, & U. Lindblom (Eds.), *Progress in pain research and management: Vol. 3. Touch, temperature, and pain in health and disease: Mechanisms and assessments* (pp. 179–191). Seattle, WA: International Association for the Study of Pain Press.

Borg, K., & Lindblom, U. (1986). Increase of vibration threshold during wrist flexion in patients with carpal tunnel syndrome. *Pain, 26,* 211–219.

Bouhassira, D., Attal, N., Willer, J.-C., & Brasseur, L. (1999). Painful and painless peripheral sensory neuropathies due to HIV infection: A comparison using quantitative sensory evaluation. *Pain, 80,* 265–272.

Boureau, F., Doubrère, J. F., & Luu, M. (1990). Study of verbal description in neuropathic pain. *Pain, 42,* 145–152.

Bowsher, D. (1992). Acute herpes zoster and postherpetic neuralgia: Effects of acyclovir and outcome of treatment with amitriptyline. *British Journal of General Practice, 42,* 244–246.

Bowsher, D. (1993). Sensory change in postherpetic neuralgia. In C. P. N. Watson (Ed.), *Pain research and clinical management: Vol. 8. Herpes zoster and postherpetic neuralgia* (pp. 97–107). Amsterdam: Elsevier.

Bruehl, S., Harden, R. N., Galer, B. S., Saltz, S., Bertram, M., Backonja, M., Gayles, R., Rudin, N., Bhugra, M. K., & Stanton-Hicks, M. (1999). External validation of IASP diagnostic criteria for complex regional pain syndrome and proposed research diagnostic criteria. *Pain, 81,* 147–154.

Caraceni, A., Zecca, E., Martini, C., & De Conno, F. (1999). Gabapentin as an adjuvant to opioid analgesia for neuropathic cancer pain. *Journal of Pain and Symptom Management, 17,* 441–445.

Carlsson, A. M. (1983). Assessment of chronic pain: I. Aspects of the reliability and validity of the visual analogue scale. *Pain, 16,* 87–101.

Carter, G. T., Jensen, M. P., Galer, B. S., Kraft, G. H., Crabtree, L. D., Beardsley, R. M., Abresch, R. T., & Bird, T. D. (1998). Neuropathic pain in Charcot-Marie-Tooth disease. *Archives of Physical Medicine & Rehabilitation, 79,* 1560–1564.

Casey, K. L., Beydoun, A., Boivie, J., Sjolund, B., Holmgren, H., Leijon, G., Morrow, T. J., & Rosen, I. (1996). Laser-evoked cerebral potentials and sensory function in patients with central pain. *Pain, 64,* 485–491.

Chan, A. W., MacFarlane, I. A., Bowsher, D., Wells, J. C., Bessex, C., & Griffiths, K. (1990). Chronic pain in patients with diabetes mellitus: Comparison with a non-diabetic population. *The Pain Clinic, 3,* 147–159.

Cheng, W.-Y., Jiang, Y.-D., Chuang, L.-M., Huang, C.-N., Heng, L.-T., Wu, H.-P., Tai, T.-Y., & Lin, B. J. (1999). Quantitative sensory testing and risk factors of diabetic sensory neuropathy. *Journal of Neurology*, *246*, 394–398.

Clark, W. C. (1974). Pain sensitivity and the report of pain: An introduction to sensory decision theory. *Anesthesiology*, *40*, 272–287.

Clark, W. C., & Yang, J. C. (1983). Applications of sensory decision theory to problems in laboratory and clinical pain. In R. Melzack (Ed.), *Pain measurement and assessment* (pp. 15–25). New York: Raven Press.

Coderre, T. J., Katz, J., Vaccarino, A. L., & Melzack, R. (1993). Contribution of central neuroplasticity to pathological pain: Review of clinical and experimental evidence. *Pain*, *52*, 259–285.

Defrin, R., Ohry, A., Blumen, N., & Urca, G. (1999). Acute pain threshold in subjects with chronic pain following spinal cord injury. *Pain*, *83*, 275–282.

Dellemijn, P. L. I., Fields, H. L., Allen, R. R., McKay, W. R., & Rowbotham, M. C. (1994). The interpretation of pain relief and sensory changes following sympathetic blockade. *Brain*, *117*, 1475–1487.

Devor, M., & Wall, P. D. (1981). Plasticity in the spinal cord sensory map following peripheral nerve injury in rats. *Journal of Neuroscience*, *1*, 679–684.

Diabetes Control and Complications Trial Research Group. (1995). The effect of intensive diabetes therapy on the development and progression of neuropathy. *Annals of Internal Medicine*, *122*, 561–568.

Dubuisson, D., & Melzack, R. (1976). Classification of clinical pain descriptions by multiple group discriminant analysis. *Experimental Neurology*, *51*, 480–487.

Duncan, G. H., Bushnell, M. C., & Lavigne, G. J. (1989). Comparison of verbal and visual analogue scales for measuring the intensity and unpleasantness of experimental pain. *Pain*, *37*, 295–303.

Dworkin, R. H. (1997a). Pain and its assessment in herpes zoster. *Antiviral Chemistry and Chemotherapy*, *8*(Suppl. 1), 31–36.

Dworkin, R. H. (1997b). Toward a clearer specification of acute pain risk factors and chronic pain outcomes. *Pain Forum*, *6*, 148–150

Dworkin, R. H. (1999, October). *Anticonvulsant efficacy in neuropathic pain and its relationship to pain quality*. Paper presented at the annual meeting of the American Pain Society, Fort Lauderdale, FL.

Dworkin, R. H., Carrington, D., Cunningham, A., Kost, R. G., Levin, M. J., McKendrick, M. W., Oxman, M. N., Rentier, B., Schmader, K. E., Tappeiner, G., Wassilew, S. W., & Whitley, R. J. (1997). Assessment of pain in herpes zoster: Lessons learned from antiviral trials. *Antiviral Research*, *33*, 73–85.

Dyck, P. J. (1988). Detection, characterization, and staging of polyneuropathy: Assessed in diabetics. *Muscle and Nerve*, *11*, 21–32.

Dyck, P. J. (1993). Quantitative sensory testing: A consensus report from the Peripheral Neuropathy Association. *Neurology*, *43*, 1050–1052.

Dyck, P. J., Bushek, W., Spring, E. M., Karnes, J. L., Litchy, W. J., O'Brien, P. C., & Service, F. J. (1987). Vibratory and cooling detection thresholds compared with other tests in diagnosing and staging diabetic neuropathy. *Diabetes Care*, *10*, 432–440.

Dyck, P. J., Davies, J. L., Litchy, W. J., & O'Brien, P. C. (1997). Longitudinal assessment of diabetic polyneuropathy using a composite score in the Rochester Diabetic Neuropathy Study cohort. *Neurology*, *49*, 229–239.

Dyck, P. J., Dyck, P. J. B., Kennedy, W. R., Kesserwani, H., Melanson, M., Ochoa, J., Shy, M., Stevens, J. C., Suarez, G. A., & O'Brien, P. C. (1998). Limitations of quantitative sensory testing when patients are biased toward a bad outcome. *Neurology*, *50*, 1213.

Dyck, P. J., Karnes, J. L., Gillen, D. A., O'Brien, P. C., Zimmerman, I. R., & Johnson, D. M. (1990). Comparison of algorithms of testing for use in automated evaluation of sensation. *Neurology*, *40*, 1607–1613.

Dyck, P. J., Karnes, J. L., O'Brien, P. C., Litchy, W. J., Low, P. A., & Melton, L. J., III. (1992). The Rochester Diabetic Neuropathy Study: Reassessment of tests and criteria for diagnosis and staged severity. *Neurology*, *42*, 1164–1170.

Dyck, P. J., Kratz, K. M., Lehman, K. A., Karnes, J. L., Melton, L. J., III, O'Brien, P. C., Litchy, W. J., Windeband, A. J., Smith, B. E., Low, P. A., Service, F. J., Rizza, R. A., & Zimmerman, B. R. (1991). The Rochester Diabetic Neuropathy Study: Design, criteria for types of neuropathy, selection bias, and reproducibility of neuropathic tests. *Neurology*, *41*, 799–807.

Dyck, P. J., Litchy, W. J., Lehman, K. A., Hokanson, J. L., Low, P. A., & O'Brien, P. C. (1995). Variables influencing neuropathic endpoints: The Rochester Diabetic Neuropathy Study of healthy subjects. *Neurology*, *45*, 1115–1121.

Dyck, P. J., Melton, L. J., III, O'Brien, P. C., & Service, F. J. (1997). Approaches to improve epidemiological studies of diabetic neuropathy: Insights from the Rochester Diabetic Neuropathy Study. *Diabetes*, *46*(Suppl. 2), S5–S8.

Dyck, P. J., Peroutka, S., Rask, C., Burton, E., Baker, M. K., Lehman, K. A., Gillen, D. A., Hokanson, J. L., & O'Brien, P. C. (1997). Intradermal recombinant human nerve growth factor induces pressure allodynia and lowered heat-pain threshold in humans. *Neurology*, *48*, 501–505.

Dyck, P. J., Zimmerman, I., Gillen, D. A., Johnson, D., Karnes, J. L., & O'Brien, P. C. (1993). Cool, warm, and heat-pain detection thresholds: Testing methods and inferences about anatomic distribution of receptors. *Neurology*, *43*, 1500–1508.

Dyck, P. J., Zimmerman, I. R., Johnson, D. M., Gillen, D., Hokanson, J. L., Karnes, J. L., Gruener, G., & O'Brien, P. C. (1996). A standard test of heat-pain responses using CASE IV. *Journal of the Neurological Sciences*, *136*, 54–63.

Eide, P. K., & Rabben, T. (1998). Trigeminal neuropathic pain: Pathophysiological mechanisms examined by quantitative assessment of abnormal pain and sensory perception. *Neurosurgery*, *43*, 1103–1110.

Eisenberg, E., Alon, N., Ishay, A., Daoud, D., & Yarnitsky, D. (1998). Lamotrigine in the treatment of painful diabetic neuropathy. *European Journal of Neurology*, *5*, 167–173.

Fields, H. L., & Rowbotham, M. C. (1994). Multiple mechanisms of neuropathic pain: A clinical perspective. In G. F. Gebhart, D. L. Hammond, & T. S. Jensen (Eds.), *Progress in pain research and management: Vol. 2. Proceedings of the 7th World Congress on Pain* (pp. 437–454). Seattle, WA: International Association for the Study of Pain Press.

Fields, H. L., Rowbotham, M., & Baron, R. (1998). Postherpetic neuralgia: Irritable nociceptors and deafferentation. *Neurobiology of Disease*, *5*, 209–227.

First, M. B., Gibbon, M., Spitzer, R. L., & Williams, J. B. W. (1997). *Structured clinical interview for DSM-IV Axis I disorders–Clinician Version (SCID-CV).* Washington, DC: American Psychiatric Press.

Forsyth, P.A., Balmaceda, C., Peterson K., Seidman, A.D., Brasher, P., & DeAngelis, L.M. (1997). Prospective study of paclitaxel-induced peripheral neuropathy with quantitative sensory testing. *Journal of Neuro-Oncology, 35,* 47–53.

Fruhstorfer, H., Lindblom, U., & Schmidt, W. G. (1976). Method for quantitative estimation of thermal thresholds in patients. *Journal of Neurology, Neurosurgery and Psychiatry, 39,* 1071–1075.

Galer, B. S. (1998). Painful polyneuropathy. *Neurologic Clinics, 16,* 791–811.

Galer, B. S., Bruehl, S., & Harden, N. (1998). IASP diagnostic criteria for complex regional pain syndrome: A preliminary empirical validation study. *Clinical Journal of Pain, 14,* 48–54.

Galer, B. S., & Jensen, M. P. (1997). Development and preliminary validation of a pain measure specific to neuropathic pain: The Neuropathic Pain Scale. *Neurology, 48,* 332–338.

Galer, B. S., & Jensen, M. P. (1999). Neglect-like symptoms in complex regional pain syndrome: Results of a self-administered survey. *Journal of Pain and Symptom Management, 18,* 213–217.

Galer, B. S., Hendersen, J., Perander, J., & Jensen, M. (in press). Course of symptoms and quality of life measurement in complex regional pain syndrome: A pilot survey. *Journal of Pain and Symptom Management.*

Galer, B. S., Miller, K. V., & Rowbotham, M. C. (1993). Response to intravenous lidocaine infusion differs based on clinical diagnosis and site of nervous system injury. *Neurology, 43,* 1233–1235.

Goldberg, J. M., & Lindblom, U. (1979). Standardised method of determining vibratory perception thresholds for diagnosis and screening in neurological investigation. *Journal of Neurology, Neurosurgery and Psychiatry, 42,* 793–803.

Gracely, R. H., & Kwilosz, D. M. (1988). The Descriptor Differential Scale: Applying psychophysical principles to clinical pain assessment. *Pain, 35,* 279–288.

Green, D. M., & Swets, J. A. (1966). *Signal detection theory and psychophysics.* New York: Wiley.

Greenspan, J. D., & McGillis, S. L. B. (1991). Stimulus features relevant to the perception of sharpness and mechanically evoked cutaneous pain. *Somatosensory and Motor Research, 8,* 137–147.

Gruener, G., & Dyck, P. J. (1994). Quantitative sensory testing: Methodology, applications, and future directions. *Journal of Clinical Neurophysiology, 11,* 568–583.

Harden, R. N., Bruehl, S., Galer, B. S., Saltz, S., Bertram, M., Backonja, M., Gayles, R., Rudin, N., Bhugra, M. K., & Stanton-Hicks, M. (1999). Complex regional pain syndrome: Are the IASP diagnostic criteria valid and sufficiently comprehensive? *Pain, 83,* 211–219.

Holland, N. R., Stocks, A., Hauer, P., Cornblath, D. R., Griffin, J. W., & McArthur, J. C. (1997). Intraepidermal nerve fiber density in patients with painful sensory neuropathy. *Neurology, 48,* 708–711.

Holroyd, K. A., Holm, J. E., Keefe, F. J., Turner, J. A., Bradley, L. A., Murphy, W. D., Johnson, P., Anderson, K., Hinkle, A. L., & O'Malley, W. B. (1992). A multi-center evaluation of the McGill Pain Questionnaire: Results from more than 1700 chronic pain patients. *Pain, 48,* 301–311.

Iadarola, M. J., Max, M. B., Berman, K. F., Byas-Smith, M. G., Coghill, R. C., Gracely, R. H., & Bennett, G. J. (1995). Unilateral decrease in thalamic activity observed with positron emission tomography in patients with chronic neuropathic pain. *Pain, 63,* 55–64.

Jensen, M. P., & Karoly, P. (1992). Self-report scales and procedures for assessing pain in adults. In D. C. Turk & R. Melzack (Eds.), *Handbook of pain assessment* (pp. 135–151). New York: Guilford Press.

Jensen, M. P., Karoly, P., & Braver, S. (1986). The measurement of clinical pain intensity: A comparison of six methods. *Pain, 27,* 117–126.

Jensen, M. P., Miller, L., & Fisher, L. D. (1998). Assessment of pain during medical procedures: A comparison of three scales. *Clinical Journal of Pain, 14,* 343–349.

Jensen, M. P., Turner, J. A., & Romano, J. M. (1994). What is the maximum number of levels needed in pain intensity measurement? *Pain, 58,* 387–392.

Koltzenburg, M. (1995). Stability and plasticity of nociceptor function and their relationship to provoked and ongoing pain. *Seminars in the Neurosciences, 7,* 199–210.

Koltzenburg, M. (1996). Afferent mechanisms mediating pain and hyperalgesias in neuralgia. In W. Jänig & M. Stanton-Hicks (Eds.), *Progress in pain research and management: Vol. 6. Reflex sympathetic dystrophy: A reappraisal* (pp. 123–150). Seattle, WA: International Association for the Study of Pain Press.

Koltzenburg, M. (1998). Painful neuropathies. *Current Opinion in Neurology, 11,* 515–521.

Koltzenburg, M., Lundberg, L. E. R., & Torebjörk, H. E. (1992). Dynamic and static components of mechanical hyperalgesia in human hairy skin. *Pain, 51,* 207–219.

Koltzenburg, M., Torebjörk, H. E., & Wahren, L. K. (1994). Nociceptor modulated central sensitization causes mechanical hyperalgesia in acute chemogenic and chronic neuropathic pain. *Brain, 117,* 579–591.

Kremer, E., Atkinson, J. H., & Ignelzi, R. J. (1981). Measurement of pain: Patient preference does not confound pain measurement. *Pain, 10,* 241–248.

Kurvers, H. A., Jacobs, M. J., Beuk, R. J., van den Wildenberg, F. A., Kitslaar, P. J., Slaaf, D. W., & Reneman, R. S. (1996). The spinal component to skin blood flow abnormalities in reflex sympathetic dystrophy. *Archives of Neurology, 53,* 58–65.

LaMotte, R. H., Lundberg, L. E., & Torebjork, H. E. (1992). Pain, hyperalgesia, and activity in nociceptive C units in humans after intradermal injection of capsaicin. *Journal of Physiology, 448,* 749–764.

LaMotte, R. H., Shain, C. N., Simone, D. A., & Tsai, E. F. (1991). Neurogenic hyperalgesia: Psychophysical studies of underlying mechanisms. *Journal of Neurophysiology, 66,* 190–211.

LaMotte, R. H., & Thalhammer, J. G. (1982). Response properties of high-threshold cutaneous cold receptors in the primate. *Brain Research, 244,* 279–287.

Lang, E., Spitzer, A., Pfannmüller, D., Claus, D., Handwerker, H., & Neundörfer, B. (1995). Function of thick and thin nerve fibers in carpal tunnel syndrome before and after treatment. *Muscle and Nerve, 18,* 207–215.

Light, A. R., & Perl, E. R. (1993). Peripheral sensory systems. In P. J. Dyck, P. K. Thomas, J. W. Griffin, P. A. Low, & J. F. Poduslo (Eds.), *Peripheral neuropathy* (3rd ed., pp. 149–165). Philadelphia: Saunders.

Martin, J. H., & Jessell, T. M. (1991). Modality coding in the somatic sensory system. In E. R. Kandel, J. H. Schwartz, & T. M. Jessell (Eds.), *Principles of neural science* (3rd ed., pp. 341–352). Norwalk, CT: Appleton & Lange.

Masson, E. A., Hunt, L., Gem, J. M., & Boulton, A. J. M. (1989). A novel approach to the diagnosis and assessment of symptomatic diabetic neuropathy. *Pain, 38,* 25–28.

Max, M. B. (1990). Towards physiologically based treatment of patients with neuropathic pain. *Pain, 42,* 131–133.

Max, M. B. (1991). Neuropathic pain syndromes. In M. Max, R. Portenoy, & E. Laska (Eds.), *The design of analgesic clinical trials* (pp. 193–219). New York: Raven Press.

Max, M. B., Lynch, S. A., Muir, J., Shoaf, S. E., Smoller, B., & Dubner, R. (1992). Effect of desipramine, amitriptyline, and fluoxetine on pain in diabetic neuropathy. *New England Journal of Medicine, 326,* 1250–1256.

McCleane, G. (1999). 200 mg daily of lamotrigine has no analgesic effect in neuropathic pain: A randomised, double-blind, placebo controlled trial. *Pain, 83,* 105–107.

Melzack, R. (1975). The McGill Pain Questionnaire: Major properties and scoring methods. *Pain, 1,* 277–299.

Melzack, R. (1983). Appendix B: McGill Comprehensive Pain Questionnaire Interviewer Guide. In R. Melzack (Ed.), *Pain measurement and assessment* (pp. 10A–14A). New York: Raven Press.

Melzack, R. (1987). The short-form McGill Pain Questionnaire. *Pain, 30,* 191–197.

Melzack, R., Terrence, C., Fromm, G., & Amsel, R. (1986). Trigeminal neuralgia and atypical facial pain: Use of the McGill Pain Questionnaire for discrimination and diagnosis. *Pain, 27,* 297–302.

Merskey, H., & Bogduk, N. (Eds.). (1994). *Classification of chronic pain: Descriptions of chronic pain syndromes and definitions of pain terms* (2nd ed.). Seattle, WA: International Association for the Study of Pain Press.

Meyerson, B. A. (1997). Pharmacological tests in pain analysis and in prediction of treatment outcome. *Pain, 72,* 1–3.

Nurmikko, T., & Bowsher, D. (1990). Somatosensory findings in postherpetic neuralgia. *Journal of Neurology, Neurosurgery and Psychiatry, 53,* 135–141.

Oaklander, A. L., Romans, K., Horasek, S., Stocks, A., Hauer, P., & Meyer, R. A. (1998). Unilateral postherpetic neuralgia is associated with bilateral sensory neuron damage. *Annals of Neurology, 44,* 789–795.

Price, D. D., Bush, F. M., Long, S., & Harkins, S. W. (1994). A comparison of pain measurement characteristics of mechanical visual analogue and simple numerical rating scales. *Pain, 56,* 217–226.

Rowbotham, M., Harden, N., Stacey, B., Bernstein, P., & Magnus-Miller, L. (1998). Gabapentin for the treatment of postherpetic neuralgia: A randomized con-trolled trial. *Journal of the American Medical Association, 280,* 1837–1842.

Rowbotham, M. C., Petersen, K. L., & Fields, H. L. (1998). Is postherpetic neuralgia more than one disorder? *Pain Forum, 7,* 231–237.

Rowbotham, M. C., Yosipovitch, G., Connolly, M. K., Finlay, D., Forde, G., & Fields, H. L. (1996). Cutaneous innervation density in the allodynic form of post-herpetic neuralgia. *Neurobiology of Disease, 3,* 205–214.

Simone, D. A., Sorkin, L. S., Oh, U., Chung, J. M., Owens, C., LaMotte, R. H., & Willis, W. D. (1991). Neurogenic hyperalgesia: Central neural correlates in responses of spinothalamic tract neurons. *Journal of Neurophysiology, 66,* 228–246.

Stacey, B., Rowbotham, M., Harden, N., Magnus-Miller, L., & Bernstein, P. (1999, August). *Effects of gabapentin (Neurontin) on pain quality in patients with postherpetic neuralgia (PHN).* Poster session presented at the Ninth World Congress on Pain, Vienna.

Triplett, B., & Ochoa, J. (1990). Contemporary techniques in assessing peripheral nervous system function. *American Journal of EEG Technology, 30,* 29–44.

Veldman, P. H. J. M., Reynen, H. M., Arntz, I. E., & Goris, R. J. A. (1993). Signs and symptoms of reflex sympathetic dystrophy: Prospective study of 829 patients. *Lancet, 342,* 1012–1016.

Vestergaard, K., Nielsen, J., Andersen, G., Ingeman-Nielsen, M., Arendt-Nielsen, L., & Jensen, T.S. (1995). Sensory abnormalities in consecutive, unselected patients with central post-stroke pain. *Pain, 61,* 177–186.

Walsh, T. D. (1984). Re: Practical problems in pain measurement [Letter]. *Pain, 19,* 96–98.

Watson, C. P. N., & Babul, N. (1998). Efficacy of oxycodone in neuropathic pain: A randomized trial in postherpetic neuralgia. *Neurology, 50,* 1837–1841.

Wiesenfeld-Hallin, Z., Hao, J.-X., & Xu, X.-J. (1997). Mechanisms of central pain. In T. S. Jensen, J. A. Turner, & Z. Wiesenfeld-Hallin (Eds.), *Progress in pain research and management: Vol. 8. Proceedings of the 8th World Congress on Pain* (pp. 575–589). Seattle, WA: International Association for the Study of Pain Press.

Wolfe, G. I., Baker, N. S., Amato, A. A., Jackson, C. E., Nations, S. P., Saperstein, D. S., Cha, C. H., Katz, J. S., Bryan, W. W., & Barohn, R. J. (1999). Chronic cryptogenic sensory polyneuropathy: Clinical and laboratory characteristics. *Archives of Neurology, 56,* 540–547.

Woolf, C. J., Bennett, G. J., Doherty, M., Dubner, R., Kidd, B., Koltzenburg, M., Lipton, R., Loeser, J. D., Payne, R., & Torebjork, E. (1998). Towards a mechanism-based classification of pain? *Pain, 77,* 227–229.

Woolf, C. J., & Decosterd, I. (1999). Implications of recent advances in the understanding of pain pathophysiology for the assessment of pain in patients. *Pain,* Suppl. 6, S141–S147.

Woolf, C. J., & Mannion, R. J. (1999). Neuropathic pain: Aetiology, symptoms, mechanisms, and management. *Lancet, 353,* 1959–1964.

Woolf, C. J., Shortland, P., & Coggeshall, R. E. (1992). Peripheral nerve injury triggers central sprouting of myelinated afferents. *Nature, 355,* 75–78.

Yarnitsky, D. (1997). Quantitative sensory testing. *Muscle and Nerve, 20,* 198–204.

Yarnitsky, D., & Ochoa, J. L. (1990). Studies of heat pain sensation in man: Perception thresholds, rate of stimulus rise and reaction time. *Pain, 40,* 85–91.

Zaslansky, R., & Yarnitsky, D. (1998). Clinical applications of quantitative sensory testing (QST). *Journal of Neurological Sciences, 153,* 215–238.

Ziegler, D., Hanefeld, M., Ruhnau, K. J., Meissner, H. P., Lobisch, M., Schutte, K., Gries, F. A., & the ALADIN Study Group. (1995). Treatment of symptomatic diabetic peripheral neuropathy with the anti-oxidant alpha-lipoic acid: A 3-week multicentre randomized controlled trial (ALADIN Study). *Diabetologia, 38,* 1425–1433.

APPENDIX 27.A. NEUROPATHIC PAIN SCALE

Instructions: There are several different aspects of pain which we are interested in measuring: pain **sharpness, heat/cold, dullness, intensity,** overall **unpleasantness,** and **surface vs. deep** pain.

The distinction between these aspects of pain might be clearer if you think of taste. For example, people might agree on how *sweet* a piece of pie might be (the *intensity* of the sweetness), but some might enjoy it more if it were sweeter while others might prefer it to be less sweet. Similarly, people can judge the loudness of music and agree on what is more quiet and what is louder, but disagree on how it makes them feel. Some prefer quiet music and some prefer it more loud. In short, the *intensity* of a sensation is not the same as how it makes you feel. A sound might be unpleasant and still be quiet (think of someone grating their fingernails along a chalkboard). A sound can be quiet and "dull" or loud and "dull."

Pain is the same. Many people are able to tell the difference between many aspects of their pain: for example, *how much* it hurts and *how unpleasant* or annoying it is. Although often the intensity of pain has a strong influence on how unpleasant the experience of pain is, some people are able to experience more pain than others before they feel very bad about it.

There are scales for measuring different aspects of pain. For one patient, a pain might feel extremely hot, but not at all dull, while another patient may not experience any heat, but feel like their pain is very dull. We expect you to rate very high on some of the scales below and very low on others. We want you to use the measures that follow to tell us exactly what you experience.

1. Please use the scale below to tell us how **intense** your pain is. Place an "×" through the number that best describes the intensity of your pain.

No pain   The most **intense** pain sensation imaginable

0	1	2	3	4	5	6	7	8	9	10

2. Please use the scale below to tell us how **sharp** your pain feels. Words used to describe "sharp" feelings include "like a knife," "like a spike," "jabbing," or "like jolts."

Not sharp   The most **sharp** sensation imaginable ("like a knife")

0	1	2	3	4	5	6	7	8	9	10

3. Please use the scale below to tell us how **hot** your pain feels. Words used to describe very hot pain include "burning" and "on fire."

Not hot   The most **hot** sensation imaginable ("on fire")

0	1	2	3	4	5	6	7	8	9	10

4. Please use the scale below to tell us how **dull** your pain feels. Words used to describe very dull pain include "like a dull toothache," "dull pain," "aching," and "like a bruise."

Not dull   The most **dull** sensation imaginable

0	1	2	3	4	5	6	7	8	9	10

5. Please use the scale below to tell us how **cold** your pain feels. Words used to describe very cold pain include "like ice" and "freezing."

Not cold   The most **cold** sensation imaginable ("freezing")

0	1	2	3	4	5	6	7	8	9	10

(cont.)

6. Please use the scale below to tell us how **sensitive** your skin is to light touch or clothing. Words used to describe sensitive skin include "like sunburned skin" and "raw skin."

Not sensitive

The most **sensitive** sensation imaginable ("raw skin")

0	1	2	3	4	5	6	7	8	9	10

7. Please use the scale below to tell us how **itchy** your pain feels. Words used to describe very itchy pain include "like poison oak" and "like a mosquito bite."

Not itchy

The most **itchy** sensation imaginable ("like poison oak")

0	1	2	3	4	5	6	7	8	9	10

8. Which of the following best describes the **time** quality of your pain? Please check only one answer.

( )   I feel a background pain *all of the time* **and** occasional flare-ups (break-through pain) *some of the time*.
      Describe the background pain: _____
      Describe the flare-up (break-through) pain: _____

( )   I feel a single type of pain *all the time*.
      Describe this pain: _____

( )   I feel a single type of pain only *sometimes*. Other times, I am pain-free.
      Describe this occasional pain: _____

9. Now that you have told us the different physical aspects of your pain, the different types of sensations, we want you to tell us overall how **unpleasant** your pain is to you. Words used to describe very unpleasant pain include "miserable" and "intolerable." Remember, pain can have a low intensity but still feel extremely unpleasant, and some kinds of pain can have a high intensity but be very tolerable. With this scale, please tell us how **unpleasant** your pain feels.

Not unpleasant

The most **unpleasant** sensation imaginable ("intolerable")

0	1	2	3	4	5	6	7	8	9	10

10. Lastly, we want you to give us an estimate of the severity of your *deep* versus *surface* pain. We want you to rate each location of pain separately. We realize that it can be difficult to make these estimates, and most likely it will be a "best guess," but please give us your best estimate.

HOW INTENSE IS YOUR *DEEP* PAIN?

No **deep** pain

The most **intense deep** pain sensation imaginable

0	1	2	3	4	5	6	7	8	9	10

HOW INTENSE IS YOUR *SURFACE* PAIN?

No **surface** pain

The most **intense surface** pain sensation imaginable

0	1	2	3	4	5	6	7	8	9	10

Note. From Galer, B. S., and Jensen, M. P. (1997). Development and preliminary validation of a pain measure specific to neuropathic pain: The Neuropathic Pain Scale. *Neurology, 48,* 332–338. Copyright 1997 by Lippincott Williams & Wilkins. Reprinted by permission of Lippincott Williams & Wilkins.

Chapter 28

Complex Regional Pain Syndrome

STEPHEN BRUEHL
HERBERT G. STEGER
R. NORMAN HARDEN

Complex regional pain syndrome (CRPS) is a perplexing pain disorder that has been the subject of misunderstanding, misdiagnosis, and mistreatment. Originally recognized as a distinct pain syndrome during the American Civil War by Weir Mitchell (Mitchell, Morehouse, & Keen, 1864), it is characterized by pain in excess of what would be expected given the degree of injury, in combination with signs of autonomic nervous system dysfunction (e.g., sweating or skin temperature or color changes). It has in the past often been mislabeled as a psychogenic pain condition (Ochoa & Verdugo, 1995) due to its unusual pain characteristics, such as a seemingly nonanatomical stocking or glove pain distribution and severe pain in response to touch (i.e., allodynia), as well as the severe pain behavior (e.g., extreme guarding of the affected limb) and intense emotional distress frequently displayed by patients (Bruehl & Carlson, 1992; Bruehl, Husfeldt, Lubenow, Nath, & Ivankovich, 1996; Lynch, 1992). Despite its seemingly unusual clinical presentation, basic research over the past 20 years has clearly demonstrated that CRPS is a pain syndrome reflecting actual pathophysiology, rather than reflecting purely *psychopathological* processes (Arnold, Teasell, MacLeod, Brown, & Carruthers, 1993; Drummond, Finch, & Smythe, 1991; Harden et al., 1994; Kurvers et al., 1996, 1998; Moriwaki et al., 1997; Price, Bennett, & Rafii, 1989; Roberts, 1986; Woolf, Shortland, & Coggeshall, 1992).

As we will detail below, psychological (e.g., emotional distress) and behavioral factors (e.g., learned disuse) are likely to interact with the pathophysiological mechanisms underlying the disorder to determine the severity of CRPS signs and symptoms, and possibly contribute to maintenance of the syndrome (Bruehl & Carlson, 1992; Bruehl, Husfeldt, et al., 1996; Harden et al., 1994). Given the likely interactions between physiological and psychological factors in CRPS, an integrated multidisciplinary assessment and treatment approach is particularly important. In this chapter, we provide an overview of the clinical characteristics of CRPS and current issues in medical assessment of the disorder. We also provide a brief summary of the pathophysiology of CRPS. We then present an overview of the role of psychological factors in the etiology and maintenance of the condition, followed by a summary of a multidisciplinary assessment approach for CRPS, with a focus on the unique psychological aspects of this condition.

MEDICAL DIAGNOSTIC ISSUES

One of the major barriers in the past to improved understanding and treatment of CRPS was the lack of agreement regarding diagnosis of the disorder. Prior to 1994, the syndrome was known by a variety of names, including *neuroalgodystrophy, shoulder–hand syndrome,* and *reflex neurovascular dystrophy,* with *reflex sympathetic dystrophy* (RSD) and *causalgia* being the most common diagnostic terms (Harden, 1994; Stanton-Hicks, 1990). Because of the variety of names for the syndrome, the absence of any widely accepted diagnostic criteria, and the numerous sets of idiosyncratic diagnostic criteria used by various research groups, the basic science and clinical research conducted regarding CRPS tended not to generalize broadly beyond the research group conducting the research (Bruehl et al., 1999; Harden et al., 1999). The clear need for standardized, agreed-upon diagnostic criteria was recognized and addressed in 1993 through a Dahlem-type think tank ("the Orlando Conference") sponsored by the International Association for the Study of Pain (IASP; Stanton-Hicks et al., 1995).

The Orlando Conference brought together experts with both clinical and research expertise regarding the syndrome. The product of this meeting was the consensus-derived set of standardized diagnostic criteria ultimately published in the official pain diagnostic taxonomy of the IASP in 1994 (Merskey & Bogduk, 1994). Acknowledging the problem of frequently inaccurate clinical assumptions associated with the existing names for the syndrome (e.g., RSD), the developers of the IASP diagnostic criteria chose a new name for the disorder that was intended to be descriptive, while not implying a specific pathophysiology for the disorder: complex regional pain syndrome.

According to the current IASP diagnostic criteria (summarized in Table 28.1), CRPS typically affects a limb rather than the trunk, and is considered to be the result of a specific trauma or immobilization of the limb. The presence of a known inciting event, however, is not *required* for diagnosis of CRPS, reflecting the clinical reality that for a small proportion of patients (fewer than 5% of cases, based on data from the Bruehl et al. [1999] and Harden et al. [1999] studies), the condition appears to develop spontaneously. For a patient to receive a diagnosis of CRPS, three general criteria must be met: (1) an abnormality in pain processing, (2) evidence for some type of autonomic dysfunction, and (3) the absence of other disorders that could account for the observed syndrome. Regarding the first criterion, a patient must display persistent pain *that is disproportionate to the inciting event*. This pain must be associated with evidence of a pain-processing abnormality, as reflected in the presence of allodynia (normally nonpainful stimuli such as touch are perceived as painful) and/or hyperalgesia (mild pain stimuli such as light pinprick are perceived as intensely painful). In

TABLE 28.1. International Association for the Study of Pain (IASP) Diagnostic Criteria for Complex Regional Pain Syndrome (CRPS)

1. The presence of an initiating noxious event, or a cause of immobilization.
2. Continuing pain, allodynia, or hyperalgesia with which the pain is disproportionate to any inciting event.
3. Evidence at some time of edema, changes in skin blood flow, or abnormal sudomotor activity in the region of pain.
4. This diagnosis is excluded by the existence of conditions that would otherwise account for the degree of pain and dysfunction.

Associated signs and symptoms of CRPS listed in IASP taxonomy but not used for diagnosis

1. Atrophy of the hair, nails, and other soft tissues.
2. Alterations in hair growth.
3. Loss of joint mobility.
4. Impairment of motor function, including weakness, tremor, and dystonia.
5. Sympathetically-maintained pain may be present.

Note. From Harden et al. (1999). Copyright 1999 by the International Association for the Study of Pain. Reprinted by permission.

addition to evidence of abnormal pain processing, a diagnosis of CRPS also requires evidence of some type of autonomic nervous system dysfunction. This dysfunction may take several forms, including bilateral asymmetry in skin color, skin temperature, sweating, and/or edema. For example, asymmetry of more than $1.2\,°C$ in the affected extremity relative to the unaffected extremity is not unusual among patients with CRPS (Bruehl, Lubenow, Nath, & Ivankovich, 1996). The current criteria additionally describe two subtypes of CRPS: CRPS type I (reflex sympathetic dystrophy) and CRPS type II (causalgia), characterized respectively by the absence or presence of a known nerve injury in the affected area.

Although the adoption of these standardized, consensus-based IASP criteria for CRPS has been a step forward, the criteria were not empirically validated before their publication (Bruehl et al., 1999; Harden et al., 1999; Stanton-Hicks et al., 1995). The lack of validation of the current criteria does present problems regarding the diagnostic assessment of CRPS. For example, validation research to date reveals one primary weakness of these consensus-based criteria: Although displaying very high diagnostic sensitivity, they appear to have only modest specificity. The current criteria have a specificity of only .36 in distinguishing between CRPS and other neuropathic pain conditions of known non-CRPS etiology (Bruehl et al., 1999). Related work indicates that nearly 40% of patients with painful diabetic neuropathy might be misdiagnosed with CRPS according to the current criteria if the etiology of the diabetic neuropathy were unclear (Galer, Bruehl, & Harden, 1998). For clinical purposes, sensitivity (i.e., being able to detect the disorder when it is present) is extremely important. On the other hand, the issue of specificity (i.e., minimizing false-positive diagnoses) is quite important for selecting research samples, as well as for minimizing unnecessary, potentially invasive treatments. The clinical implication of high sensitivity at the expense of specificity is that CRPS may be overdiagnosed and ultimately overtreated. Such overdiagnosis must be balanced with the equally undesirable consequences of failing to identify clinically relevant syndromes and to treat patients adequately.

Research is currently being conducted to address the issue of improving the IASP criteria for CRPS in a way that maintains high diagnostic sensitivity while improving diagnostic specificity (Bruehl et al., 1999; Galer et al., 1998; Harden et al., 1999). Ultimately, this research may lead to improved assessment of the disorder. To date, this validation research suggests that the signs and symptoms of CRPS form several distinct subgroups that can be detected via statistical pattern recognition techniques such as factor analysis (Harden et al., 1999). Results from a factor analysis of a large database of patients with CRPS are summarized in Table 28.2 (Harden et al., 1999). This analysis revealed a unique set of signs and symptoms indicating abnormality in pain processing. Skin color and temperature changes form a second distinct subset of signs and symptoms that is indicative of vasomotor dysfunction, with a third subset of signs and symptoms reflecting edema and sudomotor dysfunction (e.g., sweating changes). Each of these subsets of signs and symptoms is incorporated in the current criteria, although the distinct vasomotor and sudomotor/edema subsets are combined into a single criterion in the IASP taxonomy (one problem potentially contributing to poor specificity; Bruehl et al., 1999; Harden et al., 1999).

One issue in the clinical assessment of CRPS is the fact that a number of clinical characteristics not currently reflected in the CRPS diagnostic criteria have been described in the older literature as being cardinal features of RSD (Bruehl et al., 1999; Harden et al., 1999; Stanton-Hicks et al., 1995). For example, various signs of motor dysfunction (e.g., dystonia, tremor) have been described as important characteristics of this disorder (Galer, Butler, & Jensen, 1995; Schwartzman & Kerrigan, 1990; Wilson, Low, Bedder, Covington, & Rauck, 1996). In addition, trophic features have been described in the older RSD literature as being important clinical features of the syndrome (e.g., changes in hair or nail growth, development of "shiny" skin). Factor analysis indicates that these characteristics form a distinct subset of CRPS signs and symptoms that does not overlap with the three other subgroups described above (Harden et al., 1999). The extent to which inclusion of motor and trophic features in any revision of the CRPS diagnostic criteria would improve diagnostic accuracy is currently being investigated.

In summary, patients diagnosed with CRPS according to the current IASP criteria may appear with a very limited set of symptoms, such as a unilateral region of persistent pain with hyperalgesia and unilateral edema that cannot be ac-

TABLE 28.2. Factors (and Factor Loadings) Resulting from Principal-Components Analysis of Diagnostic and Associated Signs and Symptoms of CRPS

Factor 1	Factor 2	Factor 3	Factor 4
Hyperalgesia Signs (.75) Hyperesthesia Symptoms (.78)	Temperature Asymmetry Symptoms (.68) Color Change Signs (.67) Color Change Symptoms (.52)	Edema Signs (.69) Sweating Asymmetry Signs (.62) Edema Symptoms (.61)	Decreased Range of Motion Signs (.81) Decreased Range of Motion Symptoms (.77) Motor Dysfunction Signs (.77) Motor Dysfunction Symptoms (.61) Trophic Symptoms (.52) Trophic Signs (.51)

Note. As expected, allodynic signs loaded most strongly on Factor 1 (.44), but did not meet the criteria for inclusion in the factor (>.50). From Harden et al. (1999). Copyright 1999 by the International Association for the Study of Pain. Reprinted by permission.

counted for by any non-CRPS mechanism. Traditional clinical experience based on older diagnostic criteria for RSD, however, suggests that the patient with "true" CRPS is likely to have a more florid presentation, including a region of intense allodynia resulting in overprotectiveness of the limb; unilateral edema with bluish, cool, and "shiny" skin in the affected region; loss of strength and range of motion in the affected limb; and noticeable changes in hair or nail growth in the affected side compared to the unaffected side (Gibbons & Wilson, 1992; Kozin, Ryan, Carerra, Soin, & Wortmann, 1981). The psychological issues described below, in patients with CRPS, are increasingly likely to be observed in severe form with more florid presentations of the CRPS syndrome.

PATHOPHYSIOLOGY

An understanding of the pathophysiology of CRPS provides an important rationale for assessing several important characteristics of and functional effects of CRPS. Although the pathophysiology of CRPS remains to be fully elucidated, the literature suggests that a number of factors are involved in producing the syndrome (Harden, 1994). In the initial period following peripheral nerve injury, it is known that sympathetic hypofunction occurs, resulting in a warm, red extremity (Birklein, Riedl, Claus, & Neudorfer, 1998). Diminished sympathetic efferent activity results in up-regulation of peripheral catecholaminergic receptors (Harden et al., 1994; Kurvers et al., 1995, 1998). The resulting supersensitivity to circulating catecholamines produces exaggerated vasoconstriction (Arnold et al., 1993; Baron & Maier, 1996; Harden et al., 1994; Kurvers et al., 1995, 1998), leading to the characteristic cool, blue extremity seen in cases of CRPS beyond the acute stage.

Another factor contributing to CRPS is that neuromas developing following peripheral nerve injury can result in spontaneous firing in nociceptive afferents (Gracely, Lynch, & Bennett, 1992), leading to persistent nociceptive input to the central nervous system. Additional evidence suggests that following nerve injury, peripheral nociceptive and non-nociceptive afferents become sensitive to adrenergic excitation, leading to increased firing in these afferents in the presence of sympathetic discharge or circulating catecholamines (Harden et al., 1994; Sato & Perl, 1991). This becomes particularly important, given the central nervous system changes that occur following peripheral nerve injury and ongoing nociceptive input.

A pathological alteration in central signal processing occurs that is maintained by persistent nociceptive input; this altered central processing contributes to the pain-processing abnormalities of CRPS (Gracely et al., 1992). One mechanism underlying altered central processing may be that following peripheral nerve injury, the terminals of large myelinated Aβ fibers (which normally convey touch) begin rewiring into lamina II of the spinal dorsal horn, an area that is normally the termination point of nociceptive C fibers (Woolf et al., 1992). This is one means by which allodynia, in which touch is perceived is painful, may occur.

In summary, a vicious cycle may be created in which altered central processing leads to increased pain, which in turn provokes catecholamine release, with these catecholamines contributing to peripheral vasoconstriction and micronutrient deficits, as well as increased stimulation of peripheral nociceptors and non-nociceptive afferents, thus maintaining the nociceptive input. The role of central changes in CRPS has even been hypothesized to extend to the brain, with one study finding evidence for medullary dysfunction in patients with CRPS (Thimineur, Sood, Kravitz, Gudin, & Kitaj, 1998). Although the exact nature of the central changes in CRPS are still being clarified (Harden et al., 1994), the fact that centralization of CRPS occurs over time is suggested by the observation that positive responsiveness to sympathetic blockade becomes less likely with increasing duration of CRPS (Harden et al., 1999; Wang, Johnson, & Ilstrup, 1985).

Another important pathophysiological mechanism underlying CRPS is the sometimes profound disuse of the affected extremity that develops in an effort to avoid stimuli that may trigger hyperalgesia and allodynia. Although disuse itself clearly contributes to the development of some of the trophic changes (e.g., to the hair, skin, and nails) in patients with CRPS, it is unclear whether it is the *sole* cause of these changes, given that the presence of such changes does not appear to be related to increased pain duration as might be expected (Harden et al., 1999). Another pathological consequence of pain-avoidant disuse relates to the central signal-processing alterations noted above. Specifically, learned disuse of the affected extremity eliminates the normal tactile and proprioceptive input from the extremity that may be necessary to restore normal central signal processing (Carlson & Watson, 1988; Stanton-Hicks et al.,

1998). Failure to use the affected extremity also prevents desensitization, ultimately prolonging heightened pain sensitivity rather than limiting it as the patient hopes. In summary, pain-related learned disuse may contribute directly to trophic changes in CRPS, and may interact with other pathophysiological mechanisms to prevent the patient from ending the vicious cycle described above that maintains the primary features of CRPS.

SECONDARY CONDITIONS

Some patients with CRPS report that they believe the condition may be spreading, often from a distal limb to more proximal areas, but sometimes even to the contralateral limb. Although an actual spreading of CRPS from one extremity to another is theoretically possible, given the putative central nervous system changes described above, it appears to be relatively rare. Often when CRPS is appearing to spread in the upper extremities, the newly developed symptoms may be best explained on the basis of myofascial pain syndrome developing in the proximal extremity or the contralateral side secondary to pain behavior (e.g., extreme guarding, "movement phobia"), or postural or gait abnormalities associated with the CRPS-affected limb (Travell & Simons, 1983). In one series of 41 patients with CRPS, myofascial pain syndrome (as indicated by presence of muscular tender points) was identified in 61% of patients as a contributor to the pain syndrome (Rashiq & Galer, 1999). The extent to which "spreading" reflects these secondary conditions rather than actual CRPS must be assessed through careful evaluation of the observable signs (e.g., bracing, spasm, trigger points, hyperalgesia, edema) that may be detected in the area of "spreading," rather than reliance on patient impressions that "CRPS is spreading." This latter concept is unfortunately popular, and is often dramatically promulgated in support groups and lay literature.

ROLE OF PSYCHOLOGICAL FACTORS

As noted above, patients with CRPS often have been labeled as having psychogenic pain, due to their unusual, often "nonanatomical" presentation, which can include extreme guarding of the affected limb, intense distress, a stocking or glove pattern of pain, and minimal or no known injury. Psycho-

logical antecedents therefore have often been cited as etiologically significant in the condition. A review of the literature regarding this issue (Bruehl & Carlson, 1992) indicates that such etiological assumptions are common. However, the uncontrolled nature of much of the research used to support this conclusion is often not appreciated (Bruehl & Carlson, 1992). For example, retrospective work by Van Houdenhove (1986) reported a strong relationship between onset of CRPS and a contemporaneous "affective loss, separation, or a loss of self-esteem" among a series of 32 patients with CRPS. The fact that this sample consisted entirely of psychiatric referrals for "pain aggravated by psychological factors" seriously limits conclusions that can be drawn. Egle and Hoffmann (1990) similarly reported that in a series of 12 patients with CRPS, one or more significant life stressors were identified as occurring in the 6 months prior to the onset of CRPS. Neither of the case series addresses the possibility that any random sample of healthy individuals might be able to identify a significant stressor of some type occurring during any 6-month period.

Despite the limitations of uncontrolled case series studies, similar findings have been reported in a study using a case–control design (Geertzen, de Bruijn, de Bruijn-Kofman, & Arendzen, 1994). Geertzen and colleagues (1994) compared 24 patients with CRPS to 42 patients without CRPS who were scheduled to undergo elective hand surgery. Results indicated that 80% of the CRPS group had experienced a stressful life event in the 2 months before or 1 month after the initiating trauma, compared to only 20% of the control group. Although these results are intriguing, the conclusions that can be drawn are limited by the study's retrospective design (Geertzen et al., 1994).

To date, there is only one published prospective study examining a possible causal connection between antecedent psychological state and onset of CRPS (Zachariae, 1964). Forty-seven male patients without CRPS who were undergoing surgery for Dupuytren's contracture were assessed by a psychiatrist preoperatively. Based on these presurgical psychiatric judgments regarding "psychiatric risk factors," the author reported 91% accuracy in predicting postsurgical CRPS-type complications following the surgery (Zachariae, 1964). These seemingly impressive results must be tempered by the vague nature of the psychiatric judgments (e.g., "sthenic," "martyr type," "unstable," "ambitious," "self-pitying"). Surprisingly, no prospective follow-up studies have been published.

An ongoing prospective study of patients in our clinic of patients undergoing total knee arthroplasty has provided intriguing preliminary findings regarding possible psychological risk factors for CRPS. Among 18 patients with 6-month follow-up data, 5 have developed CRPS-type symptoms (including hyperesthesia and/or hyperalgesia, and edema, color, or temperature asymmetries). When body mass, age, and CRPS status at baseline were controlled for, higher scores on the Beck Depression Inventory (BDI) appeared useful for identifying those more likely to develop CRPS. Specifically, BDI scores accurately predicted 92% of the patients without CRPS and 60% of the patients with CRPS, for an overall classification accuracy of 83% ($p < .08$). Statistical significance is precluded by the small sample size; however, these results would be consistent with depression as a risk factor in at least some cases of postsurgical CRPS. Although these limited prospective data are provocative, the overall methodological limitations of the existing literature indicate that drawing a casual connection between psychological events and onset of CRPS is premature (Bruehl & Carlson, 1992; Lynch, 1992).

Although not implying causation, some studies suggest that patients with CRPS may be more emotionally distressed than patients with pain but without CRPS. For example, Geertzen and colleagues (1994) compared patients with and without CRPS who were awaiting elective hand surgery. Male patients with CRPS were found to be more anxious than their counterparts without CRPS, and female patients with CRPS were more depressed than their counterparts without CRPS. Hardy and Merritt (1988) also found elevated symptoms of depression, anxiety, and interpersonal sensitivity in a sample of nine patients with CRPS compared to eight patient controls with pain but without CRPS. Consistent with the data above, Bruehl, Husfeldt, and colleagues (1996) found that patients with CRPS reported greater phobic anxiety and depression compared to patients with low back pain when potential confounds such as pain intensity and duration were statistically controlled for. Work in progress using the new CRPS criteria in a separate sample has replicated the finding of greater affective distress in patients with CRPS than in patients with low back pain (Bruehl, Harden, & Cole, 2000). Of potentially greater interest is the finding of a significantly stronger relationship between emotional distress and pain intensity that was observed in patients with CRPS compared to patients with low back pain in both the Bruehl, Husfeldt, and colleagues study and recent unpublished work.

A significant relationship between pain intensity and psychological distress would be expected within the gate control theory of pain (Melzack & Wall, 1965). The fact that the pain–distress relationship is significantly stronger in patients with CRPS than in patients with low back pain might be consistent with a greater role for emotional distress in the maintenance and expression of CRPS symptoms. However, it is interesting to note that at least one prospective study has demonstrated that premorbid depressive symptoms predict development of musculoskeletal pain 10 years later (Leino & Magni, 1993).

Given this prospective finding, and the preliminary prospective data in patients with total knee arthroplasty noted above, it is interesting to consider the possibility that the stronger pain–distress relationship noted among patients with CRPS relative to patients with low back pain (Bruehl, Husfeldt, et al., 1996; Bruehl et al., 2000) may indicate a greater role for emotional distress in development of CRPS signs and symptoms. This possibility must remain speculative at this time, given the nonprospective nature of the CRPS studies published. Reversing direction of causality, an alternative interpretation of the data above is that for a given level of pain, patients with CRPS are more distressed than patients with low back pain because of the more negative implications of CRPS pain (e.g., it signals that CRPS is progressive and untreatable).

The data above suggesting that patients with CRPS are more distressed relative to comparable patients without CRPS are not definitive, and many factors such as sample selection criteria, demographic confounds, referral patterns to clinics, and specific psychometric measures used may have influenced the pattern of findings. In contrast to the studies discussed above, several others have failed to find evidence of elevated distress among patients with CRPS compared to patients with radiculopathy (Haddox, Abram, & Hopwood, 1988) and patients with headache and low back pain (DeGood, Cundiff, Adams, & Shutty, 1993). Other study findings are mixed, with Ciccone, Bandilla, and Wu (1997) noting that patients with CRPS reported more somatic symptoms of depression than patients with local neuropathy, but that patients with CRPS did not differ from patients with low back pain.

Research using structured diagnostic interview methodology appears to be consistent with the findings of Haddox and colleagues (1998) and DeGood and colleagues (1993). Monti, Herring, Schwartzman, and Marchese (1998) found no differences in incidence of Axis I disorders, noting that patients with CRPS and patients with disc-related radicular pain exhibited Axis I disorders (predominantly depression) at similar rates (24% vs. 20%, respectively).

The few studies using personality measures have failed to demonstrate personality characteristics that are consistently associated with CRPS (Nelson & Novy, 1996; Zucchini, Alberti, & Moretti, 1989). Nelson and Novy (1996) reported that patients with CRPS scored higher on scale 9 (Mania) of the Minnesota Multiphasic Personality Inventory (MMPI) than patients with myofascial pain; yet the patients with CRPS scored *lower* on scales 1 (Hypochondriasis), 2 (Depression), 3 (Hysteria), and 7 (Psychasthenia). In contrast, Zucchini and colleagues (1989) reported that patients with CRPS displayed more frequent elevations on scales 1–3 of the MMPI, compared to a group of patients without CRPS but with brachial plexus injury. Monti and colleagues (1998), using structured diagnostic interviews, found that the incidence of personality disorders was not significantly different between their sample of 25 patients with CRPS and 25 patients with disc-related radiculopathy. Interpretation of these latter data are complicated by the fact that an interview for personality disorders was only conducted if no Axis I disorder was identified.

In summary, the data do not support any unique personality pattern associated with CRPS compared to other types of pain. However, the existing literature suggests the possibility that patients with CRPS may be more distressed than comparable patients with non-CRPS pain. Emotional distress may also be more strongly related to pain intensity in CRPS than in non-CRPS conditions. Although there have been several studies supporting distress differences between patients with CRPS and patients with other pain, other studies fail to support such differences. Additional research is needed to clarify these issues, particularly studies using prospective designs. Given the present state of knowledge, it is likely to be most appropriate to employ an interactive, psychophysiological model when one is considering the role of psychological factors in onset and maintenance of CRPS.

Stress and emotional distress are associated with alterations in adrenergic activity (see, e.g., Abelson et al., 1991; Charney et al., 1990). For example, it is known that stress results in increased adrenergic responsiveness to excitatory stimulation in the locus coeruleus (Charney et al., 1990). Thus

chronic stress could result in systemic adrenergic overresponding to both intense pain and psychologically aversive stimuli. Consistent with this idea, work in our clinic indicated that among 16 patients with CRPS, levels of plasma epinephrine correlated positively and significantly with distress as reflected on the BDI, as well as with certain personality characteristics as reflected on scales 1 (Hypochondriasis), 3 (Hysteria), and 6 (Paranoia) of the MMPI (Bruehl, Harden, Kee, & Cole, 1998).

As described above, it is believed that sympathetic hypofunction following traumatic injury results in adrenergic receptor hypersensitivity in the affected extremity, producing supersensitivity to systemic catecholamines and thereby leading to a cool, bluish extremity. Adrenergic activity is also hypothesized as being involved in the development of pain-processing abnormalities in CRPS (Roberts, 1986). Therefore, systemic adrenergic overresponding resulting from stress could interact with sensitized adrenergic receptors in the affected extremity to produce some of the characteristic CRPS symptoms. Stress-induced adrenergic overresponding, by contributing to pain-processing abnormalities (e.g., allodynia) at the site of injury, could also help maintain the altered central processing in CRPS that appears to be induced by persistent nociceptive input (Gracely et al., 1992). In such a scenario, psychological stress or distress is neither necessary nor sufficient for development of CRPS, but can interact with the physiological changes resulting from traumatic injury to produce the syndrome (Bruehl & Carlson, 1992; Van Houdenhove et al., 1992). Altered adrenergic functioning associated with psychological factors is one element contributing to the vicious cycle described in Figure 28.1.

Whether or not psychological factors are involved in the etiology of CRPS, it is clear that once CRPS has developed, the presence of elevated stress or emotional distress would exacerbate symptoms through mechanisms such as those described above.

MEDICAL ASSESSMENT

Although a cursory reading of the literature might give the reader the impression that objective diagnostic tests are crucial to the assessment and diagnosis of CRPS, in fact the role of such tests is mainly adjunctive to support data obtained in the history and physical examination. Tests such as thermography (Bruehl, Lubenow, et al., 1996), triple-phase bone scintigraphy (Zyluk & Birkenfeld, 1999), and diagnostic sympathetic blocks (Verdugo

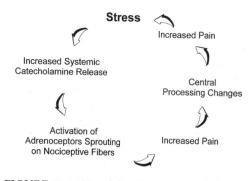

FIGURE 28.1. Hypothesized manner in which stress interacts with expression of CRPS.

& Ochoa, 1994) in theory may provide useful information about vasomotor function, trophic changes, and sympathetic mediation of pain, respectively. Several studies suggest the potential utility of thermography in CRPS (Bruehl, Lubenow, et al., 1996; Gulevich et al., 1997). However, conceptual and methodological problems frequently limit the interpretability of such tests (see, e.g., Baron, Levine, & Fields, 1999; Verdugo & Ochoa, 1994). In particular, the interpretability of diagnostic sympathetic blocks in clinical practice is complicated by a high rate of placebo responding. Verdugo and Ochoa (1994) reported in a controlled study that more patients with CRPS responded with decreased pain after placebo than with pharmacological sympathetic blockade. Even when methodological issues such as these are minimized, available diagnostic tests are not definitive because CRPS pathophysiology remains insufficiently clear to justify treating any test as a "gold standard" (Bruehl et al., 1999; Harden et al., 1999).

THE HISTORY AND PHYSICAL EXAMINATION

With the utility of diagnostic tests limited, a carefully conducted medical history and physical examination becomes crucial for effective diagnosis of CRPS. It is important for reasons of generalizability across clinical and research settings that the IASP criteria, rather than the numerous previous nonstandardized diagnostic schemes, be used for purposes of clinical diagnosis. Therefore, the ultimate purpose of the history and physical examination is to determine whether or not a patient meets the IASP diagnostic criteria for CRPS (Merskey & Bogduk, 1994). The IASP diagnostic criteria for CRPS are summarized in Table 28.1; areas to be

addressed in the history and physical examination are summarized in Table 28.3.

One issue often encountered by clinicians in attempting to make a criterion-based diagnosis of CRPS is the relative importance of self-reported symptoms obtained during the history versus objective signs observed during the physical examination. If interpreted literally, the IASP criteria for CRPS would allow diagnosis solely based upon patient self-reports of symptoms (e.g., "evidence at some time of [autonomic dysfunction]"). The possibility that patients may overreport symptoms must be considered in relying upon symptoms alone for making a diagnosis of CRPS (i.e., some patients may indicate that they experience every symptom that they are asked about during the history). Research to date, however, indicates that patient self-reports do appear to have diagnostic utility (Bruehl et al., 1999; Galer et al., 1998; Harden et al., 1999). Specifically, the relative frequencies of objective signs observed during the physical examination and the corresponding patient self-reported symptoms appear to be similar, although the corresponding symptoms are always reported by patients at a higher rate (Harden et al., 1999). This may reflect the phasic nature of the features of CRPS; color or temperature changes may be quite labile, and therefore a patient has greater opportunity to observe such changes than does a clinician in a brief examination. Although these data suggest that both the history and physical examination can be important parts of making a criterion-based CRPS diagnosis, the clinician should be cautious about diagnosing CRPS in the absence of *any* confirming objective signs (Bruehl et al., 1999; Galer et al., 1998; Harden et al., 1999).

Because the fourth diagnostic criterion for CRPS requires the exclusion of any other reasonable diagnostic explanation for the presenting signs and symptoms, it is critical that the diagnostic process begin with a careful general medical history and physical examination. The relevant "rule-outs" and conditions that can masquerade as CRPS include regional infections, poorly healing trauma, peripheral vascular disease, localized collagen vascular disease, and peripheral neuropathy. Another important rule out to consider is a central neuropathic process such as stroke, which very often presents with signs and symptoms consistent with CRPS, and is commonly called the *shoulder–hand syndrome*. Characteristic presentations of each of these processes are well known, and objective testing has been established that is definitive for mak-

TABLE 28.3. Summary of Medical Assessment in Patients with CRPS

I. A criterion-based diagnosis should be made according to current IASP criteria, using both objective signs *and* subjective symptoms.

II. Rule out all non-CRPS disorders that could account for the observed syndrome.

III. Identify initiating event (spontaneous onset is rare but possible).

IV. Assess signs and symptoms used in diagnosis; be cautious about leading questions.
   A. Pain reports must be in excess of known pathology in quality and/or quantity.
      1. "Burning" pain is common but *not* clearly pathognomonic for CRPS.
      2. Assess reports of excessive sensory sensitivity in affected region (e.g., in response to cold weather, touch of clothing).
      3. Test for allodynia: Pain in response to nonpainful stimuli (cool water bottle, light stroking).
      4. Test for hyperalgesia: Excessive pain in response to mildly painful stimulation (light pinprick).
   B. Assess for self-reports or objective signs of autonomic abnormalities (may be phasic, so not always observable in clinic).
      1. Vasomotor changes: Skin color (blue, red, mottled) or temperature (warmer or cooler) asymmetry or changes.
         a. Thermography may be used to support temperature assessment.
      2. Sudomotor changes: Sweating asymmetry or changes (increased or decreased).
         a. Use smooth-handled instrument or tissue to assess bilateral differences.
      3. Edema: Noticeable unilateral edema in the affected region.
         a. Can assess with tape measure or volumetry.

V. Assess other associated characteristics of CRPS that are not used in diagnosis but that may reflect severity of disuse or dysfunction.
   A. Trophic changes to hair (increased or decreased growth), nails (ridging, cracking), or skin tissue (thin or shiny appearance).
   B. Movement dysfunction: Decreased range of motion, weakness, clumsiness, or tremor.

VI. Assess for secondary myofascial pain syndrome.

Note. Pharmacological sympathetic blockade, thermography, triple-phase bone scintigraphy, and other objective tests are *not* definitive for diagnosis of CRPS.

ing the diagnosis in most of these non-CRPS syndromes. The description below focuses on the elements of the history and physical examination focused directly on CRPS.

The medical history in patients with CRPS should begin with an attempt to identify the initiating event. Although occasionally no antecedent trauma can be identified in patients with CRPS (fewer than 5% of cases in Harden et al., 1999), usually a history of local trauma can be elicited. The most common initiating traumas include fracture, surgery, or a crush injury. Less frequently, initiating events may include a history of some sort of trauma to the vascular system (e.g., a traumatic venipuncture); damage to muscles, ligaments, tendons, or nerves; or an immobilization resulting from casting. In an occasional patient, a history of central neurological damage can be elicited (i.e., spinal cord injury or brain lesion) that appears temporally related to onset of the CRPS symptoms.

The second criterion for CRPS diagnosis includes ongoing pain that is disproportionate to the inciting event, as well as presence of hyperalgesia and/or allodynia. Patients will often relate a history of "burning," "aching," or "stinging" types of pain. A "burning" quality in particular appears to be common in many types of neuropathic pain, being reported by more than two-thirds of patients with a variety of neuropathic pain conditions (Harden et al., 1999). Determination of whether a pain complaint is in excess of the extent of injury is necessarily confounded by the fact that pain complaints, as a form of pain behavior, are subject to modification by learning and reinforcement (e.g., so-called *secondary gain* factors; Fordyce et al., 1973). The clinician must use judgment in determining whether a patient's pain complaint is exaggerated due to financial or legal reinforcers, or rather reflects a legitimate complaint of severe pain in excess of the known trauma.

Patients' self-reports of hyperesthesia in their daily lives should be assessed, including pain in response to nonpainful stimuli (allodynia) and excessive pain experienced in response to mildly painful stimuli (hyperalgesia). For example, a patient may report that he or she always wears gloves when going outside, because air that is the slightest bit cool makes the affected hand hurt. Patients' reports of sensory abnormalities such as these during their daily lives may provide support for a CRPS diagnosis. However, the clinician should be aware that some patients are highly educated regarding the types of symptoms patients with CRPS *are supposed to report* (e.g., obtained through contact with support groups, attorneys, or other healthcare providers). For pain as well as the other characteristic symptoms of CRPS, therefore, supporting evidence should be sought in the physical examination.

Regarding the third criterion for diagnosing CRPS, the history should also assess patient reports of symptoms that are consistent with autonomic disturbance. Specifically, a patient may report vasomotor changes, reflected in a limb that will change temperature and color—often going through a phase in which the limb is hot and red, but more chronically presenting as cold and blue relative to the unaffected side (Harden, 1994). Patients may report parallel changes in sudomotor activity as well, with patients often giving a history of the limb beginning as being dry and later becoming very sweaty relative to the unaffected side. It is not unusual for patients to report that these symptoms of autonomic dysfunction are episodic.

Although trophic changes are now considered associated symptoms and not formally used in the IASP diagnostic system, patients may also report such changes, including increased or decreased hair growth, changes in their fingernails (such as ridging or cracking), and changes in the skin (such as a thin, shiny appearance). Patients may also relate a difficulty in movement, such as decreased range of motion or a feeling of stiffness in the affected joints. Other motor symptoms patients may report include weakness, stiffness, clumsiness, rigidity, or tremor. For some patients, these motor symptoms are just as distressing as the pain-related symptoms, since the motor problems may interfere more in ability to carry out important activities—particularly, for example, if the work of a patient with upper-extremity CRPS requires use of fine motor skills.

It is important to corroborate the patients' symptom reports during the physical examination to the greatest extent possible (Bruehl et al., 1999; Harden et al., 1999). For determining whether a patient meets the second criterion (abnormal pain sensation) for CRPS, a sensory examination is critically important, and either hyperesthesia or hypoesthesia needs to be recorded. Presence of hypoesthesia may be suggestive of sensory nerve impairment, possibly supporting a diagnosis of CRPS type II (causalgia). Tactile and temperature allodynia should be assessed in all patients. The examiner can assess tactile allodynia by using a finger to apply a light stroking motion to the patient's affected area. Temperature allodynia can be assessed easily by using warm and cool test tubes of water. In these tests, allodynia is present if the light stroking motion (tactile) or the moderately cool or warm test tubes (temperature) elicit a painful response. In addition to assessing allodynia, assessment of hyperalgesia is also impor-

tant for CRPS diagnosis, and this can be performed by conducting a light prick of the skin using a sterile pin. Although healthy individuals do not find this pinprick uncomfortable, a patient with hyperalgesia will display a notable pain response or report that the pain sensation lasts longer than the stimulus.

In order to determine whether a patient meets the third criterion for CRPS (evidence of autonomic dysfunction), another focus of the physical examination should be on assessing autonomic signs. To assess vasomotor function, the color and temperature of the affected limb should be compared to those of the same region on the asymptomatic side. The presentation in the affected limb can range from a red, inflamed-looking, dry extremity to a cold, blue, sweaty extremity. With regard to temperature, color, and sweating changes, bilateral asymmetry is consistent with CRPS. Temperature differences can be assessed grossly with the dorsum of the examiner's hand. With regard to color, the presence of significant, unequivocal changes in color (either reddish or bluish as described above) in the affected area compared to the unaffected side is consistent with CRPS. Alteration in sweating can be assessed by running a smooth-handled instrument over the skin and noting whether the instrument slides more easily on one side than the other, or by determining rate or degree of soaking of a facial tissue applied to the region.

The presence of edema can be assessed quantitatively either with a tape measure (comparing the circumference of the affected and unaffected side at various landmarks) or, preferably, via volumetry, in which the volume of water in a basin displaced by the affected versus the unaffected side is compared. Because a patient with temperature allodynia may be resistant to participating in this latter procedure, due to the likely temperature differential between the water and the patient's skin, water should be at or near body temperature.

Clinical experience indicates that the above-described "bedside" tests for CRPS are reasonable means to assess the presence of CRPS signs and make diagnoses in clinical practice. However, there are no data regarding the reliability of these bedside tests as carried out in a clinical setting. Although simple determination of the presence or absence of a CRPS characteristic (e.g., allodynia) is more likely to be reliable than are more elaborate determinations (Janig, 1991), the possibility of less than ideal reliability of these clinical assessment procedures does present one rationale for supplementary testing. Assessment via quantitative sensory testing, thermography, sympathetic skin response, and similar techniques can help provide quantitative support for the judgments made during the bedside assessment. (For a detailed description of quantitative sensory testing, see Dworkin, Nagasako, & Galer, Chapter 27, this volume.)

A number of signs commonly associated with CRPS in the past are no longer used in diagnosis; however, an assessment of these signs may provide valuable information on the severity of the condition. For example, it is recommended that an examination of the affected extremity be carried out to check for alterations in hair growth and changes in skin consistency relative to the unaffected side. Examination for changes such as brittle, cracked, or ridged nails on the affected side compared to the unaffected side is also recommended. Signs of movement disorder that appear to be associated with CRPS have often been neglected in assessment, although current research would indicate that it is a statistically prevalent problem (Galer et al., 1998; Harden et al., 1999). Therefore, it is recommended that motor abnormalities in bulk, tone, and power be elicited if possible, and that difficulties with range of motion, contractures, and any abnormal posturing be noted. Accurate formal assessment of strength and range of motion in patients with CRPS is often difficult due to extreme guarding and pain-limited testing; therefore, results of these assessments may often reflect more patient tolerance and fear than actual abilities. Galer and colleagues (1995) have reported observations that patients with CRPS may develop a unilateral motor neglect syndrome similar to that observed following stroke, and they suggest a test for signs of this syndrome. If identified, such a syndrome may provide one focus of treatment for physical and occupational therapy.

Frequently patients will develop myofascial pain syndrome of the musculature surrounding the joint supporting the affected limb, due to abnormal posturing and bracing. Signs and symptoms of this syndrome include deep, "achy" pain in a regional location that is often associated with muscle spasm and detectable trigger points in taut bands of muscle. Procedures for identifying muscular trigger points are described in detail elsewhere (Travell & Simons, 1983; see also Gerwin, Chapter 26, this volume). Postural abnormalities can be due to myofascial pain syndrome as well as CRPS. It is critically important to identify and aggressively treat myofascial pain along with CRPS in order to achieve optimal treatment outcomes.

PSYCHOSOCIAL ASSESSMENT

Given the medical complexity of CRPS and the role that psychological factors may play in exacerbating or maintaining the condition, close integration of the medical and psychological assessment is recommended. Such an approach should increase the likelihood of positive treatment outcomes. A critical component of a thorough psychosocial assessment of patients with CRPS is a careful clinical interview. Use of standardized questionnaires to supplement the clinical interview is recommended, particularly for purposes of providing objective feedback to patients, assisting in treatment planning, and tracking clinical outcomes. Because most psychometric instruments commonly used in the population with chronic pain are reviewed and critiqued in detail elsewhere in this volume, this section provides only brief summaries of instruments likely to be most useful in the assessment of patients with CRPS. The section focuses primarily on the psychological issues that are particularly important to assess in the clinical interview of a patient with CRPS (summarized in Table 28.4).

As in assessment of all patients with chronic pain, the presence of comorbid psychiatric disorders, such as depression or generalized anxiety, should be assessed (see Sullivan, Chapter 15). Given the catecholaminergic correlates of such disorders (Charney et al., 1990), their identification provides an important treatment target that may reduce symptom severity. Mood disorders are likely to be at least as common in patients with CRPS as they are in patients with other pain conditions. Estimates suggest a prevalence of clinical depression in patients with chronic pain of at least 25%–30% (Atkinson, Slater, Patterson, Grant, & Garfin, 1991; Katon, Egan, & Miller, 1985), whereas the prevalence of anxiety disorders, such as panic disorder, in this population is at least 10% (Atkinson et al., 1991; Katon et al., 1985). These data are consistent with the only study of psychiatric comorbidity in patients with CRPS, which reported a prevalence of 24% for Axis I disorders in these patients (Monti et al., 1998).

Although questionnaires should not be used in place of a clinical interview for diagnosing these disorders, the BDI (Beck, Ward, Mendelson, Mock, & Erbaugh, 1961) and the Center for Epidemiological Studies–Depression scale (Radloff, 1977) have proven useful in medical populations for assessing depressive symptoms. Similarly, the State–Trait Anxiety Inventory (STAI; Spielberger,

TABLE 28.4. Summary of Psychological Assessment Issues in Patients with CRPS

I. Assess for specific, comorbid psychiatric disorders that may affect treatment.
   A. Depression, panic disorder, generalized anxiety disorder, and PTSD are most common.
   B. These disorders are likely to occur at least as frequently in CRPS as in other pain conditions.
II. Assess for psychological factors that may contribute to CRPS symptoms.
   A. General emotional arousal (depression, anxiety, fear, anger).
   B. Life stressors (major life events and daily hassles).
III. Assess pain.
   A. Examine persistence, intensity, and temporal pattern of pain.
   B. Assess for allodynia (temperature, touch) and its severity.
   C. Assess fear of pain.
IV. Assess degree of pain avoidance and allodynia avoidance behaviors and their functional impact.
   A. Severe guarding, bracing, disuse.
   B. Agoraphobia.
   C. Level of perceived disability and impairment in daily activities.
V. Assess social environment.
   A. Adequacy of social support.
   B. Significant others' responses to pain behaviors.
      1. Solicitous responses may reinforce disuse.
      2. Hostile responses may add to patient's distress and increase pain.
VI. Assess treatment-relevant cognitions.
   A. Beliefs regarding CRPS.
      1. Common misconceptions: It is untreatable, inherently progressive, and will spread throughout the body (i.e., catastrophic cognitions).
   B. Beliefs regarding meaning of the pain.
      1. Common misconceptions: Pain signals damage; "if it hurts, don't do it."
   C. Beliefs regarding how treatment should progress.
      1. Common misconceptions: Sympathetic blocks are curative; treatments that exacerbate pain temporarily cannot be valuable.
   D. Embarrassment about having CRPS.
      1. Belief that others assume it is psychogenic pain.
VII. Assess health behaviors; use of caffeine and tobacco may exacerbate CRPS symptoms.

Gorsuch, & Lushene, 1970) has proven useful as a measure of generalized anxiety symptoms.

Instruments less commonly used in the population with pain are available to assess symptoms of other anxiety disorders, such as posttraumatic stress disorder (PTSD; see, e.g., Keane, Caddell, & Taylor, 1988). Except in research settings, however, PTSD and panic disorder may best be assessed by using specific prompts in the clinical interview; patients may be reluctant to admit panic attacks or posttraumatic stress symptoms because they fear they may be "crazy," given the somewhat unusual symptoms of these disorders and the unusual presentation of CRPS. Anxiety disorders such as panic disorder should be assessed in all patients with CRPS, since such disorders can be associated with substantially increased severity of CRPS pain through catecholaminergic mechanisms. In the case of panic disorder, increased pain itself can serve as the focus for increased catastrophic cognitions, which may then provoke panic attacks. For similar reasons, because of the hyperarousal generally associated with PTSD, symptoms of this disorder should be assessed routinely in all posttraumatic cases of CRPS; it is not uncommon, given the traumatic nature of many CRPS-related injuries.

In addition to assessing the presence of specific psychiatric disorders, it is particularly important to assess the frequency and intensity of any form of emotional arousal, whether it is depression, anxiety, fear, or anger, given the potentially exacerbating role of such emotions in CRPS pain intensity (Bruehl, Husfeldt, et al., 1996). Although good measures for depression and anxiety with normative data in medical and pain populations are available (e.g., the BDI and STAI), questionnaires to assess other aspects of mood have not been normed in these populations. In addition to the specific emotions noted above, it is also important to consider the affective component of patients' pain—the degree of patient suffering—in addition to the sensory intensity of the pain. Some patients may report extremely elevated affective pain intensity, thus indicating a high level of pain-related suffering, which may occur even in the presence of relatively low levels of sensory pain intensity. The sensory and affective components of pain can be assessed easily with the short form of the McGill Pain Questionnaire (Melzack, 1987; see Melzack & Katz, Chapter 3).

As with patients' emotional state, a thorough assessment of ongoing life stress should be conducted. This assessment should include both major stressors and "daily hassles," since both of these forms of stress independently affect functioning (Rowlinson & Felner, 1988). Given the catecholaminergic effects of stress (Charney et al., 1990), each of these sources of stress becomes a potential target of psychological treatment that, if better controlled, may reduce the severity of the CRPS pain. As noted above, because it is possible that stressors could play an etiological role in development of CRPS, it may be important to assess stressors occurring at the time of onset of the condition. This assessment should be conducted carefully, since some patients may misinterpret it as questioning the validity of their physical symptoms. A reasonable way to frame this issue to a patient may be as an attempt to identify the degree to which psychophysiological factors, which can be presented to the patient as stress-related adrenergic activity, may have contributed to onset of the condition after the patient's injury. Although causation should not be inferred, identification of major stressors that appear strongly related to onset of the condition may identify additional issues to be addressed in treatment.

Type and quality of pain should also be assessed. Although descriptions of the pain and observed pain behavior can clearly be influenced by operant factors such as litigation (Dush, Simons, Platt, Nation, & Ayres, 1994; Solomon & Tunks, 1991), it is important to remember that even in legitimate cases of CRPS, the pain behavior may appear somewhat exaggerated. Reasons for this apparent exaggeration are described below.

Although the presence of allodynia is likely to be assessed in the medical evaluation, an assessment of the presence and type of allodynia during the psychosocial assessment is also important, with a focus on its functional effects. Allodynia can occur in response to stimuli such as touch and temperature, which can occur independently. Patients with cold allodynia may avoid leaving the house during certain types of weather conditions, or may constantly wear winter clothing on the affected body part to ensure that it does not become cool. Patients with tactile allodynia report that even the touch of clothing is painful. This has led to extreme pain behaviors in some patients, such as the person who insisted on wearing short pants in the middle of the Chicago winter because the touch of clothing on his lower extremities was too painful. Clearly, such extreme pain behaviors are likely to interfere with functioning in a variety of ways. Tactile allodynia can also result in what appears to be a form of agoraphobia, although in this case the patient avoids crowded places due to fears that others may "bump into" the affected extremity and cause a severe increase in pain. Movement avoidance due to fear of pain is likely to develop not only in response to allodynia-related exacerbations of pain, but also in response to the underlying persistent CRPS pain and the hyperalgesia. The effects of chronic avoidance of movement and avoidance of public places can contribute to depression by reducing sources of positive reinforcement available to the patient and interfering with most meaningful activities. Therefore, specific details regarding the daily activities the patient does and does not perform, and whether the patient attributes areas of inactivity to pain avoidance, should be obtained to facilitate treatment planning.

Standardized assessment of the functioning of patients with CRPS may be useful for helping "objectify" a patient's deconditioning or disuse compared to other patients, as well as for tracking treatment progress for patients. The Pain Disability Index (Tait, Pollard, Margolis, Duckro, & Krause, 1987) is a simple measure of perceived disability in seven key areas of functioning. Another useful instrument is the West Haven–Yale Multidimensional Pain Inventory (WHYMPI; Kerns, Turk, & Rudy, 1985). Among the WHYMPI subscales, activity levels in several areas and general activity level are assessed. Use of patient scores in reference to normative data provided by the WHYMPI scoring program (Rudy, 1989) can be useful for identifying those patients with extreme inactivity problems. The WHYMPI scoring program, by classifying patients into the empirically derived categories of Adaptive Copers, Dysfunctional, and Interpersonally Distressed, can also be useful for more general assessment of overall patient adaptation to the pain condition (Rudy, 1989; see also Jacob & Kerns, Chapter 19, and Turk & Okifuji, Chapter 21).

Often accompanying the functional disability in CRPS, the intense fear of pain that may result from CRPS may be particularly important to address in treatment. A vicious cycle is frequently observed in which anxiety regarding pain, through its effects on catecholamines, exacerbates the pain intensity, thereby reinforcing patients' beliefs and anxiety that any use of the affected extremity is detrimental to their well-being. This learned vicious cycle of activity avoidance can be difficult for patients to escape. Over 60% of patients with CRPS report limitations in activities of daily living, with pain reported to be the primary contributor to diminished functioning in these patients (Geertzen et al., 1998). Given the importance of remobilization, desensitization, and normalized use of the affected limb (Carlson & Watson, 1988; Stanton-Hicks et al., 1998), this vicious cycle resulting from fear of pain can be a significant barrier to effective treatment of CRPS. In some patients this fear of pain and movement may reach the level of a true phobia, and in some cases it can result in a generally elevated somatic focus. Although some clinicians may assume that this somatic focus is the *cause of* a patient's intense pain, it is equally likely that this somatic focus is the *result* of CRPS pain.

Although formal psychometric assessment of the fear-of-pain construct has not been common in the past, the Pain Anxiety Symptoms Scale (PASS; McCracken, Zayfert, & Gross, 1992) may prove useful, particularly with patients who have CRPS. This scale provides normative data on patients with chronic pain for several important areas of pain-related anxiety, including fearful appraisal, avoidant responses, physiological anxiety, and cognitive anxiety (McCracken et al., 1992). The importance of addressing fear of pain and movement in patients with CRPS to achieve treatment success suggests that use of an instrument such as the PASS may be helpful for treatment planning.

In light of the frequency of learned disuse and intense somatic focus in CRPS, observation of pain behaviors during the clinical evaluation is an important part of judging the degree of pain/activity avoidance the patient is experiencing (see Keefe, Williams, & Smith, Chapter 10). For example, if the right upper extremity is affected, does the patient shake the examiner's hand upon greeting him or her? Does the patient use the dominant hand, if it is the one affected, to complete questionnaires? Does the patient hold the affected upper extremity as if in a sling? Does the affected extremity move normally when the patient is walking? Are any other behavioral anomalies noted (such as the short pants worn in winter by the patient noted above)? Some patients exhibit such severe disuse of the affected extremity that some researchers have hypothesized that a unilateral neglect (comparable to that observed following stroke) may develop in some cases of CRPS (Galer et al., 1995).

The problem of learned disuse may be exacerbated further by well-intentioned solicitous responses from family members (Lousberg, Schmidt, & Groenman, 1992). Given the severity of pain complaints and pain behaviors in patients with CRPS, it is not surprising that family members and friends often take over the household and other daily responsibilities of these patients. Although CRPS is no different from any other pain condition in this respect, the disuse that is reinforced by significant others is typically the primary focus of treatment in CRPS. As noted above, disuse may be an important pathophysiological mechanism in development and maintenance of CRPS. Disrupting the environmental reinforcers that may help maintain CRPS-related disuse is a crucial component in the ultimate success of efforts to get a patient to remobilize and desensitize the affected extremity. For this reason, it is particularly important during the clinical interview to include fam-

ily members, and to assess the responses of family members to the patient's pain behaviors. Quantitative assessment of a patient's perceptions of responses of significant others to pain behavior is provided as part of the WHYMPI (Kerns et al., 1985), thus permitting comparison of individual patients' results to normative data.

Other important areas to assess are the patients' beliefs regarding CRPS, the meaning of the pain, and about treatment. The first of these areas may be particularly important, since the anxiety resulting from strongly held negative beliefs is likely to exacerbate pain. Specific beliefs to assess include those regarding what causes the condition (many patients have been told that it is psychogenic); what the pain signifies (e.g., doing more damage); and what the prognosis is; particularly regarding whether it is invariably progressive, incurable, and likely to spread to the unaffected side. Beliefs regarding the meaning of the pain may interfere substantially with treatment. Patients who strongly believe that "if it hurts, don't use it," are unlikely to respond well to treatments intended to remobilize and desensitize the affected limb, and are highly susceptible to deconditioning problems. A similar problematic belief is a strong patient focus on passive treatments, as opposed to active treatments. The best example of this is when patients develop a belief (often unintentionally fostered by those performing passive, palliative treatment modalities such as sympathetic blocks) that passive treatment alone will be sufficient to manage or overcome CRPS—or, more problematically, a belief that experiencing any increased pain during treatment is unacceptable.

Although many physicians who perform passive treatment modalities (e.g., blocks) understand the importance of the active component of treatment (e.g., physical and occupational therapy), patients may selectively attend to a physician's desire to palliate pain, and mistake this for the unrealistic goal of "curing" the pain. The patient's beliefs about how treatment should progress can be strongly shaped by the physician's treatment philosophy. Patients with CRPS who are actively engaged in block-focused treatments therefore may tend to react negatively to suggestions of a more rehabilitation-focused treatment as an alternative.

One source of erroneous or exaggerated beliefs among patients with CRPS is the Internet. Some physicians who treat CRPS have posted Web sites containing negative information regarding CRPS that is not backed up by the research literature or clinical experience. For example, one physician-run Web site implies that without immediate treatment (presumably at the physician's office), CRPS is invariably progressive and likely to spread throughout the body if not stopped. The advertising goal for such claims may be obvious to some, but to many fearful patients without adequate sources of accurate information to counteract these claims, such misinformation can intensify fear (and ultimately pain intensity) regarding the disorder. Similar problems with only partially accurate or completely inaccurate information is often found on patient-run support group Web sites, newsgroups, and chat rooms as well.

One area often neglected in assessment of patients with pain that is relevant to CRPS is the degree of patient embarrassment about the condition. Patients may have been led by their clinicians or insurance companies to believe that their CRPS is a psychogenic problem, and they may be very embarrassed in situations requiring that they explain their condition to others. Since allodynia can result in extreme pain behavior but is otherwise invisible, such behavior may look "crazy" to others, and may be difficult for patients to explain to individuals without a medical background. Given that the other symptoms of CRPS (such as color changes or sweating changes) may be phasic rather than tonic, patients with CRPS may at times appear to have no objective evidence of the disorder other than the pain behavior.

Assessment of health behaviors should not be neglected as part of a comprehensive assessment of CRPS. In particular, smoking and caffeine may be relevant to CRPS. One study based on a case series, as well as theoretical reasons, suggests that smoking may serve as one factor contributing to exacerbated CRPS symptoms through its adrenergic effects (An, Hawthorne, & Jackson, 1988). Patients with CRPS were found to smoke at a rate (68%) significantly higher than a comparable group of medical control patients without pain (An et al., 1988). Although there are no published data regarding the effects of caffeine in CRPS, it may also be a factor contributing to severity of CRPS symptoms in some patients, given its stimulant effects. Identification of heavy use of either of these substances could serve as a target for behavioral intervention to address the severity of CRPS symptoms.

PERSONALITY ASSESSMENT

Measures of personality, particularly the MMPI, have often been used for assessment in the popu-

lation with chronic pain as a whole (see Bradley & McKendree-Smith, Chapter 16). As noted earlier, the available studies do not suggest that patients with CRPS display a unique personality pattern (Nelson & Novy, 1998; Zucchini et al., 1989). Therefore, it is likely that the MMPI—the most common personality measure used in the population with non-CRPS pain—would be of similar utility in the population with CRPS. The research literature, however, indicates that elevations on the "neurotic triad" (MMPI scales 1–3) are quite frequent in any population with pain (Bradley & Van der Heide, 1984), and hence the differential utility of the MMPI may be questionable in many cases. Furthermore, studies have been mixed regarding the predictive utility of the MMPI regarding outcomes, particularly with invasive treatments (Uomoto, Turner, & Herron, 1988). Overall, the cost of routine use of the MMPI is relatively high in terms of patient time and resistance to testing, given the length of the test (567 items); there thus appears to be little justification for using this instrument on a routine basis. It may, however, prove useful in limited patient situations when specific referral questions are being considered (e.g., does a patient have a psychotic disorder?).

The utility of assessment of specific personality characteristics with more focused instruments is unclear. For example, hostility has been shown to be associated reliably with signs of adrenergic hyperreactivity (Contrada & Krantz, 1988). Given this physiological correlate of hostility, this personality characteristic may be relevant to assess, in view of the theoretical impact of local adrenergic receptor supersensitivity on CRPS symptoms (Kurvers et al., 1998). There have been no published reports of research using measures such as the Cook Medley Hostility Scale in patients with pain, or, more specifically, in patients with CRPS.

BIOFEEDBACK ASSESSMENT

Since the typical biofeedback thermode assesses only a limited body area, thermal biofeedback equipment is unlikely to be particularly valuable in assessing patients with CRPS, although it may be useful in treatment of these patients. However, electromyogram (EMG) biofeedback equipment may be useful in the complete assessment of patients with CRPS. Specifically, for upper-extremity CRPS, surface EMG assessment of the proximal extremity and the shoulder/neck area may be useful for identifying patterns of guarding and bracing. Similar assessment in the proximal lower extremity and low back in cases of lower-extremity CRPS may also be useful. If elevated muscular tension is identified in the areas in which patients complain of "spreading" CRPS, the objective feedback provided by surface EMG equipment can be invaluable in helping patients understand the concept of myofascial pain secondary to chronic guarding-related muscular tension as an alternative to "spreading" of the underlying CRPS. Such use of biofeedback equipment can help the clinician begin to address a patient's preconceived beliefs. EMG assessment then can be used in efforts to reframe the patient's problem in a way that is more treatable (see Flor, Chapter 5).

CONCLUSIONS

The development in 1994 of internationally agreed-upon diagnostic criteria for CRPS has improved the clinical recognition of the disorder, although the current diagnostic criteria may lead to overdiagnosis. The four key components of CRPS appear to be pain-processing abnormalities, vasomotor dysfunction, sudomotor dysfunction and edema, and motor and trophic changes. Because knowledge of the pathophysiology of CRPS is not entirely complete, there are no definitive diagnostic tests for the syndrome. Conducting a thorough history and physical examination to assess each of the four key components is necessary for proper diagnosis. A role for psychological factors in the etiology of CRPS has been proposed, although there are no adequate prospective studies to support this hypothesis. There is mixed evidence for these patients' being unique with regard to their levels of distress compared to patients with other types of chronic pain. It appears that psychological factors such as life stress and emotional distress do, at the very least, contribute to CRPS symptom severity, most likely through their effects on catecholamines. Psychosocial assessment should be integrated closely with the medical assessment of patients with CRPS. Given the likely importance of pain-related disuse of the affected extremity in development of the condition, psychosocial assessment should be particularly careful in assessing the cognitive and behavioral components of activity avoidance, particularly beliefs about CRPS and its treatment.

REFERENCES

Abelson, J. L., Glitz, D., Cameron, O. G., Lee, M. A., Bronzo, M., & Curtis, G. C. (1991). Blunted growth hormone responses to clonidine in patients with generalized anxiety disorder. *Archives of General Psychiatry, 48*, 157–162.

An, H. S., Hawthorne, K. B., & Jackson, W. T. (1988). Reflex sympathetic dystrophy and cigarette smoking. *Journal of Hand Surgery, 13*, 458–460.

Arnold, J. M. O., Teasell, R. W., MacLeod, A. P., Brown, J. E., & Carruthers, S. G. (1993). Increased venous alpha-adrenoceptor responsiveness in patients with reflex sympathetic dystrophy. *Annals of Internal Medicine, 118*, 619–621.

Atkinson J. H., Slater, M. A., Patterson, T. L., Grant, I., & Garfin, S. R. (1991). Prevalence, onset, and risk of psychiatric disorders in men with chronic low back pain: A controlled study. *Pain, 45*, 111–121.

Baron, R., Levine, J. D., & Fields, H. L. (1999). Causalgia and reflex sympathetic dystrophy: Does the sympathetic nervous system contribute to generation of pain? *Muscle and Nerve, 22*, 678–695.

Baron, R., & Maier, C. (1996). Reflex sympathetic dystrophy: Skin blood flow, sympathetic vasoconstrictor reflexes, and pain before and after surgical sympathectomy. *Pain, 67*, 317–326.

Beck, A. T., Ward, C. H., Mendelson, M., Mock, J. E., & Erbaugh, J. K. (1961). An inventory for measuring depression. *Archives of General Psychiatry, 4*, 561–571.

Birklein, F., Riedl, B., Claus, D., & Neudorfer, B. (1998). Pattern of autonomic dysfunction in time course of complex regional pain syndrome. *Clinical Autonomic Research, 8*, 79–85.

Bradley, L. A., & Van der Heide, L. H.. (1984). Pain-related correlates of MMPI profile subgroups among back pain patients. *Health Psychology, 3*, 157–174.

Bruehl, S., & Carlson, C. R. (1992). Predisposing psychological factors in the development of reflex sympathetic dystrophy: A review of the empirical evidence. *Clinical Journal of Pain, 8*, 287–299.

Bruehl, S., Harden, R. N., & Cole, P. (2000) *Complex regional pain syndrome: Psychological differences relative to non-CRPS pain patients.* Unpublished manuscript.

Bruehl, S., Harden, R. N., Galer, B. S., Saltz, S., Bertram, M., Backonja, M., Gayles, R., Rudin, N., Bughra, M., & Stanton-Hicks, M. (1999). External validation of IASP diagnostic criteria for complex regional pain syndrome and proposed research diagnostic criteria. *Pain, 81*, 147–154.

Bruehl, S., Harden, R. N., Kee, W., & Cole, P. (1998, October). *Relationship between plasma catecholamines and psychological functioning in patients with complex regional pain syndrome.* Paper presented at the 17th Annual Meeting of the American Pain Society, San Diego, CA.

Bruehl, S., Husfeldt, B., Lubenow, T., Nath, H., & Ivankovich, A. D. (1996). Psychological differences between reflex sympathetic dystrophy and non-RSD chronic pain patients. *Pain, 67*, 107–114.

Bruehl, S., Lubenow, T., Nath, H., & Ivankovich, O. (1996). Validation of thermography in the diagnosis of reflex sympathetic dystrophy. *Clinical Journal of Pain, 12*, 316–325.

Carlson, L. K., & Watson, H. K. (1988). Treatment of reflex sympathetic dystrophy using the stress-loading program. *Journal of Hand Therapy*, 149-153.

Charney, D. S., Woods, S. W., Nagy, L. M., Southwick, S.M., Krystal, J. H., & Heninger, G. R. (1990). Noradrenergic function in panic disorder. *Journal of Clinical Psychiatry*, 51(Suppl. A), 5-10.

Ciccone, D. S., Bandilla, E. B., & Wu, W. (1997). Psychological dysfunction in patients with reflex sympathetic dystrophy. *Pain*, 71, 323-333.

Contrada, R. J., & Krantz, D. S. (1988). Stress, reactivity, and type A behavior: Current status and future directions. *Annals of Behavioral Medicine*, 10, 64-70.

DeGood, D. E., Cundiff, G. W., Adams, L. E., & Shutty, M. S. (1993). A psychosocial and behavioral comparison of reflex sympathetic dystrophy, low back pain, and headache patients. *Pain*, 54, 317-322.

Drummond, P. D., Finch, P. M., & Smythe, G. A. (1991). Reflex sympathetic dystrophy: The significance of differing plasma catecholamine concentrations in affected and unaffected limbs. *Brain*, 114, 2025-2036.

Dush, D. M., Simons, L. E., Platt, M., Nation, P. C., & Ayres, S. Y. (1994). Psychological profiles distinguishing litigating and nonlitigating pain patients: Subtle, and not so subtle. *Journal of Personality Assessment*, 62, 299-313.

Egle, U. T., & Hoffmann, S. O. (1990). Psychosomatische zusammenhange bei sympathischer reflexdystrophie (Morbus Sudeck). *Psychotherapie, Psychosomatik, Medizinische Psychologie*, 40, 123-135.

Fordyce, W. E., Fowler, R. S., Lehmann, J. F., DeLateur, B. J., Sand, P. L., & Trieschmann, R. B. (1973). Operant conditioning in the treatment of chronic pain. *Archives of Physical Medicine and Rehabilitation*, 54, 399-408.

Galer, B., Bruehl, S., & Harden, R. N. (1998). IASP diagnostic criteria for complex regional pain syndrome (CRPS): A preliminary empirical validation study. *Clinical Journal of Pain*, 14, 48-54.

Galer, B. S., Butler, S., & Jensen, M. P. (1995). Case report and hypothesis: A neglect-like syndrome may be responsible for the motor disturbance in reflex sympathetic dystrophy (complex regional pain syndrome-1). *Journal of Pain and Symptom Management*, 10, 385-391.

Geertzen, J. H. B., de Bruijn, H., de Bruijn-Kofman, A. T., & Arendzen, J. H. (1994). Reflex sympathetic dystrophy: Early treatment and psychological aspects. *Archives of Physical Medicine and Rehabilitation*, 75, 442-446.

Geertzen, J. H. B., Dijkstra, P. U., van Sonderen, E. L. P., Groothoff, J. W., ten Duis, H. J., & Eisma, W. H. (1998). Relationship between impairments, disability, and handicap in reflex sympathetic dystrophy patients: A long-term follow-up study. *Clinical Rehabilitation*, 12, 402-412.

Gibbons, J. J., & Wilson, P. R. (1992). RSD score: Criteria for the diagnosis of reflex sympathetic dystrophy and causalgia. *Clinical Journal of Pain*, 8, 260-263.

Gracely, R. H., Lynch, S. A., & Bennett, G. J. (1992). Painful neuropathy: Altered central processing maintained dynamically by peripheral input. *Pain*, 51, 175-194.

Gulevich, S. J., Conwell, T. D., Lane, J., Lockwood, B., Schwettmann, R. S., Rosenberg, N., & Goldman, L. B. (1997). Stress infrared teletherthermography is useful in the diagnosis of complex regional pain syndrome, type I (formerly reflex sympathetic dystrophy). *Clinical Journal of Pain*, 13, 50-59.

Haddox, J. D., Abram, S. E., & Hopwood, M. H. (1988). Comparison of psychometric data in RSD and radiculopathy. *Regional Anesthesia*, 13, 27.

Harden, R. N. (1994). Reflex sympathetic dystrophy and other sympathetically-maintained pains. In J. M. Conry & B. H. Horman (Eds.), *Anesthesia for orthopedic surgery* (pp. 367-372). New York: Raven Press.

Harden, R. N., Bruehl, S., Galer, B. S., Saltz, S., Bertram, M., Backonja, M., Gayles, R., Rudin, N., Bughra, M., & Stanton-Hicks, M. (1999). Complex regional pain syndrome: Are the IASP diagnostic criteria valid and sufficiently comprehensive? *Pain*, 83, 211-219.

Harden, R. N., Duc, T. A., Williams, T. R., Coley, D., Cate, J. C., & Gracely, R. H. (1994). Norepinephrine and epinephrine levels in affected versus unaffected limbs in sympathetically maintained pain. *Clinical Journal of Pain*, 10, 324-330.

Hardy, M. A., & Merritt, W. H. (1988, July-September). Psychological evaluation and pain assessment in patients with reflex sympathetic dystrophy. *Journal of Hand Therapy*, 155-164.

Janig, W. (1991). Experimental approaches to reflex sympathetic dystrophy and related syndromes. *Pain*, 46, 241-245.

Katon, W., Egan, K., & Miller, D. (1985). Chronic pain: Lifetime psychiatric diagnoses and family history. *American Journal of Psychiatry*, 142, 1156-1160.

Keane, T. M., Caddell, J. M., & Taylor, K. L. (1988). Mississippi Scale for Combat-Related Posttraumatic Stress Disorder: Three studies in reliability and validity. *Journal of Consulting and Clinical Psychology*, 56, 85-90.

Kerns, R. D., Turk, D. C., & Rudy, T. E. (1985). The West Haven-Yale Multidimensional Pain Inventory (WHYMPI). *Pain*, 23, 345-356.

Kozin, F., Ryan, L. M., Carerra, G. F., Soin, J. S., & Wortmann, R. L. (1981). The reflex sympathetic dystrophy syndrome: III. Scintigraphic studies, further evidence for the therapeutic efficacy of systemic corticosteroids, and proposed diagnostic criteria. *American Journal of Medicine*, 70, 23-30.

Kurvers, H. A. J. M., Daemen, M., Slaaf, D., Stassen, F., Van den Wildenberg, F., Kitslaar, P., & de Mey, J. (1998). Partial peripheral neuropathy and denervation induced adrenoceptor supersensitivity. *Acta Orthopaedica Belgica*, 64, 64-70.

Kurvers, H. A. J. M., Hofstra, L., Jacobs, M. J. H. M., Daemen, M. A. R. C., Van den Wildenberg, F. A. J. M., Kitslaar, P. J. E. H. M., Slaaf, D. W., & Reneman, R. S. (1996). Reflex sympathetic dystrophy: Does sympathetic dysfunction originate from peripheral neuropathy? *Surgery*, 119, 288-296.

Kurvers, H. A. J. M., Jacobs, M. J. H. M., Beuk, R. J., Van den Wildenberg, F. A. J. M., Kitslaar, P. J. E. H. M., Slaaf, D. W., & Reneman, R. S. (1995). Reflex sympathetic dystrophy: Evolution of microcirculatory disturbances in time. *Pain*, 60, 333-340.

Leino, P., & Magni, G. (1993). Depressive and distress symptoms as predictors of low back pain, neck-shoulder pain, and other musculoskeletal morbidity: A 10 year follow-up of metal industry employees. *Pain*, 53, 89-94.

Lousberg, R., Schmidt, A. J. M., & Groenman, N. H. (1992). The relationship between spouse solicitousness and pain behavior: Searching for more experimental evidence. *Pain*, *51*, 75–79.

Lynch, M. (1992). Psychological aspects of reflex sympathetic dystrophy: A review of the adult and paediatric literature. *Pain*, *49*, 337–347.

McCracken, L. M., Zayfert, C., & Gross, R. T. (1992). The Pain Anxiety Symptoms Scale: Development and validation of a scale to measure fear of pain. *Pain*, *50*, 67–73.

Melzack, R. (1987). The short form of the McGill Pain Questionnaire. *Pain*, *30*, 191–197.

Melzack, R., & Wall, P. D. (1965). Pain mechanisms: A new theory. *Science*, *150*, 971–979.

Merskey, H., & Bogduk, N. (Eds.). (1994). *Classification of chronic pain: Descriptions of chronic pain syndromes and definitions of pain terms* (2nd ed.) Seattle, WA: International Association for the Study of Pain Press.

Mitchell, S. W., Morehouse, G. R., & Keen, W. W. (1864). *Gunshot wounds and other injuries of the nerves*. New York: Lippincott.

Monti, D. A., Herring, C. L., Schwartzman, R. J., & Marchese, M. (1998). Personality assessment of patients with complex regional pain syndrome type I. *Clinical Journal of Pain*, *14*, 295–302.

Moriwaki, K., Yuge, O., Tanaka, H., Sasaki, H., Izumi, H., & Kaneko, K. (1997). Neuropathic pain and prolonged regional inflammation as two distinct symptomatological components in complex regional pain syndrome with patchy osteoporosis: A pilot study. *Pain*, *72*, 277–282.

Nelson, D. V., & Novy, D. M. (1996). Psychological characteristics of reflex sympathetic dystrophy versus myofascial pain syndromes. *Regional Anesthesia*, *21*, 202–208.

Ochoa, J. L., & Verdugo, R. J. (1995). Reflex sympathetic dystrophy: A common clinical avenue for somatoform expression. *Neurologic Clinics*, *13*, 351–363.

Price, D. D., Bennett, G. J., & Rafii, A. (1989). Psychophysical observations on patients with neuropathic pain relieved by sympathetic block. *Pain*, *36*, 273–288.

Radloff, L. (1977). The CES-D scale: A self-report depression scale for research in the general population. *Applied Psychological Measurement*, *1*, 385–401.

Rashiq, S., & Galer, B. S. (1999). Proximal myofascial dysfunction in complex regional pain syndrome: A retrospective prevalence study. *Clinical Journal of Pain*, *15*, 151–153.

Roberts, W. J. (1986). A hypothesis on the physiological basis for causalgia and related pains. *Pain*, *24*, 297–311.

Rowlinson, R. T., & Felner, R. D. (1988). Major life events, hassles, and adaptation in adolescence: Confounding in the conceptualization and measurement of life stress and adjustment revisited. *Journal of Personality and Social Psychology*, *55*, 432–444.

Rudy, T. E. (1989). *Multiaxial assessment of pain: Multidimensional Pain Inventory computer program user's manual, Version 2.1*. Pittsburgh, PA: University of Pittsburgh.

Sato, J., & Perl, E. R. (1991). Adrenergic excitation of cutaneous pain receptors induced by peripheral nerve injury. *Science*, *251*, 1608–1610.

Schwartzman, R. J., & Kerrigan, J. (1990). The movement disorder of reflex sympathetic dystrophy. *Neurology*, *40*, 57–61.

Solomon, P., & Tunks, E. (1991). The role of litigation in predicting disability outcomes in chronic pain patients. *Clinical Journal of Pain*, *7*, 300–304.

Spielberger, C. D., Gorsuch, R. L., & Lushene, R. E. (1970). *Manual for the State–Trait Anxiety Inventory*. Palo Alto, CA: Consulting Psychologists Press.

Stanton-Hicks, M. (1990). *Pain and the sympathetic nervous system*. Boston: Kluwer.

Stanton-Hicks, M., Baron, R., Boas, R., Gordh, T., Harden, N., Hendler, N., Koltzenburg, M., Raj, P., & Wilder, R. (1998). Complex regional pain syndromes: Guidelines for therapy. *Clinical Journal of Pain*, *14*, 155–166.

Stanton-Hicks, M., Janig, W., Hassenbusch, S., Haddox, J. D., Boas, R., & Wilson, P. (1995). Reflex sympathetic dystrophy: Changing concepts and taxonomy. *Pain*, *63*, 127–133.

Tait, R. C., Pollard, C. A., Margolis, R. B., Duckro, P. N., & Krause, S. J. (1987). The Pain Disability Index: Psychometric and validity data. *Archives of Physical Medicine and Rehabilitation*, *68*, 438–441.

Thimineur, M., Sood, P., Kravitz, E., Gudin, J., & Kitaj, M. (1998). Central nervous system abnormalities in complex regional pain syndrome (CRPS): Clinical and quantitative evidence of medullary dysfunction. *Clinical Journal of Pain*, *14*, 256–267.

Travell, J. G., & Simons, D. G. (1983). *Myofascial pain and dysfunction: The trigger point manual. The upper extremities*. Baltimore: Williams & Wilkins.

Uomoto, J. M., Turner, J. A., & Herron, L. D. (1988). Use of the MMPI and MCMI in predicting outcome of lumbar laminectomy. *Journal of Clinical Psychology*, *44*, 191–197.

Van Houdenhove, B. (1986). Neuroalgodystrophy: A psychiatrist's view. *Clinical Rheumatology*, *5*, 399–406.

Van Houdenhove, B., Vasquez, G., Onghena, P., Stans, L., Vandeput, C., Vermaut, G., Vervaeke, G., Igodt, P., & Vertommen, H. (1992). Etiopathogenesis of reflex sympathetic dystrophy: A review and biopsychosocial hypothesis. *Clinical Journal of Pain*, *8*, 300–306.

Verdugo, R. J., & Ochoa, J. L. (1994). Sympatheticallymaintained pain: I. Phentolamine block questions the concept. *Neurology*, *44*, 1003–1010.

Wang, J. K., Johnson, K. A., & Ilstrup, D. M. (1985). Sympathetic blocks for reflex sympathetic dystrophy. *Pain*, *23*, 13–17.

Wilson, P. R., Low, P. A., Bedder, M. D., Covington, E. C., & Rauck, R. L. (1996). Diagnostic algorithm for complex regional pain syndromes. In W. Janig & M. Stanton-Hicks (Eds.), *Progress in pain research and management. Vol. 6: Reflex Sympathetic Dystrophy: A reappraisal* (pp. 93–105). Seattle, WA: International Association for the Study of Pain Press,

Woolf, C. J., Shortland, P, & Coggeshall, R. E. (1992). Peripheral nerve injury triggers central sprouting of myelinated afferents. *Nature*, *355*, 75–78.

Zachariae, L. (1964). Incidence and course of posttraumatic dystrophy following operation for Dupuytren's contracture. *Acta Chirurgica Scandinavica*, Suppl. 336, 7–51.

Zucchini, M., Alberti, G., & Moretti, M. P. (1989). Algodystrophy and related psychological features. *Functional Neurology*, *4*, 153–156.

Zyluk, A., & Birkenfeld, B. (1999). Quantitative evaluation of three-phase bone scintigraphy before and after the treatment of post-traumatic reflex sympathetic dystrophy. *Nuclear Medicine Communications*, *20*, 327–333.

Chapter 29

Chronic Pelvic Pain

URSULA WESSELMANN

Chronic pelvic pain is a common and debilitating problem that can significantly impair a woman's quality of life. Patients with chronic pelvic pain are usually evaluated and treated by gynecologists, gastroenterologists, urologists, and internists. Although these patients seek medical care because they are looking for help to alleviate their pelvic discomfort and pain, in many cases the only focus is on finding and possibly treating the underlying pelvic disease, and these patients often undergo many diagnostic tests and procedures. However, often the examination and workup remain unrevealing, and no specific cause of the pain can be identified. At this point, patients are frequently told that no etiology for their chronic pain syndrome can be found and that nothing can be done. Some patients are then referred to psychologists or psychiatrists to be evaluated for an underlying psychological etiology, since nothing organic has been identified that could explain their symptoms. Although these patients are often depressed, rarely are the chronic pelvic pain syndromes the only manifestation of a psychiatric disease.

In these cases it is important to recognize not only that pain is a symptom of pelvic disease, but that the patient is suffering from a chronic visceral pain syndrome, where "pain" is the prominent symptom. Knowledge of the clinical characteristics of visceral pain will guide the health care provider in making a diagnosis of chronic pelvic pain and in sorting it out from the lump diagnosis of idiopathic pain (Wesselmann, 1999b). Once the diagnosis of chronic pelvic pain is made, treatment should be directed toward symptomatic pain management. This conceptualization of chronic pelvic pain is very important, because chronic pelvic pain is a treatable condition! Despite the challenge inherent in the management of chronic pelvic pain, many patients can be treated successfully (Wesselmann, 1999a). Effective treatment modalities are available to lessen the impact of pain and offer reasonable expectations of an improved functional status.

The focus of this chapter is on chronic nonmalignant pelvic pain. Another very important topic is chronic pelvic pain due to cancer, and the reader is referred to an excellent review of this topic (Brose & Cousins, 1992). In this chapter I provide an overview of the definitions of chronic pelvic pain syndromes, review current knowledge of the epidemiology and pathophysiology of pelvic pain, and then discuss clinical approaches to the patient presenting with chronic pelvic pain.

DEFINITIONS

Definitions are important, if a body of reliable information is to be built up in the scientific literature that will eventually lead to a better understanding of the pathophysiology and management of chronic pelvic pain. At present, one of the major problems of research into chronic pelvic pain is the lack of agreed-upon definitions, which would allow comparison between studies (Beard, 1998).

In the gynecological literature, a definition of *chronic pelvic pain* as noncyclic pelvic pain of greater than 6 months' duration that is not relieved by nonnarcotic analgesics has been proposed (Reiter, 1990b). This definition is, however, very problematic (Beard, 1998). It defines chronic pelvic pain in relation to the response to analgesic treatment. Immediately, one sees the problems inherent in this definition (which was, however, carefully considered, as it appeared in a guest editorial on chronic pelvic pain): Would a patient with chronic pelvic pain who responds to opioids be diagnosed with chronic pelvic pain, but a patient who responds to tricyclic antidepressants not?

The International Association for the Study of Pain defines *chronic pelvic pain without obvious pathology* as chronic or recurrent pelvic pain that apparently has a gynecological origin but for which no definitive lesion or cause is found (Merskey & Bogduk, 1994). This definition has not been widely used in the literature (Beard, 1998; Campbell & Collett, 1994). The problems with this definition are that (1) it implies absence of pathology, which is not necessarily the case; and (2) it also excludes cases in which pathology is present but not necessarily the cause of pain. In fact, the relationship of pain to the presence of pathology is often unclear in women with chronic pelvic pain.

I refer here to *chronic pelvic pain* as pelvic pain in the same location for at least 6 months (American College of Obstetricians and Gynecologists [ACOG], 1996; Campbell & Collett, 1994). This broad definition acknowledges that many chronic pain states begin with a nociceptive process, although that event may go unrecognized or unremembered.

EPIDEMIOLOGICAL FACTS

Chronic pelvic pain is a common problem among women. Overall, a woman has about a 5% risk of having chronic pelvic pain in her lifetime. In patients with a previous diagnosis of pelvic inflammatory disease, this risk is increased fourfold (approximately 20%) (see Ryder, 1996).

A study of epidemiological data from the United States showed that 14.7% of women in their reproductive ages reported chronic pelvic pain (Mathias, Kuppermann, Liberman, Lipschutz, & Steege, 1996). Extrapolating to the total female population gave an estimated 9.2 million women suffering from chronic pelvic pain in the United States alone. Fifteen percent of the women reporting chronic pelvic pain in the Mathias and colleagues (1996) study also reported time lost from work, and 45% reported reduced work productivity. In the United States, 10% of outpatient gynecological consultations are for chronic pelvic pain (Reiter, 1990a), and 40% of laparoscopies are performed for chronic pelvic pain (Howard, 1993). Chronic pelvic pain is listed as the indication for 12%–16% of hysterectomies performed in the United States, accounting for approximately 80,000 procedures annually. However, approximately 25% of women referred for evaluation of chronic pelvic pain have previously undergone a hysterectomy *without* the resolution of symptoms (see Milburn, Reiter, & Romberg, 1993). Estimated medical costs for outpatient visits for chronic pelvic pain in the United States are $881.5 million per year (Mathias et al., 1996). The personal cost to affected women in terms of years of suffering, disability, marital/couple discord, loss of employment, and unsuccessful medical intervention can be calculated less easily. Unfortunately, epidemiological studies on chronic pelvic pain have not been reported from populations outside the United States (Zondervan et al., 1998).

NEUROBIOLOGY OF THE PELVIS

The visceral structures that may give rise to pain in the pelvic region in women belong to the genitourinary system (terminal part of the ureters, urinary bladder, pelvic urethra, ovaries, fallopian tubes, uterus, and vagina), the gastrointestinal system (sigmoid colon and rectum), and the associated pelvic vasculature and lymphatic structures. A detailed review of the neurobiology of the pelvis is provided elsewhere (Burnett & Wesselmann, 1999). In the clinical context, when one is assessing a patient with chronic pelvic pain, it is important to recall that the pelvis is innervated by both divisions of the autonomic nervous system (the sympathetic and parasympathetic divisions), as well as by the somatic and sensory nervous systems. In a broad anatomical view, dual projections from the thoraco-lumbar and sacral segments of the spinal cord carry out this innervation, converging primarily into discrete peripheral neuronal plexuses before distributing nerve fibers throughout the pelvis (Figure 29.1). The visceral afferents traveling in the sympathetic trunk have cell bodies in the thoraco-lumbar distribution, and those that travel with the parasympathetic fibers have cell bodies in the sacral dorsal root ganglia. Both visceral sensory pathways play a role in pelvic sensations and reflexes.

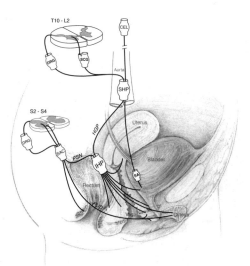

FIGURE 29.1. Schematic drawing showing the innervation of the pelvis in females. Although this diagram attempts to show the innervation in humans, much of the anatomical information is derived from animal data. CEL, celiac plexus; DRG, dorsal root ganglion; HGP, hypogastric plexus; IHP, inferior hypogastric plexus; PSN, pelvic splanchnic nerve; PUD, pudendal nerve; SA, short adrenergic projections; SAC, sacral plexus; SCG, sympathetic chain ganglion; SHP, superior hypogastric plexus; Vag., vagina. From Wesselmann, Burnett, and Heinberg (1997). Copyright 1997 by the International Association for the Study of Pain. Reprinted by permission.

Within the pelvis, the inferior hypogastric plexus is the major autonomic neuronal relay center, serving to integrate sympathetic and parasympathetic output. The distribution of innervation provided by the inferior hypogastric plexus includes the genital and reproductive tract structures, the urinary bladder, the urethra, the distal ureter, the internal anal sphincter, and the rectum. The dorsal root ganglion cells at the sacral and thoracolumbar level are the first of numerous relays of sensory neurons that transmit painful sensations from the pelvic cavity to the brain. Ascending visceral spinal pathways include the spino-thalamic and spino-reticular tract. Research has highlighted the dorsal column pathway as an important pathway for visceral sensations (Hirshberg, Al-Chaer, Lawand, Westlund, & Willis, 1996).

Somatic neuronal outflow to the pelvis is represented by the sacral nerve roots, which form the sacral plexus. Through this plexus, the pudendal nerve diverges, which carries efferent and afferent innervation and also receives postganglionic axons from the caudal sympathetic chain.

In general, sensations from the pelvic viscera are conveyed within the sacral parasympathetic system, with a far lesser contribution from the sympathetic thoraco-lumbar system (Jänig & Koltzenburg, 1993). Neuropeptide release appears to account for perineal sensations (Jänig & Koltzenburg, 1993). Numerous peptides have been associated with afferent pathways of the pelvic viscera, although a preponderance of evidence supports the roles of substance P and calcitonin-gene-related peptide as primary chemicals released from these sensory neurons (Dail, 1993; De Groat, 1987) .

CHRONIC PELVIC PAIN: A VISCERAL PAIN SYNDROME

Pelvic pain belongs to the category of visceral pain. Nowhere is the relationship of visceral pain to tissue damage less well understood than in the female pelvis. At least one-third of patients with chronic pelvic pain have no obvious pelvic pathology (Rapkin, 1990). There has been rapid progress in visceral pain research over the last 10 years, however (Gebhart, 1995; McMahon, Dmitrieva, & Koltzenburg, 1995). For the patient who presents with chronic pelvic pain, this has several implications. As the pathophysiological mechanisms of visceral pain explored in animal models provide an explanation for some of the clinical phenomena observed in patients, additional, revived, and new concepts of visceral pain have emerged: (1) A spectrum of different insults can lead to chronic visceral pain; (2) different underlying pathogenic pain mechanisms may require different pain treatment strategies for patients presenting with visceral pain; and (3) multiple different pathogenic pain mechanisms may coexist in the same patient presenting with visceral pain, requiring several different pain treatment strategies (perhaps concomitantly) to provide relief (Wesselmann, 1999a). This approach has allowed a holistic and mechanism-based approach to some of the chronic visceral pain syndromes that were previously labeled as psychogenic, since the underlying etiology could not be defined via currently available diagnostic techniques.

In the clinical context, when one is assessing a patient with chronic pelvic pain, several features of visceral pain are important to keep in mind: Visceral pain is a diffuse sensation that cannot be precisely localized. Pain in one viscus cannot be easily differentiated from pain originating in another viscus, and this often makes the differential diagnosis very complicated. Visceral pain presents with two components: true visceral pain, which is pain deep in the pelvic cavity, and referred visceral pain to somatic structures, such as muscle and skin (Head, 1893). Secondary hyperalgesia usually develops at the referred site (Giamberardino & Vecchiet, 1994). When one is examining and treating a patient with pelvic pain, it is important to consider all these aspects of pelvic pain. For example, the muscular component (referred pain) of pelvic pain can be so prominent that the chronic pelvic pain syndrome may be confused with a muscular pain problem or with back pain. The patient should be asked about all components of the pain. For the health care provider evaluating and treating a patient with pelvic pain, this approach will be helpful; it will allow him or her to look at the global picture of pelvic dysfunction, rather than "chasing" one aspect of the chronic pain syndrome out of context.

SEX DIFFERENCES IN PAIN AND GONADAL HORMONES

Chronic pelvic pain is mainly a pain syndrome of women in their reproductive years. The first onset of such pain is rarely reported in preadolescent girls or postmenopausal women, although pelvic pain can persist after a women has reached menopause or after all internal female reproductive organs have been removed surgically. Thus it seems that women are particularly likely to develop chronic pelvic pain during certain chronobiological stages (Berkley, 1997b). We are just beginning to realize the influence of the hormonal milieu on pain and the response to analgesic interventions in women and men during different reproductive stages. More research in this area is definitely needed.

BARRIERS TO ASSESSMENT AND TREATMENT

There are multiple barriers to good pain control for patients with chronic pelvic pain on both sides of the health care relationship—patients and health care providers. The subjective symptom of pain in patients with chronic pelvic pain, in the setting of a clinical presentation where the etiology often cannot be identified, or where treatment of an identified organic pathology (in many cases, surgical extirpation of the female reproductive organs) does not result in pain relief, is commonly viewed with skepticism: There is no "legitimate" reason for the

pain. Patients, health care providers, and the patients' friends and family members are all often frustrated by the puzzling clinical picture, and in many cases the patients give up on seeking pain relief once they have had a few frustrating experiences. Patients with chronic pelvic pain then often isolate themselves, feeling that nobody understands their pain and that nobody can help them, which drives them into further isolation. This frequently cumulates in a situation where there is no support system and no plan for how to manage the pain. An increase in pain therefore results in an emergency situation, which often cannot be adequately dealt with. Thus a vicious cycle develops. Recognizing that chronic pelvic pain presents with the typical features of chronic visceral pain, and thus putting this chronic pain syndrome into context with other chronic visceral pain syndromes, should have an important impact on how pain is understood by the patients, the health care providers, and the patients' communities (family members, workplace, friends). Education in this area will be an important first step toward better assessment of chronic pelvic pain.

A recent British study examined medical attitudes toward the treatment of women with chronic pelvic pain (Selfe, Van Vugt, & Stones, 1998). Scores for *pathology* (the tendency for physicians to see their major role as the detection of pathology) were lower among younger gynecologists. A sex difference just failed to reach statistical significance. This study also raised the question of *complexity*, relating to the idea of chronic pelvic pain as a difficult condition to treat, both in general and with regard to specific patients. This difficulty generates either a negative emotional response in the physician, or, by contrast, a heightened sense of satisfaction at dealing effectively with it. When patients present with chronic pelvic pain, more intellectual and emotional resources are required on the part of physicians both to consider other treatment options and to overcome more emotional reactions that could block more lateral or creative thinking.

Furthermore, the differential diagnosis of chronic pelvic pain is usually quite complex, since the symptoms are often diffuse and not specific. Most efforts of health care personnel are spent on identifying an underlying possible etiology. In addition, although many guidelines have been published on diagnosing and treating nonmalignant and malignant pelvic disease, no specific guidelines exist so far on the assessment and management of visceral pain, and physicians and other health care providers are left without any concepts on the approach to the patient with chronic pelvic pain. Further education at the graduate and postgraduate level is urgently needed to overcome this barrier, which is due to a lack of knowledge.

Another barrier is the fact that chronic pelvic pain has a direct impact on a patient's sexual life; moreover, the area of the body where the pain is experienced is often considered taboo. Both the patient and the health care provider may feel uncomfortable discussing pain of the pelvis. Location of pain may be a significant predictor for appraisals of pain and disclosure of pain complaints. Klonoff, Landrine, and Brown (1993) have demonstrated that subjects asked to imagine pain in their genitals appraised themselves as more ill than if they were asked to imagine chest, stomach, head, or mouth pain. Furthermore, subjects reported that they would be least likely to disclose genital pain and would be more worried, depressed, and embarrassed by pain in the genitals than by pain in any other area of the body.

PSYCHOLOGICAL AND PSYCHOSOCIAL ASPECTS

The literature examining psychological factors in pelvic pain has been reviewed in detail elsewhere (Fry, Crisp, & Beard, 1997; Grace, 1998; Savidge & Slade, 1997; Wesselmann, Burnett, & Heinberg, 1997).

Although psychological research on factors such as depression, anxiety, and a history of physical and/or sexual abuse has been conducted in patients with pelvic pain syndromes, much of this research is hampered by lack of appropriate control groups (utilizing patients with other types of pain), small sample size, and samples without significant self-selection factors (e.g., patients referred for psychological evaluation, patients in tertiary clinics). Many studies on chronic pelvic pain, depression, and sexual function have neglected to examine whether the psychological findings were likely to be preexisting or reactive, and it is not possible to draw conclusions about the role of these factors in the cause of the complaint. Depression and an impaired sexual life would not be surprising or necessarily indicative of psychopathology in a woman with many years of chronic pelvic pain. The important questions are (1) whether this patient was depressed and had an impaired sexual life before the chronic pain syndrome started; and (2) whether her mood and sexual life returned to

normal after successful therapy for the chronic pain syndrome. Further research in this area is clearly needed.

APPROACHES TO CHRONIC PAIN SYNDROMES OF THE PELVIC CAVITY

Women with chronic pelvic pain of the pelvic cavity complain about deep pain either unilaterally, bilaterally, or in the midline, often radiating to the low back, anterior abdominal wall, buttocks, hips, perineal area, and anterior thighs. Associated symptoms may include dyspareunia and changes in bowel and urinary habits. The pain syndrome can be exacerbated by postural changes such as walking. Pelvic pain can be cyclic (related to the menstrual cycle), intermittent, or continuous.

Chronic pelvic pain is often thought to be primarily of gynecological origin. However, it is important to keep in mind that all other structures in the pelvic cavity—including the urinary tract, the lower gastrointestinal tract, and the pelvic blood vessels—have to be included in the differential diagnosis. Other possible etiologies to be considered include musculoskeletal, neurological, and psychiatric etiologies. Thus the differential diagnosis is complicated, and a thorough workup is necessary (Table 29.1).

Localization of the source of pain is often difficult or inaccurate, because of the overlapping innervation pattern of the pelvic organs. It is important to understand that in many patients different etiologies of pelvic pain may not appear in "pure" form, but rather in various mixtures with varying contributions to a woman's total discomfort. Given the extensive convergence of visceral afferent input on the spinal cord level and in the neuronal plexuses of the pelvis demonstrated in animal studies (Cervero, 1994; Jänig, Schmidt, Schnitzler, & Wesselmann, 1991; Wesselmann & Lai, 1997), it would not be surprising if a chronic pain syndrome in one area of the pelvis could trigger the development of chronic pain and dysfunc-

TABLE 29.1. Possible Etiologies of Chronic Pelvic Pain

Gynecological	Gastrointestinal
Extrauterine	Musculoskeletal
Uterine	Neurological
Urological	Psychiatric

tion in another area of the pelvis via altered central mechanisms. Some patients present with "more than one pelvic pain": An example is the strong covariation of menstrual and bowel symptoms, and the overlap in the diagnoses of dysmenorrhea and functional bowel disorders (Moore, Barlow, Jewell, & Kennedy, 1998).

Since history and physical examination often do not allow a clinician to identify an etiology for the chronic pain syndrome, laparoscopy has been the routine tool in the investigation of chronic pelvic pain for many years. Laparoscopy is an important tool for diagnostic confirmation, histological documentation, and patient reassurance (Parsons & Stovall, 1993). However, it is important to realize that fewer than 50% of patients are helped by diagnostic or therapeutic laparoscopy, suggesting that laparoscopy is neither the ultimate investigation method nor the ultimate treatment for chronic pelvic pain (Howard, 1993). Pelvic pain is unique, because a patient may have severe pelvic pathology such as adhesions or endometriosis with little or no pain; in contrast, another patient may have severe pain but minimal pelvic pathology (Ryder, 1996).

Studies on the impact of the experience of chronic pelvic pain in the months following negative laparoscopy have shown that most patients were dissatisfied with the quantity and quality of information they were given, and that despite having continued pain, most did not receive further medical care. Many patients felt they were not believed and were not given any help in the management of their chronic condition (Stewart & Slade, 1998). It is important for the physician and the patient to recognize not only the importance but also the limitations of laparoscopy for the diagnosis of chronic pelvic pain. Despite several reports in the gynecological literature in support of this issue over the last several years, this has not been translated successfully into clinical practice yet.

The workup of the patient with chronic pelvic pain starts with a thorough medical history (Table 29.2). Patients with chronic pelvic pain, like patients with other types of chronic pain, may have had their history already taken multiple times and may be frustrated at having to go through the details again. On the other hand, in today's health care environment, it is often difficult for a health care provider to take the time to go through the extensive history of a patient with chronic pain. However, a detailed history is key to formulating a diagnosis and treatment plan, and all efforts to accomplish this are worthwhile. This may mean that the

TABLE 29.2. History of the Patient with Chronic Pelvic Pain

Onset of pain?
Duration of pelvic pain syndrome?
Pain intensity?
Pain character?
Is the pain continuous, intermittent, or cyclic?
Any precipitating events?
Location of pain (unilateral, bilateral, in midline)?
Radiation of pain (low back, anterior abdominal wall, buttocks, hips, perineal area, anterior thighs)?
Associated bowel changes?
Associated changes in urinary habits?
Dyspareunia?
Any other associated symptoms?
Aggravating factors?
Relieving factors?
Progression of symptoms?
Response to prior treatment?
Influence of the pelvic pain syndrome on mood?
Influence of the pelvic pain syndrome on function and interactions (personal life, family life, work, sexual life)?

patient has to come back for repeat office visits to complete the initial history taking. The history focuses on the intensity, character, temporal pattern, duration, location, and radiation of the pain, as well as precipitating and relieving factors. Specific attention is paid to associated changes in bowel, urinary, and sexual function. A review of systems should also include neurological and musculoskeletal functions. Associated symptoms such as anorexia, constipation, and fatigue should be evaluated. The patient should be asked about the influence of the chronic pelvic pain syndrome on her mood, and on her functioning in various aspects of her life (personal life, family life, workplace, sexual life). Given the diversity of possible etiologies, a thorough review of all previous consultations and previous diagnostic and therapeutic interventions is imperative, in order to decide whether further diagnostic workup is required. As in other chronic pain conditions, psychosocial and behavioral assessment is an essential part of the evaluation of chronic pelvic pain. A psychological interview, conducted by a psychologist or psychiatrist experienced in chronic pain management, should be part of the initial evaluation process (see Sullivan, Chapter 15, and Bradley & McKendree-Smith, Chapter 16, this volume).

The physical evaluation is focused on the area of pain and includes a general physical, neurological, musculoskeletal, and pelvic examination.

Procedures during the physical examination that provoke or exacerbate the pelvic pain are carefully noted. Areas of hyperalgesia and trigger points are documented.

Depending on the patient's symptoms and the result of the physical examination, consultations with other specialists in gynecology, gastroenterology, urology, orthopedics, and neurology, as well as further diagnostic evaluations, may be indicated before a symptomatic pain treatment plan can be established. When to stop looking further for a macroscopic abnormality that could account for the chronic pelvic pain syndrome, and when to stop treating a pelvic pathology when the treatment of that pathology is not resulting in pain relief (implying that the pathology identified is not related to the chronic pelvic pain problem), are difficult decisions that need to be tailored to the individual patient. In fact, these are decisions that many health care providers and patients avoid. It is important to call a halt to investigation once it is clearly negative (Drife, 1993). It is unlikely that if a thorough evaluation of a chronic pelvic pain problem has not identified any pelvic pathology, further diagnostic tests or repeating the same diagnostic tests will uncover an organic pathology. This caveat has to be raised especially for invasive diagnostic procedures, where the risk to the patient may be greater than the likelihood of discovering something new.

Outcome measures for the treatment of chronic pelvic pain include a reduction of pain intensity in the pelvic cavity and in the referred zone; improvement of associated changes in bowel, urinary, and sexual function; improved mood; and improvement of the patient's functional status in her personal life, in her family life, at her workplace, and in her sexual life. Different outcome measures have different importance for individual patients, and it is important to discuss this as a treatment plan is established.

Surgical Approaches

Traditionally, surgical approaches to the treatment of chronic pelvic pain have been very common. Failure to achieve pain relief after surgical procedures has often resulted in more aggressive surgical efforts, driven by the hypothesis that a surgically curable lesion might have been missed earlier. However, long-term success after surgical procedures is often disappointing when pelvic pain is *the only indication* for surgery (Parsons & Stovall,

1993). Many patients with chronic pelvic pain have already undergone several surgical diagnostic and therapeutic procedures without any pain relief. In these patients further surgical procedures should be very carefully considered, since it is less likely that further surgery will result in pain relief after previous surgical approaches have already failed. Because of the uncertain role of endometriosis and pelvic adhesions in the etiology of chronic pelvic pain, nonsurgical treatment options should be explored first, and surgical therapy for chronic pain should be limited to the treatment of surgically correctable etiologies (ACOG, 1996). In cases where a surgically correctable etiology can be identified, it is often assumed that surgical correction will result in pain relief. However, it is important for the physician and the patient to have realistic expectations—that is, to understand that the chronic pain syndrome may be improved or cured, but also may be unchanged or worsened by the procedure (Carleson, Miller, & Fowler, 1994).

Pharmacological Approaches

Despite the fact that chronic pelvic pain is a very common chronic pain syndrome, very little is known about effective pharmacological treatment for it. Further research on the mechanisms of chronic pelvic pain and controlled clinical trials are desperately needed to design improved pharmacological treatment strategies. Despite these limitations and the obvious need for improvement, pharmacological treatment strategies that have mainly been evaluated at present for other chronic pain syndromes can be successfully applied to patients with chronic pelvic pain. Several different pharmacological classes of medications have been demonstrated to be effective in alleviating pain in patients with chronic pain syndromes (Galer, 1995; Wesselmann & Raja, 1997): nonsteroidal anti-inflammatory drugs (NSAIDs), antidepressants, anticonvulsants, local anesthetics, antiarrhythmics, and opioids. Very few studies have focused specifically on the treatment of chronic pelvic pain (Beresin, 1986; Walker, Roy-Byrne, Katon, & Jemelka, 1991). These few studies suggest, that pelvic pain syndromes can be successfully treated with medications commonly used to treat other chronic pain syndromes.

The principal guidelines for pharmacological management of chronic pelvic pain are similar to those for the pharmacological treatment of other chronic pain states. Although clinical trials and case reports on the pharmacological management of chronic pain syndromes provide general guidelines as to which drug to choose, currently we have no method to predict which drug is most likely to alleviate pain in a given patient. The goal of pharmacotherapy is to find a medication that provides significant pain relief with minimal side effects. It is important for the patient to understand the limitations of this "trial-and-error" method of prescribing drugs. Adequate trials should be performed for each drug prescribed, and only one drug should be titrated at a time, because obviously the effects of a certain drug on pain scores cannot be assessed otherwise. The starting dose should always be the smallest tablet available, and titration should occur at frequent intervals, guided by pain scores and side effects. This requires frequent contact between the patient and the pain clinic during the titration period. It is important for the patient and the physician to understand that some side effects will actually improve as the patient takes a drug for several weeks. If these side effects are not intolerable, the patient should be guided through this period.

Regional Anesthesia Approaches

Peripheral nerve and abdominal plexus blocks have been advocated as diagnostic and therapeutic interventions for women suffering from chronic pelvic pain. Over the last 10 years, there has been a new interest in neurolytic superior hypogastric plexus blocks for the treatment of chronic pelvic pain associated with cancer (de Leon-Casasola, Kent, & Lema, 1993; Plancarte, de Leon-Casasola, El-Helaly, Allende, & Lema, 1997). Pain relief following neurolytic blockade of the superior hypogastric plexus may be due to interruption of the afferent pathways from the pelvic organs, or to interruption of the sympathetic outflow to the pelvic organs, as in sympathetically maintained pain syndromes (Wesselmann & Raja, 1997). These regional anesthesia techniques, which have been frequently used for patients with visceral pain due to cancer, have also been suggested as diagnostic tools and therapeutic interventions for women with chronic nonmalignant pelvic pain (McDonald, 1993; Wechsler, Maurer, Halpern, & Frank, 1995).

Patients with chronic pelvic pain after previous surgery to the abdominal area frequently describe the pain as radiating to the abdominal wall, groin, or perineal area. In these cases pelvic pain may be due to entrapment of the ilioinguinal, ilio-hypogastric, genitofemoral, or pudendal nerves, and the chronic pain syndrome can often be managed by repeated local anesthetic blocks to these nerves spaced out over time.

Trigger Point Injections, Transcutaneous Electrical Nerve Stimulation, and Acupuncture

Myofascial pain of the extremities or of the upper trunk has been shown to respond to trigger point injections (Travell & Rinzler, 1952). A typical characteristic of chronic pelvic pain is that patients may present not only with deep pelvic pain, but also with referred pain to somatic structures. Some physicians have reported marked pain relief in patients with chronic pelvic pain when trigger point injections were made to areas of referred muscle pain (trigger points in the abdominal wall, as well as sacral, perineal, and vaginal areas) (Slocumb, 1984). Further research is necessary to assess which patients might be good candidates for this approach and what the frequency of the trigger point injections should be over time (especially since some patients report that these injections are initially quite painful when given to the sacral, perineal, and vaginal areas).

Transcutaneous electrical nerve stimulation (TENS), in contrast to almost all other treatment strategies available, has no side effects. This treatment modality has been shown to be effective in some patients with primary dysmenorrhea (Lundeberg, Bondesson, & Lundström, 1985; Milsom, Hedner, & Mannheimer, 1994), and also in patients with noncyclic chronic pelvic pain (ACOG, 1996).

Acupuncture has been used for many centuries in Asia to control pain. Anecdotal reports, where acupuncture has been used as part of a multidisciplinary treatment approach, indicate an effective role for the management of chronic pelvic pain (Kames, Rapkin, Naliboff, Afifi, & Ferrer-Brechner, 1990).

Physical Therapy Approaches

Muscle pain in the referred zone is a typical component of chronic pelvic pain. Physical therapy helps to decrease musculoskeletal pain, and it can improve mobility. It is an important aspect of a multidisciplinary approach to the treatment of chronic pelvic pain (Baker, 1993).

Vascular Approaches

Venous congestion is a common finding in some patients with chronic pelvic pain (Beard, Highman, Pearce, & Reginald, 1984). Medroxyprogesterone acetate has been shown to reduce pelvic pain and venous congestion in such patients (Farquhar et al., 1989); however, the response was only short-term. There was a high relapse rate after treatment was stopped. Bilateral oophorectomy combined with hysterectomy and hormone replacement therapy has been suggested for those who have failed to respond to medical treatment (Beard et al., 1991). More recently, transcatheter embolization of lumbo-ovarian varices has been described as a safe technique offering symptomatic relief in selected patients with chronic pelvic pain due to pelvic congestion (Capasso et al., 1997; Sichlau, Yao, & Vogelzang, 1994).

Neurosurgical Approaches

In the early European literature, pelvic denervation was frequently advocated for chronic pelvic pain, including dysmenorrhea (Jaboulay, 1899; Ruggi, 1899). These surgical techniques became less popular as NSAIDs, as well as hormonal therapy, became available for the treatment of dysmenorrhea. Recently, with the widespread use of laparascopic surgery, there has been a new interest in pelvic denervation (presacral neurectomy and amputation of the uterosacral ligaments) for chronic pelvic pain. However, the literature is controversial regarding the pain relief achieved with these procedures. Although some studies claim a high success rate (Zullo et al., 1996), others have failed to prove that presacral neurectomy is effective (Vercellini, Fedele, Bianchi, & Candiani, 1991). It will be important to provide more detailed descriptions of patients who respond and do not respond to these procedures, in order to identify patients who might benefit from this approach. It has been suggested that a diagnostic superior hypogastric plexus block might predict whether a surgical presacral neurectomy will result in long-lasting pain relief (Steege, 1998). On a cautionary note, the function of the hypogastric plexus in humans has not been researched in detail, because—in contrast to the function of somatic nerves—this is difficult to study in an experimental setting. Careful attention to pelvic function (including sensation, motility such as colonic motility, and sexual function) is necessary to evaluate for possible side effects of surgical pelvic denervation. These might not be as obvious as in the somatic domain, where transection of a peripheral nerve results in motor and sensory deficits that can easily be observed and quantified.

If the clinical picture suggests entrapment of a nerve (pudendal nerve—perineal pain; ilioinguinal or iliohypogastric nerve—groin pain; genitofemoral nerve—lower abdominal and perineal pain) accounting for the chronic pelvic pain syndrome, surgical neurolysis of entrapped nerves may be indicated (Harms, DeHaas, & Starling, 1987; Robert et al., 1993, 1998). Early diagnosis of nerve entrapment seems to be an important factor in achieving pain relief with neurolysis. Diagnostic nerve blocks with local anesthetic help to confirm the diagnosis.

Limited midline myelotomy has been advocated for the relief of malignant pelvic pain (Hirshberg et al., 1996), based on very promising results in a limited number of patients with cancer. The purpose of this procedure is to disrupt ascending nociceptive signals from the pelvic organs traveling in the medial part of the posterior columns. Further research on the function of this pathway in animal studies is in progress. It is important to assess which other functions this pathway might have in addition to mediating nociceptive signals from the pelvis, before this procedure can be considered as one of the treatment options for patients with chronic nonmalignant pelvic pain (Berkley, 1997a; Gybels, 1997). One caveat is that myelotomy is an irreversible procedure, and there is no placebo control. Isolated case reports from a time when surgical procedures for pain relief involving the dissection of tracts used to be quite common have documented that success in surgery may not require cutting the tracts (Nathan, 1985).

Psychological Approaches

Psychological treatment should be made part of the treatment plan early. Psychological factors, if not addressed, may endanger the success of any other treatment modality. Patients who have experienced chronic pain often remain anxious, are impatient, and have unrealistic expectations about a "quick cure." Frequently used psychological techniques include relaxation techniques, biofeedback, psychotherapy, and group therapy (Rosenthal, 1993). Clinical outcome studies are necessary to assess which might be the best approach for different subgroups of patients with chronic pelvic pain.

SUMMARY

It is important for both patients and physicians to realize that chronic visceral pain syndromes do exist (and are in fact quite common), and that chronic pelvic pain presents with the typical features of chronic visceral pain. In this chapter I have outlined clinical approaches to patients with chronic pelvic pain (see Table 29.3 for a summary). These patients are a heterogeneous population, and therefore attempts to ascribe all cases to a particular cause or mechanism will undoubtedly fail (ACOG, 1996; Campbell & Collett, 1994). The relationship of pain to the presence of pathology is often unclear. Pelvic pain may have several components (visceral, muscular, vascular, and neuropathic), and this multifaceted presentation has to be taken into account when one is evaluating and treating patients with chronic pelvic pain. Chronic pelvic pain is truly a multidisciplinary problem whose diagnosis and management require the concerted effort of a multidisciplinary team (ACOG, 1996). Women with chronic pelvic pain have often drifted from

one physician to another without a clear diagnosis and without much improvement—a frustrating process for the patients and their treating physicians, and an expensive process for the health care system. Educating patients with chronic pelvic pain and their health care providers about currently available treatment strategies will be an important step forward, since many are not aware of options that currently exist. Further research is necessary to assess the pathophysiological mechanisms underlying chronic pelvic pain, in order to develop new and improved treatment strategies targeted to the pathophysiological mechanisms.

ACKNOWLEDGMENTS

The writing of this chapter was supported by National Institutes of Health Grants No. RO1 NS36553 (National Institute of Neurological Disorders and Stroke, Office of Research for Women's Health) and No. R21 DK57315 (National Institute of Diabetes and Digestive and Kidney Diseases); by the National Vulvodynia Association; and by the Blaustein Pain Research Foundation.

TABLE 29.3. Approaches to the Patient with Chronic Pelvic Pain

What is the etiology of the chronic pelvic pain syndrome?

- History
  What diagnostic evaluations have been done so far?
  Are further diagnostic tests necessary?
  Which pain management strategies have been tried in the past, and what was the outcome of these interventions?
  What is the patient currently using for pain relief? Does it reduce pain and improve the quality of life?
- Physical examination
- Psychological assessment
- Discuss fertility concerns as they relate to pain treatment strategies

Etiological treatment possible?

- Start specific treatment
- Taper off symptomatic pain treatment as tolerated

Etiological treatment not possible?

- Continue and improve symptomatic pain management
  Surgical approaches
  Pharmacological approaches
  Regional anesthesia approaches
  Trigger point injections, TENS, acupuncture
  Physical therapy
  Vascular approaches
  Neurosurgical approaches
  Psychological therapy

REFERENCES

American College of Obstetricians and Gynecologists (ACOG). (1996, May). ACOG Technical Bulletin No. 223: Chronic pelvic pain. *International Journal of Gynecology and Obstetrics, 54,* 59–68.

Baker, P. K. (1993). Musculoskeletal origins of chronic pelvic pain: Diagnosis and treatment. *Obstetrics and Gynecology Clinics of North America, 20,* 719–742.

Beard, R. W. (1998). Chronic pelvic pain. *British Journal of Obstetrics and Gynaecology, 105,* 8–10.

Beard, R. W., Highman, J. W., Pearce, S., & Reginald, P. W. (1984). Diagnosis of pelvic varicosities in women with chronic pelvic pain. *Lancet, ii,* 946–949.

Beard, R. W., Kennedy, R. G., Gangar, K. F., Stones, R. W., Rogers, V., Reginald, P. W., & Anderson, M. (1991). Bilateral oophorectomy and hysterectomy in the treatment of intractable pelvic pain associated with pelvic congestion. *British Journal of Obstetrics and Gynaecology, 98,* 988–992.

Beresin, E. (1986). Imipramine in the treatment of chronic pelvic pain. *Psychosomatics, 27,* 294–296.

Berkley, K. J. (1997a). On the dorsal columns: Translating basic research hypotheses to the clinic. *Pain, 70,* 103–107.

Berkley, K. J. (1997b). Sex differences in pain. *Behavioral and Brain Sciences, 20,* 371–380.

Brose, W. G., & Cousins, M. J. (1992). Gynaecologic pain. In M. Coppleson (Ed.), *Gynaecologic oncology: Fundamental principles and clinical practice* (2nd ed. pp. 1439–1479). Edinburgh: Churchill Livingstone.

Burnett, A. L., & Wesselmann, U. (1999). Neurobiology of the pelvis and perineum: Principles for a practical approach. *Journal of Pelvic Surgery, 5,* 224–232.

Campbell, F., & Collett, B. J. (1994). Chronic pelvic pain. *British Journal of Anaesthesia, 73,* 571–573.

Capasso, P., Simons, C., Trotteur, G., Dindelinger, R. F., Henroteaux, D., & Gaspard, U. (1997). Treatment of symptomatic pelvic varices by ovarian vein embolization. *Cardiovascular and Interventional Radiology, 20,* 107–111.

Carleson, K. J., Miller, B. A., & Fowler, F. J., Jr. (1994). The Maine Women's Health Study: II Outcomes of non-surgical management of leiomyomas, abnormal bleeding, and chronic pelvic pain. *Obstetrics and Gynecology, 83,* 566–572.

Cervero, F. (1994). Sensory innervation of the viscera: Peripheral basis of visceral pain. *Physiological Reviews, 74,* 95–138.

Dail, W. G. (1993). Autonomic innervation of male reproductive genitalia. In C. A. Maggi (Ed.), *Nervous control of the urogenital system* (pp. 61–101). Chur, Switzerland: Harwood Academic.

De Groat, W. C. (1987). Neuropeptides in pelvic afferent pathways. *Experientia, 43,* 801–812.

de Leon-Casasola, O. A., Kent, E., & Lema, M. J. (1993). Neurolytic superior hypogastric plexus block for chronic pelvic pain associated with cancer. *Pain, 54,* 145–151.

Drife, J. O. (1993). The pelvic pain syndrome. *British Journal of Obstetrics and Gynaecology, 100,* 510–511.

Farquhar, C. M., Rogers, V., Franks, S., Pearce, S., Wadsworth, J., & Beard, R. W. (1989). A randomized controlled trial of medroxyprogesterone acetate and psychotherapy for the treatment of pelvic congestion. *British Journal of Obstetrics and Gynaecology, 96,* 1153–1162.

Fry, R. P. W., Crisp, A. H., & Beard, R. W. (1997). Sociopsychological factors in chronic pelvic pain: A review. *Journal of Psychosomatic Research, 42,* 1–15.

Galer, B. S. (1995). Neuropathic pain of peripheral origin: Advances in pharmacologic treatment. *Neurology, 45,* S17–S25.

Gebhart, G. F. (1995). Visceral nociception: Consequences, modulation and the future. *European Journal of Anesthesiology, 12,* 24–27.

Giamberardino, M. A., & Vecchiet, L. (1994). Experimental studies on pelvic pain. *Pain Reviews, 1,* 102–115.

Grace, V. M. (1998). Mind/body dualism in medicine: The case of chronic pelvic pain without organic pathology. *International Journal of Health Services, 28,* 127–151.

Gybels, J. M. (1997). Commissural myelotomy revisited. *Pain, 70,* 1–2.

Harms, B. A., DeHaas, D. R., & Starling, J. R. (1987). Diagnosis and management of genitofemoral neuralgia. *Neurosurgery, 102,* 583–586.

Head, H. (1893). On disturbances of sensation with special reference to the pain of visceral disease. *Brain, 16,* 1–113.

Hirshberg, R. M., Al-Chaer, E. D., Lawand, N. B., Westlund, K. N., & Willis, W. D. (1996). Is there a pathway in the posterior funiculus that signals visceral pain? *Pain, 67,* 291–305.

Howard, F. M. (1993). The role of laparoscopy in chronic pelvic pain: Promise and pitfalls. *Obstetrical and Gynecological Survey, 48,* 357–387.

Jaboulay, M. (1899). Le traitement de la nevralgie pelvienne par la paralysie du sympathique sacre. *Lyon Medicine, 90,* 102–108.

Jänig, W., & Koltzenburg, M. (1993) Pain arising from the urogenital tract. In C. A. Maggi (Ed.), *Nervous control of the urogenital system* (pp. 525–578). Chur, Switzerland: Harwood Academic.

Jänig, W., Schmidt, M., Schnitzler, A., & Wesselmann, U. (1991). Differentiation of sympathetic neurons projecting in the hypogastric nerve in terms of their discharge patterns in cats. *Journal of Physiology (London), 437,* 157–179.

Kames, L. D., Rapkin, A. J., Naliboff, B. D., Afifi, S., & Ferrer-Brechner, T. (1990). Effectiveness of an interdisciplinary pain management program for the treatment of chronic pelvic pain. *Pain, 41,* 41–46.

Klonoff, E. A., Landrine, H., & Brown, M. (1993). Appraisal and response to pain may be a function of its bodily location. *Journal of Psychosomatic Research, 37,* 661–670.

Lundeberg, T., Bondesson, L., & Lundström, V. (1985). Relief of primary dysmenorrhea by transcutaneous electrical nerve stimulation. *Acta Obstetrica et Gynecologica Scandinavica, 64,* 491–497.

Mathias, S. D., Kuppermann, M., Liberman, R. F., Lipschutz, R. C., & Steege, J. F. (1996). Chronic pelvic pain: Prevalence, health-related quality of life, and economic correlates. *Obstetrics and Gynecology, 87,* 321–327.

McDonald, J. S. (1993). Management of chronic pelvic pain. *Obstetrics and Gynecology Clinics of North America, 20,* 817–838.

McMahon, S. B., Dmitrieva, N., & Koltzenburg, M. (1995). Visceral pain. *British Journal of Anaesthesiology, 75,* 132–144.

Merskey, H., & Bogduk, N. (Eds.). (1994). *Classification of chronic pain* (2nd ed.). Seattle, WA: International Association for the Study of Pain Press.

Milburn, A., Reiter, R. C., & Romberg, A. T. (1993). Multidisciplinary approach to chronic pelvic pain. *Obstetrics and Gynecology Clinics of North America, 20,* 643–661.

Milsom, I., Hedner, N., & Mannheimer, C. (1994). A comparative study of the effect of high-intensity transcutaneous nerve stimulation and oral naproxen on intrauterine pressure and menstrual pain in patients with primary dysmenorrhea. *American Journal of Obstetrics and Gynecology, 170,* 123–129.

Moore, J., Barlow, D., Jewell, D., & Kennedy, S. (1998). Do gastrointestinal symptoms vary with the menstrual cycle? *British Journal of Obstetrics and Gynaecology, 105,* 1322–1325.

Nathan, P. W. (1985). Success in surgery may not require cutting the tracts. *Pain, 22,* 317–319.

Parsons, L. H., & Stovall, T. G. (1993). Surgical management of chronic pelvic pain. *Obstetrics and Gynecology Clinics of North America, 20,* 765–778.

Plancarte, R., de Leon-Casasola, O. A., El-Helaly, M., Allende, S., & Lema, M. J. (1997). Neurolytic superior hypogastric plexus block for chronic pelvic pain associated with cancer. *Regional Anesthesia, 22,* 562–568.

Rapkin, A. J. (1990). Neuroanatomy, neurophysiology, and neuropharmacology of pelvic pain. *Clinical Obstetrics and Gynecology, 33,* 119–129.

Reiter, R. C. (1990a). A profile of women with chronic pelvic pain. *Clinical Obstetrics and Gynecology, 33,* 130–136.

Reiter, R. C. (1990b). Chronic pelvic pain [Editorial]. *Clinical Obstetrics and Gynecology, 33*, 117–118.

Robert, R., Brunet, C., Faure, A., Lehur, P. A., Labat, J. J., Bensignor, M., Leborgne, J., & Barbin, J. Y. (1993). La chirurgie du nerf pudental lors de certaines algies perineales: Evolution et resultats. *Chirurgie, 119*, 535–539.

Robert, R., Prat-Pradal, D., Labat, J. J., Bensignor, M., Raoul, S., Rebai, R., & Leborgne, J. (1998). Anatomic basis of chronic perineal pain: Role of the pudendal nerve. *Surgical Radiology and Anatomy, 20*, 93–98.

Rosenthal, R. H. (1993). Psychology of chronic pelvic pain. *Obstetrics and Gynecology Clinics of North America, 20*, 627–642.

Ruggi, C. (1899). *La simpatectomia addominale utero-ovarica come mezzo di cura di alcune lesioni interne degli organi genitali della donna*. Bologna, Italy: Zanichelli.

Ryder, R. M. (1996). Chronic pelvic pain. *American Family Physician, 54*, 2225–2232.

Savidge, C., & Slade, P. (1997) Psychological aspects of chronic pelvic pain. *Journal of Psychosomatic Research, 42*, 433–444.

Selfe, S. A., Van Vugt, M., & Stones, R. W. (1998). Chronic gynecological pain: An exploration of medical attitudes. *Pain, 77*, 215–225.

Sichlau, M. J., Yao, J. S. T., & Vogelzang, R. L. (1994). Transcatheter embolotherapy for the treatment of pelvic congestion syndrome. *Obstetrics and Gynecology, 83*, 892–896.

Slocumb, J. C. (1984). Neurological factors in chronic pelvic pain: Trigger points and the abdominal pelvic pain syndrome. *American Journal of Obstetrics and Gynecology, 149*, 536–543.

Steege, J. F. (1998). Superior hypogastric block during microlaparascopic pain mapping. *Journal of the American Association of Gynecological Laparascopy, 5*, 265–267.

Stewart, P., & Slade, P. (1998). Comparative study of pelvic and non-pelvic pain: The prevalence of chronic pelvic pain. *British Journal of Obstetrics and Gynaecology, 105*, 1335–1342.

Travell, J., & Rinzler, S. H. (1952). The myofascial genesis of pain. *Postgraduate Medicine, 11*, 425–427.

Vercellini, P., Fedele, L., Bianchi, S., & Candiani, G.B. (1991). Pelvic denervation for chronic pain associated with endometriosis: Fact or fancy? *American Journal of Obstetrics and Gynecology, 165*, 745–749.

Walker, E. A., Roy-Byrne, P. P., Katon, W. J., & Jemelka R. (1991). An open trial of nortriptyline in women with chronic pelvic pain. *International Journal of Psychiatric Medicine, 21*, 245–252.

Wechsler, R. J., Maurer, P. M., Halpern, E. J., & Frank, E. D. (1995). Superior hypogastric plexus block for chronic pelvic pain in the presence of endometriosis: CT techniques and results. *Radiology, 196*, 103–106.

Wesselmann, U. (1999a). A call for recognizing, legitimizing and treating chronic visceral pain syndromes. *Pain Forum, 8*, 146–150.

Wesselmann, U. (1999b). Pain—the neglected aspect of visceral disease [Editorial]. *European Journal of Pain, 3*, 189–191.

Wesselmann, U., Burnett, A. L., & Heinberg, L. J. (1997). The urogenital and rectal pain syndromes. *Pain, 73*, 269–294.

Wesselmann, U., & Lai, J. (1997). Mechanisms of referred visceral pain: Uterine inflammation in the adult virgin rat results in neurogenic plasma extravasation in the skin. *Pain, 73*, 309–317.

Wesselmann, U., & Raja, S. N. (1997). Reflex sympathetic dystrophy/causalgia. *Anesthesiology Clinics of North America, 15*, 407–427.

Zondervan, K. T., Yudkin, P. L., Vessey, M. P., Dawes, M. G., Barlow, D. H., & Kennedy, S. H. (1998). The prevalence of chronic pelvic pain in women in the Unread Kingdom: A systematic review. *British Journal of Obstetrics and Gynaecology, 105*, 93–99.

Zullo, F., Pellicano, M., DeStefano, R., Mastrantonio, P., Mencaglia, L., Stampini, A., Zupi, E., & Busacca, M. (1996). Efficacy of laparoscopic pelvic denervation in central-type chronic pelvic pain: A multicenter study. *Journal of Gynecological Surgery, 12*, 35–40.

Chapter 30

How to Assess Cancer Pain

KAREN O. ANDERSON
KAREN L. SYRJALA
CHARLES S. CLEELAND

Poorly controlled pain has such deleterious effects on a patient with cancer and the patient's family that its proper management should have the highest priority in the routine care of anyone with cancer. Not only do mood and quality of life deteriorate in the presence of pain, but pain has adverse effects on such measures of disease status as appetite and activity (Cleeland, 1984). Pain of severe intensity may be a primary reason why both patients and their families decide to abandon treatment, or even why patients decide to actively end their lives. The fear of uncontrolled pain is a key motivator behind the movement to legalize euthanasia and physician-assisted suicide for patients with terminal illnesses (Back, Wallace, Starks, & Pearlman, 1996).

There is strong evidence that the majority of patients can get pain relief if adequate treatment is provided. Studies of the World Health Organization's (WHO's) guidelines for cancer pain relief (WHO, 1986) indicate that 70%–90% of patients are relieved if this simple protocol for oral analgesic medications is followed (Grond et al., 1999; Shug, Zech, & Dorr, 1990; Ventafridda, Tamburini, Caraceni, DeConno, & Naldi, 1987; Zech, Grond, Lynch, Hertel, & Lehmann, 1995). When oral analgesics are not effective, a variety of supplemental pain management techniques can provide control. It is estimated that approximately 95% of patients with cancer could be free of significant pain (Foley, 1985). Unfortunately, despite the current

availability of treatment, multiple studies document undertreatment of pain (Cleeland et al., 1994; Vainio & Auvinen, 1996; Zenz, Zenz, Tryba, & Strumpf, 1995; Zhukovsky, Gorowski, Hausdorff, Napolitano, & Lesser, 1995). A study completed in the Eastern Cooperative Oncology Group (ECOG) surveyed over 1,300 outpatients with recurrent or metastatic cancer (Cleeland et al., 1994). Sixty-seven percent of the patients had pain or were being treated for pain with daily analgesics. Of those patients with pain, 42% were prescribed analgesics that were less potent than recommended by the WHO guidelines. One of the most important predictors of inadequate pain management was the discrepancy between a patient and a physician in their estimates of pain severity.

Although there are multiple barriers to good pain control for patients with cancer, inadequate assessment is the most obvious. Unrecognized pain will not be treated, and pain whose severity is underestimated will not be treated aggressively enough. Over 800 ECOG-affiliated physicians responded to a survey designed to determine their knowledge and practice of cancer pain management (Von Roenn, Cleeland, Gonin, Hatfield, & Pandya, 1993). Only half of these physicians felt that pain management was good or very good in their own practice settings. Survey respondents ranked a list of potential barriers to optimal cancer pain management in terms of how the barriers impeded pain management in their own practice settings. By far the most frequently identified barrier was lack of pain assessment; 76% of respondents rated inadequate assessment as one of the top barriers to good pain management. Patient reluctance to report pain, intimately related to inadequate assessment, was the next most frequently cited barrier. Similarly, a recent survey of physicians in the Radiation Therapy Oncology Group found that poor pain assessment and patient reluctance to report pain were identified as the top barriers to optimal pain management (Cleeland, Janjan, Scott, Seiferheld, & Curran, 2000).

Despite the recognition that it is important, formal pain assessment is rarely practiced in most cancer care settings. It is rarely practiced for a number of reasons. Health care providers do not have the time to fully assess pain and its impact, and providers often do not have the skills necessary to adequately assess pain and pain treatment effects. Pain assessment is not a standard part of patient appointments, and other priorities supplant symptom evaluation. When providers do ask about pain, they rarely attempt to quantify the severity of the pain or to document its characteristics and determinants. Even more rare is any attempt to assess the impact that pain is making on a patient's emotional, social, or functional status.

In this chapter we examine some of the methodological and practical issues in the assessment of cancer pain and its impact. We describe a "minimal data set" of information needed for treatment planning, and suggest how pain questionnaires might be used to improve assessment. Although our focus is on the clinical assessment of pain, we describe how similar pain assessment procedures can be used in such areas as clinical trials, quality assurance, and prevalence surveys. We deal here only with information that can be obtained by questionnaires, interview, and observation of the patient; however, pain assessment should include a medical evaluation and the possible addition of appropriate diagnostic procedures. A retrospective survey of patients with cancer (Gonzales, Elliot, Portenoy, & Foley, 1991) found that two-thirds of patients referred for pain assessment had new (and often treatable) pathology diagnosed as a result of the medical evaluation and follow-up.

PREVALENCE OF CANCER PAIN

Cancer is a generic term, applied to a variety of different diseases that have in common mutation of cell development leading to unregulated prolif-

eration of cell growth, which in turn results in invasion and metastases. The primary site and cell type of a cancer dictates many of its features, including rate of development; response to anticancer therapies; common sites of metastatic spread of disease; and the location, course, and quality of pain. An international study of patients with advanced cancer found that one-half of patients with lung and breast cancer had at least moderate pain. Prevalence of moderate or severe pain was highest in the gynecological cancers, head and neck cancers, and prostate cancer (Vainio & Auvinen, 1996).

Clinicians have long been aware that the majority of patients with cancer who are near the end of life will need pain management, but less attention has been paid to the problem of pain prior to the end stage of disease. Surveys of patients with nonmetastatic disease (Daut & Cleeland, 1982) and newly diagnosed cancers (Vuorinen, 1993) indicate that from 5% to 24% of patients demonstrate cancer-related pain. Studies of patients with metastatic disease found that between 60% and 80% of patients experience pain (Cleeland et al., 1994; Cleeland, Gonin, Baez, Loehrer, & Pandya, 1997; Portenoy, 1989). Many cancers that were painless at onset will be associated with a high prevalence of pain as the disease progresses. Breast cancer is an excellent example of this. Although it is rarely painful in the early stages, at least half of those affected report pain after metastatic spread of their disease (Cleeland et al., 1994; Foley, 1979). Of the patients who achieve a cure, a substantial percentage will have indefinite periods of treatment-related pain (Andrykowski et al., 1999). For example, surveys of women who undergo breast cancer surgery reveal a high incidence of postmastectomy and postlumpectomy pain (Smith, Bourne, Squair, Phillips, & Chambers, 1999; Wallace, Wallace, Lee, & Dobke, 1996). Because at least 60% of patients now survive cancer, while many live longer with more aggressive treatments, greater numbers of patients have to face extended periods of coping with pain from their cancer or its treatments (American Cancer Society, 1999).

PHYSICAL BASIS OF CANCER PAIN

Pain in patients with cancer can be due to diverse causes (Payne, 1990; Portenoy, 1999). Furthermore, multiple pain sources often coexist. Since treatment will be determined by the etiology of the pain, establishing the physical cause of the pain is an important goal of assessment. In a prospective study of over 2,000 patients with cancer referred to a pain service, 70% of the patients had pain due to multiple sources (Grond, Zech, Diefenbach, Radbruch, & Lehmann, 1996). In this study, the sources of pain were classified as (in decreasing frequency) soft tissue invasion, bone pain, nerve damage or infiltration, and visceral pain. Other studies have found that bone pain and visceral pain are the most frequent etiologies of cancer pain (Banning, Sjogren, & Henriksen, 1991; Caraceni, Portenoy, & Working Group of the IASP Task Force on Cancer Pain, 1999; Foley, 1979).

Many patients will have pain caused by cancer treatments (Caraceni et al., 1999; Chapman, Kornell, & Syrjala, 1987; Grond et al., 1996). By necessity, cancer treatment is destructive, whether it takes the form of surgery, chemotherapy, or radiation therapy. Pain is often the product of these destructive procedures. Some treatment-related pain is time-limited, while in other cases a more permanent treatment-related pain syndrome such as peripheral neuropathy may develop. Although pain generally becomes worse with progress of the disease, pain can also improve if the disease is responsive to anticancer therapies, such as chemotherapy, radiotherapy, or biological therapies.

An important distinction needs to be made between primary *nociceptive pain* (pain caused by stimulation of pain receptors) and *neuropathic pain* (painful sensations that are caused by an injury or dysfunction of peripheral or central nervous system structures). Many cancer pain syndromes involve both neuropathic and nociceptive pain (Martin & Hagen, 1997). Since pain syndromes that include neuropathic pain and syndromes involving only nociceptive pain often respond to different pharmacological interventions, it is crucial to specify the types of pain involved in each clinical circumstance.

THE CONTEXT OF CANCER PAIN ASSESSMENT

Historically, most pain assessment procedures were developed for patients with pain due to nonmalignant causes (Syrjala & Chapman, 1984). Pain assessment evolved along with the development of multidisciplinary pain clinics that, for the most part, treated patients with reasonably stable pain complaints. These patients commonly reported pain as their primary health problem. The assessment of pain due to cancer requires some reorientation, dictated by the nature of the disease, the types of

pain that cancer causes, and the medical and psychosocial context of having cancer. The dynamic and progressive nature of both the disease and its treatment must be integrated concurrently with treatment of the pain. In this context of multiple symptoms, potential organ system and metabolic instabilities, and an intense focus on disease treatment, management of pain can be a moving target, with treatment needs changing rapidly and dramatically.

Because most pain assessment procedures have evolved from the needs of patients with chronic stable pain, it is important to point out some major differences between the majority of patients seen in traditional pain clinics and those seen in cancer treatment settings. Patients seen in multidisciplinary pain clinics most often freely complain of pain, and some treatment programs are designed to reduce the frequency and tenacity of pain complaints because of the negative social consequences of persistent pain reporting.

In contrast, patients with cancer frequently underreport pain and pain severity. A number of patient-related barriers to the assessment of cancer pain have been identified (Thomason et al., 1998; Ward et al., 1993; Ward & Hernandez, 1994). Patients with cancer often do not want to be labeled as complainers, do not want to distract their health care providers from attending to their cancer, or are afraid that their pain means that the cancer is getting worse (Hodes, 1989; Ward et al., 1993). Some patients are fatalistic and believe that pain is an inevitable part of having cancer. Patients are often concerned about having to take potent opioids because they fear that they will become addicts, will be thought of as addicts, will lose control, or will have unmanageable side effects (Ersek, Kraybill, & Du Pen, 1999; Ward et al., 1993). Not surprisingly, in the context of multiple drugs and dosing schedules, other frequently reported barriers include forgetting to take pain medications, high cost, and limited availability of medications (Ersek et al., 1999; Thomason et al., 1998). Some patients are also concerned that they will become tolerant to the effects of analgesics, and therefore that the drugs will be ineffective when the disease progresses (Cleeland, 1989b; Dar, Beach, Barden, & Cleeland, 1992; Ward et al., 1993).

Another major treatment goal for the traditional pain clinic is an increase in patient function and a decrease in negative emotional states. Many patients with noncancer pain are depressed, and it is easy to see how depressed mood may perpetuate their pain. However, only a minority of individuals with cancer-related pain will report significantly depressed mood (Shacham, Dar, & Cleeland, 1984). For those who are depressed, their mood often improves markedly when adequate pain control is established. Psychosocial factors interact to a relatively small extent in predicting incidence and severity of cancer pain (Syrjala & Chapko, 1995). When pain (and not disease) limits function in patients with cancer, significantly improved function will frequently accompany pain relief.

TARGETS OF PAIN ASSESSMENT

For the patient with cancer, what do we need to know about pain in order to plan treatment? In assessing the pain itself, we depend in large measure on patient self-report. In this realm, we need first to know the location for each pain and how severe it is. Guidelines for cancer pain treatment from the Agency for Health Care Policy and Research, the American Pain Society, the National Comprehensive Cancer Network, and the WHO all use a determination of pain severity as the primary item of information in specifying treatment (American Pain Society, 1999; Grossman, Benedetti, Payne, & Syrjala, 1999; Jacox et al., 1994; WHO, 1986, 1996). The recommended analgesics change in type and increase in potency as pain increases in severity.

Location and severity are not the only assessments needed to guide treatment that can be obtained by subjective report. Models of treatment that use a wide range of therapies (such as coanalgesic medications or behavioral interventions) demand more self-report data than pain location and intensity alone. Patients need to be able to report the quality of their pain. They do this by using various descriptors—words such as "aching," "cramping," or "burning."

The temporal pattern (onset, duration, predictability, aggravating factors) of the pain is also important. Is it constant, constant with intermittent exacerbations, or only episodically severe? Information on pain quality and pattern, together with information on the location of the pain, are helpful in determining the physical bases or mechanisms of the pain. Information on physical mechanisms will be useful for choosing among a wide range of analgesic drugs available. Mechanism identification also helps to determine whether nondrug options, including stimulatory, abla-

tive, and cognitive-behavioral measures, should be considered.

An adequate pain assessment will go beyond information on pain characteristics and physical mechanisms. Information about the impact of pain on activities essential to living can be as valuable as severity ratings by indicating the extent to which pain causes disruptions in daily life. Some patients are reluctant to report their pain as severe. A patient who reports pain severity of 3 on a scale of 0–10, but is unable to sleep or walk, may need treatment as urgently as another patient who reports pain at a level of 8. We need to know whether pain interferes with sleep, activity, work, appetite, sociability, and mood. If so, perhaps treatment of pain in isolation will restore these areas of functioning. On the other hand, pain may have persisted for so long that additional treatment options, such as the use of antidepressant medications or supportive and behavioral interventions, need to be employed.

Comprehensive treatment plans also need to be based on information about a patient's and family's beliefs about cancer pain treatment. In many cases, beliefs or experience with analgesic medications will have been established in the patient's or family members' minds. As noted above, these beliefs can determine whether patients will take prescribed medications or whether family members will inhibit or discourage pain treatments. To address these barriers, we must assess the beliefs and past experiences of the patient and family caregivers in regard to pain treatment.

Finally, a medical workup is needed. Most patients have already been treated for pain. We need information about the pain history—how long the pain has existed, what aggravates or alleviates the pain, what treatments did not work or did work, and (for treatments that worked) how long they were effective. A physical exam is required, along with relevant laboratory and imaging tests that are essential to determining etiology, mechanisms, and therefore treatment. Other symptoms also need to be evaluated. Pain treatment frequently causes side effects, and many common symptoms in patients with cancer can confound pain treatment.

PAIN ASSESSMENT MATERIALS

Using standardized, reliable, and validated pain assessment instruments minimizes many patient reporting biases and assists clinicians and researchers in obtaining complete and reliable information. Using pain scales that assign a metric to pain intensity and interference makes pain more of an "objective" symptom, similar to other signs and symptoms such as blood pressure and heart rate. When pain is "measured" in this way, patients feel freer (and more obligated) to report pain presence and severity. Standard measurement also readily allows patients to indicate when treatment is not working. Patients are sometimes less concerned about acknowledging continued severe pain than about implying failure of a treatment attempted by staff members who care for them. "How is your medication working?" provokes a response of "Fine" or "OK" from a patient who wants to please, whereas "Rate your pain from 0 to 10" does not require the patient to judge the success or failure of the health care provider's treatment. Thus assigning a metric to pain allows for monitoring the effectiveness of pain treatment.

Using pain questionnaires or pain measurement scales can also minimize staff time demands and biases. Several recent studies have found that minority patients with cancer are at risk for undertreatment of their pain (Cleeland et al., 1994, 1997). For example, Cleeland and colleagues (1997) found that 65% of a sample of African American and Hispanic outpatients with cancer pain were not receiving adequate analgesic medications, as compared to 38% of a sample of nonminority patients. Using established pain measurement tools reduces the introduction of staff biases related to language, cultural variables, or the unfamiliar style of an individual patient.

One of the greatest, though often unrecognized, values of instruments that a patient can complete just before seeing the health care provider is that this method greatly reduces the amount of staff time required for the assessment process. The medical staff can use the extra time to pursue the specific needs of an individual patient based on the patient's responses to the questionnaire.

Pain Scales

Several ways of scaling the severity or intensity of pain and associated symptoms have been advocated (see Jensen & Karoly, Chapter 2, this volume). Numerical Rating Scales (NRSs) are the most widely used, and are easily adaptable to both clinical and research needs. They typically measure pain severity by asking the patient to select a number from 0 to 10 (an 11-point scale) to represent how severe the pain is. The numbers can be arrayed along a

horizontal line from left to right, with 0 labeled "no pain" and 10 labeled with a phrase such as "pain as bad as can be." Since pain due to cancer can be quite variable over a day, patients can be asked to rate their pain at the time of responding to the questionnaire, and also at its "worst," and "usual" over the last 24 hours.

Verbal Rating Scales (VRSs) have the longest history in pain research (Lasagna, 1980). The patient is asked to pick a category, such as "none," "mild," "moderate," "severe," or "excruciating," that best describes severity. Pain relief can be categorized in a similar way, such as "none," "slight," "moderate," "lots," or "complete." As a research tool, a VRS is limited by unequal distances between descriptors and its dependence on language comprehension.

Visual Analogue Scales (VASs) are often used in clinical research comparing the effectiveness of analgesic drugs and other pain treatments (Wallenstein, 1984). In using a VAS, the patient makes a judgment as to how much of the length of a 10-cm line is equivalent to the severity of the pain. One end of the line represents "no pain" and the other end some concept such as "pain as bad as you can imagine." The advantages of a VAS are the ability to repeat measurement with less influence of past measures than with recall of a number or word, and the potentially infinite number of points on the line. The disadvantages of the VAS are the need to have someone measure the line and the greater number of patients who have difficulty completing this type of pain assessment (Chapman & Syrjala, 2001; Ferraz et al., 1990).

In clinical settings, these three scales of severity approach equivalency (De Conno et al., 1994; Jensen, Karoly, & Braver, 1986), so that ease of use becomes the primary factor in scale selection. All three measures are highly intercorrelated, although the NRS and VAS are most highly correlated with one another (Syrjala, 1987). In clinical trials, the NRS has been found to be more reliable than the VAS, especially with less educated patients (Ferraz et al., 1990). With very sick patients, oral versions of the NRS are easily administered, although the written form is acceptable to most patients. Certain subsets of patients, particularly the elderly and very young, as described below, can have difficulty with the NRS, VAS, or VRS. For these groups, severity scales using faces are effective. Guidelines for pain assessment increasingly recommend the NRS, given its ease of use with the largest proportion of patients.

Pain Questionnaires

There are several pain measurement instruments that incorporate most of the relevant questions and can help to standardize pain assessment. These instruments are short enough to be considered for routine clinical use with patients who have cancer, but have established reliability and validity for research purposes as well. The Brief Pain Inventory (BPI; Cleeland, 1989a) was designed to assess pain in patients with cancer (see Appendix 30.A). Using 0–10 NRSs, the BPI asks patients to rate the severity of their pain at its "worst," "least," "average," and "now." Again using NRSs, in this case with 0 being "no interference" and 10 being "interferes completely," the BPI asks for ratings of how much pain interferes with mood, walking, general activity, work, relations with others, sleep, and enjoyment of life. The BPI also asks patients to indicate the location of their pain on a pain drawing, and asks about treatments for pain and the extent of pain relief. In a somewhat longer form, the BPI provides a list of descriptors to help the patient describe pain quality. The short form of the BPI is widely used for frequent pain monitoring in clinical settings and in clinical trials.

A short form of the McGill Pain Questionnaire (SF-MPQ) has been developed (Melzack, 1987; see aslo Melzack & Katz, Chapter 3, this volume) for assessments using verbal descriptors. The main component of the SF-MPQ consists of 15 descriptors (11 in the sensory domain, 4 in the affective domain) that are rated on an intensity scale as 0 = "none," 1 = "mild," 2 = "moderate," or 3 = "severe." Three pain scores are derived from the sums of the intensity ratings of the sensory, affective, and total descriptors. The SF-MPQ also includes the Present Pain Intensity (PPI) index of the standard MPQ and a VAS. VASs have been adapted for repeated clinical use in the Memorial Pain Assessment Card (MPAC; Fishman et al., 1987). The MPAC consists of three VASs, for pain intensity, pain relief, and mood, and one VRS. The MPAC and SF-MPQ are valuable scales, but do not include all of the core information we have defined as necessary for a brief but complete assessment of cancer pain. Missing components are the location of pain, impact, pattern, and pain history.

A one-page checklist can summarize the core information needed in clinical care. The example provided in Appendix 30.B includes the basic components of assessment necessary if cancer pain intensity is 4 or above on the 0–10 "worst pain" scale: severity of worst and usual pain, location of pain(s), quality, pattern, impact, and other symptoms. This brief form has been used effectively to facilitate patients' communication with health care providers (Syrjala et al., 1996). The form takes only a few minutes to complete, requires no writing, and provides the basic information needed, saving face-to-face time for focusing on problems rather than on routine assessment. A second checklist can be used to readily indicate which beliefs might disrupt patient adherence with pain treatment (see Appendix 30.C).

Patient and Family Education

Patient and family education is usually not thought of as part of the assessment process, but it is a natural corollary and consequence of adequate assessment. For patients with cancer pain, it is critical to recognize the reluctance they may have to report pain and to contact their health care providers if they do not get pain relief. Patients must be active partners in their pain assessment and treatment. They need to be made aware that many myths about addiction, rapid development of tolerance, and unmanageable side effects associated with opioid analgesics do not apply to the majority of patients with cancer. They have to be assured that in most instances pain relief can be obtained, and that it is part of the health care professional's role to provide that relief.

Assessment is the first step in education. Patients learn how to use numbers and descriptions to report pain. In this process, they learn that their information is essential to determining proper treatment. They see that the outcome of assessment is improved treatment, and this facilitates ongoing communication with their health care providers.

Assessment, along with educating patients about cancer pain, improves the outcome of pain treatment. Several randomized clinical trials with patients who had cancer and were experiencing pain found that brief education on pain management produced significant reductions in pain intensity ratings (De Wit et al., 1997; Syrjala et al., 1996). Many tools exist to assist clinicians in rapid education of patients; therefore, this effort ultimately saves time and improves treatment outcome.

PAIN ASSESSMENT PROCEDURE

Working within the typical limitations of a cancer treatment setting, pain assessment needs to be focused on those aspects of pain that will lead to differential treatment decisions. Rarely will there be the professional time or patient acceptance or endurance to complete the type of assessment typically done in multidisciplinary pain clinics. It may be helpful to think of cancer pain assessment in terms of a decision analysis model. Some branches of the decision tree need not be followed if appropriate screening does not indicate a treatment need. We have broken the assessment procedure into three steps. Although we would consider a comprehensive assessment to include screening at all steps, we have assigned step 1 the highest priority.

Step 1: Assessing Pain Severity

Standard assessment of the multidimensional aspects of cancer pain makes it clear that pain severity is the primary factor determining the impact of pain on the patient and the urgency of the treatment process. Many adults, both with and without cancer, function quite effectively with a background level of pain that does not seriously impair them. As pain severity increases, however, it passes a threshold beyond which it cannot be ignored and becomes disruptive to many aspects of a patient's life. At very high levels, pain becomes a primary focus of attention and prohibits most non-pain-related

activity (Serlin, Mendoza, Nakamura, Edwards, & Cleeland, 1995). Figure 30.1 presents the method for assessment of pain severity.

Simple pain scales make it possible to assess pain on each outpatient contact and at least once every 24-hour period for a patient in the hospital (or more frequently if pain is severe). Since pain in cancer is often progressive, sometimes rapidly so, pain assessment is a recursive procedure. The model presented should be thought of as being repeated until optimal pain control is achieved. In Figure 30.1, we have defined *mild, moderate,* and *severe* pain as ranges of patient response to a numerical rating of pain at its "worst" or "usual." These categories of pain severity are based on the degree of interference with function associated with each category (Serlin et al., 1995).

Mild pain (1–4 "worst" pain; 1–3 "usual" pain) that is previously untreated may call for a "mild" analgesic (acetaminophen or a nonsteroidal anti-inflammatory) or a "moderate" analgesic (such as hydrocodone or oxycodone) (Grossman et al., 1999). This is the optimal time for education about the need to report pain when it occurs, when it gets worse, or if it is not relieved by current treatment. A mild pain level requires the least assessment, since it causes the least interference with function. However, the clinician must evaluate the nature of the pain problem. In clinical practice, it is valuable to also assess the impact of pain

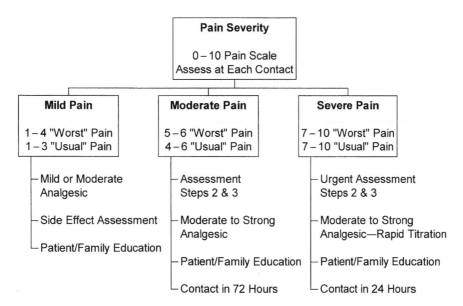

FIGURE 30.1. Step 1: Assessment of cancer pain.

when the level is 3 or 4, since a small proportion of patients will underrepresent their pain levels. Also, if the pain etiology and syndrome are understood, the clinician can determine whether the pain is likely to be progressive or subject to frequent exacerbations.

Moderate pain (5–6 "worst" pain, 4–6 "usual" pain) mandates steps 2 and 3 of the assessment process and calls for a more aggressive analgesic program. Since pain at this level impairs multiple areas of function, a follow-up contact should be made within 72 hours to assess the efficacy of the pain treatment provided. For patients at home, this requires a phone call.

When pain is *severe* (7–10 "worst" or "usual" pain), the protocol is similar to that for moderate pain, except that the analgesic selection and titration need to be aggressive, and follow-up contact (reassessment) needs to occur more quickly—within 24 hours after the initial assessment is made. In some cases, pain at this level constitutes a pain emergency and mandates hospital admission for more rapid medical workup and intravenous (IV) analgesic titration.

Step 2: Assessing Pain Characteristics

Information about aspects of cancer pain other than its severity will help refine treatment plans. Much of this information can also be gathered through the use of standard questionnaires, which guide the patient's subjective reports of these additional characteristics. Further information will need to be obtained by clinical interview. The essential elements of step 2 are presented in Figure 30.2.

Pain Location

Aiding the patient in describing the location(s) of the pain he or she is experiencing is an essential part of pain assessment. This is most easily accomplished by asking the patient to mark on a body drawing the location(s) of pain. The patient is given front and back views of a human figure and is asked to shade in his or her areas of pain. This can provide a wealth of information about possible physical mechanisms contributing to the pain. It may also help to determine why pain is more of a problem with particular movements or positions. For example, patients may draw the pain in the distribution of a particular nerve, suggesting that the mechanism of pain is tumor impingement on that nerve.

Temporal Pattern of the Pain

Not all cancer pain remains at a constant level over a 24-hour period. Whereas most pain is felt constantly, with periodic increases, some pain occurs only episodically. Some patients will have significant *incident pain*, or exacerbation of their pain with movement. Incident pain is common when the pathological process responsible for the pain is influenced by movement or position (e.g., pain in the back or near a joint). Some types of pain (especially neuropathic pain) may have periods when pain spontaneously becomes more intense. These

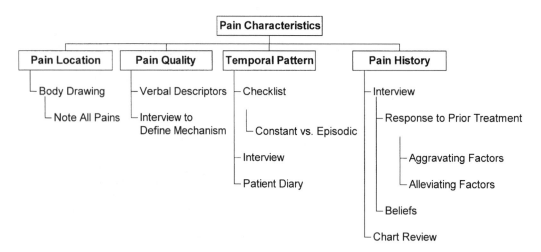

FIGURE 30.2. Step 2: Assessment of cancer pain.

periodic increases in pain are often referred to as *breakthrough pain*, defined as a transitory increase in pain occurring in the context of stable baseline pain (Portenoy & Hagen, 1990). It is standard practice to include additional analgesia for the patient to take during breakthrough or incident episodes, or even before episodes if it is possible to anticipate when they will occur. For some patients, however, the presence of breakthrough pain consistently prior to the next around-the-clock dose of medication may indicate only that the dose or potency of the analgesic is inadequate (Petzke, Radbruch, Zech, Loick, & Grond, 1999).

The temporal pattern of pain is often clearly described by the patient in an interview. Some checklists, such as those in Appendix 30.B, provide this information. If patients are unsure of the pattern or timing of increased pain, it may be necessary to have them rate their pain along with medication use in a log book or diary for a 1- to 7-day period to determine its pattern.

Pain Quality

Pain of different etiologies produces differences in the patient's subjective experience of the pain (see Table 30.1). For example, pain caused by destruction of nerve pathways may be described as "numb," "pins and needles," "burning," or "shooting." Pain from tumor destruction of soft tissue or bone is often described as "aching." Some pain problems can be mixed and include multiple characteristics (Grossman et al., 1999). Establishing the qualities of a pain is an essential part of establishing the physical basis of the pain, which will in turn determine the types of therapies to be used. For example, neuropathic pain is often less responsive to opioid medications than nociceptive pain and may be relieved by other types of medications, such as antidepressants or anticonvulsants.

TABLE 30.1. Verbal Descriptors of Pain

Neuropathic etiology	Somatic etiology	Visceral etiology
Burning	Aching	Cramping
Shooting	Throbbing	Gnawing
Pins and needles	Stabbing	Sharp
Numb	Pressure/heavy	Aching
"Electric"		

People often find it difficult to describe their pain spontaneously. Word lists of potential descriptors can help a patient portray pain quality. Some questionnaires, such as the long form of the BPI, the SF-MPQ, and the Patient Pain Checklist in Appendix 30.B, include lists of words for the patient to select from.

Pain History

The patient's response to prior pain treatment and prognosis are additional variables that need to be considered in both patient management and clinical research. When one is assessing response to prior analgesic treatments, the patient's adherence to his or her prescribed analgesic medications must be determined, along with beliefs that might dictate future adherence. A recent study of outpatients with cancer-related pain found that patients adhered to their opioid therapy only 62%–72% of the time at all study time points (Du Pen et al., 1998). Nonadherence was significantly correlated with higher levels of symptom distress and lower quality-of-life scores. In interviews examining why patients did not take analgesics prescribed, side effects were the most common reasons, but other beliefs such as addiction fear also influenced patient choices (Ersek et al.,1999). Thus it is important to determine whether a patient has taken or plans to take his or her analgesic medications as prescribed, and if not, why. Patients may not understand their analgesic regimen or the importance of taking pain medication on a regular basis, or cost may inhibit use. Careful assessment of the reasons for nonadherence can identify targets for patient education.

Treatments that have been tried or other factors that alleviate or aggravate pain can help to determine both pain etiology and the next treatment steps. For example, patients who have more pain while lying down might be helped with elevated bed positions, special beds, or other physical therapies that can greatly enhance quality of sleep, waking, and pain relief.

Patients who have been adherent to aggressive analgesic regimens but whose pain has been refractory present difficult management problems. Pain that is severe and changing rapidly may require immediate laboratory and imaging studies to diagnose fracture, infection, obstruction, epidural metastases, or other medical emergencies. Patients whose pain does not respond to oral medications or patients with unacceptable side effects may require alternate routes of analgesic administration (epidural, intrathecal, subcutaneous). Such patients will obviously require greater clinical assessment. Prognosis, concurrent symptoms, ongoing disease treatment, and organ system complications may influence pain treatment choices. For example, if pain has a predictable course as a result of cancer therapy, treatment methods may anticipate that course (e.g., use of IV patient-controlled analgesia with an opioid at the start of mucositis pain).

Step 3: Assessing Pain Impact

Step 3 of pain assessment (see Figure 30.3) measures the degree to which pain interferes with areas of the patient's life, and the degree to which other symptoms or problems interact with pain to disrupt the patient's pain relief or functioning. The suggested assessment methods are again tailored to elicit information that will lead to specific treatment recommendations. Whenever pain is moderate to severe or pain is concurrent with other symptoms, an effective intervention for pain control should be based on evaluation of more than pain severity and pain mechanism. As examples, if a patient suffers from uncontrolled nausea, an oral opioid may exacerbate nausea. The patient therefore may require an antiemetic a half-hour before the opioid, or, alternatively, the patient may need a nonoral route of administration. If a patient has relatively good pain control, but only when he or she is lying down, treatment may be inadequate. A review of only pain severity and mechanism might inappropriately indicate adequate treatment has been prescribed. As these examples demonstrate, step 3 assessments for chronic cancer pain can provide valuable information even when pain appears mild on initial screening.

Assessing Quality of Life

Innumerable studies have defined the extent to which unrelieved cancer pain broadly affects a patient's quality of life (QOL), from physical function to sleep, mood, and social interaction. *Health-related QOL* has been defined as the perceived value of life as modified by impairments, functional states, perceptions, and social opportunities influenced by disease, injury, treatment, or policy (Patrick & Erickson, 1993). The measurement of QOL for patients with cancer has received much research attention during the past decade and is part of the context in which cancer pain must be understood.

The BPI provides a synopsis of areas of pain interference with functioning. A recent study of Chinese patients with cancer found that pain interference ratings on the BPI were significantly correlated with ratings on a standardized QOL questionnaire (Wang et al., 1999). Moreover, pain intensity ratings were a significant predictor of QOL, even after disease severity was controlled for. The BPI interference items provide valuable information related to QOL and may be adequate in many cases. However, the BPI does not indicate the extent to which functioning or QOL is impaired by nonpain factors.

Extensive work has been done to define and test measures of QOL related to cancer (Cella, 1996; Moinpour, 1994; Spilker, 1996). The results of these efforts can now benefit the clinician or researcher by vastly reducing the patient burden demanded to measure separately each of the QOL domains that may interact with pain assessment and treatment. Although it is beyond the scope of this chapter to review the entire field of instruments available to measure QOL, several measures have been selected for review. The measures described

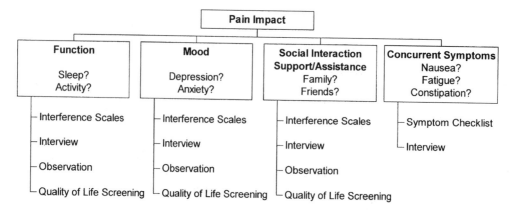

FIGURE 30.3. Step 3: Assessment of cancer pain.

below include evaluation of physical functioning, psychological status, social relationships, and (in most cases) symptoms. These domains have been identified repeatedly as minimum requirements for adequate QOL assessment (Cella, 1994; Gill & Feinstein, 1994; O'Boyle & Waldron, 1997). These domains also coincide with those listed under step 3 of our pain assessment model: functioning, mood, social interaction, and concurrent symptoms.

The European Organization for Research and Treatment of Cancer Quality of Life Questionnaire (EORTC-QLQ; Aaronson, Bullinger, & Ahmedzai, 1988) has 28 items plus 2 global QOL items. Disease- or problem-specific modules (e.g., a lung cancer supplement) can be added to the scale (Bergman, Aaronson, Ahmedzai, Kaasa, & Sullivan, 1994). The core questionnaire includes functional and symptom subscales, an overall QOL assessment, and a question about financial concerns. The EORTC-QLQ has good psychometric properties and has been used successfully in clinical trials with patients who have cancer (Aaronson et al., 1993; Herndon et al., 1999). Advantages of the scale include its careful, conceptually based construction and its conciseness.

The Functional Assessment of Cancer Therapy (FACT) measurement system is a comprehensive group of scales that measure health-related QOL in patients with cancer or other chronic illnesses (Cella et al., 1993). The 34–item general version (FACT-G) contains five subscales that assess physical, functional, social/family, and emotional well-being, and the patient's relationship with the physician. Other subscales may be added to the FACT-G to address issues specific to a disease site, treatment, or symptom. The FACT-G instrument and the multiple available subscales demonstrate good reliability and validity (Cella et al., 1993).

Several psychometrically sound QOL instruments were developed from the Medical Outcomes Study (MOS). Two broad QOL tools are the 36-Item Short-Form Health Survey (SF-36) and the 12-Item Short-Form Health Survey (SF-12) (Ware, Kosinski, & Keller, 1995; Ware & Sherbourne, 1992). These instruments include sections assessing physical functioning, role functioning, social functioning, mental health, health perceptions, and pain. The SF-36 is reliable and has been validated in widely diverse populations (Stewart & Ware, 1992; Wang et al., 1999). Similarly, the SF-12 demonstrates sound psychometric properties, although the subscale scores may be less reliable due to the limited number of items. A particular advantage of these scales is the avail-ability of normative data for comparison with research samples.

One of the above-described QOL measures will provide a good screening tool to determine factors that may be interacting with pain problems. Such a screening tool will indicate the further need to assess mood, concurrent symptoms, social support, or function. A QOL scale can be combined with the BPI and a symptom assessment instrument (see below) to evaluate patients with moderate to severe pain. In the areas of psychological functioning and concurrent symptoms, one of the QOL scales alone is unlikely to be sufficient to determine treatment needs, but it should be adequate to identify the need for further follow-up.

Function

The measures described above—the BPI, FACT, EORTC-QLQ, and SF-36 or SF-12—are designed to assess function in particular detail. The BPI measures function related to pain; the other measures do not assign a source for interference with function, measuring instead the level of activity a patient is able to perform. Both aspects of function may be relevant if a patient is ambulatory and likely to be living with pain for some time.

Mood

The majority of patients with cancer adjust to the stresses of the disease and its symptoms without diagnosable anxiety, depression, or other psychiatric disorders (Derogatis et al., 1983; Shacham et al., 1984). However, patients with pain report significantly more depression and anxiety than do those without pain (Ahles, Blanchard, & Ruckdeschel, 1983; Glover, Dibble, Dodd, & Miaskowski, 1995; Heim & Oei, 1993). Among the many symptoms possible during the course of cancer, mood disorders can be among the most difficult to identify. Difficulty in recognizing mood disruptions results from the similarity of presentation of some mood symptoms and common disease-related somatic complaints such as fatigue and weight loss. An assessment of mood can be cursorily accomplished with the QOL measures or the BPI. If these measures suggest that mood disturbance exists, we recommend further assessment of mood, either with one of the many available highly standardized tools or with a clinical interview.

In our experience, assessment of mood in patients with cancer and pain requires a focus on the affective components of mood disturbance, with somewhat more cautious evaluation of cognitive and behavioral components, and with awareness of (but not emphasis on) somatic components. It can be difficult, if not impossible, to be certain of the etiology of somatic symptoms; thus empirical approaches are sometimes needed. In other words, if pain is moderate or severe, it should be treated first, and then other possible pharmacological or organic contributors to mood should be evaluated. Next, the psychological symptoms should be treated, even if medical complications or disease progression contribute to the symptoms.

Social Interaction

Social relationships are acknowledged to be very important to the functioning and well-being of patients with cancer (Dunkel-Shetter, 1984; Wortman, 1984). Nonetheless, social support has been one of the most difficult areas for investigators to measure (Moinpour et al., 1989). In our experience, patients with cancer tend to rate their supports very positively, resulting in a ceiling effect for measurement. The QOL instruments or the BPI provide an initial screen of social support or pain interference with social interaction. A clinician assessing a patient with moderate to severe pain will want to also consider the availability of a family caregiver to assist the patient with prescribed treatments and to provide help if needed. Knowing the availability of assistance and support, as well as the beliefs of family members related to pain treatment, can be as important as the assessment of the patient.

Concurrent Symptoms

Patients with both cancer and pain are liable to have other symptoms that need management and complicate the treatment picture. The negative side effects of analgesic drugs are numerous, especially if aggressive side effect prophylaxis and management are not included in treatment plans. These side effects can be more disturbing than pain and can entirely disrupt even the best analgesic plan, resulting in patient nonadherence (Ersek et al., 1999). The most common negative side effects of analgesic treatment include constipation, nausea, fatigue, and sedation. These must be assessed routinely.

Cancer, especially as it advances, will produce fatigue, weakness, cachexia, and often cognitive deficits. Disease treatment will produce fatigue, along with tissue damage and possibly nausea and vomiting. These symptoms can produce pain or other unpleasant alterations in somatic sensations (Chapko, Syrjala, Schilter, Cummings, & Sullivan, 1989). Other symptoms, regardless of their etiology, can negatively affect mood and function, as can pain itself.

Many symptoms can be treated, either pharmacologically or behaviorally. At a minimum, a checklist of potential concurrent symptoms, such as the M. D. Anderson Symptom Inventory (Cleeland et al., 2000) or the Memorial Symptom Assessment Scale (Portenoy et al., 1994), needs to be included at this step of assessment. As with pain, it is important to evaluate these symptoms over time in order to monitor changes in severity and response to treatment. Successful treatment of pain requires concurrent treatment of other symptoms.

Interview Assessment of Pain Impact

The physical exam is a cornerstone of pain assessment. As part of this exam, a clinician can gather information on physical, emotional, and social functioning from an interview format. The advantages of an interview are that some patients will feel more understood or perceive fewer burdens with this format. In addition, an area in which a patient indicates no disruption does not have to be pursued. The danger is, of course, the converse: An area may be missed because either the interviewer or the patient determines that no problem exists, thus short-circuiting the evaluation. Suicidal ideation is a risk for patients with severe uncontrolled pain and can best be assessed in an interview.

The interview can also be used to screen for individual factors that might interact with pain or its treatment, beliefs that would disrupt treatment, or a history of heavy drug or alcohol use. Individuals with active or past substance abuse or dependence should not be denied appropriate treatment for their pain, and experience indicates that their pain can be managed successfully with appropriate medications and methods. The purpose of screening is to identify patients who may need additional psychosocial assessment and treatment, as well as monitoring of their analgesia and medication use.

OBSERVATION OF PAIN IMPACT

Observation measures within the field of cancer have historically focused on global measures of functioning. The most well-known of these is the Karnofsky Performance Status (Karnofsky, Abelmann, Craver, & Burchenal, 1948), but other, similar 5- or 10-point global assessments are available, such as the ECOG Performance Status scale (Morrow et al., 1981; Oken et al., 1982; Spitzer et al., 1981; Zubrod et al., 1960). These scales have good interrater reliabilities, but are not useful for specifying difficulties or determining treatment needs. Their primary value seems to be as outcome measures for clinical trials. Observer ratings are also available for more specific activities of daily living (Selby, Chapman, Etazadi-Amoli, Dalley, & Boyd, 1984; Spector, 1990), for behaviors related to coping with pain (Wilkie, Keefe, Dodd, & Copp, 1992), and for well behaviors (Chapko, Syrjala, Bush, Jedlow, & Yanke, 1991). These measures are less psychometrically well described. We would suggest observer ratings only in cases where patients are unable to provide their own self-report or in combination with self-report.

PAIN ASSESSMENT IN CHILDREN WITH CANCER

In most clinical settings, pain assessment in children with cancer is even more neglected than in adults with cancer (Ljungman et al., 1996). Assessment is often more difficult because the assessment has to be tailored to the developmental stage of the child. There is a consensus, however, that age-appropriate assessment techniques exist that are reliable and well validated (Beyer & Wells, 1989; McGrath, 1990; see also McGrath & Gillespie, Chapter 6). The WHO (1998) has developed guidelines for the assessment and treatment of cancer-related pain in children. These guidelines recommend regular assessment and documentation of a child's pain level as an essential vital sign. As for an adult, treatment recommendations are based on the child's pain level.

The assessment of pain in infants often relies on physiological measures and observer reports of behaviors that indicate probable pain. Developmentally appropriate pain intensity measures can be used with toddlers and preschool children. Various types of pain intensity measures are available for young children, including pain thermometers (Jay, Ozolins, Elliott, & Caldwell, 1983), color scales (Eland, 1981), and facial scales (McGrath et al., 1996). Children over the age of 5 also can be given standard NRSs and VASs (McGrath et al., 1990). VRSs may be more difficult for children to use.

A number of facial scales have been administered to children from the ages of 2 to adolescence (Beyer, 1984; Bieri, Reeve, Champion, Addicoat, & Ziegler, 1990; P. A. McGrath, de Veber, & Hearn, 1985). A facial scale usually consists of a series of drawings of faces or pictures whose expressions range from neutral or smiling to sad and suffering (see, e.g., the Faces Pain Scale in Figure 30.4). Children are asked to select a face that describes how their pain feels. Pediatric patients with cancer are able to use a facial scale to rate their pain intensity (P. A. McGrath et al., 1985).

Parents and health care providers often are asked to provide ratings of children's pain. However, multiple studies have found poor agreement between parent or provider ratings and children's self-reports of pain (Chambers et al., 1998; Manne, Jacobsen, & Redd, 1992; Miser, Dothage, Wesley, & Miser, 1987). A child's self-report of pain should be considered the "gold standard" of pediatric pain assessment, as it is with an adult, and should be used whenever possible. However, behavioral observations are critical in pain assessment of very young children and in children who do not have the ability to report their pain due to disability or disease. When behavioral observations are necessary, the use of a standardized system and trained raters is recommended. Several reliable, valid behavioral observation methods have been developed for the assessment of pediatric behaviors related

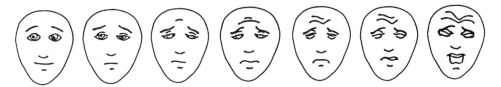

FIGURE 30.4. Faces Pain Scale for use with children, elderly patients, and any other patients unable to complete NRSs. Reprinted from *Pain, 41,* D. Bieri, R. A. Reeve, G. D. Champion, L. Addicoat, and J. B. Ziegler, The Faces Pain Scale for the self-assessment of the severity of pain experienced by children: Development, initial validation, and preliminary investigation for ratio scale properties, 139–150. Copyright 1990, with permission from Elsevier Science.

to pain, such as crying, clinging, and reduction in normal activity (Gauvain-Piquard et al., 1991; P. J. McGrath et al., 1985; Tarbell, Cohen, & Marsh, 1992).

The three steps of assessment outlined in this chapter should work equally well for children, with the provisions recommended by the WHO (1998) guidelines. In addition, a special panel of the American Academy of Pediatrics has suggested that a Pain Problem List be formulated for every child with cancer (McGrath et al., 1990). The goal of this list is to identify problems amenable to treatment, and to be sure that the multiple sources and dimensions of pain are addressed.

PAIN ASSESSMENT IN ELDERLY PATIENTS WITH CANCER

Sixty percent of all cancers occur in persons aged 65 years and older (Yancik, 1997). Because the prevalence of cancer increases with age, many elderly individuals have to deal with this life-threatening illness and its related symptoms. Several recent studies have found that elderly patients are at risk for undertreatment of cancer-related pain. In a survey of outpatients with metastatic cancer who were experiencing pain, Cleeland and colleagues (1994) found that patients 70 years of age and older were more likely to receive inadequate analgesics than younger patients. Similarly, a survey of over 13,000 nursing home residents with cancer found that 26% of the patients experiencing daily pain received no analgesics (Bernabei et al., 1998).

The undertreatment of cancer pain in the elderly is often due to lack of assessment or inadequate assessment. In the nursing home study by Bernabei and colleagues (1998), regular pain assessments were not included in most patient charts. However, 86% of the patients, including cognitively impaired individuals, were able to verbally report pain to the research staff. Similarly, Ferrell, Ferrell, and Rivera (1995) found that 83% of elderly patients in a nursing home setting could complete at least one pain intensity scale.

The three steps of assessment outlined in this chapter apply to elderly as well as younger patients. However, many elderly patients require careful instruction and practice in the use of pain assessment instruments. Prior to assessing pain, all elderly patients should be screened to identify any sensory, motor, and/or cognitive deficits that affect their ability to report pain and related symptoms (see Gagliese, Chapter 7, and Hadjistavropoulos, von Baeyer, & Craig, Chapter 8). Pain scales should be printed with large letters and scales to accommodate patients with limited visual abilities. The Faces Pain Scale (Figure 30.4) can be used for individuals who have difficulty understanding NRS or VAS formats (Herr, Mobily, Kohout, & Wagenaar, 1998). Pain assessment instruments can also be administered in an oral format for patients who have visual or motor impairments that prevent completion of paper-and-pencil measures. Clinicians and researchers should be aware of possible hearing and visual impairments and assess whether elderly patients are able to comprehend instructions (Herr & Mobily, 1991). When cognitive deficits are severe and prevent self-report of pain, observation of pain-related behaviors is an alternative strategy. An observation system to assess pain behaviors in elderly nursing home patients is a promising approach that needs further development (Weiner, Peterson, & Keefe, 1999).

In sum, the measurement of pain in elderly patients with cancer involves special considerations and challenges that researchers and clinicians are beginning to address. The substantial growth of the elderly population mandates continued work in this area.

OTHER APPLICATIONS OF CANCER PAIN MEASUREMENT

Cancer pain measurement forms the basis of several applications in addition to clinical assessment, including the epidemiology of cancer pain, efforts to assure the quality of pain management, and the conduct of clinical trials examining the effectiveness of cancer pain treatments. A brief review of these areas will illustrate the application of pain assessment techniques.

Epidemiology of Cancer Pain

Attempts to estimate the number of patients with cancer and pain, and to determine the impact and severity of this pain, depend upon accurate pain assessment. Studies published in the last 10 years using pain severity rating scales have documented that pain continues to be a problem for large numbers of patients with metastatic cancer (Caraceni et al., 1999; Cleeland et al., 1994, 1997; Grond et al., 1996). These studies have forced us to reevaluate the association between disease stage and the onset of pain due to cancer. In the past, pain was typically associated with end stage cancers, but we now realize that significant pain can be present for long periods of time, with a majority of patients with metastatic disease having pain at this level (Cleeland et al., 1994). Even if we exclude patients who survive cancer but have persistent posttreatment pain, the numbers of patients with cancer who have significant pain will be in the hundreds of thousands. Prevalence studies have demonstrated that cancer pain is a national health problem of the highest priority and have influenced national and international health policy planning (Jacox et al., 1994; WHO, 1986, 1996).

Pain Measurement for Quality Assurance

Patients with cancer should be guaranteed the best possible pain management; therefore, poorly treated pain is a quality assurance issue. The development of specific practice guidelines for pain management has led to quality assurance standards for pain treatment (American Pain Society, 1999; Jacox et al., 1994). In addition, the Joint Committee on Accreditation of Healthcare Organizations has developed standards for the assessment and management of pain. Hospitals and other health care facilities are expected to demonstrate compliance with these standards when they are reviewed for accreditation. The standards include the regular assessment and recording of patients' pain levels. Pain assessment tools provide a method for routine monitoring and charting of pain in the hospital or clinic setting. NRSs seem best suited for easy tracking of pain.

Innovative educational programs have been developed to improve pain assessment and treatment in health care institutions. A model pain management program for the treatment of cancer pain included formation of a quality improvement team, staff education, pain rounds, and focus groups to discuss cancer pain (Bookbinder et al., 1996). Procedures were established for monitoring pain assessment and treatment, as well as triggers for automatic review of pain management procedures. Following implementation of the model program, improvements were found in patients' satisfaction with pain treatment and nurses' knowledge of pain management.

The Cancer Pain Role Model Program, developed by the Wisconsin Cancer Pain Initiative in 1990, has trained over 1,000 health care professionals in the United States (Janjan et al., 1996; Weissman & Dahl, 1995; Weissman, Griffie, Gordon, & Dahl, 1997). Health care professionals who participate in the program receive intensive education in cancer pain management and are asked to develop an action plan to facilitate improved pain assessment and treatment in their own institutions.

Clinical Trials Applications

A major barrier to cancer pain treatment has been a lack of controlled clinical trials in cancer pain management. Most of our information about the effectiveness of analgesics has come from the single-dose acute analgesic assay model (Wallenstein, 1984). In this model, a test drug and a standard or placebo drug are studied in randomized, double-blind designs. These elegant single-dose studies have provided the basis for judging the comparative effectiveness of various analgesics.

Patients with cancer-related pain typically take repeated doses of analgesics on a long-term basis. Controlled clinical trials of longer duration are necessary to evaluate the effectiveness of analgesics, nonpharmacological interventions for pain control, and treatments involving multiple methods (Cleeland et al., 1986). Several recent studies evaluating cancer pain treatments provide examples of well-designed clinical trials of longer duration than single-dose studies. These clinical trials have successfully employed psychometrically sound pain assessment instruments at multiple time points (Du Pen et al., 1999; Syrjala et al., 1996; Trowbridge et al., 1997). For example, one such randomized trial evaluated the effectiveness of a pain education intervention, using a videotape, a written handbook, and a brief face-to-face review, for ambulatory patients with advanced cancer (Syrjala et al., 1996). Pain was assessed 1, 3, and 6 months after the intervention with the BPI. The results demonstrated that educating patients about pain and teaching them how to report pain to their health care providers improved pain control and communication about pain for the intervention group. Another clinical trial evaluated the inclusion of pain assessment information from the BPI in the charts of patients in the intervention group (Trowbridge et al., 1997). The physicians who treated the patients in the intervention group were more likely to increase analgesic doses, and the patients were more likely to report a decrease in the incidence of pain, as compared to patients in a standard treatment control group.

Clinical trials in cancer pain management generate the need for some special considerations. Since cancer pain is progressive, often rapidly so, planning for the duration of the trial must consider the possibility that disease progression will obscure real differences in the treatments being contrasted. Furthermore, enrolling patients with pain that is severe enough to demonstrate treatment effects usually requires selection of patients with pain from advanced disease. Missing data due to illness and mortality become major factors in study design and outcome analysis that can seriously hinder evaluation of treatment efficacy (Du Pen et al., 1998; Syrjala et al., 1996).

CONCLUSION

Although most patients with cancer-related pain should be able to get pain relief, the pain of many such patients is poorly managed. Inadequate pain assessment is most often the reason. In the typical cancer care setting, health care professionals rarely have training in pain assessment, nor do they have time for the assessment typical in multidisciplinary pain clinics. Patients may be too ill to endure lengthy assessment procedures or may not complain about their pain. Recognizing these constraints, we have presented three steps of assessment. Components at each step are designed to lead to treatment decisions. Where possible, the assessment is structured around questionnaires designed for the patient with cancer. These questionnaires minimize patients' and health care professionals' biases and time, while standardizing the assessment process. Steps 2 and 3 of the assessment need to be followed if pain intensity is 4 or above on a 0–10 scale or if screening suggests a potential treatment need.

In clinical practice, an assessment based on questionnaires needs to be supplemented by interview of the patient (with, if possible, the primary family caregiver), as well as by observation and medical examination. Proper assessment based on subjective report needs the full cooperation of the patient, yet patients with cancer may be reluctant to complain of pain or other symptoms. To be full partners in their pain assessment and treatment, patients need education about their rights to symptom relief and the availability of effective treatment, as well as exploration of barriers that may inhibit assessment or use of treatment.

Cancer pain is dynamic and ever-changing. Although sometimes pain improves with tumor regression, cancer remission, or conclusion of treatment, pain often becomes progressively worse, requiring more aggressive use of pain therapy. Once a patient develops pain, assessment needs to be repeated regularly. The steps presented in the model have additional applications outside of clinical assessment. They can be used effectively in studies of the epidemiology of cancer pain, in quality assurance, and in clinical trials examining the effectiveness of pain treatments.

ACKNOWLEDGMENTS

Charles S. Cleeland's and Karen O. Anderson's work on this chapter was supported by Grant No. DAMD17-94-J-4233 from the U.S. Army Medical Research and Materiel Command; by Grants No. CA64766 and No. CA26582 from the National Cancer Institute; and by Grant No. SIG #21 from the American Cancer Society. Karen L. Syrjala's work was supported by grants from the National Cancer Institute: No. CA63030, No. CA78990, No. CA68139, and No. DE12731.

REFERENCES

Aaronson, N. K., Ahmedzai, S., Bergman, B., Bullinger, M., Cull, A., Duez, N. J., Filiberti, A., Flechtner, H., Fleishman, S. B., & de Haes, J. C. (1993). The European Organization for Research and Treatment of Cancer QLQ-C30: A quality-of-life instrument for use in international clinical trials in oncology. *Journal of the National Cancer Institute, 85*, 365–376.

Aaronson, N. K., Bullinger, M., & Ahmedzai, S. (1988). A modular approach to quality-of-life assessment in cancer clinical trials. *Recent Results in Cancer Research, 111*, 231–249.

Ahles, T. A., Blanchard, E. B., & Ruckdeschel, J. C. (1983). The multidimensional nature of cancer-related pain. *Pain, 17*, 277–288.

American Cancer Society. (1999). *Cancer facts and figures.* Atlanta, GA: Author.

American Pain Society. (1999). *Principles of analgesic use in the treatment of acute pain and cancer pain.* Glenview, IL: Author.

Andrykowski, M. A., Curran, S. L., Carpenter, J. S., Studts, J. L., Cunningham, L., McGrath, P. C., Sloan, D. A., & Kenady, D. E. (1999). Rheumatoid symptoms following breast cancer treatment: A controlled comparison. *Journal of Pain and Symptom Management, 18*, 85–94.

Back, A. L., Wallace, J. I., Starks, H. E., & Pearlman, R. A. (1996). Physician-assisted suicide and euthanasia in Washington State: Patient requests and physician responses. *Journal of the American Medical Association, 275*, 919–925.

Banning, A., Sjogren, P., & Henriksen, H. (1991). Pain causes in 200 patients referred to a multidisciplinary cancer pain clinic. *Pain, 45,* 45-48.

Bergman, B., Aaronson, N. K., Ahmedzai, S., Kaasa, S., & Sullivan, M. (1994). The EORTC QLQ-LC13: A modular supplement to the EORTC Core Quality of Life Questionnaire (QLQ-C30) for use in lung cancer clinical trials. *European Journal of Cancer, 30A*(5), 635-642.

Bernabei, R., Gambassi, G., Lapane, K., Landi, F., Gatsonis, C., Dunlop, R., Lipsitz, L., Steel, K., Mor, V., & SAGE Study Group. (1998). Management of pain in elderly patients with cancer. *Journal of the American Medical Association, 279,* 1877-1882.

Beyer, J. E. (1984). *The Oucher: A user's manual and technical report.* Evanston, IL: Hospital Play Equipment.

Beyer, J. E., & Wells, N. (1989). The assessment of pain in children. *Pediatric Clinics of North America, 36,* 837-854.

Bieri, D., Reeve, R. A., Champion, G. D., Addicoat, L., & Ziegler, J. B. (1990). The Faces Pain Scale for the self-assessment of the severity of pain experienced by children: Development, initial validation, and preliminary investigation for ratio scale properties. *Pain, 41,* 139-150.

Bookbinder, M., Coyle, N., Kiss, M., Goldstein, M. L., Holritz, K., Thaler, H., Gianella, A., Derby, S., Brown, M., Racolin, A., Ho, M. N., & Portenoy, R. K. (1996). Implementing national standards for cancer pain management: Program model and evaluation. *Journal of Pain and Symptom Management, 12,* 334-347.

Caraceni, A., Portenoy, R. K., & Working Group of the IASP Task Force on Cancer Pain. (1999). An international survey of cancer pain characteristics and syndromes. *Pain, 82,* 263-274.

Cella, D. F. (1994). Quality of life: Concepts and definitions. *Journal of Pain and Symptom Management, 9,* 186-192.

Cella, D. F. (1996). Quality of outcomes: Measurement and validation. *Oncology, 10,* 233-244.

Cella, D. F., Tulsky, D. S., Gray, G., Sarafian, B., Linn, E., Bonomi, A., Silberman, M., Yellen, S. B., Winicour, P., Brannon, J., Eckberg, K., Lloyd, S., Purl, S., Blendowski, C., Goodman, M., Barnicle, M., Stewart, I., McHale, M., Bonomi, P., Kaplan, E., Taylor, S. IV, Thomas, C. R., Jr., & Harris, J. (1993). The Functional Assessment of Cancer Therapy scale: Development and validation of the general measure. *Journal of Clinical Oncology, 11,* 570-579.

Chambers, C. T., Reid, G. J., Craig, K. D., McGrath, P. J., & Finley, G. A. (1998). Agreement between child and parent reports of pain. *Clinical Journal of Pain, 14,* 336-342.

Chapko, M. K., Syrjala, K. L., Bush, N., Jedlow, C., & Yanke, M. R. (1991). Development of a behavioral measure of mouth pain, nausea, and wellness for patients receiving radiation and chemotherapy. *Journal of Pain and Symptom Management, 6,* 15-23.

Chapko, M. K., Syrjala, K. L., Schilter, L., Cummings, C., & Sullivan, K. (1989). Chemoradiotherapy toxicity during bone marrow transplantation: Time course and variation in pain and nausea. *Bone Marrow Transplantation, 4,* 181-186.

Chapman, C. R., Kornell, J. A., & Syrjala, K. L. (1987). Painful complications of cancer diagnosis and therapy. In C. H. Yarbro & D. B. McGuire (Eds.), *Cancer pain: Nursing management* (pp. 47-67). Orlando, FL: Grune & Stratton.

Chapman, C. R., & Syrjala, K. L. (2001). Measurement of pain. In J. D. Loeser, S. Butler, D. C. Chapman, & D. C. Turk (Eds.), *Bonica's management of pain* (3rd ed., pp. 310-328). Philadelphia, PA: Williams & Wilkins.

Cleeland, C. S. (1984). The impact of pain on the patient with cancer. *Cancer, 54,* 2635-2641.

Cleeland, C. S. (1989a). Measurement of pain by subjective report. In C. R. Chapman & J. D. Loeser (Eds.), *Issues in pain measurement* (pp. 391-403). New York: Raven Press.

Cleeland, C. S. (1989b). Pain control: Public and physicians' attitudes. In C. S. Hill, Jr., & W. S. Fields (Eds.), *Advances in pain research and therapy* (Vol. 11, pp. 81-89). New York: Raven Press.

Cleeland, C. S., Gonin, R., Baez, L., Loehrer, P., & Pandya, K. J. (1997). Pain and treatment of pain in minority outpatients with cancer. The Eastern Cooperative Oncology Group minority outpatient pain study. *Annals of Internal Medicine, 127,* 813-816.

Cleeland, C. S., Gonin, R., Hatfield, A. K., Edmonson, J. H., Blum, R. H., Stewart, J. A., & Pandya, K. J. (1994). Pain and its treatment in outpatients with metastatic cancer. *New England Journal of Medicine, 330,* 592-594.

Cleeland, C. S., Janjan, N. A., Scott, C. B., Seiferheld, W. F., & Curran, W. J. (2000). Cancer pain management by radiotherapists: A survey of Radiation Therapy Oncology Group physicians. *International Journal of Radiation Oncology, Biology, and Physics, 47,* 203-208.

Cleeland, C. S., Mendoza, T. R., Wang, X. S., Chou, C., Harle, M. T., Morrissey, M., & Engstrom, M. (2000). Assessing symptom distress in cancer: The M. D. Anderson Symptom Inventory. *Cancer, 89,* 1634-1646.

Cleeland, C. S., Rotondi, A., Brechner, T., Levin, A., MacDonald, N., Portenoy, R., Schutta, H., & McEniry, M. (1986). A model for the treatment of cancer pain. *Journal of Pain and Symptom Management, 1,* 209-215.

Dar, R., Beach, C. M., Barden, P. L., & Cleeland, C. S. (1992). Cancer pain in the marital system: A study of patients and their spouses. *Journal of Pain and Symptom Management, 7,* 87-93.

Daut, R. L., & Cleeland, C. S. (1982). The prevalence and severity of pain in cancer. *Cancer, 50,* 1913-1918.

De Conno, F., Caraceni, A., Gamba, A., Mariani, L., Abbattista, A., Brunelli, C., La Mura, A., & Ventafridda, V. (1994). Pain measurement in cancer patients: A comparison of six methods. *Pain, 57,* 161-166.

Derogatis, L. R., Morrow, G. R., Fetting, J., Penman, D., Piasetsky, S., Schmale, A. M., Henrichs, M., & Carnicke, C. L. M., Jr. (1983). The prevalence of psychiatric disorders among cancer patients. *Journal of the American Medical Association, 249,* 751-757.

De Wit, R., van Dam, F., Zandbelt, L., van Buuren, A., van der Heijden, K., Leenhouts, G., & Loonstra, S. (1997). A pain education program for chronic cancer pain patients: Follow-up results from a randomized controlled trial. *Pain, 73,* 55-69.

Dunkel-Schetter, C. (1984). Social support and cancer: Findings based on patient interviews and their implications. *Journal of Social Issues, 40,* 77-98.

Du Pen, S. L., Du Pen, A. R., Polissar, N., Hansberry, J., Kraybill, B. M., Stillman, M., Panke, J., Everly R., & Syrjala, K. (1999). Implementing guidelines for cancer pain management: Results of a randomized controlled clinical trial. *Journal of Clinical Oncology, 17,* 361–370.

Eland, J. M. (1981). Minimizing pain associated with prekindergarten intramuscular injections. *Issues in Comprehensive Pediatric Nursing, 5,* 362–372.

Ersek, M., Kraybill, B. M., & Du Pen, A. R. (1999). Factors hindering patients' use of medications for cancer pain. *Cancer Practice, 7*(5), 226–232.

Ferraz, M. B., Quaresma, M. R., Aquino, L. R., Atra, E., Tugwell, P., & Goldsmith, C. H. (1990). Reliability of pain scales in the assessment of literate and illiterate patients with rheumatoid arthritis. *Journal of Rheumatology, 17,* 1022–1024.

Ferrell, B. A., Ferrell, B. R., & Rivera, L. (1995). Pain in cognitively impaired nursing home patients. *Journal of Pain and Symptom Management, 10,* 591–598.

Fishman, B., Pasternak, S., Wallenstein, S. L., Houde, R. W., Holland J. C., & Foley, K. M. (1987). The Memorial Pain Assessment Card. A valid instrument for the evaluation of cancer pain. *Cancer, 60,* 1151–1158.

Foley, K. M. (1979). Pain syndromes in patients with cancer. In J. J. Bonica & V. Ventafridda (Eds.), *Advances in pain research and therapy* (Vol. 2, pp. 59–75). New York: Raven Press.

Foley, K. M. (1985). Treatment of cancer pain. *New England Journal of Medicine, 313,* 84–95.

Gauvain-Piquard, A., Rodary, C., Francois, P., Rezvani, A., Kalifa, C., Lecuyer, N., Cosse, M., & Lesbros, R. (1991). Validity assessment of DEGR[R] scale for observational rating of 2–6year-old child pain. *Journal of Pain and Symptom Management, 6,* 171.

Gill, T. M., & Feinstein, A. R. (1994). A critical appraisal of the quality-of-life measurements. *Journal of the American Medical Association, 272,* 619–626.

Glover, J., Dibble, S. L., Dodd, M. S., & Miaskowski, C. (1995). Mood states of oncology outpatients: Does pain make a difference? *Journal of Pain and Symptom Management, 10,* 120–128.

Gonzales, G. R., Elliott, K. J., Portenoy, R. K., & Foley, K. M. (1991). The impact of a comprehensive evaluation in the management of cancer pain. *Pain, 47,* 141–144.

Grond, S., Radbruch, L., Meuser, T., Sabatowski, R., Loick, G., & Lehmann, K. A., (1999). Assessment and treatment of neuropathic cancer pain following WHO guidelines. *Pain, 79,* 15–20.

Grond, S., Zech, D., Diefenbach, C., Radbruch, L., & Lehmann, K. A. (1996). Assessment of cancer pain: A prospective evaluation in 2266 cancer patients referred to a pain service. *Pain, 64,* 107–114.

Grossman, S. A., Benedetti, C., Payne, R., & Syrjala, K. L. (1999). NCCN Practice Guidelines for cancer pain. *Oncology, 13*(11A), 33–44.

Heim, H. M., & Oei, T. P. S. (1993). Comparison of prostate cancer patients with and without pain. *Pain, 53,* 159–162.

Herndon, J. E., Fleishman, S., Kornblith, A. B., Kosty, M., Green, M. R., & Holland J. (1999). Is quality of life predictive of the survival of patients with advanced nonsmall cell lung carcinoma? *Cancer, 85,* 333–340.

Herr, K. A., & Mobily, P. R. (1991). Pain assessment in the elderly: Clinical considerations. *Journal of Gerontology Nursing, 17,* 12–19.

Herr, K. A., Mobily, P. R., Kohout, F. J., & Wagenaar, D. (1998). Evaluation of the Faces Pain Scale for use with the elderly. *Clinical Journal of Pain, 14,* 29–38.

Hodes, R. L. (1989). Cancer patients' needs and concerns when using narcotic analgesics. In C. S. Hill & W. S. Fields (Eds.), *Advances in pain research and therapy* (Vol. 11, pp. 91–99). New York: Raven Press.

Jacox, A., Carr, D. B., Payne, R., Berde, C. B., Breitbart, W., Cain, J. M., Chapman, C. R., Cleeland, C. S., Ferrell, B. R., Finley, R. S., Hester, N. O., Hill, C. S., Jr., Leak, W. D., Lipman, A. G., Logan, C. L., McGarvey, C. L., Miaskowski, C. A., Mulder, D. S., Paice, J. A., Shapiro, B. S., Silberstein, E. B., Smith, R. S., Stover, J., Tsou, C. V., Vecchiarelli, L., & Weissman, D. E. (1994). *Management of cancer pain: Clinical practice guideline No. 9.* (DHHS Publication AHCPR No. 94-0592). Rockville, MD: U.S. Department of Health and Human Services.

Janjan, N. A., Martin, C. G., Payne, R., Dahl, J. L., Weissman, D. E., & Hill, C. S. (1996). Teaching cancer pain management: Durability of educational effects of a role model program. *Cancer, 77,* 996–1001.

Jay, S. M., Ozolins, M., Elliott, C. H., & Caldwell, S. (1983). Assessment of children's distress during painful medical procedures. *Health Psychology, 2,* 133–147.

Jensen, M. P., Karoly, P., & Braver, S. (1986). The measurement of clinical pain intensity: A comparison of six methods. *Pain, 27,* 117–126.

Karnofsky, D. A., Abelmann, W. H., Craver, L. F., & Burchenal, J. H. (1948). The use of the nitrogen mustards in the palliative treatment of carcinoma. *Cancer, 1,* 634–656.

Lasagna, L. (1980). Analgesic methodology: A brief history and commentary. *Journal of Clinical Pharmacology, 20,* 373–376.

Ljungman, G., Kreuger, A., Gordh, T., Berg, T., Sorensen, S., & Rawal, N. (1996). Treatment of pain in pediatric oncology: A Swedish nationwide study. *Pain, 68,* 385–394.

Manne, S. L., Jacobsen, P., & Redd, W. H. (1992). Assessment of acute pediatric pain: Do child self-report, parent ratings, and nurse ratings measure the same phenomenon? *Pain, 48,* 45–52.

Martin, L. A., & Hagen, N. A. (1997). Neuropathic pain in cancer patients: Mechanisms, syndromes, and clinical controversies. *Journal of Pain and Symptom Management, 14,* 99–117.

McGrath, P. A. (1990). *Pain in children.* New York: Guilford Press.

McGrath, P. A., de Veber, L. L., & Hearn, M. T. (1985). Multidimensional pain assessment in children. In H. L. Fields, R. Dubner, F. Cervero, & L. E. Jones (Eds.), *Advances in pain research and therapy* (Vol. 9, pp. 387–393). New York: Raven Press.

McGrath, P. J., Beyer, J., Cleeland, C. S., Eland, J., McGrath, P. A., & Portenoy, R. (1990). American Academy of Pediatrics Report of the Subcommittee on Assessment and Methodologic Issues in the Management of Pain in Childhood Cancer. *Pediatrics, 86,* 814–817,

McGrath, P. J., Johnson, G., Goodman, J. T., Schillinger, J., Dunn, J., & Chapman, J. A. (1985). CHEOPS: A behavioral scale for rating postoperative pain in children. In H. L. Fields, R. Dubner, F. Cervero, & L. E. Jones (Eds.), *Advances in pain research and therapy* (Vol. 9, pp. 395–402). New York: Raven Press.

McGrath, P. J., Seifert, C. E., Speechley, K. N., Booth, J. C., Stitt, L., & Gibson, M. C. (1996). A new analogue scale for assessing children's pain: An initial validation study. *Pain, 64,* 435–443.

Melzack, R. (1987). The short-form McGill Pain Questionnaire. *Pain, 30,* 191–197.

Miser, A. W., Dothage, J. A., Wesley, R. A., & Miser, J. S. (1987). The prevalence of pain in a pediatric and young adult cancer population. *Pain, 29,* 73–83.

Moinpour, C. M. (1994). Measuring quality of life: An emerging science. *Seminars in Oncology, 21,* 48–60.

Moinpour, C. M., Feigl, P., Metch, B., Hayden, K.A., Meyskens, F. L., Jr., & Crowley, J. (1989). Quality of life end points in cancer clinical trials: Review and recommendations. *Journal of the National Cancer Institute, 81,* 485–495.

Morrow, G. R., Feldstein, M., Adler, L. M., Derogatis, L. R., Enelow, A. J., Gates, C., Holland, J., Melisaratos, N., Murawski, B. J., Penman, D., Schmale, A., Schmitt, M., & Morse, I. (1981). Development of brief measures of psychosocial adjustment to medical illness applied to cancer patients. *General Hospital Psychiatry, 3,* 79–88.

O'Boyle, C. A., & Waldron, D. (1997). Quality of life issues in palliative medicine. *Journal of Neurology, 244*(Suppl. 4), 18–25.

Oken, M. M., Creech, R. H., Tormey, D. C., Horton, J., Davis, T. E., McFadden, E. T., & Carbone, P. P. (1982). Toxicity and response criteria of the Eastern Cooperative Oncology Group. *American Journal of Clinical Oncology, 5,* 649–655.

Patrick, D. L., & Erickson, P. (1993). Assessing health-related quality of life for clinical decision-making. In S. R. Walker & R. M. Rosser (Eds.), *Quality of life assessment: Key issues for the 1990s* (pp. 11–64). London: Kluwer.

Payne, R. (1990). Pathophysiology of cancer pain. In K. M. Foley, J. J. Bonica, V. Ventafridda, & M. V. Callaway (Eds.), *Advances in pain research and therapy* (Vol. 16, pp. 13–26). New York: Raven Press.

Petzke, F., Radbruch, L., Zech, D., Loick, G., & Grond, S. (1999). Temporal presentation of chronic cancer pain: Transitory pains on admission to a multidisciplinary pain clinic. *Journal of Pain and Symptom Management, 17,* 391–401.

Portenoy, R. K. (1989). Cancer pain: Epidemiology and syndromes. *Cancer, 63,* 2298–2307.

Portenoy, R. K. (1999). Managing cancer pain poorly responsive to systemic opioid therapy. *Oncology, 13*(Suppl. 2), 25–29.

Portenoy, R. K., Thaler, H. T., Kornblith, A. B., Lepore, J. M., Friedlander-Klar, H., Kiyasu, E., Sobel, K., Coyle, N., Kemeny, N., Norton, L., & Scher, H. (1994). The Memorial Symptom Assessment Scale: An instrument for the evaluation of symptom prevalence, characteristics, and distress. *European Journal of Cancer, 30A,* 1326–1336.

Portenoy, R. K., & Hagen, N. A. (1990). Breakthrough pain: Definition, prevalence and characteristics. *Pain, 41,* 273–281.

Selby, P. J., Chapman, J. A. W., Etazadi-Amoli, J., Dalley, D., & Boyd, N. F. (1984). The development

of a method for assessing the quality of life of cancer patients. *British Journal of Cancer, 50,* 13–22.

Serlin, R. C., Mendoza, T. R., Nakamura, Y., Edwards, K. R., & Cleeland, C. S. (1995). When is cancer pain mild, moderate or severe?: Grading pain severity by its interference with function. *Pain, 61,* 277–284.

Shacham, S., Dar, R., & Cleeland, C. S. (1984). The relationship of mood state to the severity of clinical pain. *Pain, 18,* 187–191.

Shug, S. A., Zech, D., & Dorr, U. (1990). Cancer pain management according to WHO analgesic guidelines. *Journal of Pain and Symptom Management, 5,* 27–32.

Smith, W. C. S., Bourne, D., Squair, J., Phillips, D. O., & Chambers, W. A. (1999). A retrospective cohort study of post mastectomy pain syndrome. *Pain, 83,* 91–95.

Spector, W. D. (1990). Functional disability scales. In B. Spilker (Ed.), *Quality of life assessments in clinical trials* (pp. 133–143). New York: Raven Press.

Spilker, B. (1996). *Quality of life and pharmacoeconomics in clinical trials.* Philadelphia: Lippincott-Raven.

Spitzer, W. O., Dobson, A. J., Hall, J., Chesterman, E., Levi, J., Shepherd, R., Battista, R. N., & Catchlove, B. R. (1981). Measuring the quality of life of cancer patients: A concise QL-Index for use by physicians. *Journal of Chronic Disease, 34,* 585–597.

Stewart, A. L., & Ware, J. E. (Eds.). (1992). *Measuring functioning and well-being: The Medical Outcomes Study approach.* Durham, NC: Duke University Press.

Syrjala, K. L. (1987). *The measurement of pain: Cancer pain management.* Orlando, FL: Grune & Stratton.

Syrjala, K. L., Abrams, J. R., Cowan, J., Hansberry, J., Robison, J., Cross, J., Roth-Roemer, S., Williams, A., DuPen, S., Stillman, M., Cleeland, C. S., & Fredrickson, M. (1996). *Is educating patients and families the route to relieving cancer pain?* Paper presented at the International Association for the Study of Pain 8th World Congress on Pain, Vancouver, British Columbia, Canada.

Syrjala, K. L., & Chapko, M. E. (1995). Evidence for a biopsychosocial model of cancer treatment-related pain. *Pain, 61,* 69–79.

Syrjala, K. L., & Chapman, C. R. (1984). Measurement of clinical pain: A review and integration of research findings. In C. Benadetti, C. R. Chapman, & G. Moricca (Eds.), *Advances in pain research and therapy* (Vol. 7, pp. 71–101). New York: Raven Press.

Tarbell, S. E., Cohen, I. T., & Marsh, J. L. (1992). The Toddler–Preschooler Postoperative Pain Scale: An observational scale for measuring postoperative pain in children aged 1–5. Preliminary report. *Pain, 50,* 273–280.

Thomason, T. E., McCune, J. S., Bernard, S. A., Winer, E. P., Tremont, S., & Lindley, C. M. (1998). Cancer pain survey: Patient-centered issues in control. *Journal of Pain and Symptom Management, 15,* 275–284.

Trowbridge, R., Dugan, W., Jay, S. J., Littrell, D., Casebeer, L. L., Edgerton, S., Anderson J., O'Toole, J. B. (1997). Determining the effectiveness of a clinical-practice intervention in improving the control of pain in outpatients with cancer. *Academic Medicine, 72,* 798–800.

Vainio, A., & Auvinen, A. (1996). Prevalence of symptoms with advanced cancer: An international collaborative study. *Journal of Pain and Symptom Management*, *12*, 3–10.

Ventafridda, V., Tamburini, M., Caraceni, A., DeConno, F., & Naldi, F. (1987). A validation study of the WHO method for cancer pain relief. *Cancer, 59*, 850–856.

Von Roenn, J. H., Cleeland, C. S., Gonin, R., Hatfield, A. K., & Pandya, K. J. (1993). Physician attitudes and practice in cancer pain management. A survey from the Eastern Cooperative Oncology Group. *Annals of Internal Medicine, 119*, 121–126.

Vuorinen, E. (1993). Pain as an early symptom in cancer. *Clinical Journal of Pain, 9*, 272–278.

Wallace, M. S., Wallace, A. M., Lee, J., & Dobke, M. K. (1996). Pain after breast surgery: A survey of 282 women. *Pain, 66*, 195–205.

Wallenstein, S. (1984). Measurement of pain and analgesia in cancer patients. *Cancer, 53*(Suppl. 10), 2260–2264.

Wang, X. S., Cleeland, C. S., Mendoza, T. R., Engstrom, M. C., Liu, S., Xu, G., Hao, X., Wang, Y., & Ren, X. S. (1999). The effects of pain severity on health-related quality of life. *Cancer, 86*, 1848–1855.

Ward, S. E., Goldberg, N., Miller-McCauley, V., Mueller, C., Nolan, A., Pawlik-Plank, D., Robbins, A., Stormoen, D., & Weissman, D.E. (1993). Patient-related barriers to management of cancer pain. *Pain, 52*, 319–324.

Ward, S. E., & Hernandez, L. (1994). Patient-related barriers to management of cancer pain in Puerto Rico. *Pain, 58*, 233–238.

Ware, J. E., Kosinski, M., & Keller, S. D. (1995). *SF-12: How to score the SF-12 Physical and Mental Health Summary Scales*. Boston: Health Institute, New England Medical Center.

Ware, J. E., & Sherbourne, C. S. (1992). The MOS 36-Item Short-Form Health Survey (SF-36): I. Conceptual framework and item selection. *Medical Care, 30*, 473–483.

Weiner, D., Peterson, B., & Keefe, F. (1999). Chronic pain-associated behaviors in the nursing home: Resident versus caregiver perceptions. *Pain, 80*, 577–588.

Weissman, D. E., & Dahl, J. L. (1995). Update on the cancer pain role model education program. *Journal of Pain and Symptom Management, 10*, 292–297.

Weissman, D. E., Griffie, J., Gordon, D. B., & Dahl, J. L. (1997). A role model program to promote institutional changes for management of acute and cancer pain. *Journal of Pain and Symptom Management, 14*, 274–279.

Wilkie, D. J., Keefe, F. J., Dodd, M. J., & Copp, L. A. (1992). Behavior of patients with lung cancer: Description and associations with oncologic and pain variables. *Pain, 51*, 231–240.

World Health Organization (WHO). (1986). *Cancer pain relief*. Geneva: Author.

World Health Organization (WHO). (1996). *Cancer pain relief and palliative care*. Geneva: Author.

World Health Organization (WHO). (1998). *Cancer pain relief and palliative care in children*. Geneva: Author.

Wortman, C. B. (1984). Social support and the cancer patient: Conceptual and methodological issues. *Cancer, 53*(Suppl. 10), 2339–2360.

Yancik, R. (1997). Cancer burden in the aged: An epidemiologic and demographic overview. *Cancer, 80*, 1273–1283.

Zech, D. F. J., Grond S., Lynch, J., Hertel, D., & Lehmann, K. A. (1995). Validation of World Health Organization Guidelines for cancer pain relief: A 10-year prospective study. *Pain, 63*, 65–76.

Zenz, M., Zenz, T., Tryba, M., & Strumpf, M. (1995). Severe undertreatment of cancer pain: A 3-year survey of the German situation. *Journal of Pain and Symptom Management, 10*, 187–191.

Zhukovsky, D. S., Gorowski, E., Hausdorff, J., Napolitano, B., & Lesser, M. (1995). Unmet analgesic needs in cancer patients. *Journal of Pain and Symptom Management, 10*, 113–119.

Zubrod, C. G., Schneiderman, M., Frei, E., Brindley, C., Gold, G. L., Shnider, B., Oviedo, R., Gorman, J., Jones, R., Jr., Jonsson, U., Colsky, J., Chalmers, T., Ferguson, B., Dederick, M., Holland, J., Selawry, O., Regelson, W., Lasagna, L., & Owens, A. H., Jr. (1960). Appraisal of methods for the study of chemotherapy of cancer in man: Comparative therapeutic trial of nitrogen mustard and triethylene thiophosphoramide. *Journal of Chronic Disease, 11*, 7–33.

APPENDIX 30.A. BRIEF PAIN INVENTORY (SHORT FORM)

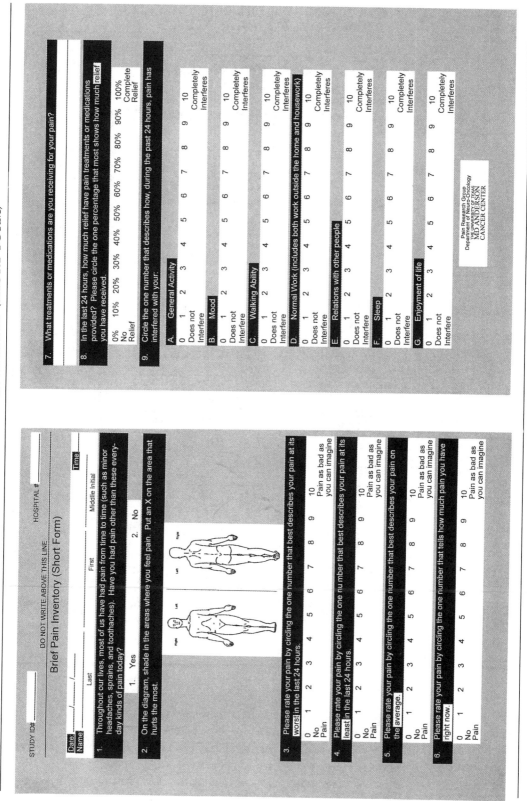

Note. Copyright 1991 by Charles S. Cleeland. Reprinted by permission.

APPENDIX 30.B. PATIENT PAIN CHECKLIST:
THINGS TO TELL YOUR DOCTOR

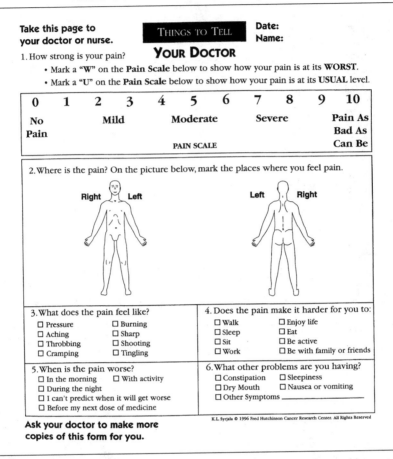

Take this page to your doctor or nurse.

THINGS TO TELL YOUR DOCTOR

Date:
Name:

1. How strong is your pain?
   - Mark a "W" on the **Pain Scale** below to show how your pain is at its **WORST**.
   - Mark a "U" on the **Pain Scale** below to show how your pain is at its **USUAL** level.

0	1	2	3	4	5	6	7	8	9	10
No Pain		Mild			Moderate		Severe			Pain As Bad As Can Be

PAIN SCALE

2. Where is the pain? On the picture below, mark the places where you feel pain.

Right   Left   Left   Right

3. What does the pain feel like?
   - ☐ Pressure   ☐ Burning
   - ☐ Aching   ☐ Sharp
   - ☐ Throbbing ☐ Shooting
   - ☐ Cramping   ☐ Tingling

4. Does the pain make it harder for you to:
   - ☐ Walk   ☐ Enjoy life
   - ☐ Sleep   ☐ Eat
   - ☐ Sit   ☐ Be active
   - ☐ Work   ☐ Be with family or friends

5. When is the pain worse?
   - ☐ In the morning   ☐ With activity
   - ☐ During the night
   - ☐ I can't predict when it will get worse
   - ☐ Before my next dose of medicine

6. What other problems are you having?
   - ☐ Constipation   ☐ Sleepiness
   - ☐ Dry Mouth   ☐ Nausea or vomiting
   - ☐ Other Symptoms _____

Ask your doctor to make more copies of this form for you.

K.L. Syrjala © 1996 Fred Hutchinson Cancer Research Center. All Rights Reserved

Note. By Karen J. Syrjala, PhD. Copyright 1996 by Fred Hutchinson Cancer Research Center. Reprinted by permission.

APPENDIX 30.C. PATIENT CHECKLIST OF BELIEFS

Circle "Yes" for any question that you **sometimes wonder** about. Circle "No" if the question is **not a concern** to you.

I WONDER:

Yes	No	Can I become addicted to pain medicine?
Yes	No	If I take strong pain medicines now, will they still work for me if my pain gets worse?
Yes	No	Should I be strong and not lean on pain medicines?
Yes	No	Does taking strong pain medicine like morphine mean that I am going to die soon?
Yes	No	Will the side effects of pain medicine be worse than the pain?
Yes	No	If a pain medicine doesn't work for me, are there other medicines that might work better?
Yes	No	Will my doctor know how my pain is even if I don't tell him or her?
Yes	No	If I talk about pain or other symptoms, will it take my doctor away from treating my disease?

Part VI

METHODOLOGICAL ISSUES

Chapter 31

Epidemiological and Survey Methods: Assessment of Chronic Pain

MICHAEL VON KORFF

Assessment of chronic pain status in survey and epidemiological research typically relies on respondent recall of pain status during a defined time period spanning weeks or months. Recent research supports the validity of retrospective report of pain intensity, persistence, and associated disability for at least a 3-month recall period. Rigorous studies assessing the validity of retrospective report of pain in relation to daily diary data have shown better pain recall than suggested by prior research based on small samples of patients at pain clinics. There is now support for the validity of (1) ratings of average or usual pain intensity on a 0–10 scale; (2) report of days with pain in the prior 3 months; and (3) ratings of interference with activities due to pain and self-report of days of activity limitation. Within this context, measures appropriate for survey research that assess pain intensity, persistence, and disability during a 1- to 6-month time interval are reviewed.

CONTEXT

Reports of a National Institutes of Health Consensus Development Conference (1986) and of the National Academy of Sciences (Osterweis, Kleinman, & Mechanic, 1987) have called for increased epidemiological and health services research concerning chronic pain conditions. More recently, the International Association for the Study of Pain has published a comprehensive monograph on the epidemiology of pain, reviewing prevalence surveys for most common chronic pain conditions (Crombie, Croft, Linton, Le Resche, & Von Korff, 1999). Although the prevalence of most common chronic pain conditions has been studied, less is known about the extent to which these conditions are associated with mild, moderate, or severe disability on a population basis, or about the distribution of chronic pain by important risk indicators (including age, gender, and lifestyle factors). This chapter considers issues of pain assessment that arise in conducting morbidity surveys to estimate the prevalence and the associated disability burden of chronic/recurrent pain conditions. Special attention is paid to brief methods of assessing pain and associated disability suitable for use in population surveys.

EPIDEMIOLOGICAL MEASURES AND THEIR RELEVANCE TO PAIN RESEARCH

Epidemiologists use various measures of disease occurrence and risk to measure the distribution, determinants, and natural history of disease. A comprehensive discussion of the application of epidemiological methods to the study of chronic pain is presented elsewhere (Von Korff, 1999).

603

Prevalence

Measures of pain *prevalence* quantify the proportion of a population with a condition at a given point in time (point prevalence rate), the proportion of persons affected by the condition during a defined period of time (period prevalence rate), or the proportion of a population affected over their lifetimes (lifetime prevalence rate). The numerator of a prevalence rate is the number of persons with the condition in the defined time period, while the denominator is the number of persons in the population or the population sample being studied. Prevalence estimates from survey data are an essential means of estimating the extent and burdens of chronic pain on a population basis.

Incidence

Measures of *incidence* quantify the probability or rate of onset of a condition among persons with no prior history. An incidence rate is the ratio of the number of onset events divided by the observed number of person-years the individuals under study were at risk of developing the condition. Kleinbaum, Kupper, and Morgenstern (1982) provide a thorough discussion of incidence and prevalence measures.

Relationships between Prevalence, Incidence, and Duration

The clinical course of chronic pain is frequently episodic (Von Korff, Dworkin, Le Resche, & Kruger, 1988). It has been shown that the steady-state prevalence of a chronic episodic condition is approximated by the product of its incidence rate, the average duration of episodes, and the average number of episodes over the course of the illness (Von Korff & Parker, 1980). This steady-state equation provides a basis for understanding the different ways in which prevalence rates can differ between two population groups. Differences in prevalence rates do not necessarily indicate differences in risk of developing a chronic pain condition, but may reflect differences in duration or recurrence. This chapter focuses on methods that may be useful for assessing differences in the burden of chronic/recurrent pain in population surveys; it does not address methods for measuring onset rates or clinical course of chronic pain.

MEASUREMENT BIASES IN EPIDEMIOLOGICAL RESEARCH

Sources of bias in survey research have been extensively studied (Bradburn, Rips, & Shevell, 1987; Cannel, 1977; Converse & Traugott, 1986). They include measurement bias in questionnaires and a variety of reporting biases, as well as sample biases such as undercoverage (persons missed by the sampling method) and nonresponse (persons refusing interview or not contacted).

Recall bias is a significant issue in epidemiological research concerning pain, because it is often necessary to ask respondents whether they have experienced an anatomically defined pain condition over some defined period of time (e.g., 2 weeks, 3 months, 6 months, 1 year). Means, Nigram, Zarrow, Loftus, and Donaldson (1989), in a monograph on autobiographical memory for health-related events, drew a distinction between *semantic memory* and *episodic memory*. Semantic memory is conceptually structured information resistant to interference from other memory traces. Episodic memory is a temporally ordered set of autobiographical events that can be more difficult to retrieve. It is important, from both a substantive and a methodological standpoint, to know what features of a chronic pain condition (e.g., persistence, intensity, interference, meaning, disability) lead to encoding of the pain condition as a semantic or as an episodic memory. If more severe, disabling, and longer-lasting pain conditions are more likely to be encoded as semantic memory, then the accuracy of recall of such pain conditions may be adequate for a recall interval of 3, 6, or 12 months. However, episodic pain conditions that are less persistent or less severe may be more likely to be forgotten.

In an epidemiological survey, it is often necessary to ask respondents whether they have experienced pain at a given anatomical site. It is not possible to ask follow-up questions about intensity, persistence, and disability until the respondent has reported the presence of the pain condition of interest. Based on research showing that memory for doctor visits decays rapidly with increasing time since a visit (Cannel, 1977), an important issue is how long a recall period should be employed in asking subjects about chronic pain conditions. There are tradeoffs for short versus long reporting intervals (Von Korff & Dworkin, 1989). A short reporting period, all else being equal, should minimize forgetting of pain conditions if the subject is not experiencing pain at the time of the interview. However, a short reporting period may not yield as reliable an estimate of a subject's characteristic chronic pain status because of the large within-subject variability in pain status over time. For example, in assessing chronic pain status it may be more informative to know that a subject has experienced back pain on 90 days in the prior 6 months than that the person has experienced pain on 7 days in the prior 2 weeks, even though 2-week recall may be more accurate than 6-month recall.

Other cognitive processes are relevant to the recall of pain in survey research. *Forward telescoping* is a tendency for respondents to report events that occurred before the reference period as having occurred during the reference period. This may be particularly problematic in studies estimating first-onset rates of pain conditions. If subjects tend to report first onset as more recent than it actually was, incidence rate estimates could be substantially inflated. There is evidence that this phenomenon occurs for recall of mental disorder onset (Simon & Von Korff, 1995). Carey, Garrett, Jackson, Sanders, and Kalsbeek (1995) studied recall of back pain among 235 patients with back pain who had made a health care visit for such pain 4 to 16 months earlier. In this study, there was evidence that episodes of back pain occurring more than 8 months before the interview tended to be recalled as occurring more recently than they actually occurred, suggesting that forward telescoping does occur.

In addition to the sources of bias encountered in surveys, investigators conducting longitudinal studies need to be aware of additional sources of bias, including loss to follow-up, missing data, and measurement biases introduced by repeated measurement. Missing data and loss to follow-up can substantially reduce sample size in a longitudinal survey, particularly if observations are made on more than two occasions. Such losses are generally not random; thus they may introduce an important source of bias. Measures that may be biased by repeated measurement or that may "drift" over time also present problems in longitudinal studies, as do unreliable measures.

ASSESSMENT OF CHRONIC PAIN STATUS IN A DEFINED TIME INTERVAL

Epidemiological and survey research on chronic pain typically requires assessment of the characteristic level and pattern of pain and associated disability over a period of time, rather than assessment of an individual's pain status only at a particular point in time. Determining a person's characteristic chronic pain status is made difficult by the large across-time variability in individual pain status, as well as the diverse sources of variation in pain measurement. Variation in pain measurement may be due to the measurement method such as the scale or questions used (see Jensen & Karoly, Chapter 2, this volume), the scaling of responses, the length of the recall period, the method of prompting for condition or anatomical site, and the method of administration (e.g., personal interview, self-administered questionnaire, telephone interview). Additional variation may be due to timing of measurements: the number of times pain status is measured, time of day, day of week, and timing of administration in relation to milestones in the natural history of the condition or treatment seeking. Context of pain measurement may also contribute to variation (e.g., work, home, health care or research settings).

Figure 31.1 depicts a hypothetical time course of frequently measured pain ratings, as might be obtained in a daily diary study. With continuous measurement, it would be possible to estimate any summary measure of this pain intensity curve, such as the percentage of time in pain, average pain intensity when in pain, or the area under the pain intensity curve. Figure 31.1 also depicts continuous measurement of the occurrence of associated disability (as indicated by the arrows above the pain intensity curve). Possible summary measures of interference with activities include the average level of disability or cumulative measures such as disability days.

In most epidemiological studies, continuous measurement of pain status and associated disability is not possible. Rather, it is necessary to rely on the retrospective report of key parameters of pain status over a defined time period, such as 3 or 6 months. Key parameters of pain status include the number of days a patient experiences the pain condition of interest, the mean pain intensity level when in pain, the mean level of interference with life activities, and the number of days of interference with daily activities (Von Korff, Ormel, Keefe, & Dworkin, 1992).

The area under the curve of the pain intensity graph could be estimated by the product of average pain intensity and the total duration of pain. This suggests that pain severity might be estimated by the product of pain intensity and duration, as in "headache index"-type measures (Von Korff, Lipton, & Stewart, 1994). However, there is evidence that pain intensity and pain dura-

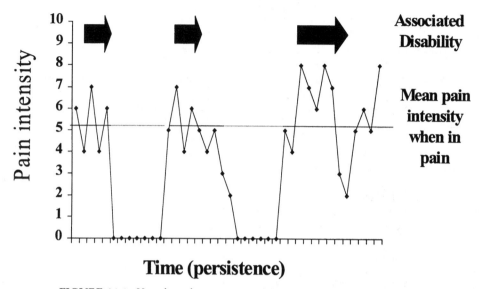

FIGURE 31.1. Hypothetical time course of frequently measured pain ratings.

tion are often not highly correlated (Von Korff et al., 1992), and that they have additive rather than multiplicative effects on other measures of pain impact (e.g., disability, medicine use, depression) (Von Korff et al., 1994). For this reason, it is useful to view persistence (or chronicity) and intensity as independent facets of pain status. In contrast, there is substantial evidence that measures of pain intensity and of pain-related interference with activities scale together, forming an underlying continuum of pain severity.

RELIABILITY AND VALIDITY OF RETROSPECTIVE REPORT OF PAIN

Over the past decade, careful empirical studies have provided new information on the reliability and validity of retrospective report of pain intensity, persistence and associated disability. Although these studies suggest that retrospective pain report is not perfect, the good news is that well-crafted questions about pain status for a 3-month recall period can yield valid data. In 1992, the National Center for Health Statistics published a methodological monograph on the assessment of pain in health surveys by respondent recall (Salovey et al., 1992). This research consisted of experiments designed to investigate factors influencing accurate recall of pain and associated activity limitations. The investigators reached the following conclusions:

Compared with the literature reviewed at the start of this paper, which reported, for the most part, considerable inaccuracy in recall of pain among small samples of patients undergoing treatment in pain clinics, recall among our subjects across most of the studies would be better characterized by its accuracy. Overall, we were impressed by how well subjects could report on their pain retrospectively. When biases in retrospective report were observed, they tended to be in the direction of overestimating rather than underestimating prior levels of pain.

The severity of prior pain, its impact on daily activities and behaviors related to the pain problem are all recalled approximately equally well and seem to be equally stable over time among individuals with chronic pain problems. Survey researchers who seek more informative data than that provided by mere intensity ratings should feel comfortable querying respondents about these other pain related behaviors.

One systematic source of bias in pain ratings is created by severity of pain at the time of recall. Controlling for original levels of pain and the amount that pain fluctuates during the applicable time period, greater pain at recall was associated with overestimating of prior pain experience. Survey researchers asking questions about prior experiences with pain may wish to include questions about current levels of pain as well.

Mood may not be a major influence on pain recall, at least not under the specific circumstances investigated here. (Salovey et al., 1992, p. 26)

This important monograph questions the oft-held assumption that recall of pain is substantially inaccurate. This suggests that a more productive stance may be to investigate how to improve the reliability and validity of the retrospective report of pain intensity, persistence, and associated disability.

VALIDITY OF RECALL OF ANATOMICALLY DEFINED PAIN

In an epidemiological survey, as noted earlier, it is often necessary to ask subjects about whether they have experienced pain at a particular anatomical site (e.g., back pain, headache) during a defined time period (e.g., 3 months, a year). It is not possible to ask follow-up questions about intensity, persistence, and disability until the subject has reported the presence of the pain condition of interest.

Research by the National Center for Health Statistics provides estimates of the probability of recall of selected chronic conditions known to have been present in the prior year because they were treated (Madow, 1973). For example, diabetes, sinusitis, and hypertension were recalled by more than 80% of treated patients, while asthma, headache, and arthritis were recalled by more than 60% of treated patients. This research showed that the agreement of self-report and medical records data increased with the number of visits for a chronic condition and was higher if a subject had received medicines for the condition. This suggests that pain conditions with greater impact are more salient, and thus more likely to be remembered and reported. Experience with asking questions about chronic conditions also suggests that they are much more likely to be reported when subjects are asked about a list of specific conditions than when they are asked a general question about chronic illness. Higher yield in pain surveys will be achieved if subjects are asked about each anatomically defined pain condition of interest than if a general question about the occurrence of pain (not anatomically defined) is asked.

In a study of high utilizers of health care who had made a health care visit for back pain within the prior year (Von Korff, 1991), it was found that recall was high (88%) if the visit had occurred within the prior 6 months, but was lower (73%) if the visit had occurred more than 6 months before the interview. Persons with multiple visits were more likely to recall their back pain episode (92%) than were persons with a single visit (69%). Depressed persons were more likely to recall their back pain episode (91%) than were nondepressed persons (74%), particularly among persons whose visit was more than 6 months before the interview (88% vs. 57%). In a survey of 235 patients with back pain who had made visits for the pain, Carey and colleagues (1995) found that 79% reported having had back pain when asked 4 to 16 months after their visit. These results suggest that ability to recall prior episodes of pain is adequate, particularly if the episode occurred within the prior 6 months and has a significant impact.

VALIDITY OF RETROSPECTIVE REPORT OF AVERAGE PAIN INTENSITY

Salovey and colleagues (1992) reported correlations between different retrospective measures of pain intensity for the prior 2 weeks and 2 weeks of hourly pain ratings for persons undergoing assessment at a pain treatment center. They found the following correlations with the mean of the hourly pain ratings: current pain, $r = .74$; usual pain, $r = .83$; worst pain, $r = .68$; and least pain, $r = .87$. De Wit and colleagues (1999) conducted a diary study of 159 patients with cancer and found correlations of .80 or higher between 1-week recall of average pain intensity and estimates of average pain intensity from a daily diary. Jensen, Turner, Turner, and Romano (1996) compared retrospective ratings of usual, least, worst and current pain to hourly pain ratings made by 40 patients with chronic pain over a period of 6 to 14 days. They reported the following correlations between diary estimated average pain and alternative measures based on patient recall: least pain, $r = .81$; usual pain, $r = .78$; current pain, $r = .64$; and worst pain, $r = .64$. They found that composite measures tended to produce modest increases in these correlations. In a subsequent study, Jensen, Turner, Romano, and Fisher (1999) found that single and composite pain measures were similar in their ability to detect change in pain status, but that composite pain measures showed greater across time correlation (stability). We (Stewart, Lipton, Simon, Liberman, & Von Korff, 1999) carried out a 3-month daily diary study in a population sample of 132 patients with migraine. We found high correlations between diary-based estimates of pain status and retrospective report of average pain intensity ($r = .74$).

Across these validity studies, retrospective report of average or usual pain intensity showed a high correlation with diary-based estimates of average pain intensity. In a population survey, a report of least pain is likely to provide a poor estimate of average pain because, unlike a sample of patients at a pain clinic, the large majority of subjects will have pain-free days. Similarly, current pain intensity ratings have a high proportion of 0 scores in community samples in which episodic pain conditions predominate. Given the favorable results of several validity studies, there appears to be sufficient empirical support for using measures of average or usual pain intensity for up to a 3-month recall period. Research suggests that pain intensity measures on a 0–10 scale provide adequate discrimination (Jensen, Karoly, O'Riordan, Bland, & Burns, 1989; Jensen, Turner, & Romano, 1994). However, there is evidence that increasing the number of occasions on which pain intensity is measured, up to three times per day for 4 days, can increase the reliability and validity of estimates of average pain (Jensen & McFarland, 1993). There is also evidence that composite measures of pain intensity (e.g., composites of average, least, worst, and current pain) can yield modest improvements in measurement properties relative to a single rating (Dworkin et al., 1990; Jensen et al. 1996, 1999).

VALIDITY OF RETROSPECTIVE REPORT OF DAYS WITH PAIN

There has been less research evaluating the validity of retrospective report of days with pain over a fixed period of time than for average pain intensity. Salovey and colleagues (1992) reported a correlation of .70 between subject recall of the number of days in the prior 2 weeks with a pain rating greater than 5 and a diary-based estimate. In our 3-month daily diary study, we (Stewart, Lipton, Simon, et al., 1999) reported a correlation of $r = .67$ between diary data on days with headache and 3-month recall of days with headache.

These results are encouraging regarding the validity of recall of days with pain over an extended period of time, but more research is needed. For purposes of differentiating persons with chronic versus recurrent or acute pain conditions, it can be questioned whether a 3-month reporting period is sufficient. The International Headache Society Headache Classification Committee (1988) defines chronic headache as headaches occurring on at least half the days in a 1-year period. Similarly, persistent back pain has been defined as back pain present on at least half the days in a 6-month period (Von Korff & Saunders, 1996). This suggests the poten-

tial utility of asking about pain days over a 6-month or 1-year time frame, even though daily diary studies to validate self-report over these longer time periods are probably not feasible.

VALIDITY OF RETROSPECTIVE REPORT OF DISABILITY ASSOCIATED WITH PAIN

There are three widely used types of questions for asking about disability associated with pain. One form of question asks respondents to rate the degree of interference with daily activities due to pain during a defined or indefinite time period (Kerns, Turk, & Rudy, 1985). A variation on this form asks respondents to rate the percentage reduction in ability to perform an activity (Stewart, Lipton, Kolodner, Liberman, & Sawyer, 1999). A second form of question, typically with a yes–no response format, asks about limitations in activities due to pain (Roland & Morris, 1983). A third format asks about days of activity limitation during a 3- or 6-month time period when the subject was unable to carry out usual activities due to pain (Von Korff et al., 1992). There is considerable support for the internal consistency and convergent validity of these kinds of questions (see below). However, there are few studies that have validated recall of pain-related disability in relation to daily diary measures.

In a population-based study of patients with migraine, we (Stewart, Lipton, Simon, et al., 1999) found a correlation of $r = .62$ between diary and retrospective report of percent reduced effectiveness at work. We reported a correlation of $r = .48$ between recall of lost work days due to headache and the corresponding diary-based measure. We observed that questions about activity limitation days with lower yield had lower correlation between recall and diary-based measures than questions with higher yield. A second validity study evaluated revised questions about activity limitation days (Stewart et al., 1999). This study yielded the correlations between a 3-month daily diary and retrospective report shown in Table 31.1.

Although there is a need for more research, these results from daily diary studies, in combination with prior research evaluating the internal consistency and convergent validity of pain disability measures, suggest that retrospective report of interference with daily activities provides useful information. Information on internal consistency and convergent validity is presented in the

TABLE 31.1. Correlation of 3-Month Retrospective Report and Mean of 3-Month Daily Diary Estimate

Retrospective report	Pearson's correlation with daily diary estimate
Number of days missed work or school due to headache	.60
Work/school days productivity reduced by half due to headache	.67
Days missed household work due to headache	.63
Days productivity in household work reduced by half due to headache	.61
Days missed family, social, or leisure activities due to headache	.61

Note. Data from Stewart and Lipton (1999).

remainder of this chapter, which discusses specific pain measures. Future research comparing retrospective report to employer records of absenteeism and work performance would be particularly useful.

BRIEF PAIN AND DISABILITY MEASURES FOR SURVEY RESEARCH

This section provides the items, response scales, and scoring rules for three brief methods of assessing dysfunctional chronic pain: the 36-Item Short-Form Health Survey (SF-36) Bodily Pain subscale, the Graded Chronic Pain Scale (GCPS), and the Migraine Disability Assessment Scale (MIDAS). Although the MIDAS was developed for use with patients who have headache, and has only been validated in this population, the scale appears

potentially useful for assessing disability for pain conditions other than headache.

The SF-36 Bodily Pain Scale

The SF-36 and its variant forms (e.g., the SF-20 and SF-12) are the most widely used general-purpose health status assessment instruments in the United States (Ware, 1993). One of the subscales of the SF-36 assesses pain. This two-item scale assesses pain intensity and interference with activities in the past 4 weeks.

Items and Scoring

Items for the SF-36 Bodily Pain subscale (Ware, 1993), adapted from a longer scale developed by Sherbourne (1992), are provided in Figure 31.2.

1. How much bodily pain have you had during the past 4 weeks?

	None	Very mild	Mild	Moderate	Severe	Very severe
	1	2	3	4	5	6
(Item value for scoring)	(6.0)	(5.4)	(4.2)	(3.1)	(2.2)	(1.0)

2. During the *past 4 weeks*, how much did bodily pain interfere with your work, including both work outside the home and housework?

	Not at all	A little bit	Moderately	Quite a bit	Extremely
	1	2	3	4	5
(Item value for scoring)	(6 or 5)*	(4)	(3)	(2)	(1)

*Note: Item 2 is scored 6 if item 1 is "none" and 5 otherwise.

Scoring rules:
1. Add item values for scoring for items 1 and 2.
2. Subtract the lowest possible score (= 2) from the item total.
3. Divide by the possible raw score range (= 10).
4. Multiply by 100.

FIGURE 31.2. The 36-Item Short-Form Health Survey (SF-36) Bodily Pain subscale. From Ware (1993). Copyright 1993 by the Health Institute, New England Medical Center. Reprinted by permission.

Detailed instructions for scoring the Bodily Pain subscale are reported elsewhere (Ware, 1993). If both items are answered, the scoring rules are summarized in Figure 31.2. The final item scores (see Figure 31.2) are summed, and the lowest possible raw score (i.e., 2) is subtracted from the sum. This result is divided by the possible range of the scale (i.e., 10). The result is then multiplied by 100 to determine the transformed scale score. The transformed Bodily Pain subscale score can range from 0 to 100, where a score of 100 indicates no pain, and a score of 0 indicates the most severe score that is possible.

Reliability and Validity

The test–retest reliability of the Bodily Pain subscale has been estimated to be .78 at a 2-week interval (Brazier et al., 1992). The internal consistency has been estimated to be between .79 and .96 across numerous studies (Ware, 1993). The validity of the Bodily Pain subscale has been assessed by showing that decreasing scores are strongly related to unemployment due to work, and by studies showing that it is correlated with other measures of pain severity and functional disability (Ware, 1993). For example, the Bodily Pain subscale showed a correlation of –.55 with the Pain subscale of the Nottingham Health Profile, and a correlation of –.45 with the Physical Mobility scale of the same instrument (Brazier et al., 1992).

Strengths and Limitations

An advantage of the SF-36 Bodily Pain subscale is that normative data are available (Ware, 1993). Based on a survey of a U.S. population sample of adults ($n = 2,474$) in the noninstitutionalized population, the mean Bodily Pain score was 75.2 ($SD = 23.7$). In this sample, the quartiles of the distribution were as follows: 75th percentile, 100 (least severe); 50th percentile, 74; and 25th percentile, 61. Age- and sex-specific population norms, and norms for various disease groups, are also published (Ware, 1993). For example, the norms for a sample with back pain are as follows: mean = 59.3 ($SD = 24.6$); 75th percentile, 82; 50th percentile, 61; and 25th percentile, 41. In addition to its wide use, extensive assessment of psychometric properties, and the availability of normative data, additional advantages of the SF-36 Bodily Pain subscale are its short length (two items) and its inclusion in a broader health status assessment. With these advantages come a few disadvantages.

The Bodily Pain subscale does not include any prompts for pain site, so its sensitivity to recurrent pain problems with limited impact may be problematic. Since the questions do not relate pain intensity and interference to a specific anatomical location, it has limited suitability for assessing condition-specific severity. Finally, it does not include an assessment of the chronicity or persistence of pain.

Graded Chronic Pain Scale

The GCPS was developed to provide a brief, simple method of grading the severity of chronic or recurrent pain for use in general population surveys and studies of patients with pain in primary care settings (Von Korff et al., 1992). The GCPS measures an underlying severity continuum defined by pain intensity and interference with daily activities. This severity continuum is comparable to the underlying dimension of severity measured by the Bodily Pain subscale of the SF-36. The GCPS has a hierarchical structure, supported by a form of analysis similar to Guttman scaling, in which lower levels of severity are differentiated by pain intensity and higher levels of severity are differentiated by interference with activities. This structure suggests that patients at higher levels of severity, defined by moderate to severe interference with activities, can show improvement by reductions in disability even if pain intensity (or persistence) is not reduced. In contrast, improvements at lower levels of severity (with low levels of interference with activities) require reductions in pain intensity.

Analyses carried out in developing the scale suggested a threshold effect for pain intensity. Respondents with moderate to severe interference with activities (grades III and IV) almost always reported intensity ratings of 50 or greater on a 0–100 scale measuring characteristic pain intensity. In other words, high pain intensity levels were a necessary (but not sufficient) condition for the presence of moderate to severe disability. This suggests that modest reductions in pain intensity may have substantial effects in reducing interference with functioning, if pain intensity is reduced below the threshold level necessary for disability.

Although pain persistence per se is not used in assigning a pain grade, a measure of pain days in the prior 6 months is included in the item set administered. Experience has shown that pain days provides useful information that supplements pain grade (Von Korff et al., 1992).

Items and Scoring

The GCPS items for grading chronic pain status are provided in Figure 31.3. The pain intensity items in this scale were formatted to permit administration by personal interview, by telephone interview, or by self-administration. The average of the three pain intensity items is used to measure characteristic pain intensity (Dworkin et al., 1990). The disability days item and the 0–10 ratings of interference with activities were adapted from prior epidemiological research (Von Korff et al., 1988;

Ask the following questions about the anatomically defined pain site (or sites) of interest, or the most bothersome site of pain identified by filter questions (see Figure 31.4).

1. On about how many days have you had [*anatomical site*] pain in the last six months?

Pain days
_____

If pain not present in the prior six months, skip the remaining questions.

2. How intense is your [*anatomical site*] pain right now, where 0 is "no pain" and 10 is "pain as bad as could be"?

No pain										Pain as bad as could be
0	1	2	3	4	5	6	7	8	9	10

3. In the past six months (or three months), how intense was your worst pain rated on a 0 to 10 scale where 0 is "no pain" and 10 is "pain as bad as could be"?

No pain										Pain as bad as could be
0	1	2	3	4	5	6	7	8	9	10

4. On days you have had pain in the last six months (or three months), how would you rate your average pain on a 0 to 10 scale where 0 is "no pain" and 10 is "pain as bad as could be"?

No pain										Pain as bad as could be
0	1	2	3	4	5	6	7	8	9	10

5. About how many days in the last six months (or three months) have you been kept from your usual activities (work, school, or housework) because of [*anatomical site*] pain?

Disability days
_____

6. In the past six months (or three months), how much has [*anatomical site*] pain interfered with your daily activities rated on a 0 to 10 scale where 0 is "no interference" and 10 is "unable to carry on any activities"?

No interference										Unable to carry on any activities
0	1	2	3	4	5	6	7	8	9	10

7. In the past six months (or three months), how much has [*anatomical site*] pain interfered with your ability to take part in recreational, social and family activities where 0 is "no interference" and 10 is "unable to carry on any activities"?

No interference										Unable to carry on any activities
0	1	2	3	4	5	6	7	8	9	10

8. In the past six months (or three months), how much has [*anatomical site*] pain interfered with your ability to work (including housework) where 0 is "no interference" and 10 is "unable to carry on any activities"?

No interference										Unable to carry on any activities
0	1	2	3	4	5	6	7	8	9	10

FIGURE 31.3. Graded Chronic Pain Scale (GCPS). Copyright 1992 by Michael Von Korff.

Von Korff, Dworkin, & Le Resche, 1990) and from ratings of interference with social and work activities from the West Haven–Yale Multidimensional Pain Inventory (Kerns et al., 1985.

The GCPS is designed to assess intensity, interference with activities, and persistence for pain at a specific anatomical location (e.g., back pain, headache). The pain days question (item 1) can be used to identify respondents who have not had the pain condition of interest in the prior 6 (or 3) months, and to skip them out of the remaining questions (items 2 through 8). Sometimes it is not possible to administer the GCPS questions for every pain problem that is present. In these situations, the questions provided in Figure 31.4 may be used to elicit whether the respondent has had pain at different anatomical locations in the past 6 months. If the respondent reports pain in more than one location, then the site of pain that has been the most bothersome is determined, and the GCPS questions are asked for that site. Alternatively, the GCPS questions can be asked separately for each of the body sites for which pain is reported, providing grading information for each anatomical site for which pain is present.

The GCPS questions were initially developed with a 6-month reporting period. Subsequently, they have been administered with a 3-month reporting interval (Von Korff et al., 1998) and with a 1-month reporting interval (Underwood, Barnett, & Vickers, 1999). A shorter reporting interval is useful in situations where respondents are being followed over time to assess change (e.g., in a study of clinical course or a clinical trial). For example, if patients are being interviewed every 3 months, then a 3-month reporting interval would be appropriate. Pain grade can be determined easily for a 3-month reporting interval by multiplying the activity limitation days item by 2 and scoring all other items in the same way as the 6-month version (see Figure 31.5). However, experience suggests that 3-month grading tends to yield a larger percentage of patients at grades III and IV than 6-month grading does.

Classification criteria for grading chronic pain status are provided in Figure 31.5. The GCPS grades the severity of the pain condition into five ordered categories: grade 0, pain-free; grade I, low intensity, low interference; grade II, high intensity, low interference; grade III, moderate interference with activities; grade IV, severe interference with activities. For patients with higher levels of disability, grading does not consider pain intensity scores. The ordered categories facilitate analysis of the spectrum of severity of chronic/recurrent pain in general population and primary care samples.

---

1. In the past six months, did you have:

	No	Yes	Don't know
a. Back pain?	1	2	8
b. Neck pain?	1	2	8
c. Headache or migraine?	1	2	8
d. Stomach ache or abdominal pain?	1	2	8
e. Joint pain in your arms, hands, legs, or feet?	1	2	8
f. Chest pain?	1	2	8
g. Facial ache or pain (in the jaw or the joint in front of the ear)?	1	2	8

(If more than one pain problem, ask Q2; otherwise skip.)

2. Which pain bothered you the most in the past six months?

a.	Back	1
b.	Neck	2
c.	Headache	3
d.	Abdominal	4
e.	Joint	5
f.	Chest	6
g.	Facial	7
	Don't know	8

If more than one pain problem reported, ask pain-grading questions about the pain problem at the anatomical site that bothered the respondent the most in the last six months. If "several" pain problems were most bothersome, ask person to pick one for pain-grading questions.

FIGURE 31.4. Questions used to identify a single anatomical site for GCPS questions. Copyright 1992 by Michael Von Korff.

SCORING

Characteristic pain intensity is a 0 to 100 score derived from questions 2–4;

Mean [pain right now, worst pain, average pain] × 10

Disability score is a 0 to 100 score derived from questions 6–8;

Mean [daily activities, social activities, work activities] × 10

Disability days is from question 5. If using the 3-month version, multiply disability days by 2 before calculating disability points.

DISABILITY POINTS Add the indicated points for disability days (question 5) and for disability score.			
Disability score		Disability days (question 5) (If using 3-month version, multiply disability days by 2)	
0–29	0 points	0–6 days	0 points
30–49	1 point	7–14 days	1 point
50–69	2 points	15–30 days	2 points
70+	3 points	31+ days	3 points

GRADED CHRONIC PAIN CLASSIFICATION	
PAIN-FREE	
Grade 0	No pain problem (prior six months or three months).
LOW INTERFERENCE	
Grade I *Low intensity*	Characteristic pain intensity less than 50 and fewer than 3 disability points.
Grade II *High intensity*	Characteristic pain intensity of 50 or greater and fewer than 3 disability points.
HIGH INTERFERENCE	
Grade III *Moderately limiting*	3–4 disability points, regardless of characteristic pain intensity.
GRADE IV *Severely limiting*	5–6 disability points regardless of characteristic pain intensity.

CHRONICITY CLASSIFICATION Nonpersistent pain	1–89 pain days (question 1)
Persistent pain	90–180 pain days (question 1)

FIGURE 31.5. Scoring rules and classification criteria for the GCPS. Copyright 1992 by Michael Von Korff.

Patients reporting pain on at least half the days in a 6-month time period on the pain days question (item 1) are classified as having persistent pain, which is an independent descriptor of chronic pain status.

The GCPS can also be used to provide continuous measures of pain intensity (average pain intensity, characteristic pain intensity), of inter-

ference with activities (disability score), and of chronicity (pain days). These continuous measures are more suitable for assessing the effectiveness of interventions in clinical trials than the ordered categories of the GCPS, because the ordered categories are likely to be less responsive to change. The continuous measures of pain intensity, disability, and chronicity may also be useful in situations where distinct measures of pain intensity, disability, and chronicity are needed (e.g., as predictor variables in multivariate analyses, or in analyses of how different components of chronic pain status change with time).

Reliability and Validity

The items used to grade chronic pain status have been evaluated in a large population survey with a 3-year follow-up and in large samples of primary care patients with pain (Von Korff et al., 1992). It has not been evaluated in a population attending a pain clinic. The grading criteria for the GCPS may limit its utility in such populations, where most patients are likely to fall at grades III and IV. Its prognostic value at 3-year follow-up has been reported for a general population sample (Von Korff et al., 1992). Site-specific normative data have been reported for primary care patients with back pain, headache, and temporomandibular disorder (TMD) pain, and for a population sample of adult health maintenance organization (HMO) enrollees. Table 31.2 provides the distribution of pain grades for these samples.

The GCPS has also been used and evaluated in pain surveys carried out in diverse settings in the United States and Europe. In its initial validation, we (Von Korff et al., 1992) showed that the GCPS was associated with an independent measure of pain-related disability, with use of health care and medicines for pain, with severity of depressive symptoms, with frequent use of doctor visits and opioids for pain, and with unemployment in samples of primary care patients with back

pain, headache, and TMD pain. The GCPS was also shown to be associated with increased likelihood of a poor functional outcome 1 and 3 years later. In this initial work, it was shown that the pain intensity and disability items formed a unidimensional scale with good psychometric properties. Based on the Pearson correlations of the seven items used in the GCPS, the internal consistency (Cronbach's alpha) was .84 for patients with back pain, .79 for patients with headache, and .84 for patients with TMD pain.

Smith and colleagues (1997) validated the GCPS in a postal survey of 293 persons drawn from a general practice roster (see also Purves et al., 1998). They confirmed that the GCPS was a unidimensional scale, with an internal consistency coefficient (Cronbach's alpha) of .91. The eigenvalue of the first factor was 4.80, while remaining factors all had eigenvalues of less than 0.85. Chronic pain grade showed a correlation of –0.84 with the Bodily Pain scale of the SF-36, and correlations of –.49 to –.65 with the Physical Function, Social Function, Physical Role, and Emotional Role scales of the SF-36 (these correlations are negative because a lower score indicates greater disability on the SF-36, whereas a higher grade indicates greater disability on the GCPS). The GCPS was also found to be significantly associated with use of health care and medicines for pain in this study.

A study of the GCPS was reported by Penny, Purves, Smith, Chambers, and Smith (1999) in a random sample of 3,605 persons drawn from general practice registers, supplemented by 3,335 persons drawn from a list of persons filling repeated prescriptions for analgesic medications. This study

TABLE 31.2. Percentage of Subjects at Each GCPS Pain Grade for Patients with Back Pain, Headache, and TMD Pain, and for a Population Sample of Adult HMO Enrollees

Grade	Back pain	Headache	TMD pain	Population sample
0. Pain-free	0.0%	0.0%	0.0%	42.3%
I. Low intensity, low interference	34.9%	29.7%	40.7%	19.9%
II. High intensity, low interference	27.9%	40.1%	43.5%	22.0%
III. Moderate interference	20.0%	20.2%	10.5%	13.1%
IV. Severe interference	17.2%	10.0%	5.4%	2.6%
(Sample size)	(1,213)	(779)	(397)	(803)

Note. Patients with pain were assessed 1–3 weeks after an initial visit.

showed a strong relationship between the GCPS and each of the subscales of the SF-36. This study also showed significant relationships between the GCPS and each of the dimensions of the Glasgow Pain Scale (including frequency, intensity, coping, emotional, and restriction).

Underwood and colleagues (1999) compared the GCPS and the Roland and Morris Disability Scale (Roland & Morris, 1983) for patients with back pain. They tested a version of the GCPS with a 1-month reporting period. They reported internal consistency coefficients of .91 for the characteristic pain scale and .89 for the disability score. They assessed test–retest reliability with intraclass correlation coefficients based on a readministration at 1–2 weeks, and reported an intraclass correlation of .82 for pain intensity and .85 for disability score. They reported high correlations of these GCPS subscales with the SF-36 Bodily Pain scale (–.67 for pain intensity and –.76 for disability score) and with the SF-36 Physical Function subscale (–.64 for pain intensity and –.72 for disability score).

Strengths and Limitations

The reliability and validity of the GCPS have now been established by several research groups in diverse populations. Some normative data are available for general population samples (Elliot, Smith, Penny, Smith, & Chambers, 1999) and for primary care samples of patients with back pain, headache, and TMD pain (Von Korff et al., 1992). The GCPS is an efficient means of assessing and comparing the severity of different chronic/recurrent pain conditions. It can be used either as an ordinal scale (pain grade) or as a set of continuous measures of pain intensity, interference with activities, and persistence. It is unclear whether the GCPS is appropriate for differentiating severity of pain in patients at pain clinics, as it has been normed on general population and primary care samples. Unlike the MIDAS (see below), the GCPS scores do not have a direct interpretation (e.g., lost time equivalents).

Migraine Disability Assessment Scale

The MIDAS, developed by Stewart, Lipton, Whyte, and colleagues (1999), assesses headache-related disability. The items in the MIDAS are provided in Figure 31.6. It is intended for clinical, health services, and epidemiological applications. The MIDAS score separately assesses lost time in each of three domains: work, chores, and nonwork activities.

Items and Scoring

The MIDAS score is calculated from five items asking about disability associated with headache in the prior 3 months. It has two additional items assessing average pain intensity and headache days. Responses to each question are scaled in units of days missed (work or school, household work, and nonwork activities) or the number of days during which productivity was reduced by half or more in the prior 3 months (work or school and household work). The MIDAS was constructed to provide simple and readily interpretable scoring. It estimates lost work day equivalents, but it only requires addition to score (not multiplication or division). The MIDAS score is estimated by simply adding the number of days for the first five MIDAS questions. The score is classified into grades by using the cut points in Figure 31.6. The MIDAS also obtains number of headache days and average pain intensity, but these items do not contribute to the MIDAS score. Like the GCPS, the MIDAS places patients in four grades. A score of 0–5 (grade I) indicates little or no disability; a score of 6–10 (grade II) reflects mild disability; a score of 11–20 (grade III) indicates moderate disability; and a score of 21+ (grade IV) reflects severe disability.

Reliability and Validity

The correlation of the overall MIDAS score with the corresponding estimate based on daily diary data was estimated to be .63. Information on the correlation of individual items with daily diary data has been provided in preceding sections of this chapter. The test–retest reliability of the MIDAS score is .84 (Stewart, Lipton, Whyte, et al., 1999). The internal consistency (Cronbach's alpha) estimated in this study was .83. Research has been carried out assessing its association with other disability measures, but has not yet been reported.

Strengths and Limitations

Advantages of the MIDAS are that it has been rigorously validated among a population sample of patients with headache in relation to daily diary data; it is easy to score; and its score has a direct clinical meaning. Disadvantages are that it has only been used in populations with headache, although it could readily be adapted to assessing disability for other pain conditions. Its responsiveness to change has not been assessed.

1. On how many days in the last three months did you miss work or school because of your headaches?

2. On how many days in the last three months was your productivity at work or school reduced by half or more because of your headaches? (Do not include days you counted in question 1 where you missed work or school.)

3. On how many days in the last three months did you not do household work because of your headaches?

4. How many days in the last three months was your productivity in household work reduced by half or more because of your headaches? (Do not include days you counted in question 3 where you did not do household work.)

5. On how many days in the last three months did you miss family, social, or leisure activities because of your headaches?

A. On how many days in the last three months did you have a headache? If a headache lasted more than one day, count each day.

B. On a scale of 0 to 10, on average how painful were these headaches (where 0 is not pain at all and 10 is pain as bad as can be)?

MIDAS Scoring Rules

Grade	Definition	MIDAS score
I	Little or no disability	0–5
II	Mild disability	6–10
III	Moderate disability	11–20
IV	Severe disability	20 +

FIGURE 31.6. Migraine Disability Assessment Scale (MIDAS). Copyright 1999 by W. F. Stewart and R. B. Lipton.

SUMMARY

This chapter has paid special attention to recent advances in brief measures of pain-related disability suitable for use in epidemiological and survey research. The measures are suitable for both cross-sectional surveys and longitudinal studies that assess the course of chronic pain over time. These measures are not appropriate for assessing the onset (incidence) of anatomically defined pain conditions or the onset of chronic pain in general, which involves special measurement issues beyond the scope of this chapter. Methodological studies now suggest that recall of key parameters of chronic/recurrent pain (average intensity, interference with

activities, activity limitation days, and days with pain) have acceptable levels of validity for at least a 3-month recall period. This suggests that self-report pain measures with an extended recall period can yield useful information on the distribution and burden of chronic pain in population samples. Further research is needed to better understand the nature and magnitude of measurement biases that are produced by these kinds of self-report measures, and to determine how the validity of self-report measures can be improved. However, available research provides strong support for the reliability and validity of brief self-report measures of pain severity based on assessment of pain intensity and interference with daily activities.

ACKNOWLEDGMENT

This work was supported by a grant from the National Institutes of Health (No. P01 DE08773).

REFERENCES

Bradburn, N. M., Rips, L. J., & Shevell, S. K. (1987). Answering autobiographical questions: The impact of memory and influence on surveys. *Science, 236,* 157–161.

Brazier, J. E., Harper, R., Jones, N. M., O'Cathain, A., Thomas, K. J., Usherwood, T., & Westlake, L. (1992). Validating the SF-36 Health Survey questionnaire: New outcome measure for primary care. *British Medical Journal, 305,* 160–164.

Cannel, C. F. (1977). *A summary of research studies of interviewing methodology, 1959–1970* (Vital and Health Statistics: Series 2. Data Evaluation and Methods Research, No. 69, DHEW Publication No. HRA 77-1343). Washington, DC: U.S. Government Printing Office.

Carey, T. S., Garrett, J., Jackman, A., Sanders, L., & Kalsbeek, W. (1995) Reporting of acute low back pain in a telephone interview: Identification of potential biases. *Spine, 20,* 787–790.

Converse, P. E., & Traugott, M. W. (1986). Assessing the accuracy of polls and surveys. *Science, 234,* 1094–1098.

Crombie, I. K., Croft, P. R., Linton, S. J., Le Resche, L., & Von Korff, M. (Eds.). (1999). *Epidemiology of pain.* Seattle, WA: International Association for the Study of Pain Press.

De Wit, R., van Dam, F., Hanneman, M., Zabndbelt, L., van Buuren, A., van der Heijden, K., Lennhouts, G., Loonstra, S., & Abu-Saad, H. H. (1999). Evaluation of the use of a pain diary in chronic cancer pain patients at home. *Pain, 79,* 89–99.

Dworkin, S. F., Von Korff, M., Whitney, C. W., Le Resche, L., Dicker, B. G., & Barlow, W. (1990). Measurement of characteristic pain intensity in field research. *Pain,* Suppl. 5, S290.

Elliot, A. M., Smith, B. H., Penny, K. I., Smith, W. C., & Chambers, W. A. (1999). The epidemiology of chronic pain in the community. *Lancet, 354,* 1248–1252.

International Headache Society Headache Classification Committee. (1988). Classification and diagnostic criteria for headache disorders, cranial neuralgias, and facial pain. *Cephalalgia,* 8(Suppl. 7), 1–96.

Jensen, M. P., Karoly, P., O'Riordan, E. F., Bland, F., Jr., & Burns, R. S. (1989). The subjective experience of acute pain: An assessment of the utility of 10 indices. *Clinical Journal of Pain, 5,* 153–159.

Jensen, M. P., & McFarland, C. A. (1993). Increasing the reliability and validity of pain intensity measurement in chronic pain patients. *Pain, 55,* 195–203.

Jensen, M. P., Turner, J. A., & Romano, J. M. (1994). What is the maximum number of levels needed in pain intensity measurement? *Pain, 58,* 387–392.

Jensen, M. P., Turner, J. A., Romano, J. M., & Fisher, L. D. (1999). Comparative reliability and validity of chronic pain intensity measures. *Pain, 83,* 157–162.

Jensen, M. P., Turner, L. R., Turner, J. A., & Romano, J. M. (1996). The use of multiple-item scales for pain intensity measurement in chronic pain patients. *Pain, 67,* 35–40.

Kerns, R. D., Turk, D. C., & Rudy, T. E. (1985). The West Haven–Yale Multidimensional Pain Inventory (WHYMPI). *Pain, 23,* 345–356.

Kleinbaum, D. G., Kupper, L. L., & Morgenstern, H. (1982). *Epidemiologic research: Principles and quantitative methods.* Belmont, CA: Lifetime Learning.

Madow, W. G. (1973). *Net differences in interview data on chronic conditions and information derived from medical records* (Vital and Health Statistics: Series 2. Data Evaluation and Methods Research, No. 57, DHEW Publication No. HSM 73-1331). Washington, DC: U.S. Government Printing Office.

Means, B., Nigam, A., Zarrow, M., Loftus, E. F., & Donaldson, M. S. (1989). *Autobiographical memory for health-related events* (Vital and Health Statistics: Series 6. Cognitive and Survey Measurement, DHHS Publication No. PHS 89-1077). Washington, DC: U.S. Government Printing Office.

National Institutes of Health Consensus Development Conference. (1986). *The integrated approach to the management of pain* (NIH Consensus Development Conference Statement, Vol. 6, No. 3). Washington, DC: U.S. Government Printing Office.

Osterweis, M., Kleinman, A., & Mechanic, D. (1987). *Pain and disability: Clinical, behavioral and public policy perspectives.* Washington, DC: National Academy Press.

Penny, K. I., Purves, A. M., Smith, B. H., Chambers, W. A., & Smith, W. C. (1999). Relationship between the chronic pain grade and measures of physical, social and psychological well-being. *Pain, 79,* 275–279.

Purves, A. M., Penny, K. I., Munro, C., Smith, B. H., Grimshaw, J., Wilson, B., Smith, W. C., & Chambers, W. A. (1998). Defining chronic pain for epidemiologic research: Assessing a subjective definition. *The Pain Clinic, 10,* 139–147.

Roland, M., & Morris, R. (1983). A study of the natural history of back pain: I. Development of a reliable and sensitive measure of disability in low-back pain. *Spine, 8,* 141–144.

Salovey, P., Seiber, W. J., Smith, A. F., Turk, D. C., Jobe, J. B., & Willis, G. B. (1992). *Reporting chronic pain episodes on health surveys* (Vital and Health Statistics: Series 6. Cognitive and Survey Measurement). Washington, DC: U.S. Government Printing Office.

Sherbourne, C. D. (1992). Pain measures. In A. L. Stewart & J. E. Ware (Eds.), *Measuring functioning and well-being: The medical outcomes study approach* (pp. 220–234). Durham, NC: Duke University Press.

Simon, G. E., & Von Korff, M. (1995). Recall of psychiatric history in cross-sectional surveys: Implications for epidemiologic research. *Epidemiologic Reviews, 17,* 221–227.

Smith, B. H., Penny, K. I., Purves, A. M., Munro, C., Wilson, B., Grimshaw, J., Chambers, W. A., & Smith, W. C. (1997). The Chronic Pain Grade questionnaire: Validation and reliability in postal research. *Pain, 71,* 141–147.

Stewart, W. F., & Lipton, R. B. (1999). Unpublished data.

Stewart, W. F., Lipton, R. B., Kolodner, K., Liberman, J., & Sawyer, J. (1999). Reliability of the Migraine Disability Assessment score in a population-based sample of headache sufferers. *Cephalagia, 19,* 107–114.

Stewart, W. F., Lipton, R. B., Simon, D., Liberman, J., & Von Korff, M. (1999). Validity of an illness severity measure for headache in a population sample of migraine sufferers. *Pain, 79,* 291–301.

Stewart, W. F., Lipton, R. B., Whyte, J., Kolodner, K., Liberman, J. N., & Sawyer, J. (1999). An international study to assess reliability of the Migraine Disability Assessment (MIDAS) score. *Neurology, 53,* 988–994.

Underwood, M. R., Barnett, A. G., & Vickers, M. R. (1999). Evaluation of two time-specific back pain outcome measures. *Spine, 24,* 1104–1112.

Von Korff, M. (1991). Memory for pain in epidemiologic research: Effects of depression on back pain recall. *Proceedings of the 12th Annual Meeting of the Society of Behavioral Medicine,* 142.

Von Korff, M. (1999). Epidemiologic methods. In I. K. Crombie, P. R. Croft, S. J. Linton, L. Le Resche, & M. Von Korff (Eds.), *Epidemiology of pain* (pp. 7–15). Seattle, WA: International Association for the Study of Pain Press.

Von Korff, M., & Dworkin, S. (1989). Problems in measuring pain by survey: The classification of chronic pain in field research. In C. R. Chapman & J. D. Loeser (Eds.), *Advances in pain research and therapy:*

Vol. 12. Issues in pain management (pp. 519–533). New York: Raven Press.

Von Korff, M., Dworkin, S., & Le Resche, L. (1990). Graded chronic pain status: An epidemiologic evaluation. *Pain, 40,* 279–291.

Von Korff, M., Dworkin, S., Le Resche, L. & Kruger, A. (1988). An epidemiologic comparison of pain complaints. *Pain, 32,* 173–183.

Von Korff, M., Lipton, R., & Stewart, W. E. (1994). Assessing headache severity: New directions. *Neurology, 44*(Suppl. 6), S40–S46.

Von Korff, M., Moore, J. E., Lorig, K., Cherkin, D. C., Saunders, K., Gonzales, V. M., Laurent, D., Rutter, C., & Comite, F. (1998). A randomized trial of a lay-led self-management group intervention for back pain patients in primary care. *Spine, 23,* 2608–2615.

Von Korff, M., Ormel, J., Keefe, F., & Dworkin, S. F. (1992). Grading the severity of chronic pain. *Pain, 50,* 133–149.

Von Korff, M., & Parker, R. D. (1980). The dynamics of the prevalence of chronic episodic disease. *Journal of Chronic Diseases, 33,* 79–85.

Von Korff, M., & Saunders, K. (1996). The course of back pain in primary care. *Spine, 21,* 2833–2837.

Ware, J. E. (1993). *SF-36 Health Survey: Manual and interpretation guide.* Boston: Health Institute, New England Medical Center.

Chapter 32

Relying on Objective and Subjective Measures of Chronic Pain: Guidelines for Use and Interpretation

SAMUEL F. DWORKIN
JEFFREY J. SHERMAN

The need for a second edition of this book, as well as its revised organization and content, reinforces our deepening understanding of acute and chronic pain not only as an intensely negative human experience but as an intensely subjective one. Acute and chronic pain, as the many chapters of the current edition attest, is understood more clearly than ever to be multifactorial. The human pain experience is shaped as much by the impact of culture, personal, and family history and environmental encounters as by physical damage. Similarly, the expression of pain is assessed as much by subjectively measured thought, emotion, and behavior as by objectively measured biopathology associated with genetic and metabolic errors, developmental defects, tumor, trauma, or infection.

The purpose of this chapter is to present a pragmatic framework for evaluating the usefulness of selected objective and subjective measures to assess the multiple dimensions of chronic pain. We first present a heuristic model (Dworkin, Von Korff, & LeResche, 1992) for depicting the various levels at which pain-relevant variables may be measured over time. Using this overall organization, we then discuss, from a practical perspective, critical issues concerning the reliability, validity, and interpretation of pain-related measures. The principal targets of this discussion are selected issues that influence the measures we use to assess signs

and symptoms of chronic pain in research and clinical treatment settings.

As a practical matter, although both acute and chronic pain represent complex and dynamic interactions of personal experience, subjectively measured, and biological processes, chronic pain has emerged ever more clearly as encompassing more problematic assessment and management challenges than are typically associated with acute, or newly emergent, pain problems. As a result, the multidimensional assessment of chronic pain continues to present challenges resistant to ready solution.

In clinical settings, chronic pain assessment translates into assessments involving multiple biomedical and biobehavioral dimensions. Assessment in these biomedical domains reflects the aspects of pain phenomenology that are unique in different pain conditions, bodily sites, and pathophysiological processes. Assessment in the biomedical domain is accomplished typically through objective measurements (laboratory tests, diagnostic imaging) across organ system specialties (orthopedics, neurology, neurosurgery, dentistry, internal medicine) that seek to identify a physically based etiology for each pain condition. The end results of objective assessments in the biomedical domain are pain diagnoses unique to bodily sites or pathophysiological processes, such as migraine head-

619

ache, complex regional pain syndrome or trigeminal neuralgia.

By contrast, when biobehavioral assessment of chronic pain is undertaken, it is observed that the most prevalent chronic pain conditions (i.e., headache, back pain, temporomandibular disorder [TMD], fibromyalgia) have in common a set of factors arising largely independently of anatomical site or pathophysiological processes. The biobehavioral dimensions of chronic pain experience must be assessed almost exclusively through subjective measurement of pain perception, cognition, affect, behavior, and sick role. Moreover, in the biobehavioral domain, multidimensional assessment of chronic pain points to the emergence of a constellation of perceptions, emotions, and behaviors that represents a final common pathway into chronic pain suffering. The pattern of suffering for which a significant proportion of patients with chronic pain are at risk is independent of bodily sites where the chronic pain condition may be located, transcending the biomedical classification of pain conditions. It includes the following:

1. Emergence of pain severity and personal distress levels that correspond only poorly to objectively observable nature or extent of pathophysiological change.
2. Transient psychological disturbance as highly likely.
3. The emergence of clinical depression, anxiety, and somatization—the tendency to report multiple nonspecific physical symptoms and seek treatment for them.
4. Interference with ability to perform usual activities at home, work, or school.
5. Maladaptive or dysfunctional behaviors, primarily deactivation, social isolation, and poor sleep patterns.
6. Frequent use of the health care system, with potential for excessive treatment seeking and abuse of medications.

LEVELS OF PAIN MEASUREMENT

Deciding What to Measure

The first issue to be confronted relates to the multiple levels at which it is possible to measure pain—that is, deciding which of the diverse manifestations of chronic pain a measure has been designed to assess. The model depicted in Figures 32.1 and 32.2 (Dworkin et al., 1992) was developed to depict the relationships among physiological, psychological,

behavioral, and social factors that interact in chronic pain, as elaborated by influential workers in the field (Fields, 1987; Fordyce, 1976; Kleinman, 1988; Mechanic, 1986; Melzack & Wall, 1965; Parsons, 1975; Petrie, 1967; Pilowsky & Spence, 1983; Turk & Rudy, 1988).

The model depicts pain phenomenology as emerging from the subjective perception of noxious physiological events that are appraised for their personal meaning and then are acted upon through behaviors shaped by social and cultural contexts to yield the role of a patient with pain (Loeser, 1982). These processes can go on within normal limits or can be maladaptively intensified. By and large, each pain measure attempts to assess only one of these levels (e.g., pain perception), although some measures assess adaptation at multiple levels (e.g., appraisal and behavior).

An exciting direction for pain research that has opened up in the last decade promises to yield new insight into pain perception and appraisal processes. From 1991 to 1999, more than 30 studies were conducted using functional imaging of various regions of the human brain as they responded to noxious stimuli (Derbyshire, 1999; see also Flor, Chapter 5, this volume). Positron emission tomography (PET), magnetic resonance imaging (MRI), and other imaging techniques used in such studies allow us to view pain information as it is being dynamically processed by the brain. Notable in these studies has been the individual variability in response and even in which specific regions of the brain are activated during the pain experience.

The essentially ecological view we are presenting is an integration of objective, subjective, and environmental influences. The model is also dynamic; that is, it recognizes that pain states change over time, as depicted in Figure 32.2. Pain experience may be influenced by time-dependent stages of development, from infancy through childhood, adolescence, maturity, and senescence. Attention has been drawn to the special challenges encountered when investigators are attempting systematic measurement of pain in children (McGrath, 1990; see also McGrath & Gillespie, Chapter 6) and elderly persons (Parmalee, 1994; Weiner, Peterson, & Keefe, 1999; see also Gagliese, Chapter 7).

Independently, pain experience over time may be acute, recurrent, or chronic, and pain measures must be responsive to the course of pain fluctuation in its natural history or in its clinical course when treatments are provided. Our current state of knowledge leaves unresolved many aspects of the longitudinal measurement of pain.

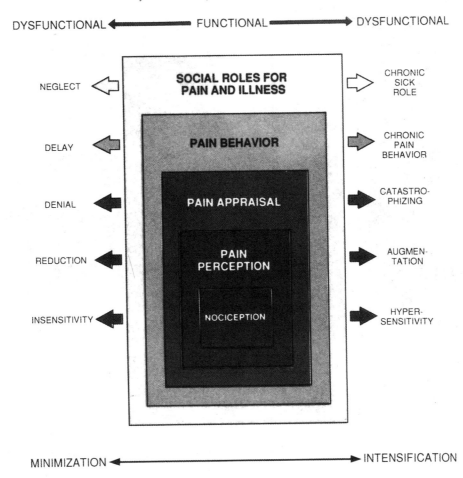

FIGURE 32.1. Ecological model for chronic pain and dysfunction: Multidimensional aspects.

Nociception and Physiological versus Clinical Measurements of Chronic Pain

Nociception

Our model assumes at the biological level that pain report is associated with information, or *signals*, being transmitted in the nervous system that have the potential for being perceived and appraised as noxious, aversive, or painful. In most settings in which human pain data are gathered, however, it is not possible to obtain information at the level of basic nociceptive processes (such as neurotransmitter concentrations or specificity of neural pathways being discharged). In clinical settings, the equivalent of the nociceptive level of measurement is the physical level of recording objective pain-related clinical signs through physical examination and, to a lesser extent, through laboratory tests. (See Polatin & Mayer, Chapter 11, and Waddell &

Turk, Chapter 23). The resultant findings, commonly labeled *signs*, are generally thought of as objective measures of the physical components of pain, since they do not appear to require subjectively derived self-report. Examples of common clinical measures include assessment of range of motion for musculoskeletal pains; use of radiographic and other imaging methods to detect abnormal structural changes; and laboratory tests for indications of painful systemic diseases, such as rheumatoid arthritis or ischemic cardiac pain. Although many of these measures are truly free of the patient's subjective report, they are not necessarily free of examiner bias when these clinical findings are interpreted, as we shall discuss below.

It has been suggested that patients with chronic pain differ in their level of sensitization to nociceptive input. Increased sensitization may be induced at peripheral sites in terms of microscopic

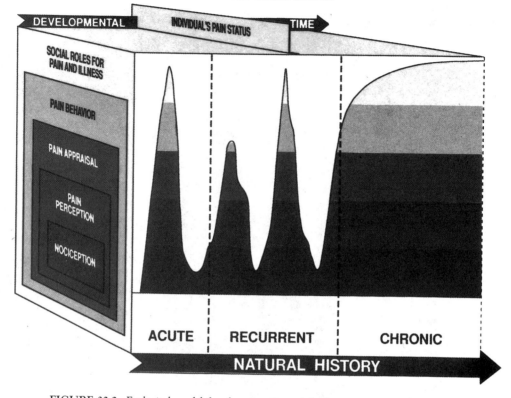

FIGURE 32.2. Ecological model for chronic pain and dysfunction: Temporal aspects.

tissue damage (Mense, Hoheisel, Kaske, & Reinert, 1997), or at the central nervous system level (e.g., central sensitization) (Mendell, 1966). Recent evidence argues for the diagnostic value of psychophysical measures of nociception and sensitization, as it appears that sensitization to nociceptive stimuli in the form of tonic heat can discriminate patients with chronic pain from healthy controls (Kleinböhl et al., 1999).

In any event, it remains one of the major enigmas of pain assessment that measurements at the physical level (typically clinical signs, in the case of patients with pain), are often inconsistent with, or inadequate to explain, subjective reports of persistent pain and suffering accompanied by frequently dysfunctional chronic pain behaviors (Sternbach, 1990).

Measuring Pain Perception

Since pain is a uniquely personal experience, the first opportunity to measure the subjective experience is at the perceptual level. At the simplest level is eliciting whether pain is present. Measurable nociceptive physiological responses presumed to reflect the presence of pain cannot be used to define whether or not a person is in pain, although they yield valuable information concerning the body's status when pain is reported. The International Association for the Study of Pain (IASP) defines *pain* as a subjective experience described in terms of bodily damage. That is, as a minimum, pain involves both perception (an internal information-processing act) and subjective report of a noxious bodily state (an overt, readily observable behavior); the formal definition of pain does not require that a pathological process be confirmed (Merskey, 1986; Merskey & Bogduk, 1994).

Most commonly, pain experience is assessed at the perceptual level using self-report measures. A distinction between the terms *sensation* and *perception* is sometimes made, but for present purposes, and especially in the context of assessing chronic pain, we prefer using the term *perception* to define assessment of pain at the level of self-reporting the physical qualities of the painful experience. Thus measurement at the level of perception in this model system attempts to assess the quality and quantity of pain by inquiring into perceived sensory attributes: intensity, location, duration (temporal qualities), and sensory qualities (e.g., sensations of "burning," "throbbing," "dull," or "sharp"). The most common measures of pain perception include Visual Analogue Scales (VASs) of pain intensity; the sensory scales of common pain measures, notably the McGill Pain Questionnaire (MPQ; Melzack, 1975); and verbal rating scales based on psychophysical methods, such as the Verbal Descriptor Scale (Gracely & Dubner, 1987) and the Pain Perception Profile (Tursky, 1976). (See Jensen & Karoly, Chapter 2; Melzack & Katz, Chapter 3; and Price, Riley, & Wade, Chapter 4.)

When pain perception is intensified beyond adaptive levels, it is often assessed as inappropriate augmentation of physical sensations (Petrie, 1967), symptom amplification (Barsky, 1979), or somatization (Simon & Von Korff, 1991). In the case of somatization, intensified pain perception may reflect a more generalized tendency to report multiple physical symptoms (e.g., numbness, tingling, shortness of breath, pounding heart), perhaps modifying the diagnostic saliency of the observed pain report (Dworkin, Von Korff, & LeResche, 1990).

Measuring Pain Appraisal

The measurement of pain perception is known to be influenced by underlying physiological processes that create large individual differences in pain thresholds and tolerance levels. In addition, pain perception is known to be heavily influenced by "higher-order" processes that characterize the cognitive and emotional appraisal of pain—what people think and feel about their pain. These pain appraisal factors include consideration of the interpersonal context in which pain is encountered (e.g., when a patient is with friends vs. alone); the emotional significance to patients of their pain (the presence of attendant anxiety or depression); and the cognitive attributions they make concerning its origins, the best way to treat the pain, and their capacity to control or otherwise cope with the pain problem (See Bradley & McKendree-Smith, Chapter 16; DeGood & Tait, Chapter 17; and Jacob & Kerns, Chapter 19.)

The cognitive and emotional influences on pain perception are well known, but are briefly summarized here as a reminder of the need to keep in mind the particular aspects of pain for which measurement is sought. The current concept of pain as multidimensional has yielded numerous measures of the cognitive (Turk & Flor, 1984) and emotional (Romano & Turner, 1985) components of pain, many of which are reflected in other chapters of this volume. When measures of cognitive appraisal reveal excessive intensification, as indicated in Figure 32.1, the patient with pain is characterized as "catastrophizing" or may be assessed as "hypochondriacal." When measures of emotional status are intensified, the patient may be assessed as clinically depressed or anxious.

Measuring Pain Behaviors

The nociceptive, perceptual, and appraisal processes underlying pain experience depicted in Figure 32.1 and discussed so far reflect intrapersonal events, or covert occurring within the individual. Overt pain behaviors—behaviors that can be measured by an observer—typically fall into two categories: (1) self-reported or verbal behaviors, as when one responds to a questionnaire or interview; and (2) nonverbal behaviors, as observed facial expressions, bodily posture, gross motor movements, and physical activities. (See Craig, Prkachin, & Grunau, Chapter 9, and Keefe, Williams, & Smith, Chapter 10.) Largely due to the efforts of Fordyce (1976) and later Keefe (Keefe & Block, 1982; Keefe, Gil, & Rose, 1986), measures of pain behavior have emerged as potent indicators of current pain status and as measures of change in response to treatment. Measuring pain in terms of observable behavior at the level of physical activity (e.g., range-of-motion studies, facial expression, activity level, and treatment-seeking behaviors) offers the possibility of assessing the status of patients with pain without recourse to subjective self-report. However, as we shall see, many behavioral measurements, although not directly involving verbal self-report, are nevertheless contingent on subjective pain experience—as, for example, when the patient is asked to "bend over and touch your toes." The range of motion, commonly thought of as a clinical sign assessed in objective units of measurement, is nevertheless often implicitly limited by the patient's subjective experience of pain symptomatology. (See Robinson, Chapter 14, on the implications of this for determining impairment ratings.)

Intensification of avoidant pain behaviors, as measured by decreased activity levels, increased pain-related interference with tasks of daily living, and excessive treatment-seeking behavior, is a major factor in assessing patients with chronic pain as dysfunctional (Von Korff, Dworkin, & LeResche, 1990). Much of pain therapy, especially in specialized pain clinics, is directed largely at modifying dysfunctional chronic pain behaviors (see Figure 32.1) (Fordyce, Roberts, & Sternbach, 1985).

The aim of such behaviorally focused therapies is to elicit measurable changes in pain behavior, principally in the form of measurably increased activity levels, with less concern for demonstrating comparable changes in self-report measures of perceived pain intensity or affect.

Others have argued that focusing primarily on measuring behavioral change, to the exclusion of assessing changes in affective status and pain attributions, does not adequately capture the full range of the pain experience (Turk, Meichenbaum, & Genest, 1983). For example, patients' beliefs about their chronic pain condition are more predictive of functioning than are either spouse/partner or and clinician ratings of pain behaviors (Jensen, Romano, Turner, Good, & Wald, 1999).

Other integrated approaches for assessing pain include assessment of the multiple dimensions depicted in Figure 32.1. The multiaxial pain assessment approach offered by Turk and Rudy (1987) is an example of a widely used approach integrating measurement of the cognitive, affective, behavioral, and interpersonal sequelae associated with chronic pain. Similarly, Jensen and colleagues (1999) recommend using instruments specifically designed to measure cognitive, behavioral, and coping strategies regarding adjustment to chronic pain. The Research Diagnostic Criteria for TMD (RDC/TMD) system (Dworkin & LeResche, 1992; see also Dworkin & Ohrbach, Chapter 25) takes a dual-axis approach to assessing persons suffering from this chronic pain syndrome. Axis I records clinical physical findings to diagnose the most common subtypes of TMD, while Axis II assesses the person's behavioral (e.g., mandibular functional disability), psychological (e.g., depression, anxiety, and somatization—the presence of nonspecific physical symptoms) and psychosocial (e.g., chronic pain grade assessing pain severity together with TMD-related interference with activities of daily living) status. Included in the RDC/TMD system is a version of the Graded Chronic Pain Scale, developed by Von Korff and colleagues (1990), which integrates measures of pain severity, pain interference, and activity limitations into a single quantitative index as a means to assess multiple dimensions of chronic pain in a theoretically integrated manner (see Von Korff, Chapter 31).

Social Roles in Chronic Pain: Measuring the Impact

The societal costs due to chronic pain are acknowledged to be very high. Both the Institute of Medicine (Osterweis, Kleinman, & Mechanic, 1987) and the U.S. Social Security Administration (1984) have labeled chronic pain as a problem of major societal significance. Attempts to measure the cost of chronic pain and chronic pain dysfunction to the U.S. economy place those societal costs at billions of dollars annually. Chronic pain behaviors are embedded in social roles for patients with pain (see Figure 32.1) that sanction temporary withdrawal from personal and work responsibilities while acknowledging the need for an appropriate increase in treatment seeking. The notion of a *sick role*, first elaborated by Parsons (1975), implies measuring the reciprocating impact of pain on both the person and the environment. The Sickness Impact Profile (Bergner, Bobbitt, Carter, & Gilson, 1981) is a measure initially developed to assess the social impact of chronic illness that has been applied to the study of impairment, disability, and dysfunction associated with chronic pain.

The intensification of the sick role for patients with chronic pain is also measured as the increased amount of lost time and expense associated with loss of productive work, together with the heightened costs of medical, surgical, and pharmacological treatment that the dysfunctional patient with chronic pain undergoes.

RELYING ON PAIN MEASURES: THE CENTRAL ISSUES OF RELIABILITY AND VALIDITY

A schematic model for organizing the levels at which pain can be assessed has been presented because we believe that evaluating pain measures for their usefulness begins with assessing which level(s) of pain (e.g., perception, appraisal, behavior) the measure purports to tap. The next step is to evaluate how well the measure actually performs. We now turn to a more detailed discussion of underlying issues that influence the performance and interpretation of pain measures, focusing specifically on the most basic properties of any measurement instrument—namely, reliability and validity. The emphasis is not on the statistical or psychometric principles and methods that underlie the measurement of pain (or any other aspect of health and illness), although statistical and psychometric issues are engaged. Rather, the focus is on sharing an approach we find useful when evaluating and interpreting chronic pain measurement methods described in the literature, or when designing studies requiring the selection of measures at one or more levels of chronic pain assessment.

Reliability and Validity: An Overview

Reliability and validity are the basic underpinnings of all pain measures because they reflect the quality, or "goodness," of a measure. An analogy commonly used to make clear the distinction between reliability and validity involves the possibilities when one is shooting at a target with a bull's-eye at its center. The shooter who is both reliable and valid hits the bull's-eye every time; the shooter who is reliable but not valid consistently hits the same point on the target, but it is not the bull's-eye; the unreliable and invalid shooter sprays bullets all over the place.

Reliability and validity indices express the extent to which we can depend on a pain measure to (1) assess current status, (2) contribute to a useful diagnosis, (3) yield rational treatment decisions, and (4) evaluate the course of a pain condition over time. *Reliability* (Anastasi, 1988) of a measure refers to consistency of measurement—the ability of a measure to yield comparable results on repeated administrations. *Replicability, reproducibility,* and *consistency* can be thought of as useful synonyms for reliability of measurement.

Classical test construction theory suggests that a score on any measure is understood to be a combination of the "true" score and some random or measurement error. The true score component reflects an examinee's status with regard to the attribute measured by the test. Measurement error is due to factors that are irrelevant to what is being measured and have an unpredictable and unsystematic effect on scores. When the measure is repeated, if measurement error is small and random, and if nothing has changed between administrations in the subjects being tested, then the initial scores will be closely related to (i.e., highly correlated with) scores on the repeated measurement, and the measure will be assessed as having high reliability. Otherwise, the reliability may be questionable. For example, a patient's rating of pain on palpation of the masseter muscle is due to both consistent nociceptive sensation (i.e., the true score) and the effects of random factors (i.e., symptom fluctuation, anxiety, attention, motivation).

Since a test's true score is not directly calculable, the reliability of the test must be estimated. We discuss several ways to estimate reliability. Each involves assessing the consistency of a test's scores over time, across parallel forms of the same test, or across different raters of the same test.

Validity (Anastasi, 1988) of a measure is often defined as the extent to which a test measures what it is supposed to measure. If reliability reflects the correlation of a measure with itself, then validity reflects the correlation of a measure with external criteria. A clinical measure such as joint palpation pain may lead to a diagnosis of joint pathology. To determine whether the measure is reliable, it may be repeated. To determine whether the joint palpation measure is valid for diagnosing joint pathology, results are compared to findings from an external criterion measure (e.g., radiographic studies of the joint), which serves as an acceptable standard of comparison. If the palpation pain measure and the radiographic interpretation agree, the palpation measure is assessed as highly valid for detecting joint pathology, since the radiograph is the so-called "gold standard."

It is obvious that reliability and validity are intimately associated. A measure that is not consistent with itself (i.e., is unreliable) cannot be consistent with some other measure (and hence is invalid). Thus the reliability of a measure places an upper limit on its validity. Statistically, reliability and validity are most often expressed as correlation coefficients. The maximum validity that can be achieved using a particular measure is the square of its reliability coefficient. It is more helpful to provide the reliability of both the measure and the external criterion.

The maximum validity that is possible can be determined as the product of the square roots of the reliability of each measure. In our example above, if the reliability of assessing joint sounds is reported as .64 and the reliability of interpreting joint radiographs is given as .81, then the maximum validity of the diagnosis using joint palpation pain as the measure and radiographic interpretation as the criterion is $.8 \times .9 = .72$. A simple approach to assessing the accuracy of prediction of this measure is to square the resulting "validity" coefficient—that is, the correlation of the measure with its criterion. In this case, about a 50% reduction ($.72^2$) in error, compared to guessing, will result when one is predicting joint pathology from the joint palpation measure (McDowell & Newell, 1987). As we shall see, many clinical measures of pain are not associated with such high levels of reliability or, perforce, validity.

Finally, it should be emphasized that reliability and validity concerns are heightened when the data being accumulated relate to subjective experience, such as when pain intensity and dysfunctional chronic pain levels are measured and where no objective standard for comparison is available. By contrast, when measurements are derived at the physiological level, reliability of measurement is generally not a problem, since measuring instruments (e.g., thermometers, electrocardiographs) that gather objective data can be calibrated to known and very high levels of reproducibility of measurement. For such objective physiological measures, reliability and validity are replaced by degree of precision and accuracy as the measurement concerns.

Reliability

Two general forms of reliability are of concern. One form assesses repeatability or consistency of a measure and has received considerable attention from those constructing pain measures (McDowell & Newell, 1987). The second form of reliability, interexaminer reliability, infrequently addressed in the pain literature, assesses whether different clinical raters or examiners assessing the same person would obtain the same results when using the same examination procedures. Intraexaminer reliability, an additional form of examiner reliability, assesses the consistency of observers with themselves on repeated trials. Intraexaminer reliability is not discussed here, because it is generally considered to be high relative to interexaminer reliability and is not viewed as a significant source of measurement error for most types of clinical research. Of importance in keeping intraexaminer reliability high is consideration that an examiner may "drift" in a particular direction with his or her ratings (i.e., may tend consistently to over- or underrate a score). To reduce this drift, regular recalibrations are recommended. Recognizing the inherent problems in clinical assessment, the World Health Organization (1971) recommends that reliability indices be routinely incorporated in all health survey reports.

Consistency or Repeatability

Consistency or repeatability, a traditional aspect of reliability, has received adequate attention in the development of pain measures (McDowell & Newell, 1987). As mentioned earlier, the most common index of consistency or repeatability is the simple correlation coefficient. Two approaches to assessing the reliability of pain measures have been employed. The first approach uses a *test–retest*

method, wherein the same measure is administered to the same group of subjects on two different occasions. The results are then correlated and expressed as a test–retest reliability coefficient. Reliability coefficients in the range of .8 or higher are considered acceptable, however test–retest coefficients of about .9 are preferred (Anastasi, 1988; McDowell & Newell, 1987). This reliability coefficient reflects the degree of stability of scores over time and is also known as the *coefficient of stability*. As a rule, the measures most commonly in use to assess the sensory, affective, coping, and other behavioral levels of pain show good reliability. For example, Scott and Huskisson (1976) reported test–retest reliability of .99 for VASs measuring pain intensity. Test–retest reliability of the Illness Behavior Questionnaire (Pilowsky & Spence, 1983), which has been used to assess maladaptive responses to chronic pain, reveals reliability coefficients of about .84, and the Back Pain Classification Scale (Leavitt, 1983) shows test–retest reliability of .86.

As many reviewers have noted, test–retest methods for assessing reliability of pain measures appear simple but are deceptively complex in interpretation. For example, in order to ensure minimal fluctuations in pain levels, repeated administrations should be close together in time. Such a procedure introduces the possibility that the repeated assessments are not independent—that is, that the subject may be remembering and then repeating the same values given in the relatively recent prior administration. When repeated administrations of the same measure are spaced further apart in time, and different values are obtained, it is difficult to separate instability of pain levels from unreliability of the measure. We return to this issue of distinguishing change or instability from unreliability of measurement when we discuss the reliability of clinical examination measures.

Test–retest reliability is useful for determining the repeatability of a measure over time, but when test results are affected by repeated testing and repeated exposure to the same test, another form of reliability is preferred. *Alternate-forms reliability* involves administration of two parallel and equivalent forms of the same test. Alternate-forms reliability is also referred to as the *coefficient of equivalence* when the two parallel forms are administered at the same time, and as the *coefficient of equivalence and stability* when a period of time separates administration of the two forms. Although many consider this the most rigorous form for estimating reliability, it is often not used, due to the difficulty in developing forms that are truly equivalent.

Internal Consistency

Partly in response to the complex issues associated with repeated administrations and developing alternate forms alluded to above, another approach to assessing reliability examines pain measures for their *internal consistency*. Internal consistency indices assess the extent to which the individual items or elements of the measure are correlated with each other, and hence presumably measuring the same thing. One form of assessing internal consistency of the items in a measure is to compare results from one-half of the measure with results from the other half.

Several methods for assessing *split-half reliability* have emerged (e.g., comparing odd- and even-numbered items). The scores on the two halves are then correlated. The most common methods for estimating internal consistency involve estimating the correlations among all possible pairs of items, using the methods derived from Kuder and Richardson and from Cronbach (Anastasi, 1988). These approaches, which assess interitem correlations, are in effect assessing the correlation between different versions of the same test. High correlations among items indicate homogeneity of the measure, which is likely to yield consistent results. Generally, acceptable levels for these internal consistency measures of reliability hover around .85, although it may be difficult to achieve these higher values when one is assessing pain at the level of dysfunctional behaviors. It must be emphasized that if a pain measure is also used to assess change over time, then high levels of consistency (e.g., reliability) are essential to be able to distinguish a real change from random fluctuations in pain. At a minimum, the measure should be able to predict itself (McDowell & Newell, 1987).

The preceding sections have discussed various aspects of consistency and repeatability of results as fundamental issues underlying measures of pain and dysfunction. For the most part, measures considered so far are identified as self-report measures or paper-and-pencil measures, because they are delivered by interview or in self-administered form. Typically, these are in the form of well-standardized scales or tests—for example, the MPQ (Melzack, 1975) and the Minnesota Multiphasic Personality Inventory (MMPI; Hathaway & McKinley, 1983) are probably the most researched for their psychometric properties—and the field of pain measurement has been reviewed favorably for the attention it pays to assessing the reliability and validity of self-report pain measures.

Examiners need to interact with patients very little in the case of self-administered pain measures. Similarly, well-standardized formats have been developed for conducting data-gathering interviews. As a result, the examiner typically has limited opportunity to bias the outcome of self-report pain measures. In marked contrast, clinical examination has multiple opportunities for successive examiners to differ in detecting, rating, and reporting clinical signs; that is, measurement of clinical findings is associated with reliability issues of a different type (Chilton, 1982; Fleiss, Slakter, Fischman, Park, & Chilton, 1979; Koran, 1975).

Consistency among Examiners: Interexaminer Reliability

A concern of paramount importance for both pain clinicians and researchers is that clinical examiners must also be reliable in their methods, or the clinical findings they generate will not be reproducible by others, and hence will not be valid for forming diagnoses and treatment plans or for evaluating treatment outcomes. As we shall see, the problem of interrater reliability in assessment of physical signs and symptoms is a generic one, not limited by any means to pain measurements. Nevertheless, it is fair to say that interexaminer reliability can be expected to be poor in many clinical areas of direct relevance to pain measurement, unless deliberate procedures are taken to ensure that when two or more clinicians examine the same patient for the same purpose, they come away with comparable sets of findings. Nor is poor interexaminer reliability limited to measuring physical signs directly from examination of patients. Studies have demonstrated that radiographic interpretation for clinical problems as diverse as detecting pulmonary lesions (Yerushalmy, 1969), dental caries, and periapical dental conditions (Reit, 1986) is associated with surprisingly low levels of interexaminer agreement.

Statistical Methods for Analyzing Reliability

Because the issues associated with interexaminer reliability in the area of pain measurement have not received adequate attention, we describe more fully some of the statistical methods used to assess interexaminer agreement. We next present data on this issue, using for these purposes Dworkin and his colleagues' studies of the reliability of examinations for TMD pain, as well as data from examinations for other painful conditions. We conclude the discussion of this topic with some recommendations to maximize interexaminer agreement among pain clinicians and researchers.

A note of caution is warranted when one is assessing the reliability between two raters. A commonly used technique for estimating this type of reliability is percentage of agreement between the two raters. This technique can lead to erroneous conclusions, because it does not take into account the level of agreement that would have occurred by chance alone. This is a particular problem for observations of scales with a high frequency of occurrence, such as pain behaviors in patients with chronic pain (i.e., groaning when bending or straightening). In cases where the behavior has a high rate of occurrence, percentage of agreement will overestimate the measure's reliability.

Two commonly used statistics that account for the rate of chance agreement between raters are the *intraclass correlation coefficient* (ICC; Shrout & Fleiss, 1979) and the *kappa statistic* (Fleiss, 1981). In fact, in certain study designs, the two have been shown to be virtually equivalent. Empirically, the particular statistic used depends upon the scale of the pain measurement. The ICC is used for continuous measurements, and the kappa statistic is used for categorical measurements. A continuous measure has, theoretically, an infinite number of possible values. A VAS for pain intensity and the amount, in millimeters, the jaw can open until pain is experienced are both examples of continuous measures. If there are only a few possible values associated with a measure, then the measure is categorical. An example of a categorical measure is the simple measure of pain coded as either "present" or "absent"; or the presence of pain can be further classified into four descriptive categories, such as "none" (scored 0), "mild" (scored 1), "moderate" (scored 2), or "severe" (scored 3), yielding a 0–3 measure of pain.

For either of these statistics, a key assumption behind reliability measures is the independence of the examiner assessments. If the measures are not independent, then it is not possible to determine how much of the agreement is due to the actual measure and how much is due to the biases of the examiners.

Intraclass Correlation. The ICC can be used to assess the agreement between two or more examiners on a continuous measure. The exact calculation of the ICC depends on the study design (Shrout & Fleiss, 1979), as well as on how the reliability results are to be interpreted and used.

There are two general study designs: (1) Each subject is evaluated by a different set of examiners, and (2) each subject is evaluated by the same set of examiners. The first case does not allow us to sort out the differences in results due to examiners, because there is no overlap between examiners and subjects. Thus the effects associated with examiners cannot be sorted out from random error.

The second design, much preferred, allows us to sort out the variability due to the subjects, the examiners, and the random error. For this second design, the formula for calculating the ICC for a group of examiners depends on the ultimate use of the examiners—that is, whether data will be analyzed for each examiner separately, or whether measurements obtained from all examiners will be pooled. For example, the longitudinal studies of TMD pain conducted by Dworkin and colleagues over a 5-year period encompassed several hundred subjects and required up to five calibrated (see below) dental hygienists/field examiners to collect measures of pain and related characteristics by performing clinical exams and interviews in the field. Each hygienist/examiner collected data from a different subset of research subjects. For the analysis phase, the investigators needed to assume that the hygienists/examiners were interchangeable, so that the data could be pooled and analyzed as a whole, rather than separately by hygienists/examiner. The reliability of our examiners was assessed by conducting several studies, already mentioned (Dworkin, LeResche, & DeRouen, 1988; Dworkin, LeResche, DeRouen, & Von Korff, 1990). High ICCs indicate that all examiners would have come up with the same measurements if they had all measured each other's subjects. For the remainder of this section, the focus is on this latter example of assessing reliability of a group of examiners calibrated to be interchangeable. If examiners are not equally reliable, then the results of a study are questionable.

Examiners will be in good agreement if for each patient (subject) evaluated, the measured responses differ very little from examiner to examiner. If, however, measures obtained by the examiners are quite discrepant, then obviously agreement is poor. The extent of agreement needs to be evaluated in light of the amount of variability observed among all the examiner measurements taken on all the subjects. If the examiners are in high agreement, then most of the variability observed among all the measurements can be attributed to subjects' having different pain experiences (plus some measurement error), rather than to differences in how examiners go about measuring pain. Examiner reliability is quantified as the proportion of variability that can be attributed to sources (subjects, errors) other than the examiners. In statistical terms, this constitutes the ratio of variances and covariances associated with subjects relative to the total observed variability and is called the ICC. The following example demonstrates the principles involved in determining and interpreting ICC.

Dworkin and his colleagues wanted to measure, in millimeters, the extent to which subjects (with and without TMD pain) could open their mouths before pain occurred. This measure was determined on $n = 25$ subjects by $k = 5$ separate examiners. To calculate the ICC, a two-way analysis of variance was performed to estimate the variability due to subjects (BMS), to examiners (JMS), and to measurement error (EMS). The following was observed:

Source of variation	Mean square error
Subjects (BMS)	434.43
Examiners (JMS)	26.30
Error (EMS)	17.89

$$ICC = \frac{BMS - EMS}{BMS + (k - 1)EMS + \dfrac{k(JMS - EMS)}{n}}$$

= .82 (estimated for illustrative purposes)

This example of intraclass correlation indicates high agreement among the five examiners. Moreover, since ICC can be thought of as a ratio of variances, it can be interpreted to represent the amount of variability explained by subjects vs. examiners. Thus, in the example above, an ICC of .82 means that 82% of the variability in measurements was due to the subjects' differing in extent of jaw opening, and that only 18% of variability in measurement (100% - 82%) was due to differences among hygienists/examiners plus measurement error. These findings can be interpreted to mean that vertical range of jaw opening was assessed with high reliability by these calibrated hygienists/examiners.

Kappa Statistic. The kappa statistic also measures the extent of agreement, but for categorical data, and does so by comparing the observed agreement between two examiners to the agreement that would be expected if the examiners merely guessed at what the measure should be. Examiners could agree just by chance alone, especially if there are

only a few choices available. If there are only two choices (e.g., "pain present" or "pain absent" in a pain clinic setting), just by guessing "present" all the time, examiners would show high agreement. However, because pain is so prevalent in this setting, the apparent agreement would not reflect high reliability of examiners.

The kappa statistic is calculated as follows:

$$\kappa = (P_o - P_e)/(1 - P_e)$$

where P_o is the actual proportion of agreement observed between two examiners and P_e is the proportion of agreement that would be expected merely by chance alone.

A low kappa can reveal poor study design when almost all subjects evaluated fall into one category, such as being largely pain-free. Such situations have a greater proportion of agreement by chance alone than does a study where a greater variety of pain levels among of subjects is being evaluated. Kappa also affords the opportunity to observe whether a particular examiner tends to disagree with other examiners in a particular direction. The following examples demonstrate some of the issues involved in the calculation and interpretation of kappa.

When 25 subjects were evaluated for presence or absence of posterior temporalis muscle pain upon palpation, the following table of results was observed:

		Examiner 2	
		Yes	No
Examiner 1	Yes	2	1
	No	1	21

Here the observed proportion of agreement, obtained by adding the values in the diagonal when both examiners found muscle pains, is 92% [(21 + 2)/25]. However, the expected agreement (calculated as for chi-square test of independence) by chance alone is 79%, which is high also. Adjusting for this chance agreement yields a kappa of .62, indicating substantial agreement between examiners 1 and 2. Now, however, suppose the following had been observed instead:

		Examiner 2	
		Yes	No
Examiner 1	Yes	1	1
	No	1	22

One observation was moved from the "Yes–Yes" to the "No–No" combination. The overall proportion of agreement would still be 92%, but the expected proportion of agreement would be 85%. This increase in the agreement expected by chance alone would be reflected in a moderate estimate of reliability, with a kappa of .47.

These examples have the same proportion of agreement (92%), and hence the same proportion of disagreement, but the kappa estimates are quite different. Thus the resulting kappa needs to be interpreted in light of the distribution of the subjects being evaluated with regard to the pain characteristic being measured.

This is to be compared with a set of 25 subjects who were varied in their actual presence or absence of pain characteristics. For example, the following might have been observed:

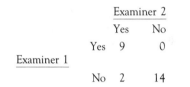

The percentage of observed agreement is still 92%, but the expected percentage agreement due to chance alone is only 52%, resulting in a kappa of .83. Such a kappa indicates "almost perfect" agreement (Landis & Koch, 1977).

Despite problems associated with interpreting kappa (all statistics are associated with problems of interpretation!), kappa remains the preferred statistic for assessing interexaminer reliability when categorical measures are being evaluated; it is especially preferred over those statistics such as percentage of agreement, which do not correct for agreement occurring by chance.

The ICC of the type considered here can range from 0 to 1. The kappa statistic can range from –1 to +1; however, the values of interest are in the range of 0 to 1. A kappa less than 0 indicates the examiners agree less often than would be expected by chance alone. If the ICC or kappa statistic is 1, then there is perfect agreement among the examiners. On the other hand, if the estimate of reliability is 0, then there is no agreement among the examiners. The general guidelines (Landis & Koch, 1977) for characterizing these reliability coefficients are as follows: .00–.20 indicates none to slight agreement, .21–.40 indicates fair agreement, .41–.60 is moderate agreement, .61–.80 is substantial agreement, and anything greater than .80 is almost perfect agreement. Our own criteria for

reliability of pain measurements obtained in our own studies are somewhat more stringent. We view ICC levels below .80 and kappa values below .60 as unacceptable levels of reliability.

The problem of attaining acceptable interexaminer agreement when conducting objective assessments of physical findings pervades virtually every domain of clinical research. For example, disagreement at about the 30% level was reported by radiologists interpreting serial radiographs for pulmonary shadows (Yerushalmy, 1969). Dentists in a reliability study of their ability to detect, radiographically, defective restorations or associated secondary caries showed levels of disagreement hovering around 34%, and comparably large variations were found in observer agreement regarding the assessment of periapical conditions and the adequacy of endodontic therapy as assessed by status of root canal fillings (Reit, 1986).

Closer to present concerns, Nelson, Allen, Clamp, and de Dombal (1979) found high levels of observer error (e.g., about 33% disagreement) in a study of the reliability and reproducibility of clinical findings in low back pain. They concluded that more precise definition and a sharper focus on what is being measured are necessary to decrease the unreliability in the examination and history data gathered to diagnose and treat back and leg pain. Stam and van Crevel (1990), in a study of the reliability of examination of non-pain-related tendon reflexes conducted with neurologists, found agreement on reflex scores as measured by ICC to be high among three examiners (ICC = .70–.88), with agreement highest for knee jerks, whereas agreement of reflex symmetry was poor, especially for the triceps (ICC = .32).

Similarly, interexaminer reliability among three chiropractors was poor for misalignment palpation (kappas hovering around .00) and was highest (kappas in the range of .57–.65) for palpation pain in soft tissues, especially in the lumbar region. The authors concluded that subjective pain reports may be gathered with more reliability than clinical spinal observations (Keating, Bergmann, Jacobs, Finer, & Larson, 1990).

In a series of reliability studies, Dworkin and his colleagues (Dworkin et al., 1988; Dworkin, LeResche, et al., 1990) reported excellent interexaminer reliability for certain clinical signs of TMD, and poor to marginal reliability for other clinical signs associated with this chronic orofacial pain condition. For example, maximum vertical range of jaw motion was a highly reliable measurement among four calibrated examiners (ICC

= .90–.98), whereas examination to detect temporomandibular joint (TMJ) sounds was associated with a marginally acceptable kappa (.62). This pattern of certain TMD signs' being associated with high interexaminer reliability whereas others are not is in substantial agreement with findings from reliability studies conducted by Liu, Alan, Clark, and Flask (1989) and Fricton and Schiffman (1986).

The relevance of these studies, taken together, is that they point to the possibility of using interexaminer reliability studies to make decisions concerning the usefulness of some clinical measurements over others. In addition, these studies have been selected to emphasize the point that reliability of clinical measurement is acknowledged to be associated with difficulties that cut across clinical disciplines and such diverse clinical examination methods as radiographic interpretation, assessment of physical findings, and even interpretation of electrocardiograms and laboratory tests (Koran, 1975). Several methods for maximizing examiner agreement are discussed below.

Obtaining Dependable Clinical Pain Measurements

Interexaminer reliability can be significantly improved by attending to several basic procedures. These procedures for obtaining reliable clinical measurements are especially relevant to clinical researchers who must communicate their methods as well as their data, to allow replication by others. Basic guidelines are available for assessing the confidence one can have in the reliability of clinical measurements (Anastasi, 1988; Chilton, 1982; Dworkin et al., 1988).

Criterion Definition. A clear definition, in measurable terms, of the clinical sign being assessed is absolutely essential. As an example, the detection of unequivocal asymmetry of knee jerks in a neurological examination was assessed in a reliability study by Stam and Van Crevel (1990), who defined reflex asymmetry as a right–left difference of at least 2 mm. Waddell and colleagues (see Waddell & Turk, Chapter 23) have been especially attentive to the need to develop clear clinical criteria and then submit them to reliability assessment. They have paid special attention to establishing criteria that distinguish among physical signs, psychological disturbance, and illness behaviors as each may be manifested in populations with chronic pain.

The need to define, in as reproducible a fashion as possible, the clinical signs being assessed should be self-evident, since it is the fundamental basis for determining reliability of measurement. In assessing reliability of measurement, it is not sufficient, for example, simply to report that "range of motion" was measured; unfortunately, the criteria for defining a clinical sign are too often stated in such vague or imprecise terms that one cannot be confident about what has been measured. Ideally, one would hope that the criterion definition results in mutually exclusive categories of clinical signs. To maximize interrater reliability, the categorical distinctions between signs must be sufficiently clear to allow examiners to select from discrete choices.

Examination Specifications. Once what is to be measured has been defined, the next step is to specify the procedures for obtaining the measurements. The assessment of reliability of clinical findings requires a set of examination procedures stated in clear behavioral terms so that methods for obtaining measurements can be reproduced by others. For example, methods for conducting an examination of muscle palpation tenderness should specify which locations on the muscle are to be palpated, what the amount and rate of pressure application should be, and whether palpation pressure is delivered digitally or through mechanical devices of specified size and type. In their own work, for example, Dworkin and colleagues found it absolutely essential to develop carefully detailed examination methods and specifications, which provide operational criteria for training examiners to conduct reliable assessments of clinical findings associated with TMD (Dworkin et al., 1988; Dworkin, Huggins, et al., 1990; Dworkin, Von Korff, & LeResche, 1990).

Calibration of Examiners. Clinical examiners, even experienced specialists, must be calibrated to the criteria being used to define the clinical variables being studied and to the examination methods used to measure those clinical variables. *Calibration of examiners* refers to specific training procedures undertaken by examiners in preparation for determining whether clinical data will be gathered in consistent fashion among the examiners. These training procedures include exposure to specific clinical criteria and examination methods all examiners will use, observing the consistency among examiners with a small sample of subjects, and using the feedback from these trial assessments to further ensure agreement on what is being measured and how the measurements are gathered.

Calibrating examiners to a common set of criteria and methods is one of the most effective ways to ensure maximum reliability of clinical measurement. It is also an approach that encounters strong initial resistance, especially among experienced clinicians, who find it difficult to believe that they need training in examination methods in order to produce reliable clinical findings. To emphasize that this phenomenon is not restricted to pain clinicians, Yerushalmy (1969) reports a fascinating series of studies involving the ability of radiologists to assess pulmonary shadows and lesions on radiographic examination. Experienced radiologists, who felt that "they knew whether a lesion was . . . fuzzy or sharply defined . . . what its shape was" (p. 390), were incredulous to learn of the difficulty in finding a reliable classification for the roentgenographic appearance of the quality of a tuberculosis pulmonary lesion.

In the studies of the reliability of clinical measurements associated with TMD pain, it was found that calibrated dental hygienists, trained to a common set of clinical criteria and examination methods by expert clinicians, were more reliable in their clinical measurements than were the clinicians themselves when each clinician went his or her own way rather than following a common set of measurement methods. Subsequent calibration of the specialist examiners significantly improved their reliability of assessment. For example, reliability of detecting TMJ sounds initially yielded a kappa of .39, which on retraining improved to an at least marginally significant level of .62. Kappa coefficients for uncalibrated examiners ranged from .13 to .54 across a broad range of clinical variables. Calibrated examiners showed a kappa range of .52–.78 for the same distribution of clinical assessments.

It should be emphasized that calibration of examiners is widely recognized as essential to maximize interrater reliability, and that the capacity to do so is completely under the control of the examiners. It is also the case that interexaminer reliability is influenced by all of the factors being reviewed here.

Selecting Appropriate Clinical Samples. When reliability estimates are provided, it is necessary to know whether an adequate representation of clinical signs was present in the sample being reported on. In a study of muscle tenderness on palpation,

Duinkerke, Luteijn, Bouman, and de Jong (1986) reported high reliability among examiners using a sample of normal, healthy volunteers, and reported excellent agreement (ranging from 83%–100%) among examiners. With Scott's pi (Scott, 1955), a measure related to kappa, it was demonstrated that the high percentage of agreement among examiners was unduly inflated for many measurements (pi ranged from .13 to 1.00), because in this instance most of the subjects did not have the clinical sign being investigated (namely, pain); most subjects were pain-free. It is clear that reliability studies must include a distribution of subjects with appropriate signs and must also include subjects without those signs, so that the reliability of appropriately detecting signs (sensitivity) when they are present and not detecting them when they are absent (specificity) can be most meaningfully assessed. This has been illustrated in the earlier section on the kappa statistic.

Assessing Unreliability versus Instability. Wherever possible, studies assessing the reliability of examiners should assure that examiners assess subjects in random order, to control for the effects of repeated examinations and the passage of time. Many clinical signs that are important to pain clinicians may vary as a function of repeated examination.

Palpation tenderness, joint sounds, and range of motion are all examples of physical signs related to several pain conditions that may yield different measurements when the first and last in a series of repetitions are compared. Thus the first examiner may discover restricted range of motion associated with a particular joint, while subsequent examiners may report more nearly adequate range of motion, as a function of repeated use of the joint associated with the repeated reliability measurements. To demonstrate this problem, pairs of examiners in the studies of TMD pain were asked to simultaneously assess the same TMJ for the presence of a clinically relevant joint sound—either a discrete click or more prolonged grating and crepitus sounds in the joint. Examiners used a "dual-headed" stethoscope to ensure that each member of the examiner pair was assessing the same joint movement. It was found that when successive pairs of examiners reported perfect intrapair agreement, on about 50% of the trials, the results obtained by each pair differed from those of the immediately preceding pair; that is, joint sounds heard by both members of one pair were different from joint sounds heard by the next pair.

We interpret the results cited above to mean that TMJ sounds can change, even over very brief periods of time, perhaps as a result of repeated observations. These findings are more consistent with instability of joint sounds than with unreliability of clinical examiners. To best control for the possibility that unreliability of examiners is confounded with instability or change in the clinical sign itself, it is essential that examiners assess subjects in random order and that each examiner assess every subject. Such practices will not eliminate instability of clinical findings, but will better disengage the confounding of interexaminer unreliability from instability of the clinical sign.

Validity

It may appear obvious that a pain measure should reflect, or be derived from, a conceptual or theoretical basis. After all, what is the measure measuring? Validity is associated with just such a question. If we are measuring pain, what do we mean by *pain*? The intended meaning of pain should be revealed by the measures used. Therefore, the validity of a pain measure is an indication of the "goodness of fit" or relevance of the pain measure to the underlying dimension of pain being assessed. The validity of a pain measure can also be interpreted by the relationship between that measure and other independently observable measures of pain.

However, as we have seen, pain is a concept invoking multiple dimensions, and as the model we have presented earlier depicts (see Figures 32.1 and 32.2), these dimensions of pain are dynamically integrated. Not surprisingly, then, validating a pain measure is much more complex than establishing its reliability (McDowell & Newell, 1987) (which, as we have seen, is not necessarily so straightforward either).

In order to evaluate whether a pain measure is measuring what it is supposed to measure, one must first consider the intended uses of the test. The intended use of a test may be to measure the extent to which a patient is familiar with a content domain or engages in a particular behavior. A test may also be used to measure the extent to which a patient possesses a particular trait. Or a test may be used to predict a patient's standing on some other criterion of concern (e.g., treatment success or failure). Considering the intended use of a test is important in determining the type of validity measure that is relevant for a particular measure.

For example, evaluating the "goodness of fit" between a pain measure and its conceptual basis is defined as establishing construct validity, and is the most intangible aspect of validity to assess. In addition to construct validity, aspects of validity usually assessed include content and criterion validity (Anastasi, 1988; Cronbach & Meehl, 1955).

Content Validity

Content validity refers to how well the specific elements, items, or questions contained in a pain measure or in a clinical procedure relate to the aims of the measure. Content validity is usually assessed informally, not statistically. The most common approach is to ask experts to furnish items or to use experts to confirm (i.e., validate) the clarity, organization, and suitability of a series of items. If experts agree that the test items constitute an adequate sample of the target domain, then the test is said to have content validity. When specific external criteria are available, item analysis statistics can be used to assess how well each item in the pain measure is related to the external measure, thus giving an index of the validity of specific items.

Criterion Validity

Criterion-related validity is of interest when the intended use of a test is to predict standing on some external criterion. Criterion-related validation indicates the effectiveness of a test in predicting an individual's performance on some other measure or activity. In this case, performance on a measure is checked against a criterion—that is, an independent measure reflecting what the original test is designed to predict.

If the criterion measure and the test being validated are completed at approximately the same time, then *concurrent validity* is being tested. Concurrent validity involves comparing the pain measure with results from a related measure that serves as a criterion for assessing a comparable aspect of the concept of pain. For example, a validity coefficient of .75 between a 4-point descriptive pain scale (the predictor) and a VAS for pain (the criterion) suggests that the 4-point descriptive pain scale has good criterion or concurrent validity. Similarly, with the MPQ as a criterion measure, correlations ranging from .60 to .63 were obtained between a pain VAS for pain intensity and the MPQ (Huskisson, 1982); this indicates that when the VAS is used as a criterion, the MPQ has adequate concurrent validity as a measure of pain intensity.

Predictive Validity

In contrast to criterion or concurrent validity, predictive validity is examined through longitudinal or prospective studies, in which changes in pain are expected, either as the result of natural history or as the result of an intervention. The idea is that if a pain measure is valid, it should predict the future course of the pain condition; for example, a measure of postoperative pain is expected to show decreases in pain intensity with the passage of time. If the comparison of baseline and subsequent pain measures does not reveal the predicted decrease, then the measure may be invalid for the assessment of postoperative pain, if postoperative pain status is theoretically assumed to change over time. When a measure has predictive validity, then the observation of comparable responses over time (e.g., two pain measure scores a week apart that are identical) allows the clinician to understand that the pain has not changed, as opposed to interpreting the comparable pain reports to mean that the measure is no good. Hence, once again, it is clear that careful attention (indicated through scientific plausibility, empirical supporting data, etc.) must be paid to selection of the external or criterion measure serving as the standard for determining whether or not the pain "really" changed. Suffice it to say that assessing the predictive validity of a pain (or any other) measure is difficult, involving complex longitudinal study designs; and so, in fact, it is rarely done.

Construct Validity

The *construct validity* of a test is the extent to which a test measures a theoretical construct or trait. In lieu of assessing how well tests predict future outcomes, pain measures can be assessed for their construct validity by sophisticated statistical methods such as factor analysis and discriminant analysis. Factor analysis, technically not usually considered under construct validity, is placed here for convenience. It is a statistical method that analyzes all the possible intercorrelations of items in a test to determine whether these items fall into groups, or factors, that are consistent with the underlying dimensions that form the conceptual basis for the test. In this sense, factor analysis may be thought of as a procedure for determining whether independent groupings of items can be discriminated from one another. Factor analysis is typically applied to multidimensional tests that were designed to measure different aspects or dimensions of the pain experience.

The MPQ is an excellent example of a multidimensional measure of pain that has as its conceptual basis the gate-control theory of pain. The MPQ purports to measure Sensory, Affective, and Evaluative dimensions of pain experience. The three-factor structure of the MPQ has been validated in some studies (Lowe, Walker, & MacCallum, 1991; see also Melzack & Katz, Chapter 3). Others argue that the items composing the three factors are highly intercorrelated (Holroyd et al., 1992; Turk, Rudy, & Salovey, 1985) and question its discriminant validity. These findings provide excellent examples of how factor-analytic studies contribute to our understanding of complicated constructs such as the concept of pain. The clearest findings relate to the validity of distinguishing between the Sensory and Affective dimensions; less agreement is reported with regard to the validity of the Evaluative dimension (McDowell & Newell, 1987).

Discriminant Analysis

Discriminant analysis is used to validate a pain measure by statistically evaluating the measure's ability to group persons (as opposed to grouping test items, as with factor analysis) according to some underlying characteristic they share. It seeks to classify individuals into mutually exclusive groups based on their responses to a series of supposedly related items or measures, and compares this new classification to a "gold standard." For example, discriminant analysis of the Back Pain Classification Scale (Leavitt & Garron, 1980) was conducted to determine the ability of the test to positively identify persons whose pain was due to psychological distress. The scale correctly classified 132 of 159 cases (83%). In a sample of patients with low back pain without organic disease, comprised of some persons who showed clinical signs of psychological disturbance and some who did not, the scale correctly classified 78% of patients into one of these two categories (i.e., those psychologically disturbed or those not showing such psychological symptoms). The MMPI Low Back scale was not as effective in discriminating between these two groups, achieving only a 37% correct classification. Discriminant analysis has also been effectively used in the validation of diagnostic criteria for psychiatric disorders, headache, and complex regional pain syndrome (Bruehl et al., 1999; Merikangas, Dartigues, Whitaker, & Angst, 1994).

Although these more sophisticated statistical methods for assessing the validity of pain measures have an intuitive appeal, it is nevertheless fair to say that assessing the validity of a measure remains at least as much an art as a science. The challenge seems even greater in the complex area of pain measurement, where the need is to uncover the relative contributions to pain experience of the physical stimulus, the characteristics of the person, and the social environment. Suggested guidelines for the construction of good validation studies emphasize the need for (1) clear statements of hypotheses and the methods used to test them; (2) inclusion of methods that demonstrate what the test does not measure, showing its ability to reject reasonable competing hypotheses, instead of being restricted to confirmations of what the test does measure; and (3) most importantly, a variety of approaches to be used, rather than relying on a single type of validation procedure.

SUMMARY AND CONCLUSION

A few key issues have been identified as most salient when clinicians or researchers are determining the extent to which they can rely on measures of pain reported in the literature. Guidelines for evaluating how well pain measures address these issues have been discussed to assist researchers and clinicians in these efforts. First and foremost, it is necessary to be clear concerning the level of pain experience being measured. Because pain is a multidimensional and complex human experience, it is now understood that relevant pain information can be assessed at the physical (biological), subjective (psychological), behavioral, and social (environmental) levels. In addition, renewed attention has been called to the temporal dimension of pain, in terms of pain as it arises in successive developmental stages and in terms of its acute, recurrent, or chronic natural history.

Broadly speaking, three classes of pain measures can be identified. One assesses physical signs of pain, reported singly or aggregated into clinical indices. A second type of pain measure assesses subjective experience, typically via self-report questionnaire or interview formats that can inquire into aspects of pain as diverse as subjective perception of pain intensity, extent of affective disturbance or somatization, cognitive appraisal of pain etiology and pain course, and social or cultural influences that shape pain interpretation and coping responses. The third class of pain measurement, and the most recent to emerge as central to our complete understanding of pain, is behavioral observation. Behavioral measures have been elaborated, notably by Keefe (Keefe & Block, 1982; Keefe et al., 1986; see also Keefe et al., Chapter 10) for assessing the extent to which pain is reflected by disturbances in gross motor movements, including physical appearance, gait, and range of motion. A more finely tuned approach has been developed by LeResche and Dworkin (1988), as well as by Craig and Prkachin (1983; see also Craig et al., Chapter 9). In this approach, the movement of facial muscles is examined to identify facial expressions of pain associated with different developmental stages; varying interpersonal contexts; and self-reported pain intensity, duration, and location.

A prime requirement of any pain measurement instrument is that it must clearly denote the level or levels of pain it has been designed to assess. This is nothing less than saying that pain measures should have a conceptual basis and be derived from a relevant body of theory. When empirical approaches are used to derive new pain measures—for example, the West Haven–Yale Multidimensional Pain Inventory (see Jacob & Kerns, Chapter 19, and Turk & Okifuji, Chapter 21) or the Graded Chronic Pain Scale (Von Korff et al., 1990; see also Von Korff, Chapter 31)—it is reasonable to expect those measures to be subjected (as the examples cited have been) to independent tests of their reliability and validity, using methods such as those discussed earlier.

The fundamental determinants of a pain measure's usefulness reside in its reliability and validity. Reliability assessment evaluates the extent to which a measure is consistent with itself. Synonyms for reliability are consistency and reproducibility. A limiting factor for the validity of a pain measure is its reliability; an unreliable measure of pain cannot be a valid one. The most common methods for assessing reliability are to examine a measure's internal consistency (Kuder–Richardson and Cronbach's alpha) and to measure its repeatability over time (test–retest reliability).

A special set of concerns arises over the reliability of clinical findings presumed to be relevant to pain. The most important concern regards interexaminer reliability. Interexaminer reliability refers to the extent to which successive clinical examiners of the same patient can be viewed as interchangeable in terms of the consistency of the data they each report. Interexaminer reliability among pain clinicians (indeed, throughout medical practice) is known to be unsatisfactory unless steps are taken to ensure that examiners use a common set of examination methods and specifications, that they have been previously calibrated in the use of these methods, and that their reliability is assessed through independent reliability studies. The issues surrounding the assessment of reliability in general and clinician reliability in particular are complex, because differences in successive measurements can be due to unreliability of examiners or instability of clinical signs due to normal biological variation, treatment effects, or disease remission or exacerbation.

Validity refers to what a test measures and how well it measures what it purports to measure. Thus it informs us about what can be inferred from test scores. Informally, the definition of validity is expressed as "Does the test measure what it is supposed to?" The validity of the MPQ, for example, rests on its ability to measure several related but unique dimensions of pain deduced from a theoretical conceptualization (the gate control theory) of pain as multidimensional. The validity of any measure cannot be assessed by a single method or in a single study. The essence of establishing the validity of any instrument to measure pain is that the measurement of its validity must be approached from several perspectives: The measure must be relevant to a conceptual dimension of pain (construct validity); experts must agree that the components of the measure follow directly from the underlying dimensions being measured (content validity); the measure must relate to independent measures of the same concept, while remaining unconfounded from other variables (concurrent validity); the measure should be predictive (predictive validity); and it should adequately discriminate those who carry the phenomenon of interest from those who do not (discriminative validity). No currently available pain measure adequately meets all of these validity criteria, but this state of affairs applies at present to all aspects of health measurement.

Finally, a great deal of attention continues to be paid to developing more sophisticated methods for improving reliability of measurement (Guyatt, Walter, & Norman, 1987; Ormel, Koeter, & van den Brink, 1989; van Belle, Uhlmann, Hughes, & Larson, 1990). Improved reliability will allow clinicians and researchers to more precisely identify components of change in health measurement corresponding to improvement of deterioration in physical or psychosocial functioning—in effect, separating observable change in clinical status from issues of reliability of measurement (van Belle et al., 1990). Examples of these approaches include approaches to reliability addressed by Chronbach's generalizability theory (e.g., see Von Korff, Chap-

ter 31). Taken together, these methods hold much promise for improving our understanding of the complexly determined and multidimensional nature of human pain experience.

REFERENCES

Anastasi, A. (1988). *Psychological testing*. New York: Macmillan.

Barsky, A. J. (1979). Patients who amplify bodily sensations. *Annals of Internal Medicine, 91*, 63–70.

Bergner, M., Bobbitt, R. A., Carter, W. B., & Gilson, B. S. (1981). The Sickness Impact Profile: Development and final revision of a health status model. *Medical Care, 19*, 787–805.

Bruehl, S., Harden, R. N., Galer, B. S., Saltz, S., Bertram, M., Backonja, M., Gayles, R., Rudin, N., Bhugra, M. K., & Stanton-Hicks, M. (1999). External validation of IASP diagnostic criteria for complex regional pain syndrome and proposed research diagnostic criteria. *Pain, 81*, 147–154.

Chilton, N. W. (1982). Reliability studies. In N. W. Chilton (Ed.), *Design and analysis in dental and oral research* (2nd ed., pp. 421–431). New York: Praeger.

Craig, K. D., & Prkachin, K. M. (1983). Nonverbal measures of pain. In R. Melzack (Ed.), *Pain measurement and assessment* (pp. 173–179). New York: Raven Press.

Cronbach, L. J., & Meehl, P. E. (1955). Construct validity in psychological tests. *Psychological Bulletin, 52*, 281–302.

Derbyshire, S. W. G. (1999, May–June). Imaging the brain in pain. *American Pain Society Bulletin*, pp. 7–9, 18.

Duinkerke, A. S., Luteijn, F., Bouman, T. K., & de Jong, H. P. (1986). Reproducibility of a palpation test for the stomatognathic system. *Community Dentistry and Oral Epidemiology, 14*, 80–85.

Dworkin, S. F., Huggins, K. H., LeResche, L., Von Korff, M., Howard, J., Truelove, E., & Sommers, E. (1990). Epidemiology of signs and symptoms in temporomandibular disorders: Clinical signs in cases and controls. *Journal of the American Dental Association, 120*, 273–281.

Dworkin, S. F., & LeResche, L. (1992). Research Diagnostic Criteria for Temporomandibular Disorders: Review, criteria, examinations and specifications, critique. *Journal of Craniomandibular Disorders: Facial and Oral Pain, 6*, 301–355.

Dworkin, S. F., LeResche, L., & DeRouen, T. (1988). Reliability of clinical measurement in temporomandibular disorders. *Clinical Journal of Pain, 4*, 89–99.

Dworkin, S. F., LeResche, L., DeRouen, T., & Von Korff, M. (1990). Assessing clinical signs of temporomandibular disorders: Reliability of clinical examiners. *Journal of Prosthetic Dentistry, 63*, 574–579.

Dworkin, S. F., Von Korff, M. R., & LeResche, L. (1990). Multiple pains and psychiatric disturbance: An epidemiologic investigation. *Archives of General Psychiatry, 47*, 239–244.

Dworkin, S. F., Von Korff, M., & LeResche, L. (1992). Epidemiologic studies of chronic pain: A dynamic-ecologic perspective. *Annals of Behavioral Medicine, 14*, 3–11.

Fields, H. (1987). *Pain*. New York: McGraw-Hill.

Fleiss, J. L. (1981). *Statistical methods for rates and proportions*. New York: Wiley.

Fleiss, J. L., Slakter, M. J., Fischman, S. L., Park, M. M., & Chilton, N. W. (1979). Inter-examiner reliability in caries trials. *Journal of Dental Research, 58,* 604–609.

Fordyce, W. E. (1976). *Behavioral methods for chronic pain and illness*. St. Louis, MO: Mosby.

Fordyce, W. E., Roberts, A. H., & Sternbach, R. A. (1985). The behavioral management of chronic pain: A response to critics. *Pain, 22,* 113–125.

Fricton, J. R., & Schiffman, E. L. (1986). Reliability of a craniomandibular index. *Journal of Dental Research, 65,* 1359–1364.

Gracely, R. H., & Dubner, R. (1987). Reliability and validity of verbal descriptor scales of painfulness. *Pain, 29,* 175–185.

Guyatt, G., Walter, S., & Norman, G. (1987). Measuring change over time: Assessing the usefulness of evaluative instruments. *Journal of Chronic Disease, 40,* 171–178.

Hathaway, S. R., & McKinley, J. C. (1983). *Manual for administration and scoring of the MMPI*. Minneapolis, MN: National Computer Systems.

Holroyd, K. A., Holm, J. E., Keefe, F. J., Turner, J. A., Bradley, L. A., Murphy, W. D., Johnson, P., Anderson, K., Hinkle, A. L., & O'Malley, W. B. (1992). A multi-center evaluation of the McGill Pain Questionnaire: Results from more than 1700 chronic pain patients. *Pain, 48,* 301–311.

Huskisson, E. C. (1982). Measurement of pain. *Journal of Rheumatology, 9,* 768–769.

Jensen, M. P., Romano, J. M., Turner, J. A., Good, A. B., & Wald, L. H. (1999). Patient beliefs predict patient functioning: Further support for a cognitive-behavioural model of chronic pain. *Pain, 81,* 95–104.

Keating, J. C., Bergmann, T. F., Jacobs, G. E., Finer, B. A., & Larson, K. (1990). Interexaminer reliability of eight evaluative dimensions of lumbar segment abnormality. *Journal of Manipulative and Physiological Therapeutics, 13,* 463–469.

Keefe, F. J., & Block, A. R. (1982). Development of an observation method for assessing pain behavior in chronic low back pain patients. *Behavior Therapy, 13,* 363–375.

Keefe, F. J., Gil, K. M., & Rose, S. C. (1986). Behavioral approaches in the multidisciplinary management of chronic pain: Programs and issues. *Clinical Psychology Review, 6,* 87–113.

Kleinböhl, D., Hölzl, R., Möltner, A., Rommel, C., Weber, C., & Osswald, P. M. (1999). Psychophysical measures of sensitization to tonic heat discriminate chronic pain patients. *Pain, 81,* 35–43.

Kleinman, A. (1988). *The illness narratives: Suffering, healing and the human condition*. New York: Basic Books.

Koran, L. M. (1975). The reliability of clinical methods, data and judgments (first of two parts). *New England Journal of Medicine, 293,* 642–646.

Landis, J. R., & Koch, G. G. (1977). The measurement of observer agreement for categorical data. *Biometrics, 33,* 159–174.

Leavitt, F. (1983). Detecting psychological disturbance using verbal pain measurement: The Back Pain Classification Scale. In R. Melzack (Ed.), *Pain measurement and assessment* (pp. 79–84). New York: Raven Press.

Leavitt, F., & Garron, D. C. (1980). Validity of a back pain classification scale for detecting psychological disturbance as measured by the MMPI. *Journal of Clinical Psychology, 36,* 186–189.

LeResche, L., & Dworkin, S. F. (1988). Facial expressions of pain and emotions in chronic TMD patients. *Pain, 35,* 71–78.

Liu, C., Alan, S., Clark, G., & Flack, K. V. (1989). Reliability of a method of detecting TMJ sounds [Abstract]. *Journal of Dental Research, 68,* 232.

Loeser, J. D. (1982). Concepts of pain. In M. Stanton Hicks & R. Boas (Eds.), *Chronic low back pain* (pp. 145–148). New York: Raven Press.

Lowe, N. K., Walker, S. N., & MacCallum, R. C. (1991). Confirming the theoretical structure of the McGill Pain Questionnaire in acute clinical pain. *Pain, 46,* 53–60.

McDowell, I., & Newell, C. (1987). *Measuring health*. New York: Oxford University Press.

McGrath, P. A. (1990). *Pain in children: Nature, assessment, and treatment*. New York: Guilford Press.

Mechanic, D. (1986). Illness behavior: An overview. In S. McHugh & T. M. Vallis (Eds.), *Illness behavior: A multidisciplinary model* (pp. 101–110). New York: Plenum Press.

Melzack, R. (1975). The McGill Pain Questionnaire: Major properties and scoring methods. *Pain, 1,* 277–299.

Melzack, R., & Wall, P. D. (1965). Pain mechanisms: A new theory. *Science, 150,* 971–979.

Mendell, L. M. (1966). Physiological properties of unmyelinated fiber projections to the spinal cord. *Experimental Neurology, 16,* 316–332.

Mense, S., Hoheisel, U., Kaske, A., & Reinert, A. (1997). Muscle pain: Basic mechanisms and clinical correlates. In T. S. Jensen, J. A. Turner, & Z. Wiesenfeld-Hallin (Eds.), *Progress in pain research and management: Vol. 8. Proceedings of the 8th World Congress on Pain* (pp. 479–496). Seattle, WA: International Association for the Study of Pain Press.

Merikangas, K. R., Dartigues, J. F., Whitaker, A., & Angst, J. (1994). Diagnostic criteria for migraine: A validity study. *Neurology, 44*(Suppl. 4), S11–S16.

Merskey, H. (1986). Classification of chronic pain: Descriptions of chronic pain syndromes and definitions of pain terms. *Pain,* Suppl. 3, S1–S225.

Merskey, H., & Bogduk, N. (Eds.). (1994). *Classification of chronic pain* (2nd ed.). Seattle, WA: International Association for the Study of Pain Press.

Nelson, M. A., Allen, P., Clamp, S. E., & de Dombal, F. T. (1979). Reliability and reproducibility of clinical findings in low-back pain. *Spine, 4,* 97–100.

Ormel, J., Koeter, M. W. J., & van den Brink, W. (1989). Measuring change with the General Health Questionnaire (GHQ): The problem of retest effects. *Social Psychiatry and Psychiatric Epidemiology, 24,* 227–232.

Osterweis, M., Kleinman, A., & Mechanic, D. (1987). *Pain and disability: Clinical, behavioral and public policy perspectives*. Washington, DC: National Academy Press.

Parmalee, P. A. (1994). Assessment of pain in the elderly. *Annual Review of Gerontology and Geriatrics, 14,* 281–301.

Parsons, T. (1975). The sick role and the role of the physician reconsidered. *Milbank Memorial Fund Quarterly, 53,* 257–278.

Petrie, A. (1967). *Individuality in pain and suffering.* Chicago: University of Chicago Press.

Pilowsky, I., & Spence, N. D. (1983). *Manual for the Illness Behaviour Questionnaire (IBQ)* (2nd ed.). Adelaide, Australia: University of Adelaide.

Reit, C. (1986). On decision making in endodontics: A study of diagnosis and management of periapical lesions in endodontically treated teeth. *Swedish Dental Journal*, Suppl. 41, 1–30.

Romano, J. M., & Turner, J. A. (1985). Chronic pain and depression: Does the evidence support a relationship? *Psychological Bulletin, 97,* 18–26.

Scott, J., & Huskisson, E. C. (1976). Graphic representation of pain. *Pain, 2,* 175–184.

Scott, W. A. (1955). Reliability of context analysis: The case of nominal scale coding. *Public Opinion Quarterly, 19,* 321–325.

Shrout, P. E., & Fleiss, J. L. (1979). Intraclass correlations: Uses in assessing rater reliability. *Psychological Bulletin, 86,* 420–428.

Simon, G. E., & Von Korff, M. (1991). Somatization and psychiatric disorder. *American Journal of Psychiatry, 148,* 1494–1500.

Social Security Administration. (1984). *National study of chronic pain syndrome.* Washington, DC: Office of Disability.

Stam, J., & van Crevel, H. (1990). Reliability of the clinical and electromyographic examination of tendon reflexes. *Journal of Neurology, 237,* 427–431.

Sternbach, R. A. (1990). *The psychology of pain.* New York: Raven Press.

Turk, D. C., & Flor, H. (1984). Etiological theories and treatments for chronic back pain: II. Psychological models and interventions. *Pain, 19,* 209–233.

Turk, D. C., Meichenbaum, D., & Genest, M. (1983). *Pain and behavioral medicine: A cognitive-behavioral perspective.* New York: Guilford Press.

Turk, D. C., & Okifuji, A. (1997). What factors affect physicians' decisions to prescribe opioids for chronic pain patients? *Clinical Journal of Pain, 13,* 330–336.

Turk, D. C., & Rudy, T. E. (1987). Towards a comprehensive assessment of chronic pain patients. *Behaviour Research and Therapy, 25,* 237–249.

Turk, D. C., & Rudy, T. E. (1988). Toward an empirically derived taxonomy of chronic pain patients: Integration of psychological assessment data. *Journal of Consulting and Clinical Psychology, 56,* 233–238.

Turk, D. C., Rudy, T. E., & Salovey, P. (1985). The McGill Pain Questionnaire reconsidered: Confirming the factor structure and examining appropriate uses. *Pain, 21,* 385–397.

Tursky, B. (1976). The development of pain perception profile: A psychophysical approach. In M. Weisenberg & B. Tursky (Eds.), *Pain: New perspectives in therapy and research* (pp. 171–194). New York: Plenum Press.

van Belle, G., Uhlmann, R. F., Hughes, J. P., & Larson, E. B. (1990). Reliability estimates of changes in mental status performance in senile dementia of the Alzheimer type. *Journal of Clinical Epidemiology, 43,* 589–595.

Von Korff, M., Dworkin, S. F., & LeResche, L. (1990). Graded chronic pain status: An epidemiologic evaluation. *Pain, 40,* 279–291.

Weiner, D., Peterson, B., & Keefe, F. (1999). Chronic pain-associated behaviors in the nursing home: Resident versus caregiver perceptions. *Pain, 80,* 577–588.

World Health Organization. (1971). *Oral health surveys: Basic methods.* Geneva: Author.

Yerushalmy, J. (1969). The statistical assessment of the variability in observer perception and description of roentgenographic pulmonary shadows. *Radiology Clinics of North America, 7,* 381–392.

Chapter 33

Assessment of Treatment Outcomes in Clinical Practice: A Survival Guide

AKIKO OKIFUJI
DENNIS C. TURK

Several terms and concepts have come into vogue that stir considerable consternation among clinical practitioners—*evidence-based medicine* (EBM), *cost-effectiveness, cost–benefit analysis*, and *patient satisfaction*. The ideas underlying these concepts are not particularly new and can generally be thought of as *accountability*. Of particular concern to health care providers is the economic implication that approval or reimbursement for clinical services will be dependent on the availability of evidence that the proposed treatment is both clinically effective and cost-effective.

A cynic might believe that third-party payers really do not care about clinical effectiveness, but only worry about cost: "How much will it cost, and what is it worth to us?" On the contrary, managed care organizations (MCOs) are increasingly becoming concerned with patient satisfaction, as volume of members (euphemistically referred to as "covered lives") is essential for them to maintain their profitability and survival. Thus, much as they might wish otherwise, they will not be able to focus solely on the bottom line, but will have to consider clinical outcomes and patients' satisfaction.

With the focus on evidence-based medicine and cost containment, health care providers are caught between Scylla and Charybdis. That is, they find themselves between two equally hazardous and onerous alternatives. On the one hand, they are required to maintain the volume of patient flow and thus have less time to spend with each individual patient, potentially reducing the quality of care and patient satisfaction. On the other, they are expected to have evidence available to justify their treatments. Collecting outcome data requires time and effort—the very resources of which health care providers are acutely short.

One appealing solution to the time crunch is reliance on published data produced by others as the evidence to support the proposed treatment. Unfortunately, much of medicine is not based on well-controlled clinical trials, but rather on consensus and clinical experience. For example, the Agency for Health Care Policy and Research Panel on Acute Low Back Problems in Adults (Bigos et al., 1994) concluded that there were only a few empirical studies available for any treatment for acute back problems, and that none of the 57 treatments discussed had sufficient evidence for its efficacy based on "multiple relevant and high-quality studies."

Even if the outcome data are available, this does not totally obviate the problem, as it takes time to keep up with the explosion of research. It is not possible for any one person to keep up with all the new developments in health care. It is estimated that a general practitioner would be required to read 19 articles a day, 365 days per year, to keep pace with the current medical advances (Sackett, Rosenberg, Gray, Haynes, & Richardson, 1996).

639

One of the organized attempts to assimilate outcome information for practitioners is the Cochrane Collaboration, an international collaborative group. The aim of the Cochrane Collaboration is to facilitate and disseminate EBM through volunteer efforts with which outcomes are systematically reviewed, compiled, and placed on a website support by the Cochrane Collaboration. With some exception, the Cochrane Collaboration looks for randomized controlled trials (RCTs) as one of the preferred if not required methodological factors to be included as "evidence." The reviews provide information on the clinical efficacy of a given treatment for a given disorder. But for such reviews to be conducted, there must be a sufficiently large number of RCTs (and, in some instances, case series) believed to be of high quality. It takes time for innovative treatments to acquire sufficient published data to permit systematic reviews.

Results from the clinical trials can guide clinical hypotheses by presenting the probability of the efficacy of the particular treatment. The number of patients included in systematic reviews is substantial. It is important for us to remind ourselves, however, that the *average* patient in a large sample does not tell us much about *our* patients. The availability of systematic reviews offers an excellent point of departure for consideration among treatment alternatives. One of the problems, however, may be that reports of clinical trials often fail to address the day-to-day clinical and social nuances that are critical in decision making about a specific patient. No one has the prototypical "average" patient (Charlton, 1995; Smith, 1995).

The majority of clinicians, through experience and practice, develop extensive expertise in clinical judgment. It has been the medical tradition and "gold standard," and it still is the bread and butter of much of clinical practice. Compared to the probability-driven outcome results in peer-reviewed journals, experience-driven clinical wisdom feels more in tune with reality. Thus despite the increasing numbers of evidence-based clinical guidelines (and many more consensus-based, best-practice clinical guidelines, some of which may be produced by organizations with vested interests and thus lack credibility for third-party payers), many practitioners continue to rely on their own judgment when making decisions about their individual patients. However, unless they evaluate the outcomes of their judgment, their practice fails to provide the critical feedback needed to contribute to clinical pathways and guidelines and to experimentally driven EBM.

In the absence of published evidence to support treatments, health care providers cannot avoid the need to collect evidence on patients in their own practice that can demonstrate the effectiveness of the treatments for which they expect to be reimbursed. Most health care professionals are highly driven to provide appropriate clinical care because of their desire to help people, which is why they entered the health professions. Only a relative handful have the experience and expertise, let alone time, to conduct studies that will demonstrate the clinical effectiveness and cost-effectiveness of each of the array of treatments they prescribe, provide, and perform.

In this chapter, we provide some suggestions for how you as a clinician can include program evaluation as a part of your practice efficiently, even without excessive training in research design and statistics. We discuss the meanings of the terms that are being used by third-party payers, to provide some insights into how they are used. We provide detailed information regarding how you can acquire the types of evidence that are being demanded by third-party payers. Throughout, we remain cognizant of the issue of limited resources and recommend efficient strategies that will enable you to obtain the necessary data without becoming overwhelmed with excessive and unrealistic demands.

THIRD-PARTY PAYERS' CONCERNS ABOUT THE COSTS OF PAIN

From the perspective of third-party payers, chronic pain is expensive in many ways: the costs for multiple diagnostic workups, treatments, health care providers, and indemnity payments. The sheer number of people with chronic pain is huge, and costs per patient are staggering. So it should not be surprising that pain has become a four-letter word—a red flag to those who are asked to pay for the seemingly endless services recommended. We need to adopt their perspective for a moment as we consider whether they are justified in this. The health care provider tends to take the perspective of his or her patients, but this somewhat myopic view results in relatively small numbers. Third-party payers tend to think in terms of groups, and consequently in much larger numbers. These individual or small-group versus large-group perspectives lead to very different considerations. The health care provider rightly keeps his or her patients in mind as treatments are prescribed. Third-party payers focus on large volumes and related costs that they must incur.

According to a recent market analysis, approximately 3,900 pain programs and solo practitioners treat 4.8 million Americans suffering from various types of pain disorders annually (Marketdata Enterprises, 1999). These programs routinely use a number of treatment modalities, ranging from invasive interventions (e.g., surgery) to conventional pharmacology (e.g., nonsteroidal anti-inflammatory drugs) to physical therapy (e.g., ultrasound, diathermy, chiropractic) to multi-disciplinary rehabilitation programs. Frymoyer (1990) noted that over 250,000 lumbar surgeries are performed in the United States each year at a cost averaging $15,000 per surgery. More recently, J. D. Loeser (personal communication, February 7, 2000) estimated that the numbers have reached 350,000 at a cost of $25,000 for each operation. Multiplying these numbers, we can derive estimates that expense for lumbar surgery range from $3.75 to $6.25 billion per year. In 1995, Marketdata Enterprises estimated that over 176,500 patients with chronic pain were treated at pain rehabilitation facilities each year at an average cost of $8,100, or over $1.4 billion per year. The expenditures for other treatments (chiropractic, physical therapy, nerve blocks, analgesic medications, etc.) to treat pain, not to mention indemnity costs, are difficult to estimate, but they surely run into additional billions of dollars.

Viewing the figures on prevalence and cost makes it is somewhat easier to understand the consternation of third-party payers when they consider patients with chronic pain. If they are being asked to pay such astronomical costs, then they have every right to be concerned with outcomes: "Does payment for such expensive treatments lead to significant cost savings?" We have an obligation to them and our patients to demonstrate that the treatments we provide are both clinically effective and cost-effective.

Baldly stated, many third-party payers are considerably skeptical regarding expensive and often unproven treatments for patients with chronic pain. Are their suspicions that pain management is expensive and ineffective warranted? The data are limited, but nevertheless there are studies that are suggestive. One thing is certain, however: We need to do a better job of disseminating and communicating the relevant information about clinical outcomes that is available. At the same time, it is imperative for survival that we generate and obtain evidence on outcomes that payers feel are impor-

tant (cost savings) as well as on clinical outcomes such as symptomatic improvement. The only way for us to persuade the skeptics of the value of our pain management approaches is to demonstrate evidence of their cost-effectiveness and clinical effectiveness, based upon reasonable outcome assessment.

TERMINOLOGY

As the health care system becomes more complex, the nature of outcomes from the delivery of clinical care becomes more complex likewise. We have already alluded to a number of important terms and concepts, and we need to clarify these and others. When we speak of the benefits of a particular treatment, we need to clarify to what exactly we are referring. There are several definitions of outcomes in treating patients with pain that need to be understood. Clinical *efficacy* refers to the benefit to patients in a defined population when an intervention is applied for a given medical problem under *controlled*, experimental conditions. *Effectiveness* can be defined as the clinical benefit when *average* clinicians provide the treatment under *average* (i.e., realistic) conditions. Although the two concepts are similar, an intervention can be efficacious but ineffective.

For a treatment to be effective, several things must take place: The treatment itself must have a therapeutic effect; the treatment must be delivered in the appropriate manner; and the patient must comply with the prescribed regimen (e.g., take medication on schedule, perform exercises as directed). In controlled environments, care and monitoring of the treatment protocol include selection of patients, careful screening of patients, and rigorous adherence to the inclusion and exclusion criteria. Patients, as subjects of a research study, receive support, are given attention, and know they are participating in a study (the so-called "Hawthorne effect"). Each of these "nonspecific" effects, along with the active ingredient of the treatment, can contribute to the outcomes. Tight controls on both clinicians' and patients' behaviors are less likely to occur in daily clinical practice. This may explain why the results of effectiveness studies are often less impressive then those in originally published efficacy studies.

The terms *efficacy* and *effectiveness* are often confused and used interchangeably. In the strict sense (Feinstein, 1983; Schwartz & Lellouch, 1967), the outcome of efficacy studies should be condition-specific, with the hypothesized therapy mechanisms modifying the severity of the given symptoms. On the other hand, the effectiveness studies may not necessarily include a double-blind procedure or a placebo; rather, they include a range of outcomes that are considered to be affected by the treatment, regardless of hypothesized mechanisms. When the clinical trials for chronic pain are considered, the majority of the studies probably fall somewhere between these two types, with pharmacological studies leaning toward the efficacy side and rehabilitation studies leaning toward the effectiveness side. The distinction is a fuzzy one, but nevertheless, we should be aware that the direct comparisons of the results from different types of clinical trials may not be meaningful.

Efficiency of treatment refers to the level of resources required to produce benefit. For example, prescription of opioid medication can be compared to multidisciplinary rehabilitation. The expenses of an office and one health care provider, a physician, and routine follow-up are all that are required in the former case, whereas a comprehensive rehabilitation program is likely to include expenses for physical and occupational therapists, psychologists, vocational rehabilitation counselors, and related space and equipment. In determining efficiency, it is important to factor in the cost of treatment required to produce a desirable outcome. In the simplest case, if two treatments produce the same outcome, then the less costly treatment is the more efficient and will be preferred (at least by third-party payers).

Three types of analysis of clinical efficiency may be conducted. In a *cost-effectiveness analysis*, outcome measures related to morbidity and mortality are reported in "natural units," such as years of life saved and functional status (e.g., disability status, days absent from work, return to work [RTW], health care utilization). Thus, for example, in a meta-analysis of multidisciplinary rehabilitation outcomes studies, Flor, Fydrich, and Turk (1992) reported a 50% reduction in disability following rehabilitation. Comparing these results to alternative treatments (e.g., surgery, implantable technologies, chiropractic) would permit a comparison of the cost-effectiveness of the interventions. It would also be important, as we have noted, to factor in the cost of the treatment. Table 33.1 includes an illustrative example. Thus, in the cost-effectiveness analysis example contained in Table 33.1, the more expensive treatment is actually more cost-effective.

TABLE 33.1. Efficiency Analyses of Pain Treatment: Comparisons between Treatment X and Treatment Y for 100 Patients Receiving Each Treatment

	Treatment X	Treatment Y
Treatment cost/pt.	$5,000	$25,000
Total cost	$500,000	$2,500,000
Cost-effectiveness analysis		
RTW	10%	60%
Cost/RTW	$50,000	$41,667
Cost–utility analysis		
Pre-tx. QALY	.1	.1
Post-tx. QALY	.4	.6
Cost for improving 0.1 QALY/patient	$1,667	$5,000
Cost–benefit analysis		
Pre-tx. annual health care cost	$10,000	$10,000
Post-tx. annual health care cost	$5,000	$2,000
Cost–benefit ratio	5,000:5,000	25,000:8,000
Cost for saving $1,000 in health care per patient	$1,000	$3,125

Note. RTW, return to work; QALY, quality-adjusted life year.

In a *cost–utility analysis*, outcomes tend to include less "objective," patient-focused measures. Utility is the value assigned by a patient on a level of health status, measured in a standard unit. Common utility measures include patient satisfaction and self-report scores of functional ability, pain, and mood. Another interesting utility measure is the concept of *quality-adjusted life years*. To date, this measure has not been reported in studies evaluating the efficacy or effectiveness of treatments for pain. Quality-adjusted life years integrate quantity and quality of human lives. One year at perfect health equals 1.0 quality-adjusted life year. Suppose that a patient, because of a pain condition, rates his or her health status as 30% of "perfect" health (premorbid health); this would be equal to .30 quality-adjusted life year. This concept has the advantage of using a consistent unit with the incorporation of patients' own judgment across studies. In the cost–utility example in Table 33.1, the more expensive treatment truly costs more to produce an equivalent improvement in quality-adjusted life years per patient, and thus the less expensive treatment may be preferred.

In a *cost–benefit analysis*, all outcomes are converted into monetary units. Outcomes or benefits include reductions in the indirect costs of disorders, such as productivity gains, changes in health care utilization, and reduced disability payments resulting from the treatment.

Examination of the example of cost–benefit analysis in Table 33.1 shows that the more expensive treatment has a higher (i.e., less favorable) cost-benefit ratio. In considering the costs and benefits of multidisciplinary pain rehabilitation, we calculated the cost of (1) screening patients, some of whom did not receive the treatment, and (2) the cost of the treatment to produce a specific outcome. We (Turk & Okifuji, 1998) compared the cost-benefit ratio of multidisciplinary pain rehabilitation

to that of surgery and found that the multidisciplinary pain centers had a ratio 21 times more favorable than that of surgery. Moreover, we did not factor the cost of iatrogenic problems that may follow surgery (Long, Filtzer, Ben Debba, & Hendler, 1988) into our alanysis.

To summarize, then, Table 33.1 illustrates the results of the three types of analyses (cost-effectiveness, cost-utility, and cost–benefit) for two hypothetical treatments, X and Y. As you can see, the level of efficiency depends upon what type of analysis one employs. Treatment Y is substantially (five times) more expensive than treatment X. Treatment Y seems also to be more costly when health care utilization and quality-of-life (QOL) costs are concerned, and costs more to produce equivalent quality-adjusted life years from the patient's perspective. However, the cost for returning one patient to work is less for treatment Y ($41,667) than for treatment X ($50,000). Thus, for the important outcome RTW, treatment Y may be regarded as the more efficient selection despite the overall cost.

OUTCOME PARAMETERS

What Is Important for Whom?

When you follow a patient with pain from the initial evaluation through discharge, how do you establish whether the treatment was a "success"? Do you rely on the patient's reports of pain reduction, objective measures of functional outcomes, or reduction in unscheduled visits because of pain flareups? All of these are important, and there are other criteria as well. It is important to realize that different constituent groups (e.g., patients, referral sources, health care providers, MCOs, workers' compensation carriers) may have different criteria upon which they base the answer to this question of success (see Table 33.2).

TABLE 33.2. Criteria of Success for Whom?

Outcome	Person or organization
Pain elimination/reduction	Patient, health care provider
Reduction in medication	Referring physician
Reduction in health care utilization	MCO, workers' compensation carrier
RTW, off-time loss	Workers' compensation carrier
Increased activity	Patient, health care provider
Closure of disability claim	Governmental and private third-party payers
Patient satisfaction	Patient, MCO, referring physician

Pain Reduction or Elimination

One obvious criterion of success is pain reduction. If you ask a patient what he or she views as a successful outcome, it will most likely be elimination or significant reduction of pain (Deathe & Helmes, 1993). There are a number of procedures available to measure pain severity (see Jensen & Karoly, Chapter 2, this volume). Many of these are appropriate for persistent pain or acute pain, but what about episodic pain? For example, migraine episodes occur at intervals. If you ask a patient to rate his or her pain between attacks, these ratings may be biased by the patient's current, pain-free state compared to his or her ratings during a headache (see Haythornthwaite & Fauerbach, Chapter 22, this volume). Patients can be asked to rate the severity of pain with different time parameters, such as current pain and worst or average pain in the past week.

It may be useful to have patients keep diaries, so that they can rate the severity of a pain at specified times in an interval and the duration of episodic pain such as headaches. Headaches can be measured with three related but not identical parameters—severity, frequency, and duration (Budzynski, Stoyva, Adler, & Mullaney, 1973; see also Andrasik, Chapter 24). One way to summarize these parameters as an index score is to compute a *headache index*—that is, the sum of all pain intensity ratings divided by the sum of the number of days recorded. Another parameter to consider is the frequency of headache attacks. This can be calculated by dividing the number of headache-free days by the number of days monitored. Duration of headaches can also be recorded. The summed duration of the headaches is then divided by the frequency for the period of days recorded.

Recently, clinical researchers have become increasingly aware of the problems and biases associated with the retrospective assessment of pain and other symptoms (see Haythornthwaite & Fauerbach, Chapter 22). Often we ask patients to rate the frequency or severity of pain (symptoms) over a defined period of time. In other words, our assessment of pain symptoms depends heavily upon patients' ability to recall their pain—say, in the past 2 weeks. To deal with problems of forgetting and memory biases, some investigators have provided patients with daily diaries or sets of cards that they mail in each day with the record of pain and other relevant information (e.g., sleep, activity) (Salovey et al., 1992). With recent advances in portable computers, several research studies have made use of palmtop computers that "page" patients at preset intervals and ask them to provide responses to a set of questions (Affleck et al., 1999; Stone, Broderick, Porter, & Kaell, 1997). The computers store the patients' responses, which may later be connected to desktop computers (or to telephone lines so that the data are uploaded to a desktop computer) and then directly entered in the commercially available database software (e.g., spreadsheets). Thus as the technology evolves, the real-time assessment of pain and related symptoms become possible, helping us collect pain data that are probably more accurate representations of pain problems in patients' daily lives than retrospective reports are.

Patient Satisfaction

The importance of both treating patients' problems and treating patients as consumers of clinical services has been gaining attention. The importance of patient satisfaction is underscored by its relation to patients' tendency to stay with treatment (Nguyen, Attkisson, & Stegner, 1983), adhere to prescriptions (Linn, Linn, & Stein, 1982), and maintain an active role in treatment (Ware, Snyder, Wright, & Davies, 1983). From an MCO's perspective, it is also important to note that patients' satisfaction has been related to staying in prepaid health plans (Ware et al., 1983) and less to health care consumption (McCracken, Klock, Mingay, Asbury, & Sinclair, 1997). Satisfaction of patients with the clinical services received is a part of the quality assurance of the care delivery (American Pain Society Commission on Quality Assurance Standards, 1991). Thus the feedback from your patients not only will help you review their progress, but also will help accrediting organizations (e.g., Commission on Accreditation of Rehabilitation Facilities, 1995) and third-party payers to evaluate your clinical practice.

It may seem reasonable to assume that pain reduction is a necessary prerequisite for high level of patient satisfaction. However, patient satisfaction goes beyond just pain reduction. Several studies (see, e.g., Miaskowski, in press; Pekarik & Wolff, 1996) have reported that even when pain and other symptoms are not significantly reduced, patients may express satisfaction with their health care providers. This appears to occur when (1) patients perceive that clinicians did their best in implementing the treatment; (2) the process was interpersonally pleasant; and (3) they acquire some skills and knowledge that they can use to manage problems in the future, even if pain cannot be completely eliminated.

In addition to pain reduction, patients mention their concerns with the way pain interferes with functional activities and their lack of life satisfaction, which is often manifested as depressed mood. Approximately 50% of patients with chronic pain are significantly depressed (Romano & Turner, 1985), and satisfaction is negatively associated with depression (McCracken et al., 1997).

At this point, the term *satisfaction* is rather loosely defined. One dimension of satisfaction is a patient's view of how helpful an intervention has been. Several groups have developed self-report inventories designed to assess this dimension (e.g., Chapman, Jamison, & Sanders, 1996). In addition to reduction in pain, McCracken and colleagues (1997) found that patients' confidence and trust in their physicians, as well as convenience factors (e.g., the amount of waiting time for the appointment and in the clinic, the return of telephone calls, and difficulty finding the clinic), were all predictors of satisfaction. Further studies need to clarify the contributions of other dimensions of patient satisfaction to the overall quality of care.

A concept that is related to satisfaction is QOL. The concept of QOL has arisen as the advances in health care have made it essential to consider not just survival and longevity, but also the quality of one's lifetime. QOL is a highly personal variable, entirely dependent upon an individual's own evaluation of his or her well-being in multiple domains of life. Thus QOL is a relative and reflective concept—one that varies with a patient's culture and personal history, as well as his or her health status (i.e., pain severity).

Many pain conditions adversely and severely affect QOL. Some common features of QOL include the perceived quality of functional ability (e.g., ability to perform activities of daily living), coping and adaptation, and health status. Some treatments, especially those with a strong emphasis on rehabilitation, tend to directly modify the levels of QOL. There are a number of standardized measures to assess these factors. Some are disorder-specific, such as the Fibromyalgia Impact Questionnaire (FIQ; Burckhardt, Clark, & Bennett, 1991) for fibromyalgia syndrome (FMS) or the Quality of Life Questionnaire–Cancer 36 (Sigurdardottir, Brandberg, & Sullivan, 1996) for cancer. Others are generic, such as the West Haven–Yale Multidimensional Pain Inventory (WHYMPI;

Kerns, Turk, & Rudy, 1985) or the 36-Item Short-Form Health Survey (SF-36; Ware & Sherbourne, 1992). Still others involve individualized assessment protocols (e.g., Ruta, Garratt, Leng, Russell, & MacDonald, 1994). The first two types are not necessarily developed as QOL measures, but are considered to tap into some dimensions of QOL in patients with pain. The significance of QOL as an outcome cannot be overstated. At times, patients and family members report that the improvement of QOL is more important than symptom remission. If there is an adverse effect of the treatment, pain may be reduced, but QOL deteriorates. Since the concept of QOL itself is rooted in patients' core values about their lives, clinicians' understanding of what is important to patients' lives can help them direct the emphasis of the treatment as well as evaluate the personally relevant merit of the treatment to the patients.

Reduction in Health Care Utilization

Earlier we have described the tremendous costs associated with health care to alleviate pain. MCOs and other third-party payers are particularly concerned about the magnitude and costs of health care services consumed by patients with chronic pain. Thus, from their perspective, a successful treatment outcome would consist of a demonstration of a significant reduction in health care consumption and costs following treatment. In short, the importance of assessing health care utilization is twofold. On one hand, reduction in health care use may be indicative of improved health. On the other hand, lower health care use can be translated into cost savings, such as in a cost–benefit analysis. In the current health care environment, where resource allocation dictates practice, it is imperative that we be able to demonstrate that our treatments do help save money. Major health care variables may be divided into four types: (1) surgical treatment, (2) medication use, (3) other medical costs (e.g., doctor visits, X-rays), and (4) nonmedical health care costs (e.g., alternative medicine, biofeedback). These variables are probably most important to third-party payers in determining whether a treatment "works" on a pain condition.

Medication Reduction

The appropriate use of opioid medication for patients with chronic pain is a controversial topic, and detailed discussion is beyond the scope of this chapter (see Turk, 1996). Prior to the mid-1980s, the use of what has come to be called chronic opioid therapy was usually avoided for patients with chronic pain. Debate about the long-term use of opioids for patients with chronic noncancer pain has been a recurring theme (Portenoy, 1996; Turk, 1996). However, reduction in medication, particularly opioid analgesics, remains the primary rationale for numerous referrals of patients with chronic pain to rehabilitation programs (Deathe & Helmes, 1993). From the standpoint of the third-party payer, there is a cost to medication and the regular physician monitoring. Thus, from their perspective, demonstrating evidence for therapeutic effects of opioids becomes critical; if such drugs are found to be ineffective, reduction of analgesic medication rates is an important consideration in evaluating the effectiveness of a treatment.

Assessing changes in medication may be a relatively easy task for an individual patient. The nature and dosage of medication from pretreatment to posttreatment and follow-up can be readily calculated. When many patients are being assessed in the aggregate, however, the nature of different drugs being consumed may be difficult to compare. For example, one patient may be taking three Percocet tablets a day, and another may be using transdermal fentanyl patches. There are a number of medication conversion tables that make it possible to compare medications on a common metric (although rarely do they compare the costs and benefits of different opioids). One option is to report the average percentage reduction across patients when the dosages and nature of the drugs are converted to a standard unit potency.

Based on a meta-analysis of 65 published studies covering 3,089 patients with chronic pain who received treatment at pain rehabilitation programs, Flor and colleagues (1992) reported that 50% of patients were taking opioid medication upon entering these programs. Following treatment, a substantial number of these patients were no longer taking any medication for pain. More impressive is a report from a long-term follow-up study (18 months to 10 years; Guck, Skultety, Meilman, & Dowd, 1985) that the percentage of patients taking opioids following treatment at a rehabilitation program was 22% compared to 61% before treatment. In contrast, 53% of patients who had spinal fusions for back pain continued to require analgesic medications at the follow-up (Lehmann et al., 1987). Although there are limitations in the comparisons that can be made across studies with different samples, the results of studies of different treatments that use similar outcome measures can provide useful comparisons.

Reduction in the Number of Treatments for Pain

Several studies have reported reduction in health care costs following treatment for patients with chronic pain. If untreated, chronic pain requires intensive consumption of health care resources, estimated yearly at $34,000 per person (Simmons, Avant, Demski, & Parisher, 1988). A reduction in pain-related intensive clinic visits and other utilization of health care resources should be one of the indicators for treatment success. For example, if one can demonstrate a 36% reduction in pain-related clinic visits at a health maintenance organization during the first year following treatment at a pain rehabilitation program (as reported by Caudill, Schnable, Zuttermeister, Benson, & Friedman, 1991), this figure can be used to calculate the cost savings that would accrue after taking into consideration the cost of the treatment, and thereby the argument in favor of the treatment can be greatly enhanced.

It is possible to compare outcomes of different treatments in terms of health care utilization. For example, Cassisi, Sypert, Salamon, and Kapel (1989) reported that only 8% of patients with low back pain treated in a pain rehabilitation program went on to receive additional surgery for their pain in the year following treatment, compared to 46% of patients receiving standard care who subsequently received surgery for their pain during the follow-up year. In this case, we can convert expenditures for operations to perform a cost–benefit analysis of the two treatments. If we assume that the average cost of lumbar surgery was $15,000 (Frymoyer, 1990), the comparative costs of rehabilitation versus standard care would be as follows: $45,000 (3 surgeries @ $15,000) versus $270,000 (18 surgeries @ $15,000), or a savings of $225,000 with rehabilitation in 1 year. Of course, it is necessary to factor in the cost of the treatment. Even if we adjust the figure with the treatment costs, however, the saving is substantial. These are the types of data that are needed to convince third-party payers that they should provide coverage for the treatment proposed.

Increases in Functional Activities and RTW

An important criterion of success is increased functional activities following treatment, since most patients with chronic pain have drastically reduced most physical activities and spend the majority of their time in sedentary activity. Not only are health care providers and third-party payers concerned about increased activity, but also patients have indicated that they are more satisfied with treatment when they are able to increase their activities (McCracken et al., 1997).

In the meta-analysis by Flor and colleagues (1992), rates of activity (broadly and variously defined) for patients who were treated in pain rehabilitation programs increased significantly, with 65% of treated patients demonstrating increases in functional activities, compared to 35% significantly improving activity levels following standard care. One study (Peters, Large, & Elkind, 1992) comparing activity levels of patients treated at a pain rehabilitation program to those of patients receiving standard care (broadly defined) reported substantial improvement in activity levels in the former and deterioration in those receiving standard care. A large number (58%) of patients with back pain report worsening of functional ability following surgery (Gallon, 1989). Earlier we noted that chronic opioid therapy is being reconsidered, and a number of studies have reported significant pain reductions accompanying this mode of treatment. This might seem a positive outcome; however, none of these studies has reported any improvement in functional activities, with some even reporting deterioration in some patients (Kjaersgaard-Andersen et al., 1990; Zenz, Strumpf, & Tryba, 1992). These data are quite telling in terms of how treatment actually affects patients' daily lives, and such data need to be communicated thoroughly to those who have decision-making power for treatment selection.

In some populations with chronic pain (e.g., pain due to work-related injury), the variable of RTW, discussed earlier, may be one of the most influential in demonstrating the effectiveness of the intervention. At first, the RTW variable seems to be a simple dichotomous factor; however, evaluation of RTW may be complex. Does RTW mean return to the former job (full-time or part-time), a modified job for the same employer, or a different job for a different employer? How should we consider patients who are currently being retrained or those who are actively seeking employment? What about people who return to work for a brief time period and then have a recurrence and take additional time off work? These questions make it difficult to make use of RTW as an appropriate outcome by which to measure success.

The problem gets even worse, because a number of factors influence RTW in patients with chronic pain, other than physical capability and work readiness. These include (1) physical demands of the job, (2) job availability, (3) regional variation in the job market, (4) availability of job accommodations, (5) marketability of patients' skills, (6) extent of wage replacement, and (7) financial incentives. Given that a choice exists and all other factors are comparable, whom would you be more likely to hire—a person who has been on disability for a work-related injury for the past 3 years, or a person with no such history? Finding an employer may be particularly difficult for patients who have long histories of chronic pain and job skills that are predicated on high degrees of physical exertion. Indeed, a recent report (Fishbain, Cutler, Rosomoff, Khalil, & Steele-Rosomoff, 1999) found that RTW intention for patients with chronic pain was better predicted by job-related variables than by pain-related variables. Similarly, the critical factor in predicting RTW seems to be the availability of a job to which an injured worker can return (Dworkin, Handlin, Richlin, Brand, & Vannucci, 1985).

Unfortunately, even with the concerns raised, some third-party payers will use RTW as the sole or primary criterion on which to base success. So, despite its limitations, RTW needs to be considered as an outcome measure. A number of studies have reported significant increases in RTW following treatment of patients with chronic pain. The most successful treatments appear to be rehabilitation and functional restoration programs, where figures suggest that approximately 50% of patients do return to work (Cutler et al., 1994; Flor et al., 1992). Approximately 71% of patients with back pain treated in rehabilitation programs return to work, compared to 44% of patients receiving standard care (Feuerstein, Menz, Zastowny, & Baron, 1994). Studies of patients with multiple back surgeries have rather poor outcomes when it comes to RTW. For example, North, Campbell, and colleagues (1991) reported that only 21% of those not working prior to repeat back surgery returned to work postoperatively. The results are little better for implantation of a spinal cord stimulator: Only about 25% of patients return to work following implantation (North, Ewend, Lawton, Kidd, & Piantadosi, 1991) and in a study conducted in Belgium, only 5% returned to work 1 year following implantation of the stimulator (Kupers et al., 1996).

Increases in functional activities are particularly important outcome criteria for patients who are homemakers, retirees, or elderly persons. For these patients, RTW is an inappropriate criterion on which to base success. Other indices of activity increases can be used, such as comparison of the number of hours sitting, standing, walking, and lying down. Patient diaries can be used to record these activities. There are also a number of functional activity measures (see Battié & May, Chapter 12) that have been shown to correlate highly with functional capacity examinations performed by physical therapists (Deyo, 1988).

Reduction in Disability Payments

The societal costs of chronic pain, including the health care utilization and disability costs, are prohibitively high. For example, between $11 and 43 billion is spent for disability compensation for back pain alone (Frymoyer & Durett, 1997). Pain accounts for 25% of all sick days, totaling approximately 50 million lost work days in 1995, with an estimated $3 billion price tag (Louis Harris and Associates, 1996). Patients may not view reduction in expenditures for disability payments as a primary goal, but workers' compensation carriers, self-insurers, and government agencies that pay disability (e.g., the Social Security Administration, federal employee insurance carriers) view this outcome as extremely significant in determining the effectiveness of any therapeutic intervention.

Like the RTW variable, however, a claim closure is not necessarily clinically determined. Claim closures for many patients with chronic pain are dependent on subjective reports rather than objective pathology, putting more weight on administrative judgment in determining the disability status. Societal and organizational pressures to facilitate closures may be growing as available financial resources decline. Thus the value of the closures of disability claims may be a reflection of various factors, including clinical status, organizational norms and pressure to close claims, the zeal of claim managers, and fiscal policies.

Some studies have demonstrated a significant reduction in the percentage of patients receiving disability payments following treatment. For example, in the meta-analysis of patients treated in rehabilitation-oriented pain treatment facilities cited previously, Flor and colleagues (1992) reported a 50% reduction in cases receiving disability. These figures should be viewed as quite significant by those agencies that are paying for disability.

In summary, then, various outcome criteria can be used to evaluate the clinical effectiveness, cost-effectiveness, and cost–benefit ratio of any treatment (i.e., pain, patient satisfaction, QOL, emotional distress, health care utilization, functional activities, and disability rates). The importance of the outcomes in determining the success will vary, depending on who is asked. Consequently, health care providers need to collect outcome data on each of these. Several factors should govern the methods selected to assess each of these outcomes.

FACTORS TO CONSIDER IN SELECTING MEASURES OF OUTCOME

In performing assessment for clinical trials or routine clinical care, health care providers should consider feasibility, patient acceptance, efficiency, sensitivity to treatment effects, clinical utility, and meaningfulness of any outcome (see Dworkin, Nagasako, Hetzel, & Farrar, Chapter 34). We briefly discuss each of these.

Feasibility

Feasibility refers to the ability to obtain the necessary outcome data. For example, if you wished to demonstrate that the number of unscheduled health care visits declined in the 6 months following treatment compared to the 6 months preceding treatment, it is essential that there be an efficient mechanism to obtain this information. Ideally, patients' medical records should be scrutinized; this may not be possible in a private clinic, but it may be much more easily accomplished in MCOs, Department of Veterans Affairs medical centers, or state workers' compensation agencies. Patient reports may be readily obtainable, and therefore, feasible, but of questionable reliability.

Sometimes what is ideal is simply unrealistic. Consider assessment of pain behaviors—those overt communications of pain, distress, and suffering (see Keefe, Williams, & Smith, Chapter 10). Pain behaviors have been shown to provide important information about the impact of responses of significant others on the maintenance of disability. Thus one outcome that might be considered is reduction in pain behaviors. Ideally, patients' behaviors should be observed in multiple settings, including those outside the clinic setting. This is important, as the clinic is not a natural setting, and patients may not provide representative behavioral samples when they know they are being observed by a health care provider. Since it is not generally feasible for health care providers to observe patients' behavior consistently in multiple settings, they must rely on enlisting significant others. This may be reasonable for patients living in a marital or other couple relationship, but may not be practical for those who do not live with a significant other.

Patient Acceptance

Patient Acceptance is associated with patient burden. There is a finite amount of information that can be obtained from a patient. Excessive demands involving lengthy questionnaires may alienate patients and decrease their willingness to provide accurate information. There is a huge and growing (indeed, metastasizing) number of psychological measures, each of which by itself might provide useful information, but the burden of completing every one described throughout this volume would be unacceptable and unrealistic. Thus the health care professional who wishes to make use of self-report measures must keep the demands within some reasonable limits.

In addition to the patient demand created by multiple measures, the nature of the questions included in self-report scales needs to be considered. If the questions do not have *face validity* (i.e., they are not credible for the patient), he or she may not respond in a valid fashion or may refuse to comply with the request. Consider the Minnesota Multiphasic Personality Inventory (MMPI), the most widely used self-report measure used by psychologists to evaluate patients with pain (Piotrowski, 1997). The first edition of the MMPI includes 556 true–false items that often bear no obvious relation to chronic pain. How does a patient with pain view this questionnaire and the health care professional who requests him or her to complete it? For example, consider a few items from the original MMPI to which the patient is asked to respond "true" or "false": "I do not read every editorial in the newspaper every day," "I would like to be a singer," "I used to like drop-the-handkerchief," "Everything is turning out just like the prophets of the Bible said it would." We are not questioning the potential of empirically derived tests such as the MMPI to provide clinically meaningful information; rather, we are raising the issue of patient acceptance. Some patients

may object actively or passively, feeling that the questions are irrelevant at best and demeaning at worst. As a self-test, we encourage anyone who plans to use a self-report questionnaire to read each item and to consider how a patient might react to items with low face validity.

Efficiency

Efficiency refers to whether the assessment information can be easily obtained. For any measures being considered, the most efficient means of obtaining the information should be used. For example, if depression is considered an important outcome, if two measures are available to assess depression that have equal reliability and validity, and if appropriate normative data are available for both, then the shorter of the two would be the preferred measure. We have already referred to the original MMPI, with its more than 500 questions. Patients may take 2–4 hours to complete this instrument. If it were shown that a measure with comparable psychometric properties consisted of 30 questions and required 15 minutes to complete, then, other things being equal, the shorter instrument should be selected as the more efficient.

Sensitivity to Treatment Effects

Sensitivity to treatment effects refers to whether the outcome criterion selected is one that is likely to change in a meaningful way following treatment. If a measure is not sensitive to treatment effects, then it would be inappropriate to select it as a criterion upon which to base a judgment of such effects. Consider the case of FMS. One of the diagnostic criteria for the research classification of FMS is the presence of pain upon palpation of at least 11 of 18 specific locations, known as *tender points*. The number of tender points is usually determined by the patient's responding "Yes" or "No" to the question of whether a specific point is painful following palpation by 4 kg of force. Change in the number of tender points might be considered an outcome measure to use to determine whether drug X is effective in treating FMS. The dichotomous judgment "Yes or No," however, provides little range and therefore little opportunity to determine small changes. Selecting change in the number of tender points as a criterion for treatment success might be setting the stage for failure. One alternative that has been suggested is to ask patients to rate the pain severity of each point following palpation on an 11-point scale anchored by "no or minimal pain" and "worst pain I can imagine," and then averaging the pain severity score (Okifuji, Turk, Sinclair, Starz, & Marcus, 1997). An 11-point range is more likely to be sensitive to change than the absolute number of tender points.

Clinical Utility

Clinical utility concerns how meaningful the assessment information is going to be. Is the measure appropriate for use as an outcome criterion? For example, if we wished to determine the effectiveness of biofeedback to improve coping with pain, assessment of range of motion or percentage of patients who reach maximum medical improvement might not be appropriate outcome criteria. However, if the treatment being evaluated was a functional restoration rehabilitation program, then these measures would be appropriate. The outcome criteria selected should be relevant to the intervention being evaluated. We should also note that improvement in one outcome criterion does not infer improvement in any other. Research has repeatedly demonstrated that impairment, disability, and pain are only modestly correlated (Turk, Okifuji, Sinclair, & Starz, 1996; Waddell, 1987).

There is a definite advantage to using a standard set of outcome factors, even if some unique measures are appropriate, given the nature of particular pain disorders. If identical or comparable data sets are collected, problems associated with the pooling and integration of findings will be much reduced. Efforts have been made by the American Pain Society and the American Academy of Pain Medicine to develop standardized protocols that will permit multicenter trials and the aggregation of data across sites.

Several sets of measures to use have been recommended. For example, Deyo and colleagues (1998) have recommended the use of standardized measurements in six core areas as the standardized set of outcome variables for evaluating low back pain treatments in a range of clinical settings. These six areas are pain, function, well-being, work disability, social disability, and satisfaction with care. A number of other outcome criteria can be used to determine whether a treatment is effective, in addition to those suggested. These include pain reduction, improvement in mood, increase in activity, reduction in consumption of opioid medications, RTW, reduction in health care utilization,

and closure of disability cases. Table 33.3 includes a set of outcomes and relevant questions and measures that can be used.

There is no doubt that the efficacy of clinical trials needs to be evaluated with large samples and most rigorous methodological considerations. However, how do we derive information on what to do with a particular patient? Statistical differences between groups, however impressive *p* values (statistical significance) may be, do not provide information about any individual patient—or, as we note in the next section, about the clinical significance of the outcomes (Feinstein & Horwitz, 1997). The literature only provides us with the evidence that a particular intervention *is likely to be effective* for an average patient with a particular pain problem.

Yet another factor that needs to be taken into consideration when one is determining the effectiveness of any treatment is that of additional costs that the treatment may incur. For example, most invasive treatments can produce iatrogenic problems that may need to be treated and therefore add a cost to the original treatment. Some treatments require continuing monitoring by health care professionals or repeated treatments (physical therapy, chiropractic manipulations, nerve blocks); the accompanying costs of these for an individual patient may seem relatively modest, but when summed across many patients can be large (Turk & Okifuji, 1998).

As noted earlier, all clinicians, through experience and practice, develop extensive expertise in clinical judgment and proficiency. Compared to the probability-driven outcome results in peer-reviewed journals, experience-driven clinical wisdom feels more in tune with reality. Thus, despite the increasing numbers of research-based clinical guidelines (and many more consensus-based, best-practice guidelines), many practitioners continue to rely on their own clinical judgment when making decisions about their individual patients. Inconsistent applications of research-based guidelines result in the absence of outcome feedback and fail to become a part of experience-driven outcomes that practitioners accumulate on a day-to-day basis.

Clinical versus Statistical Significance

One final point to note before we proceed to a systematic discussion of data collection in a clinical setting is the distinction between *clinical significance* and *statistical significance*. When we consider outcomes, we should acknowledge that the concepts

TABLE 33.3. Key Outcome Criteria and Recommended Assessment Methods

Factors	Questions/measures
Pain	Examples: Numerical Rating Scale (NRS) (see Jensen & Karoly, Chapter 2) Box Rating Scale (see Jensen & Karoly, Chapter 2) McGill Pain Questionnaire, short form (Melzack, 1987; see Melzack & Katz, Chapter 3) West Haven–Yale Multidimensional Pain Inventory (WHYMPI), scale 1 (Kerns et al., 1985; see Jacob & Kerns, Chapter 19) Number, frequency, duration of pain episodes
Function	Examples: WHYMPI, section 3 (Activity scales) Oswestry Low-Back Pain Disability Questionnaire (Fairbank et al., 1980; see Battié & May, Chapter 12) Pain Disability Index (Pollard, 1984)
Perceived impact	Examples: WHYMPI Interference scale (scale 2) Arthritis Impact Measurement Scale (Meenan et al., 1980) WHYMPI, Activity scales 9–12
Health care utilization	Medication use Treatments from health care professionals Number of unscheduled, pain-related visits to health care professionals Number of hospitalizations for pain Number of surgeries for pain
Emotional distress	Examples: Beck Depression Inventory (BDI; Beck et al., 1961) Center for Epidemiological Studies–Depression scale (CES-D; Radloff, 1977) WHYMPI, Affective Distress scale (scale 4)
Satisfaction with care	"Over the course of treatment for your pain, how would you rate your overall medical care?" "Would you recommend your health care professional or the treatment you received for a friend or relative with a similar pain problem?" Pain Service Satisfaction Test (PSST; McCracken et al., 1997)

are related but not identical. A treatment may produce improvements that are statistically significant but not clinically meaningful to patients. For example, provided the sample size is large enough, a treatment that produces a 25% reduction in pain may be statistically significant, but this may not be clinically significant if patients define a satisfactory outcome as 50% reduction in pain.

Our judgment of the treatment efficacy based upon clinical trials is probability-oriented. If the treatment yields results indicating that there is less than a 5% chance that the treated group is not different from the untreated group, researchers consider the treatment to have a significant effect. Now suppose that you decide to employ treatment X, which we consistently see producing statistically

significant differences for the treatment group. You see the pain scores of five patients 3 months after starting the treatment, as described in Table 33.4. Should you or should you not continue with this treatment? How can we determine whether the results are clinically meaningful?

Earlier we have described parameters that have been used in evaluating the outcomes of treatments for headaches. The clinical and statistical effects of a headache treatment can be determined by viewing statistical differences in the headache index before and after treatment. By convention, a 50% reduction in the headache index has come to be accepted as clinically meaningful. Similar conventions can be adopted for any outcome criterion. If we subscribe to this 50% rule, the treatment has achieved clinical significance only for patient C in Table 33.4. However, note that his patient still reported higher level of pain than all but patient A. Alternatively, one may consider achieving an absolute level to be clinically significant. If we declare that a pain score of 3 or less is clinically important, then this treatment has been effective for patients B and D in Table 33.4. However one decides to define the clinical significance, the criterion should be based on a reasonable clinical rationale.

When you want to report the results to nonclinical decision makers (e.g., insurers, administrators), there are at least two ways the results of clinical trials may be reported. The average change is commonly presented in published studies. It is also reasonable to report on the percentage of patients who have shown clinical significant improvements on any particular outcome criterion, according to consensually agreed-upon levels (e.g., a 50% reduction in pain). More sophisticated statistical approaches such as the reliability-of-change index (Jacobson et al., 1984) are also available, but may only be effective with an audience that has some background understanding of empirical research.

DATA COLLECTION IN CLINICAL SETTINGS

It is not feasible or pragmatic to expect that the methodological rigor required for published efficacy studies can be used in office practice. The data collection in daily practice should emphasize the characteristics that we have described above: It should be feasible, acceptable to patients, efficient, clinically useful, and sensitive to treatment. The data collection process also must not require excessive time or effort from the care provider or the supporting staff of the clinic, or it will not be included in standard practice.

The recent advances in computer technology may aid the data collection process. Form-scanning devices, hand-held devices, touch screens, and wireless communication systems are a few such advances that can contribute to the ease of data collection and management. These devices will require initial investment of cost and labor, but once the system is set up, they should automate the data collection process with very little paperwork.

As noted above, there are many dimensions and factors that contribute to pain disorders, making the assessment complex and cumbersome. For the simplified data collection in a clinical setting, we recommend several. Basically, we suggest having two domains of data on patients with pain: patient-focused clinical information, and the socioeconomic impact of pain.

Process Data

Although the contribution of clinical process to improve the quality of care cannot be overstated, very little attention (or funding) has been given to this topic. Process measures were initially developed during the early 20th century to assure the quality of manufacturing products, with the assumption that a better process would prevent faulty products and thereby would improve efficiency (Gillies, 1997). In health care research, *process* generally refers to the quality of the implementation of "how well it was done." The intentions of measuring process is to detect a lack of appropriate action and to prevent inappropriate action from taking place during the early stage of treatment, promoting early remedial actions to optimize the validity of a clinical trial (Crombie & Davies, 1998).

In pain medicine, such process variables include adherence to a prescribed regimen (e.g., medication intake, exercise at home), treatment format (e.g., individual vs. group format, size of group), timing (e.g., every week vs. every other week, 4 weeks

TABLE 33.4. Changes in Pain Scores for Five Hypothetical Patients 3 Months after starting Treatment X

	Pretreatment	Posttreatment	Change	Change %
Patient A	8	6	2	25%
Patient B	4	3	1	25%
Patient C	10	5	5	50%
Patient D	3	2	1	33%
Patient E	5	4	1	20%

Note. 0 = no pain, 10 = worst pain.

vs. 10 weeks), and other treatment parameters. For example, exercise is considered one of the most critical components in rehabilitating patients with chronic pain, but its effectiveness depends heavily upon patients' compliance with the exercise regimen (Wigers, Stiles, & Vogel, 1996). As another example, the same treatment may be delivered over different time intervals (Bruera et al., 1999; Rowe & Craske, 1998).

Another important process measure in the current climate of cost containment is resource allocation. The evaluation of process will help us identify the critical resources to be allocated and the unnecessary resources that we can eliminate, thereby improving the efficiency of the treatment without compromising outcome.

Hypothetical Example

The exact nature of these outcome variables and the assessment tools vary across diagnoses. We use a case of a patient diagnosed with FMS to illustrate. FMS is characterized by widespread pain, generalized hyperalgesia, fatigue, sleep disturbance, emotional distress, and functional limitation (Wolfe et al., 1990). As noted earlier, the classification of FMS requires hyperalgesic response to digital palpation of at least 11 of 18 designated *tender points* (Wolfe et al., 1990). No pathology is known at this time, and thus the targets of treatments are signs and symptoms, including the number of painful tender points, pain severity, and fatigue. In addition, patients with FMS report significantly compromised QOL (Burckhardt, Clark, & Bennett, 1993). The QOL assessment should include more global measures of emotional and functional well-being. In this example, we use two standardized scales for QOL—one specific to FMS, the other a more generic health-related QOL measure.

We summarize the outcome variables in Table 33.5. As a pragmatic solution for collecting data in a busy practice with limited resources, we suggest the assessment of these variables with the simplest possible assessment tools, such as numerical rating scales or visual analogue scales. If more comprehensive resources are desirable, various assessment tools (the majority of which are described throughout this handbook) are available.

Health care utilization is a very important factor for FMS, since the long history of suffering from multiple symptoms tends to facilitate avid consumption of health care resources (Bombardier & Buchwald, 1996). Health care utilization can be converted into monetary units targeting analgesic use, as well as other medical and nonmedical treatment costs (see, e.g., Bell, Kidd, & North, 1997). Disability and RTW are dichotomous, but the status of these variables at each assessment stage should be recorded. Service satisfaction is a utility measure that can help the clinician to evaluate and improve the quality of care. Lastly, the clinician's impression of the patient's adherence to the treatment regimen is an important process variable. If compliance is low, the clinician needs to identify the parameters of treatment that need to be reevaluated. (We must be cautious in assessing adherence, however; patients may be reluctant to report that they have been nonadherent, especially to a health care provider who is treating them.)

When should it be determined that the treatment has sufficiently benefited the patient? In general, outcome research includes initial evaluation, posttreatment evaluation at the end of the treatment, and follow-ups. The follow-ups are critical in understanding not only the maintenance of treatment gain, but also the impact of treatment efficacy upon various aspects of the patient's life. For example, determining whether the treatment has had any positive impact upon reduction of health care cost or RTW will require some duration of time following the completion of the treatment. Measuring multiple variables across multiple domains of a pain disorder over time is important, because (1) values of different variables may change at different times, and (2) some improvement in some domains may be necessary to promote improvement in other domains. Figure 33.1 on page 655 displays a sample form for assessing outcomes for patients with FMS at pretreatment, posttreatment, and two follow-ups.

Reliance on Group Averages to Establish Treatment Success

If your practice is a part of a group, or if you participate in a multicenter study and thereby increase the speed with which you can obtain an adequate sample size, you may decide that there should be a systematic data collection. When you are evaluating data and presenting the results, the realistic and plausible approach is to focus on group averages to determine the success of a treatment, as the majority of clinical outcome studies have done. One problem with reliance on group averages is that it does not let us ask this question: For whom was the treatment effective? Thus, for example, if we

TABLE 33.5. Major Outcome Domains for Pain Treatment: Example for Fibromyalgia Syndrome (FMS)

Domains	Examples	Measurement tools, examples
Symptoms	• Pain severity	NRS; WHYMPI (Pain Severity scale)
	• Tender points	Mean tender point pain severity
	• Fatigue	NRS (0–100)
	• Sleep	NRS (0–100)
	• Satisfaction rating	NRS (0–100); PSST(McCracken et al., 1997)
Patient satisfaction		
	• Fibromyalgia Impact Questionnaire (FIQ)	Standardized questionnaire
QOL		
	• Activities	Standardized questionnaire (WHYMPI Activity scales)
Functional activities		
	• Self-report/records/claims adjuster	Yes–no
RTW		
	• Medication use	Quantity and cost (% reduction)
Health care utilization	• Surgical intervention	Number and cost
	• Medical intervention	Number and cost
	• Nonmedical intervention	Number and cost
	• Hospitalization for pain	Number and cost
	• Unscheduled pain-related physician visits	Self-report or review of records
	• Verbal questioning	Yes–no and amount
Disability compensation		

Note. NRS, Numerical Rating Scale.

determine that treatment X leads to a statistically significant reduction in health care utilization, we cannot determine whether there are patients with certain characteristics who were most likely to benefit. This is important information, as the most favorable cost-benefit ratio would derive from being able to predict the characteristics of patients who have the greatest probability of benefiting from treatment.

Consider the case of spinal cord stimulation. We noted earlier that about 25% of patients who have spinal cord stimulators implanted return to work. Several physical criteria are used by surgeons and anesthesiologists to determine whether a patient is a good candidate for implantation of a stimulator. A number of insurance companies are cognizant of this issue and require presurgical psychological screening prior to implantation in an attempt to increase the positive outcomes. If RTW is an important outcome criterion, we would like to know the characteristics of those patients who do return to work following implantation. As predictive variables are identified for positive outcomes, we will be better able to prescribe treatments for those with the greatest possibility of a positive

result. We will also be able to make use of these predictive data to design treatments that meet relevant patient characteristics (physical, psychosocial, and behavioral), rather than providing the same treatment to all patients with the same diagnosis. This is especially an issue with chronic pain, as so many of the most common diagnoses (e.g., chronic low back pain, FMS, temporomandibular disorders, chronic headache, pelvic pain) are likely to consist of heterogeneous groups of patients (Turk, 1990).

CONCLUDING COMMENTS

Make no mistake about it: The survival of pain medicine will not be possible without our knowing the effects of what we do *and* effectively communicating them to nonclinical, business-minded professionals. In this chapter, we have provided a pragmatic introduction to treatment evaluation that can provide you with data to demonstrate effectiveness and viability of your practice. Assessments of outcomes (i.e., did a treatment work?) and process (i.e., how well did it do?) need to be included in such evaluations.

Patient name:
Clinic ID:
Diagnosis: Fibromyalgia syndrome

Interventions	Pre-tx. (date)	Post-tx. (date)	Follow-up 1 (date)	Follow-up 2 (date)
Pain: NRS (0–100)				
Tender points (mean severity = 0–180)				
Fatigue: NRS (0–100)				
Tx. credibility: VAS (0–10)				
Service satisfaction: NRS (0–100) or PSST				
FIQ score				
MPI scale scores (list all)				
Working (yes–no)				
Analgesic use costs ($ per month)				
Medical costs ($ per month)				
Alternative tx. costs ($ per month)				
Disability (yes–no)				
Compliance impression: VAS (0–10)				

Notes:

FIGURE 33.1. Example of data collection template for patients with FMS. NRS, Numerical Rating Scale.

There are two types of outcome evaluations. The terms *efficacy* and *effectiveness* are often mixed in our literature with no clear distinction. Strictly speaking, we test efficacy if we want to know whether a treatment has any "true" effects beyond nonspecific effects. Thus the controlling extraneous variables become extremely important in effi-cacy studies to tease apart treatment effect and nonspecific effects with rigorously refined methodology (e.g., double-blind conditions, placebo control). The testing of hypotheses underlying the study should be based upon the mechanisms of intervention upon symptoms. On the other hand, effectiveness study should address whether the treatment works in a realistic environment. In the regular clinical settings, the goal is not to find out whether mechanism-based manipulation ("treatment") has effects, but to evaluate whether a given treatment improves the condition for *any* reasons. These are two separate questions. Some treatments may be efficacious but ineffective; other treatments may be nonefficacious but effective.

Systematic reviews (e.g., the Cochrane Collaboration) have been introduced as a premier vehicle for presenting clinical data. These reviews depend largely upon efficacy studies for their evidence. What is needed as a next step is testing efficacious treatments in actual clinical settings. The accumulation of effectiveness data should serve as critical feedback to these reviews, to allow investigators to determine the feasibility and actual clinical impact of innovations in pain medicine.

We have also discussed the two major components of outcome assessment: patient-focused clinical data and socioeconomic data. The diverse areas that need to be covered in evaluation of pain treatment reflect the multidimensional nature of pain. Our recommendations in this chapter may be considered as a bare minimum for outcome studies. However, we believe that more pervasive efforts at data collection within the clinical arena are critical to the survival of pain medicine, and thus that practical solutions are needed. We hope that this chapter will serve as a guide to setting up a systematic outcome evaluation protocol. Such efforts will help reduce the research–practice gap and the adversarial provider–payer gap currently experienced in pain medicine.

ACKNOWLEDGMENTS

Preparation of this chapter was supported in part by Research Grant No. R21 AR46077 from the National Institute of Arthritis and Musculoskeletal and Skin Diseases to Akiko Okifuji, and by Research Grants No. R01 AR44724 from the National Institute of Arthritis and Musculoskeletal and Skin Diseases and No. P01 HD33989 from the National Institute of Child Health and Human Development to Dennis C. Turk.

REFERENCES

Affleck, G., Tennen, H., Keefe, F. J., Lefebvre, J. C., Kashikar-Zuck, S., Wright, K., Starr, K., & Caldwell, D. S. (1999). Everyday life with osteoarthritis or rheu-

matoid arthritis: Independent effects of disease and gender on daily pain, mood, and coping. *Pain, 83,* 601–609.

American Pain Society Commission on Quality Assurance Standards. (1991). American Pain Society quality assurance standards for relief of acute pain and cancer pain. In M. Bond, J. Charlton, & C. Woolf (Eds.), *Proceedings of the VIth World Congress on Pain* (pp. 185–189). Amsterdam: Elsevier.

Beck, A. T., Ward, C. H., Mendelson, M., Mock, J., & Erbaugh, J. (1961). An inventory for measuring depression, *Archives of General Psychiatry, 4,* 561–571.

Bell, G. K., Kidd, D., & North, R. B. (1997). Cost-effectiveness analysis of spinal cord stimulation in treatment of failed back surgery syndrome. *Journal of Pain and Symptom Management, 13,* 286–295.

Bigos, S., Bowyer. O., Braen, G., Brown, K., Deyo, R., Haldeman, S., Hart, J., Johnson, E., Keller, R., Kido, D., Liang, M., Nelson, R., Nordin, M., Owen, B., Pope, M., Schwartz, R., Stewart, D., Susman, J., Triano, J., Trip, L., Turk, D., Watts, C., & Weinstein, J. (1994). *Acute low back problems in adults. Clinical Practical Guidelines No. 14* (AHCPR Publication No. 95-0642). Rockville, MD: Agency for Health Care Policy and Research, Public Health Service, U.S. Department of Health and Human Services.

Bombardier, C. H., & Buchwald, D. (1996). Chronic fatigue, chronic fatigue syndrome, and fibromyalgia: Disability and health-care use. *Medical Care, 34,* 924–930.

Bruera, E., Belzile, M., Neumann, C. M., Ford, I., Harsanyi, Z., & Darke, A. (1999). Twice-daily versus once-daily morphine sulphate controlled-release suppositories for the treatment of cancer pain: A randomized controlled trial. *Supportive Care in Cancer, 7,* 280–283.

Budzynski, T. H., Stoyva, J. M., Adler, C. S., & Mullaney, D. J. (1973). EMG biofeedback and tension headache: A controlled outcome study. *Psychosomatic Medicine, 35,* 484–496.

Burckhardt, C. S., Clark, S. R., & Bennett, R. M. (1991). The Fibromyalgia Impact Questionnaire: Development and validation. *Journal of Rheumatology, 18,* 728–733.

Burckhardt, C. S., Clark, S. R., & Bennett, R. M. (1993). Fibromyalgia and quality of life: A comparative analysis. *Journal of Rheumatology, 20,* 475–479.

Cassisi, J., Sypert, G., Salamon, A., & Kapel, L. (1989). Independent evaluation of a multidisciplinary rehabilitation program for chronic low back pain. *Neurosurgery, 25,* 877–883.

Caudill, M., Schnable, R., Zuttermeister, P., Benson, H., & Friedman, R. (1991). Decreased clinic use by chronic pain patients: Response to behavioral medicine intervention. *Clinical Journal of Pain, 7,* 305–310.

Chapman, S. L., Jamison, R. N., & Sanders, S. H. (1996). Treatment Helpfulness Questionnaire: A measure of patient satisfaction with treatment modalities provided in chronic pain management programs. *Pain, 68,* 349–361.

Charlton, B. G. (1995). Evidence based medicine: Megatrials are subordinate to medical science. *British Medical Journal, 311,* 257; discussion, 259.

Commission on Accreditation of Rehabilitation Facilities. (1995). *Standard manual for organizations serving people with disabilities.* Tucson, AZ: Author.

Crombie, I. K., & Davies, H. T. (1998). Beyond health outcomes: The advantages of measuring process. *Journal of Evaluation in Clinical Practice, 4,* 31–38.

Cutler, R. B., Fishbain, D. A., Rosomoff, H. L., Abdel-Moty, E., Khalil, T. M., & Rosomoff, R. S. (1994). Does nonsurgical pain center treatment of chronic pain return patients to work?: A review and meta-analysis of the literature. *Spine, 19,* 643–652.

Deathe, A. B., & Helmes, E. (1993). Evaluation of a chronic pain programme by referring physicians. *Pain, 52,* 113–121.

Deyo, R. A. (1988). Measuring the functional status of patients with low back pain. *Archives of Physical Medicine and Rehabilitation, 69,* 1044–1053.

Deyo, R. A., Battie, M., Beurskens, A. J., Bombardier, C., Croft, P., Koes, B., Malmivaara, A., Roland, M., Von Korff, M., & Waddell, G. (1998). Outcome measures for low back pain research. A proposal for standardized use. *Spine, 23,* 2003–2013. (Published erratum appears in *Spine,* 1999, *24,* 418.)

Dworkin. R. H., Handlin, D. S., Richlin, D. M., Brand, L., & Vannucci, C. (1985). Unraveling the effects of compensation, litigation and employment on treatment response in chronic pain. *Pain, 23,* 49–49.

Fairbank, J. C. T., Couper, J., Davies, J. B., & O'Brien, J. P. (1980). The Oswestry Low-Back Pain Disability Questionnaire. *Physiotherapy, 66,* 271–273.

Feinstein, A. R. (1983). An additional basic science for clinical medicine: IV. The development of clinimetrics. *Annals of Internal Medicine, 99,* 843–848.

Feinstein, A. R., & Horwitz, R. I. (1997). Problems in the "evidence" of "evidence-based medicine." *American Journal of Medicine, 103,* 529–535.

Feuerstein, M., Menz, L., Zastowny, T., & Baron, B. (1994). Chronic back pain and work disability: Vocational outcomes following multidisciplinary rehabilitation. *Journal of Occupational Rehabilitation, 4,* 229–252.

Fishbain, D. A., Cutler, R. B., Rosomoff, H. L., Khalil, T., & Steele-Rosomoff, R. (1999). Prediction of "intent," "discrepancy with intent," and "discrepancy with nonintent" for the patient with chronic pain to return to work after treatment at a pain facility. *Clinical Journal of Pain, 15,* 141–150.

Flor, H., Fydrich, T., & Turk, D. C. (1992). Efficacy of multidisciplinary pain treatment centers: A meta-analytic review. *Pain, 49,* 221–230.

Frymoyer, J. W. (1990). Magnitude of the problem. In J. M. Weinstein & S. W. Wiesel (Eds.), *The lumbar spine* (pp. 1–14). Philadelphia: Saunders.

Frymoyer, J. W., & Durett, C. (1997). The economics of spinal disorders. In J. W. Frymoyer (Ed.), *The adult spine* (2nd ed., pp. 143–150). Philadelphia: Lippincott-Raven.

Gallon, R. (1989). Perception of disability in chronic back pain patients: A long-term follow-up. *Pain, 37,* 67–75.

Gillies, A. (1997). *Improving the quality of patient care.* Chichester, England: Wiley.

Guck, T. P., Skultety, F. M., Meilman, P. W., & Dowd, E. T. (1985). Multidisciplinary pain center follow-up study: Evaluation with a no-treatment control group. *Pain, 21,* 295–306.

Jacobson, N. S., Follette, W. C., Revenstorf, D., Baucom, D. H., Hahlweg, K., & Margolin, G. (1984). Variability in outcome and clinical significance of behavioral marital therapy: A reanalysis of outcome data. *Journal of Consulting and Clinical Psychology, 52,* 497–504.

Kerns, R. D., Turk, D. C., & Rudy, T. E. (1985). The West Haven–Yale Multidimensional Pain Inventory (WHYMPI). *Pain, 23,* 345–356.

Kjaersgaard-Andersen, P., Nafei, A., Skov, O., Madsen, F., Andersen, H. M., Kroner, K., Hvass, I., Gjoderum, O., Pedersen, L., & Branebjerg, P. E. (1990). Codeine plus paracetamol versus paracetamol in longer-term treatment of chronic pain due to osteoarthritis of the hip: A randomised, double-blind, multi-centre study. *Pain, 43,* 309–318.

Kupers, R., Van den Oever, R., Van Houdenhove, B., Van Houdenhove, B., Van Mechelen, W., Hepp, B., Nuttin, B., & Gybels, J. (1996). Spinal cord stimulation in Belgium: A nationwide survey on the incidence, indications and therapeutic efficacy by the health insurer. *Pain, 56,* 211–217.

Lehmann, T. R., Spratt, K. F., Tozzi, J. E., Weinstein, J. N., Reinarz, S. J., el-Khoury, G. Y., & Colby, H. (1987). Long-term follow-up of lower lumbar fusion patients. *Spine, 12,* 97–104.

Linn, M. W., Linn, B. S., & Stein, S. R. (1982). Satisfaction with ambulatory care and compliance in older patients. *Medical Care, 20,* 606–614.

Long, D. M., Filtzer, D. L., Ben Debba, M., & Hendler, N. M. (1988). Clinical features of the failed-back syndrome. *Journal of Neurosurgery, 69,* 61–71.

Louis Harris and Associates. (1996). *Pain and absenteeism in the workplace: A study of full-time employees and employee benefit managers.* New York: Author.

Marketdata Enterprises (1995). *Chronic pain management programs: A market analysis.* Valley Stream, NY: Author.

Marketdata Enterprises. (1999). *Pain management programs: A market analysis.* Tampa, FL: Author.

Miaskowski, C. (in press). Factors that influence patient satisfaction with pain management. *Pain Reviews.*

McCracken, L. M., Klock, P. A., Mingay, D. J., Asbury, J. K., & Sinclair, D. M. (1997). Assessment of satisfaction with treatment for chronic pain. *Journal of Pain and Symptom Management, 14,* 292–299.

Meenan, R. F., Gertman, P. M., & Mason, J. H. (1980). Measuring health status in arthritis: The Arthritis Impact Measurement Scales. *Arthritis and Rheumatism, 25,* 146–152.

Melzack, R. (1987). The short-form McGill Pain Questionnaire. *Pain, 30,* 191–197.

Nguyen, T. D., Attkisson, C. C., & Stegner, B. L. (1983). Assessment of patient satisfaction: Development and refinement of a service evaluation questionnaire. *Evaluation and Program Planning, 6,* 299–313.

North, R. B., Campbell, J. N., James, C. S., Conover-Walker, M. K., Wang, H., Piantadosi, S., Rybock, J. D., & Long, D. M. (1991). Failed back surgery syndrome: 5-year follow-up in 102 patients undergoing repeated operation. *Neurosurgery, 28,* 685–690.

North, R. B., Ewend, M. G., Lawton, M. T., Kidd, D. H., & Piantadosi, S. (1991). Failed back surgery syndrome: 5-year follow-up after spinal cord stimulator implantation. *Neurosurgery, 28,* 692–699.

Okifuji, A., Turk, D. C., Sinclair, J. D., Starz, T. W., & Marcus, D. A. (1997). A standardized manual tender point survey: I. Development and determination of a threshold point for the identification of positive tender points in fibromyalgia syndrome. *Journal of Rheumatology, 24,* 377–383.

Pekarik, G., & Wolff, C.B. (1996). Relationship of satisfaction to symptom change, follow-up adjustment, and clinical significance. *Professional Psychology: Research and Practice, 27,* 202–208.

Peters, J., Large, R. G., & Elkind, G. (1992). Follow-up results from a randomised controlled trial evaluating in- and outpatient pain management programmes. *Pain, 50,* 41–50.

Piotrowski, C. (1997). Assessment of pain: A survey of practicing clinicians. *Perceptual and Motor Skills, 86,* 181–182.

Pollard, C. A. (1984). Preliminary validity study of the Pain Disability Index. *Perceptual and Motor Skills, 59,* 974.

Portenoy, R. K. (1996). Opioid therapy for chronic non-malignant pain: A review of the critical issues. *Journal of Pain and Symptom Management, 11,* 203–217.

Radloff, L. S. (1977). The CES-D scale: A self-report depression scale for research in general populations. *Applied Psychological Measurement, 1,* 385–401.

Romano, J. M., & Turner, J. A. (1985). Chronic pain and depression: Does the evidence support a relationship? *Psychological Bulletin, 97,* 18–34.

Rowe, M. K., & Craske, M. G. (1998). Effects of an expanding-spaced vs. massed exposure schedule on fear reduction and return of fear. *Behaviour Research and Therapy, 36,* 701–717.

Ruta, D. A., Garratt, A. M., Leng, M., Russell, I. T., & MacDonald, L. M. (1994). A new approach to the measurement of quality of life. The Patient-Generated Index. *Medical Care, 32,* 1109–1126.

Sackett, D. L., Rosenberg, W. M., Gray, J. A., Haynes, R. B., & Richardson, W. S. (1996). Evidence based medicine: What it is and what it isn't. *British Medical Journal, 312,* 71–72.

Salovey, P., Seiber, W. J., Smith, A. F., Turk, D. C., Jobe, J. B., & Willis, G. B. (1992). *Reporting chronic pain episodes on health surveys* (Vital and Health Statistics: Series 6. Cognitive and Survey Measurement, No. 6). Washington, DC: U.S. Government Printing Office.

Schwartz, D., & Lellouch, J. (1967). Explanatory and pragmatic attitudes in therapeutical trials. *Journal of Chronic Disease, 20,* 637–648.

Sigurdardottir, V., Brandberg, Y., & Sullivan, M. (1996). Criterion-based validation of the EORTC QLQ-C36 in advanced melanoma: The CIPS questionnaire and proxy raters. *Quality of Life Research, 5,* 375–386.

Simmons, J., Avant, W., Demski, J., & Parisher, D. (1988). Determining successful pain clinic treatment through validation of cost effectiveness. *Spine, 13,* 24–34.

Smith, B. H. (1995). Evidence based medicine. Quality cannot always be quantified [Letter; comment]. *British Medical Journal, 311,* 258.

Stone, A. A., Broderick, J. E., Porter, L. S., & Kaell, A. T. (1997). The experience of rheumatoid arthritis pain and fatigue: Examining momentary reports and correlates over one week. *Arthritis Care and Research, 10,* 185–193.

Turk, D. C. (1990). Customizing treatment for chronic pain patients: Who, what, and why. *Clinical Journal of Pain, 6,* 255–270.

Turk, D. C. (1996). Clinicians' attitudes about prolonged use of opioids and the issue of patient heterogeneity. *Journal of Pain and Symptom Management, 11,* 218–230.

Turk, D. C., & Okifuji, A. (1998). Efficacy of multidisciplinary pain centers: An antidote to anecdotes. *Ballière's Clinical Anesthesiology: International Practice and Research, 12,* 103–120.

Turk, D. C., Okifuji, A., Sinclair, J. D., & Starz, T. W. (1996). Pain, disability, and physical functioning in subgroups of patients with fibromyalgia. *Journal of Rheumatology, 23,* 1255–1262.

Waddell, G. (1987). A new clinical model for the treatment of low-back pain. *Spine, 12,* 632–644.

Ware, J. E., Jr., & Sherbourne, C. D. (1992). The MOS 36-Item Short-Form Health Survey (SF-36). I. Conceptual framework and item selection. *Medical Care, 30,* 473–483.

Ware, J. E., Jr., Snyder, M. K., Wright, W. R., & Davies, A. R. (1983). Defining and measuring patient satisfaction with medical care. *Evaluation and Program Planning, 6,* 247–263.

Wigers, S. H., Stiles, T. C., & Vogel, P. A. (1996). Effects of aerobic exercise versus stress management treatment in fibromyalgia: A 4.5 year prospective study. *Scandinavian Journal of Rheumatology, 25,* 77–86.

Wolfe, F., Smythe, H. A., Yunus, M. B., Bennett, R. M., Bombardier, C., Goldenberg, D. L., Tugwell, P., Campbell, S. M., Abeles, M., Clark, P., Fam, A. G., Farber, S. J., Fiechtner, J. J., Franklin, C. M., Gatter, R. A., Hamatin, D., Lessard, J., Lichtbroun, A. S., Masi, A. T., McCain, G. A., Reynolds, W. J., Romano, T. J., Russell, I. J., & Sheon, R. P. (1990). The American College of Rheumatology 1990 Criteria for the Classification of Fibromyalgia. Report of the Multicenter Criteria Committee. *Arthritis and Rheumatism, 33,* 160–172.

Zenz, M., Strumpf, M., & Tryba, M. (1992). Long-term oral opioid therapy in patients with chronic non-malignant pain. *Journal of Pain and Symptom Management, 7,* 69–77.

Chapter 34

Assessment of Pain and Pain-Related Quality of Life in Clinical Trials

ROBERT H. DWORKIN
ELNA M. NAGASAKO
RODERICK D. HETZEL
JOHN T. FARRAR

In a classic text, Pocock (1984) has defined a clinical trial as "any form of *planned experiment* which involves patients and is designed to elucidate the most appropriate treatment of future patients with a given medical condition. Perhaps the essential characteristic of a clinical trial is that one uses results based on a limited *sample* of patients to make inferences about how treatment should be conducted in the general *population* of patients who will require treatment in the future" (p. 1; original emphasis). With respect to this definition, the "medical conditions" that we examine include not only painful conditions, but also any disorder in which pain is one of the symptoms being assessed. Clinical trials that include pain and related symptoms as outcomes require reliable, responsive, and valid measures of these purely subjective phenomena. In discussing clinical trials of the efficacy and effectiveness of pain therapies, we consider drugs and also psychological interventions, nerve blocks, surgery, physical therapy, acupuncture, or any other procedure that can be used to treat pain or a condition in which pain is an important symptom. Indeed, the same issues are applicable to clinical trials of combination treatments as well, whether the treatments are of the same type (e.g., two drugs) or of different types (e.g., nerve blocks and physical therapy).

We begin by reviewing the types of clinical trials and research designs that are most commonly used. Next, we discuss the different components of a comprehensive pain assessment, emphasizing those aspects that are especially relevant in clinical trials. Issues specific to data capture and the specifics of when and how to conduct pain assessments are considered. Finally, we discuss the analysis and interpretation of pain data in a clinical trial, again emphasizing issues that are especially relevant in the assessment of pain.

GENERAL ISSUES

The Goal of the Clinical Trial

The first issue that must be considered in assessing pain in a clinical trial is to identify the goal of the trial—specifically, the question (or questions) about a treatment or a medical condition that the trial is intended to answer. Max (1991, 1994a) has emphasized the importance of distinguishing between *pragmatic* and *explanatory* clinical trials (Schwartz & Lellouch, 1967). Pragmatic clinical trials have the goal of answering practical questions about patient care. For example, do sympathetic nerve blocks relieve pain in patients with complex regional pain syndrome (CRPS)? These trials are typically designed to reflect clinical practice to the greatest extent possible, and decisions about various features of the trial are guided by the clinical situation that the results of the trial are intended to inform. Such decisions include the treatment, its dosage and length, inclusion and exclusion criteria for patients, types of control or comparison groups, methods used for assessing outcome, and data analysis and its interpretation. The selection criteria for a pragmatic trial should closely reflect the range of patients actually seen in clinical practice; the treatment parameters should be those that are clinically realistic; and the benefit should be large enough to be considered clinically important.

The goal of an explanatory clinical trial is to answer a question about the etiology of a disease, the mode of action of a treatment, or both. The methodological features of an explanatory trial are selected to maximize the likelihood that the trial will answer a specific question about the mechanisms of disease or treatment and without regard to the realities of the clinical situation. Therefore, the inclusion criteria are likely to be more restrictive so that the sample of patients is relatively homogeneous, and the parameters of treatment may be more tightly controlled and demanding.

With respect to the assessment of pain, a pragmatic trial typically emphasizes the beneficial effects of the treatment on patients with the condition being studied. Such trials are therefore more likely to include ratings by patients of their satisfaction, treatment preference, and global improvement. Psychological distress and quality of life are also typically assessed, reflecting the multidimensional nature of pain and its diverse impacts. The assessment of pain in explanatory trials is more likely to include laboratory-based outcomes, such as the impact of treatment on quantitative sensory testing or the relationships between pain relief and drug plasma concentrations. Such treatment effects may be of less clinical importance.

Of course, answering a question about the efficacy of a treatment and answering a question about the mechanism of its action are not mutually exclusive. However, these two different goals generally require different outcome measures. Studies with both goals must be carefully planned to ensure that the two competing outcomes do not interfere with each other. Most clinical trials funded by government or private foundations have explanatory goals, which are frequently also accompanied by pragmatic goals. Industry funds mostly prag-

matic studies, with the primary intention of ultimately submitting the data collected on safety and efficacy to a regulatory agency.

Types of Clinical Trials

Clinical trials of new treatments can be further divided with respect to the different phases of research. These phases are most often used in considering studies designed to meet requirements for regulatory approval. Before being approved for human use, new potential analgesic drugs are studied in animals for safety, efficacy, and toxicity. *Phase I* studies are the first to involve humans. Usually conducted in small numbers of typically healthy volunteers, these studies are designed to provide preliminary information on drug safety, pharmacokinetics, and acceptable dosage range but typically do not examine efficacy.

If the drug is found to be safe and adequately tolerated in Phase I studies, *Phase II* trials are conducted to explore the dosage that can be tolerated, typically in a relatively small number of patients with the disease of interest (e.g., 30–125 patients). Although these studies are often done without a control group, and outcomes again focus on issues of safety and pharmacokinetics, measures are frequently included that will provide initial efficacy data. In an open trial, in which both patients and investigators are aware that the patients are receiving a new treatment, the *absence* of a treatment effect makes it quite unlikely that the treatment will demonstrate efficacy in a double-blind, placebo-controlled trial (unless the sample of patients studied is refractory or unrepresentative; Quitkin, 1999). Because the experiences of pain and pain relief are subjective, and because of the importance of placebo effects in pain treatment response (Turner, Deyo, Loeser, Von Korff, & Fordyce, 1994), the presence of a treatment effect in an uncontrolled trial is not conclusive. Instead, it provides a basis for conducting a randomized double-blind study in which efficacy is evaluated more rigorously. Although Phase II clinical trials may be conducted at a single site, they are more often conducted at a relatively small number of different sites.

Phase III clinical trials are conducted if the results of Phase II studies demonstrate that the new treatment is relatively safe and possibly efficacious in patients, and has a tolerable level of side effects. These are large studies involving a substantial number of patients (often 200 or more from multiple centers). Ideally, the new treatment is compared both with a placebo and with an established treatment, but most often one or the other of these approaches is chosen. The purpose is to demonstrate that the investigational treatment has a greater efficacy than placebo or is equivalent to a known treatment, but with a better side effect profile. Safety and tolerability of the treatment continue to be carefully evaluated. Phase III trials must be methodologically rigorous. These trials should be randomized and controlled, are usually conducted on a double-blind basis, and are often independently monitored to confirm adherence to the protocol and validity of the data collection. The number of subjects required will depend mostly on the normal variation of the primary outcome measure in the untreated population and the size of the clinical effect that is to be tested. Although small clinical effects may be of interest in drug development and in consideration of adjuvant therapies, most trials should be designed to detect an effect that will be of clinical importance to the target population.

Phase III trials require substantial resources because of the number of patients studied, and great attention must be paid to ensuring adequate statistical power—that is, a large enough number of patients—to demonstrate that the results are statistically significant (typically defined as the results not being likely to occur by chance more than 1 time out of 20). It is important to remember that statistical significance is necessary but not sufficient to demonstrate a meaningful outcome from a clinical trial. Even the smallest and most insignificant of clinical effect sizes can be shown to be statistically significant if the sample size is large enough. To be clinically useful, a Phase III trial must show both statistical significance and an effect size large enough to be clinically important. In the United States, Phase III trials are the "pivotal" clinical trials that are required for Food and Drug Administration (FDA) approval of a new treatment or a new indication for an old treatment. Ideally, all potential uses for a specific treatment will undergo the rigors of a large, randomized, double-blind, controlled clinical trial. Unfortunately, this is often not the case.

Phase IV clinical trials are conducted after approval of a drug is obtained and are generally targeted at determining long-term safety. Although it can take longer, it is possible for a new drug to be approved for use after a 3- to 5-year period of being tested in fewer than 1,000 people who have generally been carefully screened not to have serious contraindications to the use of the treatment. As such, even fatal side effects that occur in less than 1 out of 100 patients or that take longer than 5 years to develop cannot be detected during the initial testing phase. Interactions between the new treatment and the large number of other therapies that many sicker patients will use in combination with it will also not be known from the initial evaluation. Therefore, careful long-term monitoring is vital to protect the safety of the general population. The term *Phase IV* is sometimes also used to refer to studies of the new treatment in other diseases or in different patient populations (e.g., a trial to examine the efficacy of an antiepileptic drug in patients with radicular low back pain). To provide meaningful results, such studies should ideally be designed as Phase III primary efficacy trials. Sometimes a number of smaller, underpowered studies can be combined via the statistical techniques of meta-analysis to provide more accurate information. However, in order to be valid, the outcomes of each study must be comparable, which is often difficult or impossible. Phase IV trials can be conducted either by industry or by independent investigators.

Types of Pain and Types of Patients

Pain can be either a *primary endpoint*, as in a clinical trial of a pain therapy, or a *secondary endpoint*. As a secondary endpoint, pain can be a side effect of a primary therapy (e.g., postoperative pain, toxic neuropathy from chemotherapy) or a beneficial outcome of a therapy that is disease-modifying (e.g., multiple sclerosis pain following interferon treatment). Pain is often categorized in many different ways, some of which are more useful than others. An important primary distinction is between *acute* and *chronic* pain. Acute pain refers to conditions such as postoperative pain or short-lived pain associated with various diseases (e.g., acute herpes zoster) and injuries (e.g., limb fracture). It is a ubiquitous experience, simple in concept and easier to diagnose than chronic pain, with treatments that are generally effective and a course that is well-defined and usually relatively short.

Although clearly related to acute pain, chronic pain has become accepted as a distinct phenomenon over the past 30 years (Sternbach, 1974). Chronic pain is conventionally defined as pain that persists beyond the normal time of healing (Merskey & Bogduk, 1994). Pain can also be considered chronic at the point when the individual realizes that the pain will be a persistent part of his or her life for the foreseeable future. With chronic pain, there is generally no consistently effective therapy for the underlying disease process, no clearly effective long-term therapy, and a much more complex interplay between the physiological inputs of the painful process (nociception) and the central processes that shape an individual's perception and response to that input. Important factors are the individual's mood, coping mechanisms, memories and expectations, and level of function. Although these factors can also influence a patient's response to acute pain, the extended period of exposure in the chronic situation often leads to important changes in these factors over time, which must be carefully considered in any clinical trial of chronic pain. Chronic pain can also be divided into recurrent acute pain (such as migraine headaches, pain from kidney stones, or sickle cell crises), which can come and go over a lifetime; persistent pain that is related to an underlying disease such as rheumatoid arthritis or cancer; and chronic pain syndromes where the underlying process is not as well understood, such as failed back surgery syndrome or chronic nerve injury pain.

Another major classification is based on the presumed etiology of the pain—namely, *nociceptive somatic* pain versus *neuropathic* pain. Somatic pain is related to stimulation of specialized nociceptors in somatic tissue. It is the type of pain experienced by all animals and is often described as throbbing, aching, or pressure. Neuropathic pain is defined as pain that is related to aberrant somatosensory processing in the peripheral or central nervous system. It is usually a consequence of damage to pain nerve fibers themselves or to central nervous system control mechanisms. It is often described as a burning, shooting, dysesthetic pain, with a quality that the patient finds unfamiliar. *Visceral* pain is often classified separately, because it is a teleologically older system and the nerve fibers run with the autonomic nervous system innervation of the internal organs. However, there are specialized nerve endings (somatic pain), and these nerve fibers can also be directly damaged (neuropathic pain) as a result of disease, physical trauma, or nerve entrapment. Visceral pain is often described as a poorly localized, diffuse, or crampy pain.

These definitions of types of pain suggest a pathophysiology, and therefore a possible focus for treatment and the measurement of appropriate outcomes. However, given the nature of most chronic human diseases, it is often very difficult to be sure of the exact type of pain a patient is experiencing (Portenoy, 1991). Most chronically ill patients have a pain syndrome with both somatic and neuropathic components. Of course, an attempt should be made to classify these painful diseases or pain syndromes with respect to as many of these distinctions as are applicable. For example, low back pain that is chronic, nonmalignant, and non-neuropathic will be treated quite differently from back pain that results from metastatic disease compressing nervous system tissue.

In selecting the patients with pain who are to be included in a clinical trial, investigators often carefully specify the type of pain and pain syndrome, so as not to dilute or confuse the outcome of the trial and to ensure that the measurement tools are appropriate. In addition, they must pay attention to the impact of specifying other features of the pain. For many studies, the duration and intensity of the pain (worst, least, or average) are important components of the inclusion criteria. Although a minimum level of pain intensity at baseline is required in order to have the ability to demonstrate an improvement, specifying too high a level will increase the effect of regression to the mean (Meinert & Tonascia, 1986). To focus the study or to eliminate patients who may have an increased risk from the study, investigators in clinical trials often restrict enrollment based on other characteristics, including age, sex, language, other medical conditions, previous treatments or treatment response, concomitant treatments, known allergies, history of psychiatric disorders, alcohol or drug abuse, and (in women) pregnancy and the ability to conceive. Although restricting the study population is often appropriate, the effect is to reduce the generalizability of the results.

Research Design Issues

Various research designs are relevant to clinical trials of treatments for pain. In addition, specific methodological issues must be considered. Max, Portenoy, and Laska (1991) and McQuay and Moore (1998) review much of this material and provide excellent resources for anyone undertaking a clinical trial in which pain is either a primary or a secondary endpoint. General discussions of the design and analysis of clinical trials are provided by Pocock (1984), Piantadosi (1997), and Chow and Liu (1998). Ginsburg (1999) presents a useful introduction to the practical aspects of conducting industry-sponsored clinical trials. Kraemer (1992) reviews methods for evaluating medical tests and discusses a variety of sophisticated assessment issues, many of which have seldom been addressed in the assessment of pain. Senn (1997) discusses statistical issues in the design and analysis of clinical trials, and in a separate volume focuses on the particular statistical issues raised by trials using a crossover design (Senn, 1993). Finally, Begg and colleagues (1996) present a checklist and flow diagram of the information regarding research design, methods and procedures, data analysis, and generalizability that should be included in reports of clinical trials. These can be used not only when one is publishing the results of a trial, but also when one is designing a clinical trial to ensure that adequate attention will be given to documenting the manner in which the trial is actually conducted (as well as when one is evaluating the published report of a trial).

It is beyond the scope of this chapter to comprehensively discuss the often complex issues raised by the various clinical trial research designs. In general, there is a consensus that the randomized, double-blind, placebo-controlled clinical trial is the "gold standard" for evaluating the efficacy of a pain therapy. Given the ethical issues related to treating patients with pain, the placebo group is sometimes replaced with a comparison treatment group. In such a trial, patients are randomly assigned to receive either the treatment that is being investigated or the control treatment. Successful randomization of a large enough group of patients will control for all the baseline factors, both known and unknown, resulting in groups that are identical except for the study treatment.

The most rigorous studies employ a parallel-group design in which patients are assigned to only one treatment group. In situations where the treatment effect has a relatively short and predictable pharmacokinetic and biological half-life, and the disease remains constant, a crossover design can be used in which patients are first administered one treatment, followed by a washout period and then the second treatment. Open-label studies, in which patients receive treatments that are known to them as well as to the investigator, can be useful in suggesting potentially beneficial treatments and in monitoring for long-term side effects. However, they are never definitive in demonstrating the true efficacy or side effect rate. Studies can be designed specifically to examine the effects of a single dose of the treatment (including nonpharmacological treatments such as acupuncture), or to evaluate long-term effects on patients receiving multiple doses or sessions of the treatment.

In the evaluation of most investigational analgesic drugs, the design currently favored by the FDA is the randomized, double-blind, parallel-group, placebo-controlled trial. "Blinding" is of prime importance; typically, the placebo in a drug study is inert but should appear identical to the investigational drug in color, shape, size, taste, and even odor. Many of the drugs that provide pain relief have noticeable side effects, such as sedation, in a substantial proportion of patients. It has been suggested that trials investigating such drugs cannot be truly double-blind, because the patient, the investigator, or both often become aware that the patient is receiving the active treatment as a result of side effects. One solution to this concern is to use an "active placebo" that has no analgesic activity but that matches, as closely as possible, the side effect profile of the investigational treatment. For example, in trials of tricyclic antidepressants in the treatment of chronic pain, drugs that cause sedation and dry mouth but that have no analgesic effects have been used as active placebos (see, e.g., Kieburtz et al., 1998; Max et al., 1987).

Ideally, the blinding should be tested by asking patients and investigators to guess which groups the patients were in. In a properly blinded study, the guess rate should be close to 50%. However, it is vital also to assess the reasons patients think they were in a particular group. If the primary reason given is that the treatment they took was effective, the guess rate would be expected to approximate the rate of efficacy. In a clinical trial of a highly effective treatment, patients' responses that they could tell which group they were in because of the beneficial effect are evidence for the efficacy of the treatment and not an indication of poor blinding. It is only when patients are able to guess their group correctly based on unrelated factors that the blinding should be questioned.

The use of active placebos in studies of analgesic and adjuvant medications can be an effective strategy for maintaining the double-blind feature of a clinical trial. This remains somewhat controversial, however. It has recently been suggested that "the available evidence does not provide a compelling case for the necessity of an active placebo" in studies of the effects of antidepressant medications (Quitkin, 1999, p. 834). Given the difficulty of identifying suitable active placebos for many analgesic trials, it is important to determine whether active placebos are also unnecessary in clinical trials of analgesic and adjuvant medications—and, if so, in which types of trials.

The problems of blinding and the credibility of control treatments are considerably more difficult in trials of nonpharmacological treatments. For example, in trials of cognitive-behavioral therapy, it is difficult to design a control condition. However, it is important to remember that the purpose of blinding and randomization is to ensure that the treatment and control groups differ only in the treatment being tested. Therefore, the selection of the control condition will depend substantially on what component or group of components of the treatment is to be studied. If the intention is to study the effect of behavioral therapy, in which such nonspecific factors as increased attention, motivation, and activity level are considered integral components of the treatment, then a no-treatment comparison group is appropriate. If the intention is to try to isolate the specific features of the behavioral therapy, then the control condition must include all of the nonspecific features of the behavioral therapy in order to be appropriate. The latter situation is generally much more difficult to accomplish. Comparison groups that have been used in clinical trials of nonpharmacological treatments include no-treatment, waiting-list, and standard-care groups. Such methods, of course, are often not double-blind, or even single-blind, which raises important issues regarding the validity and interpretation of the results.

Another strategy that is commonly used is comparison with a control condition that is expected to have a weaker effect but that is credible to both the patient and the individual administering it. For example, physical therapy for patients with low back pain may be compared with sessions of passive immersion in a warm bath that are matched in duration, number, and frequency to the physical therapy sessions. Although this is not a truly blinded comparison, some of the nonspecific effects can be mitigated by keeping both the patients and individuals administering the bath therapy unaware of the study's hypothesis, and by employing an evaluator or data collector who is scrupulously kept unaware of the patients' group assignments. A major problem is that it is possible that the control treatment could have a separate specific beneficial effect on the patients' pain, making it more difficult to demonstrate the efficacy of the study therapy. A practical implication of the selection of a partially effective therapy for the control or comparison group is that a larger sample of patients is needed, because the clinical difference to be detected is smaller than when the control group receives a placebo treatment. A much larger sample of patients is required to demonstrate that the efficacies of two active treatments are nearly equivalent. The sample size is primarily determined by the size of the difference in clinical outcome that one wants to detect.

The nature of the control condition in a randomized controlled trial can also raise difficult ethical concerns. Compared to some other areas of medicine, the ethics of using placebo controls in studies with individuals who are suffering from pain has been infrequently discussed. An obvious concern is whether it is ethical to use placebo controls in pain studies when it is hypothesized that patients receiving placebo treatment will experience more pain than those receiving the investigational treatment. Several approaches to addressing this concern have been employed. These include the use of active treatment controls that are expected to provide at least some pain relief, but that may or may not be inferior to the investigational treatment. In addition, rescue analgesics can be provided to all patients when pain relief is needed and can then be examined as one of the outcome measures. It has also been suggested that crossover designs address this concern, but the placebo period in such research designs could still be considered unethical (if rescue medication is not made available).

There is no completely satisfactory solution to the problem of placebo groups in pain research, because there is no consensus regarding the standard of care for many pain conditions. For this reason, the principle of *equipoise* (Freedman, 1987) provides only a partial guide to the ethics of placebo and other comparison groups in pain research. Equipoise exists when the balance of possible benefits and risks is equal between the groups being compared in a trial. However, this evaluation can vary depending on whether it is made from the perspective of the individual investigator, the consensus of experts who are knowledgeable about the latest advances in basic and clinical research and their possible treatment implications, the community providers who treat the vast majority of patients with pain, or the patients considering participation in the trial (Alderson, 1996; Chard & Lilford, 1998; Lilford & Jackson, 1995).

Another issue raised by clinical trials in which pain is the primary endpoint is whether the study design includes matching of treatments to particular patient characteristics (Turk, 1990; Woolf & Mannion, 1999; see also Turk & Okifugi, Chapter 21, this volume). To some extent this is a question of the inclusion and exclusion criteria, but it also raises more complicated research design issues, such as whether patients should be assigned to different treatment groups within a trial based on their neurobiological or psychological characteristics (or both). As Turk and Okifuji (1998) have suggested, clinical trials may be conducted to examine treatments "provided in a modular fashion, in which separate components are woven into an overall treatment regimen based on individual patient characteristics" (p. 10). They note that patients with back pain, for example, may all require physical therapy, but that subgroups of these patients may also require additional treatment modules, such as for psychological treatment of depression. The extent to which it is possible to match different treatments to different subgroups of patients within a single clinical trial, or whether this can only be done across a series of trials, remains unclear.

Dose–response and concentration–response relationships can be an important complication in efficacy trials. Much more is known about these relationships for some analgesics (e.g., opioids) than for others (e.g., antidepressants; Max, 1994b). Especially in chronic pain trials, individual variation in absorption, metabolism, and physiological distribution of the study medication can substantially increase the underlying variability in patients' responses, increasing the number of patients necessary to detect a significant difference. One solution is to include a titration phase, in which the dose of study medication is increased until a patient's pain is adequately controlled or until he or she experiences side effects, as is frequently done in clinical practice.

Studies of the combination of more than one treatment for pain have also received limited attention. Clinical trials of combinations of opioid analgesics with nonsteroidal anti-inflammatory drugs (NSAIDs) and related medications have been conducted for many years (Beaver, 1984; Max, 1994c), but there are few studies examining combinations of other drugs used in the treatment of pain—for example, tricyclic antidepressants and anticonvulsants (Max, 1994b). Even rarer are studies examining the benefits of combining different modes of treatments—for example, cognitive-behavioral therapy combined with a drug, compared with the drug and cognitive-behavioral therapy each administered alone. Studies using variants of this design have been a major focus of research on the treatment of psychiatric disorders (including depression, schizophrenia, and anxiety disorders) for over 20 years, and it is surprising and unfortunate that so little effort has been devoted to this type of clinical trial in research on the treatment of patients with chronic pain (see Pilowsky & Barrow, 1990, for an instructive example of such a research design in the treatment of chronic "psychogenic" pain).

In discussions of clinical trials, a distinction is often made between *efficacy* and *effectiveness* trials (see, e.g., Piantadosi, 1997), although some clinical trials combine elements of both. To this point, we have emphasized research issues that are particularly relevant to clinical trials intended to demonstrate the efficacy of a treatment for pain. Efficacy trials test the hypothesis of whether or not there are beneficial effects of treatment in a group of patients, and the methods and procedures are tightly controlled and standardized. In such studies, threats to the internal validity of the study (e.g., the integrity of the double blind or the inclusion and exclusion criteria) are minimized to the greatest extent possible, so that treatment effects or biological mechanisms can be evaluated accurately. Effectiveness trials, on the other hand, are conducted to test the value of a treatment as applied in the "real world," in which, for example, some patients do not take all the pills they are prescribed or miss some of the treatment sessions. Because of the increased baseline variability, such trials are typically larger than efficacy trials, and there is often less control of methods and procedures. In these studies, external validity and generalizability are emphasized, and the trial is designed so that conclusions about the value of the treatment as it is actually used in the population can be drawn. A simple example of this distinction would be a comparison of two NSAIDs, which are found to have equivalent efficacy in a Phase III trial but differ in their effectiveness in a large Phase IV trial in the community because one has poorer taste and larger pills, reducing the number of patients who take it consistently.

Finally, we must consider the issues of the *reliability*, *validity*, and *responsiveness* of the measures to be used in a clinical trial. Reliability and validity are covered elsewhere in this volume, but responsiveness is a specific characteristic of measurement tools that are useful in measuring change over time or between clinical states. At issue is whether or not a measurement tool is sensitive enough to detect a response when a real difference occurs. As an obvious example, a "yes" or "no" answer to the question "Do you have pain?" will be substantially less responsive than an answer indicated on a 5- or 7-point scale, since patients must be completely free of pain to change from a "yes" to a "no" answer. Responsiveness issues can be much more subtle than this, especially in complex multidimensional questionnaires, such as those used to measure quality of life (Beurskens, de Vet, & Koke, 1996; Deyo, Diehr, & Patrick, 1991).

One problem occurs because of confusion over the appropriate use of a particular measure. Instruments that discriminate between groups are not necessarily equally good at evaluating change over time in the same groups. For example, discriminating patients likely to have depression from those without depression may well depend on questions that elicit past medical history, which would not be expected to change over time, no matter how effectively a patient is treated. The reader is referred to other sources for a more complete consideration of these issues (Guyatt, Walter, & Norman, 1987; Streiner & Norman, 1995).

COMPONENTS OF A COMPREHENSIVE PAIN ASSESSMENT

Numerous variables can be assessed in a clinical trial of a treatment that is expected to have a beneficial effect on pain. A valuable means of selecting which of these variables to include in a trial is to consider the results of recent studies seeking to identify the different dimensions that must be assessed to comprehensively evaluate patients in pain. Although some of these studies have examined chronic pain, their results are also relevant to the assessment of acute pain. However, the relative emphasis on these different components of the pain experience will differ in clinical trials of chronic and acute pain.

The results of three studies in which exploratory and confirmatory factor analyses were used to examine the assessment of patients with chronic pain suggest that three relatively independent dimensions are required to capture the multidimensionality of the pain experience (De Gagné, Mikail, & D'Eon, 1995; Holroyd, Malinoski, Davis, & Lipchik, 1999; Mikail, DuBreuil, & D'Eon, 1993). These dimensions are pain severity, psychological distress (e.g., anxiety, depression), and disability (or, conversely, functional capacity). The results of these studies also suggest that coping and social support contribute important information, indicating that it may be worthwhile to examine these psychosocial features in a comprehensive assessment of chronic pain (Jensen, Turner, Romano, & Karoly, 1991). The importance of pain severity, distress, and disability is further supported by the results of studies in which patients with chronic pain have been classified into different subtypes

based on their characteristics and outcome (see, e.g., Jamison, Rudy, Penzien, & Mosley, 1994; Klapow et al., 1993, 1995; Turk & Rudy, 1988, 1990; see also Turk & Okifugi, Chapter 21). In addition to these dimensions of the pain experience, for a comprehensive assessment of pain in a clinical trial, attention must be paid to the assessment of potential covariates (i.e., demographic variables and concurrent medical conditions and treatments) as well to global measures of treatment response (e.g., patient satisfaction and improvement).

Covariates and Other Variables Assessed at Enrollment

Demographic Variables

Various demographic characteristics of patients enrolled in clinical trials must be routinely assessed. Depending on the condition being examined, age (e.g., in postherpetic neuralgia), sex (e.g., in CRPS), and other demographic variables may be important covariates that must be examined in analyses of the data. The education, occupation (including homemaker or student), and employment status of a patient may also play a role in treatment outcome (see, e.g., Dworkin, Handlin, Richlin, Brand & Vannucci, 1985; Tait, Chibnall, & Richardson, 1990). For employment status, it can be important to determine whether or not there has been any impact of pain (e.g., working full-time, working part-time, or changed job because of pain). In trials of chronic pain syndromes, the status of workers' compensation benefits should be assessed: Specifically, are such benefits pending, ongoing, or resolved (see, e.g., Fishbain, Goldberg, Labbe, Steele, & Rosomoff, 1988; Rohling, Binder, & Langhinrichsen-Rohling, 1995)? Whether patients are receiving any other government or private insurance benefits for disability, and whether any litigation is pending, ongoing, or completed (e.g., for medical malpractice or a motor vehicle accident), should also be recorded (see, e.g., Dworkin et al., 1985; Tait et al., 1990).

Past and Present Medical Conditions and Treatments

In many clinical trials in which pain is examined, it is very important to record as much detail as possible regarding each patient's medical status. This information should include all past and present illnesses and injuries, as well as all past and present medical and nonmedical treatments for these conditions. There is a consensus that chronic pain is a complex biopsychosocial phenomenon, and it is especially important in clinical trials of chronic pain syndromes to obtain information about past and present psychiatric disorders and treatments, especially depression, suicide, substance abuse or dependence, and posttraumatic stress disorder (see, e.g., Dworkin & Caligor, 1988; Dworkin & Gitlin, 1991; Fishbain, Cutler, Rosomoff, & Rosomoff, 1997). Such disorders are often included in the exclusion criteria for a trial, and are also important because they may increase the risk of chronicity (Dworkin, 1997b) and the utilization of medical care (Mechanic, Cleary, & Greenley, 1982). In trials of chronic pain, as much detail as possible should also be recorded regarding any pain the patient has experienced in addition to the pain being examined in the trial. The presence (or history) of one or more other pain complaints may be not only one of the exclusion criteria for a trial but also an important covariate, because individuals with multiple pain complaints appear to have an increased risk of psychological distress and disability (see, e.g., Dworkin, Von Korff, & LeResche, 1990).

Expectation of Improvement

Patients being enrolled in a clinical trial—or beginning therapy at a clinic, for that matter—almost always have expectations about their likelihood of benefiting from a treatment they are about to undertake. A patient's response to a treatment intervention is due to specific treatment effects as well as to other nonspecific and placebo effects. There is little doubt that expectation of improvement is a major nonspecific effect, and that those who expect to obtain relief are more likely to improve than those who doubt that they will benefit from treatment. The explanation for the effects of expectation on treatment response is unknown. However, because expectation can be such an important determinant of treatment response, it is often worth assessing in clinical trials, especially those in which two different active treatments are being compared.

Pain-Related Variables

Pain Intensity

Many measures of pain intensity are available, and these are comprehensively reviewed by Jensen and Karoly in Chapter 2, as well as elsewhere in this

volume. These measures may be grouped into three broad types: Verbal Rating Scales (VRSs; e.g., "none," "mild," "moderate," "severe"); Numerical Rating Scales (NRSs; e.g., an 11-point scale anchored by "no pain" and "worst pain imaginable"); and Visual Analogue Scales (VASs; e.g., a 10-cm line anchored by "no pain" and "pain as bad as it could be"). There are some measures of pain intensity that combine aspects of more than one of these types of measures (e.g., the Descriptor Differential Scale [DDS]; Gracely & Kwilosz, 1988), and a few others that do not fit readily into one of these categories (e.g., facial scales).

Each of these types of measures has been used in clinical trials evaluating the effects of a treatment on pain. For example, two recent clinical trials of chronic neuropathic pain used an 11-point NRS as the primary endpoint (Backonja et al., 1998; Rowbotham, Harden, Stacey, Bernstein, & Magnus-Miller, 1998), and two recent clinical trials of low back pain used the DDS as the primary endpoint (Atkinson et al., 1998, 1999). This variability reflects the lack of consensus about the optimal method of assessing pain intensity in a clinical trial. Even though several studies in the literature have compared different pain intensity measures, most of these measures are highly correlated with each other (see, e.g., De Conno et al., 1994), and little is known regarding their differential responsiveness to treatment effects and their overall suitability in different types of clinical trials. This is an especially important area for future research, given evidence that even assessments of the simple presence or absence of pain can vary dramatically, depending on the specific pain measure used (e.g., Kornguth, Keefe, & Conaway, 1996).

Jensen and colleagues have conducted a series of studies comparing different measures of pain intensity in chronic pain (Jensen, Karoly, & Braver, 1986; Jensen, Turner, & Romano, 1994) and acute pain (Jensen, Karoly, O'Riordan, Bland, & Burns, 1989; Jensen, Miller, & Fisher, 1998). On the basis of the results of these studies and other research, Jensen and Karoly (Chapter 2) have recommended against using VASs as primary measures of pain intensity—in part because some patients, particularly elderly persons, have difficulty understanding and using these measures (cf. Duncan, Bushnell, & Lavigne, 1989; Price, 1999; Price, Bush, Long, & Harkins, 1994). It appears that NRSs are used more accurately by subjects, and that a 21-point scale with numbers ranging from 0 to 100 in multiples of 5 may be the optimal method of assessing pain intensity (see, e.g., Jensen et al., 1998). This is certainly consistent with clinical experience, because patients often respond with two adjacent numbers when administered a 0–10 NRS orally, and indicate a point midway between two adjacent numbers when administered an 11-point NRS in written form.

Since the publication of a seminal chapter by Melzack and Casey (1968), the distinction between sensory and affective aspects of pain has become one of the fundamental features of theory and research on the assessment of both clinical and experimental pain (Fernandez & Turk, 1992; Price, 1999). There are numerous methods available for separately assessing sensory and affective pain intensity, including approaches based on VASs, NRSs, and VRSs (see, e.g., Gracely, McGrath, & Dubner, 1978a, 1978b; Price et al., 1994; Smith, Gracely, & Safer, 1998), as well as specific measures of the affective component of pain (see, e.g., Jensen, Karoly, & Harris, 1991). However, attention to this distinction has not been a prominent feature of pain assessment in clinical trials.

One problematic aspect of assessing these components of pain in a clinical trial is that sensory and affective pain ratings may be subject to various demand characteristics when both are made at the same point in time (Fernandez & Turk, 1994). Separating when and varying in what order these ratings are made may reduce these demand characteristics (Fernandez & Turk, 1994). However, using such an approach to assess sensory and affective components of pain presents a challenge in clinical trials, in which treatment is expected to reduce pain intensity over time. Another important and unresolved question involves the convergent and discriminant validity of measures of the sensory and affective components of pain, evidence of which was not found in a recent study of three different approaches to assessing these components of pain (Holroyd et al., 1996).

In addition to the sensory intensity and affective unpleasantness of pain, other distinctions should be considered in conducting assessments of pain intensity. One example that has important implications in clinical trials is the distinction between *incident pain* (i.e., movement-associated pain) and ongoing pain that is not evoked by activity. For example, the Western Ontario and McMaster Universities Osteoarthritis Index, a multidimensional measure designed for studies of patients with arthritis, assesses pain during walking and stair climbing (Bellamy, Buchanan, Goldsmith, Campbell, & Stitt, 1988). Certainly, assessments of pain intensity need to reflect the types of pain

experienced by the patients enrolled in a trial, and different types of pain may be more or less responsive to a given treatment (see, e.g., Smith, Guralnick, Gelfand, & Jeans, 1986).

Pain Location, Frequency, and Duration

Relatively little attention has been devoted to the systematic assessment of pain location and area, pain frequency, and pain duration in clinical trials. In the clinic, a common approach to assessing pain location and area is to ask patients to indicate the area of their pain on drawings of the front and back of the human body. Although such drawings may be analyzed in various ways, including total area of pain and number of body regions affected, the reliability and validity of such measures in reflecting improvement in clinical trials are unclear. The areas of allodynia and hyperalgesia have begun to be assessed as secondary endpoints in recent clinical trials of such chronic neuropathic pain syndromes as postherpetic neuralgia, CRPS, and painful diabetic neuropathy. If changes with treatment are found, these studies will probably increase interest in the assessment of the area and location of pain in future clinical trials.

In evaluating treatment response in a clinical trial, it is also important to assess the temporal pattern of pain. Depending on the specific condition, pain can be constant, intermittent, or recurrent, and periodic increases of pain intensity can be either spontaneous or triggered. The specific information obtained during a trial regarding the temporal pattern of pain will therefore be determined by the particular type of pain being studied. Unfortunately, the frequency and duration of intermittent pain have typically not been assessed systematically in clinical trials (except for headache), although it would appear especially relevant in syndromes in which paroxysmal sharp and shooting pain is prominent. When measured, these aspects of pain have typically been assessed on an ad hoc basis (see, e.g., Attal et al., 2000). Several examples of questions for assessing pain frequency and duration that could be modified to address the goals of a particular clinical trial are provided by Von Korff (Chapter 31). For example, patients could be asked to indicate the typical duration of their pain (e.g., a few minutes, several minutes but less than an hour, several hours) or the number of days since their last assessment that they have had pain (e.g., if patients are assessed weekly, response options could include 1 or 2 days, about half the time, almost every day, or every day).

Two novel approaches to examining the overall duration of pain have recently been introduced in the context of studying pain in clinical trials of acute herpes zoster and postherpetic neuralgia, and these approaches could be used in other pain syndromes with a variable overall duration (e.g., postoperative pain). One of these involves simply counting the total number of days that the patient has "zoster-associated" pain from the onset of herpes zoster to the end of the trial (see, e.g., Wood, 1995; Wood, Kay, Dworkin, Soong, & Whitley, 1996). Although this approach is elegant in its simplicity, because no distinction is made between the acute pain of herpes zoster and the chronic pain of postherpetic neuralgia, important differences between the two may not be revealed (Dworkin, 1997a).

The second approach involves assessing what has been termed the *burden of pain* (Dworkin et al., 1997; Lydick, Epstein, Himmelberger, & White, 1995; Oxman, 1994). This approach can be used to examine the continuum of pain from onset to the end of the trial. Pain intensity (e.g., on a 0–10 scale) is plotted against total duration of the trial in days, and the resulting measure of pain burden is the total area under the curve. This approach could also be used to take into account the distinction between acute and chronic pain. Depending on the definition of postherpetic neuralgia, the curve could be divided at the 30-day or 3-month point to give separate measures for acute pain burden and postherpetic neuralgia pain burden. Combining pain intensity and duration in this manner in a single measure, however, yields similar levels of pain burden in patients with intense pain that resolves relatively quickly and patients with mild pain that lasts a long time; these may or may not be equivalent in the patients' experience of pain relief.

Pain Quality

The assessment of different pain qualities is an integral component of the assessment of pain. In clinical trials, it is important to assess pain quality as well as pain intensity, because a given treatment intervention may alter specific qualities of pain while not having a significant impact on pain intensity. For the past 25 years, the preeminent method for systematically assessing the quality of a patient's pain has been the McGill Pain Questionnaire (MPQ; see Melzack & Katz, Chapter 3), which is available in many languages. The MPQ includes a categorical VRS of present pain intensity, as well as sensory, affective, and evaluative descriptors of pain; these can be scored in a variety of ways, most typically for Total, Sensory, and Affective scores (Melzack, 1975; Melzack, Katz, & Jeans, 1985).

The reliability and validity of this measure have been extensively documented, and the MPQ has been used frequently in the assessment of all types of acute and chronic pain. For example, studies have used the MPQ not only to evaluate the specific qualities of pain syndromes (see, e.g., Bhala, Ramamoorthy, Bowsher, & Yelnoorker, 1988; Reading, 1982; Reading & Newton, 1977), but also to assess differences in the treatment response of different types of pain within a group of patients (see, e.g., Flor, Haag, Turk, & Koehler, 1983; Smith et al., 1986). Although there continues to be a lack of consensus on the discriminant validity of the MPQ subscales (Donaldson, 1995; Holroyd et al., 1992, 1996; Lowe, Walker, & MacCallum, 1991; Turk, Rudy, & Salovey, 1985), theoretical considerations regarding the dimensions of pain assessed by the MPQ (Fernandez & Turk, 1992; Gracely, 1992; Melzack, 1985) and the lack of a suitable alternative provide support for its continuing use in pain research, including clinical trials.

Because the MPQ can be relatively time-consuming for some patients, Melzack (1987) has developed the short-form McGill Pain Questionnaire (SF-MPQ), which is not only completed more quickly by patients but is a more easily understood measure. The SF-MPQ includes both a VAS and the same categorical VRS as the MPQ to assess pain intensity, as well as 15 pain descriptors that are each rated by the patient on a 0–3 scale of pain severity (an important advantage over the MPQ, which only records presence or absence). Initial studies using the SF-MPQ examined postsurgical, labor, and musculoskeletal pain (Melzack, 1987). More recently, it was used in the two largest randomized, controlled clinical trials conducted to date in patients with chronic neuropathic pain, in which treatment-associated changes in the SF-MPQ Total, Sensory, and Affective scores (Backonja et al., 1998; Rowbotham et al., 1998) and in each of the 11 Sensory descriptors and 4 Affective descriptors (Dworkin, 1999; Stacey, Rowbotham, Harden, Magnus-Miller, & Bernstein, 1999) were examined.

The results of numerous studies demonstrate the value of the MPQ and SF-MPQ in the assessment of pain in clinical trials. For assessing pain, the greatest value of these measures may lie less in their Total, Sensory, and Affective scores and more in the specific Sensory descriptors that are assessed. A similar conclusion was reached by the investigators of a multicenter study of the MPQ in 1,700 patients with chronic pain, who concluded that combining the MPQ descriptors into these subscales may seriously limit the information obtained, because "information concerning the specific pain qualities endorsed by the patient is lost" (Holroyd et al., 1992, p. 309). Recent efforts to select a parsimonious set of MPQ descriptors of sensory pain quality may provide the basis for another shortened version of the MPQ that retains the validity of the MPQ but provides more information than the SF-MPQ (Fernandez & Towery, 1996; Towery & Fernandez, 1996).

Because of the dominance of the MPQ and SF-MPQ as methods for assessing pain quality, few other instruments are available for this purpose. Tursky, Jamner, and Friedman (1982) developed the Pain Perception Profile, but this measure has been used infrequently in pain research. There are thus relatively few data available that can be used to compare the responses of different samples of patients, whether with the same or with different types of pain (Holroyd et al., 1996).

The MPQ and the SF-MPQ were developed to be applicable in the assessment of all types of acute and chronic pain. One of the disadvantages of casting such a wide net is that pain qualities that are specific to particular types of pain are not as comprehensively assessed as may be required. Galer and Jensen (1997) have developed the Neuropathic Pain Scale (NPS), a questionnaire specifically designed to assess the different qualities of neuropathic pain (see Dworkin, Nagasako, & Galer, Chapter 27). The NPS has been used to compare pain quality in different neuropathic pain syndromes (Carter et al., 1998; Galer & Jensen, 1997) and to assess treatment response to intravenous lidocaine and phentolamine infusions in patients with peripheral and central neuropathic pain (Galer & Jensen, 1997). It is likely that such efforts to develop measures of pain quality designed for specific pain syndromes will continue.

Pain Relief

Direct assessment of pain relief was motivated by the concern that categorical pain intensity scales may not present patients with enough response options to optimally distinguish changes in pain intensity. As Max and Laska (1991) have noted, patients who believe that a particular intervention reduced their pain from "greater than severe" to "below severe but well above moderate" must choose the "severe" category for both the pre- and posttreatment ratings. Portenoy (1991) has noted that some patients have difficulty discriminating between differences in pain intensity resulting from treatment, but are more able to evaluate the degree of pain relief they obtained. Portenoy has further suggested that pain relief and pain intensity may represent separate and distinct components of the pain experience, noting that pain relief was found to be more closely associated with mood than with pain intensity among patients with cancer pain (Fishman et al., 1987).

Like pain intensity, pain relief can be assessed with VRS, NRS, and VAS measures. In each format, the patient is asked to indicate the amount of pain relief he or she has experienced over a given time period. Categorical pain relief scales provide a range of verbal descriptors for the patient to choose from (e.g., "pain worse," "no pain relief," "slight pain relief," "moderate pain relief," "a lot of pain relief," and "complete pain relief"). VAS and NRS measures of pain relief typically present a 100-mm line or an 11-point scale in which the ends are labeled with verbal descriptors of the extremes of pain relief (e.g., "no pain relief at all" and "complete pain relief").

Assessments of pain relief may refer to the overall level of pain, or separate assessments may be made for different types of pain. Pain may be specified by location (e.g., deep vs. cutaneous incisional pain following cesarean section; Smith et al., 1986) or by provoking stimulus and duration (e.g., ongoing, paroxysmal, or touch-evoked pain in postherpetic neuralgia; Watson & Babul, 1998). Although such distinctions are typically used for pain intensity ratings, they may be made in using measures of pain relief as well.

Pain relief ratings have been made at hourly (see, e.g., Morrison, Daniels, Kotey, Cantu, & Seidenberg, 1999), daily (see, e.g., Galer, Rowbotham, Perander, & Friedman, 1999; Watson & Babul, 1998), and weekly (see, e.g., Watson, Vernich, Chipman, & Reed, 1998) intervals. Pain relief scales have also been used as global measures at the end of multiweek trials (see, e.g., Kieburtz et al., 1998; Max et al., 1992; Nelson, Park, Robinovitz, Tsigos, & Max, 1997). Because the direct assessment of pain relief implicitly requires the comparison of current levels of pain intensity with recollections of previous pain, it should be noted that differences have been found between pain intensity ratings made at the time point of interest and pain intensity ratings made retrospectively.

Studies of experimental pain (Price et al., 1999) and chronic pain (Linton & Melin, 1982) have found that ratings of present pain were lower than ratings of recollected pain made later. This suggests that the longer the time period over which relief is assessed, the more pain relief serves as a global measure, incorporating other factors in addition to any changes in pain intensity. Moreover, the reliability of pain relief data generally decreases as study length and design complexity increase (Max & Laska, 1991).

Treatment response can also be measured in quantities derived from pain intensity scores. Rather than using a pain relief scale, trials that assess pain intensity may use the change from baseline as an endpoint (see, e.g., Ehrich et al., 1999; Rowbotham et al., 1998). Pain intensity difference (PID) scores are defined as the difference between the reported intensity and the pain intensity at baseline (see Table 34.1). PID scores can be calculated from a variety of formats for assessing pain intensity, such as VAS and VRS measures (Littman, Walker, & Schneider, 1985).

The onset, offset, and total duration of pain relief are also important quantities to assess in many clinical trials. *Onset* is defined as the point in time at which a "clinically significant amount of pain relief" occurs. Similarly, *offset* is the point at which relief is no longer significant (Laska, Siegel, & Sunshine, 1991), and *duration* is then the interval between these two times. Like pain relief, these quantities may be assessed directly or through calculations using measurements over time. Often the time course of treatment effects is estimated through statistical comparison of the treatment arms. The first point at which significant differences in an outcome measure occur is used as an estimate of onset. Another approach is to examine the time to a given amount of pain relief (e.g., time to a PID greater than or equal to 1; Morrison et al., 1999).

These indirect approaches have been criticized for using magnitude comparisons to infer time domain properties, with rescue medication use and withdrawals acting to distort the estimates of onset time (Laska et al., 1991). One method for direct assessment of time course is provided by Laska and colleagues (1991). Patients are given two stopwatches that are started at drug administration, and are asked to stop one watch at the onset of pain relief and to stop the other watch when significant relief no longer occurs. Duration is then calculated from the two directly measured times.

In addition to separate measures of the magnitude and duration of pain relief, summary measures have been devised that combine these two quantities. It has been argued that these measures are more sensitive in studies of longer duration than are measures of relief alone. Combining relief magnitude and duration into a single score is commonly done by estimating the area under the relevant time–effect curve. The summed pain intensity differences (SPID) score uses the time-weighted sum of the PID scores. This is equivalent to the area under the plot of PIDs over time. The total pain relief (TOTPAR) score uses the time-weighted sum of the pain relief scores. This is equivalent to the area under a plot of relief scores over time.

Few studies have directly compared these different measures of pain relief. Littman and colleagues (1985) conducted a comparison of a VRS pain relief measure with VRS and VAS pain intensity measures. Pain intensity differences from the VRS intensity scale (PID), pain intensity differences from the VAS (PAID), and cumulative measures from the pain relief scale (TOTPAR), summed PID (SPID), and summed PAID (SPAID) scores were also examined. The relief score, PID, and PAID were highly correlated at 1 hour ($r = $.84–.88), as were the the cumulative measures (TOTPAR, SPID, SPAID) at 6 hours ($r = $.90–.93). The authors compared the statistical significance of these relationships among the relief measures at 1 hour (pain relief, PID, PAID) and among the cumulative measures, and did not find consistent differences in sensitivity. The lowest p values were associated with the TOTPAR (among cumulative measures) and pain relief (among the 1-hour scores). The use of the magnitude of p values to infer the responsiveness of measures (i.e., the effect size) is problematic, however, especially when all of the comparisons are statistically significant.

For subjects with the same PID but different baseline intensities, the amount of pain relieved is a different percentage of the total pain (i.e., for a given PID value, a subject with more intense baseline pain has a smaller fraction of his or her pain relieved than a subject with less baseline pain). Furthermore, the maximum PID that a study can demonstrate is limited by the pain intensity level at baseline. Subjects with complete relief of pain will have PIDs equal to their baseline pain intensity; those with low baseline pain will have low PIDs regardless of the effects of the treatment. One potential solution is to use the percentage of change.

TABLE 34.1. Measures of Pain Intensity and Relief

Measure	Abbreviation	Definition	Formula
Time between ratings	Δt	Time between current and previous ratings	
Total duration	T	Time between final rating and baseline	
Relief rating	R(t)	Relief rating at time t	
Maximum relief rating	R_{max}	Relief rating corresponding to complete relief	
Pain intensity rating	P(t)	Pain intensity rating at time t	
Pain intensity difference	PID(t)	Difference between baseline pain intensity and current pain intensity	P(0) – P(t)
	PAID(t)	PID calculated using Visual Analogue Scale (VAS) scores	
Summed pain intensity differences	SPID	Sum of time-weighted PID scores; the sum of the PID scores multiplied by the interval between ratings	Σ PID(t) $\times$ Δt; Σ (P(0) – P(t)) $\times$ Δt
	SPAID	SPID calculated using VAS scores	
Total pain relief	TOTPAR	Sum of time-weighted relief scores; sum of the relief scores multiplied by the interval between ratings	Σ R(t) $\times$ Δt
Theoretical maximum SPID	maxSPID	Maximum possible SPID for a given study; SPID if complete relief was obtained over the entire study duration	P(0) $\times$ T
Theoretical maximum TOTPAR	maxTOTPAR	Maximum possible TOTPAR for a given study; TOTPAR if complete relief was obtained over the entire study duration	R_{max} $\times$ T
Percentage of theoretical maximum SPID	%maxSPID	Actual SPID as a percentage of the theoretical maximum SPID	SPID/maxSPID $\times$ 100
Percentage of theoretical maximum TOTPAR	%maxTOTPAR	Actual TOTPAR as a percentage of the theoretical maximum TOTPAR	TOTPAR/maxTOTPAR $\times$ 100
Number of patients with greater than 50% relief	>50%maxTOTPAR	Number of patients with an actual TOTPAR greater than half of the theoretical maximum TOTPAR	

Price, McGrath, Rafii, and Buckingham (1983) have recommended that the scale be considered as a ratio scale for chronic pain, and a recent study has shown that a 33% change had a high degree of association with patients' not needing additional medication to treat episodes of pain (Farrar, Portenoy, Berlin, Kinman, & Strom, 2000).

Quantities normalized to the maximum score possible are attempts to address this problem and allow comparisons across studies (Cooper, 1991; Moore, Moore, McQuay, & Gavaghan, 1997). The %maxSPID accounts for the baseline intensity rating and normalizes the SPID score to the maximum SPID score possible (i.e., the SPID score if the treatment had provided complete relief). The TOTPAR

can also be normalized to the maximum possible TOTPAR or %maxTOTPAR, with a value of 33% again providing the closest association with not requiring additional medication (Farrar et al., 2000). Pain relief data can also be summarized in a dichotomous form. One measure in early use was the division of subjects into groups with >50% pain relief and <50% pain relief, but recent data suggest that it is better to divide subjects into those with moderate or better pain relief and those with less than moderate pain relief (Farrar et al., 2000). Although these scores have appeared to provide more sensitive measures of analgesic effects in clinical trials, they combine time and magnitude information. If precise estimates of temporal quantities such as onset and offset are important, separate measures for these quantities should be used.

One application for dichotomous measures is in the area of meta-analysis (Moore et al., 1997). Many trials report data in the form of mean values (e.g., mean %maxTOTPAR) for the different treatment conditions. However, because pain data is often asymmetrically distributed, the use of means can be misleading (McQuay, Carroll, & Moore, 1995). Consequently, to compare different studies, an alternate statistic is necessary that can be derived from these mean values but that more accurately reflects the trial data. The number of patients with 50% relief as defined by a TOTPAR score >50% of maximum has been shown to be a measure that can be used for meta-analyses in this manner. An analysis of data from over 4,700 patients with acute pain demonstrated that the number of patients with >50%maxTOTPAR could be reliably calculated from SPID, VAS SPID, TOTPAR, and VAS TOTPAR means (Moore et al., 1997). The use of the dichotomous >50%maxTOTPAR measure allows the inclusion of a wider range of studies into meta-analyses.

The possible inadequacies of using 50% pain relief as a sole measure of treatment outcome have recently been examined from the perspective of studies of neurosurgical interventions (Seres, 1999). Rather than a critique of this particular dichotomous measure of pain relief, the major argument appears to be the inadequacy of using a simple threshold of pain relief to reflect meaningful improvements in overall quality of life. Of course, this issue—the relative importance of pain relief and improvements in other domains in evaluating the effects of pain treatments—is the reason we and many others believe that an adequate assessment of all types of chronic pain and many types of acute pain must be multidimensional.

Treatment Adherence and Rescue Medications

> If the criterion of adequate analgesia is that a patient is not requesting more analgesic, phenothiazines could be said to "spare" narcotics. But if the patient is asked how bad the pain is, the reply generally will indicate that the phenothiazine does not seem to be improving the situation . . .
> —BEAVER (1984, p. 48)

It is important to record the extent and duration of all pain-related treatments during the course of a clinical trial—not only the treatment being investigated, but concomitant treatments as diverse as rescue analgesics and visits to a chiropractor. This is a straightforward task in single-dose analgesic trials that preclude the concurrent use of other medications during the course of the trial, but is more difficult in longer trials that allow the concurrent use of other medications and treatments. Turk and Rudy (1991) have discussed treatment adherence in the context of evaluating the efficacy of chronic pain treatment, emphasizing multidisciplinary pain clinics. From the perspective of clinical trials of medications, four issues are important: the determination of study drug intake for the assessment of compliance; the assessment of concomitant medication usage during the trial; the measurement of analgesics used as rescue medications; and, where applicable, the assessment of medication usage as an outcome after the conclusion of the clinical trial.

Various methods can be used to assess whether patients are adhering to the study protocol and taking the prescribed doses of an investigational medication at the designated intervals. For example, patient adherence can be measured by self-report, with patients being required to record the time they take each dose of their medication in a pain diary. Another method of assessing patient adherence is to count the number of pills remaining in the bottle or blister package at various points during the course of the protocol. Such methods may be subject to inaccuracies of various sorts, but are commonly used due to their ease of implementation.

Many studies allow previously prescribed medications to be continued throughout the clinical trial. Often dosage stabilization is required before patients are allowed to enroll in the trial (Nelson et al., 1997; Rowbotham et al., 1998). Alternatively, changes in the use of concomitant analgesic medications can be considered an outcome measure. One method of assessing changes in medication use is described by Kieburtz and colleagues (1998) in their report of a clinical trial of amitriptyline and mexiletine in patients with HIV-related painful neuropathy. Concomitant medications were assigned to categories based on the World Health Organization (WHO) analgesic ladder, with steps ranging from no medication (step 0) to "stronger preparations of opioids such as morphine, fentanyl, hydromorphone, or methadone" (step 3). Medication use was classified as "increased" if the highest WHO step increased or if there was an increase in total opioid dose. Medication usage was classified as "decreased" if the highest WHO step decreased or if there was a decrease in total opioid dose. Changes in dosage of acetaminophen and NSAIDs were not considered when making these determinations. This method of assessing changes in medication usage from baseline to the end of a clinical trial allows comparisons between groups based on the number of patients in the three categories of "increased," "no change," and "decreased."

The results of a clinical trial are also affected by the use of rescue medications and withdrawal from the study due to inadequate pain relief. Withdrawals due to inadequate pain relief or for other reasons are usually dealt with by conducting analyses of the intention-to-treat sample as well as of those subjects who completed the trial. As discussed later in this chapter, the criteria used to define the intention-to-treat group can vary in clinical trials. The percentage of patients who withdraw due to lack of treatment effectiveness may also be treated as an endpoint (see, e.g., Bensen et al., 1999; Ehrich et al., 1999).

Max and Laska (1991) note that many different approaches have been used in the analysis of data when rescue medications are allowed in a clinical trial. Among these are simply leaving pain and pain relief ratings at their reported values at the times rescue medications have been used; setting pain relief ratings to their lowest possible value when rescue medications are used; and setting pain intensity ratings either to their highest possible value or to their baseline value at the time of rescue. As these authors recognize, the assignment of arbitrary data values is a problematic undertaking—one that can lead to invalid conclusions, depending on the number of patients involved and other considerations. One alternative is to treat rescue medication use itself as an outcome. Quantities such as time until use and amount used can be assessed (Ehrich et al., 1999; Morrison et al., 1999).

Many authors have noted that different patients use rescue medications to achieve varying levels of analgesia. It is also quite clear that the use of rescue medications is affected by both patients' and care providers' beliefs about this use, perhaps especially when the rescue medications are opioid analgesics. Because of this, composite measures have been proposed that combine rescue medication usage and pain intensity ratings into a single score. One method for arriving at a composite score was described by Lehmann (1990), who used the product of rescue medication dose (per kilogram of body weight per hour) and retrospective pain

scores (assessed by a category scale ranging from "no pain" to "discontinuation due to inefficacy") to compare analgesic consumption across opioids and surgery types.

Another method of combining pain and analgesic use (Silverman, O'Connor, & Brull, 1993) has been used in some studies of postsurgical pain (see, e.g., Katz et al., 1996; Reinhart et al., 1996). In this approach, rank orders are used to combine pain ratings and medication usage into a single score. Rankings of patients based on pain rating and analgesic use are converted into percentage differences from the mean rank. The pain percentage difference and the medication percentage difference are added to produce a summed percentage difference for each patient.

One recent ingenious study design completely circumvented the difficult question of how to evaluate rescue medication effects on pain ratings by using time-to-exit as the primary outcome measure (Galer et al., 1999). This enriched-enrollment study used a two-period crossover design to compare a topical lidocaine patch and a vehicle control patch. Patients enrolled in the trial had previously reported successful pain control using the lidocaine patch on an open-label basis and had been using this treatment until study initiation. During the trial, the degree of pain relief was rated daily, and the criterion for transition to the second treatment period was a decrease by two or more levels in a patient's pain relief ratings for 2 consecutive days. A long time spent in a given treatment period indicated a sustained level of pain relief and high efficacy; conversely, a short time until exit indicated low efficacy in this design. In this manner, the subjects were able to switch treatments and receive pain relief (or exit the trial entirely) when their relief was not adequate. This research design made it possible to evaluate placebo response in a manner that did not deny patients pain relief.

The ongoing usage of pain medications after treatment may be used as an outcome measure. For example, studies evaluating outcome in patients treated in chronic pain management programs have used the combination of medication usage, activity level, and pain intensity to assess outcome (Malec, Cayner, Harvey, & Timming, 1981; Peters, Large, & Elkind, 1992). Scales such as the Medication Quantification Scale (MQS; Steedman et al., 1992) allow the quantification of medication use in chronic pain patients based on dosage and medication class. The MQS rates medication classes based on potential beneficial and detrimental effects; a net detriment weight (1–6) is assigned to each class. Dosage levels are rated on a 0–4 scale relative to the standard therapeutic range (<1 dose/week, subtherapeutic dose, low therapeutic dose, high therapeutic dose, supratherapeutic dose). The combination of detriment weights and dosages yields a single measure of medication usage.

Pain Behavior

The pain-related behavior that is often manifested by those suffering from pain—for example, grimacing, guarding, and (especially in infants and children) crying—has played a very important role in both the conceptualization and treatment of chronic pain (Fordyce, 1976; Keefe & Dunsmore, 1992; Turk & Flor, 1987). Several measures have been developed to assess such behaviors (see, e.g., Feuerstein, Greenwald, Gamache, Papciak, & Cook, 1985; Keefe & Hill, 1985), and they are reviewed elsewhere in this volume (see McGrath & Gillespie, Chapter 6, and Keefe, Williams, & Smith, Chapter 10). Because of the prominence of the concept of pain behavior in the multidisciplinary and psychological treatment of chronic pain, studies of the efficacy of these treatment approaches have used such measures in the evaluation and prediction of treatment outcome (see, e.g., Connally & Sanders, 1991; Peters et al., 1992; Turner & Jensen, 1993).

Studies of the efficacy of other treatment approaches for pain (e.g., drugs, nerve blocks) have generally not examined pain behavior. There are several reasons for this, not the least of which is a fundamental question about the intended effects of treatment interventions for patients with pain. Certainly, what patients desire first and foremost from such an intervention is pain relief, and then secondarily a return to premorbid quality of life. From this perspective, a reduction in pain behavior has little value as an endpoint in a clinical trial, although it may have theoretical implications regarding the experience of pain and its consequences.

Physical Examination Findings and Quantitative Sensory Testing

Measures that quantify pain-related physical and physiological responses can provide valuable additional information in the comprehensive assessment of pain (these measures are reviewed in detail elsewhere in this volume). Various aspects of the physical examination can be standardized to yield measures of outcome that can be used in clinical trials. It is possible to examine, for example, trunk strength and lumbar range of motion in low back pain (see, e.g., Cassisi, Robinson, O'Conner, & MacMillan, 1993; Shirley, O'Connor, Robinson, & MacMillan, 1994), jaw opening in temporomandibular disorder (see, e.g., Dworkin et al., 1994), upper-extremity range of motion in CRPS (see, e.g., Oerlemans, Oostendorp, de Boo, & Goris, 1999), and tender point pain in fibromyalgia (see, e.g., Burckhardt, Mannerkorpi, Hedenberg, & Bjelle, 1994).

In studies of neuropathic pain, increasing attention has been paid to developing standardized methods for assessing allodynia and hyperalgesia (see, e.g., Attal, Brasseur, Chauvin, & Bouhassira, 1999). Quantitative sensory testing, in which thresholds and stimulus–response curves for innocuous and painful stimuli are measured (see Dworkin et al., Chapter 27), has also been used to assess the effects of treatments on peripheral and central pain pathways (see, e.g., Eisenberg, Alon, Ishay, Daoud, & Yarnitsky, 1998).

Psychophysiological responses associated with pain and presumed to reflect its sensory intensity or affective unpleasantness (or both) have also been included in clinical trials (see Flor, Chapter 5), especially in studies of acute pain and experimentally induced pain. Such measures have examined autonomic nervous system (e.g., heart rate, respiration rate, blood pressure) as well as central nervous system (e.g., electroencephalography, positron emission tomography, functional magnetic resonance imaging) responses to pain. In clinical trials involving electromyographic (EMG) biofeedback, either as a single treatment (see, e.g., Flor et al., 1983) or as one component in a multidisciplinary pain program (see, e.g., Peters & Large, 1990), changes in EMG levels have also been examined. It should be noted that many of these psychophysiological measures have not been studied extensively; as a consequence, their validity as indicators of the patient's experience of pain is not well established.

Perhaps because many measures of physical and physiological responses have the appearance of being more "objective" than measures of pain and pain relief, less attention has been paid to measurement issues in their assessment, including reliability and validity (Rudy, Turk, Brena, Stieg, & Brody, 1990; Rudy, Turk, & Brody, 1992; see also Dworkin & Sherman, Chapter 32).

This is unfortunate, because inadequacies in the quality of physical and physiological assessments will markedly diminish the validity of the results obtained in studies using these measures.

Quality-of-Life Variables

In recent years, the assessment of quality of life has become an essential component of the assessment of treatment response in clinical trials. Turk, Rudy, and Sorkin (1993), Portenoy (1991), and many others have noted that in clinical trials examining pain, the effectiveness of a particular treatment is determined not only by the degree of pain reduction, but also by improvement in psychological status and daily functioning. It is important to emphasize that although it is certainly important to examine quality of life in clinical trials of psychological interventions, it is often just as important to assess it in trials of other treatments as diverse as physical therapy (see, e.g., Hope & Forshaw, 1999) and drugs (see, e.g., Backonja et al., 1998; Rowbotham et al., 1998). For example, a drug or other treatment that both relieves pain and improves quality of life has greater value than one that only relieves pain. Alternatively, if the dosages of a drug that provide optimal pain relief reduce quality of life because of side effects, then the drug will possess limited clinical value.

Measures of psychological function and disability are most often examined in clinical trials as a component of the assessment of treatment response, but such measures can also be included as covariates in analyses of pain relief (see, e.g., Syrjala, Cummings, & Donaldson, 1992). In addition, depending on the specific pragmatic and explanatory goals of a clinical trial, measures of pain-related coping and beliefs, dysfunctional cognitions, self-efficacy, social support, and stressful life events can be examined as putative mediators—or moderators (Baron & Kenny, 1986)—of treatment outcome (e.g., Turner & Jensen, 1993). The assessment of these psychosocial variables is discussed by DeGood and Tait in Chapter 17.

In the remainder of this section, we briefly discuss the assessment in clinical trials of two broad domains of quality of life—psychological distress (vs. well-being) and disability—that are reviewed in detail elsewhere in this volume. The effects of treatment on health care utilization (see, e.g., Flor et al., 1983) and the cost–benefit relationships of treatment (see, e.g., Okifuji, Turk, & Kalauokalani, 1999), including pharmaco-

economic issues, are examined in a growing number of clinical trials; the assessment of these aspects of treatment is discussed by Okifuji and Turk in Chapter 33.

Psychological Distress (vs. Well-Being)

The association between both acute and chronic pain and psychological distress is well documented (Gatchel & Turk, 1999). The results of numerous studies suggest that higher levels of pain are usually associated with higher levels of psychological distress, particularly depression, anxiety, and anger (see Bradley & McKendree-Smith, Chapter 16). In addition, there is considerable comorbidity between chronic pain syndromes and various psychiatric disorders, including mood, anxiety, and substance use disorders (Dworkin & Caligor, 1988; Dworkin & Gitlin, 1991; see also Sullivan, Chapter 15). The nature of the causal pathways accounting for these relationships is an important question for research on the pathogenesis of chronic pain, but is often less relevant in the assessment of psychological and psychiatric status in clinical trials. For example, whether depression causes pain or pain causes depression, a treatment that alleviates both is much desired from a pragmatic perspective.

From an explanatory perspective, however, it is important to determine whether or not reported pain relief is a direct consequence of treatment or is secondary to an improvement in psychological distress (or sleep or energy). The assessment of mood has therefore been particularly important in the investigation of drugs that have psychological effects, particularly antidepressants. For example, Max (1994b) has concluded that the antidepressant properties of tricyclic antidepressants do not explain their analgesic effects. This conclusion was based on comparing clinical trials that did and did not include depressed patients and on the absence of significant relationships between pain relief and mood and mood improvement within these trials (as well as on possibly different antidepressant and analgesic dose–response relationships). Clearly, if the investigation of such indirect mechanisms of pain relief is a goal, then appropriate measures should be used throughout the course of a clinical trial to assess potential changes in psychological function.

The presence of considerable psychological distress in some patients with acute pain and many patients with chronic pain also presents a challenge when one is assessing symptoms such as fatigue, sleep disturbance, weight loss, reduced activity level, and memory or concentration difficulties: Should these symptoms be considered consequences of pain or symptoms of psychological distress and psychiatric disorder? Although this question has been much discussed in the psychiatric literature with respect to the diagnosis of depression in medically ill patients, no satisfactory resolution of it has emerged. In the majority of studies, such symptoms are viewed as reflecting psychological distress or psychiatric disorder, even though it is quite plausible that they are a result of an ongoing physical disorder.

Methods for assessing psychological distress and psychiatric symptoms can be divided into those that use a questionnaire completed by the patient and those that rely on ratings provided by an investigator, which are often based on an interview. For many of the symptoms of psychological distress that are assessed in clinical trials of pain, both types of measures are available. For example, the Beck Depression Inventory (Beck, Ward, Mendelson, Mock, & Erbaugh, 1961) and the Center for Epidemiologic Studies–Depression scale (Radloff, 1977) are both designed to be completed by patients, whereas the Hamilton Depression Rating Scale (HDRS; Hamilton, 1960) consists of ratings by a clinician or other trained investigator. It is known that the interrater reliability and the coverage of relevant information of such measures are greatly improved when the ratings are made on the basis of structured interviews (e.g., see Williams, 1988, for the HDRS).

Measures of psychological distress that can be used in clinical trials either assess a single symptom—for example, depression, anxiety, or anger—or consist of subscales that purport to measure several such symptoms. The Symptom Checklist-90 Revised (Derogatis, 1983) and the Profile of Mood States (McNair, Lorr, & Doppleman, 1971; Shacham, 1983) are two examples of questionnaires that include several different subscales, each assessing a separate symptom dimension; both have been used in recent pain research and clinical trials (see, e.g., Kieburtz et al., 1998; Watson & Babul, 1998; Williams, Urban, Keefe, Shutty, & France, 1995). The discriminant validity of the subscales of questionnaires such as these has not been adequately demonstrated. Because of this, it is possible that subscale scores on many if not all of these questionnaires are simply redundant measures of psychological distress.

Although the psychiatric diagnoses of patients are much less commonly a part of clinical trials than questionnaire and interview assessments of various aspects of psychological function, some trials evaluate such diagnoses; this is most often done because one or more psychiatric disorders are exclusion criteria. The traditional approach to making such diagnoses is to conduct open-ended clinical interviews, but state-of-the-art assessments of psychiatric disorder use structured psychiatric interviews such as the Structured Clinical Interview for DSM-IV (First, Gibbon, Spitzer, & Williams, 1997). These measures provide reliable and valid psychiatric diagnoses, but they all require substantial training prior to their administration, as well as considerably more time from patients and investigators than self-report questionnaires.

Disability

In addition to psychological distress, assessments of the impact of a treatment on quality of life routinely include measures of disability and functional impairment. Such measures typically assess physical, social, and role disability, and evaluate such diverse aspects of a patient's life as sleep, strength, social relationships, and the ability to carry out activities of daily living (e.g., cooking dinner, working); many of these measures also include items designed to assess psychological distress. The major decision to be made in assessing the impact of a treatment on these aspects of quality of life involves whether a generic or a disease-specific measure will be used. The tradeoffs between these two approaches have important implications for the interpretation of the results of a trial. Disease-specific measures of disability are designed to evaluate the impacts of a specific condition (e.g., ability to wear shoes in individuals with diabetic neuropathy). Such specific effects of a disorder may be missed by a generic measure, and disease-specific measures may therefore be more likely to reveal changes in disability that are a consequence of treatment. In addition, responses on disease-specific measures will generally not reflect the quality-of-life impacts of comorbid conditions, which may confound the interpretation of changes in quality of life occurring over the course of a trial when generic measures are used. Generic measures, however, make it possible to compare the quality-of-life and public health impacts of a disorder and its treatment with those of different conditions.

This distinction between generic and disease-specific quality-of-life measures is somewhat oversimplified, because there are also measures at intermediate levels of generality—for example, specific to chronic illness or chronic pain—in addition to those that are specific to a particular pain syndrome. Of course, more than one type of measure may be used within a trial, but this inclusive approach comes at the cost of increased patient burden.

In clinical trials of treatments for pain, each of these types of measures have been used. The 36-Item Short-Form Health Survey (SF-36; Ware & Sherbourne, 1992) and the Sickness Impact Profile (SIP; Bergner, Bobbitt, Carter, & Gilson, 1981) are examples of disability measures that are applicable across a broad range of medical and psychosocial disorders, and that have been used in assessing patients with pain and in evaluating their treatment response (see, e.g., Backonja et al., 1998; Follick, Smith, & Ahern, 1985; Solomon, 1997). The Chronic Illness Problem Inventory (Kames, Naliboff, Heinrich, & Schag, 1984) is a more specific measure than these generic measures, designed to assess the impact of *chronic* illnesses, which has also been used for patients with pain (see, e.g., Romano, Turner, & Jensen, 1992).

At an even more specific level are disability measures that have been developed to assess chronic pain and that can be used with heterogeneous samples of patients with such pain, as well as with more homogeneous samples of patients suffering from a particular pain syndrome. These measures vary in the depth of their coverage, from brief measures with several items that each assess a different type of disability (e.g., the Pain Disability Index; Tait, Chibnall, & Krause, 1990) to more comprehensive measures with multiple subscales. Foremost among the latter is the West Haven–Yale Multidimensional Pain Inventory (WHYMPI; Kerns, Turk, & Rudy, 1985; Turk & Rudy, 1990; see also Jacob & Kerns, Chapter 19, and Turk & Okifuji, Chapter 21). The WHYMPI consists of three sections (the experience of pain and its impact, the responses of others, and participation in daily activities) comprising 12 specific subscales (e.g., Affective Distress, Social Activities). At the most specific level are measures of disability that have been designed for a particular type of pain. For example, there are measures designed to evaluate quality of life in patients with low back pain (see, e.g., Daltroy, Cats-Baril, Katz, Fossel, & Liang, 1996; Roland & Morris, 1983), arthritis (see, e.g., Bellamy et al., 1988; Bombardier & Raboud, 1991), fibromyalgia (see, e.g., Burckhardt, Clark, & Bennett, 1991), and headache (see, e.g., Jacobson, Ramadan, Aggarwal, & Newman, 1994; Stewart, Lipton, Simon, Liberman, & Von Korff, 1999).

The validity of quality-of-life measures has been evaluated by examining their relationships with pain severity, analgesic use, psychological distress, and treatment response, and by determining whether these measures distinguish between different levels of pain severity (see, e.g., Bombardier & Raboud, 1991; Mauskopf, Austin, Dix, & Berzon, 1994). Given the variety of measures that can be used in the assessment of disability in patients with pain, and their different levels of specificity, it is unfortunate that there are so few studies comparing the reliability and validity of one measure with another (e.g., see Jensen, Strom, Turner, & Romano, 1992, for a comparison of the generic SIP with the Roland and Morris scale for low back pain). There are also relatively few studies that have compared the incremental validity of quality-of-life measures (Mauskopf, Austin, Dix, & Berzon, 1995)—that is, the degree to which different measures add to the information obtained from other measures in predicting treatment response or disease course and prognosis. Little attention has been paid to the clinical significance of quality-of-life changes (Guyatt, Feeny, & Patrick, 1993; Lydick & Epstein, 1993), and it is therefore unknown what magnitude of a statistically significant treatment response on, for example, the SF-36 in a patient with postherpetic neuralgia (Rowbotham et al., 1998) reflects a meaningful difference to the patient.

Adverse Events and Side Effects

The importance of monitoring adverse events and side effects in the evaluation of new drugs has long been recognized and is a component of all clinical trials of medication. Max and Laska (1991) have noted that common analgesic side effects (e.g., gastrointestinal distress, cognitive dysfunction, sedation) can limit the dosage of analgesic that can be realistically prescribed. Side effects may be assessed via open-ended questions (see, e.g., see Nelson et al., 1997) or by inquiry about specific expected side effects (see, e.g., Max et al., 1992; Watson & Babul, 1998; Watson et al., 1998). It is well known that providing patients with lists of specific symptoms results in a considerably greater incidence of reported side effects (in both active drug and placebo groups) than the use of such open-ended questions as "How are you feeling?" and "Have you had any medical changes or problems since your last visit?" In studies of opioid analgesics and benzodiazepines, the Addiction Research Center Inventory provides a comprehensive assessment of specific drug effects, such as euphoria, sedation, and psychotomimetic effects (Jasinski, Martin, & Sapira, 1967).

Patients can also rate the severity of their side effects. As with measures of pain intensity, a variety of different rating scales can be used, including VRS, NRS, and VAS formats. It is also important for the investigator to evaluate whether the reported adverse events or side effects are associated with the study medication. These judgments are typically recorded with rather crude categorical scales (e.g., "possible," "probable," "definite"), and the interjudge reliability of such evaluations must surely be quite low.

Overall Measures of Outcome

Because the number of measures that can be included in clinical trials of treatments expected to provide pain relief is so large, it is not surprising that investigators have developed measures that combine one or more of the variables discussed above, or that seek to summarize the patient's overall response to treatment. The benefits of such methods of assessing pain treatment response are considerable. A global measure of outcome could capture the effects of treatment on pain and its adverse impacts on the patient's quality of life, and would thereby provide an ideal primary endpoint in many studies of acute and chronic pain. The risks of such approaches are also substantial. Although conceptually appealing, combining measures that may themselves have inadequate reliability and validity, or using elegant but possibly unreliable ratings of global treatment response, could make it more difficult to find treatment effects.

Combined Measures of Pain Severity and Quality of Life

Various attempts have been made to develop outcome measures that combine one or more pain-related measures, typically pain intensity, with one or more measures of quality of life. Some of these measures simply include ratings of both pain intensity and disability in a single scale (see, e.g., Gatchel, Polatin, & Mayer, 1995; Million, Nilsen, Jayson, & Baker, 1981). Other investigators have developed sets of criteria for evaluating "successful outcome": For example, the patient must be employed or otherwise occupied and active at least 8 hours each day; must not have had pain-related hospitalizations or surgeries since treatment; and

must not be receiving compensation or disability benefits, or taking opioid analgesics or psychotropic medications (Guck, Skultety, Meilman, & Dowd, 1985; Roberts & Reinhardt, 1980).

Yet another approach has been to develop categorical classifications of patients based on patterns of responses to measures of pain severity and quality of life. For example, Turk and Rudy (1988, 1990) have classified patients with pain based on their WHYMPI responses into three groups: Dysfunctional, Interpersonally Distressed, and Adaptive Copers (see also Jamison et al., 1994). Similarly, Von Korff, Ormel, Keefe, and Dworkin (1992; see also Smith et al., 1997) have graded patients with chronic pain into four groups based on the severity of their pain and disability. These classifications of patients with chronic pain can be used in clinical trials, not only to predict treatment response, but also as measures of treatment outcome (see, e.g., Dworkin et al., 1994; Turk, Okifuji, Sinclair, & Starz, 1998). By examining improvement in pain classification, this approach provides a primary endpoint whose clinical significance can be readily interpreted.

Global Improvement

Global measures of outcome in clinical trials provide an assessment of the net beneficial effect of treatment, including both the magnitude of pain relief and improvements in quality of life, as well as any negative effects. Responses on these measures may combine degree of pain relief with the impact of side effects, convenience of dosing, and other aspects of treatment. Given the important role that side effects play in patient satisfaction with drug treatment, such measures can be useful for judging the clinical acceptability of treatments that achieve significant pain relief at the cost of pronounced side effects.

Global ratings may use patient ratings or clinician ratings, and may have a variety of formats. The Patient Global Impression of Change (PGIC) and Clinician Global Impression of Change (CGIC) are 7-point category rating scales of overall status that range from "very much improved" to "very much worse" (Guy, 1976). The PGIC asks the patient to choose the option that best describes "any change which you have experienced since beginning the study medication" while the CGIC asks the clinician for a rating of "any change in the patient which you have observed since beginning the study medication." These measures have been used in recent assessments of analgesics in various chronic pain syndromes (Backonja et al., 1998; Rowbotham et al., 1998). The PGIC and CGIC ratings take into account all change, regardless of whether or not the individual making the rating (patient or clinician) believes it is due to the treatment. The interrater reliability of ratings such as the CGIC is rarely assessed; as Turk and colleagues (1993) note, "it must be assumed that an outcome measure is unreliable until proven otherwise," which is "particularly true for the ratings of success made by health care providers" (p. 5).

Other approaches to the global assessment of treatment response include ratings of patient satisfaction, ratings of change attributed to the therapy, and global ratings of disease state from which changes from baseline can be calculated. These ratings differ in the degree of emphasis given to rating the treatment's performance (e.g., degree of response to treatment, helpfulness or usefulness of treatment) versus the patient's feelings about the treatment (e.g., satisfaction, preference).

Measures of satisfaction may simply ask whether or not the patient is satisfied (Watson et al., 1998) or may use a categorical rating scale ranging, for example, from "extremely dissatisfied" to "extremely satisfied" (see, e.g., Turner & Jensen, 1993). An indirect method for the assessment of satisfaction is having the patient rate the likelihood of recommending the treatment to a friend (Dworkin et al., 1994). In crossover trials, satisfaction may be assessed by asking which treatment phase the patient preferred (Watson & Babul, 1998). Such assessments of treatment preference should, of course, be made under double-blind conditions. In some trials, inquiry about preference has been limited to those patients who had good responses to both drugs (see, e.g., Watson et al., 1998).

Global ratings of the treatment may also focus on change attributable to the treatment by assessing the overall evaluation of the therapy (e.g., on a scale ranging from "poor" to "excellent"; Morrison et al., 1999) and the helpfulness of the therapy (e.g., on a scale ranging from "not at all helpful" to "extremely helpful"; Dworkin et al., 1994). Patients' assessment of their degree of treatment response has also been evaluated, using category scales (e.g., on a scale ranging from "excellent" to "none"; Ehrich et al., 1999) and percentage scales (Watson et al., 1998). In crossover trials, the patients can also be asked to indicate which phase provided the best relief (Galer et al., 1999).

Global measures of treatment response have also been derived from patient and clinician ratings of a patient's overall disease state. In recent clinical trials of celecoxib in rheumatoid arthritis (Simon et al., 1999) and osteoarthritis (Bensen et al., 1999), and of rofecoxib in osteoarthritis (Ehrich et al., 1999), patients and clinicians made global assessments of disease status at baseline and at intervals throughout the study. Both categorical (Bensen et al., 1999; Ehrich et al., 1999; Simon et al., 1999) and VAS (Ehrich et al., 1999) formats were used, and the change from baseline was then calculated. Measures may also be combined to provide a composite rating that explicitly considers a variety of factors. Watson and colleagues (1998) divided patients into categories based on "clinical effectiveness." A classification of "excellent" clinical effectiveness corresponded to patients who had no pain, disability, insomnia, or depression, and who had tolerable side effects and expressed satisfaction with their degree of pain relief. Categories of "good" effectiveness, "improved but unsatisfactory," and "unchanged" were similarly constructed based on criteria for pain severity and relief, side effect tolerability, depression, insomnia, disability, and expression of satisfaction.

DATA CAPTURE

Clinical trials have a number of different phases, depending on their type. Some trials have a *run-in* period, which is used to exclude patients from the trial for various reasons. These include lack of compliance with the requirements of the protocol (e.g., keeping diaries of daily pain ratings), beneficial response to placebo (excluding such individuals increases the statistical power and efficiency of the trial), lack of beneficial response to the trial drug (an *enriched-enrollment* design), and presence of adverse effects from the trial drug (Pablos-Méndez, Barr, & Shea, 1998). A run-in period can also be used to make the results of the trial applicable to clinical practice—for example, by determining dosage equivalence when patients are changed from one drug to another.

Clinical trials of pain treatments typically have a baseline period, and this should include observations of the patients' pain levels made on several occasions (Max, 1991). This phase of a trial can be important because it makes it possible to analyze the difference between pain levels during the baseline and pain levels following treatment; as discussed above, such data can be examined using absolute differences or percentage change. In clinical trials of analgesic medications, the beginning of the phase of active treatment (the point at which patients are randomly assigned to conditions in a randomized trial) may include a period in which the dosage of the medication is titrated to a designated therapeutic dosage (in some trials, titration can be stopped at a dosage below the target if side effects prevent further escalation).

A very important consideration in clinical trials of treatments for chronic pain is the length of the treatment period. The major factor in determining the length of the treatment phase is the investigator's belief about the length of time needed for the investigational treatment to demonstrate a beneficial effect. For some treatments, this may be a single session (e.g., a lidocaine infusion in neuropathic pain), whereas with other treatments, several weeks of sessions (e.g., physical therapy in low back pain) or medication (e.g., tricyclic antidepressants in fibromyalgia) may be required. With chronic pain syndromes, longer durations of treatment are desirable to evaluate whether any beneficial effects of the treatment are maintained over time; this is, of course, important in patients who have a chronic condition and are not likely to improve spontaneously.

At the end of the treatment phase, some trials include a phase during which the treatment is tapered. This is most common in studies of medications that should not be discontinued abruptly, such as opioid analgesics. But studies of psychological and physical therapies may also include a phase at the end of the treatment period in which the frequency of treatment is decreased, as a means of extending the overall duration of treatment or of ensuring that patients continue to practice what they have learned during the initial, more intense phase of treatment.

There are two major reasons why clinical trials have a follow-up period during which patients are studied after treatment has ended. In medication trials, a follow-up period is needed to evaluate late adverse events associated with treatment. Follow-up periods are also required in trials of treatments expected to have beneficial effects that persist after treatment has ended. Such treatments include psychological and physical therapies, which in modifying patients' adjustment to their pain can have an enduring beneficial effect, as well as nerve blocks and other treatments that by providing short-term pain relief are thought to attenuate factors maintaining chronic pain. Although there are few examples for chronic pain, a medication could also have an enduring beneficial effect, and in this sense it would be a "disease-modifying"

rather than a symptomatic treatment for a chronic pain syndrome (e.g., a drug that abolished central sensitization).

The duration of the follow-up period is an important consideration when the enduring effects of treatment are assessed in a clinical trial. Longer follow-up periods make it possible to demonstrate that beneficial effects are maintained well beyond treatment cessation, which provides very compelling support for the efficacy of the treatment. The disadvantages of a long follow-up period, however, are (1) that it places a burden on both investigators and patients; and (2) that by increasing the percentage of patients who are lost to follow-up, it may decrease the generalizability of the results of the trial (Turk et al., 1993).

How to Assess

To this point, we have reviewed diverse measures of assessing pain and pain-related quality of life in clinical trials. We have said little, however, about the specific methods used for administering these measures. For example, is a measure of pain intensity or depression obtained by giving patients a questionnaire to complete, reading the questions to patients in a face-to-face interview; reading the questions to patients over the telephone; having patients enter their responses on a device kept in their possession (e.g., a palmtop computer or personal digital assistant); having patients respond by voice or by touch tones to recorded prompts after dialing into a central phone number or after an automatically generated telephone call to them; or having patients enter their responses over the internet (e.g., to an e-mailed questionnaire or at a designated Web site)?

There are obvious constraints in selecting from this long but not complete list of methods. For example, a VAS measure of pain intensity cannot be administered over the telephone or to subjects who cannot indicate their pain with a written response (either because of limited motor function or because of the specific assessment situation—e.g., during a surgical procedure). Nevertheless, in most situations investigators have a variety of options available, and there are unfortunately relatively few studies that have compared the reliability and validity of these different methods. Moreover, the reliability and validity of these methods probably vary as a result of what is being assessed; it would not be surprising if responses to questions about, for example, depression or sexual disability differ, depending on whether they are made in a face-to-face interview or on a questionnaire.

The results of the few studies that have compared different methods of collecting the types of data discussed in this chapter suggest that more attention to these considerations is required. For example, although it was originally stated that the MPQ should be read aloud to patients in an interview (Melzack, 1975; see also Melzack & Katz, Chapter 3), most studies have adapted it for administration as a paper-and-pencil questionnaire, despite data suggesting that the two formats differ (see, e.g., Klepac, Dowling, Rokke, Dodge, & Schafer, 1981). Likewise, in the assessment of health-related quality of life, responses to the SF-36 have been found to vary according to whether they are collected in telephone interviews, in face-to-face interviews, or by self-administration (Weinberger et al., 1994; Weinberger, Oddone, Samsa, & Landsman, 1996). As the investigators noted, some of their results were troubling. In comparisons of the physical, social, emotional, and mental health domains, face-to-face interviews "provided a more optimistic picture of health than did self-administration" (Weinberger et al., 1996, p. 139). Although it is tempting to assume that the reports of poorer quality of life when the SF-36 was self-administered are more veridical, it is also possible that patients exaggerated their disability when completing the SF-36 by themselves, to ensure that their impersonal questionnaire responses would receive adequate attention.

In addition to differences in reliability and validity, the different methods of administering measures of pain and pain-related quality of life can vary in such characteristics as expense, time required, response rate, error rate, and need for interviewer training. The preferences of patients may also differ; for example, patients overwhelmingly preferred face-to-face administration of the SF-36 to telephone interviews and self-administration (Weinberger et al., 1996). Although such differences in patient preference do not necessarily translate to different patterns of results (cf. Kremer, Atkinson, & Ignelzi, 1981), the extent to which patients prefer different methods of administration could have a considerable impact on subject retention in clinical trials.

When to Assess

Additional important questions regarding the administration of the measures discussed in this chapter are these: At what frequency should they be administered, and what instructions should be given to patients regarding the time window to be used when making their responses? Assessments will generally be made more frequently in relatively short-term studies of acute pain and single administrations of a treatment than in longer-lasting studies of chronic pain with multiple treatment doses or sessions. Pain, in particular, can be rated every several minutes, hours, days, weeks, or months. Certainly, the choice among these alternatives will often be determined by the specific treatment and type of pain being examined in a clinical trial. However, there are many situations in which investigators must decide among these options, and there is unfortunately not a great deal of guidance in the literature in making this decision.

Ratings of pain made on an hourly basis provide a comprehensive assessment of a patient's characteristic pain and its fluctuations (see, e.g., Jamison & Brown, 1991; Jensen & McFarland, 1993; Kerns, Finn, & Haythornthwaite, 1988). Although hourly pain ratings (Flor et al., 1983) and five-times-daily pain ratings (Nelson et al., 1997) have been used in clinical trials, ratings made this frequently would seem to be impractical in many trials lasting more than several days. In clinical trials of chronic pain, the choice is typically between requiring patients to rate their pain every day in a diary or once each week, typically during an office visit; pain ratings can also be made on a fortnightly or monthly basis. In daily diary ratings, both "pain in the past 24 hours" and "pain today" have been used as instructions for making ratings. Our preference is to use the latter (made close to bedtime), because if "pain in the past 24 hours" is used as the time window, some patients may attempt to average in their pain during sleep.

Whether ratings are made on a daily or weekly basis, a choice must be made between asking patients to rate their current (i.e., pain right now), usual (average), worst, or least pain. It has been established that a rating of current pain is not adequate if the primary goal of the assessment is to obtain information about previous levels of pain (Jensen & McFarland, 1993). Although recall of past pain is influenced by present pain (see, e.g., Smith et al., 1998), the results of several studies suggest that the average of hourly ratings of pain is more strongly associated with later ratings of least and usual pain than with later ratings of worst and current pain (Jensen, Turner, Turner, & Romano, 1996; Salovey, Smith, Turk, Jobe, & Willis, 1993). Redelmeier and Kahneman (1996), however, found that patients' memories of painful medical procedures (i.e., colonoscopy, lithotripsy) rated within an hour of the procedure were predicted best by pain at the worst part of the procedure and at the end of the procedure. Unexpectedly, various composites of ratings of current, usual, least, and worst pain do not seem to be better at evaluating treatment response than the individual ratings themselves, but the composites do demonstrate somewhat greater test–retest stability (Jensen, Turner, Romano, & Fisher, 1999).

The results of these studies provide limited guidance with respect to choosing the most valid and efficient method of characterizing pain intensity in patients with ongoing pain. Some investigators have required patients to make daily diary ratings of average, worst, and least pain in the past 24 hours, as well as weekly ratings of average, worst, and least pain over the preceding week. This practice places a burden on both patients and investigators, and the likelihood of type I errors is increased because of the multiple comparisons possible when such data are analyzed. In a recent study of 200 patients with low back pain, Bolton (1999) examined intraclass correlation coefficient (ICC) measures of agreement between the average of 28 pain ratings made four times daily for 7 days and single ratings made the next day of current pain intensity and usual, least, and worst pain during the previous week. The single rating of usual pain in the previous week was a more accurate measure of the actual average of the daily pain ratings (ICC = .82) than the three other single pain ratings. The agreement between the actual average pain and various composites of the four single measures was also examined, and was greatest with a composite that was the average of all four single measures (ICC = .86). Because the composite measures require more time for a patient to complete and for data entry and analysis, the author concluded that a rating of usual or average pain over the previous week would "appear to be the single most practical and valid measure of a patient's pain intensity over this period of time in this patient group" (Bolton, 1999, p. 537).

DATA ANALYSIS

In this section, we briefly discuss several often controversial issues that arise in the analysis and interpretation of data from clinical trials. Although these issues have received limited attention in clinical trials examining pain, it is unfortunately beyond the scope of this chapter to discuss them in depth.

Matching the Analysis to the Hypothesis and the Data

An important and often neglected issue is the importance of using the correct analysis to answer the appropriately framed question. Specifically, it is as important to determine the correct analysis a priori as it is to specify a specific hypothesis a priori. Like the hypothesis, the type of analysis that is appropriate should be based on the underlying physiology and the expected response to treatment, not simply on the shape of the distribution of the data after the study has been completed. At one extreme, if the data are normally distributed and the study treatment is expected to have a largely uniform effect, then a mean and standard deviation are most appropriate. At the other extreme, if responses are most likely to come from a bimodal distribution (e.g., potential responders and potential nonresponders), and the effect of the treatment will vary according to a patient's underlying potential to respond, then an analysis of the proportion of responders may be more appropriate.

In addition, the analysis should provide the appropriate information for the question being addressed by the clinical trial. If the question is "How many patients get better to a clinically important degree?", then an analysis of the proportion of patients who achieve a clinically important response is appropriate, using statistical tests for categorical data. If the question is "On average, how much will a patient improve?", then statistical tests for ordinal data may be appropriate. In practice, it is very valuable to present both analyses in a publication and allow the reader to determine which is more useful.

Intention-to-Treat versus Efficacy-Evaluable Analyses

The most conservative *intention-to-treat* analysis examines all patients enrolled in a trial, regardless of whether they meet all of the inclusion and exclusion criteria and whether they have received even a single dose or session of the treatment. In some trials, a modified intention-to-treat analysis is used— for example, only analyzing data from patients if they have taken at least one dose of the study medication or if they have the appropriate diagnosis. *Efficacy-evaluable* analyses examine data from those patients who would be expected to benefit from the treatment—that is, those who have the diagnosis for which the treatment is intended, and who have received an amount of the treatment that could be expected to have a beneficial effect (in other words, patients whose participation in the trial was "per protocol").

Intention-to-treat analyses more closely reflect the real situation outside of the clinical trial setting, and such analyses are typically required by regulatory authorities for approval of medications. However, including patients who do not have the relevant disorder (e.g., patients who appear to have herpes zoster but whose laboratory test results change the diagnosis to herpes simplex), or who are less likely to derive benefit from therapy because of noncompliance, makes it difficult to evaluate the true effects of a treatment. Hence efficacy-evaluable analyses are valuable in determining whether a treatment can have beneficial effects when it is administered as intended (Sheiner & Rubin, 1995). All criteria for excluding patients from the efficacy-evaluable analyses should be prospectively defined; such analyses could exclude, for example, noncompliant patients and other protocol violations (e.g., patients who take prohibited concomitant medications). Similarly, if the intention-to-treat analysis will not include all patients enrolled in the trial, the criteria used should also be prospectively defined (e.g., subjects who "had evidence of taking at least 1 dose of study medication and provided at least 1 follow-up efficacy assessment"; Rowbotham et al., 1998, p. 1838).

Statistically significant evidence of efficacy may be found in analyses of an efficacy-evaluable subsample and not in intention-to-treat analyses of the entire sample of patients enrolled in a trial. When this occurs, it may be because patients who are unlikely to receive benefit have been included in the intention-to-treat analysis. In such instances, the efficacy-evaluable analysis may yield a more accurate assessment of the potential beneficial effects of the treatment. It can be expected, however, that the direction of differences in efficacy between treatment conditions should be the same for both intention-to-treat and efficacy-evaluable analyses.

Primary versus Secondary Endpoints

It is generally advisable and sometimes required that an investigator identify the primary endpoint and distinguish it from the secondary endpoints when designing a clinical trial. As we have discussed above, a measure of improvement in pain severity is often the primary endpoint in a clinical trial of a treatment for a pain condition. The other

components of the pain experience, including the impact of pain on psychosocial functioning and disability, are then considered secondary endpoints. Assessments of pain and related variables are secondary endpoints in a clinical trial of a condition in which pain is not the symptom or sign targeted by the treatment (e.g., a disease-modifying treatment for diabetes that might also improve painful diabetic neuropathy). This distinction between primary and secondary endpoints is necessary for determining the statistical power and required sample size of the clinical trial. By identifying the specific outcome that the treatment is intended to improve, this distinction also addresses the problem of multiple comparisons when a study examines the effects of a treatment on multiple outcomes. A planned statistical test of the hypothesis that treatment has a beneficial effect on the primary endpoint does not require correction for multiple comparisons, whereas multiple significance tests of the effects of treatment on the secondary endpoints may require such correction.

Adjusting for Covariates and Subgroup Analyses

Adjusting for factors that have been shown to have an influence on the primary endpoint has become a feature of many recent clinical trials. It is generally recognized that adjusting for covariates in this manner can have a profound effect on the results. Consequently, it is important to consider whether all potential covariates should be included in adjusted analyses of efficacy; whether only those covariates that are found to be significantly associated with the endpoint should be included; or whether only those prospectively defined covariates that have been found to significantly affect the endpoint in prior research should be included. This question is important, because the greater the number of covariates to be included in the analyses, the larger the sample size must be to ensure that the effect of each covariate is determined accurately.

Covariate analyses are valuable for examining factors that predict prolonged pain and better therapeutic response. For pivotal trials, however, such analyses should be few in number and prospectively identified, with adjustments made for multiple comparisons if necessary. For example, older age and greater pain severity at enrollment have both been found to be associated with prolonged herpes zoster pain in a large number of studies, and because of these robust associations it has been recommended that adjustments for these two covariates be made routinely in all clinical trials of herpes zoster pain (Dworkin et al., 1997).

Related to the question of adjusting for covariates is the value of separately analyzing data from subgroups of patients. The major argument in favor of conducting such analyses is that if subgroups differ in their treatment response, analyses of one group may detect differences that are less apparent in analyses of the data from all patients. Viewing the results of the subgroup analyses in conjunction with the analyses of the entire sample may therefore provide a more complete picture of treatment efficacy. This potential advantage of a subgroup analysis can be offset by the loss in statistical power resulting from analyzing a smaller number of patients. In addition, patients in the different treatment conditions may be less comparable in their baseline characteristics when analyses of subgroups are conducted. Subgroup analyses have been considered acceptable, provided that the groups are specified in advance of data analysis and can be shown to be balanced with respect to important covariates (Dworkin et al., 1997).

INTERPRETING THE RESULTS

After the design, implementation, data collection, and data analysis are completed, we are left to interpret the results of the clinical trial. No matter what analysis has ultimately been used to test the a priori hypothesis, the result is a summary statistic or effect size and a test of the probability that the results occurred by chance (i.e., their statistical significance). Both of these numbers are necessary, but the appropriate interpretation of the results depends almost entirely on the size of the effect that is detected. Although necessary, statistical significance remains only a test of probability and is of no direct importance to patient care. The definition and defense of the clinical importance of the results of a clinical trial will depend on the characteristics of the disease being treated. For example, a 5% difference in patients' pain ratings may be of almost no clinical importance, whereas a 5% increase in survival from a myocardial infarction may be of substantial interest and clinical importance. The primary problem is that it is not always obvious what constitutes a clinically important difference. Even in situations where it is possible to obtain a highly reliable and valid objective measure, such as blood pressure, determining what

cutoff point or level of change will constitute an important difference can be difficult. This does not relieve researchers of the responsibility of making this determination. Factors involved in this decision include the following:

1. The clinical question that the trial has been designed to answer.
2. The risks of not treating the disease (self-limited to fatal).
3. The benefits gained from the treatment (cure or amelioration of symptoms).
4. The risks of the treatment (side effects: none to severe).
5. Whose perspective is being considered in evaluating clinical importance: the patient, the patient's family, the physician, the insurance company, or society.

Ultimately, when a clinician is faced with an individual patient, the decision about the clinical importance of a result is a yes–no choice: The clinician must choose either to use a treatment or not. To adequately fulfill their responsibility in interpreting the results of clinical trials, authors must present their data in a way that can be applied to the clinical encounter. This means providing data that are useful at the level of the individual patient and guidance about the clinical importance of the treatment, taking into account all of the factors listed above.

To be most useful, these issues should be considered in the original design of the study. In particular, the outcome measures should be of clinical relevance, and the analysis should be planned to provide usable information. In pain management trials, a number of specific issues must be considered—many of which are also discussed in other chapters in this volume, but that are briefly summarized here from the perspective of the interpretation of clinical trial data.

First, pain is a symptom, and there are no fully objective measures of pain. Pain is inherently subjective, and pain measures, no matter how quantitative they may appear, reflect the subjective responses of patients. Our goal in treating pain is to make patients feel better by ameliorating the symptom, while trying to avoid the sometimes substantial side effects of the therapies we have available. Ultimately, only a patient is able to decide whether the effect of a treatment is sufficiently important to warrant continuing treatment, taking into account all of the factors involved. Therefore, the best outcome measure would be an unbiased assessment of patients' perceptions of their level of improvement with treatment. Although none of the measures currently available can be said to be truly unbiased, the global response and the need for additional pain medication are examples of measures that should be considered.

Second, we must consider that the perception and report of pain involve more than changes in the number of nociceptors being stimulated. Rather, the perception of pain is influenced by a number of other cognitive processes, including affective state, previous experience, level of expectation, understanding of etiology, and coping ability. The importance of measuring these other factors in understanding underlying processes and representative measures are discussed in detail above and in other chapters in this volume. However, such additional data should be analyzed whenever possible, to provide information about the types of patients who will respond to the therapy being studied and to provide a more comprehensive picture of their response. For example, this may include the development of prediction rules or, at the very least, careful presentation of the clinical importance of different treatment effects. It is also important to remember that in considering what constitutes a clinically important outcome in clinical trials of pain therapies, these separate components of the experience of pain can be combined using mathematical models that reflect patient behavior. However, it would also be reasonable to argue that a patient's perception is the best model for integrating these various factors and for deciding whether a treatment is of sufficient value to be continued.

Third, because of the large interperson variability in responses on pain and symptom scales, it is important to consider methods for determining clinical importance at the level of the individual. This usually involves a decision about the degree of intraperson change that should be considered adequate pain relief. One approach is to use a measure (e.g., deciding to continue treatment) that provides a dichotomous outcome directly related to clinical importance. A second approach would be to try to attribute a level of clinical importance to changes in more traditional pain measures. Various methods have been devised to try to accomplish this task, although none of them are completely satisfactory (Farrar et al., 2000).

Fourth, group means are often used in summarizing the results of a clinical trial. Whether or not this is the most appropriate analysis is controversial and clearly depends on the nature of the

trial. However, it is generally true that a mean value does not provide a unique solution to the question of how many patients will obtain clinically important benefit from a particular treatment. An analysis of the proportion of patients that obtain a fixed level of improvement provides additional information that is highly clinically relevant. Because it is often difficult to obtain agreement on the exact level of change in pain intensity or pain relief that is clinically important, it may be appropriate to present the proportion of responders at several clinically relevant levels, along with the corresponding level of significant side effects, to allow a reader to decide whether the treatment is of sufficient value to be useful in his or her practice.

In summary, it is a truism that pain is a subjective experience. The implication of this for the assessment of pain in clinical trials is that to be adequate, an assessment of pain must address this subjective experience by asking patients to describe their pain using reliable, valid, and responsive measures. Knowledge of the pathophysiology of the pain system and the interaction between the central and peripheral nervous systems has increased, leading to a greater understanding of the mechanisms of specific painful conditions. A consensus has also emerged that extended nociceptive input in chronic pain patients is usually accompanied by a complex interaction between the sensory aspects of pain and diverse psychological and social processes. In addition, understanding of the methods involved in the design, conduct, and analysis of clinical trials continues to expand. It is important that careful consideration be given to all of these factors as we move forward toward the day when pain can be adequately treated for all patients.

REFERENCES

Alderson, P. (1996). Equipoise as a means of managing uncertainty: Personal, communal and proxy. *Journal of Medical Ethics, 22,* 135–139.

Atkinson, J. H., Slater, M. A., Wahlgren, D. R., Williams, R. A., Zisook, S., Pruitt, S. D., Epping-Jordan, J. E., Patterson, T. L., Grant, I., Abramson, I., & Garfin, S. R. (1999). Effects of noradrenergic and seratonergic antidepressants on chronic low back pain intensity. *Pain, 83,* 137–145.

Atkinson, J. H., Slater, M. A., Williams, R. A., Zisook, S., Patterson, T. L., Grant, I., Wahlgren, D. R., Abramson, I., & Garfin, S. R. (1998). A placebo-controlled randomized clinical trial of nortriptyline for chronic low back pain. *Pain, 76,* 287–296.

Attal, N., Brasseur, L., Chauvin, M., & Bouhassira, D. (1999). Effects of single and repeated applications of a eutectic mixture of local anaesthetics (EMLA) cream on spontaneous and evoked pain in post-herpetic neuralgia. *Pain, 81,* 203–209.

Attal, N., Gaude, V., Brasseur, L., Dupuy, M., Guirimand, F., Parker, F., & Bouhassira, D. (2000). Intravenous lidocaine in central pain: A double-blind, placebo-controlled, psychophysical study. *Neurology, 54,* 564–574.

Backonja, M., Beydoun, A., Edwards, K. R., Schwartz, S. L., Fonseca, V., Hes, M., LaMoreaux, L., & Garofalo, E. (1998). Gabapentin for the symptomatic treatment of painful neuropathy in patients with diabetes mellitus: A randomized controlled trial. *Journal of the American Medical Association, 280,* 1831–1836.

Baron, R. M., & Kenny, D. A. (1986). The moderator-mediator variable distinction in social psychological research: Conceptual, strategic, and statistical considerations. *Journal of Personality and Social Psychology, 51,* 1173–1182.

Beaver, W. T. (1984). Combination analgesics. *American Journal of Medicine, 77,* 38–53.

Beck, A. T., Ward, C. H., Mendelson, M., Mock, J., & Erbaugh, J. (1961). An inventory for measuring depression. *Archives of General Psychiatry, 4,* 561–571.

Begg, C., Cho, M., Eastwood, S., Horton, R., Moher, D., Olkin, I., Pitkin, R., Rennie, D., Schulz, K. F., Simel, D., & Stroup, D. F. (1996). Improving the quality of reporting of randomized controlled trials: The CONSORT statement. *Journal of the American Medical Association, 276,* 637–639.

Bellamy, N., Buchanan, W. W., Goldsmith, C. H., Campbell, J., & Stitt, L. W. (1988). Validation study of WOMAC: A health status instrument for measuring clinically important patient relevant outcomes to antirheumatic drug therapy in patients with osteoarthritis of the hip or knee. *Journal of Rheumatology, 15,* 1833–1840.

Bensen, W. G., Fiechtner, J. J., McMillen, J. I., Zhao, W. W., Yu, S. S., Woods, E. M., Hubbard, R. C., Isakson, P. C., Verburg, K. M., & Geis, G. S. (1999). Treatment of osteoarthritis with celecoxib, a cyclooxygenase-2 inhibitor: A randomized controlled trial. *Mayo Clinic Proceedings, 74,* 1095–1105.

Bergner, M., Bobbitt, R. A., Carter, W. B., & Gilson, B. S. (1981). The Sickness Impact Profile: Development and final revision of a health status measure. *Medical Care, 19,* 787–805.

Beurskens, A. J., de Vet, H. C., & Koke, A. J. (1996). Responsiveness of functional status in low back pain: A comparison of different instruments. *Pain, 65,* 71–76.

Bhala, B. B., Ramamoorthy, C., Bowsher, D., & Yelnoorker, K. N. (1988). Shingles and postherpetic neuralgia. *Clinical Journal of Pain, 4,* 169–174.

Bolton, J. E. (1999). Accuracy of recall of usual pain intensity in back pain patients. *Pain, 83,* 533–539.

Bombardier, C., & Raboud, J. (1991). A comparison of health-related quality-of-life measures for rheumatoid arthritis research. *Controlled Clinical Trials, 12*(Suppl.), S243–S256.

Burckhardt, C. S., Clark, S. R., & Bennett, R. M. (1991). The Fibromyalgia Impact Questionnaire: Development and validation. *Journal of Rheumatology, 18,* 728–733.

Burckhardt, C. S., Mannerkorpi, K., Hedenberg, L., & Bjelle, A. (1994). A randomized, controlled clinical trial of education and physical training for women with fibromyalgia. *Journal of Rheumatology, 21,* 714–720.

Carter, G. T., Jensen, M. P., Galer, B. S., Kraft, G. H., Crabtree, L. D., Beardsley, R. M., Abresch, R. T., & Bird, T. D. (1998). Neuropathic pain in Charcot–Marie–Tooth disease. *Archives of Physical Medicine and Rehabilitation, 79,* 1560–1564.

Cassisi, J. E., Robinson, M. E., O'Conner, P., & MacMillan, M. (1993). Trunk strength and lumbar paraspinal muscle activity during isometric exercise in chronic low-back pain patients and controls. *Spine, 18,* 245–251.

Chard, J. A., & Lilford, R. J. (1998). The use of equipoise in clinical trials. *Social Science and Medicine, 47,* 891–898.

Chow, S. C., & Liu, J. P. (1998). *Design and analysis of clinical trials: Concept and methodologies.* New York: Wiley.

Connally, G. H., & Sanders, S. H. (1991). Predicting low back pain patients' response to lumbar sympathetic nerve blocks and interdisciplinary rehabilitation: The role of pretreatment overt pain behavior and cognitive coping strategies. *Pain, 44,* 139–146.

Cooper, S. A. (1991). Single-dose analgesic studies: The upside and downside of assay sensitivity. In M. Max, R. Portenoy, & E. Laska (Eds.), *Advances in pain research and therapy* (Vol. 18, pp. 117–124). New York: Raven Press.

Daltroy, L. H., Cats-Baril, W. L., Katz, J. N., Fossel, A. H., & Liang, M. H. (1996). The North American Spine Society lumbar spine outcome assessment instrument. *Spine, 21,* 741–749.

De Conno, F., Caraceni, A., Gamba, A., Mariani, L., Abbattista, A., Brunelli, C., La Mura, A., & Ventafridda, V. (1994). Pain measurement in cancer patients: A comparison of six methods. *Pain, 57,* 161–166.

De Gagné, T. A., Mikail, S. F., & D'Eon, J. L. (1995). Confirmatory factor analysis of a four-factor model of chronic pain evaluation. *Pain, 60,* 195–202.

Derogatis, L. R. (1983). *SCL-90-R: Administration, scoring, and procedures manual* (2nd ed.). Towson, MD: Clinical Psychometric Research.

Deyo, R. A., Diehr, P., & Patrick, D. L. (1991). Reproducibility and responsiveness of health status measures. Statistics and strategies for evaluation. *Controlled Clinical Trials, 12*(Suppl.), S142–S158.

Donaldson, G. W. (1995). The factorial structure and stability of the McGill Pain Questionnaire in patients experiencing oral mucositis following bone marrow transplantation. *Pain, 62,* 101–109.

Duncan, G. H., Bushnell, M. C., & Lavigne, G. J. (1989). Comparison of verbal and visual analogue scales for measuring the intensity and unpleasantness of experimental pain. *Pain, 37,* 295–303.

Dworkin, R. H. (1997a). Pain and its assessment in herpes zoster. *Antiviral Chemistry and Chemotherapy, 8,* 31–36.

Dworkin, R. H. (1997b). Which individuals with acute pain are most likely to develop a chronic pain syndrome? *Pain Forum, 6,* 127–136.

Dworkin, R. H. (1999). *Anticonvulsant efficacy in neuropathic pain and its relationship to pain quality.* Paper presented at the meeting of the American Pain Society, Fort Lauderdale, FL.

Dworkin, R. H., & Caligor, E. (1988). Psychiatric diagnosis and chronic pain: DSM-III-R and beyond. *Journal of Pain and Symptom Management, 3*, 87–98.

Dworkin, R. H., Carrington, D., Cunningham, A., Kost, R. G., Levin, M. J., McKendrick, M. W., Oxman, M. N., Rentier, B., Schmader, K. E., Tappeiner, G., Wassilew, S. W., & Whitley, R. J. (1997). Assessment of pain in herpes zoster: Lessons learned from antiviral trials. *Antiviral Research, 33*, 73–85.

Dworkin, R. H., & Gitlin, M. J. (1991). Clinical aspects of depression in chronic pain patients. *Clinical Journal of Pain, 7*, 79–94.

Dworkin, R. H., Handlin, D. S., Richlin, D. M., Brand, L., & Vannucci, C. (1985). Unraveling the effects of compensation, litigation, and employment on treatment response in chronic pain. *Pain, 23*, 49–59.

Dworkin, S. F., Turner, J. A., Wilson, L., Massoth, D., Whitney, C., Huggins, K. H., Burgess, J., Sommers, E., & Truelove, E. (1994). Brief group cognitive-behavioral intervention for temporomandibular disorders. *Pain, 59*, 175–187.

Dworkin, S. F., Von Korff, M., & LeResche, L. (1990). Multiple pains and psychiatric disturbance: An epidemiologic investigation. *Archives of General Psychiatry, 47*, 239–244.

Ehrich, E. W., Schnitzer, T. J., McIlwain, H., Levy, R., Wolfe, F., Weisman, M., Zeng, Q., Morrison, B., Bolognese, J., Seidenberg, B., & Gertz, B. J. (1999). Effect of specific COX-2 inhibition in osteoarthritis of the knee: A 6 week double blind, placebo controlled pilot study of rofecoxib. Rofecoxib Osteoarthritis Pilot Study Group. *Journal of Rheumatology, 26*, 2438–2447.

Eisenberg, E., Alon, N., Ishay, A., Daoud, D., & Yarnitsky, D. (1998). Lamotrigine in the treatment of painful diabetic neuropathy. *European Journal of Neurology, 5*, 167–173.

Farrar, J. T., Portenoy, R. K., Berlin, J. A., Kinman, J. L., & Strom, B. L. (2000). Defining the clinically important difference in pain outcome measures. *Pain, 88*, 287–294.

Fernandez, E., & Towery, S. (1996). A parsimonious set of verbal descriptors of pain sensation derived from the McGill Pain Questionnaire. *Pain, 66*, 31–37.

Fernandez, E., & Turk, D. C. (1992). Sensory and affective components of pain: Separation and synthesis. *Psychological Bulletin, 112*, 205–217.

Fernandez, E., & Turk, D. C. (1994). Demand characteristics underlying differential ratings of sensory versus affective components of pain. *Journal of Behavioral Medicine, 17*, 375–390.

Feuerstein, M., Greenwald, M., Gamache, M. P., Papciak, A. S., & Cook, E. W. (1985). The Pain Behavior Scale: Modificiation and validation for outpatient use. *Journal of Psychopathology and Behavioral Assessment, 7*, 301–315.

First, M. B., Gibbon, M., Spitzer, R. L., & Williams, J. B. W. (Eds.). (1997). *Structured Clinical Interview for DSM-IV Axis I Disorders–Clinician Version (SCID-CV).* Washington, DC: American Psychiatric Press.

Fishbain, D. A., Cutler, R., Rosomoff, H. L., & Rosomoff, R. S. (1997). Chronic pain-associated depression: Antecedent or consequence of chronic pain? *Clinical Journal of Pain, 13*, 116–137.

Fishbain, D. A., Goldberg, M., Labbe, E., Steele, R., & Rosomoff, H. (1988). Compensation and non-compensation chronic pain patients compared for DSM-III operational diagnoses. *Pain, 32*, 197–206.

Fishman, B., Pasternak, S., Wallenstein, S. L, Houde, R. W., Holland, J. C., & Foley, K. M. (1987). The Memorial Pain Assessment Card: A valid instrument for the evaluation of cancer pain. *Cancer, 60*, 1151–1158.

Flor, H., Haag, G., Turk, D. C., & Koehler, H. (1983). Efficacy of EMG biofeedback, pseudotherapy, and conventional medical treatment for chronic rheumatic back pain. *Pain, 17*, 21–31.

Follick, M. J., Smith, T. W., & Ahern, D. K. (1985). The Sickness Impact Profile: A global measure of disability in chronic low back pain. *Pain, 21*, 67–76.

Fordyce, W. E. (1976). *Behavioral methods for chronic pain and illness.* St. Louis, MO: Mosby.

Freedman, B. (1987). Equipoise and the ethics of clinical research. *New England Journal of Medicine, 317*, 141–145.

Galer, B. S., & Jensen, M. P. (1997). Development and preliminary validation of a pain measure specific to neuropathic pain: The Neuropathic Pain Scale. *Neurology, 48*, 332–338.

Galer, B. S., Rowbotham, M. C., Perander, J., & Friedman, E. (1999). Topical lidocaine patch relieves postherpetic neuralgia more effectively than a vehicle topical patch: Results of an enriched enrollment study. *Pain, 80*, 533–538.

Gatchel, R. J., Polatin, P. B., & Mayer, T. G. (1995). The dominant role of psychosocial risk factors in the development of chronic low back pain disability. *Spine, 20*, 2702–2709.

Gatchel, R. J., & Turk, D. C. (Eds.). (1999). *Psychosocial factors in pain: Critical perspectives.* New York: Guilford Press.

Ginsberg, D. (Ed.). (1999). *The investigator's guide to clinical research.* Boston: CenterWatch.

Gracely, R. H. (1992). Evaluation of multi-dimensional pain scales. *Pain, 48*, 297–300.

Gracely, R. H., & Kwilosz, D. M. (1988). The Descriptor Differential Scale: Applying psychophysical principles to pain assessment. *Pain, 35*, 279–288.

Gracely, R. H., McGrath, P., & Dubner, R. (1978a). Ratio scales of sensory and affective verbal pain descriptors. *Pain, 5*, 5–18.

Gracely, R. H., McGrath, P., & Dubner, R. (1978b). Validity and sensitivity of ratio scales of sensory and affective verbal pain descriptors: Manipulation of affect by diazepam. *Pain, 5*, 19–29.

Guck, T. P., Skultety, F. M., Meilman, P. W., & Dowd, E. T. (1985). Multidisciplinary pain center follow-up study: Evaluation with a no-treatment control group. *Pain, 21*, 295–306.

Guy, W. (1976). *ECDEU assessment manual for psychopharmacology* (DHEW Publication No. ADM 76-338). Washington, DC: U.S. Government Printing Office.

Guyatt, G. H., Feeny, D. H., & Patrick, D. L. (1993). Measuring health-related quality of life. *Annals of Internal Medicine, 118*, 622–629.

Guyatt, G. H., Walter, S., & Norman, G. (1987). Measuring change over time: Assessing the usefulness of evaluative instruments. *Journal of Chronic Diseases, 40*, 171–178.

Hamilton, M. (1960). A rating scale for depression. *Journal of Neurology, Neurosurgery and Psychiatry, 23*, 56–62.

Holroyd, K. A., Holm, J. E., Keefe, F. J., Turner, J. A., Bradley, L. A., Murphy, W. D., Johnson, P., Anderson, K., Hinkle, A. L., & O'Malley, W. B. (1992). A multi-center evaluation of the McGill Pain Questionnaire: Results from more than 1700 chronic pain patients. *Pain, 48*, 301–311.

Holroyd, K. A., Malinoski, P., Davis, M. K., & Lipchik, G. L. (1999). The three dimensions of headache impact: Pain, disability and affective distress. *Pain, 83*, 571–578.

Holroyd, K. A., Talbot, F., Holm, J. E., Pingel, J. D., Lake, A. E., & Saper, J. R. (1996). Assessing the dimensions of pain: A multitrait-multimethod evaluation of seven measures. *Pain, 67*, 259–265.

Hope, P., & Forshaw, M. J. (1999). Assessment of psychological distress is important in patients presenting with low back pain. *Physiotherapy, 85*, 563–570.

Jacobson, G. P., Ramadan, N. M., Aggarwal, S. K., & Newman, C. W. (1994). The Henry Ford Hospital Headache Disability Inventory (HDI). *Neurology, 44*, 837–842.

Jamison, R. N., & Brown, G. K. (1991). Validation of hourly pain intensity profiles with chronic pain patients. *Pain, 45*, 123–128.

Jamison, R. N., Rudy, T. E., Penzien, D. B., & Mosley, T. H., Jr. (1994). Cognitive-behavioral classifications of chronic pain: Replication and extension of empirically derived patient profiles. *Pain, 57*, 277–292.

Jasinski, D. R., Martin, W. R., & Sapira, J. D. (1967). Antagonism of the subjective, behavioral, pupillary, and respiratory depressant effects of cyclazocine by naloxone. *Clinical Pharmacology and Therapeutics, 9*, 215–222.

Jensen, M. P., Karoly, P., & Braver, S. (1986). The measurement of clinical pain intensity: A comparison of six methods. *Pain, 27*, 117–126.

Jensen, M. P., Karoly, P., & Harris, P. (1991). Assessing the affective component of chronic pain: Development of the Pain Discomfort Scale. *Journal of Psychosomatic Research, 35*, 149–154.

Jensen, M. P., Karoly, P., O'Riordan, E. F., Bland, F., Jr., & Burns, R. S. (1989). The subjective experience of acute pain: An assessment of the utility of 10 indices. *Clinical Journal of Pain, 5*, 153–159.

Jensen, M. P. & McFarland, C. A. (1993). Increasing the reliability and validity of pain intensity measurement in chronic pain patients. *Pain, 55*, 195–203.

Jensen, M. P., Miller, L., & Fisher, L. D. (1998). Assessment of pain during medical procedures: A comparison of three scales. *Clinical Journal of Pain, 14*, 343–349.

Jensen, M. P., Strom, S. E., Turner, J. A., & Romano, J. M. (1992). Validity of the Sickness Impact Profile Roland scale as a measure of dysfunction in chronic pain patients. *Pain, 50*, 157–162.

Jensen, M. P., Turner, J. A., & Romano, J. M. (1994). What is the maximum number of levels needed in pain intensity measurement? *Pain, 58*, 387–392.

Jensen, M. P., Turner, J. A., Romano, J. M., & Fisher, L. D. (1999). Comparative reliability and validity of chronic pain intensity measures. *Pain, 83*, 157–162.

Jensen, M. P., Turner, J. A., Romano, J. M., & Karoly, P. (1991). Coping with chronic pain: A critical review of the literature. *Pain, 47*, 249–283.

Jensen, M. P., Turner, L. R., Turner, J. A., & Romano, J. M. (1996). The use of multiple-item scales for pain intensity measurement in chronic pain patients. *Pain, 67*, 35–40.

Kames, L. D., Naliboff, B. D., Heinrich, R. L., & Schag, C. C. (1984). The Chronic Illness Problem Inventory: Problem-oriented psychosocial assessment of patients with chronic illness. *International Journal of Psychiatry in Medicine, 14*, 65–75.

Katz, J., Clairoux, M., Redahan, C., Kavanagh, B. P., Carroll, S., Nierenberg, H., Jackson, M., Beattie, J., Taddio, A., & Sandler, A. N. (1996). High dose alfentanil pre-empts pain after abdominal hysterectomy. *Pain, 68*, 109–118.

Keefe, F. J., & Dunsmore, J. (1992). Pain behavior: Concepts and controversies. *American Pain Society Journal, 1*, 92–100.

Keefe, F. J., & Hill, R. W. (1985). An objective approach to quantifying pain behavior and gait patterns in low back pain patients. *Pain, 21*, 153–161.

Kerns, R. D., Finn, P., & Haythornthwaite, J. (1988). Self-monitored pain intensity: Psychometric properties and clinical utility. *Journal of Behavioral Medicine, 11*, 71–82.

Kerns, R. D., Turk, D. C., & Rudy, T. E. (1985). The West Haven–Yale Multidimensional Pain Inventory (WHYMPI). *Pain, 23*, 345–356.

Kieburtz, K., Simpson, D., Yiannoutsos, C., Max, M. B., Hall, C. D., Ellis, R. J., Marra, C. M., McKendall, R., Singer, E., Dal Pan, G. J., Clifford, D. B., Tucker, T., Cohen, B., & the AIDS Clinical Trial Group 242 Protocol Team. (1998). A randomized trial of amitriptyline and mexiletine for painful neuropathy in HIV infection. *Neurology, 51*, 1682–1688.

Klapow, J. C., Slater, M. A., Patterson, T. L., Atkinson, J. H., Weickgenant, A. L., Grant, I., & Garfin, S. R. (1995). Psychosocial factors discriminate multidimensional clinical groups of chronic low back pain patients. *Pain, 62*, 349–355.

Klapow, J. C., Slater, M. A., Patterson, T. L., Doctor, J. N., Atkinson, J. H., & Garfin, S. R. (1993). An empirical evaluation of multidimensional clinical outcome in chronic low back pain patients. *Pain, 55*, 107–118.

Klepac, R. K., Dowling, J., Rokke, P., Dodge, L., & Schafer, L. (1981). Interview vs. paper-and-pencil administration of the McGill Pain Questionnaire. *Pain, 11*, 241–246.

Kornguth, P. J., Keefe, F. J., & Conaway, M. R. (1996). Pain during mammography: Characteristics and relationship to demographic and medical variables. *Pain, 66*, 187–194.

Kraemer, H. C. (Ed.). (1992). *Evaluating medical tests: Objective and quantitative guidelines.* Newbury Park, CA: Sage.

Kremer, E., Atkinson, J. H., & Ignelzi, R. J. (1981). Measurement of pain: Patient preference does not confound pain measurement. *Pain, 10*, 241–248.

Laska, E. M., Siegel, C., & Sunshine, A. (1991). Onset and duration: Measurement and analysis. In M. Max, R. Portenoy, & E. Laska (Eds.), *Advances in pain research and therapy* (Vol. 18, pp. 691–698). New York: Raven Press.

Lehmann, K. A. (1990). Patient-controlled analgesia for postoperative pain. In C. Benedetti, C. R. Chapman, & G. Giron (Eds.), *Advances in pain research and therapy* (Vol. 14, pp. 297–324). New York: Raven Press.

Lilford, R. J., & Jackson, J. (1995). Equipoise and the ethics of randomization. *Journal of the Royal Society of Medicine, 88*, 552–559.

Linton, S. J., & Melin, L. (1982). The accuracy of remembering chronic pain. *Pain*, *13*, 281–285.

Littman, G. S., Walker, B. R., & Schneider, B. E. (1985). Reassessment of verbal and visual analog ratings in analgesic studies. *Clinical Pharmacology and Therapeutics*, *38*, 16–23.

Lowe, N. K., Walker, S. N., & MacCallum, R. C. (1991). Confirming the theoretical structure of the McGill Pain Questionnaire in acute clinical pain. *Pain*, *46*, 53–60.

Lydick, E., & Epstein, R. S. (1993). Interpretation of quality of life changes. *Quality of Life Research*, *2*, 221–226.

Lydick, E., Epstein, R. S., Himmelberger, D., & White, C. J. (1995). Area under the curve: A metric for patient subjective responses in episodic diseases. *Quality of Life Research*, *4*, 41–45.

Malec, J., Cayner, J. J., Harvey, R. F., & Timming, R. C. (1981). Pain management: Long-term follow-up of an inpatient program. *Archives of Physical Medicine and Rehabilitation*, *62*, 369–372.

Mauskopf, J. A., Austin, R., Dix, L. P., & Berzon, R. A. (1994). The Nottingham Health Profile as a measure of quality of life in zoster patients: Convergent and discriminant validity. *Quality of Life Research*, *3*, 431–435.

Mauskopf, J. A., Austin, R., Dix, L. P., & Berzon, R. A. (1995). Estimating the value of a generic quality-of-life measure. *Medical Care*, *33*, AS195–AS202.

Max, M. B. (1991). Neuropathic pain syndromes. In M. Max, R. Portenoy, & E. Laska (Eds.), *Advances in pain research and therapy* (Vol. 18, pp. 193–219). New York: Raven Press.

Max, M. B. (1994a). Divergent traditions in analgesic clinical trials. *Clinical Pharmacology and Therapeutics*, *56*, 237–241.

Max, M. B. (1994b). Antidepressants as analgesics. In H. L. Fields & J. C. Liebeskind (Eds.), *Pharmacological approaches to the treatment of chronic pain: New concepts and critical issues* (pp. 229–246). Seattle, WA: International Association for the Study of Pain Press.

Max, M. B. (1994c). Combining opioids with other drugs: Challenges in clinical trial design. In G. F. Gebhart, D. L. Hammond, & T. S. Jensen (Eds.), *Proceedings of the 7th World Congress on Pain* (pp. 569–586). Seattle, WA: International Association for the Study of Pain Press.

Max, M. B., Culnane, M., Schafer, S. C., Gracely, R. H., Walther, D. J., Smoller, B., & Dubner, R. (1987). Amitriptyline relieves diabetic neuropathy pain in patients with normal or depressed mood. *Neurology*, *37*, 589–596.

Max, M. B., & Laska, E. M. (1991). Single-dose analgesic comparisons. In M. Max, R. Portenoy, & E. Laska (Eds.), *Advances in pain research and therapy* (Vol. 18, pp. 55–95). New York: Raven Press.

Max, M. B., Lynch, S. A., Muir, J., Shoaf, S. E., Smoller, B., & Dubner, R. (1992). Effects of desipramine, amitriptyline, and fluoxetine on pain in diabetic neuropathy. *New England Journal of Medicine*, *326*, 1250–1256.

Max, M. B., Portenoy, R. K., & Laska, E. M. (Eds.) (1991). *Advances in pain research and therapy* (Vol. 18). New York: Raven Press.

McNair, D. M., Lorr, M., & Droppleman, L. F. (1971). *Profile of Mood States*. San Diego, CA: Educational and Industrial Testing Service.

McQuay, H., Carroll, D., & Moore, A. (1995). Variation in the placebo effect in randomized controlled trials of analgesics: All is as blind as it seems. *Pain*, *64*, 331–335.

McQuay, H., & Moore, A. (1998). *An evidence-based resource for pain*. Oxford: Oxford University Press.

Mechanic, D., Cleary, P. D., & Greenley, J. R. (1982). Distress syndromes, illness behavior, access to care and medical utilization in a defined population. *Medical Care*, *20*, 361–372.

Meinert, C.L., & Tonascia, S. (1986). *Clinical trials: Design, conduct, and analysis*. Oxford: Oxford University Press.

Melzack, R. (1975). The McGill Pain Questionnaire: Major properties and scoring methods. *Pain*, *1*, 277–299.

Melzack, R. (1985). Re: Discriminative capacity of the McGill Pain Questionnaire. *Pain*, *23*, 201–203.

Melzack, R. (1987). The short-form McGill Pain Questionnaire. *Pain*, *30*, 191–197.

Melzack, R., & Casey, K. L. (1968). Sensory, motivational and central control determinants of pain: A new conceptual model. In D. R. Kenshalo (Ed.), *The skin senses* (pp. 423–443). Springfield, IL: Charles C Thomas.

Melzack, R., Katz, J., & Jeans, M. E. (1985). The role of compensation in chronic pain: Analysis using a new method of scoring the McGill Pain Questionnaire. *Pain*, *23*, 101–112.

Merskey, H., & Bogduk, N. (Eds.). (1994). *Classification of chronic pain: Descriptions of chronic pain syndromes and definitions of pain terms* (2nd. ed.). Seattle, WA: International Association for the Study of Pain Press.

Mikail, S. F., DuBreuil, S., & D'Eon, J. L. (1993). A comparative analysis of measures used in the assessment of chronic pain patients. *Psychological Assessment*, *5*, 117–120.

Million, R., Nilsen, K. H., Jayson, M. I., & Baker, R. D. (1981). Evaluation of low back pain and assessment of lumbar corsets with and without back supports. *Annals of the Rheumatic Diseases*, *40*, 449–454.

Moore, A., Moore, O., McQuay, H., & Gavaghan, D. (1997). Deriving dichotomous outcome measures from continuous data in randomised controlled trials of analgesics: Use of pain intensity and visual analogue scales. *Pain*, *69*, 311–315.

Morrison, B. W., Daniels, S. E., Kotey, P., Cantu, N., & Seidenberg, B. (1999). Rofecoxib, a specific cyclooxygenase-2 inhibitor, in primary dysmenorrhea: A randomized controlled trial. *Obstetrics and Gynecology*, *94*, 504–508.

Nelson, K. A., Park, K. M., Robinovitz, E., Tsigos, C., & Max, M. B. (1997). High-dose oral dextromethorphan versus placebo in painful diabetic neuropathy and postherpetic neuralgia. *Neurology*, *48*, 1212–1218.

Oerlemans, H. M., Oostendorp, R. A., de Boo, T., & Goris, R. J. (1999). Pain and reduced mobility in complex regional pain syndrome: I. Outcome of a prospective randomised controlled clinical trial of adjuvant physical therapy versus occupational therapy. *Pain*, *83*, 77–83.

Okifuji, A. T., Turk, D. C., & Kalauokalani, D. (1999). Clinical outcome and economic evaluation of multidisciplinary pain centers. In A. R. Block, E. F. Kremer, & E. Fernandez (Eds.), *Handbook of pain syndromes: Biopsychosocial perspectives* (pp. 77–97). Mahwah, NJ: Erlbaum.

Oxman, M. N. (1994). *Trial of varicella vaccine for the prevention of herpes zoster and its complications (VA Cooperative Study no. 403): Vol. 1. Protocol.* San Diego, CA: Infectious Diseases Section, Veterans Affairs Medical Center.

Pablos-Méndez, A., Barr, R. G., & Shea, S. (1998). Run-in periods in randomized trials: Implications for the application of results in clinical practice. *Journal of the American Medical Association, 279,* 222–225.

Peters, J. L., & Large, R. G. (1990). A randomised control trial evaluating in- and outpatient pain management programmes. *Pain, 41,* 283–293.

Peters, J. L., Large, R. G., & Elkind, G. (1992). Follow-up results from a randomised controlled trial evaluating in- and outpatient pain management programmes. *Pain, 50,* 41–50.

Piantadosi, S. (Ed.). (1997). *Clinical trials: A methodologic perspective.* New York: Wiley.

Pilowsky, I., & Barrow, C. G. (1990). A controlled study of psychotherapy and amitriptyline used individually and in combination in the treatment of chronic intractable, 'psychogenic' pain. *Pain, 40,* 3–19.

Pocock, S. J. (Ed.). (1984). *Clinical trials: A practical approach.* New York: Wiley.

Portenoy, R. K. (1991). Cancer pain: General design issues. In M. Max, R. Portenoy, & E. Laska (Eds.), *Advances in pain research and therapy* (Vol. 18, pp. 233–266). New York: Raven Press.

Price, D. D. (Ed.). (1999). *Progress in pain research and management: Vol. 15. Psychological mechanisms of pain and analgesia.* Seattle, WA: International Association for the Study of Pain Press.

Price, D. D., Bush, F. M., Long, S., & Harkins, S. W. (1994). A comparison of pain measurement characteristics of mechanical visual analogue and simple numerical rating scales. *Pain, 56,* 217–226.

Price, D. D., McGrath, P. A., Rafii, A. & Buckingham, B. (1983). The validation of visual analogue scales as ratio scale measures for chronic and experimental pain, *Pain, 17,* 45–56.

Price, D. D., Milling, L. S., Kirsch, I., Duff, A., Montgomery, G. H., & Nicholls, S. S. (1999). An analysis of factors that contribute to the magnitude of placebo analgesia in an experimental paradigm. *Pain, 83,* 147–156.

Quitkin, F. M. (1999). Placebos, drug effects, and study design: A clinician's guide. *American Journal of Psychiatry, 156,* 829–836.

Radloff, L. S. (1977). The CES-D scale: A self-report depression scale for research in the general population. *Applied Psychological Measurement, 1,* 385–401.

Reading, A. E. (1982). A comparison of the McGill Pain Questionnaire in chronic and acute pain. *Pain, 13,* 185–192.

Reading, A. E., & Newton, J. R. (1977). A comparison of primary dysmenorrhoea and intrauterine device related pain. *Pain, 3,* 265–276.

Redelmeier, D. A., & Kahneman, D. (1996). Patients' memories of painful medical treatments: Real-time and retrospective evaluations of two minimally invasive procedures. *Pain, 66,* 3–8.

Reinhart, D. J., Wang, W., Stagg, K. S., Walker, K. G., Bailey, P. L., Walker, E. B., & Zaugg, S. E. (1996). Postoperative analgesia after peripheral nerve block for podiatric surgery: Clinical efficacy and chemical stability of lidocaine alone versus lidocaine plus clonidine. *Anesthesia and Analgesia, 83,* 760–765.

Roberts, A. H., & Reinhardt, L. (1980). The behavioral management of chronic pain: Long-term follow-up with comparison groups. *Pain, 8,* 151–162.

Rohling, M. L., Binder, L. M., & Langhinrichsen-Rohling, J. (1995). Money matters: A meta-analytic review of the association between financial compensation and the experience and treatment of chronic pain. *Health Psychology, 14,* 537–547.

Roland, M., & Morris, R. (1983). A study of the natural history of back pain: Part 1 Development of a reliable and sensitive measure of disability in low-back pain. *Spine, 8,* 141–144.

Romano, J. M., Turner, J. A., & Jensen, M. P. (1992). The Chronic Illness Problem Inventory as a measure of dysfunction in chronic pain patients. *Pain, 49,* 71–75.

Rowbotham, M., Harden, N., Stacey, B., Bernstein, P., & Magnus-Miller, L. (1998). Gabapentin for the treatment of postherpetic neuralgia: A randomized controlled trial. *Journal of the American Medical Association, 280,* 1837–1842.

Rudy, T. E., Turk, D. C., Brena, S. F., Stieg, R. L., & Brody, M. C. (1990). Quantification of biomedical findings of chronic pain patients: Development of an index of pathology. *Pain, 42,* 167–182.

Rudy, T. E., Turk, D. C., & Brody, M. C. (1992). Quantification of biomedical findings in chronic pain: Problems and solutions. In D. C. Turk & R. Melzack (Eds.), *Handbook of pain assessment* (pp. 447–469). New York: Guilford Press.

Salovey, P., Smith, A. F., Turk, D. C., Jobe, J. B., & Willis, G. B. (1993). The accuracy of memory for pain: Not so bad most of the time. *American Pain Society Journal, 2,* 184–191.

Schwartz, D. & Lellouch, J. (1967). Explanatory and pragmatic attitudes in therapeutical trials. *Journal of Chronic Diseases, 20,* 637–648.

Senn, S. (Ed.). (1993). *Cross-over trials in clinical research.* New York: Wiley.

Senn, S. (Ed.). (1997). *Statistical issues in drug development.* New York: Wiley.

Seres, J. L. (1999). The fallacy of using 50% pain relief as the standard for satisfactory pain treatment outcome. *Pain Forum, 8,* 183–188.

Shacham, S. (1983). A shortened version of the Profile of Mood States. *Journal of Personality Assessment, 47,* 305–306.

Sheiner, L. B., & Rubin, D. B. (1995). Intention-to-treat analysis and the goals of clinical trials. *Clinical Pharmacology and Therapeutics, 57,* 6–15.

Shirley, F. R., O'Connor, P., Robinson, M. E., & MacMillan, M. (1994). Comparison of lumbar range of motion using three measurement devices in patients with chronic low back pain. *Spine, 19,* 779–783.

Silverman, D. G., O'Connor, T. Z., & Brull, S. J. (1993). Integrated assessment of pain scores and rescue morphine use during studies of analgesic efficacy. *Anesthesia and Analgesia, 77,* 168–170.

Simon, L. S., Weaver, A. L., Graham, D. Y., Kivitz, A. J., Lipsky, P. E., Hubbard, R. C., Isakson, P. C., Verburg, K. M., Yu, S. S., Zhao, W. W., & Geis, G. S. (1999). Anti-inflammatory and upper gastrointestinal effects of celecoxib in rheumatoid arthritis: A randomized controlled trial. *Journal of the American Medical Association, 282,* 1921–1928.

Smith, B. H., Penny, K. I., Purves, A. M., Munro, C., Wilson, B., Grimshaw, J., Chambers, W. A., & Smith, W. C. (1997). The Chronic Pain Grade questionnaire: Validation and reliability in postal research. *Pain*, *71*, 141–147.

Smith, C. M., Guralnick, M. S., Gelfand, M. M., & Jeans, M. E. (1986). The effects of transcutaneous electrical nerve stimulation on post-cesarean pain. *Pain*, *27*, 181–193.

Smith, W. B., Gracely, R. H., & Safer, M. A. (1998). The meaning of pain: Cancer patients' rating and recall of pain intensity and affect. *Pain*, *78*, 123–129.

Solomon, G. D. (1997). Evolution of the measurement of quality of life in migraine. *Neurology*, *48*, S10–S15.

Stacey, B., Rowbotham, M., Harden, N., Magnus-Miller, L., & Bernstein, P. (1999, August). *Effects of gabapentin (Neurontin) on pain quality in patients with postherpetic neuralgia (PHN)*. Poster session presented at the Ninth World Congress on Pain, Vienna.

Steedman, S. M., Middaugh, S. J., Kee, W. G., Carson, D. S., Harden, R. N., & Miller, M. C. (1992). Chronic-pain medications: Equivalence levels and method of quantifying usage. *Clinical Journal of Pain*, *8*, 204–214.

Sternbach, R. A. (1974). *Pain patients: Traits and treatment*. New York: Academic Press.

Stewart, W. F., Lipton, R. B., Simon, D., Liberman, J., & Von Korff, M. (1999). Validity of an illness severity measure for headache in a population sample of migraine sufferers. *Pain*, *79*, 291–301.

Streiner, D. L., & Norman, G. R. (1995). *Health measurement scales: A practical guide to their development and use*. New York: Oxford University Press.

Syrjala, K. L., Cummings, C., & Donaldson, G. W. (1992). Hypnosis or cognitive behavioral training for the reduction of pain and nausea during cancer treatment: A controlled clinical trial. *Pain*, *48*, 137–146.

Tait, R. C., Chibnall, J. T., & Krause, S. (1990). The Pain Disability Index: Psychometric properties. *Pain*, *40*, 171–182.

Tait, R. C., Chibnall, J. T., & Richardson, W. D. (1990). Litigation and employment status: Effects on patients with chronic pain. *Pain*, *43*, 37–46.

Towery, S., & Fernandez, E. (1996). Reclassification and rescaling of McGill Pain Questionnaire verbal descriptors of pain sensation: A replication. *Clinical Journal of Pain*, *12*, 270–276.

Turk, D. C. (1990). Customizing treatment for chronic pain patients: Who, what, and why. *Clinical Journal of Pain*, *6*, 255–270.

Turk, D. C., & Flor, H. (1987). Pain is greater than pain behaviors: The utility and limitations of the pain behavior construct. *Pain*, *31*, 277–295.

Turk, D. C., & Okifuji, A. (1998, September–October). Directions in prescriptive chronic pain management based on diagnostic characteristics of the patient. *American Pain Society Bulletin*, pp. 5–12.

Turk, D. C., Okifuji, A., Sinclair, J. D., & Starz, T. W. (1998). Differential responses by psychosocial subgroups of fibromyalgia syndrome patients to an interdisciplinary treatment. *Arthritis Care and Research*, *11*, 397–404.

Turk, D. C., & Rudy, T. E. (1988). Toward an empirically derived taxonomy of chronic pain patients: Integration of psychological assessment data. *Journal of Consulting and Clinical Psychology*, *56*, 233–238.

Turk, D. C., & Rudy, T. E. (1990). The robustness of an empirically derived taxonomy of chronic pain patients. *Pain*, *43*, 27–35.

Turk, D. C., & Rudy, T. E. (1991). Neglected topics in the treatment of chronic pain patients: Relapse, noncompliance, and adherence enhancement. *Pain*, *44*, 5–28.

Turk, D. C., Rudy, T. E., & Salovey, P. (1985). The McGill Pain Questionnaire reconsidered: Confirming the factor structure and examining appropriate uses. *Pain*, *21*, 385–397.

Turk, D. C., Rudy, T. E., & Sorkin, B. A. (1993). Neglected topics in chronic pain treatment outcome studies: Determination of success. *Pain*, *53*, 3–16.

Turner, J. A., Deyo, R. A., Loeser, J. D., Von Korff, M., & Fordyce, W. E. (1994). The importance of placebo effects in pain treatment and research. *Journal of the American Medical Association*, *271*, 1609–1614.

Turner, J. A., & Jensen, M. P. (1993). Efficacy of cognitive therapy for chronic low back pain. *Pain*, *52*, 169–177.

Tursky, B., Jamner, L. D., & Friedman, R. (1982). The Pain Perception Profile: A psychophysical approach to the assessment of pain report. *Behavior Therapy*, *13*, 376–394.

Von Korff, M., Ormel, J., Keefe, F. J., & Dworkin, S. F. (1992). Grading the severity of chronic pain. *Pain*, *50*, 133–149.

Ware, J. E., & Sherbourne, C. D. (1992). The MOS 36-Item Short-Form Health Survey (SF-36): Conceptual framework and item selection. *Medical Care*, *30*, 473–483.

Watson, C. P. N., & Babul, N. (1998). Efficacy of oxycodone in neuropathic pain: A randomized trial in postherpetic neuralgia. *Neurology*, *50*, 1837–1841.

Watson, C. P. N., Vernich, L., Chipman, M., & Reed, K. (1998). Nortriptyline versus amitriptyline in postherpetic neuralgia: A randomized trial. *Neurology*, *51*, 1166–1171.

Weinberger, M., Nagle, B., Hanlon, J. T., Samsa, G. P., Schmader, K., Landsman, P. B., Uttech, K. M., Cowper, P. A., Cohen, H. J., & Feussner, J. R. (1994). Assessing health-related quality of life in elderly outpatients: Telephone versus face-to-face administration. *Journal of the American Geriatrics Society*, *42*, 1295–1299.

Weinberger, M., Oddone, E. Z., Samsa, G. P., & Landsman, P. B. (1996). Are health-related quality-of-life measures affected by the mode of administration? *Journal of Clinical Epidemiology*, *49*, 135–140.

Williams, D. A., Urban, B., Keefe, F. J., Shutty, M. S., & France, R. (1995). Cluster analyses of pain patients' responses to the SCL-90R. *Pain*, *61*, 81–91.

Williams, J. B. W. (1988). A structured interview guide for the Hamilton Depression Rating Scale. *Archives of General Psychiatry*, *45*, 742–747.

Wood, M. J. (1995). How should zoster trials be conducted? *Journal of Antimicrobial Chemotherapy*, *36*, 1089–1101.

Wood, M. J., Kay, R., Dworkin, R. H., Soong, S.-J., & Whitley, R. J. (1996). Oral acyclovir therapy accelerates pain resolution in patients with herpes zoster: A meta-analysis of placebo-controlled trials. *Clinical Infectious Diseases*, *22*, 341–347.

Woolf, C. J., & Mannion, R. J. (1999). Neuropathic pain: Aetiology, symptoms, mechanisms, and management. *Lancet*, *353*, 1959–1964.

Chapter 35

The Future of Imaging in Assessment of Chronic Musculoskeletal Pain

ANTHONY JONES

This chapter is intended to raise and discuss some issues concerning the role of both structural and functional imaging in pain management. The main question to be addressed in this chapter is whether both structural and physiological imaging can be used to enhance effective management of chronic pain. Arguments are presented for a much more selective use of structural imaging. A more formal and integrated organization of primary, secondary, and tertiary pain management is proposed, to allow this to happen effectively and safely. Lastly, some suggestions are made as to how physiological (functional) imaging can inform the development of more effective therapeutic strategies and underpin the development of new therapies.

Modern imaging techniques are able to provide an objective description of structure and function in patients. Structural imaging techniques such as plain radiography, computed tomography (CT), ultrasound, and magnetic resonance imaging (MRI) all provide anatomical information (at varying levels of detail) that is, apart from the data provided by ultrasound imaging, routinely static. Functional imaging techniques, which include gamma scintigraphy, single-photon emission computed tomography (SPECT), positron emission tomography (PET), functional magnetic resonance imaging (fMRI), and electrophysiological techniques (electroencephalography [EEG] and magnetoencephalography), all provide different types of imaging of physiological processes—which are by their nature dynamic.

Several comprehensive reviews of these issues have been published recently, and the points made there are not repeated here. Instead, the present discussion centers on the actual and potential use of imaging techniques to change pain therapy and management. Although this discussion focuses on my own particular interest in neuropathic and musculoskeletal pain, many of the principles can be applied more broadly.

The problem with pain is that it is the commonest cause of suffering in patients, but it can also provide an indication of serious underlying pathology. Traditionally, medical students are taught to rigorously identify the source of the nociceptive stimulus, but not much about what to do when pathology has been excluded as the causes of pain. In practice, for many types of chronic pain, it is hard to identify a nociceptive cause of the pain with any degree of certainty. At the end of a series of expensive and sometimes unpleasant investigations, a patient may therefore be no better off. Meanwhile the pain, by definition, has become more chronic. If treatment fails at this point, the patient may be labeled "a chronic pain patient." In the United Kingdom, it is common practice at this point to refer the patient to a chronic pain clinic or orthopedic clinic, which may have a waiting list of up to 1 year.

So it is probably fair to say that in general, imaging of various sorts has a tendency to delay systematic treatment of chronic pain. Such delays are likely to be minimized by rapid access to an informed and integrated combined investigation and treatment strategy for each type of musculoskeletal pain, as I propose here.

In relation to pain management, structural imaging is used mainly to exclude unexpected pathology or to identify a structural abnormality that might be the cause of a patient's pain. However, there is always a small or large leap of faith in attributing the pain to a structural abnormality. Structural imaging therefore diagnoses structural lesions that may be associated with pain, but is rarely able to diagnose the cause of pain with any level of certainty. The danger inherent in structural imaging's being used to diagnose the cause of pain is the implication that ablation (surgically or otherwise) of the structural abnormality should remove the pain. Radiotherapy for metastatic disease is probably one of the few instances in which this ablative approach works consistently. Another is, with some qualifications, hip replacement. The large numbers of patients who have experienced the failure of nonselective lumbar surgery over the last 20 years is one of many examples of the weakness of this approach. Structural imaging, apart from any radiation that may be involved, therefore carries its own inherent dangers of precipitating inappropriate therapy.

CONTRIBUTIONS OF STRUCTURAL IMAGING TO MANAGEMENT OF CHRONIC MUSCULOSKELETAL PAIN

This section describes some of the clinical issues relating to structural imaging for musculoskeletal pain.

Back Pain

What Structural Information Is Useful?

The first indispensable part of any investigation of back pain is a careful history and examination. This may seem very obvious, but an audit of imaging for this disorder in a London community hospital showed that only 5% of patients were fully examined prior to physicians' ordering a plain lumbar radiograph, 76% were partially examined, and 19% were not examined at all (Halpin, Yeoman, & Dundas, 1991). Unfortunately, it takes less time to order an investigation than to examine a patient. The guidelines for

imaging patients with back pain vary greatly, but there is a general consensus that no imaging is recommended in the first 6 weeks of an acute episode of back pain (Chisholm, 1991). Exception to this should be in the rare instance where infection or malignancy is suspected.

The distinction between chronic and acute back pain has probably been exaggerated. Up to 60% of patients with acute back pain may go on to develop chronic or recurrent back pain within the next 3 years (Rossignol, Suissa, & Abenhaim, 1992). There are at present no agreed-upon guidelines for exactly when to do any imaging on these patients. Generally, imaging is only recommended if there is clinical suspicion of infection or malignancy (the latter being commoner in elderly patients) or of progressive neurological impairment or pain. There will be such a suspicion for only a minority of patients (fewer than 10%).

Are Plain Radiographs Useful?

There is a growing consensus that plain radiography is not particularly useful in the management of back pain, apart from the diagnosis of osteoporotic collapse and ankylosing spondylitis. Some would also make an argument for its use in the diagnosis of spondylolisthesis.

However, there is some doubt about both the reliability of plain radiography in spondylolisthesis, and the effectiveness of surgical intervention based on radiographic findings. The aim of the latter is stabilization, and yet the phenomenon of instability has not been demonstrated radiographically in this condition (Butt, 1989). There is also considerable variability in the reliability of radiological diagnosis that is highly dependent on imaging protocol (Butt, 1989). Because plain radiography is considerably less sensitive than MRI in the diagnosis of spinal malignancy, it is probably not the first choice if a choice is available.

When Is MRI Necessary?

The most common clinical indication for MRI in patients with back pain is to exclude significant disc protrusion. The problem with this "hunt the pathology" approach is that it is evident from two major studies that most types of disc "pathology" occur in asymptomatic members of the population (Boden, Davis, Dina, Patronas, & Wiesel, 1990; Jenssen, Brant-Zawadzki, Obuchowski, Modic, & Malkasian, 1994). There is therefore a serious danger of inappropriate intervention based on imaging (Deyo, 2000).

The only finding that was rarely present in the asymptomatic population was an extruded disc, defined as a lesion with a definite neck to it. This is in contrast to disc protrusions, which are relatively common in pain-free individuals. The Jenssen and colleagues (1994) study also found that one expert neuroradiologist was 30% more likely than another to diagnose disc protrusion. This level of reporting variability, together with the observation of disc protrusion in over half of asymptomatic patients, suggests that disc protrusion should be regarded as a normal finding and not used as an indication for surgery.

Studies suggest that imaging studies poorly predict surgical requirement or outcome (Enzmann, 1994). Return to work is best predicted by psychological and clinical factors other than findings on MRI (Enzmann, 1994).

Deyo (1994) points out that "although surgery relieves pain in carefully selected patients with herniated discs, most patients improve without an operation" (p. 115), and also points out that MRI itself may be responsible for the increase in back surgery in the United States. In contrast, in the United Kingdom, it was found that the main effect of MRI on clinical decision making was to encourage more conservative therapy (Rankine, Gill, Hutchinson, Ross, & Williamson, 1998). This may reflect differences in baseline practice and incentives to perform back surgery in the two countries.

It is suggested that clinical and possibly psychological assessment should be the primary basis for management of back pain. Plain radiographs and MRI (if available) may be useful in a highly selected patient population. Further decisions on management should be made on the basis of clinical, psychological, and imaging assessments taken together, rather than on the basis of imaging studies alone, and perhaps only extruded discs should be considered for surgical intervention.

Joint Pain

What Essential Information Is Obtained from Joint Imaging?

It is not intended to review all types of joint pain in this section, as some general principles can be derived from the examples discussed. Joint pain is a common symptom and is usually not associated with arthritis. Only those patients with persistent or disabling symptoms should be considered for further investigation.

The key point to emphasize is that joint imaging should be used as a diagnostic aid, not as a test of whether a patient's pain is justified or not. The relationship between pain and changes on plain radiography is poor (McAlindon, 1999). The diagnosis of arthritis is predominantly based on careful history taking and clinical examination. The pattern and type of joint involvement, together with the history and a small range of blood tests (erythrocyte sedimentation rate or C-reactive protein), are usually sufficient to make a provisional diagnosis. Furthermore, specialized tests including radiographs may be required at the early stages of osteoarthritis, where the clinical manifestations may be minimal or difficult to distinguish from those of inflammatory arthritis. They may also be required in the early stages of inflammatory arthritis to confirm erosive disease where the clinical diagnosis is in doubt. If the pattern and type of joint involvement are not obvious from clinical examination, plain radiographs may be useful in clarifying these. This particularly applies to radiographs of the hands, where both the pattern and type of bony destruction can provide important additional diagnostic information. Imaging of the spine and sacroiliac joints may also be useful in patients suspected of having a seronegative spondylarthritis. This is particularly so for those without peripheral joint involvement, where the condition may be difficult to distinguish from other causes of low back pain. These conditions are particularly important to diagnose early, as the mainstay of treatment, if the disease is confined to the back and sacroiliac joints, is analgesia combined with aggressive physiotherapy and exercise. However, if there is clinical doubt, there can be little harm in recommending this anyway.

Is It Necessary to Make a Diagnosis to Manage Joint Pain?

The short answer to the question of whether a diagnosis is needed for management of joint pain is no. The principles of pain therapy are similar for any type of joint pain. However, for patients with inflammatory arthritis, where specific disease-modifying agents may be appropriate, early referral to a specialist clinic is likely to substantially affect their long-term pain and disability. Still, it should be mentioned that data from our own group and from colleagues in the United States (Escalante & del Rincón, 1999) have shown that factors such as mood state, coping strategies, and level of social support may be as important as joint destruction in determining the level of pain and disability in patients with inflammatory arthritis.

Is It Really Necessary to Make a Diagnosis in All Patients with Osteoarthritis?

The question of whether a diagnosis is needed for all patients with osteoarthritis is more difficult and has not been formally addressed. In my opinion, it is not necessary to make a diagnosis to initiate effective drug therapy for pain. However, there may be medicolegal issues centering around, for instance, the injection of steroids into a joint without a formal diagnosis.

It is unclear how patients respond to being told they have osteoarthritis. For some it may be reassuring to have a diagnosis, whereas for others it may cause inappropriate worry and time off work. There may therefore be an argument for delaying diagnosis until it becomes obvious from clinical examination alone, on the grounds that in those in whom it does not become clinically obvious are unlikely to develop severe disease anyway. This may seem like a trivial issue, but the casual use of plain radiographs has substantial resource implications.

In conclusion, plain radiographs are not really necessary in the management of arthritis pain, and probably should be reserved for cases where inflammatory arthritis (to establish a diagnosis and to assess effect rate of progression), malignancy, or other rarer pathologies are suspected, in addition to cases where joint replacement is planned.

What Is the Place of MRI?

MRI is capable of delineating detailed soft tissue abnormalities within and around joints that cannot be visualized with conventional plain radiography or CT. In terms of altering management, the detection of tendon or cartilage damage is probably the most useful application, particularly in relation to the knee and shoulder. In patients with unexplained severe pain in these joints, particularly where there is a history suggestive of avulsion injury, this is a useful additional investigation when used selectively. MRI of the hip is also useful in patients suspected of having avascular necrosis of the hip or other entheses when plain X-rays may be normal. MRI is also the investigation of choice

when bony or soft tissue malignancy is suspected in the region of a joint.

Ultrasound of both small and larger (e.g., knee and shoulder) joints is also being developed and, particularly in the case of three-dimensional ultrasound, provides remarkable structural detail. To what extent this detail will change clinical management is currently being assessed.

An Overall Strategy for Musculoskeletal Pain Management

The principles of integrating the present approach to structural imaging with musculoskeletal pain management are very simple and can be summarized as follows:

1. Commence treatment for pain in parallel to any necessary investigations.

2. Exclude serious underlying pathology by taking a thorough history and performing a detailed examination. This should exclude underlying depression and sleep disorder. Only order investigations necessary either to confirm the clinical diagnosis or to exclude possible underlying pathology that will alter the management. The nature of these investigations should be explained to the patient.

3. Decide on what the main factors maintaining the pain are, rather than trying to determine the exact source of the pain (i.e., is the pain mainly maintained by nociceptive, psychogenic, or neuropathic mechanisms?). This assessment inevitably takes place at different levels of objectivity and requires some experience. It will mainly determine which drugs should be established first.

4. Treat any underlying mood and/or sleep disorder. In my experience, this should occur prior to any other therapy; if either type of disorder is severe, patients are unlikely to respond to other types of therapy.

For mood disorder, commence amitriptyline (10 mg at night, increased to 125–150 mg slowly as tolerated over 6–8 weeks). For sleep disorder, amitriptyline should be slowly increased to a dose sufficient to provide a night's sleep with tolerable side effects, then maintained at this dose. Patients should be warned about side effects and cautioned about driving. Other nonselective tricyclic antidepressants, such as venlafaxine, may also be used in the same contexts. Venlafaxine is considerably more expensive than amitriptyline, but it does not have the antimuscarinic effects of amitriptyline.

Selective serotonin reuptake inhibitors may also be used, but they may not have the analgesic effects of the less selective agents. The current evidence is that they are no more effective as antidepressants, but are safer and do have fewer adverse effects.

5. Treat pain with evidence-based therapies if possible (for the most part, high-quality, long-term, placebo-controlled trials have not been done). Physical therapies (including physiotherapy, osteopathy or referral to a chiropractor, acupuncture, and/or other stimulation therapies) may be used where appropriate and where resources exist. Analgesics should be used as follows:

First-line: Paracetamol (acetaminophen, in the United States) in full dosage.

Second-line for psychogenically maintained pains and neuropathic pain: Amitriptyline up to antidepressant doses as outlined in point 4 above.

Second-line for nociceptive pain: Add tramadol or a mild opiate such as codeine phosphate or dextropropoxyphene.

Third-line for all types of pain: Higher-dose opiates such as dihydrocodeine, slow-release forms of morphine (sulfate), or a fentanyl patch; and/or a nonsteroidal analgesic (with or without gastroprotection, or a Cox-2 selective nonsteroidal antiinflammatory drug if indicated or funded).

6. If a patient is still in moderate to severe pain after 3–4 months' therapy, reconsider the diagnosis; this may include further imaging or reassessment of mood state and abnormal pain behavior, as well as appropriate referral.

7. For those with arthritis, consider more invasive therapies (e.g., joint injections with steroids and local anesthetics, and joint replacement) where appropriate and after the assessments above have been made. Joint injections should only be performed by those with appropriate training, but may be considered at any stage as an adjunct to the analgesic ladder.

PROPOSAL FOR EQUAL ACCESS TO SECONDARY PAIN MANAGEMENT

Where Should Chronic Pain Be Managed and by Whom?

Ideally, most chronic pain problems should be managed in primary care or jointly between primary and secondary care. However, the training or resources for this to occur are not always available. The selection of patients sent to a secondary or tertiary referral center, and the types of specialists they end up seeing, are often surprisingly arbitrary in much of Europe and the United States. This situation is clearly unsatisfactory in a number of ways.

The first problem is that many physicians and surgeons do not regard the management of chronic pain as part of their practice, so patients with chronic pain tend to bounce from one clinic to another in their quest for an opinion. The second is that many specialist pain clinics have very long waiting lists. The third is that there is usually no inventory or directory of local specialists with interests in chronic pain management that primary care physicians can refer to.

Is There a Simple Solution?

One solution is that every department of a hospital should have some specific interest in chronic pain management. A very simple strategy is to designate one or two people within each clinical specialty to deal with chronic pain referrals of a particular type (e.g., fibromyalgia and arthritis pain to rheumatology, chronic abdominal pain to gastroenterology, painful diabetic neuropathy to diabetology). The proposal is for a simple hub-and-spokes referral system, where the first hospital referral is always to the relevant department. The central hub would consist of a general chronic pain clinic, with access to pain behavior modification programs, specialist nerve blocks, and other more invasive procedures. Provision of nerve blocks and other procedures would be a tertiary referral service only. Shared protocols for different aspects of chronic pain management would need to be developed by all the involved groups, and part of this process would form the basis of regular discussions between the clinical leaders within each group and the primary health care groups. The sharing of these on local networks should also facilitate "virtual referrals" without a patient's leaving primary care.

One of the perceived barriers to such referrals is access to specialist imaging technology. This is perhaps another instance where advances in structural imaging have provided the false impression that chronic pain management is too complex for the average physician to deal with. The availability of impressive imaging technology may have mainly had the effect of increasing the distance between a patient's chronic pain symptoms and the attention of the average physician. This hub-and-spokes arrangement may begin to close that gap.

In summary, it is possible to envisage a relatively effective, non-imaging-based management strategy for musculoskeletal pain, based in primary care with rapid access to advice from secondary care. One advantage of this strategy is that it could be implemented with relatively few or no additional resources, and that it is also practical for poorer countries. Overreliance on imaging and secondary care rather than clinical assessment may have contributed to the slow progress toward these goals. The first challenge is therefore organization of care. The second is the effective use of existing therapies and acquiring the necessary evidence upon which to base this. The third major challenge is the development of more effective new therapies.

In spite of the large amounts of money devoted to the development of new therapies, progress has been slow. Much of the research of the last two decades has been based on an increased understanding of the physiology of the peripheral and spinal cord components of the nociceptive system, which has mainly been based on studies of animal models of pain. These components of the nociceptive system are moderately difficult to access in humans, and therefore it is usually only possible to partially validate these models for pain in humans. Except for non-steroidal analgesics (aspirin predates these) and possibly tricyclic antidepressants (for which the analgesic mechanisms are far from clear), no new classes of analgesics for musculoskeletal pain were developed in the 20th century. It may therefore be time to reassess our strategies for developing new analgesics.

FUNCTIONAL IMAGING

New imaging techniques have made it possible to identify the main cerebral components of the human nociceptive system. We are just beginning to understand the division of functions within this system. The development of targeted drug interventions is likely to be substantially faster over the next decade, due to the advances in compound synthesis and screening. The development of such new interventions in parallel with robust models for the function of the human nociceptive system, which can be used in late phase I trials or at the proof-of-concept phase of development, provides some exciting opportunities for more rapid and tailored analgesic development.

Why Do We Need Functional Imaging?

The experience of pain can only be defined in terms of human consciousness. As with all sensory experience, there is no way of being certain that one person's experience of pain is the same as another's. There is therefore no absolute quantification of pain experience, which can only be estimated by verbal or magnitude scaling methods. The common question as to whether functional imaging can be used to differentiate "real" from "imagined" pain needs to be approached with some caution.

Pain should not be equated with *nociception*. Nociception is the response to excitation of nociceptors. Although nociception may give rise to the experience of pain, pain may arise in the absence of nociception. Conversely, nociception may also occur in the absence of pain. Hence the terms *non-nociceptive pain* (e.g., neurogenic and psychogenic pain) and *nociceptive pain* (e.g., inflammatory pain) need to be clearly differentiated.

There is therefore a spectrum of pain experience—from pain that may closely reflect physical events in tissue, to pain that is generated without any peripheral physical input. The brain is therefore acting as a virtual reality system that may or may not be constrained by interactions with the body's internal and external environment. In order to understand these interactions, noninvasive methods for measuring cerebral responses in humans are required. Surface electrophysiological techniques have made important contributions to our understanding of early cerebral events (first 800 milliseconds) and have been reviewed elsewhere (Chen, 1993). This section concentrates on PET, with a brief mention of fMRI, both of which have temporal resolutions of seconds to minutes.

All these techniques have complementary strengths and weaknesses in the investigation of how the human brain processes nociceptive inputs and elaborates the experience of pain. There is now the exciting possibility of integrating some of these different technologies. In the interests of brevity, this discussion focuses on some of the important issues that PET imaging of human pain responses has raised, but it is not intended to be an exhaustive review of all the excellent work that has been done in this field (see Apkarian, 1995; Jones, 1992, 1999; Jones & Derbyshire, 1996).

How Can the Brain–Pain Problem Be Solved?

Nociceptive second-order projections from the dorsal horn neurons to the brain are mainly (approximately 90%) via the opposite spino-thalamic tract. Projections are mainly to the brainstem and to the medial and lateral thalamic nuclei (Apkarian & Hodge, 1989; Bowsher, 1957) (see Figure 35.1). However, there are also polysynaptic medial projections to the medial thalamic nuclei. The more medial projections and their corresponding thalamic nuclei are generally slower, with relatively poor spatial information. The lateral projections, in contrast, are somatotopic (i.e., projections are arranged in a body map) and are subserved by relatively fast transmission. The latter project to the primary and secondary somatosensory cortices and the insula (Craig, Bushnell, Zhang, & Blomqvist, 1994).

The more medial structures are considered to subserve the so-called *medial pain system*, as distinct from the projections of the lateral thalamic nuclei, which are thought to subserve the *lateral pain system* (for a more detailed discussion, see Jones, 1999; Jones & Derbyshire, 1996). Vogt and colleagues considerably extended the concept of the medial pain system by demonstrating projections of the medial thalamic nuclei to area 24 of the anterior cingulate cortex (Sikes & Vogt, 1992; Vogt, Sikes, & Vogt, 1993). The anterior cingulate cortex is an extensive area of the limbic cortex overlying the corpus callosum, which is involved in the integration of cognition, affect, and response selection (Devinsky, Morrell, & Vogt, 1995). There are also medial thalamic nociceptive projections to the prefrontal cortex (Tsubokawa, Katayama, Ueno, & Moriyasu, 1981). The descending connections of the anterior cingulate cortex to the medial thalamic nuclei and to the periaqueductal grey in the brainstem suggest that this system may also be involved in the modulation of reflex responses to noxious stimuli.

Partly because of the differences in latency of response and their respective connections, it has been suggested that the medial pain system and lateral pain systems are mainly responsible for processing chronic and acute pain, respectively (Albe-Fessard, Berkley, Kruger, Ralston, & Willis, 1985). However, from the wiring diagram (Figure 35.1), it is evident that these systems are interconnected and operate in parallel. Only at the level of the cortex do they become discrete. Stimulation or removal of somatosensory cortex in humans rarely causes or relieves pain (Devinsky et al., 1995). Indeed, damage to the spino-thalamo-cortical pathways is commonly associated with central deafferentation pain (Bowsher, 1996). Deafferentation or removal of the anterior cingulate, however, does not abolish chronic pain, but simply reduces the unpleasantness of it (Foltz & White, 1962). Further identification of the cerebral structures involved in human pain processing and of their physiological interactions has been facilitated by functional imaging techniques.

What Does PET Do?

PET is an expensive technique for measuring very small changes in concentration of introduced radioactivity in living tissues over a period of time (seconds to days, depending on the half-life of the radioisotope introduced). Depending on the tracer introduced, this provides measurements of regional tissue metabolism (regional cerebral blood flow, blood volume, or glucose metabolism) or neurochemical function (e.g., pre- and postsynaptic receptor binding, transmitter reuptake, or metabolism). Noninvasive (PET and fMRI) techniques have been extensively used to quantitate changes in blood flow in humans as indices of neuronal activity in response to physiological stimuli (Lueck et al., 1989). The underlying assumption in applying these techniques is that there is a close relationship between blood flow and neuronal function. There is good evidence from animal studies that there is such a relationship, and that changes in blood flow are closely related to neuronal energy metabolism (Raichle, 1987). These methods therefore provide the exciting possibility of defining functional neuroanatomical substrates of different internally or externally generated physiological stimuli.

What Are the Main Findings from Human PET Studies of Nociceptive Processing?

Recent PET studies in humans have identified a matrix of structures (illustrated in Figure 35.1) that respond to acute pain. It is clear from these studies that the more fronto-cortical structures, such as prefrontal and anterior cingulate cortex, are the predominant ones that respond to the suffering components of both acute pain (Casey et al., 1994; Di et al., 1994; Jones, Brown, Friston, Qi, &

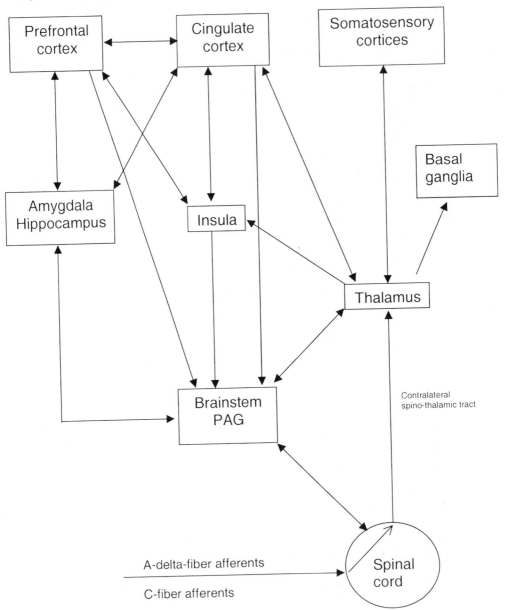

FIGURE 35.1. Schematic diagram of some of the main anatomical components of the pain matrix, and their possible functional significance. PAG, periaqueductal grey matter.

Frackowiak, 1991; Talbot et al., 1991; Vogt, Derbyshire, & Jones, 1996) and chronic pain (Hsieh, Belfrage, Stone, Hansson, & Ingvar, 1995).

Early studies suggested lateralization of these responses. However, more recent studies suggest bilateral nociceptive activation of thalamus, insula, cingulate, and prefrontal cortices (Vogt et al., 1996) in humans. These studies have also identified two main nociceptive areas (perigenual and midcingulate) within an extensive network of responsive areas in the cingulate cortex. Extensive bilateral nociceptive representation in the cingulate cortex has also now been confirmed by direct electrophysiological recording (Lenz et al., 1998) in subjects undergoing neurosurgery, as well as by fMRI studies (Jones et al., 1998; Rosen et al., 1994). The more rostral perigenual area may be more concerned with affective responses and vocalization, whereas the midcingulate region may be more concerned with executive responses such as response selection. Adjacent but discrete areas of the anterior cingulate cortex are also involved in attention (Davis, Taylor, Crawley, Wood, & Mikulis, 1996; Derbyshire, Vogt, & Jones, 1998). The bilateral cingulate responses are in keeping with observations by Sikes and Vogt (1992) of hemi- and whole-body nociceptive receptive fields in area 24 of the anterior cingulate cortex.

Some support for anterior cingulate processing of the affective components of pain comes from PET studies of patients with atypical facial pain (in which psychogenic mechanisms are thought to contribute to the perseveration of the pain). These patients showed increased anterior cingulate responses and reduced prefrontal responses to a standardized experimental pain stimulus, compared to controls (Derbyshire et al., 1994). By comparison, PET studies (using the same protocol) of patients with acute and chronic inflammatory pain have shown considerable reductions of anterior cingulate responses (Derbyshire, Jones, Collins, Feinmann, & Harris, 1999; Jones & Derbyshire, 1997). The patients with chronic inflammatory pain (rheumatoid arthritis, or RA) also demonstrated reduced subcortical responses.

These very different patterns of response in different types of chronic pain suggest that they may be subserved by different mechanisms, possibly related to differences in attention to the affective components of acute pain. The majority of patients with RA are known to have well-developed coping strategies (Keefe et al., 1991), whereas those with atypical facial and coexistent pain generally do not.

Further evidence for the importance of the anterior cingulate cortex to affective processing comes from studies where the relative intensity and unpleasantness of experimental noxious stimuli were manipulated via hypnotic suggestion. The level of unpleasantness was correlated with regional cerebral blood flow in the anterior cingulate cortex (Rainville, Duncan, Price, Carrier, & Bushnell, 1997).

From our own and other studies, it seems likely that the somatosensory cortex is involved in the sensory and discriminatory components of the pain response, such as temporal, spatial, and possibly early intensity discrimination (Hari, Kaukoranta, Reinikainen, Huopaniemie, & Mauno, 1983; Treede, Kenshalo, Gracely, & Jones, 1999). This raises the possibility that different components of pain are processed in parallel, in common with some of the main sensory modalities such as vision.

The neurochemical basis for the differences in response in the different types of chronic pain is uncertain. However, it is interesting that RA pain is associated with decreased *in vivo* opioid receptor binding in prefrontal and anterior cingulate cortex, consistent with increased occupation by endogenous opioid peptides (Jones et al., 1994). Subsequent studies on patients with trigeminal neuralgia studied before and after surgery showed similar significant and more extensive increases within cortical and subcortical projections of the medial pain system (Jones et al., 1999).

This provides evidence that the endogenous opioid system is activated in at least two types of chronic pain. The precise behavioral consequences of these phenomena are not known, but may be related to the reinforcement of coping strategies in these patients (Bandura, O'Leary, Taylor, Gauthier, & Gossard, 1987).

The exciting possibility of enhancing such responses with orally active enkephalinases has been a Holy Grail for drug development for some years. Recent developments have provided some encouragement that this may be a realistic goal (Chipkin et al., 1988). One of the problems in drug development is establishing adequate uptake in the target tissue (Cunningham et al., 1991). It is still common for expensive drug development programs to be abandoned prior to these parameters' being established in humans.

Radiolabeling of drugs with [11C] or [18F] provides a relatively cost-effective way of establishing the tissue levels of a drug after administration at an early phase of drug development (Langstrom,

Bergstrom, Hartvig, Valind, & Watanabe, 1995). The human PET studies of opioid receptor binding provide a model for phase II development of such compounds, in terms of proving concepts and establishing effective doses of the compounds. Human pain activation studies would also provide a means of establishing which components of the human nociceptive system are modulated by such compounds and comparing these findings with the effects of established analgesics such as synthetic opiates (Jones, Friston, et al., 1991).

Is There a Final Cortical Site of Integration of Nociceptive Information?

The failure of any single cortical lesion to abolish pain consistently, together with the evidence for a pain matrix from functional imaging studies, suggests that there is no final integration site or "pain center." This raises the possibility that pain is processed and possibly experienced within a distributed network or matrix of cortical and subcortical structures, as Melzack (1989, 1990) has suggested. How such parallel information is coupled, or how each noxious stimulus retains its spatial and temporal signature within this matrix, is not known. Frequency coding is one possibility, which would be most easily investigated electrophysiologically (Chen & Rappelsberger, 1994).

How Much Variability Is There?

Not surprisingly, there has been some variability of cerebral responses to pain reported by different groups and within groups (Jones, Friston, & Frackowiak, 1992; Vogt et al., 1996). Some of this is likely to be due to methodological differences related to both the type of stimulus (e.g., contact or noncontact, escapable or nonescapable) and the PET technology used. However, the psychological context and the intensity of the stimulus are likely to be as important.

The contributions of these factors are only beginning to be sorted out, but it is clear that the intensity of pain experience is most closely correlated with the pattern of cortical and subcortical activation (Derbyshire et al., 1997). Further confirmation of this comes from ingenious studies using the thermal grill illusion, in which alternating warm and cool bars at non-nociceptive temperatures are collectively experienced as painful. This type of induced pain activates the cingulate, insula, and somatosensory cortex (Craig, Reiman, Evans, & Bushnell, 1996).

One potential source of variability is the anticipation of pain. Studies employing fMRI have allowed this component to be identified as being processed in areas of the medial frontal and anterior cingulate cortex that are discrete from the nociceptive areas (Ploghaus et al., 1999). Apart from its inherent interest, this also provides a further potential target for drug development.

Can Functional Imaging Distinguish "Genuine" Pain from "Nongenuine" Pain?

The question of whether functional imaging can distinguish between "genuine" and "nongenuine" pain has been included here because of the frequency with which it is asked. In my experience, this is rarely a useful question, although it is accepted that it may have medicolegal importance. Creating the right incentives and workplace environments to encourage people to work should perhaps not be a major preoccupation of the medical profession, nor should scarce resources be devoted to it. Given the interindividual variability of nociceptive responses, it is doubtful that imaging can provide a reliable way of distinguishing "real" from "imagined" pain in an individual. However, if this is a serious goal, then the appropriate resources from insurance and government agencies should find the means to achieve it.

In short, some of the key components of the pain matrix in humans have now been identified. The precise definition of the physiological functions of each component of this matrix has only just begun, but some of the suggested functions are illustrated in Figure 35.1, which is based on human and animal studies.

SUMMARY

The contribution of structural imaging to musculoskeletal pain management is relatively limited. The benefit from technological advances in this field has probably reached a plateau. The importance of this type of imaging has perhaps been overstated by the medical profession and may have contributed to inappropriate management of patients with musculoskeletal pain. A relatively structural-imaging-independent approach to musculoskeletal pain has been suggested within an integrated and informed primary, secondary, and tertiary care system. Most of these components require relatively few resources and are therefore relevant to Third World countries.

The substantial potential for physiological imaging to help target new drug development and facilitate the early stages of clinical trials has been outlined. This will pave the way for the generation of new classes of analgesics in this new millennium.

REFERENCES

Albe-Fessard, D., Berkley, K. J., Kruger, L., Ralston, H. J., & Willis, W. D., Jr. (1985). Diencephalic mechanisms of pain sensation. *Brain Research, 356,* 217–296.

Apkarian, A. V. (1995). Functional imaging of pain: New insights regarding the role of the cerebral cortex in human pain perception. *Seminars in Neurology, 7,* 279–293.

Apkarian, A. V., & Hodge, C. J. (1989). Primate spinothalamic pathways: III. Thalamic terminations of the dorsolateral and ventral spinothalamic pathways. *Journal of Comparative Neurology, 288,* 493–511.

Bandura, A., O'Leary, A., Taylor, C. B., Gauthier, J., & Gossard, D. (1987). Perceived self-efficacy and pain control: Opioid and nonopioid mechanisms. *Journal of Personality and Social Psychology, 53,* 563–571.

Boden, S. D., Davis, D. O., Dina, T. S., Patronas, N. J., & Wiesel, S. W. (1990). Abnormal magnetic-resonance scans of the lumbar spine in asymptomatic subjects: A prospective investigation. *Journal of Bone and Joint Surgery (American), 72,* 403–408.

Bowsher, D. (1957). Termination of the central pain pathway in man: The concious appreciation of pain. *Brain, 80,* 607–622.

Bowsher, D. (1996). Central pain: Clinical and physiological characteristics. *Journal of Neurology, Neurosurgery and Psychiatry, 61,* 62–69.

Butt, W. P. (1989). Radiology for back pain. *Clinical Radiology, 40,* 1–10.

Casey, K. L., Minoshima, S., Berger, K. L., Koeppe, R. A., Morrow, T. J., & Frey, K. A. (1994). Positron emission tomographic analysis of cerebral structures activated specifically by repetitive noxious heat stimuli. *Journal of Neurophysiology, 71,* 802–807.

Chen, A. C. (1993). Human brain measures of clinical pain: A review. I. Topographic mappings. *Pain, 54,* 115–132.

Chen, A. C., & Rappelsberger, P. (1994). Brain and human pain: Topographic EEG amplitude and coherence mapping. *Brain Topography, 7,* 129–140.

Chipkin, R. E., Berger, J. G., Billard, W., Iorio, L. C., Chapman, R., & Barnett, A. (1988). Pharmacology of SCH 34826, an orally active enkephalinase inhibitor analgesic. *Journal of Pharmacology and Experimental Therapeutics, 245,* 829–838.

Chisholm, R. (1991). Guidelines for radiological investigations [Editorial]. *British Medical Journal, 303,* 797–798.

Craig, A. D., Bushnell, M. C., Zhang, E. T., & Blomqvist, A. (1994). A thalamic nucleus specific for pain and temperature sensation. *Nature, 372,* 770–773.

Craig, A. D., Reiman, E. M., Evans, A., & Bushnell, M. C. (1996). Functional imaging of an illusion of pain. *Nature, 384,* 258–260.

Cunningham, V. J., Pike, V. W., Bailey, D., Freemantle, C. A. J., Page, B. C., Jones, A. K. P., Kensett, M. J., Bateman, D., Luthra, S. K., & Jones, T. (1991). A method of studying pharmacokinetics in man at picomolar drug concentrations. *British Journal of Clinical Pharmacology, 32,* 167–172.

Davis, K., Taylor, S., Crawley, A., Wood, M., & Mikulis, D. (1996). fMRI reveals separate pain and attention related regions in the human anterior cingulate cortex. In *Proceedings of the 8th World Congress on Pain* (p. 445). Vancouver, BC, Canada: International Association for the Study of Pain Press.

Derbyshire, S. W. G., Jones, A. K. P., Collins, M., Feinmann, C., & Harris, M. (1999). Cerebral responses to pain in patients suffering acute post-dental extraction pain measured by positron emission tomography (PET). *European Journal of Pain, 3,* 103–113.

Derbyshire, S. W. G., Jones, A. K. P., Devani, P., Friston, K. J., Feinmann, C., Harris, M., Pearce, S., Watson, J. D. G., & Frackowiak, R. S. J. (1994). Cerebral responses to pain in patients with atypical facial pain measured by positron emission tomography. *Journal of Neurology, Neurosurgery and Psychiatry, 57,* 1166–1172.

Derbyshire, S. W. G., Jones, A. K. P., Gyulai, F., Clark, S., Townsend, D., & Firestone, L. L. (1997). Pain processing during three levels of noxious stimulation produces differential patterns of central activity. *Pain, 73,* 431–445.

Derbyshire, S. W. G., Vogt, B. A., & Jones, A. K. P. (1998). Pain and Stroop interference tasks activate separate processing modules in anterior cingulate cortex. *Experimental Brain Research, 118,* 52–60.

Devinsky, O., Morrell, M. J., & Vogt, B. A. (1995). Contributions of anterior cingulate cortex to behaviour. *Brain, 118,* 279–306.

Deyo, R. (1994). Magnetic resonance imaging of the lumbar spine: Terrific test or tar baby? *New England Journal of Medicine, 331,* 115–116.

Di Piero, V., Ferracuti, S., Sabatini, U., Pantano, P., Cruccu, G., & Lenzi, G. L.(1994). A cerebral blood flow study on tonic pain activation in man. *Pain, 56,* 167–173.

Enzmann, D. R. (1994).On low back pain. *American Journal of Neuroradiology, 15,* 109–113.

Escalante, A., & del Rincón, I. (1999). How much disability in rheumatoid arthritis is explained by rheumatoid arthritis? *Arthritis and Rheumatism, 42,* 1712–1721.

Foltz, E., & White, L. (1962). Pain relief by frontal cingulotomy. *Neurosurgery, 19,* 89–100.

Halpin, S. F., Yeoman, L., & Dundas, D. D. (1991). Radiographic examination of the lumbar spine in a community hospital: An audit of current practice [see comments]. *British Medical Journal, 303,* 813–815.

Hari, R., Kaukoranta, E., Reinikainen, K., Huopaniemie, T., & Mauno, J. (1983). Neuromagnetic localization of cortical activity evoked by painful dental stimulation in man. *Neuroscience Letters, 42,* 77–82.

Hsieh, J. C., Belfrage, M., Stone, E. S., Hansson, P., & Ingvar, M. (1995). Central representation of chronic ongoing neuropathic pain studied by positron emission tomography. *Pain, 63,* 225-236.

Jenssen, M., Brant-Zawadzki, M., Obuchowski, N., Modic, M., & Malkasian, D. (1994). Magnetic resonance imaging of the lumbar spine in people without back pain. *New England Journal of Medicine, 331,* 69-73.

Jones, A. K. P. (1992). Do "pain centres" exist? *British Journal of Rheumatology, 31,* 290-292.

Jones, A. K. P. (1999). The contribution of functional imaging techniques to our understanding of rheumatic pain. *Rheumatic Disease Clinics of North America, 25,* 123-152.

Jones, A. K. P., Brown, W. D., Friston, K. J., Qi, L. Y., & Frackowiak, R. S. J. (1991). Cortical and subcortical localization of response to pain in man using positron emission tomography. *Proceedings of the Royal Society of London Biological Sciences, 244,* 39-44.

Jones, A. K. P., Cunningham, V. J., Ha, K. S., Fujiwara, T., Luthra, S. K., Silva, S., Derbyshire, S., & Jones, T. (1994). Changes in central opioid receptor binding in relation to inflammation and pain in patients with rheumatoid arthritis. *British Journal of Rheumatology, 33,* 909-916.

Jones, A. K. P., & Derbyshire, S. W. G. (1996). Cerebral mechanisms operating in the presence and absence of inflammatory pain. *Annals of the Rheumatic Diseases, 55,* 411-420.

Jones, A. K. P., & Derbyshire, S. W. G. (1997). Reduced cortical responses to noxious heat in patients with rheumatoid arthritis. *Annals of the Rheumatic Diseases, 56,* 601-607.

Jones, A. K. P., Friston, K. J., & Frackowiak, R. S. (1992). Localization of responses to pain in human cerebral cortex. *Science, 255,* 215-216.

Jones, A. K. P., Friston, K. J., Qi, L. Y., Harris, M., Cunningham, V. J., Jones, T., Feinman, C., & Frackowiak, R. S. J. (1991). Sites of action of morphine in the brain. *Lancet, 338,* 825.

Jones, A. K. P., Hughes, D. G., Brettle, D. S., Robinson, L., Sykes, J. R., Aziz, Q., Hamdy, S., Thompson, D. G., Derbyshire, S. W. G., Chen, A. C. N., & Jones, A. K. P. (1998). Experiences with functional magnetic resonance imaging at 1 tesla. *British Journal of Radiology, 71,* 160-166.

Jones, A. K. P., Kitchen, N. D., Watabe, H., Cunningham, V. J., Jones, T., Luthra, S. K., & Thomas, D. G. (1999). Measurement of changes in opioid receptor binding in vivo during trigeminal neuralgic pain using [^{11}C]diprenorphine and positron emission tomography. *Journal of Cerebral Blood Flow and Metabolism, 19,* 803-808.

Keefe, F. J., Caldwell, D. S., Martinez, S., Nunley, J., Beckham, J., & Williams, D. A. (1991). Analyzing pain in rheumatoid arthritis patients: Pain coping strategies in patients who have had knee replacement surgery. *Pain, 46,* 153-160.

Langstrom, B., Bergstrom, M., Hartvig, P., Valind, S., & Watanabe, Y. (1995). Is PET a tool for drug evaluation? In D. Comar (Ed.), *PET for drug development and evaluation* (pp. 37-50). Dordrecht: Kluwer Academic.

Lenz, F. A., Rios, M., Chau, D., Krauss, G. L., Zirh, T. A., & Lesser, R. P. (1998). Painful stimuli evoke potentials recorded from the parasylvian cortex in humans. *Journal of Neurophysiology, 80,* 2077-2088.

Lueck, C. J., Zeki, S., Friston, K. J., Deiber, M. P., Cope, P., Cunningham, V. J., Lammertsma, A. A., Kennard, C., & Frackowiak, R. S. (1989). The colour centre in the cerebral cortex of man. *Nature, 340,* 386-389.

McAlindon, T. (1999). The knee. In A. D. Woolf (Ed.), *Baillière's best practice & research. Clinical rheumatology* (pp. 329-344). London: Baillière Tindall.

Melzack, R. (1989). Labat Lecture: Phantom limbs. *Regional Anesthesia, 14,* 208-211.

Melzack, R. (1990). Phantom limbs and the concept of a neuromatrix. *Trends in Neurosciences, 13,* 80-92.

Ploghaus, A., Tracey, I., Gati, J. S., Clare, S., Menon, R. S., Matthews, P. M., Nicholas, J., & Rawlins, P. (1999). Dissociating pain from its anticipation in the human brain. *Science, 284,* 1979-1987.

Raichle, M. E. (1987). Circulatory and metabolic correlates of brain function in normal humans. In F. Plum (Ed.), *American Physiology Society handbook of physiology. Section 1: The nervous sytem* (pp. 643-674). Bethesda, MD: American Physiological Society.

Rainville, P., Duncan, G. H., Price, D. D., Carrier, B., & Bushnell, M. C. (1997). Pain affect encoded in human anterior cingulate but not somatosensory cortex. *Science, 277,* 968-971.

Rankine, J. J., Gill, K. P., Hutchinson, C. E., Ross, E. R., & Williamson, J. B. (1998). The therapeutic impact of lumbar spine MRI on patients with low back and leg pain. *Clinical Radiology, 53,* 688-693.

Rosen, S. D., Paulesu, E., Frith, C. D., Frackowiak, R. S., Davies, G. J., Jones, T., & Camici, P. G. (1994). Central nervous pathways mediating angina pectoris. *Lancet, 344,* 147-150.

Rossignol, M., Suissa, S., & Abenhaim, L. (1992). The evolution of compensated occupational spinal injuries: A three-year follow-up study. *Spine, 17,* 1043-1047.

Sikes, R. W., & Vogt, B. A. (1992). Nociceptive neurons in area 24 of rabbit cingulate cortex. *Journal of Neurophysiology, 68,* 1720-1732.

Talbot, J. D., Marrett, S., Evans, A. C., Meyer, E., Bushnell, M. C., & Duncan, G. H. (1991). Multiple representations of pain in human cerebral cortex. *Science, 251,* 1355-1358.

Treede, R. D., Kenshalo, D. R., Gracely, R. H., & Jones, A. K. P. (1999). The cortical representation of pain. *Pain, 79,* 105-111.

Tsubokawa, T., Katayama, Y., Ueno, Y., & Moriyasu, N. (1981). Evidence for involvement of the frontal cortex in pain-related cerebral events in cats: Increase in local cerebral blood flow by noxious stimuli. *Brain Research, 217,* 179-185.

Vogt, B. A., Derbyshire, S., & Jones, A. K. P. (1996). Pain processing in four regions of human cingulate cortex localized with co-registered PET and MR imaging. *European Journal of Neuroscience, 8,* 1461-1473.

Vogt, B. A., Sikes, R. W., & Vogt, L. (1993). Anterior cingulate cortex and the medial pain system. In B. A. Vogt & M. Gabriel (Eds.), *Neurobiology of cingulated cortex and limbic thalamus: A comprehensive handbook* (pp. 313-344). Boston: Birkhäuser.

CONCLUSION

Chapter 36

Trends and Future Directions in Human Pain Assessment

DENNIS C. TURK
RONALD MELZACK

> When the right thing can only be measured poorly, it tends to cause the wrong thing to be measured only because it can be measured well. And it is often much worse to have good measurement of the wrong thing—especially when, as is so often the case, the wrong thing will *in fact* be used as an indicator of the right thing—than to have poor measurement of the right thing.
>
> —TUKEY (1979, p. 786)

The chapters in this volume attest to the breadth and depth of attention given to the issues involved in assessment of the person in pain. A wide range of new instruments, methods, and procedures has become available, and new ones are constantly being developed. This trend reflects the growing awareness of the importance of comprehensive and specific assessment methods. It is altogether fitting, therefore, to heed Tukey's admonition cited above and to consider the current trends and issues in human pain assessment, as well as to consider some future directions.

PAIN > SENSORY INTENSITY

It is evident from the chapters in this volume that major advances have been made in developing sophisticated instruments and procedures designed to quantify the subjective experience of pain. The question most frequently asked by physicians when a patient complains of pain is some variation of "How much does it hurt?" A great deal of attention has been given to the fact that pain is a multidimensional perception and not a simple sensation. It is the person's perception of pain rather than the nociceptive stimulus that determines the extent of pain experienced, levels of adaptation, and responses to the stimulus. Thus appropriate measurement of pain needs to include motivational-affective and cognitive-evaluative contributions.

QUANTIFICATION OF PAIN VERSUS ASSESSMENT OF THE PERSON WHO EXPERIENCES PAIN

It is apparent that the experience and report of pain are influenced by multiple factors, including cultural conditioning, expectancies, current social contingencies, and the like. Physical pathology and the resulting nociception thus constitute only one, albeit a very important, contributor to the experience of and subsequent response to pain. Rather than

707

focusing exclusively on the assessment of pain, many clinicians and investigators have urged that adequate assessment, especially of patients with chronic pain, needs to be comprehensive. Attention needs to be given to patients' beliefs, attitudes, coping resources, mood state, and behaviors as they relate to the impact of pain on daily life, as well as physical pathology. To understand a person's pain obviously requires knowledge of the various domains that influence it.

SUBJECTIVITY VERSUS OBJECTIVITY

Pain is a subjective experience. There have been ongoing efforts to develop objective measures of pain that cannot be biased by a patient. Thus investigators have attempted to develop performance tests to assess strength, lifting capacity, and trunk muscle function. However, there is little evidence that physical examination and biomechanical measurements are correlated highly with pain. Motivational and cognitive factors affect performance on these tests and cannot be separated from a person's responses. Similarly, the association between psychophysiological parameters and pain has not been demonstrated. As Sternbach (1968, p. 57) noted, "Because of the variability of responses elicited by different pain stimuli, and because of the additional variance contributed by individual differences in response-stereotype, it is difficult to specify a pattern of physiological responses characteristic of pain." It is also true that studies of the association between observable pain behaviors and self-reports of pain have provided equivocal results. These efforts have not produced the objective measures of pain that many researchers and clinicians desire.

It is important to acknowledge that we will probably never be able to evaluate pain without some reliance on patients' subjective reports. These reports are also important because they influence how patients are responded to by significant others, including health care providers. Moreover, patients' self-reports of their beliefs, mood, coping strategies, and expectations have been shown to be related to the following:

- Functional behavior (see, e.g., Jensen, Romano, Turner, Good, & Wald, 1999; Vlaeyen, Kole-Snijiders, Rotteveel, Ruesink, & Heuts, 1995).
- Return to work (see, e.g., Linton et al., 1994).

- Adjustment (Jensen, Turner, Romano, & Lawler, 1994).
- Disability (see, e.g., Turner, Jensen, & Romano, 2000).
- Use of the health care system (Flor & Turk, 1988).
- Dropping out of treatment (Coughlan, Ridout, Williams, & Richardson, 1995; Richmond & Carmody, 1999).
- Compliance with treatment (Brus, van de Laar, Taal, Rasker, & Wiegman, 1999).
- Response to treatment (see, e.g., Jensen, Turner, & Romano, 1994; Tota-Faucette, Gil, Williams, Keefe, & Goli, 1993).

We anticipate that there will be refinements in self-report measures, and that such measures will continue to be part of comprehensive assessment protocols. It is also important to realize that many of the physical measurements that are viewed as "objective" are in fact influenced by a patient's motivation, effort, and psychological state (Pope, Rosen, Wilder, & Frymoyer, 1980).

Research to date suggests that patients' performances on physical and biomechanical measures are not associated with the risk of acute pain's evolving into chronic pain (Burton, Tillotson, Main, & Jollis, 1995) or with return to work (see, e.g., Gallagher et al., 1989). Thus the hope that objective measurement based on performance, using sophisticated apparatus designed to assess functional capacity, will predict disability or will identify malingering is unlikely. Furthermore, the relationship between this performance and return to work has yet to be demonstrated. Investigators and clinicians must be cautious in not overselling these expensive pieces of equipment and advanced technologies.

GOING BEYOND THE PSYCHOMETRIC PROPERTIES OF INSTRUMENTS AND ASSESSMENT PROCEDURES

The importance of psychometric characteristics has long been acknowledged, and careful attention to reliability, validity, utility, and normative data is required for any new assessment instrument. Many chapters in this volume (e.g., Dworkin & Sherman, Chapter 32) focus a great deal of discussion on the reliability of instruments and procedures. Considerably less attention, however, has been given to the issue of validity: Is the instrument or procedure appropriate, meaningful, and useful for making specific inferences? The question is whether the test is valid for the purposes and samples for which it is to be used. Proxy measures should be demonstrated to be related to meaningful outcome criteria (e.g., health care utilization, return to work, response to treatment). Much greater effort needs to be put into demonstrating that assessment instruments and procedures are valid. In addition, they need to be evaluated regarding their clinical utility.

In a number of chapters in this volume, authors have emphasized that greater attention must be given to the combination of sets of physical information and to the processes whereby decisions are made about the extent of pathology present, the amount of impairment, the degree of disability, and the appropriateness of different treatment alternatives. Additional research is needed to demonstrate the interrelationships among pathology, impairment, disability, and pain. It is essential that research addresses how individual characteristics of patients and their social environments influence responses to impairment, development of disability, and differential responses to alternative treatment interventions (see, e.g., Romano, Turner, & Jensen, 1997).

There is also a need to demonstrate the association of various physical measures (e.g., electromyographic activity) with meaningful variables such as functional status and actual behavior (Deyo, 1988). Similarly, it is essential that the association between psychological measures and meaningful behaviors be established. What is the relationship between the frequency of rubbing a painful body part and uptime, use of the health care system, or functional capacity? Does differential responding on the Minnesota Multiphasic Personality Inventory (MMPI) correlate with specific behaviors that can be addressed in treatment? Does spinal mobility relate to disability?

One trend that can be observed is the translation of assessment instruments originally developed in one language into other languages. The fact that the questions constituting the instruments can be translated, however, does not mean that the concepts being measured are equivalent in different cultures. Consequently, the fact that an instrument has been shown to be valid for one sample of patients is not a guarantee that it is valid for another sample with different characteristics. This was demonstrated by Deyo (1984) when he showed the pitfalls of simply translating an assessment instrument into another language and assuming that

the validity of the instrument in the two languages (English and Spanish) was comparable. It is not sufficient to demonstrate that a specific assessment instrument is reliable and valid.

NORMATIVE INFORMATION

The appropriateness of tests' norms has rarely been considered in the pain literature. In the absence of normative information, the raw score on any test is meaningless. To observe that a patient with migraine headaches scores a 10 on a Visual Analogue Scale (VAS) of pain intensity conveys little or no information. However, if it is known that the average VAS pain severity score for 100 patients with migraine headache is 5.4 with a standard deviation of 1.0, this information would permit the conclusion that this patient is signifying a very high level of pain relative to other such patients. If, on the other hand, the only available normative evidence was based on patients with cancer, and their mean was 5.4 with a standard deviation of 1.0, then it is not known how the patient rated his or her pain relative to a group of patients with migraine. Is the patient's pain report atypical for sufferers from migraine? Without appropriate normative information, it will not be possible to answer this question.

In all areas of pain assessment, it is important to know the type(s) of patients for whom normative information is available, and thus the appropriateness of generalizing from the original sample(s) used to establish the reliability. In many cases, instruments that were developed for use with physically healthy or psychiatrically impaired people have been used for patients with chronic pain. This can lead to erroneous conclusions. For example, the MMPI (Main & Spanswick, 1995; see also Bradley & McKendree-Smith, Chapter 16) was originally developed to diagnose personality types associated with psychopathology.

Several studies have directly addressed concerns about the item content of the MMPI scales and interpretations of elevations of the first three scales for medical patients. Pincus, Callahan, Bradley, Vaughn, and Wolfe (1986) asked 18 rheumatologists to predict which of the 117 statements that constitute the first three MMPI scales would be answered differently by patients with rheumatoid arthritis (RA) and normal subjects, without regard to psychological status. The predictions of the rheumatologists were analyzed by actually comparing the responses of the patients with RA and the healthy subjects. The findings suggest that in patients with RA, elevated scores on the MMPI Hypochondriasis (*Hy*), Depression (*D*), and Hysteria (*Hs*) scales result from chronic disease rather than from psychological abnormality.

Naliboff, Cohen, and Yellin (1982, 1983) have demonstrated that patients with chronic pain produce MMPI profiles that are quite similar to those produced by patients with chronic illnesses such as hypertension and diabetes. These investigators have also shown that 20%–30% of the variance in patients' *Hy*, *D*, and *Hs* scale scores are determined by functional disability. Brennan, Barrett, and Garretsen (1986–1987) report that correlations between MMPI scale scores and outcome appear to be direct associations between the MMPI scales and pain-related characteristics, perhaps as a result of "artifactual" elevations due to pain-related items on these scales. When the predictive values of initial pain and disability are statistically accounted for, psychological test scores tend not to produce a further significant increment in predictability of pain clinic treatment outcome. In short, there is a strong possibility that the elevations shown by patients with pain on certain MMPI scales may be primarily a function of their disease or injury per se, its sequelae, and the medication used, rather than the experiences reflected by those same scales when they are used with psychiatric patients (Turk & Fernandez, 1995).

Before using the norms of an instrument, it is important to demonstrate the invariance of the factor structure of the new instrument for the new population. For example, Turk and Rudy (1988) demonstrated that subgroups of patients with pain could be identified based on their responses on the West Haven-Yale Multidimensional Pain Inventory (WHYMPI: Kerns, Turk, & Rudy, 1985; see also Jacob & Kerns, Chapter 19, and Turk & Okifuji, Chapter 21). The original sample consisted of a heterogeneous group of patients evaluated at a pain clinic. Would the same subgroups generalize to other medical diagnoses, or were the results idiosyncratic to the original sample of patients? Turk and Rudy (1990) demonstrated that although the mean scores on the different scales of the WHYMPI and the percentage of patients comprising each subgroup differed among patients with low back pain, headache, and temporomandibular disorder pain, the correlation matrices among the scales were invariant. Thus, although different normative values should be used for different diagnoses, the subgroups identified transcended medical and dental diagnoses, thus validating the generalizability of the patterns of the scales that characterize the subgroups.

As many chapters in this volume illustrate, measures that were never developed for samples of patients with pain, but that were used because they were readily available, are being replaced by ones that are specifically developed for and standardized (normed) on patients with specific types of pain. Future research needs to demonstrate that these pain-specific measures are both psychometrically acceptable and clinically useful.

The incremental validity of any new instrument should also be considered. That is, do the new instruments add anything to existing measures, or do they place less demand upon the patient? When two measurement instruments are shown to be measuring the same thing, the one that requires least time and therefore places least burden on the patient to complete may be preferred, all others things being equal.

PROLIFERATION OF MEASURES

The development of new assessment instruments and procedures is a laborious task requiring large samples of patients. It is all too easy to avoid this task by making use of published instruments that appear to measure constructs related to our interests (Main & Spanswick, 1995). It is also possible that the availability of instruments may shape the research questions that we ask.

The wealth of available pain assessment measures and procedures described throughout this volume can be both a blessing and a curse. Not only must the clinician or investigator choose a set of procedures to use, but he or she must also decide how to integrate the large amount of information obtained. Many questions should be considered in determining an assessment battery. What measures should be included in the assessment of a patient with pain? Have the measures been shown to be psychometrically sound? Can the information be aggregated into a single score? Are these measurements reproducible and sensitive enough to detect clinical response to therapy? Does each measure, regardless of its name, assess a unique variable, or does it merely duplicate an existing measure that has a different label but assesses the same domain? What norms are available, and are they appropriate?

Those who select from the array of assessment instruments must also ask themselves, "Assessment for what purpose—classification, diagnosis, treatment planning, decision making, prediction, outcome criteria?" (See Turk & Okifuji, Chapter 21.) Although some criteria for evaluating the appropriateness of a specific instrument cross these different purposes, this is not always the case. For example, if an investigator or clinician wishes to evaluate the efficacy of a treatment based on changes from pretreatment to posttreatment, he or she needs to be concerned about whether the instruments selected to evaluate success are subject to change. Related to this is the ability of an instrument to detect small changes. For example, the diagnostic criteria for fibromyalgia syndrome include the presence of 11 of 18 specific tender points. Positive tender points are based on the patient's dichotomous response ("yes" or "no") when asked whether he or she feels pain on palpation at each location. The range of response is quite limited on such a simple rating system, and the system may not be sensitive to small but significant changes following treatment (Okifuji, Turk, Sinclair, Starz, & Marcus, 1997).

Another important question concerns what to assess. In clinical areas there should be some relation between the instruments selected and treatment. It is unfair to ask a patient to complete a lengthy assessment battery or to submit to a large number of laboratory tests if the information collected is simply entered in the patient's file but has no impact on treatment.

Insufficient attention has been devoted to customizing treatments to important characteristics of patients (Turk, 1990; see Turk & Okifuji, Chapter 21). Several studies have identified subgroups of patients with the same medical diagnosis on the basis of psychosocial and behavioral characteristics (e.g., Riley, Robinson, & Geisser, 1999; Turk & Rudy, 1990). Only recently, however, have efforts been made to evaluate differential responses of patients to treatment for various chronic pain syndromes (Turk, Okifuji, Sinclair, & Starz, 1998; Turk, Rudy, Kubinski, Zaki, & Greco, 1996). The new measures that are described in this volume may help to answer the questions about customizing treatment.

DEVELOPMENT OF STANDARDIZED PROCEDURES

It has long been debated whether standardized instruments and methods of aggregating data are better than clinicians' judgments (Meehl, 1954). Many clinicians resist the use of standardized assessment

instruments in assessing pain, emphasizing the nuances of clinical judgment. For example, Foley (1984, p. 22) advocates that clinical assessment of a patient with cancer adhere to nine principles:

1. Believing in the patient's pain complaint.
2. Taking a careful history of the pain complaint.
3. Assessing the psychosocial status of the patient.
4. Performing a careful medical and neurological examination.
5. Ordering and personally reviewing the appropriate diagnostic procedures.
6. Evaluating the extent of the patient's disease.
7. Treating the pain to facilitate the diagnostic study.
8. Considering alternative methods of pain control during the initial evaluation.
9. Reassessing the pain complaint during the prescribed therapy.

This approach relies heavily on clinical judgment. The availability of standardized. assessment methods and strategies for aggregating data, such as those described throughout this volume, can be complementary to the clinician's judgment; the two approaches need not be viewed as mutually exclusive.

FEASIBILITY

There is a growing concern about feasibility of various assessment procedures for different samples (see Okifuji & Turk, Chapter 33). There may be an ideal measure, but one that is not appropriate. For example, it may not be possible to administer a lengthy pain questionnaire on a frequent basis to patients with pain who are in the terminal stage. Young children and patients with limited communication skills may be unable to respond to questions in the same way that "normal" adults can (see McGrath & Gillespie, Chapter 6, and Hadjistavropoulos, von Baeyer, & Craig, Chapter 8). Older people display different "pain behaviors" than younger adults and may not be able to engage in some biomechanical tests (see Gagliese, Chapter 7).

The behaviors of patients with different pain syndromes may be influenced by the nature of their diseases, and it may be inappropriate to generalize from one disease to another (cf. Keefe & Dolan, 1986; Wilkie, Keefe, Dodd, & Copp, 1992). Particular consideration must be given to the special characteristics of different populations in determining what assessment procedures can reasonably be used—for example, for patients with cancer versus low back pain. The comparability of measures that are ostensibly designed to measure the same things, but in demographically very different samples, needs to be demonstrated.

SOME NEW DIRECTIONS

The development and refinement of advanced imaging procedures (e.g., single-photon emission tomography [SPECT] and functional magnetic resonance imaging [fMRI]) have begun to provide new insights into the processing of noxious information associated with pain (see Flor, Chapter 5; Jones, Chapter 35). For example, recent studies have shown that when acute noxious stimuli are administered to normal subjects, there is activation of cerebral blood flow in multiple brain areas. The fact that many different areas respond to the same noxious stimuli supports the view that the pain experience is a distributive process not based exclusively in one location, but results from interaction among a number of distinct brain regions. Interestingly, imaging studies suggest that the patterns of activation of regions of the brain are different for chronic pain syndromes (e.g., Cesaro et al., 1991; DiPiero et al., 1991).

In Chapter 5, Flor describes procedures for using SPECT, fMRI, and other sophisticated imaging methods for research. It should not be long until these procedures are refined, and perhaps new ones will evolve that will be used for clinical assessment of pain. In the future it may be possible to use these procedures not only for diagnostic assessment, but also for evaluation of responses to treatment.

The vast majority of research on pain assessment has relied on patients with chronic pain who are treated at multidisciplinary pain centers. Yet only a small proportion of people with chronic and recurring pain are treated in such facilities. Consequently, these samples are highly selective and may not be representative of people with persistent pain. For example, epidemiological studies comparing patients treated at specialized pain clinics and those with chronic pain in the community indicate that those treated at pain centers had greater psychological distress, greater psychiatric morbidity, and lower levels of education, and that they were more likely to have experienced work-related injuries (Crook, Weir, & Tunks, 1989). Realization of the limitations of samples from pain clinics has resulted in efforts to learn more about people with persistent pain in the general community by national surveys (Leitman, Binns, & Unni, 1994), in primary care settings (Von Korff, Ormel, Keefe, & Dworkin, 1992), and in community settings (see, e.g., Drossman et al., 1988). In Chapter 31, Von Korff describes the basic features of epidemiological and survey methods that are likely to expand our understanding of chronic pain beyond the usual setting of tertiary care.

Much of the research on pain has focused on patients' retrospective self-reports. There are several problems with self-reports that may bias responses and impede the validity of our understanding of pain (see Haythornthwaite & Fauerbach, Chapter 22). Most notably, they rely on patients' memory and their ability to average information over periods of time. Retrospective recall will be influenced by the patients' current mood and pain severity. Current state will serve as an anchor for retrospective recall. Consider your own response if we asked you to provide a rating of your average fatigue over the past month. Most likely you would use your current level of fatigue as the basis for your reflections, recall, and estimate of your average fatigue. The question is thus how accurate your recall and subsequent estimate would actually be. One way to examine this question would be to compare the average ratings collecting daily over a month and to compare these with the retrospective recall.

The availability of palmtop computers has resulted in a number of studies that have attempted to assess ratings of pain, mood, activity, and fatigue on a "real-time" basis. That is, patients carry the computers with them and are paged and interviewed several times during the day. This methodology holds promise for identifying the interrelationships among pain and other important variables on an ongoing basis, and for examing the lagged effects of pain and other variables at time 1 on subsequent reports (see, e.g., Affleck et al., 1999; Lefebvre et al., 1999). We anticipate that this technology will lead to important advances in understanding the role of different variables on pain severity and will eliminate reliance on recall bias. There is a tradeoff, however, as the demand for frequent ratings may sensitize patients to their pain and influence their ratings. The sensitization effect of this approach needs to be examined.

CONCLUSIONS

It is almost a score of years since Melzack's (1983) volume on pain assessment first appeared, and almost a decade since the first edition of the current text was published. In the time since the publication of these volumes, there has been a veritable explosion of research devoted to the development of systematic techniques for measuring pain and for evaluating people who experience it. The chapters contained in this volume present the state of the art at this point in time.

As we noted in the first edition of this book, it is precarious to predict how pain assessment will evolve. In that edition we enumerated a nine-item "wish list." At this juncture it seems appropriate that we review the progress made on our list.

1. We hoped that trends in developing appropriate psychometrics for instruments and procedures developed for assessment of people in pain would escalate. Over the past decade, investigators and clinicians have adopted our concern; much more information has been published on the reliability, validity, utility, and normative data for existing and new assessment methods. In the area of physical assessment, however, there continues to be much less attention given to psychometrics, especially the intrajudge and interjudge reliability of physical examination procedures.

2. We indicated that new instruments and procedures should be developed in an effort to measure domains that are believed to be important in understanding pain and the person who experiences it. Many new procedures and measures have been developed, with greater attention being given to the role of anxiety (Vlaeyen et al., 1995) in chronic pain and readiness for treatment (Kerns, Rosenberg, Jamison, Caudill, & Haythornthwaite, 1997).

3. We called for the consolidation of instruments that might be measuring similar concepts, as well as the replacement of some by new approaches that have been demonstrated to be more appropriate (reliable, valid, less demanding on patients). Little effort has been devoted to this call, and there continue to be a large number of measures that are likely to be highly correlated. The availability of such overlap often leads to confusion among investigators who have to select from among the diversity of measures assessing similar constructs.

4. We suggested that greater emphasis should be placed on relating assessment instruments and procedures to important behavioral outcomes. As we note in this chapter, there is no question that investigators have begun to move beyond instrument development to evaluating the utility of measures and procedures in assessing important outcomes.

5. We noted that more attention needed to be given to innovative strategies for integrating diverse sets of information. Unfortunately, the issue of information integration has not received sufficient attention and continues to be an area greatly in need of research.

6. We recommended that greater emphasis should be given to prescribing treatments based on patient characteristics derived from assessment data, rather than treating all patients with pain as basically the same, or matching treatment exclusively to medical diagnosis. Some initial attempts (see, e.g., Turk et al., 1996; Turk, Okifuji, et al., 1998) have been reported, but the emphasis has continued to be on identification of subgroups without taking the next step of relating subgroups to treatments. Statistical procedures can easily be used to identify clusters or profiles of patients, but these groupings may have little clinical utility. We hope that more treatment-matching studies will be conducted to demonstrate the additive value of knowing the characteristics of patient subgroups.

7. We suggested that there was a need to demonstrate the generalizability of different instruments to new populations, rather than assuming that such instruments can be used with samples that differ from the original sample. Several studies have begun to evaluate the appropriateness of generalizing from some of the instruments that were originally developed on one population of patients with chronic pain to others (e.g., Turk, Sist, et al., 1998).

8. We suggested that recent advances in test theory (e.g., item response theory) should be used in evaluating pain assessment instruments and procedures. On this point, we have seen little progress. There continues to be a tendency to rely on classical psychometric methods.

9. We noted that we expected to see major advances in the use of sophisticated imaging procedures to advance our understanding of pain and responses to treatment. There has been an explosion of interest in brain imaging, including a few studies reporting changes in brain activity as a result of treatments (see Jones, Chapter 35).

On the whole, it appears that important strides have been taken since the first edition of this volume. There remain areas noted in our list that have not yet received sufficient attention, and that we hope will be addressed in the next decade.

One primary goal of this volume has been to provide practical and useful information for clinical investigators and health care providers. It is our hope that the discussions initiated throughout this volume will serve to inspire additional research. The continuing evolution of human pain assessment is essential for success in the search for treatments for those who continue to suffer.

ACKNOWLEDGMENTS

Preparation of this chapter was supported in part by grants from the National Institute of Arthritis and Musculoskeletal and Skin Diseases (No. AR/AI44724) and the National Institute of Child Health and Human Development (No. HD33989) awarded to Dennis C. Turk.

REFERENCES

Affleck, G., Tennen, H., Keefe, F. J., Lefebvre, J. C., Kashikar-Zuck, S., Wright, K., Starr, K., & Caldwell, D. S. (1999). Everyday life with osteoarthritis or rheumatoid arthritis: Independent effects of disease and gender on daily pain, mood, and coping. Pain, 83, 601–609.

Brennan, A. F., Barrett, C. L., & Garretson, H. D. (1986–1987). The prediction of chronic pain outcome by psychological variables. International Journal of Psychiatry in Medicine, 16, 373–387.

Brus, H., van de Laar, M., Taal, E., Rasker, J., & Wiegman, O. (1999). Determinants of compliance with medication in patients with rheumatoid arthritis: The importance of self-efficacy expectations. Patient Education and Counseling, 36, 57–64.

Burton, A. K., Tillotson, M., Main, C. J., & Hollis, S. (1995). Psychosocial predictors of outcome in acute and subchronic low back trouble. Spine, 20, 722–728.

Cesaro, P., Mann, M. W., Moretti, J. L., Defer, G., Roualdes, B., Nguyen, J. P., & Degos, J. D. (1991). Central pain and thalamic hyperactivity: A single photon emission computerized tomographic study. Pain, 47, 329–336.

Coughlan, G. M., Ridout, K. L., Williams, A. C. deC., & Richardson, P. H. (1995). Attrition from a pain management programme. British Journal of Clinical Psychology, 34, 471–479.

Crook, J., Weir, R., & Tunks, E. (1989). An epidemiological follow-up survey of persistent pain sufferers in a group family practice and specialty pain clinic. Pain, 36, 49–61.

Deyo, R. A. (1984). Pitfalls in measuring the health status of Mexican Americans: Comparative validity of the English and Spanish Sickness Impact Profile. American Journal of Public Health, 6, 560–573.

Deyo, R. A. (1988). Measuring the functional status of patients with low back pain. Archives of Physical Medicine and Rehabilitation, 69, 1044–1053.

Deyo, R. A., & Diehl, A. K. (1983). Measuring physical and psychosocial function in patients with low-back pain. Spine, 8, 635–647.

DiPiero, V., Jones, A. K. P., Iannotti, F., Powell, M., Perani, D., Lenzi, G. L., & Frackowiak, R. S. J. (1991). Chronic pain: A PET study of the central effects of percutaneous high cervical cordotomy. Pain, 46, 9–12.

Drossman, D. A., McKee, D. C., Sandler, R. S., Michell, C. M., Cramer, E. M., Lowman, B. C., & Berger, A. L. (1988). Psychosocial factors in the irritable bowel syndrome: A multivariate study of patients and non-patients with irritable bowel syndrome. Gastroenterology, 95, 701–708.

Flor, H., & Turk, D. C. (1988). Chronic pain and rheumatoid arthritis: Predicting pain and disability from cognitive variables. Journal of Behavioral Medicine, 11, 251–265.

Foley, K. M. (1984). Assessment of pain. In R. G. Twycross (Ed.), Pain relief in cancer (pp. 17–31). London: Saunders.

Gallagher, R. M., Rauh, V., Haugh, L. D., Milhous, R., Callas, P. W., Langelier, R., McClallen, J. M., & Frymoyer, J. (1989). Determinants of return-to-work among low back pain patients. Pain, 39, 55–67.

Jensen, M. P., Romano, J. M., Turner, J. A., Good, A. B., & Wald, L. H. (1999). Patient beliefs predict patient functioning: Further support for a cognitive-behavioral model of chronic pain. Pain, 81, 95–104.

Jensen, M. P., Turner, J. A., Romano, J. M., & Lawler, B. K. (1994). Relationship of pain specific beliefs to chronic pain adjustment. Pain, 57, 361–369.

Keefe, F. J., & Dolan, E. (1986). Pain behavior and pain coping strategies in low back pain and myofascial pain dysfunction syndrome patients. Pain, 24, 49–56.

Kerns, R. D., Turk, D.C., & Rudy, T. E. (1985). The West Haven–Yale Multidimensional Pain Inventory (WHYMPI). Pain, 23, 345–356.

Kerns, R. D., Rosenberg, R., Jamison, R. N., Caudill, M. A., & Haythornthwaite, J. (1997). Readiness to adopt a self-management approach to chronic pain: The Pain Stages of Change Questionnaire (PSOCQ). Pain, 72, 227–234.

Lefebvre, J. C., Keefe, F. J., Affleck, G., Raezer, L. B., Starr, K., Caldwell, D. S., & Tennen, H. (1999). The relationship of arthritis self-efficacy to daily pain, daily mood, and daily pain coping in rheumatoid arthritis patients. Pain, 80, 425–435.

Leitman, R., Binns, K., & Unni, A. (1994). McNeil National Pain Survey. New York: Louis Harris & Associates.

Linton, S. J., Althoff, B., Melin, L., Lundin, A., Bodin, L., Magi, A., Lidstrom, K., & Lihagen, T. (1994). Psychological factors related to health, back pain, and dysfunction. Journal of Occupational Rehabilitation, 4, 1–9.

Main, C. J., & Spanswick, C. C. (1995). Personality assessment and the Minnesota Multiphasic Personality Inventory, 50 years on: Do we still need our security blanket? Pain Forum, 4, 90–96.

Meehl, P. E. (1954). Clinical vs. statistical prediction. Minneapolis, MN: University of Minnesota Press.

Melzack, R. (Ed.). (1983). Pain measurement and assessment. New York: Raven Press.

Naliboff, B. D., Cohen, M. J., & Yellin, A. M. (1982). Does the MMPI differentiate chronic illness from chronic pain? Pain, 13, 333–341.

Naliboff, B. D., Cohen, M. J., & Yellin, A. M. (1983). Frequency of MMPI profile types in three chronic illness populations. Journal of Clinical Psychology, 39, 843–847.

Okifuji, A., Turk, D. C., Sinclair, J. D., Starz, T. W., & Marcus, D. A. (1997). A standardized manual tender point survey: I. Development and determination of a threshold point for the identification of positive tender points in fibromyalgia syndrome. *Journal of Rheumatology, 24,* 377–383.

Pincus, T., Callahan, L. F., Bradley, L. A., Vaughn, W. K., & Wolfe, F. (1986). Elevated MMPI scores for hypochondriasis, depression, and hysteria in patients with rheumatoid arthritis reflect disease rather than psychological status. *Arthritis and Rheumatism, 29,* 1456–1466.

Pope, M. H., Rosen, J. C., Wilder, D. G., & Frymoyer, J. W. (1980). Relation between biomechanical and psychological factors in patients with low-back pain. *Spine, 5,* 173–178.

Richmond, R. L., & Carmody, T. P. (1999). Dropout from treatment for chronic low-back pain. *Professional Psychology: Research and Practice, 30,* 51–55.

Riley, J. L., III, Robinson, M. E., & Geisser, M. E. (1999). Empirical subgroups of the Coping Strategies Questionnaire–Revised: A multisample study. *Clinical Journal of Pain, 15,* 111–116.

Romano, J. M., Turner, J. A., & Jensen, M. P. (1997). The family environment in chronic pain patients: Comparison to controls and relationship to patient functioning. *Journal of Clinical Psychology in Medical Settings, 4,* 383–395.

Sternbach, R. (1968). *Pain: A psychophyiological analysis.* New York: Academic Press.

Tota-Faucette, M. E., Gil, K. M., Williams, D. A., Keefe, F. J., & Goli, V. (1993). Predictors of response to pain management treatment: The role of family environment and changes in cognitive processes. *Clinical Journal of Pain, 9,* 115–123.

Tukey, J. W. (1979). Methodology and the statistician's responsibility for both accuracy and relevance. *Journal of the American Statistical Association, 74,* 786–793.

Turk, D. C. (1990). Customizing treatment for chronic pain patients: Who, what, and why. *Clinical Journal of Pain, 6,* 225–270.

Turk, D. C., & Fernandez, E. (1995). Personality assessment and the Minnesota Multiphasic Personality Inventory in chronic pain: Underdeveloped and overexposed. *Pain Forum, 4,* 104–107.

Turk, D. C., Okifuji, A., Sinclair, J. D., & Starz, T. W. (1998). Differential responses by psychosocial subgroups of fibromyalgia syndrome patients to an interdisciplinary treatment. *Arthritis Care and Research, 11,* 397–404.

Turk, D. C., & Rudy, T. E. (1988). Toward an empirically derived taxonomy of chronic pain patients: Integration of psychological assessment data. *Journal of Consulting and Clinical Psychology, 56,* 760–768.

Turk, D. C., & Rudy, T. E. (1990). The robustness of an empirically derived taxonomy of chronic pain patients. *Pain, 43,* 27–35.

Turk, D. C., Rudy, T. E., Kubinski, J. A., Zaki, H. S., & Greco, C. M. (1996). Dysfunctional TMD patients: Evaluating the efficacy of a tailored treatment protocol. *Journal of Consulting and Clinical Psychology, 64,* 139–146.

Turk, D. C., Sist, T. C., Okifuji, A., Miner, M. F., Florio, G., Harrison, P., Massey, J., Lema, M. L., & Zevon, M. A. (1998). Adaptation to metastatic cancer pain, regional/local cancer pain and non-cancer pain: Role of psychological and behavioral factors. *Pain, 74,* 247–256.

Turner, J. A., Jensen, M. P., & Romano, J. M. (2000). Do beliefs, coping, and catastrophizing independently predict functioning in patients with chronic pain? *Pain, 85,* 115–125.

Vlaeyen, J. W. S., Kole-Snijiders, A. M. J., Rotteveel, A., Ruesink, R., & Heuts, P. H. T. (1995). The role of fear of movement/(re) injury in pain disability. *Journal of Occupational Rehabilitation, 5,* 235–252.

Von Korff, M., Ormel, J., Keefe, F., & Dworkin, S. F. (1992). Grading the severity of chronic pain. *Pain, 50,* 133–149.

Wilkie, D. J., Keefe, F. J., Dodd, M. J., & Copp, L. A. (1992). Behavior of patients with lung cancer: Description and associations with oncologic pain variables. *Pain, 51,* 231–240.

Author Index

717

Subject Index